Praise for the *Textbook of Global Health*

"Much more than a textbook: an indispensable and exhaustively documented desk reference that belongs in the library of every global health student, researcher, and practitioner."—*American Journal of Public Health*

"For the thoughtful undergraduate or graduate student interested in understanding the complex political, social, and environmental drivers of health disparities worldwide, this is for you. In fact, this insightful, well-researched, comprehensive textbook should be required reading for anyone working in global health."
—*Clinical Infectious Diseases*

"This is a must read for those seeking to understand the structural factors, arrangements and rules generating poor health and inequities at home and across the globe."—*Occupational Medicine*

"Highly integrated, interdisciplinary, comprehensive, and unique; a serious and essential contribution to teaching and learning global health. It is refreshing and invigorating to see a text engage with the contradictions of its subject with such rigor and honesty."—*Canadian Medical Education Journal*

"Highly recommended. An incredible resource for educators, researchers and practitioners concerned with situating their work in a wider global reality."—*South African Medical Journal*

"A deep, comprehensive, and eclectic work for students, professionals, and diplomats who want to confront the current dilemmas of global health. It offers readers the pleasure of frequent consultation, as I have done since it fell into my hands a few weeks ago."—*Ciência & Saúde Coletiva*

"This book provides a forward-looking, highly exhaustive, up-to-date and balanced analysis over the unsolved issues and gaps still impairing equitable access to global health on a world scale."
—*Policies for Equitable Access to Health*

Praise for the Previous Editions

"With its all-encompassing view, clear and rich in humanist thinking and social and human commitment, this book is a stimulating contribution to all health and diplomacy professionals engaged in these new and fascinating domains of International Relations that make us more capable of changing the world into a better place to live."
—*Journal of Public Health Policy*

"I found it to be a clear, comprehensive introduction to public health's major concepts... Students praised the text's comprehensive nature: as many noted, it answered most questions they had about specific concepts, and it was extremely useful as a reference. They valued its readability and noted approvingly that it is 'written in a way that doesn't talk down to us.' They also appreciated the key questions and learning points in each chapter, which helped them focus on what was most important within the huge amount of information this book presents."
—*Medical Anthropology Quarterly*

"This is a unique book. There is probably no other written work out there available to students and professionals that focuses on health problems prevalent on a global scale, and discusses available solutions... This book has a wealth of data for decision-making committees."—*Biz India*

"The book provides excellent historic insight into international health. Very powerful observations result from the orientation to infrastructure and economics. The content builds upon traditional issues such as environmental to healthcare systems, implementation, and working in international health.... The book is an appropriate consideration for an introductory text on international health."—*Doody's*

Textbook of Global Health

FOURTH EDITION

Anne-Emanuelle Birn, MA, ScD
Professor of Critical Development Studies and Global Health,
University of Toronto, Toronto, Canada

Yogan Pillay, PhD
Deputy Director-General: HIV/AIDS, TB and Maternal,
Child and Women's Health National Department
of Health, Pretoria, South Africa

Timothy H. Holtz, MD, MPH, FACP, FACPM
Adjunct Associate Professor of Global Health, Rollins School of Public Health
Emory University, Atlanta, United States

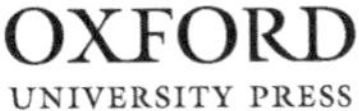
OXFORD
UNIVERSITY PRESS

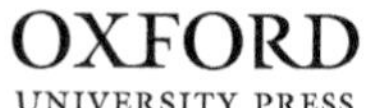

Oxford University Press is a department of the University of Oxford. It furthers the University's objective of excellence in research, scholarship, and education by publishing worldwide. Oxford is a registered trade mark of Oxford University Press in the UK and certain other countries.

Published in the United States of America by Oxford University Press
198 Madison Avenue, New York, NY 10016, United States of America.

First issued as an Oxford University Press paperback, 2018

Library of Congress Cataloging-in-Publication Data
Names: Birn, Anne-Emanuelle, 1964- author. | Pillay, Yogan, author. | Holtz, Timothy H., author.
Title: Textbook of global health / Anne-Emanuelle Birn, Yogan Pillay, Timothy H. Holtz.
Other titles: Textbook of international health
Description: Fourth edition. | Oxford ; New York : Oxford University Press, [2016] |
Preceded by Textbook of international health / Anne-Emanuelle Birn,
Yogan Pillay, Timothy H. Holtz. 2009. | Includes bibliographical references and index.
Identifiers: LCCN 2016046206 (print) | LCCN 2016048722 (ebook) |
ISBN 9780199392285 (hardback : alk. paper) | ISBN 9780199392292 (e-book) |
ISBN 9780199392308 (e-book) | ISBN 9780190916527 (paperback : alk. paper))
Subjects: | MESH: Global Health | Socioeconomic Factors | Health Policy |
International Cooperation
Classification: LCC RA441 (print) | LCC RA441 (ebook) | NLM WA 530.1 |
DDC 362.1—dc23
LC record available at https://lccn.loc.gov/2016046206

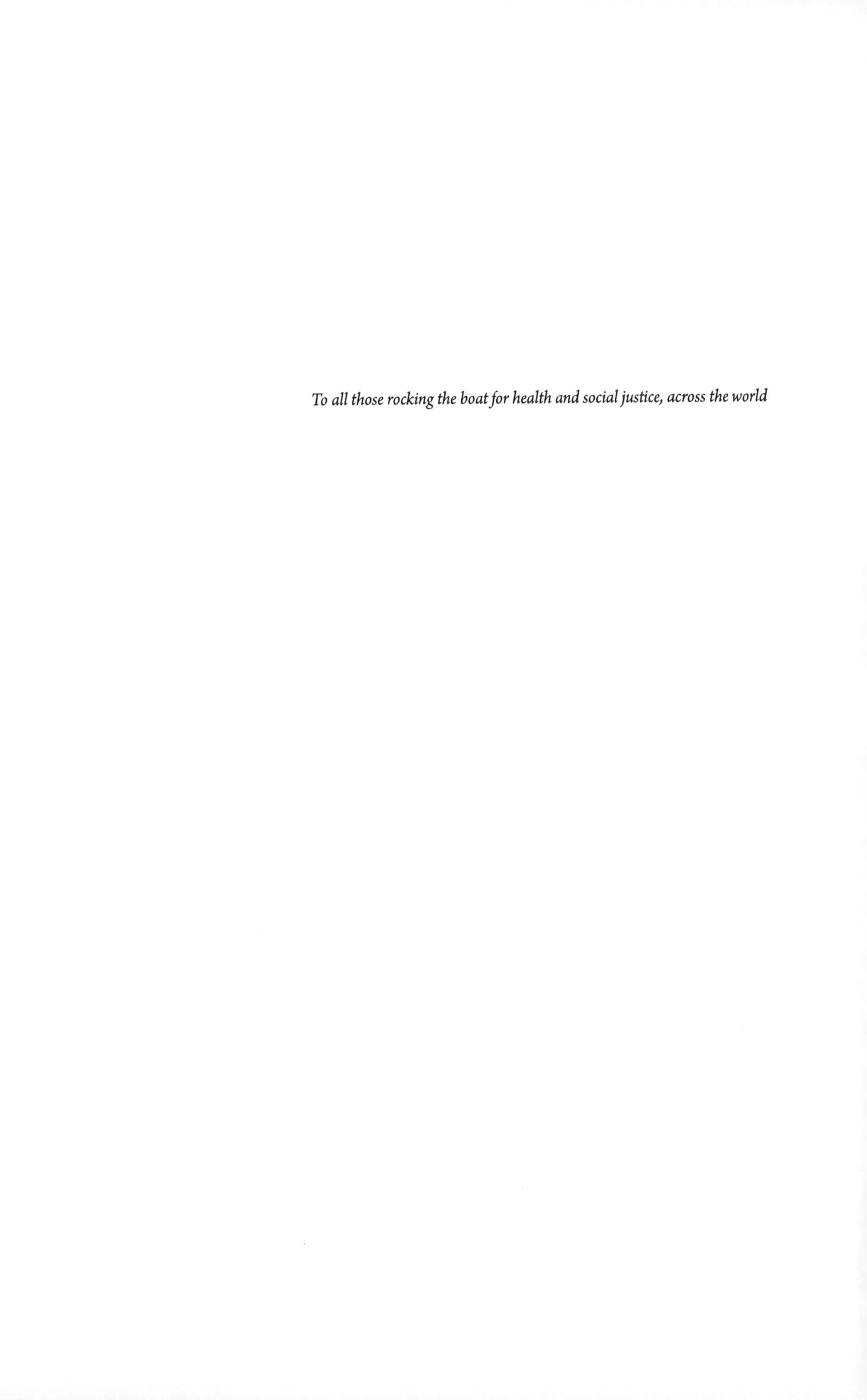

To all those rocking the boat for health and social justice, across the world

CONTENTS

LIST OF ILLUSTRATIONS: FIGURES, TABLES, AND BOXES

FIGURES

TABLES

BOXES

ACKNOWLEDGMENTS

This fourth edition of the *Textbook of Global Health*, like its immediate predecessor, is written by a trio of authors with a range of research, practice, teaching, and leadership experience in various regions of the world involving policymaking, epidemiology, international cooperation, and historical and political analysis. At different moments we have worked with and for local and national governments, NGOs, multilateral organizations, universities, and social movements.

Even with our diversity of backgrounds and work trajectories, we could not possibly have produced this volume alone. Consistent with the solidarity principles espoused herein, this volume has benefited enormously from a global collective of comrades, friends, and acquaintances who have generously shared their time, wisdom, and experience to help sharpen the analysis, relay expertise, correct misunderstandings, and improve this volume in a myriad ways. Of course, all shortcomings and errors are the authors' alone. Those who have supported us constitute a veritable global health network in and of themselves, hailing from every continent and dozens of countries.

Our heartfelt thanks go to:

Abtin Parnia
Albert Berry
Alex Scott-Samuel
Alina Salganicoff
Amit Sengupta
Andrea Vigorito
Andrew Pinto
Antonio Torres-Ruiz
Arne Rückert
Barry Levy
Beverly Bradley
Bridget Lloyd
Brook Baker
Carles Muntaner
Carlos Quiñonez
Cesar Victora
Christopher Sellers
Denis Holdenried
Denise Gastaldo
Devaki Nambiar
Donald Cole
Eduardo Siqueira
Eileen Dunne
Elia Abi-Jaoude
Ellen 't Hoen
Esperanza Krementsova
Eugenio Villar
Faraz Vahid Shahidi
Gabriela Martínez Malagón
Gregg Mitman
Hani Serag
Hans Pols
Howard Waitzkin
Ida Hellander
Ilker Kayi
Janet Rodriguez Iraola
Jannah Wigle
Jason Beckfield
Jillian Clare Kohler
Jingjing Su
Joan Benach
Joel Lexchin
John MacArthur
John Serieux
Judith Richter
Judith Teichman
Juliana Martínez Franzoni
Kathleen Ruff
Kathy Moscou
Kim Lindblade
Krista Lauer
Krista Maxwell
Lesley Doyal
Leslie London
Lída Lhotská
Matthew Anderson
Meri Koivusalo

Mira Lee
Miriam Gross
Mitch Wolfe
Nandini Oomman
Pam Dougherty
Raúl Necochea López
Rick Rowden
Ryan Isakson
S. Patrick Kachur
Samuel Yingst
Simon Szreter
Sofia Gruskin
Solomon Benatar
Sonja Olsen
Sukarma Tanwar
Suzanne Sicchia
Victoria Blackwell-Hardie
Wanda Cabella
Zinzi Bailey

We are especially grateful to colleagues (including current and former University of Toronto students) who reviewed one or two chapters of the book and shared their deep insights and suggestions:

Andrea Cortinois
Andrea Gerstenberger
Ben Brisbois
Carmen Concepción
Claudia Chaufan
Deika Mohamed
Franziska Satzinger
Gilberto Hochman
Héctor Gómez Dantés
John Pringle
José Tapia Granados
Kavita Sivaramakrishnan
Lori Hanson
Paul Hamel
Robert Chernomas
Suzanne Jackson
Ted Schrecker
Theodore Brown
William Ventres

Several former research and teaching assistants reviewed the 3rd edition of the *Textbook* and provided invaluable recommendations around what to keep, what to chuck, and how to reorganize and update. Profound appreciation goes to: Ghazal Fazli, Andrew Leyland, and Marrison Stranks.

A few people went above and beyond the call of collegiality to review multiple chapters and provide ongoing intellectual and other forms of sustenance. With neverending gratitude to these *true comrades*:

Laura Nervi, Nancy Krieger, Nikolai Krementsov, and Ramya Kumar.

Expert research and reference assistance was provided by Sarah Silverberg, Tanveer Singh, and Tanyawarin Janthiraj.

No one shared the scholarly joys and pains of this volume more than our amazing research assistant, Mariajosé Aguilera! Tireless, committed, astute, persistent, and level-headed, she pushed us incessantly to improve clarity and narrative flow, pursued every last research avenue, and challenged us to refine and substantiate our analysis in an enormously productive way. This book would have been impossible without Mariajosé's incredibly hard work, expertise, and good humor. ¡Mil y más gracias!

At Oxford University Press, Chad Zimmerman has been a variously patient and impatient editor, wise and witty almost always in the right measure, and supportive to the very end. Thank you, thank you. We also appreciate the work of Devi Vaidyanathan and the production team at Newgen.

This revision lasted far longer than we expected (involving numerous power and internet outages; perhaps a dozen pairs of broken reading/computer glasses; several kg of lost girth; and moves across 4 continents). Nobody suffered more than our families. While we know that merci, kob khun ka, xièxie, gracias, grazie, sthoothi, obrigado, nandri, danke, and spasibo are never enough, we express our thanks nonetheless, from heart and soul.

INTRODUCTION: WHY GLOBAL HEALTH?

H1N1 influenza. Diabetes. Ebola. Antimicrobial resistance. Zika. Whether in New York or New Delhi, almost every year another sensationalized potential or actual pandemic grabs global headlines and raises alarms among politicians, business executives, United Nations (UN) agencies, celebrities, humanitarian organizations, magnates, and the wider public.

To highlight just one among many, in May 2015, the Brazilian government confirmed the first locally-acquired case of Zika virus (primarily transmitted by *Aedes aegypti* mosquitoes; also communicable between humans) in the Americas. Generally causing a mild illness accompanied by fever, joint pain, and neurological symptoms, Zika was first identified in Uganda in 1947, with subsequent, likely under-reported, outbreaks in Africa, Southeast Asia, and the Pacific. The situation in Brazil escalated as evidence mounted that an upsurge in microcephaly (small head size, linked to incomplete brain development) among newborns was due to intrauterine Zika infection (Lessler et al. 2016). With the 2016 Rio de Janeiro Olympic Games approaching and the virus spreading across the Americas, Zika garnered widespread media coverage and sparked alarmism, including in some public health quarters.

By February 2016, the World Health Organization (WHO) declared Zika a "Public Health Emergency of International Concern," recommending that pregnancy be postponed among those living in or visiting areas where there is Zika virus transmission (WHO 2016a). Several governments made similar (contentious) recommendations, despite restricted access to contraception in many Latin American countries. Moreover, the focus on pregnancy prevention belies the larger context of Zika's emergence and impact (Ventura 2016). The combination of rapid urbanization, poverty, climate change, and intense deforestation—driven by logging, agribusiness, mining, and oil and gas development—has accelerated the proliferation of a range of old and new vector-borne diseases, including dengue, malaria, and chikungunya. Critically, over 90% of Brazil's 1,800 Zika-related microcephaly cases have been in the country's poor northeast region, where housing, sanitation, and public health measures are inadequate, leading mosquito breeding sites to multiply (for example in household water storage containers) and facilitating human-vector contact (Possas 2016; WHO 2016b). Although the microcephaly cases (and possible association with Guillain-Barré syndrome) are certainly worrisome—and dozens of countries throughout the Americas and the Caribbean now have Zika outbreaks—some are questioning whether global fear-mongering is over-reactive given the many other threats beyond Zika posed by the insalubrious social and economic conditions that favor its proliferation (Galea, Thea, and Annas 2016).

To be sure, global health is not simply a matter of emerging diseases and epidemic threats. Virtually every crisis has global health implications affecting up to hundreds of millions of people, whether related to financial collapse, precarious employment, wars and displacement, ecological disasters, climate change, or any other catastrophe, including due to political instability, social insecurity, and dismantling of social infrastructure, such as health care services. To name but one example, the escalating global refugee crisis, stemming from war and violence in Syria, Yemen, Afghanistan, South Sudan, and Somalia, among other countries, has led to over 65 million people being forcibly displaced from their homes as of 2015 due to conflict and persecution—the highest number ever recorded (UNHCR 2016).

Yet visible situations of crisis can also mask day-to-day problems of social injustice: preventable disease, disability, and premature death related to poor living and working conditions, limited health care access, discrimination, and, ultimately, the gross inequities across population groups due to highly skewed distribution of wealth, power, and resources among the world's over 7.5 billion people. Indeed, pervasive occupational epidemics, such as "non-traditional" chronic kidney disease linked to poor agricultural working conditions and pesticide exposure—and soaring rates of cancer and heart disease in workplaces where exploitation and the absence of labor protections feed on one another—are under-prioritized by the global health agenda despite their importance in ill health and premature mortality terms. Meanwhile, a range of (other) preventable ailments remain major killers among poor populations, notably tuberculosis (TB), HIV, child diarrhea, and malaria.

Although inequities are particularly pronounced between high-income (HIC) and low- and middle-income countries (LMICs), they are also present within countries, including wealthy ones, generating attendant negative health effects. A prime example is the high level of lead-contaminated drinking water detected in 2015 in Flint, Michigan, a US town with a majority low-income African-American population. Exposure to lead in childhood is linked to permanent cognitive damage, hearing problems, and behavioral disorders. In pregnant women it can provoke miscarriage and fetal growth problems, and in all age groups it is associated with heart, kidney, and neurological problems. Outrageously, Flint's elevated lead exposure and burgeoning health problems resulted from a deliberate local government cost-savings policy to switch the town's water supply to a known contaminated source, flagrantly violating public health and ethical standards (Hanna-Attisha et al. 2016).

Given the innumerable pressing concerns across the world, what is needed to promote global health and social justice in the 21st century? This fourth edition of Oxford University Press's *Textbook of Global Health* responds to this question by examining the field's historical origins, the patterns and underlying causes of leading health problems, distinct approaches to resolving these issues, the players and priorities of contemporary global health, as well as the development of global health as a field of study, research, and practice. We carry out this analysis paying close attention to how health, locally and globally, relates to the organization of political and economic activity, social structures and relations, and the distribution of power and control over wealth and resources.

In a nutshell, this textbook aims to:

1. Convey an understanding of global health as shaped by the interaction of global, national, regional, and local forces, processes, and conditions
2. Provide grounding in the epidemiologic, economic, political, ethical, historical, environmental, and social underpinnings of health and disease patterns within and across countries and populations
3. Show the consequences of these patterns at global, societal, and community levels
4. Present a range of transnational, national, and local approaches to improving health and effectuating change that unfold via scientific and social knowledge and practices, public health measures and health care systems, social and political movements, and overall public policymaking

This introduction proceeds with an exploration of global health's underpinnings and some of the persistent dilemmas of the field. Then we outline a critical political economy framework and provide a snapshot of the key themes, ideologies, elements of, and approaches to global health examined throughout this volume. The introduction culminates with a brief guide on how to navigate the textbook.

CONCEPTS AND FRAMEWORKS

Global health is connected to various health-related concepts (population health, social and societal determinants of health, health inequities, etc., which will be covered in later chapters), but it also draws from values and ideas around equity, solidarity, social justice, ethics, and human rights. While perhaps not always visible, these ideas have influenced global health practice, aspirations, institutions, and movements. Here we highlight a few of these notions to launch our discussion.

The Making of Global Health Today

The term *global health* is relatively recent. Its predecessor, "international health," came into use circa 1900 after sovereign countries recognized the value of intergovernmental cooperation and began to establish permanent bodies to address health issues of mutual interest, albeit in a context of intense inter-imperial competition. Imperial powers—though sometimes reluctant to exchange information with commercial and political rivals—were especially intent on fending off epidemics of deadly diseases such as cholera and plague that interrupted trade and generated social unrest (see chapter 1).

A century later, international health was recast as global health, focused on "improvement of health worldwide, the reduction of disparities, and protection of societies against global threats that disregard national borders" (Macfarlane, Jacobs, and Kaaya 2008, p. 383). Global health is meant to rise above international health's association with colonial medicine, as well as the Cold War development context (in which health cooperation was deployed in the ideological and geopolitical rivalry between US and Soviet blocs), to connote a common global experience of and responsibility for health (for a fuller discussion on competing definitions and meanings of global health, see chapter 2).

Notwithstanding the invoked distinctions, there is considerable conflation, and many similarities, between international health and global health. Some consider global health to be a collection of problems (Kleinman 2010). Many see it as an arena for ensuring domestic security from external threats, as a big business and "big data" opportunity, or as a "soft power" foreign policy instrument. Others view global health as an opportunity for institutional and career advancement, while still others see it as a domain for small nongovernmental organizations (NGOs), solidarity efforts, and struggles for health and social justice. So contested and subject to multiple interpretations is the notion of global health that many use it more as "a 'brand name' than a robust concept—a politically expedient term to denote any program dealing with health outside of [or among marginalized groups in] one's own country, while appealing to an ideal of broad reach and holistic focus" (Garay, Harris, and Walsh 2013).

Moreover, insufficient attention is given to the role of power in global health—who wields it and how it is utilized to privilege certain meanings and roles (and exclude others) and why particular actors are able to exert legitimacy to define problems and set the global health agenda (Lee 2015; Marten 2016). Some hold that "the gradual construction of a global society" based on shared sovereignty (Frenk, Gómez-Dantés, and Moon 2014, p. 96) will lead to the betterment of health outcomes globally. Missing from this stance is recognition of the role of the overarching global political order of neoliberal capitalism: policymaking is not shared democratically but skewed in favor of powerful countries and corporate interests. As such, national "sovereignty remains a safe bet, offering both a defense against the narrow self-interest of global economic forces and an advantageous context for the struggle for health" (De Ceukelaire and Botenga 2014, p. 952).

This textbook advocates for a more socially just arrangement of global health agenda-setting, especially prioritizing the health issues and underlying factors most overlooked by the leading global health actors.

Box 0-1 Some Key Concepts Related to Global Health

Health: According to the preamble to WHO's Constitution, "Health is a state of complete physical, mental, and social well-being and not merely the absence of disease or infirmity." This idealistic and expansive definition—which leaves out the important dimensions of social justice and spiritual well-being—is much cited but rarely heeded by major global health actors.

Public health: Coined in the early 19th century to distinguish government efforts from private actions around the preservation and protection of health, public health was famously defined a century later by one of the field's most prominent U.S. leaders, C.-E.A. Winslow (1920, p. 23), as:

> the science and art of preventing disease, prolonging life, and promoting physical health and efficiency through organized community efforts for the sanitation of the environment, the control of community infections, the education of the individual in principles of personal hygiene, the organization of medical and nursing service for the early diagnosis and preventive treatment of disease, and the development of the social machinery which will ensure to every individual in the community a standard of living adequate for the maintenance of health.

Because of public health's association with governmental efforts, it has also been contested/challenged through an alternative concept of collective health, which emerged in the 1970s during Brazil's dictatorship, in the context of a government that was repressive, unrepresentative, and unresponsive to the collective needs of the population. Collective health emphasizes the role and agency of ordinary people, communities, health workers, health justice organizations, and social movements in shaping and promoting health (Granda 2004).

Health and social justice: A broad term for action that strives for genuine equality, fairness, and respect among peoples and leads towards equitable distribution of power, resources, and processes affecting health and the societal determinants of health (Buettner-Schmidt and Lobo 2011; National Conference for Community and Justice et al. n.d.)

Critical Political Economy Framework

A child born today will be over 80 years old as we enter the 22nd century, that is, if they attain the life expectancy of Japan (currently the longest). Whether this child will be alive and healthy in 2100 will depend on the type of future we aspire to and the decisions made today around the environmental, social, political, and economic forces that shape our world and the forms of resistance and reshaping we engage in, from street action to organizational efforts toward building truly equitable societies and a socially just global order.

People experience good and poor health individually, but illness and death are also social phenomena shared by households, friends and kin, classmates and work colleagues, caregivers and healers, and the larger society. At the same time, the societal context—how people live, work, and recreate, and the differences between rich and poor and other kinds of dominant and subordinate social groups at national, local, and global levels—greatly affects who becomes ill (and of what diseases), disabled, or dies prematurely. Yet the majority of global health strategies focus on disease-control measures (based on behavioral and biomedical approaches to health), garnering a great deal of attention and resources for certain diseases while ignoring, or only superficially supporting, health care systems (Storeng 2014) and especially the larger societal context influencing health and health inequities.

This *Textbook of Global Health* employs a critical political economy framework to describe, explain, and analyze health in the context of the social, political, and economic structures of societies, that is, who owns what, who controls what, and how these factors are shaped by and reflect the social and institutional fabric—class, racial/ethnic/gender structures and relations, existence of a redistributive welfare state, and so on (Navarro 2009) (see chapter 3 for further explanation). Behavioral, biological, and medical/health care system factors are not excluded from this framework but rather understood as part of larger societal forces that influence health and well-being. A powerful illustration stems from the global noncommunicable disease (NCD) crisis: the growing epidemic of diabetes, for example, is typically linked to soda consumption and household food decisions. But far larger factors are also at play: with soaring and volatile prices of basic foodstuffs starting in 2007, people across LMICs had to work harder to feed their families, leaving less time for food preparation. This double effect of price hikes and time pressures ushered millions to switch from traditional to processed and packaged foods, a dietary shift that endured even after food prices stabilized (Scott-Villiers et al. 2016). (Meanwhile, the sugar industry has long sought to mask scientific evidence about the connections between sugar consumption and heart disease [Kearns, Schmidt, and Glantz 2016].)

Our critical political economy framework separates this textbook from dominant ways of understanding global health based on tackling diseases with technical tools and behavioral approaches, purveyed through programs, prescriptions, and incentives emanating centrifugally from powerful HICs, global health agencies, and, increasingly, private sector actors. In this text, we present *both* the nuts and bolts of global health, its ideologies, practices, and institutions *and* analyze and explain each topic—from health data to disease patterns, disasters, and development and health cooperation—through a critical political economy lens that contextualizes and fundamentally alters the way these issues are understood and addressed.

Other global health textbooks certainly mention the role of social (and sometimes political, but rarely world order) determinants of health as topics of interest, but these are typically presented as just another topic and remain unintegrated with the main approach. Political economy has also been reduced by some to considering political and economic variables without asking how and why power is distributed asymmetrically and in whose interest, what is the impact on health, and how the world order might be re-imagined and rearranged. This text, by contrast, makes links among factors that are often considered unconnected—such as the relation of capital flight and oppression to health—and asks tough questions that do not necessarily yield straightforward or rapid solutions, and that challenge existing local and global power relationships. In this way, the production of health, disease, and death are understood as endpoints of a constellation of influences and processes. Not only do we intend for this textbook to provide readers with a comprehensive understanding of diverse aspects of global health, we anticipate that the framework will be useful at distinct career stages. In sum, this approach may be rather different from others encountered by many students, yet (we hope) essential to forming a comprehensive and deeply critical perspective on the forces shaping global health, past and present.

OVERVIEW OF THE TEXTBOOK

Key Themes

Disease Distribution and Health Inequities

The global health field brings good news, bad news, and complicated news. At the aggregate level, health is improving, as measured by a global life expectancy higher than ever before, increasing from 52.5 years in 1960 to 71.6 years today. What is more, UN member countries came together in 2015 to endorse the Sustainable Development Goals (SDGs), heralding a new commitment to improving health and well-being on the aspirational heels of the predecessor Millennium Development Goals.

Yet health inequities have not disappeared, and many of the problems plaguing (particularly poor and marginalized) people across the globe are recurrences of diseases previously under control. Stopping yellow fever outbreaks was among the original rationales for international sanitary cooperation in the 19th century. After an effective vaccine was developed in the 1930s, the disease was believed eminently preventable. Yet existence of a vaccine is not enough: yellow fever has returned in recent years, with an initially little noticed 2016 epidemic in Angola and the Democratic Republic of Congo contributing to ballooning global yellow fever deaths of up to 50,000 annually—90% in Africa, especially in rural settings where there is little access to health services and overall social conditions are appalling.

Such resurgent diseases are not only a feature of LMICs. TB is now the world's leading infectious disease killer, with incidence (new cases per year) highest in sub-Saharan Africa. But TB incidence in the Canadian Arctic territory of Nunavut—home to a largely Inuit population—reached 300 cases per 100,000 people in 2010, 65 times higher than Canada's overall rate (Gallant, McGuire, and Ogunnaike-Cooke 2015) and exceeding the average incidence of 271 per 100,000 people in all low-income countries (WHO 2011). This represents an enormous inequity in one of the highest GDP per capita countries with a notable national health insurance system. Notwithstanding Nunavut's abundant natural resources, its Indigenous population has experienced years of crisis around inadequate housing, education, health care, and water infrastructure, atop centuries of neglect and mistreatment by the national government and a legacy of colonial oppression.

Meanwhile, key mortality inequities between countries have increased over the past few decades. In the case of maternal mortality, there is a 200-fold difference between countries with the highest and lowest maternal death rates, a doubling of the gap since 1990 (Koblinsky et al. 2016). Inequities within countries also persist. Across most settings, infant and maternal mortality are markedly higher in poorer than wealthier groups, with disparities worsening during periods of economic growth (Minujin and Delamonica 2003). In India, for example, inequality in both child mortality and malnutrition has risen over time (Chalasani 2012). Simultaneous to the lack of accessible and quality maternity care services for many women (especially displaced populations), among other groups, private sector incentives lead to excessive and unnecessary medicalization, with caesarean section rates approaching or exceeding 50% in certain Latin American and Middle Eastern countries (Miller et al. 2016).

Health is also deteriorating in several HIC settings. In the United States, life expectancy for certain middle-aged groups has dropped in recent years, linked to rises in drug and alcohol overdoses, suicide, and chronic liver disease, likely due to precarious employment and economic insecurity and their psychosocial effects (Case and Deaton 2015). In the United Kingdom, too, where social care benefits have been slashed over the past decade, life expectancy among older ages has stagnated or declined (Public Health England 2016).

At the same time, in diverse LMIC settings, there is promising news: infant mortality in Cuba and maternal mortality in Sri Lanka keep decreasing, and are respectively lower or equivalent to US rates (the United States is one of few countries worldwide where maternal mortality has risen in the past 15 years, partly reflecting high rates among African-American women) (WHO 2015). How do we reconcile the paradox of increasing inequities amid rising life expectancy overall? And what explains the favourable health results in certain LMIC settings, that is, how do some countries manage to buck the trend?

The SDGs purport to resolve the most central and intractable problems of health and well-being, but omitted from this calculus is addressing the powerful national and global financial and political forces undergirding health and social inequities. For example, SDG 5 calls for gender equality and women's empowerment, importantly citing women's equal rights to economic resources (e.g., access to land, education, and health services), as well as the role of gendered dimensions of oppression in the family and community. Yet it fails to recognize the exploitative conditions of women's labor—intertwined with factors linked to social class and race/ethnicity—that drive economic growth at the global level (Kumar, Birn, and McDonough 2016).

Health and the World Order

The association between global health and globalization—the growing worldwide circulation of business interests, people, products, ideas, and information amid greater economic integration—is a key underpinning of the field. But this is not a benign or neutral issue: although worldwide exchange and interdependence are not new, today's integration of markets, unfettered financial transactions, the concomitant spread of neoliberal ideology—favoring privatization, pro-corporate tax policy and trade and investment agreements, and the intentional shrinking of welfare state entitlements—the increasing power of transnational capital and corporations, and the reorganization of the global labor market and ratcheting down of worker and environmental protections all have enormous bearing on the lives of all, with widespread negative consequences except for elites (see chapter 9).

To name but a few effects of this neoliberal phase of capitalism, the debt crises and international financial institution (IFI)-imposed economic restructuring across LMICs since the 1980s led to decimation of social services, with repercussions still felt today, as in Liberia, Guinea, and Sierra Leone, which suffered the brunt of Ebola deaths in the 2014–2015 outbreak. In dozens of HICs and MICs, the global financial crisis of 2008 and subsequent Great Recession, with accompanying austerity and unemployment, have been associated with over 260,000 excess cancer deaths (Maruthappu et al. 2016).

Even absent crisis conditions, the ongoing effects of illicit financial flows, such as tax abuse, have resulted in trillions of dollars in lost public revenues that otherwise could have improved housing, education, water and sanitation, employment, and environmental protection for people across LMICs and HICs alike. These revenue losses, framed by national politics, including tax policy, also profoundly affect whether health care system principles of universality, accessibility, affordability, quality, and equity can be reached. The 2016 Panama paper revelations of wealthy elites sheltering their billions in tax havens offers only a glimpse at the maneuverings of corporations and wealthy elites to accumulate capital at the expense of the vast majority of people.

Furthermore, rising militarism to protect capitalist interests in natural resources—oil in the Middle East, minerals in Central Africa—as well as pursue ideological and geopolitical interests and advance the military-industrial complex itself, is among the most heinous attributes of the contemporary world order.

Also linked to globalization are climate change and environmental degradation. From drought presaging extreme food crisis for tens of millions in southern Africa (UNOCHA 2016) to global water scarcity (Mekonnen and Hoekstra 2016), fossil-fuel combustion-driven temperature changes and sea-level rises, and air and water contamination, the repercussions of environment-related health harms—associated with almost one quarter of global deaths—are almost invariably borne by the socially excluded, poor, and oppressed. Meanwhile, the main drivers of contamination and resource depletion are large-scale industry including agribusiness, mining, energy extraction and production, and chemical manufacturing, in combination with rapid urbanization and mass consumption.

At the heart of neoliberal globalization is big business, especially transnational corporations (TNCs), financial interests, and their government collaborators. To name but a few effects: land grabs displace small farmers and communities for the purpose of expanding export-oriented agriculture; mining operations contaminate precious water sources; flagrant workers' rights abuses characterize much of the garment industry; a surge in factory farming has provoked avian influenza; and transnational marketing has brought highly processed foods and sugary beverages to every corner of the world (wreaking health havoc among young and older populations alike). The power, influence, and tactics of TNCs to pursue profits invariably comes at the expense of public health and human rights.

The corporate pharmaceutical industry plays a particularly problematic role at the nexus of globalization and inequity. The global patent rules that enable Big Pharma profiteering mean that scientific improvements in medicines—HIV drugs in the recent past (whose patent protection has been challenged by transnational social movements and the courageous stances of countries like Brazil, India, and Thailand), and hepatitis C and cancer treatments currently, plus the first new TB treatment in 40 years, bedaquiline—are priced exorbitantly, feeding pharmaceutical greed while remaining out of reach for LMICs (DeAngelis 2016).

Given the complex global scenario, who bears responsibility for protecting and promoting health within and across countries? How should these entities be held accountable? What is the role of health professionals, public entities, and civil society groups in shaping health conditions and societal destiny writ large?

Actors, Agendas, Health Diplomacy, and Global (Health) Governance

The global health field is populated by a range of agencies, many staffed with young professionals seeking to make a difference. Some organizations are longstanding, including government development agencies, multilateral organizations, IFIs, universities, philanthropies, and missionary and humanitarian organizations; others are part of a newer guard of foundations, consulting firms, NGOs, business interests, and public–private initiatives. Global health and development donors provide various forms of financial and technical "aid" to so-called "recipients"; the flow of aid has traditionally been from HICs to LMICs (with a smaller contingent of South–South actors proffering the possibility of a more democratized form of cooperation).

Simultaneously, there are countless people—health educators, midwives, activists, primary health care workers, occupational hygienists, planners, community leaders, social workers, local, national, and international civil servants, entomologists, and so on—who contribute every day to addressing global health problems. Yet these key players are little recognized as they are typically not considered part of the global health scenario.

Why so many actors are engaged in global health raises questions around what they are doing and whose interests they serve. The spread of disease from one place to another is a recurring economic and political concern, in HICs often couched in racist or xenophobic rhetoric about the ills of LMICs "not reaching our shores." National security concerns around potential bioterrorist threats and the social and political menace posed by health crises—often accompanied by lurid media coverage—have helped propel global health upwards on the foreign policy agenda of many countries.

Another prime driver of geopolitical interests in global health is protection of the world economic order: neoliberal capitalism. In this sense, global health governance is concerned with disease outbreaks that could interrupt commerce, manufacturing, tourism, and other sectors that represent the interests of powerful economic actors. These concerns also shape interest in maintaining the health of military personnel, the productivity of multinational enterprises, and protecting the health of expatriate populations and travelers, as well as ensuring overall geopolitical stability.

Analysis of these drivers and motives is a recurring theme throughout the textbook, essential to comprehending both whose and which concerns set the global health agenda (Sridhar 2012) and the sources of friction between donor and "recipient" priorities. Points of contention include: tending to global health emergencies versus chronic and underlying issues; investing in single-disease campaigns versus health system strengthening; and social movement and LMIC challenges to HIC and financial elite hegemony (viz., control by dominant actors, largely unchallenged) in agenda-setting. These tensions have enormous repercussions both for the funding of WHO, whose activities are overwhelmingly controlled by donors rather than democratically representing the needs of member countries, and for LMIC national health systems, whose priorities and policies are often distorted by donors and by the interests of national elites. On rare occasions, a form of South–South health diplomacy manages to break with asymmetrical aid by organizing truly solidarity-oriented approaches to cooperation in health, such as Cuba's efforts around primary health care implementation in over 100 LMICs.

Far more prominently, global health has become big business (Deaton 2013), whether in terms of market opportunities for private health insurance and pharmaceuticals or in promoting the marriage of private enterprise and philanthropy ("philanthrocapitalism") via a wide range of public-private partnerships (PPPs) dedicated to combating diseases and malnutrition and to promoting medicines and vaccine distribution, drug development, management of hospitals, and so on. The increasing penetration of private sector actors into global health normalizes their role as legitimate "stakeholders" even as it enables the primary fiduciary obligation of companies—to maximize profits—to trump the public's health. Public-interest civil society actors have decried private sector intrusion into global health policy and governance as conflictual, unethical (e.g., transnational food corporations involved in discussions around prevention of NCDs), and impelled by self-interest (Lhotská and Gupta 2016). Yet far too many domestic and international civil servants (who serve the public) and academics (largely funded by the public) stay mute on these issues. Ultimately, global health PPPs are a double-edged sword—on one hand furnishing needed funding, on the other subjecting public matters and resources to private ends and profiteering (Velásquez 2014).

Another central facet of global health is the humanitarian response to disasters and emergencies, especially those involving large numbers of people whose lives are disrupted by ecological, economic, or military calamity. Yet many humanitarian organizations play a contradictory (and unwitting, at least on the part of front-line workers) role in assisting those experiencing the most inhumane circumstances of conflict, famine, and displacement, while often doing little to speak out or address the conditions and underlying forces that perpetuate the need for humanitarian assistance.

Mainstream Global Health versus (Transnational Global) Health Activism and Resistance

In mainstream circles, global health is often portrayed as the diffusion of ideas, practices, and technologies, principally from HICs to LMICs. Many global health efforts thereby presume that the health problems of LMICs stem from lack of resources, knowledge (including about unhealthy behaviors), and particular tools (e.g., bed nets to prevent malaria) or technologies (e.g., medications), and that it is the role of global health agencies to decide which of these to purvey and how. But such a perspective belies the countless historical and contemporary innovations and discoveries arising from LMICs, whether in surgical practice or malaria prophylaxis. To name just one current example, nearly three quarters of medications used in modern cancer care are derived from traditional medicinal plants (Prasad and Tyagi 2015).

Moreover, important as scientific advances are, the preponderance of global health actors and initiatives fail to acknowledge or understand what is perhaps the crucial factor accompanying and enabling progress in health: the role of power, access to resources, social and political relations, and the "rules of the game" in shaping patterns of health and health equity and seeking to address them. Indeed, scientific and technological innovations are often framed as the sources of global health success, whereas failures are attributed to "political interference," as if politics could be neatly separated from health and disease patterns (Lee 2015, p. 257). This is not a question of whether or not disease control interventions should be employed, but rather how and when technical interventions should be incorporated into integrated social and political approaches to improving health that involve not only "on the ground" measures, but also address the context of inequality and discrimination at all levels, global trade and financial policies, and environmental and labor standards, among other measures.

In contrast to dominant approaches, proponents of social justice perspectives consider global health to be a collective concern of ordinary people, involving their/our own advocacy (Freire 1992), supported by like-minded movements locally and in other settings, solidarity-oriented transnational efforts, and (ideally) governments *representative* of people's needs. Social justice perspectives draw from critical political economy, whereby understanding and addressing the role of oppression and the imbalanced distribution of power and resources—social, economic, political, scientific—is essential to tackling the challenges of global health. Human well-being, health, and dignity derive, accordingly, from just and equitable societies; political struggles for universal social rights and protections are thus central to global health transformation. As such, a social justice model counters neoliberal ideology guided by market (in)justice. Most global health actors pay little mind to social justice-oriented healthy societies, illustrating renowned scholar-activist Noam Chomsky's insight regarding the threat of a good example. These ideas, movements, and examples will be discussed thoroughly in the chapters ahead.

Social justice efforts often entail resistance, be it through transnational social movements or local organizations. For example, Honduran environmental activist Berta Cáceres, alongside local Indigenous communities, struggled for decades in opposition to environmentally damaging projects including the infamous Agua Zarca Dam, which would have jeopardized access to safe water, food, and medicine, violating Indigenous rights and livelihoods. In 2013, these efforts successfully halted the dam project, but in March 2016 Cáceres's unwavering activism ended when she was brutally assassinated in her home. This textbook emphasizes the great importance of similar valiant efforts around building healthy and just societies in all corners of the world, recognizing that at times they come at enormous personal cost.

On another front, in June 2016 Médecins Sans Frontières (MSF) announced it would no longer accept funding from the European Union (EU) in protest of its migration policy that prioritizes deterrence over humane and timely protection, assistance, and resettling of refugees. Despite needing resources, MSF rejected the untenable contradiction of receiving EU funding for assisting the victims of EU policies. If only more humanitarian agencies acted according to principle and took such stances against donors! This underscores the point that public health practitioners, scholars, and activists may hold a critical perspective and engage in resistance, even while maintaining affiliation with more traditional public health fields, agencies, and institutions.

Throughout the textbook we will cover illustrations of this more hopeful face of struggling for global health equity, including engaging in global health without a passport.

Box 0-2 Questions to ponder throughout the textbook

- Why have some LMICs been able to make great strides in reducing disease and mortality while certain HIC settings have persistently large health inequities?
- How is the world order (the arrangement of political and economic rules and institutions) related to the global health agenda (today or in the past)?
- What is the relationship between the distribution of power and resources— within and between countries—and patterns of morbidity and mortality?
- What should be the role of global institutions and agendas in shaping domestic and local policies concerning health and well-being?
- Should global health actors emphasize underlying causes of ill health or immediate problems? Or both?
- Who should set the global health agenda?
- What constitutes success in global health?
- Why are social justice, political economy, and health and human rights approaches left out of most mainstream global health efforts?

How to Use this Textbook

This textbook is designed for a semester-long advanced undergraduate or early-year graduate course. The chapters are meant to flow logically from week to week, but ample cross-referencing allows for material to be presented in a different order or for students to read ahead. Each chapter includes key questions for major chapter sections. The questions provide a basis for individual reflection and group discussion, as well as a helpful reading and study guide. The chapters conclude with learning points that summarize key take-home messages. Although we have done our best to provide real-time updates as the book has been in production, the global health arena is changing so rapidly that this new edition is already outdated on some dimensions. Yet even if certain details and examples are not entirely current, the book's critical political economy of health framing and the tools and methods employed to understand and analyze the field remain as relevant as ever.

The first section of the textbook (chapters 1–7) provides the basic tools for understanding global health. With multiple pressing health needs today, it may seem unexpected to find several chapters dedicated to the history of international health. Nonetheless, as we will see, contemporary patterns, priorities, and practices of global health have been signficantly shaped by past experience, making historical analysis an essential tool in understanding the field's challenges, pitfalls, and prospects. History tells stories—about who we are and how we came to be, explaining shifting and ongoing trends and contexts—offering a window on society and insight in times of crisis and change.

Chapter 1 explores the historical roots of international health, analyzing the forces and developments (including imperialism, colonialism, slavery, and industrialization) that marked international health actors and activities in the past, many of which have had lasting bearing on the field's ideas, institutions, and approaches. Chapter 2 examines dominant development ideologies in the post-World War II and Cold War contexts, the waxing and waning of the WHO as *the* international health authority and its principal activities in different eras, and the transition to global health. Chapter 3 presents the book's critical political economy of health framework, providing a theoretical and practical basis for understanding and addressing the challenges of global health in contrast to bio-behavioral models. It also examines political economy of development in foreign policy, donor-recipient relations, and the aid milieu and discusses development goals and other contemporary approaches to development, including global health governance. Chapter 4 profiles the range of agencies, actors, and activities that have populated and influenced global health in recent decades, critically reviewing the role, motivations, and impact of global health aid and of the most important global health players: IFIs, bilateral agencies, multilateral agencies, South–South arrangements, philanthropic and corporate foundations, PPPs, military actors, humanitarian agencies, NGOs, social movements, and others. Chapter 5 outlines how mortality and morbidity are measured and statistics produced, how and why health data are or are not collected, and what gaps in information must be filled in order to address global health problems and health inequities adequately. Chapter 6 provides an overview epidemiologic profile of health and disease patterns across the world, contesting traditional dichotomies of communicable and non-communicable diseases to explore the causes of ill health and premature death under conditions of: marginalization and deprivation (e.g., diarrhea, malaria, and respiratory infections); modernization and work (e.g., cardiovascular disease, cancer, and road traffic injuries and death); marginalization and modernization (e.g., TB, HIV, and diabetes); and emerging (global) social and economic patterns (e.g., MERS, avian influenza, narcotics overdoses). Chapter 7 focuses on the societal determinants/determination of health, illness, and mortality—at household, community, national, and global levels—*and* how they intertwine with, and are underscored by, health inequities, both within and across societies; it also explores the role of integrated policy approaches, such as Health in All Policies.

The next section of the textbook (chapters 8–12) analyzes global health and its ongoing challenges from a set of key lenses—the priority areas and building blocks for understanding and improving global health efforts. In chapter 8 we examine the issue of health under crisis conditions: ecological disasters; complex humanitarian emergencies; the refugee crisis; war, militarization (covering the effects of the arms industry and nuclear, chemical, and biological weapons), and civil violence (increasingly involving narcotrafficking); and the reach and limits of humanitarian assistance. Chapter 9 explores the impact of neoliberal globalization on health in HICs and LMICs alike, the role of trade and investment agreements, TNCs, and other features of contemporary capitalism in shaping overall health conditions, and the effects of labor market reorganization and poor working conditions on health. Chapter 10 reviews health concerns arising from environmental degradation affecting air, water, and land, including climate change, as well as the economic and social forces undergirding these problems: consumption-driven economies; industrial production; and polluting industries such as mining, agribusiness, and energy. It also discusses a range of current and potential responses to them at global, national, local, and social movement levels. Chapter 11 offers a comparative analysis of a range of health care systems and health reforms, and lays out principles and policies that contribute to effective and equitable health systems. Chapter 12 explores health economics, health financing, and the economics of health, explaining, analyzing, and critiquing the main tools of these fields.

The final section of the textbook (chapters 13 and 14) turns to the making of healthy policies across the world—and the roles and responsibilities of those working in the field locally, internationally, and transnationally. Chapter 13 provides a set of examples of countries and cities that have invested in inclusive, universal, and equitable policies to improve health, sometimes under trying circumstances, and discusses health promotion, and Indigenous and degrowth paradigms that can contribute to building healthy societies. These efforts are contrasted with the disease-control and targeted campaigns that continue to characterize mainstream global health and development. Chapter 14 focuses on the practice of global health: how to foster solidarity-oriented cooperation; understand, navigate, contribute to, and ethically engage in the field; and the many alternatives to mainstream approaches to global health. This final section of the textbook is also foreshadowed by the activist and advocacy efforts against neoliberal globalization highlighted in chapter 9 and against environmental injustice in chapter 10. Ultimately, the textbook presents an unfinished story: subsequent chapters remain to be written, and will be based on the aspirations and contributions of *you* collectively—as current and prospective leaders, researchers, practitioners, and activists shaping global health and social justice into the future.

Readers may be wondering about the significance of the image portrayed on this textbook's front cover of a small fishing craft bobbing on murky waters. Some may see it as portending the uncertain future of global health, with its bareness suggesting that much is missing from the field at present. Others may view this picture of a Brazilian boat named *Saúde Global* ("global health" in Portuguese) more optimistically, with bright colors enveloping a vessel open to a world of possibilities. Regardless of a priori perspective, we are about to embark on a global health voyage together, one that may take us to unexpected places and that will undoubtedly, like all journeys, leave us challenged and changed.

REFERENCES

Buettner-Schmidt K and Lobo M. 2011. Social justice: A concept analysis. *Journal of Advanced Nursing* 68(4):948–958.

Chalasani S. 2012. Understanding wealth-based inequalities in child health in India: A decomposition approach. *Social Science & Medicine* 75(12):2160–2169.

DeAngelis CD. 2016. Big Pharma profits and the public loses. *The Milbank Quarterly* 94(1):30–33.

Deaton A. 2013. *The Great Escape: Health, Wealth and the Origins of Inequality.* Princeton, NJ: Princeton University Press.

De Ceukelaire W and Botenga MJ. 2014. On global health: Stick to sovereignty. *Lancet* 383(9921):951–952.

Freire P. 1992. *Pedagogy of Hope: Reliving Pedagogy of the Oppressed.* London: Bloomsbury.

Frenk J, Gómez-Dantés O, and Moon S. 2014. From sovereignty to solidarity: A renewed concept of global health for an era of complex interdependence. *Lancet* 383(9911):94–97.

Galea S, Thea D, and Annas G. 2016. A gold medal in fear mongering. *Huffington Post Blog*, June 2.

Gallant V, McGuire M, and Ogunnaike-Cooke S. 2015. A summary of tuberculosis in Canada, 2013. *Canada Communicable Disease Report* 41(S2):2–7.

Garay J, Harris L, and Walsh J. 2013. Global health: Evolution of the definition, use and misuse of the term. *Face à face* 12 [online] http://faceaface.revues.org/745.

Granda E. 2004. ¿A qué llamamos salud colectiva, hoy? *Revista Cubana de Salud Pública* 30(2).

Hanna-Attisha M, LaChance J, Sadler RC, and Champney Schnepp A. 2016. Elevated blood lead levels in children associated with the Flint drinking water crisis: A spatial analysis of risk and public health response. *American Journal of Public Health* 106(2):283–290.

Kearns CE, Schmidt LA, and Glantz SA. 2016. Sugar industry and coronary heart disease research: A historical analysis of internal industry documents. *JAMA Internal Medicine.* [Epub ahead of print].

Kleinman A. 2010. Four social theories for global health. *Lancet* 375(9725):1518–1519.

Koblinsky M, Moyer CA, Calvert C, et al. 2016. Quality maternity care for every woman, everywhere: A call to action. *Lancet* [Epub ahead of print].

Kumar R, Birn A-E, and McDonough P. 2016. International cooperation in women's health: Critical analysis of a quarter century of paradigm shifts. In Gideon J, Editor. *Handbook on Gender and Health*. Cheltenham, UK: Edward Elgar Publishing.

Lee K. 2015. Revealing power in truth: Comment on "Knowledge, moral claims and the exercise of power in global health." *International Journal of Health Policy and Management* 4(4):257–259.

Lessler J, Chaisson LH, Kucirka LM, et al. 2016. Assessing the global threat from Zika virus. *Science* 353(6300):aaf8160.

Lhotská L and Gupta A. 2016. Whose health?: The crucial negotiations for the World Health Organization's future. *Asia & the Pacific Policy Society*, May 19.

Lima NT, Santana JP, and Paiva CHA. 2015. *Saúde Coletiva: A Abrasco em 35 anos de história*. Rio de Janeiro: Associação Brasileira de Saúde Coletiva.

Macfarlane SB, Jacobs M, and Kaaya EE. 2008. In the name of global health: Trends in academic institutions. *Journal of Public Health Policy* 29(4):383–401.

Marten R. 2016. Global health warning: Definitions wield power: Comment on "Navigating between stealth advocacy and unconscious dogmatism: The challenge of researching the norms, politics and power of global health." *International Journal of Health Policy and Management* 5(3):207–209.

Maruthappu M, Watkins J, Noor AM, et al. 2016. Economic downturns, universal health coverage, and cancer mortality in high-income and middle-income countries, 1990–2010: A longitudinal analysis. *Lancet* 388(10045):684–695.

Mekonnen MM and Hoekstra AY. 2016. Four billion people facing severe water scarcity. *Science Advances* 2(2):e1500323.

Miller S, Abalos E, Chamillard M, et al. 2016. Beyond too little, too late and too much, too soon: A pathway towards evidence-based, respectful maternity care worldwide. *Lancet* [Epub ahead of print].

Minujin A and Delamonica E. 2003. Mind the gap! Widening child mortality disparities. *Journal of Human Development* 4(3):397–418.

Navarro V. 2009. What we mean by social determinants of health. *International Journal of Health Services* 39(3):423–441.

Office of Multicultural Affairs. 2014. *Diversity and Social Justice: A Glossary of Working Definitions*. Lowell: Office of Multicultural Affairs, University of Massachusetts.

Possas C. 2016. Zika: What we do and do not know based on the experiences of Brazil. *Epidemiology and Health* 38:e2016023.

Prasad S and Tyagi AK. 2015. Traditional medicine: The goldmine for modern drugs. *Advanced Techniques in Biology and Medicine* 3(1):e108.

Public Health England. 2016. *Recent Trends in Life Expectancy at Older Ages: Update to 2014*. London: Public Health England.

Scott-Villiers P, Chisholm N, Wanjiku Kelbert A, and Hossain N. 2016. *Precarious Lives: Food, Work and Care After the Global Food Crisis*. Brighton: IDS and Oxfam International.

Sridhar D. 2012. Who sets the global health research agenda? The challenge of multi-bi financing. *PLoS Medicine* 9(9):e1001312.

Storeng KT. 2014. The GAVI Alliance and the "Gates approach" to health system strengthening. *Global Public Health* 9(8):865–879.

UNHCR. 2016. *Global Trends: Forced Displacement in 2015*. Geneva: UNHCR.

UNOCHA. 2016. *Regional Outlook for Southern Africa: Recommendations for Humanitarian Action and Resilience Response*. Geneva: UNOCHA.

Velásquez G. 2014. *Public-Private Partnerships in Global Health: Putting Business before Health?* Geneva: South Centre.

Ventura DFL. 2016. From Ebola to Zika: International emergencies and the securitization of global health. *Cadernos de Saúde Pública* 32(4):1–4.

WHO. 2011. *Global Tuberculosis Control 2011*. Geneva: WHO.

______. 2015. Global Health Observatory data repository. http://www.who.int/gho/database/en/. Accessed June 9, 2015.

______. 2016a. *Prevention of Sexual Transmission of Zika virus: Interim Guidance Update: 7 June 2016*. Geneva: WHO.

______. 2016b. *Situation Report: Zika virus, Microcephaly and Guillain-Barré syndrome: 8 September 2016*. Geneva: WHO.

Winslow C-EA. 1920. The untilled fields of public health. *Science* 51:23–33.

SOME ABBREVIATIONS AND ACRONYMS

AIDS	Acquired Immunodeficiency Syndrome
ALAMES	Latin American Social Medicine Association
ARI	Acute Respiratory (Tract) Infection
ART	Antiretroviral Therapy
ARVs	Antiretroviral Drugs
AU	African Union
BCG	Bacille Calmette-Guerin (tuberculosis vaccine)
BMGF	Bill and Melinda Gates Foundation
BRAC	Bangladesh Rehabilitation Assistance Committee
BRICS	Brazil, Russia, India, China, South Africa
BWC	Biological Weapons Convention
CBA	Cost–Benefit Analysis OR Community-Based Adaptation
CBO	Community-Based Organization
CBW	Chemical and Biological Weapons
CCTs	Conditional Cash Transfers
CDC	Centers for Disease Control and Prevention (US)
CEA	Cost-Effectiveness Analysis
CFCs	Chlorofluorocarbons
CHD	Coronary Heart Disease
CHE	Complex Humanitarian Emergency
CHW	Community Health Worker
CKD	Chronic Kidney Disease
CLTS	Community-Led Total Sanitation
CMH	Commission on Macroeconomics and Health
COPD	Chronic Obstructive Pulmonary Disease
CSDH	Commission on Social Determinants of Health
CVD	Cardiovascular Disease
CWC	Chemical Weapons Convention
DAC	Development Assistance Committee (OECD)
DAH	Development Assistance for Health
DALY	Disability-Adjusted Life Year

DFID	Department for International Development (UK)
DGH	Doctors for Global Health
DHS	Demographic and Health Survey
DoD	Department of Defense (US)
DRC	Democratic Republic of Congo
EC	Ethical Research Committee
EDCs	Endocrine Disrupting Chemicals
EIA	Environmental Impact Assessment
EPI	Expanded Programme on Immunization (WHO)
EPZ	Export Processing Zone
EQUINET	Regional Network on Equity in Health in Southern Africa
EU	European Union
EVD	Ebola Virus Disease
FAO	Food and Agriculture Organization of the UN
FCTC	Framework Convention on Tobacco Control (WHO)
FDI	Foreign Direct Investment
FENSA	Framework for Engagement with Non-State Actors (WHO)
GAVI	Global Alliance for Vaccines and Immunization, now GAVI, the Vaccine Alliance
GBD	Global Burden of Disease
GBV	Gender-Based Violence
GDP	Gross Domestic Product
GHGs	Greenhouse Gases
GNH	Gross National Happiness
GNI	Gross National Income
GNP	Gross National Product
GOBI	Growth Monitoring, Oral Rehydration, Breastfeeding, Immunization
GOBI/FFF	GOBI plus Family Planning, Female Education, Food Supplementation
GP	General Practitioner
HAI	Health Alliance International
HCP	Healthy Cities Program
HDI	Human Development Index
HIA	Health Impact Assessment
HiAP	Health in All Policies
HICs	High-Income Countries
HIPC	Heavily Indebted Poor Countries (Initiative)
HIV	Human Immunodeficiency Virus
HNP	Health, Nutrition, and Population Division (World Bank)
HPV	Human Papilloma Virus
IBFAN	International Baby Food Action Network
IBRD	International Bank for Reconstruction and Development (World Bank)
ICD	International Classification of Diseases
ICRC	International Committee of the Red Cross
IDA	International Development Association (World Bank)
IDPs	Internally Displaced Persons
IFBA	International Food and Beverage Alliance
IFIs	International Financial Institutions
IHME	Institute for Health Metrics and Evaluation
IHR	International Health Regulations
ILO	International Labour Organization (previously Office)

IMF	International Monetary Fund
IMR	Infant Mortality Rate
INGO	International Nongovernmental Organization
IPCC	Intergovernmental Panel on Climate Change
IPHU	International People's Health University
IRB	Institutional Review Board
ISDS	Investor-State Dispute Settlement
J-PAL	Abdul Latif Jameel Poverty Action Lab (MIT)
LASM	Latin American Social Medicine
LGBTQIA	Lesbian, Gay, Bisexual, Transgender, Queer, Intersex, and Asexual
LICs	Low-Income Countries
LMICs	Low- and Middle-Income Countries
LNHO	League of Nations Health Organisation
MDGs	Millennium Development Goals
MDRI	Multilateral Debt Relief Initiative
MEA	Multilateral Environmental Agreement
MERS-CoV	Middle East Respiratory Syndrome Coronavirus
MICs	Middle-Income Countries
MMR	Maternal Mortality Ratio
MMRate	Maternal Mortality Rate
MOH	Ministry of Health
MSF	Médecins Sans Frontières
MTCT	Mother-to-Child Transmission (of HIV)
NATO	North Atlantic Treaty Organization
NCDs	Noncommunicable Diseases
NGO	Nongovernmental Organization
NHS	National Health Service (UK)
NIEO	New International Economic Order
NIH	National Institutes of Health (US)
NMR	Neonatal Mortality Rate
NTDs	Neglected Tropical Diseases
OCHA	UN Office for the Coordination of Humanitarian Affairs
ODA	Official Development Assistance
OECD	Organization for Economic Cooperation and Development
OIHP	Office International d'Hygiène Publique
ORT	Oral Rehydration Therapy
OSH	Occupational Safety and Health
PAHO	Pan American Health Organization
PASB	Pan American Sanitary Bureau
PDP	Product Development Partnership
PEPFAR	President's Emergency Plan for AIDS Relief (US)
PHC	Primary Health Care
PHI	Popular Health Insurance (Mexico)
PHM	People's Health Movement
PIH	Partners In Health
PM	Particulate Matter
POPs	Persistent Organic Pollutants
PPP	Public-Private Partnership OR Purchasing Power Parity
PRGT	Poverty Reduction and Growth Trust
PRSP	Poverty Reduction Strategy Papers

R&D	Research and Development
RCT	Randomized Controlled Trial
RF	Rockefeller Foundation
SAL	Structural Adjustment Loan
SAP	Structural Adjustment Program
SARS	Severe Acute Respiratory Syndrome
SDGs	Sustainable Development Goals
SDOH	Social/Societal Determinants of Health
SEP	Socioeconomic Position OR Smallpox Eradication Programme
SES	Socioeconomic Status
SPHC	Selective Primary Health Care
SSC	South-South Cooperation
SJSSC	Social Justice-Oriented South-South Cooperation
STD	Sexually Transmitted Disease
STI	Sexually Transmitted Infection
SUS	Unified Health Care System (Brazil)
SWAp	Sector-Wide Approach
TB	Tuberculosis
TFC	Transnational Food Corporation
TNC	Transnational Corporation
TRIPS	Trade-Related Aspects of Intellectual Property Rights (Agreement)
UAEM	Universities Allied for Essential Medicines
UDHR	Universal Declaration of Human Rights
UHC	Universal Health Coverage
UN	United Nations
UNASUR	Union of South American Nations
UNCTAD	UN Conference on Trade and Development
UNDP	UN Development Programme
UNEP	UN Environment Programme
UNESCO	UN Educational, Scientific, and Cultural Organization
UNFCCC	UN Framework Convention on Climate Change
UNFPA	UN Population Fund
UN-HABITAT	UN Human Settlements Programme
UNHCR	UN High Commissioner for Refugees
UNICEF	UN Children's Fund
UNODC	UN Office on Drugs and Crime
UNRRA	UN Relief and Rehabilitation Agency
USAID	US Agency for International Development
USPHS	US Public Health Service
VA	Verbal Autopsy
WDR	World Development Report (World Bank)
WFP	World Food Programme
WHA	World Health Assembly (WHO)
WHO	World Health Organization
WSF	World Social Forum
WTO	World Trade Organization
YPLL	Years of Potential Life Lost

ABOUT THE AUTHORS

Anne-Emanuelle Birn is Professor of Critical Development Studies (UTSC) and Social and Behavioural Health Sciences (Dalla Lana School of Public Health) at the University of Toronto, where she served as Canada Research Chair in International Health from 2003 to 2013. She is widely published in North America, Latin America, Europe, and Africa; her books include: *Marriage of Convenience: Rockefeller International Health and Revolutionary Mexico* (2006); and *Comrades in Health: US Health Internationalists, Abroad and at Home* (2013). Professor Birn's honors include Fulbright and Rotary fellowships, election to the Delta Omega Public Health Honor Society, and numerous endowed lectureships across the Americas and Asia. In 2014 she was recognized among the top 100 Women Leaders in Global Health.

Yogan Pillay is Deputy Director General for HIV, Tuberculosis, and Maternal, Newborn, and Child Health Programmes in the National Department of Health, South Africa. He has 20 years' experience in the planning and implementation of health system reforms and has published widely on the topics of HIV, tuberculosis, and health systems.

Timothy H. Holtz is an Adjunct Associate Professor of Global Health at the Rollins School of Public Health at Emory University. His field experience has focused on infectious disease epidemiology and disease control, and he has worked with the U.S. Centers for Disease Control and Prevention and as a consultant to the World Health Organization. From 2002-2010 Dr. Holtz worked in southern Africa, Eastern Europe, and South America on multidrug-resistant tuberculosis control and tuberculosis/HIV program capacity building. He is an internationally recognized expert on the emerging threat of anti-tuberculosis drug resistance and was part of the team of scientists that discovered extensively drug-resistant tuberculosis (XDR TB). He has also directed an HIV prevention clinical trial research program in Thailand, and an HIV and TB technical assistance program in India. He is a founding member of Doctors for Global Health, a health and social justice nongovernmental organization with projects in the U.S., Latin America, and sub-Saharan Africa.

1

THE HISTORICAL ORIGINS OF MODERN INTERNATIONAL (AND GLOBAL) HEALTH

Key Questions:

- When and why did governments (elected, hereditary, and despotic), moneyed interests (elites, merchants, business owners, etc.), scientists and health professionals, and the public become concerned with the spread of disease from place to place?
- How were these concerns addressed?
- What were the roles of imperialism, slavery, global commerce, and industrialization in shaping international health?
- Who and what motivated the establishment of early international health agencies?

Imagine a sudden disease outbreak causing high fever, severe dehydration, debility, and a terrifying spate of deaths in otherwise healthy people. Then picture swirling rumors about the causes of the epidemic, questionable therapeutics, assertive—if seemingly ungrounded—control measures imposed by authorities, and calls for quarantine and restrictions on travel and commerce, all fueled by fear and prejudice. From the cholera pandemic ravaging Delhi, Hamburg, and New York circa 1830; to the worldwide spread of H1N1 influenza in 2009; to perennial outbreaks of insect-borne diseases—and whether communicated by microbes or mosquitoes—such epidemics serve as the most visible rationale for global health action. Yet past or present, the justifications for global health have gone far beyond stemming illness and mortality, extending into realms of economic, political, and cultural importance.

Indeed, in order to understand the organization, goals, and dilemmas of, and influences on, the arena of global health today, it is worth asking how concern with international health arose in the past. A historical perspective can help to explain various interlocking questions: how did the larger economic and political context interact with local and national/regional factors to affect the emergence, spread, consequences, and fight against diseases both domestically and globally?; what was the role of shifting paradigms and practices of science and public health?; and who were the key players driving international health activities and organizations in different eras?

To address these issues, we begin by exploring the main antecedents of modern international (and global) health, starting with the 1300s–1600s waves of Eurasian plague and early attempts to combat this pandemic. Next, we examine the rise of colonialism and the slave trade—and their health consequences—from the late 15th century onward. We then turn to the interaction of imperialism with the Industrial Revolution amid the rise of capitalism, 19th century sanitary reform movements in various settings, and their repercussions for international health. Finally, we trace the appearance and evolution of a new set of international health institutions—both intergovernmental and nongovernmental—from the mid-19th century through the

1930s. In chapter 2 we discuss political, institutional, scientific, and social developments since World War II that have further shaped contemporary institutions, ideologies, and practices of global health.

ANTECEDENTS OF MODERN INTERNATIONAL HEALTH: BLACK DEATH, COLONIAL CONQUEST, AND THE ATLANTIC SLAVE TRADE

Key Questions:

- What aspects of the Black Death made it an international as opposed to a local issue?
- What were the health dimensions of colonial invasion and occupation?
- How did the Atlantic slave trade fit into colonialism and what were its health implications?

Although the modern system of international health—involving disease surveillance, sanitary regulation, dedicated organizations, information exchange, and cross-border activities—did not emerge until the 19th century, some of its features were present long before. Preoccupation with public health started thousands of years ago in ancient Andean, Chinese, Egyptian, Ethiopian, Greco-Roman, Hindu, Khmer, Mesoamerican, Moorish, Persian, and other civilizations. All of these societies developed healing approaches, theories of disease causation, and specific tools to address health problems. Each had sophisticated engineering capacity (as evidenced in the palaces, pyramids, and temples they left behind) and many devised elaborate systems of water supply (e.g., artesian wells and aqueducts), irrigation, garbage disposal, and sewage (Koloski-Ostrow 2015). Observational and empirical skills enabled the development of botanical remedies and surgical techniques, oftentimes dispensed in combination with supernatural practices. Medical/health knowledge and beliefs mostly remained within particular societies but could also traverse from one place to another through war, conquest, trade, and exploration. Until the Middle Ages, however, health concerns and disease outbreaks rarely extended beyond limited regions, except in the case of military incursions (e.g., as per Thucydides's account of plague during the Peloponnesian war in the 5th century BCE), and the occasional ailing trader.

Plague and the Beginnings of Health Regulation

For the most part, scientific ideas, technologies, and practices in medieval Europe trailed those of other societies, particularly in the Islamic world, where influential advances were made in such areas as astronomy, surgery, theories of disease-transmission, mind-body connections, and medical institutions (Pormann and Savage-Smith 2007). European healing involved a combination of local wisdom (e.g., knowledge of medicinal herbs passed down from generation to generation and among lay practitioners, including midwives who apprenticed with other wise women) and a hierarchy of town-based practitioners, such as apothecaries, barber-surgeons, and, later in the Middle Ages, university-trained physicians (Siraisi 1990).

It was during the Middle Ages that hospitals and religious orders dedicated to healing were established in Europe, partly to care for crusaders returning from Church-sanctioned military campaigns to recapture Palestine from Muslim control. Some institutions, such as St. Bartholomew's (St. Bart's) in London, founded in 1123, still function today. From about the 13th century on, secular hospitals were also founded in many municipalities (Horden 2008).

But changes were afoot that would test sanitary localism and Europe's backwardness. As rival leaders fought for land and power (needing ever greater resources for these exploits), and merchants became interested in the riches and resources of faraway places, travel and commerce gradually increased, with microbes as companions. The congested towns of late medieval Europe had markedly lower standards of water supply, sanitation, and hygiene than prior and contemporary civilizations elsewhere, such as the Aztec Empire, and thus became excellent candidates for epidemic disease.

Plague is among the earliest documented pandemics, with two great outbreaks bracketing the Middle Ages. The first, known as the Plague of Justinian, struck in 542 CE, decimating populations throughout Eurasia. The second was the Black Death of the 14th–17th centuries, the most destructive epidemic in the history of humankind, which resulted in an estimated 100 million deaths (almost one quarter of the world's population, especially striking Asia, Europe, and the Middle East).

Surmised to have originated in wild rodents (likely in Central Asia), whose habitats were disrupted by a mix of human invasion, expansion of farming lands, and new trading patterns, what became known as the Black Death traveled by land and water along the Silk Road. It reached the Black Sea in 1346. By 1348 it had spread northward to Russia, westward to Europe, eastward toward China, and southwestward to the Middle East.

The appearance of disease was understood by some in cosmological or environmental terms; others considered it God's punishment for collective or personal sin. These interpretations motivated, variously, days of prayer and the disposal and burning of corpses and belongings. Many doctors fled the towns, and aristocrats and wealthy merchants took refuge in their country estates, as depicted in Boccaccio's mid-14th-century fictionalized account of fleeing Florentine elites, *The Decameron*. Scapegoats were sought, and many blamed Jews, who suffered greatly as a result. With half or even more of the population perishing, the entire social, economic, political, and ecclesiastical structure of Europe, particularly, was shaken to its foundations (Slack 2012).

Although its cause was unknown,[1] plague's suspected communicability led to the earliest attempts at international disease control. In 1348, believing that plague was introduced via ships, the city-state of Venice adopted a 40-day detention period for entering vessels (a policy soon copied by Genoa, Marseille, and other major ports) after which the disease was believed to remit. This practice of *quarantine*—from the Italian word for forty—was minimally effective in stopping plague. Quarantine's stricter counterpart, the *cordon sanitaire*—a protective geographic belt barring exit of people or goods from cities or entire regions—would also be used frequently in succeeding centuries. In 1403 Venice established the first *lazaretto*, a quarantine station to hold and disinfect humans and cargo. Its island location was emulated by other cities across the world.

Because the Black Death's initial appearance preceded the formation of nation-states, sanitary efforts were adopted and implemented by municipal authorities with little coordination. While word of disease spread through travelers, there was no official system of notification or cooperation between city-states. Following the first plague pandemic, many towns and cities established plague boards, sometimes made into permanent public health boards, charged with imposing the necessary measures at times of outbreak. This precursor to international health authority was, paradoxically, local and unilateral rather than international and cooperative.

Over time, new ideas evolved around plague's communicability, justifying ever-strict quarantine measures. In 1546, the Veronese physician-scholar Girolamo Fracastoro revived ancient notions of contagion in his tract on plague transmission, theorizing that "seeds of disease" could be spread either through direct contact or by dissemination into the atmosphere (Roccasalva 2008).

Though the virulence of plague lessened somewhat in the late 14th and 15th centuries, subsequent visitations of the Black Death worsened. In 1630–1631, plague killed one quarter of the population in Bologna, one third in Venice, almost half in Milan, and almost two thirds in Verona. A scant generation later, half of the inhabitants of Rome, Naples, and Genoa succumbed to the plague of 1656–1657.

Plague, of course, was not the only deadly or epidemic ailment of the Middle Ages and early modern period. Smallpox, diphtheria, measles, influenza, tuberculosis, scabies, erysipelas, anthrax, trachoma, leprosy, and nutritional deficiencies were also rife (Rosen 2015). Less familiar today, mass hysteria in a climate of superstition led to outbreaks of dancing mania (St. Vitus Dance). Ergotism, arising from fungal contamination of rye, killed or disabled large numbers of people in dozens of epidemics between the 9th and 15th centuries.

Despite stringent sanitary enforcement during plague years, concepts of cleanliness and sanitation took hold slowly in Europe's cities. Through increasingly forceful legislation and public awareness, announced via the printing press (c. 1440) and town criers, urban centers began to approach the hygienic standards reached by the Roman Empire more than a millennium earlier. Although plague boards disbanded in the 17th century, many town governments took over control of street cleaning, disposal of dead bodies and carcasses, public baths, and water maintenance. By the 18th century, cities began to employ, fitfully, a new environmental engineering approach to epidemic disease, which emphasized preventive actions including improved ventilation, drainage of stagnant water, street cleaning, reinterment, cleaner wells, fumigation, and the burial of garbage (Riley 1987).

Even before the plague fully retreated, a new economic system began to develop that would irrevocably shape worldwide patterns of disease and eventually lead to international health measures and institutions.

The Rise of European Imperialism

During the Middle Ages, classical scientific and medical knowledge was retained by Islamic scholars, who established learned settlements in Spain, Portugal, Sicily, and throughout the Middle East and North Africa (Iqbal 2012), part of centuries of tolerant coexistence of Muslims, Christians, and Jews on the Iberian peninsula. Contacts with the Muslim world opened new vistas to European eyes. Partly as a continuation of the Christian–Muslim rivalry, partly for riches and adventure, and aided by a breakdown of Eurasian dominance and technical improvements in navigation and seacraft, Western Europeans of the early 15th century embarked on a series of conquests.

Portugal and then Spain—both maritime societies with established coastal trading—were in the vanguard of these ventures. Portugal's plundering raids into North Africa and later India led to permanent garrisons serving the lucrative spice trade from the East. Meanwhile, Spain's united Catholic monarchs restored royal authority domestically, unleashing the repressive Inquisition in 1478 and driving the Moors from the Iberian peninsula. After curbing Muslim influence, they instigated Crusades-inspired military-proselytizing campaigns, coupling newfound power with greed for expensive commodities and ever more territories. Genoan Cristoforo Colombo's Spanish-sponsored expeditions "discovered" the "New World" in 1492, claiming its lands and mineral wealth for his royal patrons. Spanish and Portuguese monarchs—abetted by a series of Papal bulls—arrogantly divided control of the world and embarked upon a ruthless land grab in the Americas and into Asia.

In the 17th century, the English and Dutch challenged Iberian dominance, extending European commercial, political, and military power even further. The Westphalian system of nation-states emerged around this time, setting national boundaries and asserting sovereignty within Europe, even as European powers were violently staking territorial claims across the world. Subsequently, France, Belgium, Germany, Italy, and others became colonial overlords in Africa, with Russia, Japan, and the United States among the last to enter the imperial fray in the late 19th century. The era of imperialism roughly spanned the late 15th to the mid-20th centuries, with a few colonies persisting to the present.

Colonialism, Health, and Medicine

Imperialism was marked by transmission of diseases in multiple directions (Berlinguer 1992). Europeans carried with them influenza, typhus, smallpox, measles, and cholera. Certain kinds of malaria parasites may have been present in the Americas, but the deadly tertian (*falciparum*) malaria almost certainly came from Africa via European slave ships, as did, perhaps, hookworm and other ailments. Syphilis, conversely, was probably introduced to Europe by early Iberian explorers who acquired it in the New World (Arrizabalaga, Henderson, and French 1997).

The New World conquest stood out because of the magnitude of death as well as the mortality differential between invaders and invaded. Dire health consequences accompanied every phase and locale of imperial expansion centuries before industrialization's urban misery put public health on domestic political agendas. Though their life expectancy was perhaps 10 years longer than Europeans on the eve of conquest (Ortiz de Montellano 1990), Indigenous societies in Mesoamerica certainly experienced high death rates from violence, occasional famine, and infectious diseases (Alchon 2003). But the Spanish invasion and colonization of what is now Latin America and the Caribbean had a devastating demographic impact, currently understood to have derived from lack of previous immunity-conferring exposure to various diseases. Spanish friar Bartolomé de las Casas, a 16th century historian, sometime colonial critic, and later Bishop of Chiapas, reported that upon Colombo's arrival, the Indigenous population of the Antilles was 3,770,000; by 1518 only 15,600 people had survived warfare, forced labor, and exposure to new diseases. Cuba's Taíno, for example, were largely wiped out, with similar scenarios, if equally uncertain estimates, elsewhere.

Infamously, up to 8 million Aztecs died of smallpox during Spain's 1519–1521 conquest of Mexico, likely spread intentionally (via infested blankets) by conquistador Hernán Cortés and his soldiers (McCaa 1995). Yet subsequent mortality was far higher, as European demands for New World resources rose steeply, with ominous health consequences. Among these were: slavery and indentured servitude involving dangerous work in mines, construction, and plantations; dispossession from land and cultural heritage, jeopardizing survival; crowded living conditions; food shortages; increased trade and human movement (with attendant maladies); ecological alterations (canalization, railroads, exploitation of forests), facilitating mosquito breeding sites and malaria; and continued conflict. All told, between one third and one half of Indigenous inhabitants were killed in the late 15th and 16th centuries by the military, economic, and social dimensions of Spanish colonization (Crosby 1993).

In colonial Mexico, for instance, sanitary and living conditions and associated gastrointestinal, respiratory, and vector-borne mortality worsened markedly due to environmental changes under the Spaniards. Traditionally, the Mexica (Aztecs) kept the streets, markets, and plazas of their capital, Tenochtitlán, conspicuously clean. Potable water was brought to Tenochtitlán through aqueducts, built in the 1460s, and wastewater was carefully separated from the clean sources of Lake Texcoco surrounding the city. Solid waste was saved as fertilizer for crops. This was far more ecologically sound than the sanitary environments of European cities even hundreds of years later (Becerril and Jiménez 2007). After Tenochtitlán was destroyed and rebuilt as Mexico City under Spanish rule, Lake Texcoco was transformed into a giant cesspool: swampy landfill projects, heavy canal commerce, and inadequate sewage disposal generated frequent flooding, contamination, and mosquito breeding sites, with enormous negative health consequences (Cooper 1965).

To be sure, colonists also suffered high rates of disease, but inordinately high occupational mortality and early death among displaced Indigenous groups, bonded laborers, and African slaves meant that these groups on average lived far shorter and sicklier lives than Iberian elites (Cook 1998; Gomes 2012).

The "Columbian exchange" between Europe and the lands it invaded resulted in circulation not only of microbes but also of flora, fauna, and people, all with health implications (Crosby 1972). Early travelers brought cultivated plants from one continent to another: rice, bananas, yams, taro, and sugar from Asia; coffee and oil palm from Africa; and maize, cassava, peanuts, tomatoes, papayas, pineapples, tobacco, and potatoes from the Americas. These foods were distributed and added to diets throughout the world, improving nutrition in some cases, and resulting in perilous single-crop reliance (as with potatoes in 19th century Ireland) in others.

Imperialism entailed far more than a set of ecological encounters. Long before the emergence of modern medicine, health-related activities accompanied the colonial enterprise of invasion, occupation, and commercial exploitation. Medical practitioners, initially hired by conquistadores to protect military forces, began to be integrated into colonial authority structures. In Spain's viceroyalties, protomedicatos (i.e., medical tribunals) were set up in the 16th century to govern medical practice; license and oversee physicians, apothecaries, and surgeons; and even implement emergency measures during epidemics, sometimes in competition with the viceroy and Church (Hernández Sáenz 1997; Lanning 1985). Three centuries later, Bourbon authorities sponsored an ambitious vaccination campaign throughout the Spanish Empire (Box 1-1).

Given the paucity of therapeutic measures in the European medical armamentarium, colonizers were eager to learn from indigenous healing knowledge and began to catalog the local pharmacopeia. The earliest and most important was the *Codex Badianus* of 1552, an illustrated compendium of hundreds of medicinal herbs. Written in Nahuatl by Martín de la Cruz and translated into Latin by Juan Badiano (both Aztec men who had been trained in

Box 1-1 Smallpox Vaccination During Late Spanish Colonialism

Exemplifying the complex travels and application of medical knowledge under imperialism is Spain's Royal Philanthropic Expedition of the Vaccine organized in 1803 to prevent the very ailment that had been so destructive during conquest: smallpox. Smallpox inoculation had long been practiced by Chinese and Ayurvedic healers, who observed that previous contact with smallpox conferred protection. Inoculation—smallpox pustules ground into powder and placed in a cotton wad inside the nose—was effective if sometimes lethal. Variations on this approach were practiced in colonial Guatemala with the support of Mayan authorities (Few 2010). English surgeon Edward Jenner—observing milkmaids circa 1796—found that vaccination with cowpox (generally not deadly to humans) could prevent smallpox in humans, transforming vaccination into a safer endeavor.

In 1803 Charles IV (the Bourbon king of Spain), having lost a child to smallpox, sponsored an extraordinary vaccination expedition throughout the Spanish Empire in the Americas and the Pacific (Balaguer Perigüell and Ballester Añón 2003). The small Balmis-Salvany group (named for its director and assistant) arrived in Puerto Rico in 1804, traveling on to present-day Venezuela, Panama, Colombia, Ecuador, Peru, Chile, and Bolivia. Because there was no means of preserving the vaccine, it was administered live—arm-to-arm—maintained in the bodies of 21 Spanish orphans commandeered for the voyage, and later transferred into the arms of slaves when the supply ran out (Mark and Rigau-Pérez 2009). Smallpox vaccine, with accompanying instructions, was delivered throughout the region on foot, horseback, and along waterways.

While the effort was meant to be co-financed and supported by local authorities and physicians in the colonies, it faced opposition in Puerto Rico, Mexico, and elsewhere, because of Balmis's authoritarianism, protests against forcible vaccination, and because in some places it had been preempted by supplies arriving via the English Caribbean or other parts of Latin America (Cueto and Palmer 2014). From Mexico, Balmis's galleon left for the 2-month trip to the Spanish colony of the Philippines, where it received a more positive reception (Colvin 2012). This first mass health campaign (vaccinating perhaps half a million people) was a precursor to other conflictual colonial vaccination efforts (Bhattacharya, Harrison, and Worboys 2005) and a distant prelude to the World Health Organization's smallpox eradication campaign, conducted almost 300 years later (see chapter 2).

a Franciscan academy in Mexico City), it was produced for the Spanish emperor.

Over the centuries, colonial administrations sponsored medical faculties in leading cities, including Lima (Peru), with medical training provided as early as 1571 and establishment of a formal medical faculty in 1811; and Salvador da Bahia (Brazil) in 1808, all greatly abetted by the Catholic Church. Hundreds of hospitals were built across the continent, segregating care for colonists and native populations. Indigenous, European, and African healing traditions coexisted and a rough hierarchy of medical practitioners was established, with titled physicians serving urban elites, Catholic hospitals providing charity care, and traditional healers and midwives attending the majority of the population. There was also considerable admixture of medical paradigms, practitioners, and patients (Warren 2010).

Religious missionaries—first Catholic in the Spanish and Portuguese Empires, and, by the 19th century, increasingly Protestant, especially in Africa and Asia—played an important role in colonization (Hardiman 2006). Missionaries reached deep into rural areas, where they judged local practices and cultures and sought to inculcate Christian values, including through medicine (Greene et al. 2013). Medical missionaries typically operated on a different plane from colonial medical officials, whose priorities were controlling epidemics in ports and towns and improving worker productivity in zones rich in natural resources. For medical missionaries, who served as key points of contact with, and gathered information about, local populations, the moral "uplift" of the colonizing process took place one body and soul at a time (Vaughan 1991). Relations between colonial and missionary medics were often marked by suspicion and distrust, but also collaboration and mutual dependence, especially after 1900. Missionaries raised funds through their mother churches in Europe and North America, enabling the building of extensive networks of leprosaria and hospitals (many of which still exist), in which charity and medical and religious proselytization were intertwined, offering a humanitarian rationale for colonialism's "civilizing mission" (Vongsathorn 2012).

Colonial conquest's most fatal impact was on Indigenous populations, slaves, and bonded laborers, but European soldiers, settlers, and contract workers were also felled by endemic diseases to which they had scant resistance. Nowhere was this truer than in West Africa, the so-called "white man's grave." The Portuguese had established slaving stations along the West African coast in the 15th century, disease-ridden outposts that did not last. Multiple European groups attempting to colonize parts of Africa in subsequent centuries were decimated by dysentery (called bloody flux, among other vivid names) and malaria, including British troops posted in Sierra Leone in 1816–1837, whose crude death rate was almost 50%, some 20 times that of local populations (Curtin 1998).

Still, the hope of obtaining riches outweighed the price of sickness and death in the minds of many Europeans, especially those who profited from these exploits without leaving Europe. Gold from the Gold Coast, ivory from the Ivory Coast—to say nothing of palm oil and, above all, slaves—provided the stimulus for continued expeditions to Africa and well beyond by adventurers, soldiers, mercenaries, and traders.

The Atlantic Slave Trade

Labor—needed to extract, trade, and profit from lucrative raw materials, especially minerals and agricultural products—was central to the imperial project. Within decades of European invasion of the Americas, growing labor needs, fueled by commercial expansion, competition, and the greed of elites, could no longer be met. Many Indigenous groups had been wiped out by war, disease, displacement, and bondage; others were found "unsuitable" for labor. Meanwhile, the supply of voluntary migrants and European indentured servants and criminals was insufficient and hard to control in vast territories.

Thus, accelerating in the 16th century and until the 19th, the colonial system relied on slavery—the capture, trade, sale, reproduction, and subjection to violence and bondage of millions of human beings. Slavery was not a new phenomenon—Italian city-states, for example, used slaves to fill labor shortages following plague epidemics—but it had never before been practiced on a worldwide scale, as an institutionalized economic feature, or in such a racist manner. Europeans targeted Black Africans as the primary source of slave labor for ideological and economic reasons: Africans' physical features (e.g., darker skin color than most Europeans) facilitated slaveowner control and vigilance over escapees; Europeans perceived Africans as constitutionally suited to working in tropical climates, where most agricultural labor was needed (on plantations growing coffee, cotton, rice, sugar, indigo, tobacco and so on); and a system for capturing slaves in Africa and transporting them across the Atlantic was relatively easily implemented (Walvin 2013).

The slave trade also had an enormous impact on many African societies. In addition to the violence, social displacement, and suffering caused by centuries of slave raids, West African nation-building in states such as Mali and Songhay—involving established trade routes, salt mining, agricultural endeavors, tax collection systems, and cultural and educational institutions—was severely disrupted. Moreover, resistance to further European incursion was impeded by exacerbated societal divisions, a depleted labor pool, and warfare changes due to the introduction of muskets.

The circulation of slave labor, raw materials, and manufactured commodities followed a hugely profitable triangular route whereby slaves were traded in Caribbean and North and South American colonies for cash crops, which were then brought to Dutch,

Portuguese, French, and British ports and sold or exchanged for textiles, arms, alcohol, and metals, which in turn were sold or bartered for slaves in West African ports. Enormous profits were made at each stop.

The Atlantic slave trade between Africa and the Americas accounted for the bulk of slave traffic. Between 1502 and 1870, an estimated 11.4 million Africans were forced into bondage. Between 8 and 10 million were sent to Brazil and the Caribbean, with another 1 million to the United States and Spanish South America. Some 12% to 15% of those captured died in the "middle passage" before reaching American shores (Curtin 1968). For the survivors, life was abysmal, marked by brutal treatment, inhumane labor conditions, separation from kin, and rape and other forms of violence. Slave life expectancy in the United States before the Civil War was 21 years, approximately half that of whites. Staggeringly high infant mortality meant that half of all babies born into slavery died in their first year, compared with one fourth of non-slave infants (McCandless 2011; Steckel 2010). For those who survived into adulthood, few lived past 50. Slaves in Brazil and Caribbean colonies faced even worse fates, with labor conditions on sugar and rice plantations particularly oppressive (Bergad 2007). As long as profits were being made and the labor force reproduced, outside epidemic control imperial authorities paid limited heed to the health of slaves and other laborers. African healing and healers, by contrast, played an important and evolving role in remedying illness and addressing the physical and psychological suffering due to imperialism and slavery. As well, African healers defied colonial hierarchies, at times treating slaveholders, even as they both fiercely critiqued imperialism and interacted with it (Sweet 2011).

HEALTH, "THE TROPICS," AND THE IMPERIAL SYSTEM

Key Questions:

- Why and how did the area of tropical medicine emerge?
- What were its principal tenets?

By the 18th century, medicine and public health had become established as major ingredients in the colonization of peoples around the world, far more nefarious than their sometime portrayal as the humanitarian component of military and political ventures. Indeed, the "assumption that imperialism, whatever its other faults, at least led to an improvement in the health of the indigenous populations" (Farley 1988, p. 189) belies the various intents of colonial public health and medical measures (Box 1-2) that together helped legitimate colonialism.

Even as Indigenous healing was suppressed or banned in some settings, such as Britain's Cape Colony in Southern Africa (Phatlane 2014), colonial medicine was never all powerful: across time and space, it was contested, only selectively taken up, resisted, and overshadowed by local preferences for Indigenous medicine or complemented by pluralistic approaches (Sharma 2012). Elite physicians in 19th century Indian cities, for example, parlayed the expanding institutional medical environment to promote and rescue "traditional medicine." Within a few decades, Ayurvedic medicine gained an organized platform and was increasingly connected to nationalist aspirations (Bala 2014). In colonial Punjab, Sikh practitioners also mobilized to revive Ayurveda in scientific terms that both fit into and challenged the frames of colonial medical research and practice (Sivaramakrishnan 2006). Likewise, medical missionaries in colonial (and post-colonial) Congo did not impose Western practices of childbirth, but instead drew extensively on local knowledge to create a hybridized form of maternal health care (Hunt 1999). Thus, far from unidirectionally impinging on local healing cultures, it was European medicine—whose capacity was highly limited well into the 20th century—that had to find its place amid both medical and popular tendencies to syncretism and pluralism, with many local variations in the Americas, Asia, and Africa (Au 2011; Cueto and Palmer 2014; Digby, Ernst, and Muhkarji 2010).

By the late 1800s—as imperial powers expanded further into Asia and Africa—the East India Company and other European commercial monopolies (whose quasi-governing roles also encompassed military and administrative duties) were dissolved, bringing colonies under direct imperial control. With intensified extraction, production, and trade (and concomitant concerns around labor productivity and spread of disease), government officials, plantation owners, and merchants had a mounting (self-)interest in developing stronger medical responses, at least in colonial enclaves (Bhattacharya 2012; Greenwood 2015). Diseases spread via ship (such as cholera) and parasitic diseases associated with the tropical climates of many colonies (for example, malaria, trypanosomiasis, and leishmaniasis) all represented threats to labor productivity, the health and survival of European invaders and settlers, and trade. Calling a part of the globe "the tropics" also became a way for imperial powers to define something culturally alien to, environmentally distinct from, and potentially dangerous to Europe and other "temperate" regions (Arnold 1997; Harrison 1999).

This invention of "the tropics" and of tropical medicine emerged to address health issues considered specific to the colonies, making settings such as colonial Brazil central locales for "tropical" disease research (Furtado 2008; Stepan 2001). Much of this research shaped racialized explanations regarding susceptibility to disease, suitability for work, and possibilities for social and economic "advancement" of colonized groups (Deacon 2000; De Barros, Palmer, and Wright 2009; Dunn 2014; McCallum 2005; Peard 1999). Acclimatization arguments invariably favored the colonizer—whether providing an argument for why so many Europeans perished in their initial encounters with hot climes and dreaded diseases despite purported racial superiority; rationalizing the use of "brown labor" that could better tolerate hot, humid weather; or justifying the exploitation of regions and peoples deemed unable to escape their medico-geographic state of "backwardness" (Harrison 1996).

Notwithstanding tropical medicine's assumption that place and climate shaped disease, many ailments labeled "tropical"—such as leprosy and malaria—were (previously) endemic in temperate or cold regions. Yet even today, this inaccurate conception of "tropical" diseases as those only found, highly prevalent, or especially hard to control, in tropical and subtropical regions retains salience in medical quarters. Past and present, tropical medicine's definition (Warren 1990) leaves out the interaction of political, cultural, and economic factors (production, organization of labor, class relations, healing milieus, political and institutional oppression) with ecological conditions.

The Menace of Malaria and the Rise of Tropical Medicine

A range of diseases shaped and were shaped by the contours of imperialism. Malaria's menace to colonial expansion, for example, spanned hundreds of years. From the 16th century, the building of towns and clearing of forests, inadequate drainage and sewage disposal, and, later, new canals and train routes disrupted mosquito habitats and exacerbated malaria in much of the colonized world. Various French, British, Belgian, and Dutch attempts to establish permanent settlements in Africa and Asia were thwarted or forced to relocate due to the high death toll from malaria (Packard 2007; Yip 2009).

Box 1-2 Rationales for Colonial Health and Tropical Medicine

- Protecting imperial military forces to enable conquest
- Facilitating occupation and colonial expansion
- Making "the tropics" habitable for European and other colonial settlers
- Safeguarding commercial interests
- Improving productivity of (enslaved, indentured, coerced) workers
- Improving colonial relations and staving off unrest
- Exercising colonial power—subjugating conquered populations
- Reinforcing political and social stratification between colonizer and colonized, and asserting cultural superiority
- "Saving souls": Christianizing, missionary work, humanitarian efforts
- "Moral"/patronizing justifications for "civilizing" populations/developing economies

In the early 1600s, Jesuits in South America learned of an Indigenous malaria cure—an alkaloid in the bark of *Cinchona officinalis*, a tree native to the Andes. By the middle of the 17th century, fame of this "Jesuit bark" or *Lignum febrium* had spread throughout Europe, where it rapidly gained favor as a specific treatment for agues and fevers. Soon bark collectors almost caused the disappearance of the wild trees, though the Dutch eventually established profitable plantations in Java through careful selection, grafting, and cultivation. Quinine became a tool to protect European troops involved in 19th century imperial expansion but was used unevenly in colonial settings (Monnais 2013). The Dutch had a virtual monopoly of cinchona production until World War II when the supply was cut off, creating an incentive for development of synthetic antimalarials such as chloroquine.

Meanwhile, as of the 18th century, towns and cities in Europe and the Americas saw a retreat of malaria following implementation of environmental and sanitary measures (Dobson 1997; Knaut 1997; Rodríguez and Rodríguez de Romo 1999). Only in the late 19th century did scientific attention to malaria come to a crescendo, with imperial and private backing for budding bacteriological and parasitological research. Malaria research—discoveries of its etiology, the parasitic life-cycle, and vector and transmission patterns—was crucial to the establishment of the field of tropical medicine (Packard 2007). Scientists, medical officers, and local assistants (whose contributions went unrecognized) in colonial Algeria, Formosa, sub-Saharan Africa, and India, as well as Italy, Brazil, and Argentina, participated in the networks of colonial-imperial medicine (Alvarez 2008; Webb 2009).

One key player was Scottish physician-parasitologist Patrick Manson. After medical training, Manson was posted in the 1860s as medical officer to the Chinese Imperial Maritime Customs on Formosa (now Taiwan), charged with ship and crew inspection. He also worked at missionary hospitals on mainland China and Hong Kong. Closely observing "tropical" diseases, Manson elaborated a model of disease transmission—hypothesizing a link between parasite and mosquito vector—initially based on his observations of filariasis in the 1870s, later of malaria. Manson's work also drew from French military medical officer Charles Laveran's 1880 discovery of the malaria parasite while he was posted in the French colony of Algeria. Manson became a mentor to Englishman Ronald Ross, a surgeon with the Indian Medical Service who himself had had a bout with malaria. In 1898, under Manson's tutelage from afar, Ross described the life cycle of malaria parasites in mosquitoes and demonstrated the role played by mosquitoes in bird malaria. (Ross later pursued malaria control work in West Africa, Cyprus, the Suez Canal zone, and other reaches of the British Empire.) This discovery earned him the 1902 Nobel Prize (Laveran won it in 1907, but the competitive Ross failed to cite Manson's mentorship and also kept Italian entomologist Giovanni Grassi, who specified the role of the *Anopheles* mosquito in human transmission, from sharing the prize [Bynum 2002]).

These researchers were also instrumental in institutionalizing the tropical medicine field. When Manson returned to London in the 1890s, he became medical advisor to the Colonial Office, persuading Britain's Colonial Secretary to establish schools of tropical medicine in London (where he worked) and Liverpool (where Ross later worked) in support of imperial needs (Haynes 2001). Similarly, Laveran was a co-founder of France's *Société de pathologie exotique* in 1908.

The Trials of Trypanosomiasis

Trypanosomiasis *africana* (sleeping sickness) offers an even more telling causal connection to imperialism. Various African societies had longtime knowledge that sleeping sickness (known locally as *nagana)* attacked cattle; local populations were able to contain the disease through herding practices in wilderness areas between neighboring territories. Yet until the late 19th century, human sleeping sickness—transmitted by a tsetse fly vector parasite that attacks the immune system, then other organ systems, and finally the central nervous system, eventually killing those infected—had not been recorded in East Africa.

Amid the tumultuous European "scramble" for African colonies and imposition of international boundaries by the 1884-1885 Berlin Conference, frontier zones were destroyed and the locally-maintained ecological equilibrium dissipated. The commercial and agricultural activities of Europeans provoked an increase in tsetse fly populations and the spread of trypanosomiasis to new areas (Lyons 1992). Its probable introduction by the ruthless expedition led by Englishman Henry Morton Stanley from the Congo area to the African Great Lakes region (1874–1877) resulted in an enormous outbreak among residents of Uganda from 1900 to 1908, killing an estimated one tenth of the population, and depopulating large parts of neighboring German colonial possession Tanganyika.

Colonial medical authorities, who knew little of the disease before the European occupation of Africa, attributed high death rates from trypanosomiasis—as well as tuberculosis, malaria, and other ailments—to the poor hygiene and diet of Africans and to their purported biological debility. This paradigm located sickness in individual bodies rather than in the body politic (Turshen 1984). Political and medical officials alike failed to consider that the "civilizing" process—wars of conquest, the slave trade, the imperial division of Africa, large-scale population displacement, forced labor in industrial enterprises, environmental degradation—was driving trypanosomiasis and other epidemics (Hoppe 2003).

Instead, British, French, Belgian, and German authorities across a band of African colonies carried out research and treatment measures that were paternalistic and arrogant, if not coercive and harmful. These draconian and racist control policies included: segregating infected Africans into concentration camps; administering painful and marginally effective medications; experimenting on captive subjects; and mandating forced population removal and detention of suspected carriers. At the height of the trypanosomiasis epidemic in the early 20th century, there was considerable inter-imperial sharing among scientists, with careerist and disease control imperatives outweighing political rivalries (Neill 2012). Far from isolated instances of subjugation for epidemic control purposes, public health approaches to a multiplicity of "tropical" diseases served as tools of colonial power. At the same time, the encounters of colonial scientists with complex vernacular (local indigenous) knowledge systems challenged European understandings and the colonial disease control enterprise as a whole (Tilley 2011). As late as the 1950s, a putative trypanosomiasis preventive—a pentamidine vaccine produced by a French pharmaceutical company and known to be both deadly and of limited efficacy—was forcibly administered in French, Belgian, and Portuguese colonies. Despite these dangers, and declining trypanosomiasis mortality, the campaign followed a racialized logic that subsumed the well-being of Africans to the eradication dreams of colonial physician-scientists (Lachenal 2014). Ironically, this overstudied ailment—an archetype of colonial medico-administration—is today considered to be a "neglected" "tropical" disease (see chapter 6).

Comparative Colonial Approaches in the "Tropical" Disease Era

While colonial disease anxieties were shared (Peckham 2015), as were scientific personnel (Arnold 2015), a variety of medico-imperial approaches emerged across time and place. For example, in its West African colonies, France's "mise en valeur" civilizing mission hubristically imposed values and cultural institutions emphasizing economic development and hygiene as vehicles for advancement (Conklin 2000). In inter-war Indochina, although quinine was held up as a priority for malaria control—and even with French pharmaceutical manufacturers eager to expand the market for antimalarials in competition against German companies—this unpopular intervention was of secondary importance to doctors and residents of malarious areas and, especially, to an inertia-ridden colonial bureaucracy focused on railroad expansion, which exacerbated spread of malaria (Monnais 2013).

Belgium's notorious rule, centralized in its vast Congo colony (first under King Léopold, then under the "colonial trinity" of the state, missionaries, and private interests) built an extensive network of hospitals to treat trypanosomiasis, employing medicalization to dominate an already brutalized population (Lyons 1992).

In French Cameroon, meanwhile, an entire province plagued by trypanosomiasis was turned over to colonial doctors in a grandiose World War II-era sanitary utopia—a medical *mise en valeur* experiment. Using paternalistic public health approaches—including model villages, health screening, maternity camps, education, sport, and agricultural schemes—the doctors attempted to modernize this rural and sparsely populated era. But after some initial successes, the experiment went awry, beset by underfunding, wartime exigencies that drew workers back into rubber-tapping and mining, and a resurgence of disease (Lachenal 2010).

In the fraught domain of colonial psychiatry, too, stated intentions of assimilating French and North African Muslim patients into the same institutions using modern psychiatric methods were routed by French religious, racial, cultural, and climatic chauvinism that associated North African Muslims with violence, criminality, irrationality, and psychiatric pathology (Keller 2007).

The medical apparatus of the sprawling British Empire, by contrast, focused pragmatically on maintaining law and order, productivity, and trade, which required controlling cholera, plague, and other associated disease outbreaks (Harrison 2010), also inter-mixed with less interventionist attention. Still, Britain's perennial alarm around the commerce-interrupting spread of epidemics in and from East and South Asia spurred periods of panic-driven authoritarianism, such as during the 1894 Hong Kong bubonic plague outbreak (Peckham 2013).

Although most focused on political and commercial matters, imperial Britain also partook in a "civilizing" discourse. For example, mid-19th century British authorities recognized that addressing malaria—colonial India's leading cause of sickness and death (albeit a lesser economic priority)—would help remedy and "tame" India's "backwardness." Despite this rhetoric, the British made few inroads in malaria control and were widely criticized (Harrison 1999). At the same time, cholera provided a platform for inter-imperial exchange of knowledge and experts, and, intermittently, repressive and publicly-resisted actions (Harrison 1999). A century later, Britain's government sought to correct its parsimony, and in the 1940s increased investments in some aspects of colonial health and welfare (see chapter 2).

Germany's smaller and shorter-lived medico-colonial enterprise in Africa combined burgeoning bacteriologic and diagnostic knowhow with a moralizing discourse that was also used domestically to stem the spread of venereal disease, among others. Over time, German physicians implemented punitive measures not only on soldiers and local prostitutes, but also against wider Indigenous populations, considered licentious and morally degenerate (Walther 2013). Such moralizing was transposed to the arena of maternal and child health, which prioritized correcting perceived maternal ignorance over addressing poverty, with German colonial measures somewhat more rulebound than British counterparts (Lindner 2014).

Inter-imperial comparisons served as an important touchstone for health and medical investment in Portugal's African colonies in the early 20th century. Growing concerns around the potential economic impact of African depopulation failed to jumpstart the organization of medical efforts beyond urban enclaves. As criticism of appalling conditions in Angola and other Portuguese possessions rose in the 1920s, Portugal's fear that it would be dispossessed of its colonies due to international pressure led it to implement an extensive French-inspired medical service (Coghe 2015). Overcoming this warning, Portuguese colonial medical efforts focused on productivity of workers in plantations and extractive industries for much of the 20th century (Varanda and Cleveland 2014).

Acquiring colonies later than European countries, the United States, as we shall see, both drew from European precedents and nurtured its own prejudices. Americans vigorously applied practical, technological approaches to disease control to enable rapid economic expansion (e.g., in building the Panama Canal) and make the tropics "habitable" for white colonizers (Gorgas 1909). Even as the hygienic behavior of local populations was pathologized by occupying forces, US authorities were troubled by the psychological toll of occupation on military personnel, such as in the Philippines (Anderson 2006), all in a collapsed time frame of becoming an imperial power.

The few examples cited here only hint at the multitude of health-related effects set in motion by worldwide exploration, colonization, and commerce since the 15th century. Major demographic changes occurred, with massive forced and voluntary migration of populations in multiple directions. For example, after the British Parliament formally abolished the slave trade (1807) and then slavery (1833), Britain increasingly transferred laborers and recruited professionals (including doctors and nurses [Greenwood and Topiwala 2015]) from one part of its empire to another, explaining substantial populations of Indian ancestry in former British

Box 1-3 Imperialism, Health, and the Rubber Industry

The rubber industry offers an illustration of the interweaving of a range of imperial imperatives: military, commercial and industrial, government, scientific, and public health. When the mid-19th century process of vulcanization transformed rubber trees into a high-demand commodity (as rubber replaced leather belts in factories and subsequently became essential for vehicle tires, military equipment, medical devices, and consumer products), control of rubber plantations became paramount. In the 1850s, Britain's Royal Botanical Garden sent an agent to smuggle thousands of seedlings of the rubber tree (*Hevea brasiliensis*), native to South American rainforests, out of imperial Brazil (which was seeking to protect its share of the lucrative rubber trade). Grown in London hothouses, they became the basis for commercial plantings of rubber trees in conducive habitats, designed to give the British Empire greater control over this newly essential industry.

Conditions on the Malay Peninsula—Britain's "possession"—were ideal for growing rubber trees, and plantations were prepared in the 1890s. But the local population was sparse, and Chinese workers were deemed difficult to manage. After the abolition of the slave trade in the early 19th century, Britain sourced contract laborers from southern India (Kaur 2012). Thousands of Tamils from the Madras region already worked on Malayan coffee and sugar estates; now British authorities transferred tens of thousands more workers each year. Almost immediately, there were severe malaria, hookworm, and other health problems on the rubber estates. High mortality, low productivity, and worker unrest forced many plantations to be abandoned (Manderson 1996) and helped stimulate Britain's investments in malaria control. Parallel French efforts in colonial Indochina to cultivate rubber trees from Brazilian seeds were enabled by government-industry-science cooperation (including through efforts of Pasteurian bacteriologist Yersin; see ahead), with plantation economies generating similar labor–capital strife.

In the 1920s, the United States sought to end Britain's near monopoly on rubber, with the US Department of State strong-arming Liberia (settled by freed US slaves, then established as Africa's first republic in 1847) to grant the Firestone company a land concession to establish a massive rubber plantation to supply the auto industry, military, and other sectors. Denounced by critics as a forced labor scheme like those prevalent in African colonies, Firestone hired local laborers for only the harshest work and generated insignificant improvements in local living conditions (McBride 2002). Part of Firestone's "corporate welfare" approach was to provide medical care to employees (Mitman and Erickson 2010), who were also studied by US medical researchers. Although malaria was found to be widespread both on the rubber plantation and throughout the country, Firestone's minuscule tax contribution meant that the Liberian government had minimal resources to address health needs (McBride 2002). Liberian workers also served as "clinical material" in Firestone's 1948 film *Medicine in the Tropics* shown to US medical students.

colonies as distant as Trinidad, Fiji, South Africa, and Malaya (exemplified by Box 1-3's discussion of the rubber industry).

For hundreds of years colonial regimes sought to impose their cultural and social institutions on local societies, variously disrupting, superseding, and blending with preexisting counterparts. This is true of languages, legal systems, and medicine, including concepts of causality and treatment, and patterns of medical organization and practice. Colonizers' belief in the "civilizing" effects of medicine upon native peoples, their adherence to the notion that infectious diseases originated in the "primitive and dangerous world" of the tropics, their fascination with questions of acclimatization and racial difference (Lorcin 1999), and the hiding of diseased settlers in order to perpetuate the myth that Europeans possessed superior immunity, all attest to the centrality of health matters to imperial power. Of course, learning circulated in multiple directions, via colonial experts, shared techniques, and medical practice. As well, indigenous understandings and practices often proved superior to colonial approaches (e.g., Andean cinchona against malaria, 19th century Ayurvedic knowledge about and remedies for cholera) and informed developments in Europe and its empires.

INDUSTRIALIZATION, URBANIZATION, AND THE EMERGENCE OF MODERN PUBLIC HEALTH

Key Questions:

- What drove sanitary (subsequently renamed public health) ideas and actions during the period of industrialization?
- How did these vary across countries and empires?

At the height of the imperial grab for colonies in the 18th and 19th centuries, European countries underwent a massive transformation from largely agrarian societies, with peasants tied to the land as serfs, into urbanized capitalist industrial economies based on wage laborers. This transformation was financed by the riches amassed—and fueled by the raw materials extracted—through colonial exploits. Most European countries went stepwise from collections of fiefdoms to larger nation-states. Revolutionary movements in France, North America, and elsewhere fostered and disseminated ideas of the right to political freedom (mostly for property-owning males). Simultaneously, the largest colonial empires in history were being assembled, enslavement of millions persisted across several continents, and Europe's peasants were being forced into nightmarish urban factories, prisons, and workhouses.

The transition from feudalism to capitalism entailed vast social and demographic shifts, fundamentally altering the way people lived and died. Between 1750 and 1900 the human population doubled—despite soaring urban mortality—from about 800 million to 1.7 billion, following centuries of stagnant and sometimes declining numbers (during food shortages). Europe's feudal social divisions among monarchs and noblemen, a small artisan class, and the large peasantry gave way to new classes of merchants and industrialists (the bourgeoisie) and urban industrial workers (the proletariat) under a new capitalist economic order—based on private land ownership, competition among private enterprises, and free market (albeit regulated) principles.

The term *Industrial Revolution* denotes the period from about 1750 to 1850 during which factories and power-driven machinery were first employed for the mass production of commercial goods (drawing from innovations in engineering and chemistry), and unprecedented volumes of raw materials and consumer goods crisscrossed the world.

Increasing imperial needs and commercial exchange led to greater official patronage for science, generating new military, transport, and agricultural technologies. There were also important developments in astronomy, physics, botany, and medicine. Advances in science and technology both contributed to capitalist industrialization and were stimulated by it. The textile industry played an early role in industrializing northern Europe (first in home-based cottage industries under "proto-industrialization" [Mendels 1972]), with the flying shuttle, spinning machines, and, above all, intricate power looms enabling the production of huge quantities of cotton cloth. Textile machinery initially relied on water power, restricting the placement of mills, but after James Watt's invention of the steam engine in 1781, factories could be located at almost any site, limited only by supplies of labor, coal, and materials. The need for factory workers produced a whole new category of wage laborers drawn from peasants stripped of their land and displaced by larger, technology-reliant, and less labor-intensive farms.

The new factories generated enormous wealth for their owners, who bought raw materials at rock bottom prices from the countryside and colonies and displayed an indifference to the welfare of the workers, paying the lowest wages they could get away with, even as they invested heavily in changing technology. Safety devices were minimal and small children, sometimes literally chained to the machines, toiled from dawn to dusk in dusty, noisy, unheated, and unventilated workrooms. It would take over a century of struggle before child labor was abolished and workers were protected by welfare states through economic security, workplace safety, and social services.

The health of the population became more important with the rise of the nation-state and of the capitalist system, initially at a national level. The new political obligations to citizens (or at least the subset with voting rights) and worker health had some bearing on productivity (although the endless replenishment of workers from the impoverished peasantry, including ever younger child laborers, made this less of a priority). Still, manufacturing and trade needed to remain disease-free to operate smoothly. Health also became a question of moral and social order, as indicated in Prussian physician Johann Peter Frank's 1790 address "The People's Misery—Mother of all Disease." But then, as today, understanding of the connections between poor social conditions and ill health did not automatically translate into political action.

New Sanitary Ideas

The local particularities of industrial development shaped the policy and regulatory responses in different societies, ranging from Prussian medical policing to French social assistance to British sanitary reform. Frank's landmark, multivolume *A System of Complete Medical Police,* published between 1779 and 1827, was an embodiment of the new statist approach to public health issues.

In this time of rapid industrialization, proletarianization, and urbanization, France occupied a premier position in social and political thought. Having employed revolutionary means to overthrow the despotic, ancien régime at the end of the 18th century, France began in the 19th century to develop administrative structures and intellectual frameworks for public health research and action in advance of Britain and long before the United States. In the administrative domain, health councils were set up in major cities (starting with Paris in 1802, and reaching Lyon, Marseille, Lille, and Nantes in the 1920s) to monitor and make recommendations on sanitation of markets, public baths, sewers and cesspits, prison conditions, medical statistics, epidemics, industrial health, and food quality (Murard and Zylberman 1996).

These new administrative arrangements helped shape intellectual frameworks for public health research and policy, including a specialized journal *Annales d'hygiène publique et de médecine légale* (1829) and the Royal (later National) Academy of Medicine (1820). With new state-produced data at hand, several talented researchers began to investigate the health consequences of rapid industrialization and urbanization, building on the work of 17th century Italian physician Bernardino Ramazzini, who had examined the health problems associated with different occupations. Alexandre-Jean-Baptiste Parent-Duchâtelet undertook prodigious studies of the pathology of the city: privies, prostitution, sewers, wells, and waste. His younger colleague Louis-René Villermé uncovered the relations among mortality, urban geography, and poverty (La Berge 1992). Villermé's classic 1820s studies, published under the auspices of the Academy of Medicine, described the differential mortality of rich and poor in Paris (see chapter 5 for details). In 1840, in an inquiry into the working and living conditions of French textile workers sponsored by the Academy of Moral and Political Sciences, he discovered that all laborers suffered excessive mortality, reflecting the material misery of their lives and helping advance legislative measures against child labor. Ten years later, Ambroise Tardieu utilized these and other studies to produce a monumental, three-volume *Dictionnaire d'hygiène publique et de salubrité* (Paris: 1852–1854)—the most comprehensive analysis of public health at the time.

Though the French research regarding the health implications of industrialization, urbanization, and poverty was pathbreaking, it was action in the streets and legislative efforts—first in Britain and then elsewhere—that generated concrete sanitary reforms.

Political Unrest and Sanitary Reform

In the first half of the 19th century, industrial cities were bursting at their seams, with populations doubling, tripling, or more within a generation. Urban housing was constructed as quickly and cheaply as possible, packing dozens of people into windowless rooms. City planning was nonexistent and sanitation neglected. Early horse- and donkey-based transport systems littered streets with great volumes of manure, attracting flies (helping spread trachoma and dysentery), and causing severe disposal problems. Garbage, industrial waste, excrement, and animal carcasses were summarily dumped into rivers, lakes, and makeshift landfills. What remained behind accumulated along unpaved streets and back alleys, mixed with mud and stagnant water, and produced foul stenches and cesspools of microorganisms.

The smoke from innumerable factories and coal fires filled the air and blackened buildings and lungs alike. Despite improvements in agricultural production, nutrition was poor. Rickets became common in children rarely exposed to sunshine, and contagious diseases such as tuberculosis, diphtheria, and louse-borne typhus took a great toll. The first cholera pandemic to strike Western Europe took many thousands of lives in the early 1830s and quickly traveled to North America via shipping routes. Occupational injuries and deaths were common, as were diseases arising from unrestricted industrial use of lead, mercury, phosphorus, and other toxic substances.

Workers began to organize collective efforts to better their conditions, joined by certain middle-class social reformers who were outraged at the shocking conditions in city slums, factories, and mines. These efforts faced formidable foes in industrial owners and their political partners, but by the mid-19th century, the resistance of moneyed interests to sanitary and industrial reform was no longer tenable.

The movement for sanitary reform in Britain engendered heated debates over the role of the state and of private interests in the protection of public health, featuring most prominently Edwin Chadwick and Friedrich Engels. Chadwick, a lawyer and lifetime civil servant, authored the *Poor Law of 1834*, which drove the growth of the industrial workforce by compelling the destitute to enter urban "hellhole" workhouses instead of receiving welfare assistance in their home parishes as they had since Elizabethan times. He then turned to preventing illness (as a means of reducing welfare expenditures) in his report on the dismal health of the working class (Chadwick 1842; Hamlin 1998). Chadwick's belief in the miasmatic origins of disease—putrid air arising from festering filth—shaped his zeal for clean water, sewage, and public sanitation, measures that he believed would prevent most diseases and poverty. However, he rejected improved working conditions, wages, and food as remedies for pauperism. The notion that poverty itself was the cause of illness was, for Chadwick, unthinkable.

Meeting considerable resistance, Chadwick's 1842 report eventually formed the basis of the Public Health Act of 1848 that established the General Board of Health and authorized local medical officers and boards. In 1849, amid a lethal cholera epidemic, London physician John Snow countered the prevailing miasmatic theory by suggesting that cholera was spread by sewage-contaminated water. During an 1854 outbreak he challenged naysayers by demonstrating that contaminated drinking water from London's Broad Street pump was the source of cholera. Analyzing household and neighborhood patterns of disease distribution, he found that water drawn from the lower Thames River, after passage through the city, was far more likely to transmit cholera than water from upstream localities. Although the association was clear, the precise mechanism remained unknown to him (see ahead); moreover, despite evident social configurations of disease distribution, Snow explicitly disavowed a class analysis of contaminated water exposure, instead proposing an atomistic "risk factor" approach.

Friedrich Engels, the son of a wealthy German manufacturer sent to manage a thread factory in Manchester, revealed the horrendous living and occupational conditions of industrial workers, but with a fundamentally distinct explanatory framework from Chadwick's. In *The Condition of the Working Class in England*, Engels attributed workers' misery and ill health to the exploitation of the industrial working class under the capitalist economic system:

> When one individual inflicts bodily injury upon another, such injury that death results, we call the deed manslaughter; when the assailant knew in advance that the injury would be fatal, we call this deed murder. But when society places hundreds of proletarians in such a position that they inevitably meet a too early and an unnatural death, one which is quite as much a death by violence as that by the sword or bullet, when it deprives thousands of the necessaries of life, places them under conditions in which they

> *cannot* live—forces them, through the strong arm of the law, to remain in such conditions until that death ensues which is the inevitable consequence—knows that these thousands of victims must perish, and yet permits these conditions to remain, its deed is murder just as surely as the deed of the single individual (Engels 1845, p. 27).

Engels believed political action was necessary to redress these conditions. In 1848, Engels joined Karl Marx in penning *The Communist Manifesto,* calling for the revolutionary overthrow of the exploitative capitalist system. The same year Prussian physician Rudolf Virchow famously decried poor social and political conditions as the cause of a typhus outbreak, helping launch a social medicine approach to health and well-being (see chapter 3).

Within a few decades, important advances were made: new knowledge regarding waterborne disease transmission; sanitary engineering innovations enabling piped water supply, sewage, and drainage systems; and development of water purification techniques of filtration, chemical treatment, and chlorination. The only wanting ingredients for improved urban health were class and political struggle and transformation of existing power structures. Britain did not undergo a communist revolution, yet a combination of sanitary (later called public health) reforms and militant class struggles from the mid-19th to early 20th century resulted in marked improvements in social conditions, moderate income redistribution, and increases in life expectancy, although intractable social inequalities in health (as we will see in chapter 7) remained.

Across Europe and throughout the world, a cascade of social movements, culminating in a series of 1848 uprisings, unleashed widespread resistance to the Industrial Revolution, to imperialism, and to the concentration of wealth and power and the oppression they generated (Krieger and Birn 1998; Rapport 2008). The people of Berlin, Paris, Vienna, Palermo, Milan, Naples, Parma, Rome, Warsaw, Prague, Dakar, Budapest, and other cities rose up in protest against miserable living and working conditions; in India, the Second Sikh War demonstrated continued protest against British colonial rule. Where the protests were not brutally repressed, they resulted in some gains, including for public health. For example, the uprising in Paris led to the abdication of France's last king, Louis-Philippe, and the founding of the Second Republic, which created a public health advisory committee and established a network of local public health councils. By the 1880s, France was developing one of the world's foremost protectionist systems for mothers and children.

The appalling conditions in England were shared across industrializing societies, with distinct political contexts, institutional cultures, historical trajectories, configurations of class power, and geo-epidemiological conditions shaping particular public health tendencies in different countries (Baldwin 1999; Porter 1994). Germany's commitment to aggressive public health policies, such as compulsory vaccination and quarantines, was rooted in the need to fend off epidemics from the East, as well as to fashion a domestic politics of power—in large part to stabilize worker unrest—in a state that was late to form (Evans 1987; Weindling 1994). Britain's more laissez-faire approach drew from a long history of local and voluntary governance and a belief that its island geography protected it against epidemics (Hardy 1993; Porter 1999). In China, the political fragmentation following the 1911 Revolution meant that public health problems received isolated and disorganized attention (Yip 1995) even as the emerging realm of hybridized Chinese medicine was receptive to public health as a state (and nationalist) responsibility (Lei 2014).

Urban centers in North America had the advantage of relative newness (such as wider streets and more recent buildings), but by the middle of the 19th century the crush of immigration had rendered them as noxious as their European counterparts. New York City, for instance, grew from about 75,000 people in 1800 to more than half a million by 1850, with little attention to sanitation or safety. In 1845 John Griscom published *The Sanitary Condition of the Laboring Population of New York,* followed by Lemuel Shattuck's prophetic 1850 *Report of the Sanitary Commission of Massachusetts,* neither of which resulted in prompt legislative or sanitary actions. Apart from the short-lived National Board of Health (1879–1883), public health in the United States, other than for immigration and border control, remained largely decentralized until the Great Depression (Fee 1994).

In Latin America—by the late 19th century mostly constituted by independent republics—the sanitary authorities that had periodically mobilized to combat epidemic outbreaks during more than three centuries of Spanish and Portuguese colonialism were transformed into permanent health and hygiene boards and departments. Hampered by limited state capacity, they catered mainly to urbanites (Agostoni 2003; Carrillo 2002; Hochman and Armus 2004; Palmer 2003; Quevedo et al. 2004). Brazil's Oswaldo Cruz Institute was an exception, becoming a major research institute with both international ties and close collaboration with the national health department, leading it deep into the hinterlands to carry out disease campaigns (Benchimol 1990).

Russia, which began industrializing only in the late 19th century, had among the worst documented public health indicators. It was only with the establishment of the Soviet Union that public health became centralized, with local-level medical societies and health initiatives abolished after the 1917 Revolution (Solomon and Hutchinson 1990).

The Bacteriological Turn in Industrial and Imperial Contexts

Evolving policy changes were undergirded by the increasing scientific and technical potential of public health and medicine. From roughly 1850 to 1910, theories of miasma and vague conceptions of communicability of disease gave way to experimentally-based understandings and data regarding the genesis of infectious diseases. New knowledge and techniques were spawned by the germ theory of disease and fostered by extensive institutional developments that served imperial and industrial needs. In 1854, the same year Snow postulated cholera's waterborne transmission, University of Florence physician-scientist Filippo Pacini used his observations under the microscope to establish its cause, identifying *Vibrio cholerae* in the stools and intestines of deceased cholera patients. While Pacini's work was supported by Tuscany's Grand Duke, it was largely ignored by scientists; 30 years later, famed German bacteriologist Robert Koch (who had identified the tubercle bacillus in 1882) rediscovered the vibrio as the cause of cholera during his imperial service in Calcutta.

A flood of discoveries emanating from the world's research hubs and scientists (at the time overwhelmingly dominated by Western Europeans; only in the 1930s would the US emerge as a contending scientific metropole, upstaging Europe after WWII) identified the causal agent and basic means of transmission of almost every major bacterial and parasitic disease of humans and domestic animals. These findings, by the likes of Frenchman Louis Pasteur, Britishmen Manson and Ross, and Brazilian Carlos Chagas, among many, showcased scientific public health's new capacity, including laboratory-based verification of disease and a small but growing armamentarium of disease-control measures, such as diphtheria antitoxin, deriving from work by Emile Roux, Emil von Behring, and others. The Pasteur Institute, for example, was founded in the late 1880s with an outpouring of funds donated by a willing citizenry to support the development of legendary chemist and microbiologist Louis Pasteur's anti-rabies vaccine. The Institute quickly flourished in research and teaching realms. In 1891 Pasteur enjoined Albert Calmette—a French naval physician turned tropical medicine specialist who had served in Hong Kong and French West Africa—to become founding director of the Institute's first overseas branch in Saigon (French Indochina; today Ho Chi Minh City, Vietnam), where he studied snake venom and organized vaccine production. Pasteur Institutes were subsequently established in several dozen countries in France's colonial empire in Africa, Asia, and the Caribbean, as well as in Europe, Brazil, and the Middle East (Moulin 1996).

The research arenas, populations, and opportunities provided in and by the colonies—together with the patronage of the state, military, industrial, and commercial interests—helped build the careers and discoveries of these scientists, enabling them to test out and implement new ideas and resolve debates, with little regard for the consequences on local subjects (and rather than testing on themselves). For example, Koch carried out his cholera research in British-occupied Egypt and India; Charles Nicolle worked out typhus transmission (earning him a Nobel) as longtime director of the Pasteur Institute in French colonial Tunisia (Pelis 2006); Calmette returned to France from Saigon to develop snake anti-venom and later the Bacille Calmette-Guérin (BCG) vaccine against tuberculosis; and Franco-Swiss Alexandre Yersin worked as a physician for a shipping company out of Saigon and, sent by the Pasteur Institute to Hong Kong to investigate the 1894 plague outbreak, famously identified the bubonic plague bacillus (*Yersinia pestis*). As well, renowned German physician-scientist Paul Ehrlich used his connections with French and British colleagues working in African colonies to field-trial various chemical preparations against trypanosomiasis, which, although unsuccessful and highly unpleasant, immeasurably advanced his larger chemotherapeutic agenda (Neill 2012). Latin American-based scientists, such as Chagas, were also able to parlay their international scientific reputations to further hone their research visions at home (Kropf 2009). The evolving imperial scientific space was thus driven by, and dynamically connected, *both* social and industrial demands in metropolitan settings *and* military and commercial exigencies and experiences in colonies.

Alongside the harnessing of scientific knowledge to industrial needs and imperial power, physicians developed new diagnostic equipment, therapeutic measures, and surgical techniques (e.g., antisepsis and anesthesia). Allopathic physicians' rising professionalization fueled their efforts to displace other kinds of healers and secure increasing authority and political purview over medical education, health care provision, and (colonial) social policy.

In the realm of public health, the bacteriological revolution's influential explanatory framework and accompanying interventions began to displace prior environmentally-oriented activities. Consensus over the nature, funding, and reach of public health measures, however, was far from automatic. Public health became embroiled in the political and social struggles of the day, at times legitimating an activist state, suffering from a backlash against such interventionism, and also, paradoxically, serving purely private interests (Baldwin 1999).

The "new" public health found itself at the vortex of clashing constituencies—scientific experts striving to assert their status, reformers seeking to improve the social order, liberal industrialists eager for economic growth and bureaucrats looking to increase their purview, as well as socialists, feminists, and laborites fighting for better working and living conditions.

In colonial settings, the new public health measures were not systematically applied outside colonists' enclaves and sites of commercial importance, except in the case of epidemic emergencies, when vaccination, extermination, and quarantine were forcefully imposed. For example, the colonial state's measures against bubonic plague in India circa 1900 drew little from the new bacteriological findings, instead implementing Black Death-era style approaches (Chandavarkar 1992). Furthermore, British authorities blamed "fanatical" rumors, not repressive plague control measures, for Bombay riots and attacks on officials. Nevertheless, given colonial medical uncertainty, the plague outbreak proffered new public roles for local practitioners, with alliances of Indigenous medical practitioners helping temper colonial use of military intervention (Sivaramakrishnan 2011).

As late as 1929, Charles Nicolle erroneously attributed plague to a group of migrant laborers in French colonial Tunis, and supervised a military-enforced roundup and quarantine of hundreds of workers. Even after they were cleared, the press and public health authorities continued targeting this group as a plague reservoir (Keller 2006).

To be sure, into the 20th century there was growing attention to maternal and child health in both metropolitan and colonial settings. Measures aimed at bettering maternity, childbirth, and child welfare were at the nexus of imperial priorities around population fitness, size, and eugenic improvement, on one hand, and demands from working class and colonized groups on the other. In metropolitan and colonial settings alike, middle-class women reformers often served as gendered interlocutors for these overlapping, if divergent, demands (De Barros 2014; González 2015; Manderson 1992; Nguyen 2010). Ceylon's early and extensive implementation of measures to ensure infant and mothers' health may well have derived from its status as a "model" colony (Jones 2004), yet also reflected prevalent class-based (and racialized) assumptions in Britain.

Back and forth learning between colonial experience and the metropole not only influenced research questions and careers but also interconnected public health practices and tools, sometimes upending hierarchies in unexpected ways. Epidemic and excremental control successes in early 20th century US-controlled Philippines, for example, led doctors to turn racialized prejudices around personal hygiene into classist sensibilities, a transformation that mainland US public health did not undergo (Anderson 2006).

This flurry of developments in metropolitan and colonial public health also generated ideas, policies, technologies, and practices—and influenced debates and schemes—that would emerge in a new domain, "international health."

THE MAKING OF INTERNATIONAL HEALTH

Key Questions:

- How did health become an international concern?
- Who were the principal international health actors and institutions of the early 20th century, and what motivated their emergence?
- Why did it take European countries so long to agree to sanitary cooperation?
- What drove the Rockefeller Foundation's interest in international health? What were the pioneering elements of its approach?

By the early 19th century, intense commercial competition between empires–interacting with and compounding economic and demographic disruption—heightened the worldwide threat of cholera and other diseases. Even as individual imperial powers undertook incipient efforts to carry out surveillance and control outbreaks, the scale of interchange between, among, and beyond empires propelled demands for coordination and communication.

A confluence of factors brought epidemic fears to the fore circa 1850: (a) large-scale immigration from Europe and Asia to the Americas (Cox and Marland 2013), itself spurred by social unrest around the vast changes unleashed by industrialization and urbanization, including rural immiseration (such as the 1840s Irish famine) and political tyranny following the 1848 uprisings; and (b) the explosion of mineral extraction, manufacturing, trade, and marketing of goods in turn enabled by a revolution in transportation (e.g., steamships [invented 1810], railroads [1830]) and new routes, such as the Suez Canal (opened in 1869). The now globalized commercial system meant that an actual or potential epidemic in one part of the world could impede production, trade, consumption, and well-being elsewhere, and on a fast timetable (Harrison 2012; Ronzón 2004). A new global economic interdependence magnified the potential dangers of disease and made its control a politically charged matter that would prove complicated and trying wherever it was attempted.

The Americas First

In the Americas, independence wars against European powers in the late 18th and early 19th century were followed by a series of bloody conflicts within and between the new republics. But by century's end, cooperation, including in the sanitary realm, became a genuine possibility. Discussions and exchanges among Latin American physicians were thriving as part of regional professional, scientific, and commercial meetings on issues ranging from coffee to crime, electricity, housing, and literature (de Almeida 2006).

As elsewhere, sanitary concerns, interacting with growing commerce, affected political relations among South American countries. The profitable meat and hide-exporting economies of Argentina and Uruguay were particularly intent on fending off yellow fever outbreaks from Brazil, and the three countries initiated sanitary deliberations in the 1870s (Chaves 2009). Yellow fever had been afflicting ports and triggering quarantines of people and goods (well before the cause was identified) from Buenos Aires to Halifax since the 18th century; however, the problem had long eluded an agreed-upon response. In 1887, Brazil, Argentina, and Uruguay signed a sanitary convention detailing quarantine periods for ships harboring cholera, yellow fever, and plague. In quick succession, the Andean countries of Bolivia, Chile, Ecuador, and Peru signed the Lima Convention of 1888 (Moll 1940). Both efforts were circumscribed and short-lived due to mistrust and limited enforcement; the 1887 agreement, for example, lasted only 4 years before breaking apart (Chaves 2013).

The United States, politically ambitious and economically powerful in Latin America, had great interest in these developments. Americans joined or spearheaded Latin American interchanges, transforming them into Pan American efforts. Under the Monroe Doctrine of 1823, and amplified by US

President Theodore Roosevelt's 1904 "corollary," the United States justified military intervention across the region whenever it sensed its interests were threatened. As the world's foremost immigration destination between 1890 and 1920, the United States was also highly attentive to the entry of disease. In the late 1870s, the US Marine Hospital Service started publishing weekly bulletins with epidemic outbreak news furnished by a worldwide network of informants. An 1893 US Presidential Act obliged all immigrants and cargo ships to present certificates of health signed by the US consul and a medical officer in the departing port, and the Marine Hospital Service (later the US Public Health Service) stationed personnel in key ports in the United States (most famously Ellis Island in New York) and around the world to inspect ships and passengers for disease and to enforce quarantine (Birn 1997). Although the US government exerted little energy on domestic health matters or international cooperation in the 19th century, the organization representing US public health professionals sought to impose US sanitary interests in Latin American countries (Carrillo and Birn 2008).

The US government's attention to international health intensified with acquisition of colonies in the Caribbean and the Pacific following the 1898 Spanish-American War. The US forces invading Cuba, for example, suffered major troop losses from yellow fever, a virus causing an excruciating hemorrhagic fever that killed up to half its victims (especially those not previously exposed) within a few days. Once mostly a trade concern, it now became an imperial one. Like other colonial powers, the United States began to take on public health activities both to protect its military and colonists from "tropical" diseases and to prevent yellow fever from reaching US ports aboard merchant ships, saving the harshest measures for local Cuban populations (Espinosa 2009). Public health activities accompanying US military occupation of the Philippines (1898–1912) were particularly repressive. Amid a massive cholera outbreak, cruel quarantine measures were imposed, entire villages destroyed, and dubious medicines forcibly administered. American racialized and infantilizing prejudices blamed the outbreak on local immorality and "primitive" hygiene practices: fears that "natives" were reservoirs of disease (even if unaffected by disease) and therefore ongoing threats to American colonizers offered a rationalization for interventionist public health as a central tool of the US's paternalistic regime (Anderson 2006).

In December 1902, representatives of a dozen countries from across the Americas met at an International Sanitary Convention in Washington, DC, at the behest of the Conference of American States. Together, they formed the International Sanitary Bureau, which became the Pan American Sanitary Bureau (PASB) in 1923 and the Pan American Health Organization in 1958. The United States was the prime mover behind the founding of this first international health organization, which initially operated out of the US Public Health Service and headed until 1947 by a succession of US Surgeons-General (Bustamante 1952).

Most Latin American republics soon joined the Bureau and were represented at its quadrennial conferences. The United States was especially interested in the drafting of, and region-wide compliance with, enforceable sanitary treaties. The PASB's early years were devoted to the establishment of protocols on the reporting and control of epidemic diseases, including yellow fever, plague, and cholera, culminating in a 1924 Sanitary Code, the first Pan American treaty of any kind to be signed by all 21 member countries (Cueto 2007).

The Health Occupation of Cuba and the Panama Canal

Atop concerns connected to its burgeoning colonial empire and command of pan-American sanitary policy, the United States was decisively alerted to the importance of international health through its role in the construction of the Panama Canal. Although the building of the canal hinged upon malaria and yellow fever control, its very completion ironically raised the peril of further epidemics due to shorter shipping routes to and from Asia.

Interest in constructing a canal across the Central American isthmus was ignited as early as the 16th century, but the project was deemed impossible and abandoned until the 1870s, when French naval officers undertook a new feasibility survey. Years of complex planning and negotiations finally led to groundbreaking in 1880. But the Compagnie Universelle du Canal Interocéanique de Panama, created to oversee canal construction, allocated little funding for hygiene and sanitation, even though the region was a well-known hotbed of yellow fever. (To note: the cause and means of transmission of malaria and yellow fever were not yet fully established.) After 8 years of work, US$300 million in expenditure, the hiring of tens of thousands of workers—principally from France and Jamaica—and almost 20,000 deaths from malaria and yellow fever, the Compagnie went bankrupt, plagued by a corruption scandal, and abandoned its efforts.

US interest in taking over the canal redoubled following the Spanish-American War, which provided military impetus, imperial aspirations, and public health techniques that would enable the canal's completion. By the time negotiations with French and Panamanian authorities were concluded in 1904, the US military had had its own encounter with raging malaria and yellow fever outbreaks in Cuba.

As early as 1881, Cuban physician Carlos Finlay had proposed that yellow fever was transmitted through the bite of a mosquito (López Sánchez 1987). Most refused to believe him (although Ronald Ross's subsequent demonstration of malaria's mosquito vector did not face such skepticism). After an outbreak of yellow fever at a military garrison in US-occupied Havana in 1900, the American Yellow Fever Commission, headed by Walter Reed, conducted experiments following Finlay's ideas, using mosquitoes fed on patients and then on uninfected volunteers. The commission fully confirmed Finlay's observation and announced at the Pan American Medical Congress in Havana in 1901 that the mosquito *Stegomyia fasciata* (now called *Aedes aegypti*) was the sole vector of yellow fever. The hardy *Aedes* mosquito could last for long periods aboard ships, making it a menace to commerce (McNeill 2010).

In 1899 US Army surgeon William C. Gorgas had been appointed Chief Sanitary Officer for the Department of Cuba, organizing a system of surveillance and disease notification, designated hospital wards for the sick, camps for non-immune individuals, home fumigation, and cesspool sanitization. After the Yellow Fever Commission's findings were established in 1901, Gorgas narrowed in on mosquito-killing. He put in place a series of ordinances—enforced by a sizeable squad of men under his control—that resulted in a dramatic decline in yellow fever in Havana in a matter of months (Espinosa 2009). These rules required eliminating virtually all breeding sites by covering, screening, and/or petrolizing every water receptacle, drain, and stagnant pool in sight; daily inspection of houses and yards by an army of sanitarians; the imposition of a stiff fine on property owners found to have mosquito larvae on their premises; and the reporting and isolation of every suspected case of yellow fever. Similar measures were soon implemented in other settings, such as Brazil, where French bacteriologist Emile Marchoux devised a special screened chamber during his participation in a 1901–1905 Pasteur Institute mission that helped control a yellow fever epidemic in Rio de Janeiro (Löwy 2001; Benchimol 1999) (Figure 1-1).

After the United States took over the Panama Canal Zone in 1904, Gorgas was brought in as sanitary chief for the Isthmian Canal Commission—perhaps the most mosquito-ridden place on earth (Sutter 2009). Gorgas's military team was abetted by US Public Health Service officers overseeing quarantine, hospital and laboratory services, and elimination of rats and mosquito larvae (Stern 2005). By 1905 more than 4,000 men were employed in mosquito extermination alone. Two brigades were formed—one, aimed at yellow fever breeding sites, worked primarily around houses and settlements; the other, an *Anopheles* brigade involving teams of contract laborers from the Caribbean, cleared jungles, drained and oiled swamps, and worked to reduce this recently-confirmed malaria mosquito vector (Figure 1-2). Piped water supplies were built to replace drinking water barrels that produced clouds of mosquitoes. Houses were fumigated and screened with wire gauze. Quinine was issued both as a prophylactic against malaria and as a cure, and persons with fevers were isolated behind mosquito-proof screening.

As the engineers blasted and dredged, the war waged against *Aedes* and *Anopheles* by the sanitarians gradually brought yellow fever and malaria under control. Hailed for enabling completion of the Panama Canal, this achievement was widely touted by local health officials across North America, who sought to associate with successful public health investments. Yet the sanitary efforts largely overlooked—and the US occupation of Panama exacerbated—more pressing endemic problems for local populations, such as malnutrition, diarrhea, and tuberculosis (McBride 2002).

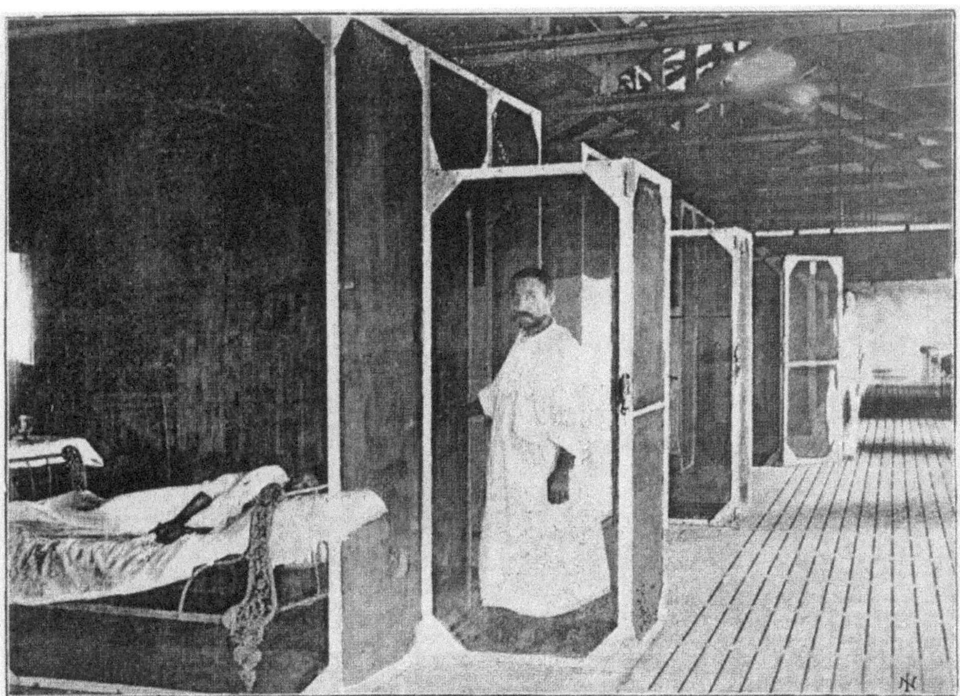

Figure 1-1: Isolating yellow fever using the Marchoux chamber, Hospital S. Sebastião, Rio de Janeiro, Brazil (photo originally published in 1909).
Source: Photo by Oswaldo Cruz, courtesy of Wellcome Library, London.

Health Cooperation in and Beyond Europe: The Long Journey from Meetings to Measures

In Europe, meanwhile, prospects for cooperation had materialized as early as the 1814–1815 Congress of Vienna, which concluded a dozen years of major conflict pitting Napoleon's French Empire against various alliances. Europe's longtime inter-imperial rivalries and perennial warfare appeared to be yielding to diplomatic approaches based on face-to-face negotiation, including regarding quarantine (Harrison 2006). But sanitary agreement would prove a tortuous process.

Decades before the yellow fever threat helped forge organization of the PASB, another ailment had emerged as a worldwide menace, shaping an even larger effort. Cholera had been endemic for centuries in the Ganges River basin; abruptly in 1818 it spread to Southeast Asia, China, Japan, East Africa, the eastern Mediterranean (Syria and Palestine), and southern Russia. Within a few years, another wave swept through Russia, where hundreds of thousands died, and into the major cities of Europe by 1831. The Middle East was not spared, and Muslim pilgrims returning from the Hajj in Mecca were blamed for carrying cholera into Egypt, North Africa, and beyond.

Cholera's emergence in Europe was intimately tied to industrialization—the acceleration of trade, together with the urban squalor accompanying urban life, facilitated its spread and increased its severity (Evans 1987). Within a year, transatlantic ships brought this terrifying disease—provoking diarrhea, vomiting, dehydration, and death within the space of a few hours—to New York, New Orleans, Montreal, and other ports, into the interior, then the Pacific Coast and Mexico in 1833, and southward to Argentina. With pandemics recurring every 15 to 20 years, moralistic responses

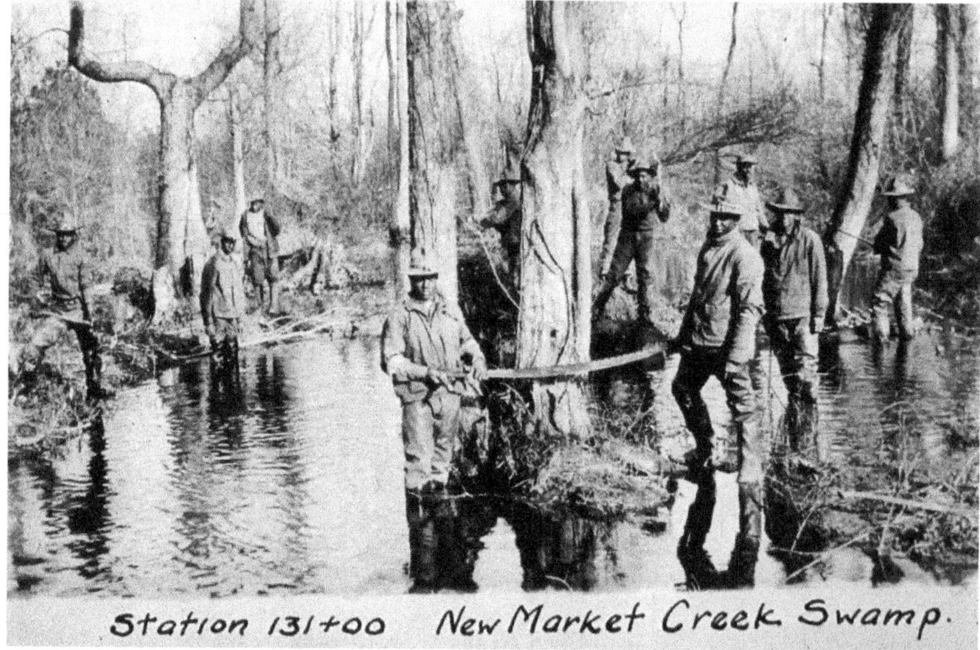

Figure 1-2: Caribbean laborers felling trees for swamp drainage and canal construction at New Market Creek Swamp, Panama, circa 1910.

Source: Courtesy of the US National Library of Medicine.

were eventually supplanted by forceful, initially local, government measures (Rosenberg 1987).

By the mid-1800s, the outbreaks of cholera compelled some sort of international action to prevent spread of the disease. Often unilaterally-imposed, *cordons sanitaires* and quarantine regulations, enforced by the military, had existed since the 14th century but were entangled in complicated calculations. With rising international commerce, such blockades were seen by producers and merchants as obstacles to trade, even as government authorities recognized their political importance. Within India, colonial authorities oscillated between harsh measures, including against Hindu pilgrims, and fears that such control might spark political unrest (Arnold 1986).

Middle Eastern authorities were among the first to act. In 1831, Egypt—then under the Ottoman Empire—set up the Council of Alexandria to protect against entry of cholera and plague, involving a complicated governance structure of domestic officials and doctors and European colonial powers permitted to enact or refuse quarantine. After Britain occupied Egypt in 1882, the Alexandria quarantine board and the Suez Canal came under British control, later affiliating with European agencies. Another Health Council based in Constantinople (Istanbul), enforced maritime quarantine in the Mediterranean under administration of Ottoman and European delegates between the late 1830s and World War I.

European powers took until 1851 to organize an International Sanitary Conference, called by France and attended by Austria, Great Britain, Greece, Portugal, Russia, Spain, Sardinia, the Papal States, Tuscany, and the Kingdom of Two Sicilies (the latter four subsequently unifying as Italy). The Paris meeting lasted 6 months, with each state represented by a diplomat and a physician. Although delegates could not agree on whether cholera was contagious, they eventually produced a lengthy convention dealing with the quarantine of ships against plague, cholera, and yellow fever. Only France, Portugal, and Sardinia ratified the document, but the latter two revoked acceptance because its 137 measures proved burdensome. A similar convention generated by a second (1859) conference went unratified.

The early conferences ended in frustration partly because there was no consensus regarding the causes and transmission of the diseases in question. A third conference, held in Constantinople in 1866, reviewed voluminous evidence on the cause of cholera, including the works of Snow and German hygienist Max von Pettenkofer (see chapter 12), and concluded that the disease was spread through what we would today call the "fecal-oral" route. At the fourth International Sanitary Conference in Vienna (1874), a proposal was made to establish a permanent International Commission on Epidemics, but was rejected (Bynum 1993). Altogether, it took some four decades for a binding sanitary convention to be passed, and 11 conferences held over more than 50 years before agreement was reached to establish a permanent international health organization.

It is not entirely surprising that international interchange among professionals and diplomats did not immediately lead to cooperation in health matters. Simultaneous to the sanitary conferences, international meetings spanning virtually every scholarly and professional domain marked a furious exchange of ideas, standards, challenges, and breakthroughs across and beyond Europe. In 1851 alone, the "Great Exhibition" of London (the first World's Fair) celebrated trade and manufacturing, and the First International Congress on Statistics was held in Brussels, followed by a demography and hygiene congress in 1852, and congresses on ophthalmology in 1857, veterinary medicine in 1863 and so on. As attested to by the rise of international journals and the exchange of correspondence in this period, professional interactions sometimes tested the dual loyalties of scientists (to their disciplines and their countries).

Likewise, that sanitary agreement seemed to trail scientific developments reflected the highly political nature of decisionmaking regarding these matters. Initially Britain resisted French overtures and remained opposed to any form of regulation of its extensive trade. Britain was ready to impose surveillance and coercive measures on Muslim pilgrims (Low 2008) and condemn the Hajj for the 1865 cholera pandemic (Afkhami 1999), but refused to implicate British trade routes. The British government went so far as to reverse its quarantine and isolation policies in India before the opening of the Suez Canal, so that the reduced transport time for trade to and from its most profitable colony would not be inconvenienced by disease-control measures (Watts 1997).

Britain's refusal to endorse cholera conventions stemmed from more than commercial self-interest: it had its own system of "intercolonial" (de facto worldwide) health arrangements of information gathering, research, and conferences, essentially precluding the need for participation in a multilateral effort with potential rivals (Maglen 2002) and enabling it to set its own rules. Into the late 19th century, for example, Britain opposed quarantine on its ships and goods in Japanese ports, going against Japan's wishes. Meanwhile, Japanese officials and physicians implemented quarantine measures in Korean ports to protect against cholera even before Japan emerged as an imperial power (Kim 2013).

The US's first involvement in the International Sanitary Conferences was its hosting, on its own initiative, of the fifth meeting in 1881. With the participation of seven Latin American countries plus China, Japan, Liberia, and the usual Europeans, the conference aimed to obtain international approval for an 1879 US law to inspect and regulate vessels en route to the United States to prevent "the introduction of contagious or infectious diseases from foreign countries." Although some delegates expressed interest in a system of mutual disease notification, the US proposal was struck down. Like Britain and Mexico, the United States instead proceeded to develop a system of epidemic informants on its own.

The sanitary conferences took on greater urgency in the 1890s: punctuated by new cholera pandemics, they resulted, finally, in international conventions in 1892 and 1893 (on cholera control along the Suez Canal and in Europe), in 1894 (specifically on the sanitary control of the Mecca pilgrimage), in 1897 on plague, and in 1903 (replacing the previous conventions) (International Sanitary Convention of Paris 1903; Textes juxtaposés 1897).

By the 1890s there were quarantine stations operated by the British in the Suez and the Ottomans near the mouth of the Red Sea (which lasted in various guises until 1956) specifically to prevent the spread of disease through the Hajj (Bulmus 2012). While quarantine was heightened in the East, Western Europe relaxed its own restrictions (Baldwin 1999) and delayed cooperation.

At long last, a 1903 agreement led to the 1907 conference in Rome that set up l'Office International d'Hygiène Publique (OIHP). Opening its doors in Paris in 1909, the OIHP was charged with collecting and disseminating public health information (especially relating to cholera, plague, and yellow fever) among participating countries, overseeing sanitary treaties, and sharing measures to tackle epidemic diseases.

A formal international health agency had finally been established. The OIHP's original 23 European members subsequently expanded to almost 60, including from the Americas and Asia. But there were no African participants, even though Ethiopia was hit hard by cholera (Echenberg 2011) (independent Liberia was also a potential attendee), a reminder that Black Africans were uniquely isolated and disregarded throughout the rise of modern international health.

With a staff of barely half a dozen people, the OIHP worked diligently and yet could hardly keep up with its stated mission. With protecting Europe from "foreign" epidemics its foremost objective, the OIHP focused on such areas as effective methods for sea crew and passenger inspection, the de-ratting of ships, an international agreement to control sexually transmitted diseases in seamen, standardization of some biological products, and a study of hospital organization.

Just as health professionals had begun to collaborate across borders, Europe's uneasy peace unraveled amid growing militarism, nationalism, and imperialist territorial and commercial rivalries. War conditions starkly revealed the limits to international cooperation. The OIHP's permanent representative committee did not meet at all during World War I (1914–1918), and the OIHP was impotent in the face of outbreaks of diseases such as typhus, which infected millions of people in war-torn Europe. Even more dramatically, the great influenza epidemic of 1918-1919 killed an estimated 50 to 100 million people worldwide, with up to half of the deaths in colonial India alone, many in areas such as Assam and Berar already suffering from famine (Killingray and Phillips 2003). Only Spain, which was not party to the war, notified international authorities about the influenza outbreak, leading to the misnomer "Spanish influenza" (Porras Gallo 1997). The OIHP could not intervene to decry or address the pandemic, and war secrecy imperatives impeded effective communication regarding the outbreak and spread of influenza among troops, including the half million US soldiers who were mobilized precisely as the epidemic was unfolding, undoubtedly exacerbating it.

The Rockefeller Foundation

Even as Europe's diplomatic crisis was threatening incipient internationalism, another development was afoot in the United States. With bureaucratization, standardization, epidemic disease control, and the safeguarding of trade beginning to be addressed through nascent multilateral institutions, international health entered a new phase, one that combined tropical medicine concerns with on-the-ground cooperation from metropolitan powers to peripheral locales. In addition to controlling disease outbreaks, cooperation offered the potential to: stimulate economic growth; stabilize colonies and emerging nation-states by helping them meet the social demands of their populations; improve diplomatic relations; expand consumer markets; and encourage the transfer and internationalizing of scientific, bureaucratic, and cultural values.

At the same time, local elites—through participation in international health activities—could be linked to the world's great powers. International health thus proffered the promise of generating goodwill and economic development in place of gunboat diplomacy and colonial repression, all the while supporting the expansion of global capitalism.

At this time a novel kind of player, the Rockefeller Foundation (RF), emerged on the international health scene as part of a new American movement—"scientific philanthropy." Heeding rags-to-riches steel magnate Andrew Carnegie's call for the wealthy to channel their fortunes to the good of society by supporting systematic social improvements—to education, public health, and community well-being[2]—rather than charity, such philanthropy also burnished the reputation of much reviled "robber barons" of American industry. Founded in 1913 by oil mogul John D. Rockefeller "to promote the well-being of mankind throughout the world," the RF virtually single-handedly popularized the concept of *international health* and was a major influence upon the field's 20th century agendas, approaches, and actions. Rockefeller, his business and philanthropic consigliere Frederick Gates (a Baptist minister), and John D. Rockefeller Jr. built upon Carnegie's ideas, expanding from hospital, church, and university donations to fund medical research and large-scale campaigns aimed at social melioration.

Public health became the ideal vehicle through which Rockefeller philanthropy could apply scientific findings to the public good while ensuring expansion of global markets. After uncovering the important part played by hookworm disease in the economic "backwardness" of the US South—and the possibilities of public health campaigns to eliminate the disease through an anti-helminthic drug and public health "propaganda"—the RF soon created an International Health Board, reorganized as the International Health Division (IHD) in 1927. The IHD befriended dozens of governments around the world by helping modernize their health institutions, promoting the importance of public health among countless populations, and preparing vast regions for investment and increased productivity. By the time of its dismantling in 1951, the IHD had spent the equivalent of billions of dollars carrying out scores of hookworm, yellow fever, and malaria campaigns, as well as efforts to control yaws, rabies, influenza, schistosomiasis, malnutrition, and other health problems, in more than 90 countries and colonies around the globe. It also sponsored some 2,500 fellows to pursue graduate study in public health, mostly in the United States and founded 25 schools of public health in North America and across the world (Cueto 1994; Farley 2004; Fee 1987).

In its trademark public health efforts, the RF pursued a narrow, biological approach to disease based on short-term, technical solutions. The RF drove the agenda of cooperation with national governments, set its temporal and geographical parameters (at times with the accompanying intention of fending off radical political movements), relied on efficient "magic bullets" against disease, and placed disease-eradication and education campaigns under the direction of its own officers (or local experts trained at RF-funded public health schools such as Johns Hopkins and Harvard), even as "recipient" governments were expected eventually to foot most of the bill for cooperative activities (Stepan 2011). To be sure, a range of in-country actors reshaped and sometimes rejected these endeavors to their own ends (Trujillo-Pagan 2013). The RF modus operandi of crediting local authorities without drawing excessive attention to itself, developed through decades of experience, helped mitigate resistance and reinforced its model (Birn and Fee 2013).

In Mexico, for instance, venerated RF-trained public health physician Miguel Bustamante, who rose to become Mexico's deputy health minister and Secretary-General of the PASB, worked with the RF but resented and withstood the imposition of US-style technical public health models, instead framing the expansion of local health units in terms of broader societal health needs (Birn 2006). The RF, for its part, was not a monolith: it changed over time and had to deal with shifting political priorities at home and abroad.

With field officers in virtually every setting in which it operated, the RF could rely on a well-honed bureaucracy to infuse its particular ideas and approaches into local efforts to institutionalize public health (Birn 2006), even as each campaign became a new experiment in international health, changing in context and refashioning the RF itself (Palmer 2010). Perhaps the greatest success attributed to the IHD was yellow fever control, involving: (a) extensive campaigns across Latin America to reduce the presence of the *Aedes aegypti* mosquito vector through use of insecticides, drainage, and larvicidal fish (Magalhães 2016); and (b) the development of the Nobel-prize winning 17D yellow fever vaccine in the mid-1930s, which showcased US scientific expertise to European rivals. While yellow fever campaigns ended costly commercial interruptions, by this time the disease was, ironically, of minor epidemiological concern in Latin America, where even during epidemics, it felled a relatively small number of people, mostly newcomers.

Indeed, in the 1920s the RF organized major campaigns against yellow fever and hookworm in Veracruz state, Mexico, although neither of these diseases was considered a priority by domestic health officials. But Veracruz was a key oil producer and agricultural center and a hotbed of agrarian rebellion, making it an attractive locale for both the RF and national political authorities. Meanwhile, Mexican public health official and local requests for campaigns against onchocercosis and tuberculosis were not heeded, for neither disease could offer an effective demonstration of the RF's disease-control model of public health: only diseases with ready technical tools (insecticides and larvicides in the case of yellow fever, and anti-helminthic drugs against hookworm) were selected, whereas both tuberculosis and onchocercosis required significant long-term social investments in housing and nutrition.

By the late 1930s, the RF claimed credit for eradicating malaria, under particular circumstances: the introduced African mosquito *Anopheles gambiae* was responsible for an immense outbreak of malignant tertian malaria in Brazil, with more than 100,000 cases and 14,000 deaths in 1938 alone. RF efforts, supported by Brazilian nation-building strongman President Getulio Vargas, eventually eradicated *A. gambiae* from Brazil after years of larval control. This demonstrated the possibility of vector eradication in the case of introduced species or on islands, as in Sardinia (Löwy 2001; Packard and Gadelha 1994; Stapleton 2004).

With its Latin American campaigns among the most active, the RF also worked in China, parts of Europe, and across the British Empire, including in Asia and various Caribbean islands. In colonial settings, the RF's small menu of rural, technical approaches differed from the tropical medicine approach Britain was trying to consolidate. Early 20th century India was a key hub for the production and worldwide dissemination of medical knowledge (Amrith 2006), amid colonial neglect of wide swaths of the rural populations. Though these efforts were complementary (and the RF was always "invited"), they sometimes engendered tense encounters.

Over several decades, the RF's stock hookworm campaign in Ceylon treated multitudinous tea estate workers, but plantation owners' refusal to invest in sanitation led workers to become repeatedly reinfected. By the 1930s, the RF was pushed by villagers and political leaders, as well as its own officers, to set up a network of health units to prevent and treat an array of diseases and address water and sanitation problems, nutrition, and school hygiene, in some ways preempting British efforts (Hewa 1995).

In India, by contrast, the RF's hookworm campaign (Figure 1-3) was met with indifference by governments, plantation owners, physicians, and villagers, even as the RF considered India to be a world reservoir of hookworm, spreading disease through its large diaspora of laborers. While the RF experimented with different treatments, it overestimated the role of the minor ailment of hookworm in instilling broad support for public health organization. The RF also failed to meet colonial administrators' expectations of wide population coverage, ultimately focusing on settings with existing agencies, such as hospitals and prisons, to ensure the work would become permanent. Only through the subsequent establishment of health units did India's lukewarm reception to the RF turn into a greater technically-oriented consciousness of health administrators (Kavadi 2016).

Simultaneous to the RF's involvement in country-by-country activities, it was also mapping out, directly and indirectly, international health's institutional framework. Its activities and organization provided the groundwork for a new international health system featuring its own bureaucracy, legitimacy, and mode of conduct. Indeed, the IHD identified its most successful contribution to be "aid to official public health organizations in the development of administrative measures suited to local customs, needs, traditions, and conditions" (LNHO 1927, p. 743). Thus, although highly influential in shaping the enduring *modus operandi* of international health through technically-based disease campaigns and transnational public health training, the RF's self-defined mark of success was its role in generating political and popular support for public health, in the creation of national public health departments across the world, and in its support for the institutionalization of international health. Even as the RF bolstered ascendant US capitalist power, it also remained open—on the

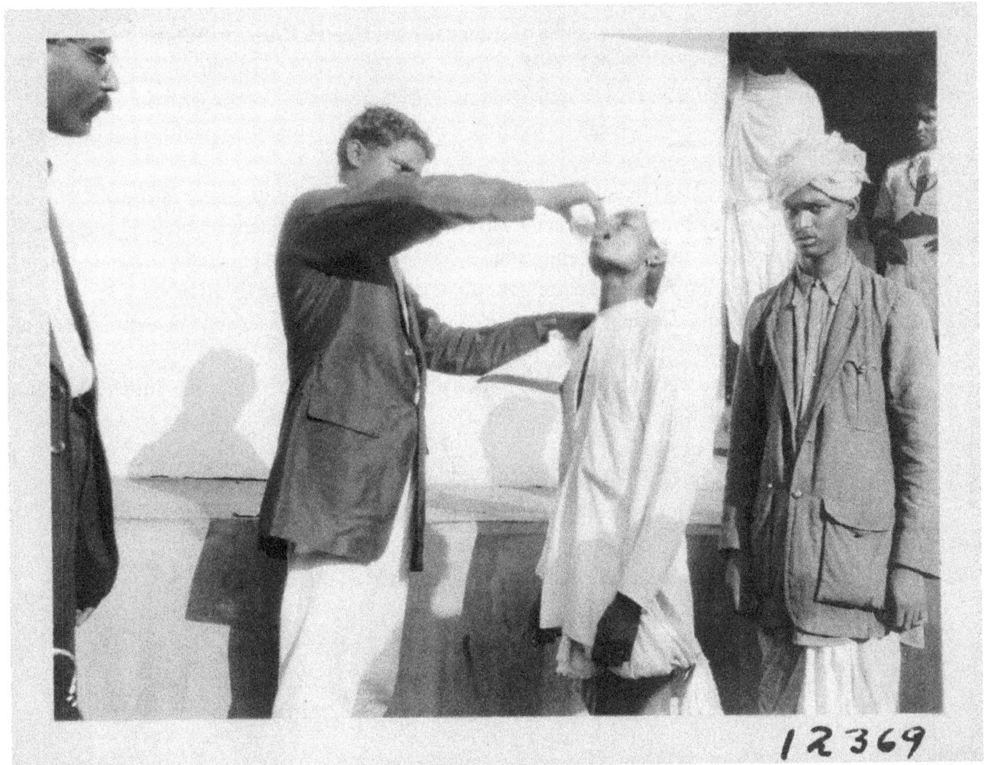

Figure 1-3: Administering hookworm treatment at Karapa (India). Rockefeller Foundation International Health Board's Cooperative Hookworm Campaign, 1920s.

Source: Courtesy of the Rockefeller Foundation, *100 Years: The Rockefeller Foundation*, accessed March 12, 2016, http://rockefeller100.org/items/show/1681.

margins—to social medicine approaches to public health that were unfolding together with progressive political developments (Birn 2014).

The new international health, as pioneered by the RF, was neither narrowly self-interested nor passively diffusionist. Instead, the RF actively sought national partnerships to spread its public health gospel via interaction with political and professional authorities and local populations. The RF's philanthropic status, its purported independence from both government and business interests, and its limited accountability enabled its success. Its work patterns included rapid demonstrations of specific disease-control methods based on proven techniques, a missionary zeal in its own officers, marshaling national commitment to public health through significant co-financing obligations, and using fellowships to mold a cadre of public health leaders (Box 1-4). It also carefully avoided disease campaigns that might be costly, overly complex, time consuming, or distracting to its technically-oriented public health model (Birn 2006).

Other US philanthropies, such as the Milbank and Commonwealth Funds and Kellogg and Ford Foundations, entered the international health arena, but none came close to the RF's purview over the field's ideologies, institutions, and practices. As per chapter 2, its strategies continue to influence the operating policies and practice of global health today, serving, like the more recent Bill and Melinda Gates Foundation, as both an arm of imperialism and an agent of change.

Box 1-4 Rockefeller Foundation Principles of International Health Cooperation

1. Agenda-setting from above: international health activities are donor-driven, with the agenda of cooperation formulated and overseen by the international agency, whether via direct in-country activities or the awarding of grants.
2. Budget incentives: activities are only partially funded by donor agencies; matching funding mechanisms require "recipient" governments to commit substantial financial, human, and physical resources to the cooperative endeavor.
3. Technobiological paradigm: activities are structured in disease-control terms based upon: (a) biological and individual behavioral understandings of disease; and (b) technical tools applied to a wide range of settings.
4. A priori parameters of success: activities are bound geographically, through time limits, by disease and intervention, and/or according to clear exit strategies in order to demonstrate efficiency and ensure visible, positive outcomes.
5. Consensus via transnational professionals: activities hinge on transnational professionals—who are trained abroad (often alongside donor agency staff) and involved in international networks—easing the local translation of cooperative endeavors.
6. On-the-ground reality check for successful implementation: adaptation of activities to local conditions, as needed.

Source: Adapted from Birn (2006, p. 270).

INTERNATIONAL HEALTH INSTITUTION-BUILDING: THE LNHO AND THE INTER-WAR YEARS

Key Questions:

- How did international health organizations evolve after World War I?
- What were their constraints?

The Great War (World War I) and the Russian Civil War, following Russia's 1917 revolution, devastated much of Europe, even as new hopes for a more just world emerged from the ashes. Institution-building took two key forms: first, the establishment of international organizations that played a strategic role in planning and marshaling expertise to address world health problems (Box 1-5), and second, the cultivation of a cooperative spirit that began to make health an international priority.

A 1920 London conference recommended that the OIHP be absorbed by the health section of the newly created League of Nations (based in Geneva). This plan was aborted by the United States (which was an OIHP member but declined to join the League of Nations) and France (which preferred to retain the Paris-based OIHP). Nevertheless, a health committee of the League of Nations was set up, initially to oversee an Epidemic Commission formed to control (and therefore protect Western Europe from) outbreaks of typhus in Russia, as well as cholera, smallpox, and other diseases in the Ottoman Empire. Permanently established in 1923, the League of Nations Health Organisation (LNHO) convened health experts and institutionalized international health, soon expanding its mission and reach well beyond the initial focus on protecting Europe's eastern flank (Borowy 2009; Weindling 1995a).

The LNHO played a vital coordinating function for an array of activities far beyond disease control, its wide charter allowing opportunistic social activism under Polish hygienist Ludwik Rajchman's widely recognized leadership (Balinska 1995). Where there had been none just 20 years before, now three official international health organizations operated more or less separately: the PASB in Washington, DC, the OIHP in Paris, and the LNHO in Geneva.

Box 1-5 Early International Health Organizations, Location, and Year of Founding/Establishment

- Pan American Sanitary Bureau, Washington, DC, 1902
- Office International d'Hygiène Publique, Paris, 1907/1909
- Oswaldo Cruz Institute, Rio de Janeiro, 1900/1908
- Rockefeller Foundation (International Health Commission/Board/Division), New York, 1913
- Save the Children, London, 1919/Geneva, 1920
- League of Nations Health Organisation, Geneva, 1920/1923
- International American Institute for the Protection of Childhood, Montevideo, 1927

Decades earlier, the first international non-governmental agency, the International Red Cross, had been founded by Jean-Henri Dunant, a Swiss national moved by witnessing the terrible suffering of soldiers in the Italian unification wars' bloody 1859 Battle of Solferino. The founding document of the Red Cross, which promoted neutral humanitarian assistance to wounded combatants, entered into force in 1865 and became known as the original Geneva Convention. The International Red Cross soon spawned a series of national Red Cross and Red Crescent organizations.

World War I and its aftermath led to both proliferation and fracturing of international health institutions. In 1919 Henry Davison, head of the wartime American Red Cross, orchestrated the establishment of the League of Red Cross Societies (LRCS) as a federation of the national societies that had attracted thousands of committed volunteers during wartime. He envisioned the League as a truly international agency that would spearhead peacetime international humanitarian cooperation to combat epidemic disease and war-induced destitution, transcending the International Red Cross's war focus (and lack of cooperation among national societies), and modeling itself after the new League of Nations. While the LRCS soon became involved in nursing education, first aid, disaster relief, community health, and youth training, Davison's dreams for a US-led humanitarian agency coordinating international health were triply dashed by the US's failure to join the League of Nations, overshadowing by the LNHO, and ongoing feuds with the International Red Cross (Hutchinson 1996).

The issue of responsibility for the health aspects of worker welfare also produced certain tensions. The International Labour Office (ILO) was founded in 1919 to protect workers and promote peace through social justice efforts. Charged by the Treaty of Versailles with guiding occupational health standards and the prevention of worker sickness, it expediently pulled back from involvement in medical matters after the LNHO's founding. Later, the ILO and LNHO heightened joint work, after Rajchman became more politically vocal and the onset of the Depression demanded greater coordination between the two agencies (Weindling 1995b).

A set of international initiatives and agencies focused on children's health and well-being also emerged in this period. In 1919 English social reformers Eglantyne Jebb and her sister Dorothy established the first modern relief agency, "Save the Children," to feed and rescue children in war-torn Germany and Austria. By 1920 they had launched the Save the Children International Union in Geneva to extend rescue efforts to children suffering from famine in Russia and elsewhere. Within a few years, Save the Children became active in Africa, providing famine aid in colonial Rwanda, and full-blown war relief to children displaced by Italy's 1935 invasion of Ethiopia (Iliffe 1987). Meantime, a rival organization, the International Association for the Protection of Child Welfare, was founded in 1921 in Brussels. In 1924, Jebb was able to get the League of Nations Assembly to adopt her "Declaration of the Rights of the Child" and to establish a child welfare committee to oversee a range of social questions relating to child protection (Marshall 1999). In 1927 the International American Institute for the

Protection of Childhood was established in Uruguay with the LNHO's support as a policy and practice clearinghouse and beacon for the Pan American Child (movement and) Congresses, which had been meeting in Latin America since 1916. The Institute brought a worldwide platform for a child rights approach to children's health and well-being in the 1930s (Birn 2012).

Even with the competing efforts and overlapping missions of these and other agencies, the LNHO became a crossroads for international health activity in the inter-war years. Rajchman's particular interest in child health, for instance, led the LNHO to carry out comparative international studies of the societal causes of infant mortality (Scarzanella 2003), and motivated him to help establish UNICEF after World War II. By the late 1920s Rajchman and the LNHO were drawing concertedly on social medicine precepts (Brown and Birn 2013) that called for the political and structural underpinnings of health to be addressed (Borowy and Hardy 2008; Zylberman 2004)—from living and working conditions to political representation—as part of the scientific basis for public health action.

The LNHO's multi-national staff and advisors pursued an ambitious agenda of epidemiologic surveillance, expert scientific research, standardization, and interchange of health personnel. Its activities were far broader than the quarantine mandates of previous decades, furthering the collection, standardization, and dissemination of vital and health statistics around the world. In matters of outbreaks and gathering epidemiological information, the office collaborated with the OIHP, albeit with tensions around turf, and the US's and Britain's attempts to rein in the LNHO. In 1926 the LNHO started publication of the *Weekly Epidemiological Record* (still produced by the World Health Organization). It also organized a branch in Singapore in 1925 to gather information on health conditions in Asia, and it held conferences around the world. Communication was carried out by (sea) mail, telegrams and, where possible, by telephone or two-way radio. Obtaining timely information about disease outbreaks in remote areas was a continuing challenge (Borowy 2009). The LNHO, like most of the public health world at the time, grappled with eugenic policies aimed at social "advancement," even as it sidestepped birth control questions (Bashford 2014; Connelly 2008).

Tensions between the LNHO and OIHP persisted and other rivalries surfaced with the PASB and a regional health governance effort in Asia (Akami 2016) contesting European control over international sanitary legislation and networks (Sealey 2011). In the end, the OIHP retained official jurisdiction over international health agreements and epidemic intelligence, and it served, in principle, as an advisory council to the LNHO. This arrangement permitted the United States, as a non-member of the League of Nations, to keep a window open to the LNHO. Various US experts served as LNHO staff members or consultants (Dubin 1995), sustaining a rising role for the United States in international health that would solidify after World War II.

Another important American connection was through the RF. The LNHO was partially modeled on the RF's International Health Board and shared many of its values, experts, and knowhow in disease control, institution-building, and educational and research work even as it challenged narrow, medicalized understandings of health. Rather than being supplanted by the LNHO, the RF became its major patron and lifeline, funding study tours, projects, and eventually its operating budget, and taking over some of its key activities during World War II (Barona 2015).

The LNHO established numerous scientific and technical commissions to: set standards for drugs and vaccines; survey medical education, medical facilities, and public health organization; and study housing, nutrition, and the health impact of the worldwide economic Depression. LNHO committees investigated and reported not only on major infectious diseases (e.g., syphilis, tuberculosis, and malaria), but also on issues such as opiates, trafficking of women, health insurance, cancer, and heart disease (Barona-Vilar and Guillem-Llobat 2015; Borowy 2009). The LNHO coordinated transnational exchanges and public health training and fostered international networks of professionals, together enabling multi-directional learning.

Using European public health problem-setting as a launching pad, the LNHO interacted with the RF, colonial powers, and sister health agencies, with experts moving transregionally and transinstitutionally. In the arena of nutrition and food policy, for example, Latin American reformers helped negotiate standard-setting among the ILO, PASB, and LNHO (Pernet 2013). Britain's inter-war "discovery" of malnutrition in Kenya and especially, India, where dietary deficiencies were linked to widespread beriberi (Worboys 1988), provoked colonial anxieties about the failure of its agricultural schemes. A British nutrition expert, brought in from the LNHO, critiqued the colonial rice economy for rural impoverishment (Amrith 2006), though colonial authorities eschewed structural explanations to focus on more technical dimensions of malnutrition.

The LNHO's studies of Depression-era rural misery and ill health in Europe were brought to a larger stage with its sponsorship of a 1937 rural hygiene conference in Bandoeng, Java (where the RF worked with Dutch colonial authorities to support rural hygiene but stopped short of addressing the causes of poverty), bringing together representatives of China, Japan, Siam (Thailand), the RF, Red Cross, and Dutch, British, and French colonies concentrated in Asia. Straddling collaboration with colonial powers and social medicine concerns with rural reconstruction, land reform, and indigenous sensitivity, Rajchman was implicitly offering solidarity with various anti-colonial and revolutionary efforts (Brown and Fee 2008).

Despite Rajchman's capable protagonism, the LNHO became mired in League of Nations politics, and budgetary constraints meant that it could realize only part of its agenda. Rajchman's left-wing proclivities became increasingly pronounced, leading him to appoint socialist Italian malariologists, take a secondment in rural revolutionary China, and publicly support the anti-fascist side in the Spanish Civil War. Accused of being a crypto-Communist, he was forced to resign in 1939 (Brown and Birn 2013). Even before the onset of World War II, operations of both the OIHP and LNHO were marred by international bickering, the chaos of worldwide Depression, and growing tensions in Europe, with resultant wavering support for health cooperation (Solomon, Murard, and Zylberman 2008).

During wartime, international health efforts continued, with an increased military focus. For example, US authorities tested (with the RF's cooperation in Mexico) and then administered the use of the insecticide DDT against louse-borne typhus in the Americas and Europe and against malarious mosquito vectors in the Pacific military theater, around military bases, and in areas of strategic military importance (Stapleton 2004). Also receiving sanitary attention were rubber- and quinine-growing regions of Brazil and the Andes, which were needed to replace Malaysian and Dutch East Indies supplies during Japanese occupation. As well, the accelerated production of newly developed sulfonamides and the antibacterial wonder drug penicillin enabled distribution to Allied soldiers in the latter years of the war. During this period, the US government also launched a large-scale cooperative sanitary effort throughout Latin America to improve diplomatic relations and forge alliances to fend off Axis influence in the region, as well as to assert its leadership in projected post-war development and rebuilding (Campos 2008). At the same time, other international health activities dwindled: the research and standardization efforts of the LNHO and the public health projects of the RF (outside the Americas) had to be suspended because of the war, only to be resurrected under a new guise in the post-war period.

CONCLUSION

Learning Points:

- The rise of modern international health was crucially shaped by the triad of military conquest, imperialism, and industrialization, forces also undergirding the development of the global capitalist economy.
- Medicine and public health accompanied conquest, facilitated and justified colonialism, and sought to mitigate certain ill effects of imperialism, slavery, and industrialization through epidemic control and diffusion of health practices.
- Enhancing productivity, safeguarding commerce, and moralizing (missionary) and civilizing ("development") concerns were at the heart of these endeavors, influenced by imperial imperatives and cultural (racial, gender, class, etc.) prejudices.
- Despite a marked asymmetry of power, Indigenous knowledge, practices, and healers, together with local populations, shaped approaches to international health, in part through resistance to them.
- The institutionalization of international health in the early 20th century was influenced by concerns around spread of epidemics and social

unrest, protection of trade, access to resources and markets, scientific diffusion, as well as charity, development, diplomacy, and solidarity.
- International (and global) health is not simply a technical arena but was (and is) intertwined with and molded by powerful social, political, economic, cultural, and scientific factors and resources.

With localized responses to the Black Death serving as a key precursor, the rise of imperialism, slavery, industrialization, and global commerce played a critical role in shaping worldwide patterns of health and disease and spurred the development of colonial medicine, tropical medicine, public health, and international health measures and institutions.

While some advocates of organized international health may have been motivated by altruistic impulses, the field's origins were particularly reflective of the political, commercial, and expansionist exigencies of the age of imperialism and the inauguration of global capitalism. International health's primary efforts were accordingly focused on: facilitating conquest and occupation; increasing worker productivity in factories, mines, and plantations in metropolitan and colonial settings; fending off social unrest; and ensuring a smooth and uninterrupted trade system. These forces and activities engendered lasting approaches to problem-setting and disease control, shaping relationships among key players and patterns of power and decisionmaking.

The historical events covered in this chapter remind us how present day global health remains embedded in structures and relations of *power* and *influence*—despite the universalist evocations of the term *global health* (Hodges 2012). This holds true for the multiple charitable, nongovernmental, multilateral, and bilateral development organizations aimed at generating and sharing seemingly apolitical health measures and policies.

In sum, this chapter and the next serve not only to lay out the background of global health but to present three key underpinnings of the field that allow us to understand how and why it operates as it does. First, as we have seen, international and global health need to be understood within a larger context of social and political ideas, institutions, and movements. That is to say, medicine and health are not neutral, purely technical domains; instead they are framed socially, economically, and culturally—in temporal and spatial terms—and politically, in terms of local, regional, international, social, economic, ideological, and institutional struggles for power.

Second, many ideas, practices, and institutions of international health that began during the colonial era were cemented in the course of the 20th century and now resonate in contemporaneous global health. This historical legacy plays out in the motives of and incentives for involvement of different actors, in specific instruments of the field such as disease campaigns and fellowships, and in the bureaucratic mechanisms of goal-setting, funding, policy implementation, and effectiveness evaluation.

Third, processes of negotiation have shaped and continue to affect global health efforts. Here the role and interplay of local actors, international networks, business interests, scientific and social practices, and health agencies can be understood as a complicated dance involving multiple partners who participate in the institutions, ideologies, politics, and practices of international and global health and in the worldwide circulation of knowledge.

With the long effort to institutionalize international health on a cooperative basis realized in the aftermath of the horrific First World War, a new optimistic focus, drawing from principles of social medicine, sought to reorient the field to address the political, structural, and social factors underlying the health of the public, blurring boundaries between domestic and global goals.

But just as international health's focus was shifting from plagues toward peoples, the LNHO's aspirations were disrupted by worldwide economic and political crises in the 1930s and the onset of World War II. As we shall see in chapter 2, after the war, a new geopolitical configuration took shape, one that initially unified international health efforts in the World Health Organization's progressive mission—drawing from the LNHO's ideals and organizational structures—yet almost immediately undermined in the context of the rise of the "international development" paradigm, decolonization struggles, and, especially, the Cold War rivalry between Western (US-led) and Eastern (Soviet-led) blocs.

NOTES

1. Debates around Black Death's pathogen have been reignited by developments in molecular biology, entomology, and forensic medicine (Cohn 2002; Green 2014; Little 2011). Long linked to bubonic plague (transmitted by *Yersinia pestis*, see p. 19) spread via rat-hosted flea bites, and associated with poor urban refuse disposal and rodent infestation, other diseases (e.g., anthrax) have also been postulated. Recent London rail excavations uncovered a mass grave from Britain's last major plague outbreak in 1665–66, enabling scientists to confirm presence of *Y. pestis* through DNA evidence. The high death toll and apparent person-to-person spread suggest that pneumonic plague (its most virulent form, communicated via aerosolized droplets after bubonic plague reaches the lungs) may also have been important (Stanbridge 2016).
2. Philanthropists partially succeeded in staving off the US welfare state: compared with European and many Latin American countries, the private and philanthropic sectors in the United States have had since the early 20th century a far greater role in the provision of social welfare—both limiting the size of the welfare state and giving private interests undemocratic purview over social welfare.

REFERENCES

Afkhami AA. 1999. Defending the guarded domain: Epidemics and the emergence of an international sanitary policy in Iran. *Comparative Studies of South Asia, Africa, and the Middle East* 19(1):122–136.

Agostoni C. 2003. *Monuments of Progress: Modernization and Public Health in Mexico City, 1876-1910*. Boulder: University Press of Colorado.

Akami T. 2016. A quest to be global: The League of Nations Health Organisation and inter-colonial regional governing agendas of the Far Eastern Association of Tropical Medicine 1910–25. *The International History Review* 38(1):1–23.

Alchon SA. 2003. *A Pest in the Land: New World Epidemics in a Global Perspective*. Albuquerque: University of New Mexico Press.

Alvarez A. 2008. Malaria and the emergence of rural health in Argentina: An analysis from the perspective of international interaction and co-operation. *Canadian Bulletin of Medical History* 25(1):137–160.

Amrith S. 2006. *Decolonizing International Health: India and Southeast Asia, 1930-65*. Basingstoke: Palgrave Macmillan.

Anderson W. 2006. *Colonial Pathologies: American Tropical Medicine, Race, and Hygiene in the Philippines*. Durham, NC: Duke University Press.

Arnold D. 1986. Cholera and colonialism in British India. *Past & Present* 113(4):118–151.

———. 1997. The place of "the tropics" in Western medical ideas since 1750. *Tropical Medicine and International Health* 2(4):303–313.

———. 2015. Globalization and contingent colonialism: Towards a transnational history of "British" India. *Journal of Colonialism & Colonial History* 16(2).

Arrizabalaga J, Henderson J, and French RK. 1997. *The Great Pox: The French Disease in Renaissance Europe*. New Haven: Yale University Press.

Au S. 2011. *Mixed Medicines Health and Culture in French Colonial Cambodia*. Chicago: University of Chicago Press.

Bala P. 2014. 'Re-constructing' Indian medicine: The role of caste in late nineteenth- and twentieth-century India. In Bala P, Editor. *Medicine and Colonialism: Historical Perspectives in India and South Africa*. London: Pickering and Chatto.

Balaguer Perigüell E and Ballester Añón R. 2003. *En el nombre de los niños: La Real Expedición Filantrópica de la Vacuna (1803-1806)*. Madrid: Asociación Española de Pediatría.

Baldwin P. 1999. *Contagion and the State in Europe 1830–1930*. New York: Cambridge University Press.

Balinska M. 1995. *Une vie pour l'humanitaire: Ludwik Rajchman, 1881–1965*. Paris: Editions la Découverte.

Barona JL. 2015. *The Rockefeller Foundation, Public Health and International Diplomacy, 1920–1945*. New York: Routledge.

Barona-Vilar JL and Guillem-Llobat X, Editors. 2015. *Sanidad internacional y transferencia de conocimiento científico*. Valencia: Universidad de Valencia.

Bashford A. 2014. *Global Population: History, Geopolitics, and Life on Earth*. New York: Columbia University Press.

Becerril JE and Jiménez B. 2007. Potable water and sanitation in Tenochtitlán: Aztec culture. *Water Science & Technology: Water Supply* 7(1):147–154.

Benchimol JL, Editor. 1990. *Manguinhos do sonho à vida - a ciência na Belle Epoque*. Rio de Janeiro: Casa de Oswaldo Cruz/Fiocruz.

———. 1999. Dos Micróbios aos Mosquitos. Rio de Janeiro: Editora Fiocruz/ UFRJ.

Bergad L. 2007. *The Comparative Histories of Slavery in Brazil, Cuba, and the United States.* Cambridge: Cambridge University Press.

Berlinguer G. 1992. The interchange of disease and health between the Old and New Worlds. *American Journal of Public Health* 82(10):1407–1413.

Bhattacharya N. 2012. *Contagion and Enclaves: Tropical Medicine in Colonial India.* Liverpool: Liverpool University Press.

Bhattacharya S, Harrison M, and Worboys M. 2005. *Fractured States: Smallpox, Public Health and Vaccination Policy in British India, 1800-1947.* New Delhi: Orient Longman.

Birn A-E. 1997. Six seconds per eyelid: The medical inspection of immigrants at Ellis Island, 1892–1914. *Dynamis* 17:281–316.

———. 2006. *Marriage of Convenience: Rockefeller International Health and Revolutionary Mexico.* Rochester, NY: University of Rochester Press.

———. 2012. Uruguay's child rights approach to health: What role for civil registration? In Breckenridge K and Szreter S, Editors. *Registration and Recognition: Documenting the Person in World History.* Oxford: Oxford University Press/British Academy.

———. 2014. Philanthrocapitalism, past and present: The Rockefeller Foundation, the Gates Foundation, and the setting(s) of the international/global health agenda. *Hypothesis* 12(1):e8.

Birn A-E and Fee E. 2013. The Rockefeller Foundation: Setting the international health agenda. *Lancet* 381(9878):1618–1619.

Borowy I. 2009. *Coming to Terms with World Health: The League of Nations Health Organisation, 1921–1946.* Frankfurt: Peter Lang.

Borowy I and Hardy A, Editors. 2008. *Of Medicine and Men: Biographies and Ideas in European Social Medicine Between the World Wars.* Frankfurt: Peter Lang.

Brown TM and Birn A-E. 2013. The making of health internationalists. In Birn A-E and Brown TM, Editors. *Comrades in Health: U.S. Health Internationalists, Abroad and at Home.* New Brunswick, NJ: Rutgers University Press.

Brown TM and Fee E. 2008. The Bandoeng Conference of 1937: A milestone of health and development. *American Journal of Public Health* 98(1):42–43.

Bulmus B. 2012. *Plague, Quarantines, and Geopolitics in the Ottoman Empire.* Edinburgh: Edinburgh University Press.

Bustamante M. 1952. Los primeros cincuenta años de la Oficina Sanitaria Panamericana. *Boletín de la Oficina Sanitaria Panamericana* 33(6):471–531.

Bynum W. 1993. Policing hearts of darkness: Aspects of the international sanitary conferences. *History and Philosophy of the Life Sciences* 15:421–434.

———. 2002. Mosquitoes bite more than once. *Science* 295(5552):47–48.

Campos AL de V. 2008. Politiques internationales (et réponses locales) de santé au Brésil: le Service Spécial de Santé Publique, 1942-1960. *Canadian Bulletin of Medical History* 25(1):111–136.

Carrillo AM. 2002. Economía, política y salud pública en el México porfiriano (1876-1910). *História, Ciências, Saúde-Manguinhos* 9(Suppl 1):67–87.

Carrillo AM and Birn A-E. 2008. Neighbours on notice: National and imperialist interests in the American Public Health Association, 1872–1921. *Canadian Bulletin of Medical History* 25(1):225–254.

Chadwick E. 1842. *Report to Her Majesty's Principal Secretary of State for the Home Department, from the Poor Law Commissioners, on an Inquiry into the Sanitary Condition of the Labouring Population of Great Britain.* London: W. Clowes and sons for H.M.S.O.

Chandavarkar R. 1992. Plague, panic and epidemic politics in India, 1896–1914. In Ranger T and Slack P, Editors. *Epidemics and Ideas: Essays on the Historical Perception of Pestilence.* Cambridge: Cambridge University Press.

Chaves CL. 2009. Políticas internacionais de saúde: o primeiro acordo sanitário internacional da América (Montevidéu, 1873). *Locus, Revista de História* 15(2):9–27.

———. 2013. Poder e saúde na América do Sul: Os Congressos Sanitários Internacionais, 1870-1889. *História, Ciências, Saúde-Manguinhos* 20:411–434.

Coghe S. 2015. Inter-imperial learning and African health care in Portuguese Angola in the interwar period. *Social History of Medicine* 28(1):134–154.

Cohn Jr SK. 2002. The Black Death: End of a paradigm. *American Historical Review* 107(3):703–738.

Colvin TB. 2012. The real expedición de la Vacuna and the Philippines, 1803–1807. In Monnais L and Cook H, Editors. *Global Movements, Local Concerns: Medicine and Health in Southeast Asia.* Singapore: National University of Singapore Press.

Conklin AL. 2000. *A Mission to Civilize: The Republican Idea of Empire in France and West Africa, 1895-1930.* Redwood City, CA: Stanford University Press.

Connelly M. 2008. *Fatal Misconceptions: The Struggle to Control World Population.* Cambridge: Belknap Harvard.

Cook ND. 1998. *Born to Die: Disease and New World Conquest, 1492–1650.* Cambridge University Press.

Cooper DB. 1965. *Epidemic Disease in Mexico City, 1716–1813: An Administrative, Social, and Medical Study.* Austin: University of Texas Press.

Cox C and Marland H, Editors. 2013. *Migration, Health and Ethnicity in the Modern World.* New York: Palgrave Macmillan.

Crosby A. 1972. *The Columbian Exchange: The Biological and Social Consequences of 1492.* Westport, CT: Greenwood Press.

———. 1993. *Ecological Imperialism: The Biological Expansion of Europe, 900–1900.* Cambridge: Cambridge University Press.

Cueto M, Editor. 1994. *Missionaries of Science: The Rockefeller Foundation and Latin America.* Bloomington: Indiana University Press.

———. 2007. *The Value of Health: A History of the Pan American Health Organization.* Rochester: University of Rochester Press.

Cueto M and Palmer S. 2014. *Medicine and Public Health in Latin America: A History.* Cambridge: Cambridge University Press.

Curtin PD. 1968. Epidemiology and the slave trade. *Political Science Quarterly* 83(2):190–216.

———. 1998. *Disease and Empire: The Health of European Troops in the Conquest of Africa.* Cambridge: Cambridge University Press.

De Almeida M. 2006. Circuito Aberto: Idéias e intercâmbios médico-científicos na América Latina nos orimórdios do século XX. *História, Ciências, Saúde – Manguinhos* 13(3):733–757.

De Barros J. 2014. *Reproducing the British Caribbean: Sex, Gender, and Population Politics after Slavery.* Chapel Hill, NC: University of North Carolina Press.

De Barros J, Palmer S, and Wright D, Editors. 2009. *Health and Medicine in the Circum-Caribbean, 1800–1968.* New York: Routledge.

Deacon H. 2000. Racism and medical science in South Africa's Cape Colony in the mid- to late nineteenth century. *Osiris* 15:190–206.

Digby A, Ernst W, and Muhkarji PB. 2010. *Crossing Colonial Historiographies: Histories of Colonial and Indigenous Medicines in Transnational Perspective.* Newcastle upon Tyne: Cambridge Scholars Publishing.

Dobson MJ. 1997. *Contours of Death and Disease in Early Modern England.* Cambridge: Cambridge University Press.

Dubin MD. 1995. The League of Nations Health Organisation. In Weindling P, Editor. *International Health Organisations and Movements, 1918–1939.* Cambridge: Cambridge University Press.

Dunn RS. 2014. *A Tale of Two Plantations: Slave Life and Labor in Jamaica and Virginia.* Cambridge: Harvard University Press.

Echenberg M. 2011. *Africa in the Time of Cholera: A History of Pandemics from 1817 to the Present.* Cambridge: Cambridge University Press.

Engels F. 1845. *The Condition of the Working Class in England.* Translated by Institute of Marxism-Leninism. 1969 edition. Moscow: Panther Books.

Espinosa M. 2009. *Epidemic Invasions: Yellow Fever and the Limits of Cuban Independence, 1878–1930.* Chicago: University of Chicago Press.

Evans R. 1987. *Death in Hamburg: Society and Politics in the Cholera Years 1830–1910.* New York: Oxford University Press.

Farley J. 1988. Bilharzia: A problem of "Native Health," 1900–1950. In Arnold D, Editor. *Imperial Medicine and Indigenous Societies.* Manchester: Manchester University Press.

———. 2004. *To Cast Out Disease: A History of the International Health Division of the Rockefeller Foundation, 1913–1951.* New York: Oxford University Press.

Fee E. 1987. *Disease and Discovery: A History of the Johns Hopkins School of Hygiene and Public Health, 1916–1939.* Baltimore: Johns Hopkins University Press.

———. 1994. Public health and the state: The United States. In Porter D, Editor. *The History of Public Health and the Modern State.* Wellcome Series in the History of Medicine. Amsterdam: Rodopi.

Few M. 2010. Circulating smallpox knowledges: Guatemalan doctors, Maya Indians, and designing Spain's royal vaccination expedition, 1780-1806. *British Journal for the History of Science* 43(4):519–537.

Furtado JF. 2008. Tropical empiricism: Making medical knowledge in colonial Brazil. In Delbourgo J and Dew N, Editors. *Science and Empire in the Atlantic World.* New York: Routledge.

Gomes F. 2012. The Atlantic demographics of Africans in Rio de Janeiro in the seventeenth, eighteenth, and nineteenth centuries: Some patterns based on parish registers. *História, Ciências, Saúde-Manguinhos* 19(Suppl 1):81–106.

González EM. 2015. Nurturing the citizens of the future: Milk stations and child nutrition in Puerto Rico, 1929–60. *Medical History* 59:177–198.

Gorgas WC. 1909. The conquest of the tropics for the white race. *Journal of the American Medical Association.* 52(25):1967–1969.

Green MH, Editor. 2014. Pandemic disease in the medieval world: Rethinking the Black Death. *The Medieval Globe* 1.

Greene J, Basilico MT, Kim H, and Farmer P. 2013. Colonial medicine and its legacies. In Farmer P, Kim JY, Kleinman A, and Basilico MT, Editors.

Reimagining Global Health: An Introduction. Berkeley: University of California Press.

Greenwood A, Editor. 2015. *Beyond the State: The Colonial Medical Service in British Africa*. Manchester: Manchester University Press.

Greenwood A and Topiwala H. 2015. *Indian Doctors in Kenya, 1895-1940*. London and New York: Palgrave MacMillan.

Hamlin C. 1998. *Public Health and Social Justice in the Age of Chadwick: Britain, 1800–1854*. New York: Cambridge University Press.

Hardiman D, Editor. 2006. *Healing Bodies, Saving Souls: Medical Missions in Asia and Africa*. Amsterdam: Rodopi.

Hardy A. 1993. Cholera, quarantine and the English preventive system, 1850-1895. *Medical History* 37:250–269.

Harrison M. 1996. "The Tender Frame of Man": Disease, climate and racial difference in India and the West Indies, 1760–1860. *Bulletin of the History of Medicine* 70(1):68–93.

———. 1999. *Climates and Constitutions: Health, Race, Environment and British Imperialism in India, 1600–1850*. New Delhi: Oxford University Press.

———. 2006. Disease, diplomacy and international commerce: The origins of international sanitary regulation in the nineteenth century. *Journal of Global History* 1(2):197–217.

———. 2010. *Medicine in an Age of Commerce and Empire: Britain and its Tropical Colonies, 1660-1830*. Oxford: Oxford University Press.

———. 2012. *Contagion: How Commerce Has Spread Disease*. New Haven: Yale University Press.

Haynes DM. 2001. *Imperial Medicine: Patrick Manson and the Conquest of Tropical Disease*. Philadelphia: University of Pennsylvania Press.

Hernández Sáenz LM. 1997. *Learning to Heal: The Medical Profession in Colonial Mexico, 1767–1831*. New York: Peter Lang.

Hewa S. 1995. *Colonialism, Tropical Disease and Imperial Medicine: Rockefeller Philanthropy in Sri Lanka*. Lanham, MD: University Press of America.

Hochman G and Armus D. Editors. 2004. *Cuídar, Controlar, Curar: Ensayos Históricos Sobre Saúde e Doença na América Latina e Caribe*. Rio de Janeiro: Fiocruz.

Hodges S. 2012. The global menace. *Social History of Medicine* 25(3):719–728.

Hoppe KA. 2003. *Lords of the Fly: Sleeping Sickness Control in British East Africa, 1900–1960*. Westport, CT: Praeger.

Horden P. 2008. *Hospitals and Healing from Antiquity to the Later Middle Ages*. Aldershot, UK: Ashgate Publishing Company.

Hunt NR. 1999. *A Colonial Lexicon of Birth Ritual, Medicalization, and Mobility in the Congo*. Durham, NC: Duke University Press.

Hutchinson JF. 1996. *Champions of Charity: War and the Rise of the Red Cross*. Boulder, CO: Westview Press.

Iliffe J. 1987. *The African Poor: A History*. Cambridge: Cambridge University Press.

International Sanitary Convention of Paris. 1903. Paper read at 11th International Sanitary Conference, Paris.

Iqbal M, Editor. 2012. *New Perspectives on the History of Islamic Science*. Aldershot, UK: Ashgate Publishing Company.

Jones M. 2004. *Health Policy in Britain's Model Colony: Ceylon, 1900–1948*. New Delhi: Orient Longman.

Kaur A. 2012. Rubber plantation workers, work hazards and health in colonial Malaya, 1900–1940. In Sellers C and Melling J, Editors. *Dangerous Trade: Histories of Industrial Hazard across a Globalizing World*. Philadelphia: Temple University Press.

Kavadi SN. 2016. Rockefeller public health in colonial India. In Winterbottom A and Tesfaye F, Editors. *Histories of Medicine and Healing in the Indian Ocean World*. New York: Palgrave Macmillan.

Keller RC. 2006. Geographies of power, legacies of mistrust: Colonial medicine in the global present. *Historical Geography* 34:26–48.

———. 2007. *Colonial Madness: Psychiatry in French North Africa*. Chicago: University of Chicago Press.

Killingray D and Phillips H, Editors. 2003. *The Spanish Influenza Pandemic of 1918-1919: New Perspectives*. New York: Routledge.

Kim JR. 2013. The borderline of 'empire': Japanese maritime quarantine in Busan c.1876-1910. *Medical History* 57(2):226–248.

Knaut AL. 1997. Yellow fever and the late colonial public health response in the port of Veracruz. *Hispanic American Historical Review* 77(4):619–644.

Koloski-Ostrow AO. 2015. *The Archaeology of Sanitation in Roman Italy: Toilets, Sewers, and Water Systems*. Chapel Hill, NC: University of North Carolina Press.

Krieger N and Birn A-E. 1998. A vision of social justice as the foundation of public health: Commemorating 150 years of the spirit of 1848. *American Journal of Public Health* 88(11):1603–1606.

Kropf SP. *Doença de Chagas, doença do Brasil: ciência, saúde e nação*. Rio de Janeiro: Editora Fiocruz, 2009.

La Berge AEF. 1992. *Mission and Method: The Early Nineteenth-Century French Public Health Movement*. Cambridge: Cambridge University Press.

Lachenal G. 2010. Le médecin qui voulut être roi. Médecine coloniale et utopie au Cameroun. *Annales. Histoire, Sciences Sociales* 65(1):121–156.

———. 2014. *Le médicament qui devait sauver l'Afrique: un scandale pharmaceutique aux colonies*. Paris: La Découverte.

Lanning JT. 1985. *The Royal Protomedicato: The Regulation of the Medical Profession in the Spanish Empire*. Durham, NC: Duke University Press.

Lei SH. 2014. *Neither Donkey Nor Horse: Medicine in the Struggle Over China's Modernity*. Chicago: University of Chicago Press.

Lindner U. 2014. The transfer of European social policy concepts to tropical Africa, 1900–50: The example of maternal and child welfare. *Journal of Global History* 9(02):208–231.

Little LK. 2011. Plague historians in lab coats. *Past and Present* 213(1):267–290.

LNHO [League of Nations Health Organisation]. 1927. *International Health Yearbook 1927* (Third Year). Geneva: WHO.

López Sánchez J. 1987. *Finlay: El hombre y la verdad científica*. La Habana: Editorial Científico-Técnica.

Lorcin PME. 1999. Imperialism, colonial identity, and race in Algeria, 1830–1870: The role of the French Medical Corps. *Isis* 90(4):653–679.

Low MC. 2008. Empire and the Hajj: Pilgrims, plagues, and pan-Islam under British surveillance, 1865–1908. *International Journal of Middle East Studies* 40(02):269–290.

Löwy I. 2001. *Virus, moustiques, et modernité: La fièvre jaune au Brésil entre science et politique*. Paris: Éditions des Archives Contemporaines.

Lyons M. 1992. *The Colonial Disease: A Social History of Sleeping Sickness in Northern Zaire, 1900–1940*. Cambridge: Cambridge University Press.

Magalhães RC da S. 2016. *A erradicação do Aedes aegypti: Febre amarela, Fred Soper e saúde pública nas Américas (1918–1968)*. Rio de Janeiro: Editora Fiocruz.

Maglen K. 2002. "The first line of defence": British quarantine and the port sanitary authorities in the nineteenth century. *Social History of Medicine* 15(3):413–428.

Manderson L. 1992. Women and the state: Maternal and child health in colonial Malaya. In Fildes VA, Marks F, and Marland H, Editors. *Women and Children First: International Maternal and Infant Welfare, 1870-1945*. London: Routledge.

———. 1996. *Sickness and the State: Health and Illness in Colonial Malaya, 1870–1940*. Cambridge: Cambridge University Press.

Mark C and Rigau-Pérez JG. 2009. The world's first immunization campaign: The Spanish smallpox vaccine expedition, 1803–1813. *Bulletin of the History of Medicine* 83(1):63–94.

Marshall D. 1999. The construction of children as an object of international relations: The Declaration of Children's Rights and the Child Welfare Committee of League of Nations, 1900–1924. *The International Journal of Children's Rights* 7:103–147.

McBride D. 2002. *Missions for Science: U.S. Technology and Medicine in America's African World*. New Brunswick, NJ: Rutgers University Press.

McCaa R. 1995. Spanish and Nahuatl views on smallpox and demographic catastrophe in the conquest of Mexico. *Journal of Interdisciplinary History* 25(3):397–431.

McCallum MJ. 2005. The last frontier: Isolation and Aboriginal health. *Canadian Bulletin of Medical History* 22(1):103–120.

McCandless P. 2011. *Slavery, Disease and Suffering in the Southern Lowcountry*. Cambridge: Cambridge University Press.

McNeill JR. 2010. *Mosquito Empires: Ecology and War in the Greater Caribbean, 1620–1914*. Cambridge: Cambridge University Press.

Mendels FF. 1972. Proto-industrialization: The first phase of the industrialization process. *The Journal of Economic History* 32(1): 241–261.

Moll A. 1940. The Pan American Sanitary Bureau: Its origin, development and achievements: A review of inter-American cooperation in public health, medicine, and allied fields. *Boletín de la Oficina Sanitaria Panamericana* 19(12):1219–1234.

Monnais L. 2013. 'Rails, Roads, and Mosquito Foes': The state quinine service in French Indochina, 1905-40. In Peckham R and Pomfret D, Editors. *Imperial Contagions: Medicine, Hygiene, and Cultures of Planning in Asia*. Hong Kong: Hong Kong University Press.

Moulin AM. 1996. Tropical without the tropics: The turning point of Pastorian medicine in North Africa. In Arnold D, Editor. *Warm Climates and Western Medicine: The Emergence of Tropical Medicine, 1500–1900*. Amsterdam: Rodopi.

Mitman G and Erickson P. 2010. Latex and blood science, markets, and American empire. *Radical History Review* 107:45–73.

Murard L and Zylberman P. 1996. *L'hygiène dans la République: La santé publique en France ou l'utopie contrariée 1870-1918*. Paris: Fayard.

Neill DJ. 2012. *Networks in Tropical Medicine: Internationalism, Colonialism and the Rise of a*

Medical Specialty, 1890–1930. Redwood City, CA: Stanford University Press.

Nguyen TL. 2010. French-educated midwives and the medicalization of childbirth in colonial Vietnam. *Journal of Vietnamese Studies* 5(2):133–182.

Ortiz de Montellano B. 1990. *Aztec Medicine, Health, and Nutrition*. New Brunswick, NJ: Rutgers University Press.

Packard RM. 2007. *The Making of a Tropical Disease: A Short History of Malaria*. Baltimore: Johns Hopkins University Press.

Packard RM and Gadelha PA. 1994. A land filled with mosquitoes: Fred L. Soper, the Rockefeller Foundation, and the *Anopheles gambiae* invasion of Brazil. *Parassitologia* 36(1–2):197–213.

Palmer S. 2003. *From Popular Medicine to Medical Populism, Doctors, Healers, and Public Power in Costa Rica 1800-1940*. Durham, NC: Duke University Press.

———. 2010. *Launching Global Health: The Caribbean Odyssey of the Rockefeller Foundation*. Ann Arbor: University of Michigan Press.

Peard J. 1999. *Race, Place, and Medicine: The Idea of the Tropics in Nineteenth-Century Brazil*. Durham, NC: Duke University Press.

Peckham R. 2013. Infective economies: Empire, panic and the business of disease. *The Journal of Imperial and Commonwealth History* 41(2):211–237.

———, Editor. 2015. *Empires of Panic: Epidemics and Colonial Anxieties*. Hong Kong University Press.

Pelis K. 2006. *Charles Nicolle, Pasteur's Imperial Missionary: Typhus and Tunisia*. Rochester, NY: University of Rochester Press.

Pernet CA. 2013. Developing nutritional standards and food policy: Latin American reformers between the ILO, the League of Nations Health Organisation, and the Pan-American Sanitary Bureau. In Kott S and Droux J, Editors. *Globalizing Social Rights: The International Labour Organization and Beyond*. London: Palgrave Macmillan.

Phatlane S. 2014. The resurgence of indigenous medicine in the age of the HIV/AIDS pandemic: South Africa beyond the 'miracle'. In Bala P, Editor. *Medicine and Colonialism: Historical Perspectives in India and South Africa*. London: Pickering and Chatto.

Pormann PE and Savage-Smith E. 2007. *Medieval Islamic Medicine*. Edinburgh University Press.

Porras Gallo MI. 1997. *Un reto para la sociedad madrileña: la epidemia de gripe de 1918-1919*. Madrid: Editorial Complutense.

Porter D, Editor. 1994. *The History of Public Health and the Modern State*. Amsterdam: Rodopi.

———. 1999. *Health, Civilization, and the State: A History of Public Health from Ancient to Modern Times*. London: Routledge.

Quevedo E, Borda C, Eslava JC, et al. 2004. *Café y Gusanos, Mosquitos y Petróleo: El Tránsito desde la Higiene hacia la Medicina Tropical y la Salud Pública en Colombia, 1873-1953*. Bogotá: Instituto de Salud Pública, Universidad Nacional de Colombia.

Rapport M. 2008. *1848: Year of Revolution*. New York: Basic Books.

Riley J. 1987. *The Eighteenth-Century Campaign to Avoid Disease*. Basingstoke, UK: Macmillan Press Ltd.

Roccasalva A. 2008. *Girolamo Fracastoro: Astronomo, Medico e Poeta Nella Cultura del Cinquecento Italiano*. Genoa: Nova Scripta.

Rodríguez ME and Rodríguez de Romo AC. 1999. Asistencia médica e higiene ambiental en la Ciudad de México, Siglos XVI-XVIII. *Gaceta Médica de México* 135(2):189–198.

Ronzón J. 2004. *Sanidad y Modernización en los Puertos del Alto Caribe 1870-1915*. Mexico: Universidad Autónoma Metropolitana, Unidad Azcapotzalco/ Grupo Editorial Miguel Angel Porrúa.

Rosen G. 2015. *A History of Public Health, Revised Expanded Edition*. Baltimore: Johns Hopkins University Press.

Rosenberg CE. 1987. *The Cholera Years: The United States in 1832, 1849, and 1866*. Chicago: University of Chicago Press.

Scarzanella E. 2003. Los pibes en el Palacio de Ginebra: Las investigaciones de la Sociedad de las Naciones sobre la infancia latinoamericana (1925–1939). *Estudios Interdisciplinarios de América Latina y el Caribe* 14(2).

Sealey A. 2011. Globalizing the 1926 International Sanitary Convention. *Journal of Global History* 6(3):431–455.

Sharma M. 2012. *Indigenous and Western Medicine in Colonial India*. New Delhi: Cambridge University Press India.

Siraisi N. 1990. *Medieval and Renaissance Medicine: An Introduction to Knowledge and Practice*. Chicago: University of Chicago Press.

Sivaramakrishnan K. 2006. *Old Potions, New Bottles: Recasting Indigenous Medicine in Colonial Punjab (1850-1945)*. New Delhi: Orient Longman.

———. 2011. Recasting disease and its environment: Indigenous medical practitioners, the plague, and politics in colonial India, 1898–1910. In Ax CF, Brimnes N, Jensen NT, and Oslund K, Editors. *Cultivating the Colonies: Colonial States and their Environmental Legacies*. Athens: Ohio University Press.

Slack P. 2012. *Plague: A Very Short Introduction*. Oxford: Oxford University Press.

Solomon SG and Hutchinson JF, Editors. 1990. *Health and Society in Revolutionary Russia*. Bloomington: Indiana University Press.

Solomon SG, Murard L, and Zylberman P, Editors. 2008. *Shifting Boundaries of Public Health: Europe in the Twentieth Century*. Rochester, NY: University of Rochester Press.

Stanbridge N. 2016. DNA confirms cause of 1665 London's Great Plague. *BBC News*, September 8.

Stapleton DH. 2004. Lessons of history? Anti-malaria strategies of the International Health Board and the Rockefeller Foundation from the 1920s to the era of DDT. *Public Health Reports* 119(2):206–215.

Steckel RH. 2010. Demography and slavery. In Paquette RL and Smith MM, Editors. *The Oxford Handbook of Slavery in the Americas*. Oxford: Oxford University Press.

Stepan NL. 2001. *Picturing Tropical Nature*. Ithaca, NY: Cornell University Press.

———. 2011. *Eradication: Ridding the World of Diseases Forever?* Ithaca, NY: Cornell University Press.

Stern AM. 2005. The Public Health Service in the Panama Canal: A forgotten chapter of US public health. *Public Health Reports* 120(6):675–679.

Sutter PS. 2009. Tropical conquest and the rise of the environmental management state: The case of U.S. sanitary efforts in Panama. In McCoy AW and Scarano FA, Editors. *Colonial Crucible: Empire in the Making of the Modern American State*. Madison: University of Wisconsin Press.

Sweet JH. 2011. *Domingos Álvares, African Healing, and the Intellectual History of the Atlantic World*. Chapel Hill: University of North Carolina Press.

Textes juxtaposés. 1897. *Conventions Sanitaires Internationales de Venise 1892-Dresde 1893-Paris 1894-Venise 1897*. Bruxelles: Hayez, Imprimeur de la Chambre de representatives.

Tilley H. 2011. *Africa as a Living Laboratory: Empire, Development, and the Problem of Scientific Knowledge, 1870-1950*. Chicago: University of Chicago Press.

Trujillo-Pagan NE. 2013. Worms as a hook for colonising Puerto Rico. *Social History of Medicine* 26(4):611–632.

Turshen M. 1984. *The Political Ecology of Disease in Tanzania*. New Brunswick, NJ: Rutgers University Press.

Varanda J and Cleveland T. 2014. (Un)healthy relationships: African labourers, profits and health services in Angola's colonial-era diamond mines, 1917–75. *Medical History* 58(1):87–105.

Vaughan M. 1991. *Curing Their Ills: Colonial Power and African Illness*. Palo Alto, CA: Stanford University Press.

Vongsathorn K. 2012. "First and foremost the evangelist?" Mission and government priorities for the treatment of leprosy in Uganda, 1927-1948. *Journal of Eastern African Studies* 6(3):544–560.

Walther DJ. 2013. Sex, public health and colonial control: The campaign against venereal diseases in Germany's overseas possessions, 1884–1914. *Social History of Medicine* 26(2):182–203.

Walvin J. 2013. *Crossings: Africa, the Americas and the Atlantic Slave Trade*. London: Reaktion Books.

Warren A. 2010. *Medicine and Politics in Colonial Peru: Population Growth and the Bourbon Reforms*. Pittsburgh: University of Pittsburgh Press.

Warren KS. 1990. Tropical medicine or tropical health: The Heath Clark lectures, 1988. *Reviews of Infectious Diseases* 12(1):142–156.

Watts S. 1997. *Epidemics and History: Disease, Power and Imperialism*. New Haven: Yale University Press.

Webb JLA. 2009. *Humanity's Burden: A Global History of Malaria*. Cambridge: Cambridge University Press.

Weindling P. 1994. Public health in Germany. In Porter D, Editor. *The History of Public Health and the Modern State*. The Wellcome Institute for the History of Medicine. Amsterdam: Rodopi.

———, Editor. 1995a. *International Health Organisations and Movements, 1918–1939*. Cambridge: Cambridge University Press.

———. 1995b. Social medicine at the League of Nations Health Organisation and International Labour Office compared. In Weindling P, Editor. *International Health Organisations and Movements 1918-1939*. Cambridge: Cambridge University Press.

Worboys M. 1988. The discovery of colonial malnutrition between the wars. In Arnold D, Editor. *Imperial Medicine and Indigenous Societies*. Manchester: Manchester University Press.

Yip KC. 1995. *Health and National Reconstruction in Nationalist China: The Development of Modern Health Services, 1928-1937*. Ann Arbor, MI: Association for Asian Studies, Inc.

———, Editor. 2009. *Disease, Colonialism, and the State: Malaria in Modern East Asian History*. Hong Kong: Hong Kong University Press.

Zylberman P. 2004. Fewer parallels than antitheses: René Sand and Andrija Stampar on social medicine, 1919–1955. *Social History of Medicine* 17(1):77–92.

2

BETWEEN INTERNATIONAL AND GLOBAL HEALTH

Contextualizing the Present

This chapter brings international health's history into the contemporary period of global health by exploring the evolution of the field's principal paradigms and actors from World War II through the post-Cold War era. We begin with an analysis of how wartime and post-war needs—combined with the creation of the United Nations (UN), late imperialism, and decolonization processes—shaped a more muscular, if still fragmented, international health authority than predecessor institutions (intergovernmental, colonial, and charitable agencies). We examine the role of Cold War and development ideologies, which together shaped relations between so-called First World (capitalist bloc) and Third World (non-aligned) countries, as well as the alternative presented by the Second World (Communist bloc), on the players, precepts, and practices of international health.

A primary lens for this exploration is the World Health Organization (WHO) and its activities; we also touch on the role of bilateral agencies, philanthropies and other private actors, nongovernmental organizations (NGOs), and some in-country efforts. We briefly discuss alternate circuits of international health exchange, including South–South cooperation and the non-aligned movement, as well as moments when the dominant approaches to international health were contested. We then turn to how the political and economic forces and shifts that started under 1980s neoliberalism and endured into and beyond the post-Cold War context of the 1990s affected the international health field and then reshaped it into global health, marked by both continuities and differences in principles and approaches.

To begin, a note on terminology, which we will revisit in greater depth towards the chapter's end. The arena now widely called global health was known as international health for much of the 20th century, in turn deriving from a prior suite of fields: international sanitary cooperation, tropical medicine, colonial medicine, and so on. These nomenclature shifts, drawing from political and cultural ideologies, as well as contemporary scientific-medical understandings, are enormously telling in their conceptual connections to the health paradigms of each period. Just as tropical and colonial medicine appellations reflected the processes, priorities, and prejudices of imperialism, and sanitary cooperation was similarly linked to the rise of trade and migration as economic and security concerns, the terms international and global health are also related to the dominant conceptions of the day (Harrison 2015).

Each term also needs to be problematized: as discussed in chapter 1, "tropical" diseases were not originary or confined to "the tropics" and "colonial" medicine was closely linked to imperial and metropolitan research and practices. Under "imperial" science, knowledge and policies circulated regionally and multidirectionally, often circumventing or even resisting prevailing power structures and flows of information (Sivaramakrishnan 2015), with European and American state authorities more reluctant to cooperate around international sanitary and medical matters than most scientists (Neill 2012). Similarly, the use of the term *international health* suggests an increasing role for interaction among national governments/sovereign states, the new UN inter-state/multilateral system, and the nations emerging from decolonization, even as the designation *World* Health Organization implied that the agency would be serving the world according to a collective and inclusive ethic. The notion of *global* health, as we explore ahead, seeks to transcend the prime role of states, optimistically implying a sharing of problems and solutions unimpeded by formal borders or national interests. Yet global health remains hegemonic (dominant and largely unquestioned) in that the term global is totalizing, both lacking context and squeezing out other possibilities. Despite assertions otherwise, global health is more "partial" health than global, given that its institutions and ideas are heavily influenced by a small number of powerful players with particular agendas. Nonetheless, it is also invoked by those who do not share these agendas, who resist and recast these global health interests, or who incorporate contrasting, local, and alternative players and concerns.

THE POST-WORLD WAR II INTERNATIONAL (HEALTH) ORDER

Key Questions:

- How did the United Nations and Bretton Woods institutions come about?
- What forces led to decolonization? What changed and what continued from the past?
- Why did post-war development initially focus on Europe and Japan?

By the 1930s international (largely intergovernmental) health activities were being shepherded by a delimited set of overlapping agencies—l'Office International d'Hygiène Publique (OIHP), League of Nations Health Organisation (LNHO), and Pan American Sanitary Bureau (PASB). Their early mandate around information-sharing, sanitary treaties, and border control activities to prevent the spread of disease via migration, transport, and commerce had burgeoned in the 1920s, with a flurry of activities covering vital statistics collection, surveillance, health commissions, expert research, training, standardization, and health policy.

While fragile, these agencies drew legitimacy from the growing public health armamentarium in fields such as bacteriology and parasitology as well as from increasing state patronage for public health in Europe and the Americas (see chapter 1).

Some of these efforts were influenced by social medicine movements, which embedded modern medicine and public health within a social and political framing of health and disease that addressed living and working conditions as central to improving health (Brown and Birn 2013). In situ cooperative public health efforts, including disease campaigns and public health training, were further amplified through the active work of multinational and humanitarian agencies (Everill and Kaplan 2013), most prominently the Rockefeller Foundation (RF), Save the Children, and Red Cross and Red Crescent societies.

International health activities also continued through colonial and military operations. As reviewed in chapter 1, for several centuries until just 70 years ago, the world—and international health—was characterized by large imperial blocks: rival powers based in Europe, later joined by North America and Japan; colonized regions (Africa, the Caribbean, much of Asia and the Pacific); and regions that were politically and economically dominated, and periodically occupied, by imperial powers, but either had gained independence in the 19th century or were never colonized (Latin America and parts of Asia). Each imperial power had its own health office, charged with control of epidemics, medical care and infrastructure for select groups, and bolstered by tropical medicine research institutes, health activities connected to industry, military occupation and bases, and the work of religious missionaries.

A New World Order (of Health and Development Institutions): UN, World Bank, International Monetary Fund

As the pre-war imperial system gave way to a new political and economic order, the international health field and its key institutions were at the confluence of, and deeply affected by, two contextual shifts: (1) the disintegration of the old imperial system and its reincorporation into a new one—involving decolonization and extensive state-building in Asia, Africa, and Latin America; and (2) the Cold War context—the political, ideological, military, and economic contest between US capitalism and Soviet communism—which lasted from 1946 to 1991. Ideologies around "development" and the place of health cooperation within it were embroiled in each of these factors, arguably framing international and global health activities to this day.

A watershed for these developments was the war itself: both the world political order and the organization of international health underwent profound changes during and in the immediate aftermath of World War II. During the war, amid combat, civilian atrocities, death, and displacement, international health institutions floundered: the LNHO, already struggling to survive during the Depression, remained isolated in Geneva, denuded of resources and staff while its rival, Paris-based OIHP, decamped to Vichy in 1939 and collaborated with the Nazis (Borowy 2008). European colonial medical offices and humanitarian agencies were focused on war needs. The RF sought to step up its efforts, organizing a separate European office for emergency relief, to aid government agencies, and to cooperate with the Red Cross and Allied powers. The RF also expanded its health work in other regions, most notably Latin America.

Meanwhile, the overwhelmingly US-funded and controlled UN Relief and Rehabilitation Administration (UNRRA), established in 1943, took over responsibility from US and other Allied military forces for providing food (distributing excess US agricultural output), shelter, medical attention, and other aid. By war's end, UNRRA was charged with the herculean task of caring for upwards of 60 million refugees and displaced persons. UNRRA's health division coordinated with the remnants of pre-war international health agencies to deliver medical relief, disease control and sanitary services, and supplies in war-torn countries, all on a massive scale. UNRRA maintained a staff of almost 1,400 health professionals from 40 countries and expenditures of up to US$80 million/year (equivalent to US$1 billion/year in 2015 dollars) for health, medicine, and sanitation (Sawyer 1947). But by 1946, it was being critiqued on multiple fronts: by Western European countries concerned about US economic encroachment, by the Soviets for failing to adequately help Eastern Europe, and by right-wing US politicians alarmed about too much aid going to Eastern Europe (Gillespie 2008; Reinisch 2013a). UNRRA was a key precursor to the UN's s soon-to-be formed specialized health agency, WHO, which absorbed its activities. But upon its demise, UNRRA's leftover budget provided start-up funding for the UN's Children's Fund (UNICEF), not WHO.

The origin of the UN system stems from the *Declaration by United Nations* of January 1, 1942, when representatives of 26 nations pledged to continue fighting against the Axis Powers. (Such agreement had been foreshadowed by the 1941 Atlantic Charter signed by US President Franklin D. Roosevelt and British Prime Minister Winston Churchill, calling for a post-war world of economic cooperation and, even, the right to sovereignty for all countries.) In 1944, a year before World War II ended, representatives of China, the Soviet Union, the United Kingdom, and the United States developed plans for the UN. A key dimension of international cooperation was maintaining financial stability to avoid repetition of the chaos and danger of worldwide Depression (and refrain from using war reparations as punishment). That year, the UN Monetary and Financial Conference in Bretton Woods, New Hampshire hosted delegates from 43 countries to help create a new global monetary system based on fixed exchange rates and smooth-running trade policies.

The United States, having sustained Britain during the war through the lend-lease system, was angling to expand its exports, secure a prime place for the dollar, and replace Britain as the world's dominant financial and imperial force (Steil 2013). While more than half of the countries and participants were from "developing" regions, their influence was overshadowed by the Anglo-American negotiations. Still, the large Latin American presence helped shape post-war ideas around state-led development, drawing from the "Good Neighbor" US–Latin American model of the 1930s, which favored a strong government role involving infrastructure-building, social investment, and economic security as a means of fending off Nazi influence (Helleiner 2014).

The Bretton Woods meeting established two key institutions: the International Monetary Fund (IMF) to focus on macroeconomic policy, short-term loans for balance of payment problems, and, eventually, provide loans conditional on adoption of anti-inflationary and debt re-payment policies; and the International Bank for Reconstruction and Development, more commonly called the World Bank, to provide loans for particular development projects in areas such as infrastructure and agriculture. The US Treasury Department, as the largest shareholder of both institutions (initially holding approximately 37% of shares, declining to around 16% more recently), has wielded substantial influence over them since their inception (Gutner 2016). Also planned was a body to govern multilateral trade (launched in 1947 as the General Agreement on Tariffs and Trade but only institutionalized in 1995 as the World Trade Organization [WTO]—see chapters 4 and 9). Then, at a special conference held in San Francisco from April to June 1945, representatives of 50 countries created the UN Charter.

The intense collaboration undertaken to defeat the Axis Powers during World War II and rebuild after the war helped US and Western European planners envision a future of international economic and political stability through new institutions and policies, even as the Soviet Union and its allies posed an alternative to capitalism, and the possibility of a nuclear war was an ever-present threat. The West's immediate concern was rebuilding industries and economies ravaged by the war and assuring monetary stability to promote orderly international investment and commerce.

Yet even before Europe's and the global economy's recovery were assured, attention turned to other realms of cooperation, with the general umbrella of the UN fostering a set of specialized agencies in the mid-1940s, including WHO, the Organization for Education, Science and Culture (UNESCO), UNICEF, the Food and Agriculture Organization (FAO, created at a 1945 Québec meeting, but envisaged two years earlier at an international conference hosted by Roosevelt), and so on (see chapter 4). These agencies represented not so much a birth as a re-birth of efforts that had begun in prior decades, albeit at a grander scale (Frey, Kunkel, and Unger 2014; Staples 2006).

Many supporters of the UN viewed international cooperation idealistically, as a means of preventing war and freeing humanity from widespread misery; sadly its mandate would prove less sanguine. The political leaders of the dominant powers that established the UN machinery harbored no such illusions (indeed, the North Atlantic Treaty Organization [NATO] was founded in 1949 to bring Western European and North American powers together in a military alliance to ensure "security" and "freedom" in the face of the Soviet bloc threat). From the start, the UN was designed to maintain the international balance of power under the control of a handful of large countries represented permanently on the Security Council (and with veto power over the General Assembly), morphing to favor US and Western European goals of staving off communism while serving economic needs. Still, the UN's staff and some member states (initially principally from Europe and the Americas), perhaps naïvely, recognized the possibilities of the UN as a catalyst for global problem-solving and positive change brokered among governments, experts, and civil society (Frey, Kunkel, and Unger 2014).

For example, US-led UNICEF, founded in 1946, initially distributed surplus US milk production to European refugees (Gillespie 2003). Soon, UNICEF was making a splash with a global BCG vaccination campaign against tuberculosis (see ahead), the beginning of its highly visible and well-oiled child-feeding and saving interventions that gave it an enormously popular worldwide public face. Despite the unpredictability of its voluntary funding model, UNICEF was able to attract millions in both government and individual donations year after year (Black 1996).

Although mythically portrayed as a quintessentially altruistic entity, the UN was faced with deep contradictions from its very inception. It initially sought to prolong and justify imperialism by serving its membership of colonial powers, laying bare the UN Charter's empty promises to colonized peoples across the world. Yet soon some of its emerging decolonized members, especially independent India under Jawaharlal Nehru's leadership, turned the UN into a vehicle for ending colonialism (Mazower 2009), waging ongoing struggles to democratize the UN and make the voices and needs of the Third World count (Prashad 2007).

Also problematic, the nascent UN served as an incubator for promulgating universal human rights (as articulated in the UN Charter), but with no clear course on the shared responsibility needed to realize them. In 1948, the UN General Assembly adopted the *Universal Declaration of Human Rights* (UDHR), which enumerated the right to life, freedom from discrimination, education, a standard of living adequate for health and well-being, and declared: "recognition of the inherent dignity and of the equal and inalienable rights of all members of the human family is the foundation of freedom, justice and peace in the world" (UN 1948).

During the debates over the UDHR's drafting and role, conflicting views emerged regarding which rights to prioritize. Whereas Western bloc countries emphasized civil and political rights (CP), Eastern bloc nations concentrated on the rights to health, food, and education (economic, social, and cultural [ESC] rights). Although various Latin American players insisted on the need for *both* political and civil rights *and* economic, social, and cultural rights (Sikkink 2014; Wright-Carozza 2003), Cold War divisions led to the eventual forging of two separate human rights treaties in these respective areas. Entering into force in 1976, these covenants revealed the hypocrisy of their advocates, who were from societies marked by human rights infringements (Meier 2013). The dichotomy lasted for decades, despite the UDHR framers' belief that CP and ESC rights were interwoven (Glendon 2001). At WHO, these tensions led to a distancing, starting in the 1950s, from its Constitutional proclamation of a right to health. As we will see, this commitment would be resurrected through the 1978 Alma-Ata declaration. Since the end of the Cold War, the longtime emphasis on CP rights has given way to greater attention to ESC rights, including the right to health (see chapters 3 and 14).

Decolonization, "Development," and Colonial Legacies in Health

Another key shift after World War II was the prolonged, often turbulent end to explicit colonialism (for many but not all colonies). As the political, social, and economic costs of maintaining empire mounted, colonialism was replaced with a less expensive and less fraught division of world power. On one side, anti-colonial movements across Asia and Africa articulated social demands and the right to self-determination; on the other, European countries, weakened by Depression and war, became increasingly ambivalent about their commitments overseas. More than simply a transfer of power, decolonization was a calculated choice and ongoing process (Duara 2003) that ended day-to-day imperial "responsibilities," while enabling Europe's continued economic dominance and political influence over former colonies.

Resistance to imperialism was transposed into the medical realm, as chronicled by Martinique-born psychiatrist Frantz Fanon, who became a medical revolutionary in the Algerian liberation movement following his training in France. Arguing that colonial medicine was not beneficial but rather another facet of colonial racism and control, he explained the perceived "irrational" behavior (mental illness) of Algerian patients as a reaction to colonialism. Fanon held that colonial mental disorders were generated by oppression and humiliation under imperial power, reasoning that revolution would change all of this (Fanon 1963).

Decolonization came first in Asia, beginning with the retreat of Japanese armies. By 1950, British rule over its colonies of India, Burma, and Ceylon (now Sri Lanka), and French control over Laos and Cambodia, had essentially ended. In the ensuing decades, dozens of African, Middle Eastern, and remaining Asian colonies achieved independence, many after bitter and bloody struggles and facing further violence in the context of displacement or inadequate negotiations over territorial divisions (as with the 1947 partition of India and Pakistan). The new countries—most stripped of resources and facing enormous social needs—generally maintained the same borders as former colonies, which had been established with little regard for historical, cultural, and political affinities (Prashad 2007).

From the start, many recently independent nation-states were tugged at from "above" by former colonial powers and intergovernmental organizations and from "below" by their own citizens with high expectations for improved social and economic conditions. With sovereignty challenged by the former imperial powers and Cold War rivals meddling in political affairs—not to mention minimal infrastructure, a skeletal civil service, shortage of trained staff in all fields, foreign companies controlling key resources, and paltry tax revenues—the new states assumed the responsibility of providing services to their populations on a highly uneven economic playing field. Modernizing aspirations were key to rationalizing the pains and pressures of development in decolonized societies, with former colonial powers summoned to participate in development efforts. There was remarkable continuity in the former powers' assumptions of cultural superiority, "often used to justify exploitative economic policies and violently abusive governance practices," with patronizing indifference to the role of colonialism in creating poverty, now considered the defining feature of the post-colonial world (Allina Pisano 2012, p. 39).

A complex of affiliations and relations emerged, marked by a mix of economic goals, destructive civil wars, solidarity, local ideas of—as well as paternalistic approaches to—development, and ongoing political and economic hegemony. Some former colonial powers ceded control less discordantly, with the expectation that national (authoritarian) elites would serve as political and economic intermediaries in the continued exploitation of labor and resources. When nationalist movements challenged such "business as usual" arrangements (as did Patrice Lumumba in Congo—see chapter 8), NATO allies were enjoined to thwart sovereign aspirations and installed more amenable, often ruthless, subordinates. The Cold War rivalry would soon play out in extended and unspeakably brutal proxy wars and dictatorships across the Third World but also through more peaceable development (and health) endeavors.

Well before decolonization, development had emerged as a priority that would span distinct periods. After World War I, imperial powers had resurrected their "dual mandate"—the notion that alongside economic exploits came their "civilizing" responsibility to advance the material and human well-being of the colonies (as per imperial conceptions)—an idea further propagated in subsequent years. Early strategies adopted in this period included some infrastructure investments outside the main cities and economic enclaves, as well as social welfare schemes, aimed, variously, at averting unrest and displaying an "ethical commitment," in addition to promoting markets and economic expansion (Hodge 2016).

Two decades later, faced with an escalating Indian independence movement and labor discontent across its colonies, Britain passed the 1940 Colonial Development and Welfare Act. Amended over ensuing decades to extend funding and programs, this policy served as a last-ditch effort to prolong increasingly resisted imperial control (Cooper 1996). In 1946, France, too, established the Fonds d'Investissements pour le Développement Économique et Social (Investment Fund for Social and Economic Development) amid the UN's emerging anti-colonialism (Atangana 2009). French authorities redoubled their inter-colonial cooperation to prevent UN interference and ensure ongoing ties with African dependencies (Pearson-Patel 2015). While the bulk of late colonial development efforts were economic, for instance large cotton-growing schemes in Sudan and Northeast Tanzania (Schuknecht 2010), this so-called "Second Colonial Occupation" also upped spending in education, housing, health care, and sanitation.

Humanitarian and medical missionary activity also expanded in various settings (Ermisch 2014; Watt and Mann 2011), drawing from post-war therapeutic developments around leprosy, for example, with treatment now administered by formally trained missionary doctors and nurses in collaboration with new UN agencies such as UNICEF (Manton 2003). The ideology of human or social development was thus not inimical to (post-)colonialism but central to its moral imperative. These tensions between economic and human development persist to the present, even as their form, emphases, and influences have shifted over time (see chapter 3).

Although many of these projects failed according to their stated aims, they served as a basis and lasting legacy for the scientific and technical bent of the post-war development project. To be sure, different political and intellectual strata within republics-to-be did not reject development, but rather considered it a perennially broken colonial promise for which there was pent-up demand; instead these groups embraced their own form of modernization that considered a range of approaches and decentered Western (and later Cold War) exigencies (Chakrabarty 2010).

India's 1946 Bhore Report provided a wide-ranging assessment of health conditions and post-independence health planning. It was led by senior Indian civil servants and physicians and advised by a remarkably progressive group of international experts. Echoing social medicine ideas from prior Indian and foreign proposals, the report emphasized the need for public health planning to integrate political, economic, environmental, and social understandings and approaches to health. Its discussion of population-wide health needs and eugenics echoed colonial and other contemporary public health concerns (Nair 2011), while its attention to rural health and education marked a departure from colonial negligence on these matters. The Bhore Report served as an enduring blueprint for domestic health organization and an influential counterpoint to dominant international health and development approaches (Amrith 2006).

Given such aspirations, Europe's imperial powers sought to cultivate renewed networks and relations with former colonies—the British Commonwealth, La Francophonie, and so on, as well as via bilateral agencies. Prior asymmetries of power were thus preserved through economic ties as well as in social (including health) arenas. Emerging "developing" states were also complicit in aiding a continued rule of experts (both former colonial and local elites) and in encouraging large-scale development projects. At times, newly liberated countries would also circumvent these structures via regional and neighboring arrangements (such as the East African Community and the South Asian Association for Regional Cooperation). As we will see, persistent unequal power relations in the UN and other agencies—and the division of Cold War spheres of influence—would be especially contested by the formation of a pan-Third World network that defied challenges to sovereignty but also sought fair entry to the UN's bona fide possibilities (even as the UN's "development decades" delivered far less than promised).

Post-war Rebuilding and the Early Cold War

Topping the US-led "liberal multilateralist" development agenda of the post-war world order was rebuilding Europe. In addition to Europe's upwards of 50 million deaths during World War II (including 20 million Soviet soldiers and civilians) and some 60 million refugees, the misery and economic slowdown of the 1930s Great Depression were still fresh memories, with measures to prevent a recurrence a high priority. Europe's redevelopment, country by country, was central to a new, more managed form of global capitalism under a Keynesian model of government monetary controls and responsive fiscal policy to ensure economic stability and mitigate capitalism's ills. At the same time, across Europe and parts of Latin America, rising post-war expectations for better working and living conditions drove strong working class movements, picking up from socialist mobilization during the Depression.

After Germany surrendered in May 1945, it was divided into four zones occupied by Britain, France, the United States, and the Soviet Union (by the 1950s Germany was split into East and West). Subject to a mix of reparations, expulsions, and disarmament mandates, Germany's nutritional, housing, and health conditions were dire. The occupying forces focused first on staving off localized epidemics to protect themselves, domestic populations, and nearby countries. Occupying forces also employed public health services to maintain order and help post-war reconstruction, balancing health needs with the perils of working with and aiding the former enemy (Reinisch 2013b).

The World Bank was the initial source of funds for Europe's reconstruction, starting with a massive loan to France for equipment, fuel, and raw materials, accounting for fully one third of the Bank's loanable funds at the time. This was followed in 1947 by the so-called "Marshall Plan" (named after the US Secretary of State), which provided a staggering US$13.3 billion (about US$141 billion today) to rebuild 17 countries in Europe over 4 years. At over 1.3% of US GDP per year—this was arguably the largest aid program ever. US industry was paradoxically a major beneficiary of this aid—goods, equipment, and transport vessels were US-made; such a domestic boon would prove a long tradition in development assistance.

These efforts were quickly tethered to the Cold War, whose beginning is marked by a 1946 speech by then former British Prime Minister Churchill citing the descent of an Iron Curtain between Eastern European countries influenced by the USSR and the "democratic" countries of Western Europe. Although conservative US legislators in ascendancy after World War II fought hard against domestic government health and social welfare spending (with the backdrop of the anti-communist fanaticism of the McCarthy era, they considered such government programs to constitute creeping socialism), they accepted US support for European recovery and welfare state expansion as necessary to lessen the influence of communist political parties (e.g., in France and Italy): Europe's economic stability was perceived as a vital buffer against Soviet influence. The renewed polarization between capitalist and communist camps—suppressed in the name of the fight against fascism—shaped both military and development aid strategies. By 1947, the ideological East-West Cold War got hotter when US President Harry Truman sent substantial military and economic aid to Greece and Turkey to fight off communist insurgents—the so-called Truman doctrine of "containment" of Soviet expansion.

The United States was also preoccupied with demilitarizing Japan to remove the power of the Meiji emperor and undo remnants of Japanese imperial claims in the Pacific. Having detonated atomic bombs that levelled the cities of Hiroshima and Nagasaki in August 1945 (see chapter 8), the US-led Allies then occupied Japan until 1952. They invested more than US$18.5 billion (in 2015 dollars) in rebuilding the devastated country (Japan experienced 2.3 million combat fatalities, 800,000 civilian deaths in air raids; and at war's end was expecting repatriation of 6 million people). Occupying forces chief US General Douglas MacArthur helped craft a remarkably progressive Constitution to ensure that Japanese society would be peaceable and democratic. Not only did Japan renounce war and create a new parliamentary system, the Constitution ensured universal suffrage, social security and public health protections, non-discrimination, academic freedom, free universal education, and workers' rights to organize and bargain collectively. Wealth and power were deconcentrated, a *maximum* wage established, and perhaps the world's most extensive land reform undertaken (Caprio and Sugita 2007). Economic redistribution, broad social welfare measures, and other societal factors help explain Japan's subsequent rapidly rising life expectancy, starting with an unprecedented jump of 14 years between 1945 and 1955 despite continued post-war poverty (Johansson and Mosk 1987).

Public health reconstruction and alleviating suffering were an important part of the US occupation. In Kyoto prefecture, for example, health activities were mostly welcomed by a population that had been spared bombings but nonetheless was in sore need of public health and preventive measures against leprosy, cholera, tuberculosis (TB), smallpox, and diphtheria, among other ailments (Nishimura 2008). But overall, particularly in areas that had been bombed, the health and welfare measures under the Allied Occupation (implemented without public consultation) were resented, and various of these—banning pensions for wounded veterans and suppressing information on the medical effects of the atomic bomb—were overturned as soon as Allied forces left Japan (Nishimura 2009). As such, the longtime US portrayal that this was a "model" health occupation (Jones et al. 2006) is a decidedly one-sided view.

In the end, colossal US investments in rebuilding post-war Europe and Japan would be a singular occurrence, linked to restoring confidence in capitalism and creating a bulwark against the Soviet bloc. Even before their economies began to grow, the countries of Western Europe joined forces with the United States in NATO, and Japan would emerge as a key strategic ally in Asia, especially after the Chinese revolution in 1949.

These geopolitical issues—decolonization politics, re-establishing a secure footing for global capitalism, and the strategic shifts under the Cold War, together with a refashioned development imperative for the countries and colonies of Africa, Latin America, and Asia—played a central role in the post-war reconfiguration of international health and would have enormous bearing on its structure and activities.

THE RISE OF THE WHO AND "THIRD WORLD" DEVELOPMENT

Key Questions:

- What was the place and role of health in the new post-war order?
- How and why did WHO's initial aspirations for addressing health become displaced?
- Who were the key players in disease campaigns?

How an international health organization would fit into the new world order was not initially charted by the dominant powers. Unlike the post-World War I urgency of addressing serious epidemics of typhus, dysentery, influenza, and other ailments, World War II military medical agencies' research on and application of a growing bevy of sanitary measures, vaccinations, vector control, plus UNRRA's efforts, meant combatant and occupied countries did not experience major disease outbreaks among troops and civilian populations (typhus and malnutrition-related mortality in concentration camps being an important exception). The era's soaring confidence in biomedicine's technical toolbox, particularly penicillin, the first real antibiotic, initially appeared to lessen the security concerns justifying cooperative disease control, even as health care systems needed to be rebuilt in war-torn countries. Yet outside a band of industrialized countries, endemic diseases, including TB, diarrhea, and malaria—linked to malnutrition, poor sanitation, and poverty—continued to take a huge toll and arguably demanded action at an international level.

Indeed, it was two progressive-minded physicians from major "developing" countries, together with Scandinavia's leading public health man, a socialist, who proposed formation of a new international health authority at the UN's founding meeting in 1945. Unbeknownst to the trio, US and UK delegations had secretly agreed that health would not be on the agenda of the San Francisco conference. But this was not to hold. A Brazilian–Chinese duo, respectively Geraldo de Paulo Souza, a prominent public health professor and government administrator, and Szeming Sze, an esteemed Chinese public health official, diplomat, and health administrator, both of whom worked with UNRRA, got backing from their home governments to jointly recommend the establishment of a specialized health agency (Cueto, Brown, and Fee 2011; Sze 1982). They, in turn, were inspired and encouraged in this proposal by Norway's famed Director-General of Public Health Karl Evang (called back from the conference to resume his duties before the proposal could be introduced), whose political radicalism interconnected with his social medicine endeavors (Ringen 1990).

The following year an inaugural international health conference convened in New York brought together over 50 of the world's leading health specialists, many of whom were advocates of social medicine, to draft the Constitution of the WHO. On April 7, 1948, following required ratification of the Constitution and funding commitments by 26 UN member states (then a majority), WHO was officially founded as the UN's hallmark specialized agency (April 7 is commemorated annually as World Health Day).

WHO was never the sole international health actor, but its designation as the field's foremost authority—as opposed to inter-war agencies' sharing of roles and turf—its enormous growth in its first few decades, and the multiplicity of actors with which it engaged (including almost all governments and major agencies involved in the field) made it the pulse of international health. Although its broadest mandate—promoting the principles in the preamble to its Constitution (Box 2-1)—was forced to take a back seat to technical cooperation, WHO remained home to the key ideas and practices of international health. Virtually all of the late 20th century debates in this field—bio-technical versus socio-political approaches, democratic versus corporate-influenced decisionmaking, and so on—played out vividly at WHO, making it a touchstone for struggles also manifest at local levels, albeit with differing aims and players.

These divisions made WHO's representative governance structure all the more striking.[1] Shaped by social medicine advocates, such as Yugoslav Andrija Štampar and Peruvian Carlos Paz Soldán, and the LNHO's earlier vision, WHO's Constitution was solidarity-minded, openly regarded health in social and political terms, and advocated a strong government role, belying the ideological divisions to come.

Despite its ambitious and patently idealistic preamble, the reality of WHO operations was more circumscribed. Even before opening its doors in 1948, WHO's Interim Commission was tasked with stemming a post-war cholera epidemic in Egypt. While this was hardly the bold effort to address the fundamental underpinnings of health as envisioned by its trio of founders, WHO proved highly effective at sourcing and distributing cholera vaccine and purveying information to the various parties. This activity also demonstrated to the dominant powers (especially the reluctant United States) WHO's utility in the emerging post-war geopolitical configuration (Deutsch 1958).

Box 2-1 Preamble to the WHO Constitution (1946)

"Health is a state of complete physical, mental and social well-being and not merely the absence of disease or infirmity.

The enjoyment of the highest attainable standard of health is one of the fundamental rights of every human being without distinction of race, religion, political belief, economic or social condition.

The health of all peoples is fundamental to the attainment of peace and security and is dependent upon the fullest co-operation of individuals and States.

The achievement of any State in the promotion and protection of health is of value to all.

Unequal development in different countries in the promotion of health and control of disease, especially communicable disease, is a common danger.

Healthy development of the child is of basic importance; the ability to live harmoniously in a changing total environment is essential to such development.

The extension to all peoples of the benefits of medical, psychological and related knowledge is essential to the fullest attainment of health.

Informed opinion and active co-operation on the part of the public are of the utmost importance in the improvement of the health of the people.

Governments have a responsibility for the health of their peoples, which can be fulfilled only by the provision of adequate health and social measures."

With the establishment of WHO, international health's enhanced, if inherited, agenda—including standard-setting, data collection, epidemiologic surveillance, training and research, emergency relief, and cooperative activities—resided in a single agency for the first time. Thanks to its growing membership of 85 countries by 1955 and over 100 in the 1960s (as decolonized nations joined), and its democratic decisionmaking structure via the annual World Health Assembly (WHA), the WHO enjoyed more legitimacy and permanence than its predecessors, which had been hampered by meager resources, limited mandates, and interagency jealousies.

However, PASB's assertive American backers forced a scheme of six regional offices (Table 4-5) to ensure that WHO headquarters would not usurp regional control. This resulted in some regional offices being stronger than others, and the entire arrangement at times weakened WHO's authority. Moreover, the US's membership in WHO was almost derailed by an embittered US Congressional debate about post-war international involvement amid the brewing Cold War and mounting domestic red-baiting (Brickman 2013), leaving public health leaders angry and embarrassed at potential repetition of the US's failure to join the League of Nations. The United States finally signed on in July 1948, following a compromise resolution permitting its withdrawal from WHO on 1 year's notice (Birn 2014). Ironically, it was the USSR delegate who formally proposed US acceptance into WHO. Meanwhile, the US Congress increasingly accepted foreign aid for health (and involvement in multilateral agencies such as WHO) as a valuable weapon in the anti-communist arsenal (Logan 1955).

Notwithstanding the dreams of true health cooperation, Cold War tensions soon surfaced: the USSR and most of its Eastern bloc allies suspended their participation in the UN, and therefore WHO, starting in early 1949 claiming (not inaccurately) that given high dues, UN agencies offered too much advice and insufficient material aid for addressing their enormous post-war rebuilding needs. Listed as non-active members, these countries returned only in 1956-1957, after the Soviet delegate announced that WHO was doing "useful work" (Siddiqi 1995, p. 108). In spite of the polarization provoked by the Cold War, there remained agreement on WHO's importance. The USSR continued to back WHO: even when it was not an active member, it furnished 6% of WHO's budget, which more than doubled to 13% by 1959 (US Congress, Senate Committee on Government Operations 1959).

Box 2-2 Eras of International Health Activity

- Meeting and Greeting, 1851–1902: early meetings and agreements on the need to share information on epidemic outbreaks and enforce quarantine during the imperial era
- Institution-Building, 1902–1939: first international health agencies established; sanitary treaties signed; incipient international health research/education; disease campaigns
- Bureaucratization and Professionalization, 1946–1970: permanent health organizations founded; large scale training of personnel; global disease campaigns in the context of the Cold War
- Contested Success, 1970–1985: vertical campaigns (e.g., smallpox) versus horizontal health and social infrastructure efforts (e.g., primary health care)
- Evidence and Evaluation, 1985–present: demand for measurable successes and "evidence-based" interventions; reinforcement of technical and cost-effective global health initiatives; renewal of countering paradigm stressing social justice, infrastructure, human rights

Source: Adapted from Birn (2009b).

The WHO's early years were marked first and foremost by its own institutional development, with rules, procedures, practices, and a set of tasks and priorities. WHO's marking of its territory and promotion of its own growth also represented international health's overall bureaucratization and professionalization in this era (Box 2-2). The WHO's staff expanded from 206 persons in 1948 to 1,481 in 1957 and 3,178 in 1967, accompanied by budget increases from US$3.8 million in 1948 to US$17.7 million in 1957, US$67.6 million in 1967, and US$187.2 million in 1978 (Beigbeder 1995; Siddiqi 1995). With approximately one third of staff based in Geneva headquarters in this period and another quarter at regional offices, bureaucratization—involving short- and long-range planning, programs and research, setting regulations and standards, convening meetings and expert committees, and overseeing evaluation activities—legitimated international health in a permanent multilateral body aimed at impartial technical cooperation for health improvement and development (Table 2-1).

Hand in hand with bureaucratic growth went the formation of professional international health cadres: policymakers and administrators, researchers, and field health workers. In its first two and a half decades, the WHO sponsored more than 50,000 fellowships, focusing on the areas of public health administration, sanitation, nursing, maternal and child health, health services, communicable diseases, and clinical medicine. WHO even provided one-time technical support for a penicillin plant in India in the 1950s, with funding from UNICEF.

The dominant approach of the international health field, with its biomedical bias, focus on disease control rather than holistic well-being, and agenda-setting by the most powerful countries (especially the United States and the United Kingdom), also became institutionalized during this era. After the Soviet bloc became inactive, the WHO was further badgered by Anglo-American interests concerned with nesting health activities within a larger anti-communist agenda (US Department of State 1979). By the late 1950s, "extrabudgetary" funding—that is, "voluntary" contributions that did not come from assessed member dues, instead bypassing the WHO's decisionmaking body—gave ever greater agenda-setting powers to large donors, most notably the United States. WHO's first director, Canadian psychiatrist Brock Chisholm, was ill-prepared to balance these tensions/influences, finding himself at loggerheads with US authorities over his support for social and economic approaches to public health (Birn 2014) and with Catholic countries over the issue of birth control (Farley 2008).

Table 2-1 Major WHO Activities

Years	Activity
1946–1948 (Interim Commission)	Control of cholera epidemic in Egypt
1947–1970s	Fellowships program, sponsoring training for more than 50,000 doctors, nurses, sanitary engineers, and other health workers
1948-1950s	International Tuberculosis Campaign (initially launched by UNICEF) to immunize children with BCG
1952–1964	Global Yaws Control Programme (with UNICEF): tested 160 million and treated 50 million people in 50 countries, resulting in 95% reduced global prevalence
1955–1969	Global Malaria Eradication Programme
1963	Codex Alimentarius created with FAO (to harmonize international standards guidelines and codes around food production, trade, and safety)
1967–1980	Smallpox Eradication Programme (SEP)
1974–	Expanded Programme on Immunization (EPI) launched, focusing on six diseases: diphtheria, pertussis, tetanus, measles, poliomyelitis, and tuberculosis
1975–	Special Programme for Research and Training in Tropical Diseases (TDR) established
1977–	Essential Drugs Program founded with publication of first *Model List of Essential Medicines*
1978	International Conference on Primary Health Care (with UNICEF) issuing *Declaration of Alma-Ata* endorsing Health for All
1981	International Code of Marketing of Breast-Milk Substitutes (with UNICEF)
1982–	Child Survival programs spearheaded by UNICEF (based on Selective Primary Health Care)
1986–	Global Programme on AIDS established
1986	Ottawa Charter for Health Promotion
1988–	Global Polio Eradication Initiative launched (original partners included Rotary International, CDC, and UNICEF, now expanded)
1990s–	Rise of public–private partnerships, e.g., Roll Back Malaria (1998–); Stop TB Partnership (2000–); GAVI, the Vaccine Alliance (2000–)
1995–	Launch of directly-observed treatment (DOTS) strategy for TB control, reaching over 65 million people through 2015
2000–2001	Commission on Macroeconomics and Health
2001–	Measles Initiative started (in partnership with the American Red Cross, UNICEF, CDC)
2003	Framework Convention on Tobacco Control adopted by the WHA

Table 2-1 Continued

Years	Activity
2003–2005	3 by 5 Initiative, aiming to get 3 million people on antiretroviral treatment by 2005
2003–2006	Commission on Intellectual Property Rights, Innovation and Public Health
2005–2008	Commission on Social Determinants of Health
2007 (1951, 1969)	Implementation of new International Health Regulations (and previous revision years)
2013–	Launch of United Nations Interagency Task Force on the Prevention and Control of NCDs (under WHO leadership)
2014–2016	Commission on Ending Childhood Obesity

Source: Adapted and updated from WHO (2008).

The principle of international activities financed through a system of matching funds became established at the WHO in 1949, when the UN's Expanded Programme of Technical Assistance (EPTA) was created to coordinate in-country cooperative efforts by the UN's specialized agencies. Funded by voluntary donations from member countries, EPTA was to cover expert consultancies and working groups, demonstration projects, professional training and fellowships, and project materials (Beigbeder 1995; Howard-Jones 1981; Siddiqi 1995). EPTA put in place a strict system of co-financing, redolent of the system of budget incentives honed by the RF. Countries "receiving" cooperation were required to fund a growing percentage of the annual costs of the project, as well as: finance all local personnel (administrative, technical, and support staff, translators and interpreters, drivers, etc.); provide and maintain offices, buildings, furniture and all materials available in the country; pay local transport, mail, and telecommunications expenses; assume health care and housing costs for local personnel carrying out cooperative activities; and cover a considerable portion of the travel and daily expenses of foreign experts.

Although EPTA was critiqued by Latin American countries, in the end most countries acceded to the conditions, because they risked exclusion from cooperation and isolation from other international health opportunities—such as fellowships and positions within WHO—if they refused or were unable to contribute. From 1950 to 1954, voluntary payments to EPTA totaled US$400 million (US$3.6 billion in 2015 dollars), with low- and middle-income countries (LMICs) contributing about 11% of the total. But further to this amount, LMICs were also required to allocate approximately US$900 million dollars (US$8 billion in 2015 dollars) for in-country expenses, straining domestic health budgets and agendas (Beigbeder 1995; Siddiqi 1995).

Grounded in evolving scientific knowhow, the WHO drew heavily on personnel, principles, and practices from prior health agencies, including colonial medical offices and some research laboratories that were being downsized and dismantled. Europeans and Americans were over-represented as permanent scientific staff, but expert committees also incorporated LMIC scientists affiliated with tropical medicine institutes.

Most important was the RF, whose top health advisors had both planned and directed UNRRA (Gillespie 2008), which in turn served as a pipeline for WHO's first generation of personnel (Cueto, Brown, and Fee 2011; Farley 2008). The RF's most direct imprint on the WHO took place through Dr. Fred Soper, who had spent almost two decades at the helm of the International Health Division's (IHD) large-scale campaigns against malaria and yellow fever in Brazil before becoming head from 1947 to 1958 of the PASB (as of 1949, WHO's regional office for the Americas, changing its name to Pan American Health Organization [PAHO] in 1958) (Birn 2014). The IHD modus operandi found further resonance in the WHO with the election and re-elections of Dr. Marcolino Candau as Director-General (1953–1973), who had worked under Soper in the IHD's campaigns in Brazil and briefly at the PASB.

Early Disease Campaigns

Perhaps the greatest shadow cast by the RF was its technical disease campaign approach (see chapter 1). Just before WHO was officially inaugurated, UNICEF had launched a massive effort to immunize millions of infants and children in Europe with BCG vaccine against TB, arguably the first truly global disease campaign. Despite misgivings about BCG's safety and efficacy, Chisholm and WHO had little choice but to agree to supervise the campaign as it was extended into the early 1950s to hundreds of millions of children in the British Caribbean, Latin America, the Middle East, North Africa, and across Asia (Altink 2014). The BCG campaign faced concerted resistance in the first LMIC to sign on, India, where concerns about BCG's soundness and appropriateness slowed vaccination down markedly amid claims of exploitation of children as guinea pigs and reliance on a quick-fix technology without sufficient attention to infrastructure and other underlying causes of TB, as per the Bhore Report (McMillen and Brimnes 2009). Notwithstanding this controversy, the BCG campaign entrenched reliance on biomedicine's panoply of technical tools, including the promise of DDT, the new wonderdrug penicillin, and yellow fever vaccine, which had been tested and employed by military forces during World War II.

Yaws

WHO's first large "demonstration" project was a campaign against yaws, a highly contagious skin and bone disease spread through treponema bacteria and accompanied by lesions and bodily disfiguration. The effort involved a disease of poverty, an effective technical tool, and a multilateral collaboration carried out in command-and-control style. In the late 1940s a long-acting penicillin formula, enabling a single-shot injection method, was tested and shown effective in Haiti. In July 1948 the government of Haiti applied to the UN Secretary General for the first UN Mission of Technical Assistance. This general assistance request, which pitched combating yaws as an issue of labor efficiency, received a positive response in just 10 days (Mohamed 2016).

A yaws campaign was launched in 1950, coordinated among WHO and PASB (together providing experts and travel costs), UNICEF (purveying medicine and vehicles), and the Haitian government (funding administrative and health personnel, office space, etc.) (Farley 2008). Its "inheritance" from the RF clearly visible, the campaign was heavily promoted by PASB director (and former RF man) Soper, who wrested control of an existing yaws effort in Haiti (first based on arsenic, then on a short-acting penicillin preparation requiring multiple treatments) from the RF and the US State Department's Institute of Inter-American Affairs (Stepan 2011).

With over half of rural Haitians infected with yaws, the campaign initially employed trained auxiliaries to administer high-dose single-injections of penicillin via mobile clinics. This method changed in 1951 to a house-to-house method in order to reach remote endemic areas. Within 3 years, nearly 1.7 million Haitians had been treated.

Consistent with the RF principle of budget incentives, the government of Haiti paid almost half the first 5 years of campaign costs of US$605,000, with PAHO footing US$200,000 and UNICEF US$580,000 (Cueto 2007b). By 1957, at the program's end, nearly the entire population of Haiti had been surveyed and/or treated for yaws. Yet virtually no attention had been paid to extreme poverty and lack of sanitation in rural areas—the underlying conditions that facilitated the disease's devastating spread. (Indeed, while the prevalence plunged in Haiti, rural misery and its attendant diseases persisted under the Duvaliers' US-backed decades-long dictatorship [see chapter 8], and despite an effective tool and campaign against yaws, the disease reappeared within a few decades.)

With the worldwide prevalence of yaws estimated at 20 million people in the 1950s and Haiti's program (along with similar efforts in Thailand, Indonesia, and the Philippines) deemed a success, WHO and UNICEF quickly extended the campaign to India, parts of Africa, Brazil, and other Latin American countries under the auspices of the 1952 WHO Global Yaws Control Programme (Asiedu, Fitzpatrick, and Jannin

2014; Muniz 2013). The program wound down in the late 1960s, having treated some 50 million people in dozens of countries, with prevalence reduced by 95% and yaws no longer a public health priority. But without addressing rural poverty, poor sanitation, inadequate housing, and weak health care systems unable to sustain surveillance, there was a resurgence of yaws in the 1970s.

Malaria

The apparent effectiveness of the yaws campaign led WHO to pursue next an even more far-reaching campaign against malaria. As discussed in chapter 1, malaria was a sometime impediment to colonization and commercial expansion (e.g., delays in construction of the Panama Canal). After the malaria vector—the *Anopheles* mosquito—was identified in the late 19th century, use of screens and bed-nets to reduce transmission became common, especially in Europe and North America. Where housing improvements were accompanied by social reforms that led to clean water and sanitation systems (eliminating reliance on water storage vessels, where mosquitoes breed), malaria was eliminated (a prime example being the Tennessee Valley in the United States) (Humphreys 2001).

Vector control was also part of the malaria-combatting armamentarium alongside the longtime use of therapeutic quinine (and in the 1930s, synthetic antimalarials). From the 1910s, government and colonial anti-malaria campaigns (often supported through RF funding) operated in the South of the United States, Latin America and the Caribbean, Southern Europe, the USSR, and South and East Asia, focusing on killing *Anopheles* mosquito larvae by draining swamps and spraying stagnant water with larvicidal oils. *Paris green*, a rodenticide initially used in Paris's sewer system, was adapted for use as an insecticide in the 1920s and widely applied to mosquito breeding sites by national and RF campaigns (Packard 2007).

But it was DDT (synthesized as a pesticide in the late 19th century), newly recognized as an insecticide, that inaugurated a novel era in malaria control. During World War II, DDT was found effective against flea and louse-borne typhus in Europe (which had proven so deadly after World War I), as well as against malaria (killing adult mosquitoes, not just larvae). Aerial spraying of DDT in the Pacific theater of World War II protected Allied troops against malaria, and DDT was also shown to work as an efficient residual household spray in campaigns in the Southern United States, Italy, West Africa (Stapleton 2004; Webb 2014), and elsewhere. DDT, together with the next generation of antimalarials able to kill malaria's *Plasmodium* parasite (and thus interrupt transmission) provided effective and inexpensive technical tools that portended malaria eradication on a global scale, with no need for complementary social investments in housing, clean water and sanitation, and drainage, which were all but abandoned in many settings.

As with campaigns against yaws and *Aedes aegypti* (the mosquito vector for yellow fever, dengue, chikungunya, and Zika viruses), among others, the Americas served as a pilot region (Magalhães 2016). With Soper heavily touting a DDT-based malaria campaign and abetted by US government pressure on WHO, Latin American efforts served as a showcase for eradication: the Brazilian government initially favored malaria control (that is, reducing malaria prevalence rather than seeking to eradicate the disease), but it was incentivized by the United States and WHO to endorse eradication (Hochman 2008). Meanwhile Venezuela's proclaimed eradication of malaria offered the final push (Litsios 1997; Stepan 2011).

In 1955, the eighth WHA, held in Mexico City, approved the Global Malaria Eradication Programme and urged member states to adopt national policies endorsing malaria eradication through large-scale DDT spraying and targeted treatment. In various countries, including Mexico, Sri Lanka, India, and Argentina (Cueto and Palmer 2014; Silva 2014), the decline of malaria thanks to a mix of housing and sanitation improvements, swamp draining, insecticides (all reducing mosquito breeding sites) and treatment, predated WHO's campaign, although observers later confused this issue. Despite disagreement about the feasibility of malaria eradication, those in the hopeful camp won out.

Such was confidence in the prospects of DDT that Kingsley Davis, one of the world's leading demographers and a vocal proponent of the so-called "demographic transition" (see chapter 3), grandiosely argued in 1956: "The main cause of the spectacular decline of mortality in Ceylon is well known. It was the use of D.D.T. as a residual spray in the control of malaria"

(Davis 1956, p. 311). Further, he argued "it seems clear" that North-South technical aid was responsible:

> . . .in underdeveloped areas since 1940 [the great reduction in mortality] has been brought about mainly by the discovery of new methods of disease treatment applicable at reasonable cost, by the diffusion of these new methods from the advanced countries to the unadvanced through international organizations and scientific communication, by international financial help furnished through international organizations and governments and private foundations, and by the use of experts and medical personnel furnished primarily by the industrial countries. The reduction could be rapid, because it did not depend on general economic development or social modernization in the underdeveloped areas. It did not depend on training local medical personnel or local research or local prosperity. It was an example of a rapid cultural diffusion of death-control techniques which did not depend on the diffusion of other cultural elements or basic changes in the institutions and customs of the people affected (Davis 1956, p. 314).

With WHO now headed by Soper's former deputy, Candau, the campaign was heavily backed by the United States (funding over 85% of the budget), which viewed it as a means of both fostering economic development and combating communism, requiring minimal political or social interference. The malaria campaign was championed by the US's new bilateral agency, the International Cooperation Administration (precursor to USAID), itself lobbied by the chemical and pesticide industry, which had seen sales dry up after World War II (Packard 2007). The US government made an inaugural US$1.5 million allocation to WHO's special malaria fund. This prompted substantial support from various Latin American countries, as well as a sizeable UNICEF contribution as part of its bankrolling of international health campaigns, including US$14 million for the Mexican campaign alone (Cueto 2007a, 2008).

Emulating World War II efforts, the campaign followed military-style phases (planning, preparation, attack, consolidation, maintenance) to achieve malaria eradication, relying heavily on DDT rather than on the previous mixed approach of drainage, spraying, and chemotherapy. Within a decade, some three dozen countries in temperate zones in Europe and the Americas—as well as in warmer endemic areas in the eastern Mediterranean, Asia, and the Pacific— were freed from malaria.

The initial focus of the campaign was interrupting transmission of the disease through spraying of DDT several times per year in every house and building during 3 to 4 years to temporarily eliminate the vector. Then, all people infected with malaria had to be identified and treated to prevent returning mosquitoes from becoming infected. Although the smallest unit of action was the human dwelling, the campaign paid little attention to social conditions or local context. In most settings, national malaria eradication teams were organized in a service parallel to the Ministry of Health, duplicating activities and often dominating health budgets, given the in-kind and monetary contributions expected from national governments.

Over time, problems of vector resistance to DDT (residual insecticides could not be used indefinitely), coupled with the campaign's indifference to basic health infrastructure, concerns regarding the top-down structure of the campaign, and environmentalists' condemnation of DDT 's harmful effect on birds and other wildlife, vividly portrayed in Rachel Carson's prophetic 1962 book *Silent Spring*, led the WHO to abandon eradication in the late 1960s in favor of a malaria control program (Packard 1998).

Incredibly, Africa—the world's most malarious region—was left out of WHO's eradication goal from the outset (Dobson, Malowany, and Snow 2000). To be sure, there was an important spray effort in South Africa, and various pilot programs in the region. By the late 1950s the Malaria Programme was carrying out field surveys across most of the continent, and funds and WHO consultants were sent to support existing colonial malaria control programs using DDT and quinine/paludrine prophylaxis. But Africa's deliberate exclusion from eradication plans stemmed from WHO's own characterization of numerous obstacles to eradication of malaria in the region, from seasonal population movements to indifference to prophylactic pills, to impatience with household disruption (Giles-Vernick and Webb

2013; Webb 2014). Focusing so narrowly on DDT thus served as both hope and curse for a post-colonial international health approach that did not want to bother with people and their living conditions (Kinkela 2011).

Again, renowned demographer Davis's observations would prove wrongheaded:

> Though in the literature on public health there is still great lip service paid to the necessity of general economic improvement and community welfare in the control of disease, the truth is that many scourges can be stamped out with none of this, just as diseases in cattle can be eliminated (Davis 1956, p. 314).

As explored in subsequent chapters, despite its shortcomings, this technology-focused ideology continues to have wide currency. Indeed, when malaria eradication was abandoned in 1969, WHO experts named vector resistance and the administrative complexity of reaching out-of-the-way populations, not any problem inherent to narrow technological reliance, as the culprits.[2]

The campaign also undermined more comprehensive national public health measures that were already in place in South Asia, Latin America, and other settings, including land reform, educational improvements, strengthened public services, rural development, sanitary measures, and health education, as well as malaria-specific efforts around irrigation, ditch draining, and medical treatment (Gómez-Dantés and Birn 2000). It also failed to take Indigenous beliefs into account (Cueto 2007a).

Some contemporaries recognized the limitations of RF-style selective, single disease approach and related vertical programs (viz. addressing one ailment at a time using technical tools and largely carried out or supervised by a specialized service with its own personnel) as opposed to an integrated, comprehensive approach (Gonzalez 1965). Subsequent recounts suggest that the campaign was doomed by its formulaic approach:

> Its chief architects misjudged the willingness of humans and malarial mosquitoes to live, eat, sleep, and generally behave according to technical assumptions. . . . The most important lesson to be learned from the programs of the 1950s was that the people of Africa, Asia, and Latin America were not a blank sheet of paper on which experts from the industrialized world could write their own version of progress (UNICEF 1996).

Still, from the perspective of many governments, malaria was a priority: approximately half of the 50 countries that launched campaigns managed to eliminate the disease by 1970, and others saw important declines (Packard 2007). In India, malaria was recognized for its effects on food production, because fertile but malarious areas were undercultivated. The calamitous 1943 Bengal famine under British rule helped motivate Indian desire and US support for malaria control several years before the global campaign began (Zimmer 2014). Consonant with the Bhore Report, however, Indian authorities favored social and economic, including nutritional, investments alongside vector control.

In the end, rather than indicate the limits of the disease eradication model, the malaria campaign only reinforced it: following this reasoning, WHO had simply picked the wrong disease and the wrong technique.

The New Development Imperative and the "Third World"

The malaria campaign was embedded in the larger politics of the day. Notwithstanding hopes on the part of many for a new post-war order based on *genuine* cooperation, the Cold War led Western and Eastern blocs to compete for power and influence throughout the developing world. International health became a pawn in this chess game, with multilateral institutions and the largest bilateral agencies calling most of the shots.

With decolonization, the major players smelled both opportunity and threat. After the United States had begun to address Europe's and Japan's problems, it returned to the rest of the world, eyeing pre-existing and new markets and sources of raw materials to fuel what was now the world's largest economy. Instead of pursuing ideas around development rooted in European colonial schemes, the swaggering American empire sought to remake development in its own guise.

In his famed 1949 inauguration speech, US President Harry Truman discussed the situation of poorer countries, including those newly decolonized, defining them as "underdeveloped areas" (essentially coining this expression and replacing the previous nomenclature of "backward" countries) (Ekbladh 2015). In Point IV of his speech Truman addressed the problem of underdevelopment in terms of a new arrangement of international relations, with the United States taking the lead in raising the living standard of the "developing" world through the provision of technical skills, knowledge, and equipment:

> More than half the people of the world are living in conditions approaching misery . . . Their poverty is a handicap and a threat both to them and to more prosperous areas . . . The material resources which we can afford to use for assistance of other peoples is limited. But our imponderable resources in technical knowledge are constantly growing and are inexhaustible . . . And, in cooperation with other nations . . . Our main aim should be to help the free peoples of the world, through their own efforts, to produce more food, more clothing, more materials for housing, and more mechanical power to lighten their burdens . . . With cooperation of business, private capital, agriculture, and labor in this country, this program can greatly increase the industrial activity in other nations and can raise substantially their standards of living. Such new economic developments should be devised and controlled to the benefit of the peoples of the areas in which they are established (Truman 1949).

As articulated in "Point IV aid programs," early post-war definitions of development centered on industrialization and modernization—considered the vehicles to enable (some) people in poorer countries to emulate the consumption patterns of people in richer countries (Cooper and Packard 1997). Western, capitalist, industrialized countries were framed as the ideal. Investments in factories, large-scale agricultural projects, and public infrastructure such as roads and dams were particularly encouraged. Accompanying these economic developments was another goal: staving off Soviet influence by offering an attractive alternative (at least for elites charged with maintaining "law and order" [Escobar 2011]).

Of course, imperial powers had long invested in colonial industry, commerce, certain social institutions, and political stability (the latter bolstering the former), and, as discussed, the United Kingdom, France, and other powers renewed their development efforts after World War II in part as a vain means to forestall decolonization. In addition, starting in 1943, the United States spent tens of millions of dollars on a Cooperative Public Health Services program of infrastructure support in Latin America, in large part to secure support for the Allied Powers during wartime. The post-war development ideology, congealed in modernization theory (Box 2-3), made even bolder claims about the paths to achieve development and its projected effectiveness in both economic (standard of living) and political (anti-communism) terms.

Before development could be taken up, however, the problem of poverty as the cause of underdevelopment in the settings targeted for investment had to be created. In the mid-1940s, the World Bank set a yardstick for poverty, overnight designating some two thirds of the world's population as poor, and justifying innumerable interventions to unleash economic growth and development. The Bank decided, rather arbitrarily, that an annual national income per capita level of $100 constituted poverty (ironically roughly twice today's global poverty line when adjusted for inflation). But unlike Europe and Japan, which were granted massive sums of US public monies to rebuild their economies and escape post-war poverty, Third World countries enjoyed only minor such investment (and experienced continued extraction of raw materials at unfair commodity prices and

> "So, poor and hungry I certainly was. But underdeveloped? I never thought—nor did anybody else—that being poor meant being 'underdeveloped' and lacking human dignity. True, there is no comfort and glory in poverty, but the whole concept of development (or underdevelopment) was totally alien to me and perhaps to most other Nepalis." (Shrestha 1995, p. 268)

Box 2-3 Development as Modernization versus Development as Dependency

Development, posited as a linear path from poverty (the post-war term now characterizing the lot of colonies and economically dominated regions) to capitalism via investment in big ticket infrastructure (e.g., dams) and industrial sectors (largely primary commodities) and adoption of Western values, was crystallized in "modernization theory." Formulated by US economist Walter W. Rostow as a succession of five societal stages of economic growth culminating in the final stage of "high mass consumption," its goal was ideological as much as economic, as announced by its subtitle: *A Non-Communist Manifesto*. Modernizing development strategies thus aimed to partner growth with democracy "in association with the non-Communist politicians and peoples" (Rostow 1960, p. 164). These ideas became the cornerstone of Kennedy's international development policy, propelling the UN's declaration of the 1960s as the first "Decade of Development" (followed by two more). Many LMIC elites, who associated modernization with progress, were also supportive (Ferguson 1999).

Contested as ahistorical, culturally biased (Eurocentric), empirically flawed, and inadequately accounting for colonial legacies, modernization theory was countered with competing understandings of development paths. Argentinean economist Raúl Prebisch argued that as long as "developing countries" were reliant on primary exports whose value declines over time relative to manufactured exports, prosperity would be stymied. Instead, import substitution industrialization, enabling the growth of domestic industries and internal markets—and already implemented by various Latin American countries—was considered fundamental to national social and economic development.

In the 1960s, modernization theory faced more radical challenges. Rejecting modernization's assumptions of industrialized countries as models to emulate, proponents of "dependency theory," including Paul Baran and André Gunder Frank, showed that Western imperialism had turned Africa, Asia, and Latin America into sources of cheap primary materials for Western development. Perpetuation of an international division of capital, resources, and profits forced *peripheral* formerly colonized countries to trade, on unfavorable terms, raw materials and agricultural exports for manufactured imports from *core* industrial, former colonial powers (Frank 1972). Moreover, elites in LMICs (dubbed the *lumpenbourgeoisie*) advanced their own class interests by maintaining this economic division—accompanied by political repression and bolstered by the economic and military power of core nations, especially the United States—at the expense of the vast majority of the population in their countries. Accordingly, "developing countries," forced to export raw materials and nonindustrial goods, were doomed to economic "backwardness." The alternative path supported by dependency theorists emphasized government ownership of industry, agrarian collectivism, and state economic planning, going well beyond Prebisch's import substitution.

exchange rates). Moreover, the state of "underdevelopment" became defined in such a way that countries' need for rescue would become a permanent condition (Escobar 2011), with development serving as a "secular theory of salvation" (Nandy 1987).

Development strategies became tied to historic, imperial, and regional groupings, such as the Colombo Plan—launched in 1951 to bring together seven British Commonwealth countries (initially Australia, Canada, Ceylon, India, New Zealand, Pakistan, and the UK) to focus on training, technical assistance, and infrastructure in South and Southeast Asia (Colombo Plan Secretariat 2011), and the Alliance for Progress, inaugurated by US President John F. Kennedy in 1961 as a "Marshall Plan" for Latin America (Taffet 2007). Aiming to prevent a repetition of Cuba's 1959 revolution, Kennedy invoked science and technology as an ambitious harness to development aims. The Alliance initially focused on literacy, economic growth, and supporting "democratic governance" but soon included significant military spending, as militant left-wing movements proliferated throughout the region.

Latin American countries officially joined the Alliance with the signing of the Charter of Punta del Este in 1961. With health considered precursor and beneficiary of economic development, the Charter's Ten-Year Public Health Plan established measurable goals for improving water access, sanitation, control of communicable diseases, and maternal and child health (all existing PAHO priorities), with national health plans oriented at integrating preventive and curative health services. The plan endorsed a lead role for PAHO, whose director, Chilean physician Abraham Horwitz, promoted a synergistic understanding of health as partner and precursor to economic development (Pires-Alves and Maio 2015). PAHO, together with WHO and the Central University of Venezuela, developed a health planning methodology to achieve Charter goals. While many countries employed the methodology, few managed to transform planning into concrete changes, in part because it focused principally on the health care sector (Gutiérrez 1975).

The development enterprise became entangled with both the decolonization process and the Cold War in various ways. Looking ahead, leaders of liberation movements pursued alliances and resources to help meet their political constituencies' claims on the state (Cooper 1996). For post-colonial governments, knowhow and resources—from economic and demographic forecasting to evaluation expertise—purveyed by a new American patron made for an attractive modernization model that differed from longstanding European paternalism.

Yet US faith in technocratic solutions to development problems yielded disastrous results in a number of settings, contradicting stated goals around social improvement (Latham 2011). As well, Americans tended toward a "recipe" approach (implementing the same technique with small variations regardless of local context): application of uniform interventions to country after country belied a diversity of experiences in "recipient" settings based on distinct colonial histories, resources, gender and cultural relations, and economic niches.

Such recipes were both pragmatic and reflected US chauvinism about the larger world, even as development actors had to negotiate an array of institutions and players. Contenders comprised both new UN agencies and former colonial interests keen to maintain political and economic ties, such as the French, who were perennially jealous of encroaching US influence in their former colonies. Starting in the 1960s the World Bank intensified its enterprise as both project sponsor and knowledge producer, collecting and analyzing wide-ranging economic and social data, including on health and population, and training thousands of LMIC experts (Goldman 2006).

The Cold War intensified the urgency of development efforts (Hodge 2016), further heightened in the context of Third World resistance to US hegemony, symbolized in the 1959 Cuban Revolution and 1960s Vietnam War. Such contestation also invited an alternative model of development from the Soviet Union and China. The USSR's experience of rapid industrialization and redistribution was admired by many Third World politicians, intellectuals, and activists and was bolstered by extensive Soviet fellowship and training programs and technical assistance (providing less cash than Western counterparts) (Engerman 2011). Many players in poor and rural countries also looked to China's model of mass mobilization for the collective good, with China's South–South cooperation efforts beginning in 1963 to Algeria, then to Tanzania and a range of other African countries in the 1970s (Liang et al. 2014; Youde 2010). To be sure, these were not permanent arrangements: alignments within the respective blocs were often tenuous and shifted a great deal based on political and economic circumstances.

In the first decade of the Point IV plan, US development aid doubled in dollar terms, going from 0.3% to more than 0.5% of GNP. As European economies were rebuilt, they also participated in official development assistance (ODA) efforts, which increased almost five-fold in the 1950s (Fuhrer 1996). World Bank loans became a key source of financing, with US$5.1 billion lent to 56 countries between 1949 and 1961—focusing on agriculture, finance, industry, energy, and infrastructure (Kapur, Lewis, and Webb 1997). However, the priority of safeguarding capitalism and fending off communist influence that fueled the redevelopment of Europe did not translate into the same fervor or dollars for Asia (except Japan), Africa, and Latin America. By the 1960s, US and European development assistance (with the exception of Nordic countries) began to drop and then stagnated, both in total and GNP percentage terms (see chapter 3 for trends since 1970).

A key development project was the "Green Revolution," launched in the 1940s through the RF's Mexican Agricultural Program. Involving a research center to produce heartier crops and incentives for farmers to utilize new tools, the program offered a blueprint for agri-technology approaches. Within ten years, investments in equipment (especially tractors) and techniques—such as crop hybridization (to resist fungi), fertilizers, pesticides, and irrigation—were hailed for increasing wheat, maize, and rice output and enabling Mexican self-sufficiency (Fitzgerald 1986). Extended to Brazil, the Philippines (where the RF established a rice institute in 1953), Indonesia, South Asia, and beyond, the Green Revolution was (named as such and) deemed a worldwide boon (except in Africa) for agricultural productivity in the late 1960s. Yet, as exemplified in India, what was portrayed as a largely US-driven agricultural effort actually involved various government sectors, national scientists, and NGOs, among other players (Unger 2014). Moreover, technology-based "success" might more appropriately be attributed to a mix of government subsidies and policy changes.

Importantly, the Green Revolution's effects were uneven. The high cost of seeds, fertilizers, irrigation, processing, and transport technologies generated indebtedness, environmental contamination, and farm loss among hundreds of thousands of smallholders as mechanization and profitable export crops replaced human labor and scaled production for domestic markets (Kerr 2012). Increased concentration of land ownership among large landholders and agribusinesses worsened rural poverty and inequality leading to millions becoming landless across Latin America, South Asia, and elsewhere (Cullather 2010). Like other development schemes, the Green Revolution also distracted from or undermined post-colonial political efforts to improve rural conditions through distribution of agrarian lands to small farmers.[3]

These post-war development initiatives had mixed results indeed (even as local elites and donor country consultants and contractors invariably benefited). New infrastructure was built, though hydropower, highway, and pipeline projects displaced large populations in India, Ghana, Nepal, Argentina, Brazil, Egypt, Nigeria, and numerous other settings (Thomas 2002). Still, improvements in health conditions, as measured through child mortality declines, were widespread, with particularly rapid improvements in places such as Sri Lanka, where there were significant investments in sanitation, education, and other social policies (see chapter 13).

Alongside big development there was also small-scale community development, aimed at convincing villagers—whether in Pakistan or Paraguay—to adapt modern agricultural methods or work together on local economic and infrastructure projects. Drawing from the inter-war Tennessee Valley Authority mega-project, US development experts transported their experience from the US South to the Global South, combining infrastructure investment with the "small development" task of changing prevailing attitudes. But when development involved, for example, DDT spraying against malaria or smallpox vaccination, community organizers in Delhi, India met with local resistance, finding attitudes difficult to change. This was not a question of "irrational" beliefs about poisonous products, but rather derived from the long experience of counterproductive colonial hygiene campaigns (Immerwahr 2015).

Meanwhile, many issues vital to the well-being of populations in LMICs—land reform, fair systems of commodity pricing, adequate housing and income—were overlooked or even exacerbated. For instance, huge investments in dirty industries—minerals and metals mining, logging, oil drilling, roads and railways—proved environmentally destructive, causing massive deforestation, and soil and water contamination, as well as increased poverty and malnutrition due to greater land concentration (Rich 2013). As well, the riches extracted from natural resources were unevenly distributed, and economic development aid often arrived in the form of arms to protect these valuable industries.

Additionally, large commitments for capital investment on the part of recipient countries and onerous debt repayments meant that the net financial flows to most LMICs were actually quite limited. Even so, various countries, especially in Latin America and Asia, sought to channel foreign assistance toward a state-led development model (Helleiner 2014) using strategies such as import substitution industrialization (Box 2-3), which sought to displace foreign imports with heightened domestic production. This had a crucial impact in various health-related domains, including pharmaceutical and equipment manufacturing.

The USSR, whose overseas aid efforts started in earnest under Nikita Krushchev's leadership in the mid-1950s, launched economic agreements with large countries like India and Indonesia, key Middle Eastern and North African countries (Iraq, Egypt, Tunisia, Algeria), Afghanistan, and other smaller countries. For the most part Third World countries initiated these relations, with the Soviets eager to reciprocate with low-interest, open-ended loans. In several countries, the Soviets built pharmaceutical plants.

Eastern bloc efforts had a smaller reach than Western counterparts, but were similarly focused on industrialization and showcase projects, albeit with a more prominent state-led role (Engerman 2011). Most notably, starting in the 1960s, Soviet-bloc university fellowships, such as those held at the famed Moscow People's Friendship University (renamed Patrice Lumumba University, after the assassinated Congolese liberation leader), trained tens of thousands of doctors, engineers, social scientists, agronomists, and other professionals from across Asia, Africa, and Latin America (with roughly one third from each region) who served as important interlocutors, enabling support for socialism (if not necessarily the Soviet variant) to thrive in distinct milieus (Rupprecht 2015). Smaller Soviet-bloc solidarity efforts across various time periods (e.g., East German hospital-building in the 1980s in countries with leftist governments, for instance Ethiopia and Sandinista Nicaragua [Borowy 2016]) were also important politically, if not economically, as well as on a human solidarity level.

As development became a pawn in the Soviet-American competition for power and influence, many Third World countries also learned to play the rivals against one another, sometimes stimulating increased aid and furthering domestic agendas, other times provoking political conflict and struggles over access to resources (Cueto 2008; Hess 2003, 2005; Hong 2015). Under Indira Gandhi, for example, India received as much or more aid from Washington as from Moscow, with both superpowers eager to accede to New Delhi's requests for foreign development assistance (Vojtech 2010). Insofar as there was expansion of needed infrastructure and social services, including education and public health, Cold War geopolitics brought certain advantages to Third World countries, in addition to the constant passage of Western and Eastern bloc experts.

But the West's effort to contain communism also led to escalating military aid (and proxy wars—see chapter 8), proliferating in response to left-wing

Box 2-4 Bilateral Assistance and the Making of Population Control as an International Health Concern

Demographic problems drew considerable international attention in the 1920s, particularly in terms of economists' views that underpopulation posed an obstacle to economic advancement (Bashford 2014). League of Nations experts, for example, were concerned that large parts of South America had few inhabitants. As well, reformers, economists, and politicians in colonial India took up population concerns in anticipation of public health dimensions of state-building (Nair 2011). In many settings, population policies revolved around the eugenic dimensions of reproduction, variously, the breeding in of "good" genes; and the breeding out of "bad" genes, via sterilization, prenuptial testing, and immigration controls. After World War II, keeping global fertility and mortality patterns in check became a burgeoning Cold War priority: demographers' prior belief that fertility patterns were a question of cultural preferences abruptly switched to confidence that birth control programs could effectively reduce population growth (see chapter 3 discussion of demographic and epidemiologic transition). WHO under Chisholm proposed sponsoring contraceptive research in the early 1950s, but this was roundly rejected, leaving the RF-funded Population Council and several UN centers to spearhead education, training, surveys, and prototype programs (Connelly 2008). Only in the 1960s would US government sponsorship of these programs become feasible in political and financial terms, abetted by alarmist fears of a global population "explosion" (Ehrlich 1969).

From 1965, USAID (founded in 1961 from a US State Department predecessor office, the International Cooperation Administration) prioritized population control among its international health activities. This entailed expanding fertility-reducing activities through aid to government programs, NGOs, and the private sector, plus supporting policymaking, evaluation, biomedical research on contraception, demographic research, and data collection. While population programs later addressed certain issues of birth spacing, reproductive health, and infant mortality, during the Cold War, US programs (together with those of the World Bank and other bilateral and private funders) were largely aimed at reducing the size of developing country populations in order to defuse revolutionary, potentially pro-Soviet, pressures. Many highly-touted USAID-sponsored sterilization and contraceptive activities were manipulative, insensitive, and coercive (Hartmann 1997). For example, in the mid-1960s, USAID funding and political lobbying shaped the mission of Peru's first population agency to go from exploring the broad connections between demographic change and development, to overseeing new birth control clinics across low-income urban areas (Necochea López 2014). In the 1970s, the government of India, long a champion of population efforts, co-sponsored infamous vasectomy camps, which operated on up to 10 thousand men per day, and sterilized over 14 million men and women by 1973 (Hodges 2006; Vicziany 1982).

To carry out these functions, USAID provided over US$9.8 billion (unadjusted) in population assistance to LMICs between its founding and the mid-2000s (PAI 2005). Nowadays, programs aimed at HIV, malaria, and other priority diseases far exceed population spending, though USAID continued to allocate almost US$6 billion between 2006 and 2015 (KFF 2015) for family planning and reproductive health and has spearheaded donor pledges of US$4.6 billion to post-2015 efforts (Fabic et al. 2015).

Population aid was also embroiled in controversies around "reproductive freedom" and abortion. Some programs were accused of following the cultural agenda of Western feminists regarding family size preferences and values around reproductive "choice." At the 4th UN population conference held in Mexico City in 1984, the US government announced a policy prohibiting support to organizations that provided or offered information on abortion (the "gag rule"). At the landmark 1994 Cairo population conference, feminists from around the world worked together to widen the scope of family planning and reproductive health to "sexual and reproductive rights," influencing the policies of many countries, including the United States (Kumar, Birn, and McDonough 2016). However, in 2001, following the election of a conservative government influenced by fundamentalist religious values, the US Bush administration reimposed the gag rule, limiting contraceptive services to millions of women around the world. The gag rule was repealed in 2009 under the Obama administration but the US government still refuses to fund abortions for family planning purposes, currently even in the case of rape, incest, or when pregnancy endangers a women's life (PAI 2015).

movements in the 1960s. Growing US and European support for brutal pro-Western leaders across the world (e.g., Stroessner in Paraguay, Habré in Chad; Suharto in Indonesia, Pahlavi in Iran) made the underlying geopolitical and ideological dimensions of Western development assistance more patent than ever (Westad 2005). The anti-communist rationale even motivated the US government to eventually sponsor a major population control effort (Box 2-4) despite considerable political reluctance. Violent US-backed military coups, such as the CIA-sponsored 1954 overthrow of the democratically-elected Guatemalan government of Jacobo Arbenz—who had legalized the Communist Party and whose land reform affected US agricultural interests—had a devastating effect on various Third World countries seeking to implement progressive social policy. Many countries did not wish to participate in these struggles, but few escaped the yoke of development and military assistance.

The "Non-Aligned" Alternative

Although the North–South development model was pervasive, alternative paradigms did emerge. The 1955 Bandung (Indonesia) Conference gathered leaders from the newly decolonized nations of Africa and Asia who sought to challenge neocolonialism in aid and instead structure cooperation "on the basis of mutual interest and respect for national sovereignty" (Bandung Conference 1955). Seven years later, the non-aligned movement (countries not aligned with the United States or the USSR) was created, and in 1964 the Group of 77 (now 134 countries) was formed—the largest intergovernmental organization of "developing" countries within the UN. The G-77 has since articulated and advocated for the collective economic needs of LMICs, such as around fair terms of trade. This concern was institutionalized at the UN through the General Assembly's Conference on Trade and Development (UNCTAD).

In the 1970s, UNCTAD gave voice to the principal project of the non-aligned movement—the formation of a New International Economic Order (NIEO), a call adopted in principle by the UN General Assembly in 1974 (though with extreme reservations by Western countries). The NIEO and its accompanying Charter of Economic Rights and Duties of States deftly employed universalist rhetoric in calling for full and permanent sovereignty over natural resources and economic activities, including the right to nationalize foreign-owned property, form primary producer cartels, and establish price supports for "developing" country commodity exports. Not only was this vision of a "dramatically 'alternative' geopolitical future" and the "right to development" taken seriously by the international community, it was "the most widely discussed transnational governance" initiative of the 1970s (Gilman 2015).

Though heavily resisted by the United States and other powerful countries, the NIEO helped shape ideas and efforts around social and economic justice (Whelan 2015), including negotiation of a Code of Conduct by the UN's Commission on Transnational Corporations (1975–1992). This effort was the NIEO's most enduring legacy, not only because it lasted a decade longer than the overall NIEO project, which fizzled with the Third World debt crisis (see ahead), but because the issue of corporate behavior in Third World countries remains as salient and debated today as it was 40 years ago (Bair 2015).

As we shall see, the NIEO served as an inspiration for the international movement for primary health care (PHC) launched in the 1970s (Centre Tricontinental, Gresea, and Editions Syllepse 2007).

A prominent experience of non-hegemonic development was spawned by the 1967 Arusha Declaration, in which Tanzania's first post-colonial President, Julius Nyerere, declared his political party's aim "to build a socialist state" (Prashad 2007). While African socialism (like Arab socialism in Gamal Abdel Nasser's Egypt) was invoked in Mali and Ghana, among other countries (often in conjunction with Pan-Africanism), these efforts sought economic equality in African cultural contexts of humanism and communalism rather than in the terms posed by European class struggle. The urgency of Nyerere's social and economic plan—*ujamaa* (Swahili for "familyhood")—calling for nationalization of industry, resettlement of the scattered rural population into villages (villagization), universal access to education and health care, and collective economic development, rather than individual wealth accumulation, resonated widely (Lal 2015).

Tanzania's "socialism in a hurry" contrasted with India's growing, if unequal, welfare state, seeking to bypass capitalist industrialization altogether. An early instance of South–South cooperation supporting socialist governments was China's building of the 1800-km-long Tanzania–Zambia railway (a project rejected by Western donors) starting in the late 1960s (Monson 2010), complemented by Chinese medical teams and hospital construction (Anshan 2011; Youde 2010).

Notwithstanding Nyerere's lofty goals, the implementation of ujamaa was marred by inadequate public engagement. African socialist dreams of justice, peace, and freedom from exploitation were derailed when Nyerere's successor was forced to accept IMF prescriptions in 1985, demonstrating how "little real political or economic freedom of maneuver" the countries of the Third World had (Prashad 2013, p. 91).

No country took on non-aligned, social justice-oriented health cooperation with greater gusto or commitment than Cuba, which has been engaged in over half a century of health diplomacy. Following a major earthquake in Chile in 1960, and even as half of Cuba's own doctors were fleeing, the Cuban government sent a team of medics to provide disaster relief. In the years that followed, Cuba cemented its South–South cooperation on the basis of solidarity and gratitude toward countries that had supported the Cuban Revolution. In 1963, despite the effects of a US embargo, Cuba sent 56 medics to Algeria to help the newly independent country meet its enormous health needs in the wake of the violent liberation struggle against France (Feinsilver 2010). All told, between 1963 and 1999, over 40,000 Cubans participated in medical missions to 83 countries, and the Cuban government provided free medical training to over 12,000 LMIC health professionals, training tens of thousands more in 9 medical faculties it helped create and 37 others it supported (Beldarraín Chaple 2006), ultimately "affect[ing] the lives of millions of people in developing countries each year" (Feinsilver 2010, p. 97). (For more details on Cuba's contemporary South–South efforts, see chapters 11 and 14.)

By the late 1970s South–South cooperation was advocated by the UN too—in an attempt to make development more inclusive (but responding to the NIEO only obliquely). The 1978 Buenos Aires Plan of Action for Promoting and Implementing Technical Cooperation among the Developing Countries, adopted by the UN General Assembly, called for self-reliance and local solutions to development problems; ironically, the meeting was hosted by Argentina, then under a repressive US-backed dictatorship. South–South cooperation would re-emerge in later decades in the context of mainstream development failures and economic crisis.

In the 1980s Nyerere returned at the international level to spearhead the South Commission (1990 report), which underscored the need for a separate Southern form of development and later inspired the formation of the India-Brazil-South Africa group (IBSA) and then the BRICS countries (Brazil, Russia, India, China and South Africa) (see chapter 4) as "locomotives of the South," (Prashad 2013, p. 10). But Southern initiatives did not necessarily represent bona fide alternatives.

While these events were unfolding in the larger development sphere, WHO was in the middle of its own tug-of-war between contrasting approaches to international health.

The Contest for International Health and the Fate of the WHO

Smallpox

Given the challenges around the malaria campaign, WHO was under considerable pressure to ensure success in its next major endeavor. Even before the malaria effort was scaled back, in 1967 WHO launched a new eradication campaign, this time against smallpox, a viral disease leading to blindness, high fever, characteristic facial pockmarks, and death of up to one quarter of people infected.

A smallpox campaign was first proposed by the Soviets in 1958 after they rejoined WHO. In part this was because although the USSR had eliminated smallpox in the 1930s, it faced the threat of reintroduction via bordering Asian countries and the thousands of Third World students it welcomed each year to pursue professional degrees. The Soviets also recognized that they could make a concrete contribution in terms of vaccine production, in contrast to US control of DDT production for the malaria campaign (Venediktov 1998). The Americans, meanwhile, projected domestic economic benefits to discontinuing smallpox vaccination, as well as foreign policy gains from the humanitarian dimensions of supporting a campaign in politically volatile settings (Manela 2014).

Smallpox presented several advantages over malaria as a target for eradication. There were millennia of experience with smallpox inoculation, practiced in ancient India and China, as well as through intermittent vaccination programs across Europe, the Americas, and other settings (Agostoni 2016) (Box 1-1). Vaccination campaigns had also spread to areas under colonial rule in Asia, Africa, and elsewhere, where they had a checkered history due to disinclination on the part of medical authorities and colonial subjects alike (Anderson 2007; Schneider 2009).

Other important factors were the lack of an animal reservoir (exclusive human-to-human transmission) and the availability of an effective freeze-dried vaccine—able to be easily delivered, by the 1960s, via rapid jet vaccinators (and in the 1970s via bifurcated needles). After pilot programs organized by the US Centers for Disease Control (CDC) in Tonga and West Africa proved effective, the Smallpox Eradication Programme (SEP) was formally inaugurated. Large teams of vaccinators, requiring minimal training, fanned out across affected countries, with the USSR providing the bulk of vaccines, and the United States—now fully cognizant of the campaign's diplomatic potential—purveying logistical and infrastructural support (Manela 2010; Reinhardt 2015).

Though there were early doubts, smallpox eradication, like malaria's, was technically feasible, albeit at a steep price, especially for national governments of endemic countries, given the limited financial support allocated to the campaign by WHO and large donors to vaccinate 1.2 billion people in some 33 countries. In 1977, the last known case of smallpox was registered (in Somalia), and in 1980 smallpox became the first disease to be declared completely eradicated.

Ironically, at the launch of the campaign, smallpox incidence and mortality had already been declining for many decades thanks to widespread use of the vaccine in most HICs and some LMICs. Not a significant health priority, smallpox was distant from the leading causes of death. Even in the most affected countries, annual smallpox deaths rarely exceeded a few thousand (outside of India and a handful of other settings, there were typically no more than a few hundred deaths per year) (Fenner et al. 1988).

WHO's SEP was headed by D.A. Henderson, director of surveillance at the CDC's Epidemic Intelligence Service. This marked the CDC's first foray into international health (Greenough 2011), a role that grew considerably over time. Echoing the same ideology and militaresque approach as the Malaria Eradication Programme, it was divided into defined, if overlapping, phases:

- *Attack phase*: Where smallpox was endemic with a substantial number of unvaccinated persons, a mass vaccination program was instituted, aiming for 100% coverage. When documented coverage reached 80% and the incidence of smallpox fell below five cases per 100,000 inhabitants, the program was considered ready to move into the next phase.
- *Consolidation phase*: At this point mass vaccination was terminated, and only new arrivals and newborns were vaccinated. Under the SEP's surveillance-containment approach, among its key innovations, surveillance activities were augmented and case detection improved, with health personnel charged with searching for active smallpox cases. Once potential cases were identified, they and their contacts, including family and neighbors, were isolated and vaccinated to prevent further spread. Where no new cases occurred for over 2 years, yet another phase was entered.
- *Maintenance phase*: Surveillance and reporting were normally shifted to the national or regional health service, and any cases detected received intensive investigation.

According to dominant accounts, the eradication of smallpox offers a dramatic tale of technological and organizational triumph over naysayers, of the single greatest public health success in history, and even of an unlikely victory of Cold War cooperation (Fenner et al. 1988; Gates 2005; Yekutiel 1981). SEP chief Henderson (2009) argued that the decade-long smallpox campaign was the greatest ever international health investment (even though smallpox was not a significant global health problem on the eve of the campaign). Importantly, the activities *not* carried out because of smallpox spending—provision of clean water, nutrition, housing, and primary care improvements—constitute missed opportunities (see chapter 12).

Arguably, the oft-repeated heroic narrative of single-minded global cooperation to eradicate smallpox is vastly oversimplified. To begin, there was no consensus over the approach or the vaccines to be used. In India, for example, there were divisions over whether or not to use an Indian-produced oral smallpox vaccine to demonstrate self-sufficiency (Bhattacharya 2006). Furthermore, wherever welfare states had begun to develop—reflecting struggles for a range of social (including health) protections throughout the Americas, Europe, and beyond—smallpox vaccination, together with other effective public health measures from diphtheria anti-toxin to garbage collection, had proliferated. Undoubtedly, in the post-colonial settings where endemic smallpox was most problematic in the 1950s and 1960s, these struggles were incipient, as subjects-turned-citizens started to make claims on newly independent states (Amrith 2006). But to say that "it was only after the World Health Organization's decision to eradicate smallpox in 1966, did the world begin to rid itself of this ancient scourge," (Roy 2010) as does a smallpox eradication commemorative volume, is a gross misstatement.

Further, while the campaign demonstrated the respective strengths of the Cold War giants—large-scale vaccine production by the Soviets and organizational knowhow on the part of the Americans (Venediktov 1998)—this account overshadows the perspective of other important but lesser players such as Canada and Scandinavian countries, not to mention the diversity of experiences and actors involved in the campaign in different settings. For example, India's concerns around Bhutan's politically sensitive role shaped the campaign there far more than did WHO (Bhattacharya 2013). Brazil's efforts, too, must be understood in the context of waxing 19th century then waning 20th century attention to smallpox vaccination that helped shape receptivity to the campaign in the 1960s, coupled with the military regime's ability to mobilize resources to serve domestic health capacity even as it was constrained by its relations with USAID and WHO (Hochman 2009).

Most pointedly, the campaign was enormously costly to the LMICs where smallpox was endemic, who had to foot two thirds of the bill (Table 2-2). Yet savings have accrued far more to HICs now that smallpox vaccination is no longer carried out (although bioterrorist threats in recent years have raised controversy, especially in the United States, around vaccinating frontline health and military personnel).

While national authorities sought to adapt the campaign to each country's circumstances, the smallpox campaign's technical approach disregarded—and was implemented at the expense of—what many local health personnel deemed to be far more pressing needs, including water and sanitation, safe housing, education, and occupational health. The campaign also caused divisions between international and national authorities and experts, as well as within countries, particularly India (Bhattacharya 2006). Moreover, it was extremely coercive in some places in South Asia, leading to resentment of public health activities, and imperiling the ability of subsequent endeavors to reach certain populations (Greenough 1995). Given these circumstances, one might ask whether the end justified the means (Birn 2011b).

The End of the Disease Eradication Model?

By the 1980s WHO was facing an internal crisis, just at the apex of its fame. Smallpox eradication, as we have seen, offered the quintessential global health parable. Yet in 1980, WHO's Director-General Halfdan Mahler (a Danish physician, first elected in 1973, and serving until 1988), portended a less-than-laudatory appraisal in his biannual report to the WHA by declaring: "Important lessons can be learned from smallpox eradication—but the idea that we should single out other diseases for worldwide eradication campaigns is not among them. That idea is tempting but illusory" (WHO 1980b, p. xii). Mahler's stated reason was that smallpox's epidemiology was "unlike that of any other disease."

Table 2-2 Costs of the Smallpox Eradication Programme

Source of Funds	Original Amount (1980 US$)	Current Amount (2015 US$)/ As % of Total
WHO regular budget	38,000,000	109,300,000/ 12%
WHO voluntary fund for health promotion	43,000,000	123,690,000/ 14%
Bilateral aid	32,000,000	92,050,000/ 10%
Estimated national expenditures	200,000,000	575,280,000/ 64%
Total (approximate)	**313,000,000**	**900,320,000**

Adapted from: WHO (1980a).

But his subtext was patent: the announcement of smallpox eradication—although "heralding the triumph of an aspiration"—was far removed from attaining the WHO Constitutional goal of making governments take "responsibility for the health of their peoples . . . by the provision of adequate health and social measures" (ibid).

Mahler's lukewarm assessment of the smallpox eradication campaign was a clear indication of the growing dissatisfaction with the WHO top-down disease-based approaches to international health, which in the 1970s began to be challenged both by member states—especially G-77 countries, which were seeking cooperative efforts that addressed health in an intersectoral fashion—and from within headquarters, under Mahler's visionary leadership (Box 2-5).

During Mahler's tenure as Director-General, the WHO initiated several programs that deviated from its signature eradication campaigns. In 1974 it began the Expanded Programme on Immunization (EPI) to cover six diseases (diphtheria, pertussis, tetanus, measles, poliomyelitis, and TB) for which proven vaccines were available. At the time only about 4% of people living in LMICs had been fully immunized against all six diseases. The goal of the EPI was

Box 2-5 Critiques of Disease Eradication Programs

The WHO focus on disease eradication campaigns has been critiqued by a variety of commentators on a number of grounds:

- They skew priorities, making local and national needs secondary to global eradication aims.
- They typically require enormous "recipient" country spending, with countries enjoined to commit significant resources in the name of "international solidarity" (Fenner et al. 1988) or subject to inappropriate incentives and aid conditionalities.
- They reinforce technical, disease-based approaches that do little to address overall health or well-being.
- They disregard the underlying and shared social etiology of many diseases and miss the synergistic possibilities of tackling the social determinants of multiple causes of ill health at once.
- They can backfire—coercion may be needed to achieve goals, generating mistrust (Keller 2006), not just against the campaign but against other public health efforts (as happened, for instance, in India, where the coercive nature of the late-stage smallpox campaign jeopardized subsequent public health efforts because many rural populations refused to participate) (Greenough 1995). Resistance to the more recent polio campaign has been similarly evidenced in Nigeria and elsewhere (Obadare 2005).
- Often they do not coordinate with health care systems and national and local authorities, leaving infrastructure to deteriorate (Bhattacharya 2006; PHM et al. 2005), with parallel and simultaneous disease programs duplicating efforts and wasting resources.
- For the majority of diseases, feasibility is highly questionable (for example, the Global Malaria Eradication Programme excluded Africa from the beginning) (Dobson, Malowany, and Snow 2000).
- They miss opportunities to prevent and/or treat other problems. The RF noted this with its multi-country hookworm campaigns in the 1910s and 1920s, in which RF officers had to disregard other, far more serious, health conditions in order to meet hookworm treatment targets (Birn 2006b).

Even disease-eradication "gurus" concur with some of these assessments (Arita, Wickett, and Nakane 2004; Goodman et al. 1998; Vastag 2003).

universal coverage, ideally in the context of primary care or maternal and child health programs, differentiating it from targeted campaigns that operated outside the realm of health care systems. In 1977, the WHO Action Programme on Essential Medicines was launched, specifying some 200 to 500 "essential drugs," including vaccines, nutrients, minerals, and vitamins, to satisfy the baseline pharmaceutical needs of almost any population (later expanded to cover health technologies), with variations for diseases of local importance in different areas. The program sought to ensure availability and affordability to those most in need (Greene 2010). Many national drug formularies drew on the *WHO Model List of Essential Medicines*, raising the ire of Big Pharma (details ahead).

But these years would most be marked by WHO's attempt at radical transformation from "vertical" approaches to horizontal (also known as *upstream*) efforts that emphasized strengthening health systems and infrastructure, and integrating technical and socio-political aspects of public health via a social medicine approach that had garnered popularity since the 1920s at the LNHO and in various countries. It was not until the late 1970s that socio-political approaches were formally articulated as a priority when the WHO's PHC approach emerged out of a decade of discussion (Litsios 2002).

Primary Health Care and the Struggle for WHO's Soul

In September 1978, WHO and UNICEF convened hundreds of high-level government (134 countries) and NGO representatives (67 organizations) at the International Conference on Primary Health Care in Alma-Ata, USSR. The *Declaration of Alma-Ata* called for health needs to be addressed as a fundamental human right through universally accessible health care services, integrated social and health measures tailored to local conditions, and by tackling the underlying economic, political, and social causes and context of health. This call for "urgent and effective national and international action to develop and implement primary health care throughout the world" in order to achieve "Health for All by the Year 2000" (WHO 1978) represented an explicit alternative to the existing disease-control modus operandi (see chapter 11 for more details).

The Alma-Ata conference and declaration entailed complex political negotiations at all levels. It used as PHC examples certain missionary efforts in India (and the 1946 Bhore Report) and, especially, China's experience with increasing access to care in rural areas through use of barefoot doctors (Fang 2015).[4] The declaration also reflected the demands of health activists (including the Christian Medical Commission [Smith and Smith 2015]) and LMICs, in part mirroring Cold War rivalries over the path the international health field would pursue (Mahler 1976a, 1976b; WHO 1978).

Not only did the declaration decry "gross inequality" within and between countries as "politically, socially, and economically unacceptable," but it invoked the non-aligned movement and G-77's call for an NIEO to undergird this new PHC orientation (Chorev 2012).

The heart of the Alma-Ata strategy—a commitment to addressing the roots of leading health problems, including food supply, basic sanitation, and social and economic inequality, from a community-based, primary-care approach—generated enormous discursive currency, but in practice it was quickly fragmented and criticized for being overtly political, too ambitious, and requiring long-term and costly approaches (Werner and Sanders 1997). In the wake of Alma-Ata, the RF sponsored a conference on "*selective* primary health care" (SPHC)—a technical approach based on vaccines and vector control—to replace the broad view of PHC (Walsh and Warren 1979; Warren 1988). SPHC's promise of efficient results led UNICEF, the WHO, and various bilateral agencies to work on a far narrower agenda than the one envisioned by the Alma-Ata declaration (Cueto 2004). The articulation of the PHC approach did not end global eradication campaigns, but may have forestalled them. (The WHA did not approve the launch of another eradication campaign [against polio] until May 1988, just 2 months before Mahler's retirement.[5])

Child Survival

Another clear indication of PHC's dislodging was UNICEF's spearheading of a "child survival revolution" based on SPHC's "cost-effective" approach. With UNICEF director James Grant (son of an eminent RF officer) as its champion, in 1984 a Task Force for Child Survival was established involving the World Bank, UNDP, WHO, and the RF. Four "main" interventions were promoted to reduce child mortality and morbidity: growth monitoring (G), oral rehydration therapy (O), breastfeeding (B), and immunization (I) against the six vaccine-preventable childhood killers (TB, diphtheria, whooping cough, tetanus, polio, and measles), overshadowing the WHO's EPI program. Collectively, this approach became known as "GOBI." Later, family planning, female education, and food supplementation were added to the original GOBI, resulting in the acronym GOBI-FFF.

Soon garnering hundreds of millions of dollars from a US Congressional appropriation and organized under UNICEF's extensive network of field offices, Child Survival was an undertaking more immediately understandable than PHC's approach of government policy reorientation and public deliberation (Cueto and Palmer 2014) (recalling that in many countries across Latin America, Africa, and Asia, there were authoritarian regimes in place that precluded public-interest civil society and democratic discussions on these matters).

Meanwhile, child survival's return to vertical approaches meant that each measure overlooked the broader social and economic context: routine growth monitoring without addressing the reasons for poor nutrition; oral rehydration therapy that sidestepped the underlying causes of diarrhea (i.e., the need to provide clean water and proper sanitation); breastfeeding programs that lacked social support; and little coordination between immunization programs and PHC efforts where they were implemented. The technical and top-down orientation of the child survival initiative was also accompanied by a focus on individual behavior change:

> The poor are charged with ignorance and inappropriate behavior, and are asked to change their life-styles to better adjust to the circumstances in which they are embedded. For example, they are asked to adjust to the realities of contaminated water by treating diarrhea, rather than being coached in methods for demanding improved waterworks from their local governments . . . We should be fully aware of the implications of doing band-aid work where major surgery is needed (Kent 1991, p. 53).

Despite these criticisms, UNICEF proclaimed that the child survival strategy contributed to a significant reduction in infant and child mortality in many LMICs (UNICEF 1996). Yet child mortality declines were steepest in the 1960s and 1970s (Ahmad, Lopez, and Inoue 2000)—well before the start of UNICEF's child survival campaign. In the end, Child Survival and other SPHC programs had mixed success (child mortality decreased much faster in settings in which community-based PHC was adopted).

Financial, Oil, and Debt Crises and the Breakdown of the Post-war Development Model, 1970s–Early 1980s

The debates over PHC took place against a backdrop of global political upheaval. Having reached its crescendo by 1960, the post-war liberal development compact was being contested through tumultuous movements across the world, ranging from Third World challenges to Western hegemony and continued imperialism, to armed struggle against authoritarian and repressive regimes propped up by the Cold War superpowers, and social mobilization against war, around civil rights and anti-racism, sexual and gender rights, economic justice, and better labor and environmental conditions. Meanwhile, in 1971, US President Richard Nixon, pressed by business interests concerned with the competitiveness of US industry, abandoned the gold standard backing for the US dollar and the worldwide fixed-rate exchange system, which had been established at Bretton Woods. US industry leaders' pinpointing of the high dollar launched a sustained battle against Keynesian economic interventions, which, although advantageous for welfare state-building, ate, they argued, into their profits.

Then, in October 1973, members of the Organization of Arab Petroleum Countries decided to cut oil supplies to countries that had supported Israel in that month's Yom Kippur War. The Organization of Petroleum Exporting Countries (OPEC), long frustrated by unchanging oil prices despite rising global inflation, seized on these events and raised the price of crude oil. The quadrupling of oil prices in 1974 led to a large stock market decline, then a boom in other commodity prices.

The increased circulation of petrodollars (US dollars earned from petroleum sales) initially brought increased access to capital in petrol-exporting countries, but many others experienced economic slowdown, inflation, public sector deficits, and an increase in unemployment.

The second oil price shock began in the lead-up to the 1979 Iranian Revolution, followed by the 1980s Iran–Iraq war, both of which severely curtailed oil exports. The real price of crude oil increased from US$8 per barrel in 1971 to US$40 in 1973 to over US$60 in 1980, generating a worldwide recession and sharp rises in interest rates.

While oil exporters benefited, many LMICs faced deepening financial problems. Countries in need of revenues to cover the high cost of oil and imports were persuaded to take ever larger loans from multilateral and commercial lenders flush with petrodollars (Nasser 2003). Governments that borrowed heavily found themselves short of foreign exchange to buy imported goods or inputs to industry and agriculture. The United States, United Kingdom, and other HICs raised interest rates to combat inflation, compounding these problems.

By the early 1980s, a full-blown debt crisis had materialized. Total LMIC debt in real 2005 dollars went from US$360.9 billion in 1970 to US$1.2 trillion in 1980, with annual debt service payments rising over 200% (World Bank 2016). Much of this debt was built on decades of irresponsible lending and borrowing practices (often at usurious interest rates) that rarely benefited the economic and social conditions of the poor and precariously positioned working and middle classes—instead lining the corrupt pockets of lenders and wealthy LMIC elites alike.

Latin America imploded first, its debt reaching US$327 billion in 1982. This led a band of countries across the continent to default on private loans in rapid succession, beginning with Mexico in 1982. Mexico's default spread a financial shockwave across the continent. As of October 1983, 27 LMICs, many in the Americas, had defaulted on their loans or were in the process of rescheduling debts. In response to mounting debt, foreign investors and commercial interests rapidly withdrew resources and finances from vulnerable countries. This capital flight, which also involved domestic financiers, further exacerbated the financial crisis (FDIC 1997; López 1998).

The 1980s are known as the "lost decade" in Latin America. Between 1980 and 1990, the poverty rate increased from 40.5% to 48.3%, not recuperating until 2004. Real wages in the formal sector fell sharply while informal employment expanded. Hyperinflation reached an average of over 400% in 1990 before starting to fall (Bértola and Ocampo 2012). In sub-Saharan Africa, per capita GDP fell by 13% during the same period (World Bank 2016), and between the early 1970s and 1990s foreign investment in Africa plunged (Bond 2006), even as hundreds of billions of dollars were siphoned out through capital flight, in a corrupt nexus of foreign investors, bankers, and domestic politicians (Ajayi and Ndikumana 2015).

These events had enormous implications for health, especially in LMICs, leaving economies shattered, soaring unemployment, and a denuding of public provision of health, education, and other social investments. International health institutions and their activities would also be drastically affected, not least by the emerging neoliberal ideological model.

Neoliberalism, Development, and the Washington Consensus

Currency liberalization, oil and debt crises, and waning interest in ODA—particularly as the Soviet Union was facing its own economic and political crises (including the 1980 invasion of Afghanistan) and no longer served as counterbalance to or justification for Washington's LMIC investment policies—opened the way for a major shift in development strategies. This shift, in turn, was shaped by a transformation in the overall economic order that had begun in the 1970s toward neoliberal capitalism.

The neoliberal transformation had hefty repercussions for development. In the late 1970s, World Bank President Robert McNamara had invited German Chancellor Willy Brandt to head a commission to resolve the "North–South" political impasse on development strategies and the NIEO. The commission called for the mutual dependence of industrialized and "underdeveloped" nations, balancing issues of trade, financial reforms, and economic integration with concerns around the environment, energy use, food and agricultural development, and aid (Brandt 1980; Independent

Commission on International Development Issues 1983). Like the Millennium Declaration 20 years later (see chapter 3), the Brandt Commission failed to address power differentials within and between countries as both the prime cause of and solution to underdevelopment. Instead it stressed enlightened self-interest and moral appeals for social justice rather than structural change in the global political economy (Navarro 1984). Released just as the debt crisis was unfolding and international financial agencies were turning to neoliberal development policies, the Brandt Commission reports were shelved.

Neoliberalism, arising initially under neoconservative governments in the United Kingdom and United States, has involved implementing "free" market ideology to return capitalism to profitability and "restore the power of economic elites" (Harvey 2005, p. 19) by overturning many of the rights, protections, and societal redistribution policies that had flourished in the post-war period and reorienting the state to favor business at the expense of public well-being (see chapter 9 for further details).

But it was unleashed in its greatest frenzy in LMICs. The IMF and World Bank began to furnish loans to debtor countries to relieve balance-of-payments deficits and the burden of servicing debt—as well as bail out the private banking sector in HICs. But the strings attached to these loans (called conditionalities) came at a high price—the implementation of "structural adjustment programs" (SAPs). SAPs and subsequent loan programs compelled major economic reforms designed to open domestic markets to foreign penetration and stimulate low-cost exports. Reforms included: drastic cuts to government spending (particularly in health, which was already a low budget priority, and other social sectors) and agricultural subsidies, labor sector reform, deregulation of industry (including mining sector reform), removal of restrictions on foreign investment, trade and financial sector liberalization, currency devaluation, and privatization of state enterprises and government services, as well as monetary policy reform.

Widely reviled, SAPs affected health through often drastic reductions in health care and other social sector services, privatization of public assets, and the introduction of user fees in the public sector. For example in Zimbabwe, as in many LMICs, spending cuts and privatization resulted in reduced access to, and poorer quality of, health care, education, and other services, disproportionately affecting women and children (Bassett 2013) (see chapter 9 for a detailed account).

The Waning of WHO (and the PHC-NIEO Approach)

For WHO, all of these developments spelled trouble. There was no doubt that the United States and other wealthy interests deemed PHC and WHO's articulated sympathy for an NIEO to be subversive, even revolutionary. Soon these parties moved to reign in WHO's advocacy and displace its flagship role in international health. An ominous sign was the 1982 vote by the WHA to freeze WHO's budget in the context of stretched public coffers. Then, in 1985, right-wing US President Ronald Reagan's administration unilaterally cut its UN-assessed contributions by 80% and withheld its WHO member dues in 1986. These measures were at least partially designed to reprimand WHO for its 1977 Essential Medicines Programme and List, opposed by leading US-based pharmaceutical companies (Brown, Cueto, and Fee 2006; Chorev 2012; Godlee 1994), as well as amplify corporate displeasure at the 1981 WHO-UNICEF International Code of Marketing of Breast-Milk Substitutes aimed at ending unethical marketing practices by infant formula companies in LMICs (Chetley 1986).

Formally, the excuse for this clawback was that WHO was inefficient, autocratic, and poorly managed (an accusation that might be leveled at virtually any bureaucracy). In reality, the opposite was true, at least in regard to PHC. PHC's endorsement of public provision of primary care contradicted neoliberal strategies to cut public sector spending, privatize state activities, and lessen regulations on worker, environmental, and consumer protections, even as state regulation was reoriented to protect private capital accumulation.

Illustrating this stance, a 1985 study published by the conservative Heritage Foundation think tank entitled: *The WHO: Resisting Third World Ideological Pressures*, advised US policymakers that the WHO's (and the UN's) mobilization against private enterprise—whether through support for generic drugs or codes of conduct for transnational corporations—had to be curbed. Accordingly, Western countries needed to "quietly and persistently insist that the Organization adhere to its technical mandate" of improving health, which for Reaganites implied expanding commercial markets in the Third World, hardly WHO's technical mandate! Moreover, referring to Health for All, the study author advised that "WHO should reexamine carefully the long-term effectiveness of specific programs" (Starrels 1985, pp. 43–44).

By the mid-1980s, WHO's role (as an intergovernmental entity at the heart of international health agenda-setting and activities) fundamentally changed. Its dues plummeted, and its mission was dispersed among other UN agencies not subject to democratic policymaking processes. Already on the sidelines of the UNICEF-led SPHC and child survival effort, it was upstaged by the World Bank in health financing and reform, and, in 1996, displaced by UNAIDS in addressing the HIV epidemic. PHC was underfunded in the context of the US's all-out assault on WHO. As we shall see in subsequent chapters, however, PHC and the Alma-Ata principles have inspired new movements in recent years.

By the early 1990s, less than half of WHO's budget came from annual member state dues subject to "democratic" WHA decisions. Instead, donors, who by now included a variety of private corporations and philanthropies in addition to member countries, increasingly shifted WHO's budget away from dues-funded activities to a priori assignment of funds to particular programs and approaches, growing to 50% of the total WHO budget in the early 1990s and, incredibly, close to 80% today.

Once the Cold War ended, the anti-communist rationale for Western bloc support for WHO disappeared (WHO faced unprecedented invective targeting its perceived bureaucratic inefficiency in a 1994 *BMJ* series penned by its current editor-in-chief [Godlee 1994]), leaving in its wake the promotion of trade, the commodification of health, disease surveillance, and health security as justifications for international health, all priorities of powerful countries and wealthy interests (Kassalow 2001; Ollila 2005). By this time, apart from its role—usually underfunded—addressing surveillance, notification, and control of resurgent infectious diseases (e.g., TB), and, especially, pandemics, (e.g., influenza), WHO was no longer at the heart of international health activities, as had been stipulated in its 1948 Constitution.

In the 1990s, the World Bank stepped in to fill the vacuum intentionally created by the defunding of WHO. The Bank, pushing for cost-effective reforms and privatization of health care services, had a far larger health budget than WHO, and many bilateral agencies simply bypassed WHO in their international health activities (Banerji 1999). The WHO hobbled along thanks to its tethering to a panoply of public–private partnerships (PPPs), alliances, and initiatives (Brown, Cueto, and Fee 2006). These entities shrewdly drew on WHO for legitimacy, inviting its input and providing circumscribed funding, but were controlled by actors lacking public accountability. This granted business interests such as pharmaceutical corporations a major, arguably unjustified, role in international public health policymaking (Richter 2004). Throughout the 1990s international health spending—in the UN system and as part of development spending generally—was stagnating, and the future of WHO and the entire field seemed to be in question. We pick up on the contemporary dimensions of the field, starting circa 2000, in chapters 3 and 4.

Of course, WHO was far from the only player in international health over this period: in many ways, bilateral players, UNICEF and other UN agencies, big and small NGOs, missionaries, and many other groups have collectively had a greater global presence than WHO (Mann Wall 2015; Packard 2016) (see chapter 4). Still, the waxing and waning of WHO was emblematic of international health's possibilities and problems. At least through the 1980s, WHO had served as the beacon of much international health activity. What transpired next would revamp the international health scene once again, albeit retaining certain features from the past, just as international health's transition from the imperial era to the Cold War era involved both continuity and change.

STRADDLING INTERNATIONAL AND GLOBAL HEALTH

- Why did the term *global health* come about and who favors its use?
- What are the continuities and discontinuities between international and global health?
- How does a historical understanding shed light on current global health debates?

As the Cold War was melting away circa 1990, an accompanying transition took place in the overarching appellation applied to the times—from an era of polarization to one of globalization. While only the most ahistorical and ideologically foolhardy heralded globalization as marking the undeniable triumph of market capitalism (Fukuyama 1992)—and despite globalization's patent rationale for neoliberal economic policies (Chernomas and Sepehri 2002)—the term has become omnipresent in vernacular and academic discourse alike.

The health arena has certainly not been immune to these developments. Since the mid-1990s a cascade of institutions and individuals have seized upon the vogue of globalization to rechristen the field of international health as global health, furthering a variety of agendas, be they idealistic, opportunistic, or driven by realpolitik (Cueto and Zamora 2006). Motivated in part to distance the field from Cold War associations, this new term has been adopted broadly over the past two decades, implying a shared global susceptibility to, experience of, and responsibility for (ill) health. In its more collective guise, global health refers to health and disease patterns in terms of the interaction of global, national, and local forces, processes, and conditions in political, economic, social, and epidemiologic domains. Notwithstanding the invoked distinctions—there is a jumbled understanding of the "global" in global health (Bozorgmehr 2010; Rowson et al. 2012) and considerable conflation between international and global health—the "new" global health bears many similarities to its international health predecessor (Birn 2011a) (Table 2-3).

The term *global health* had been employed on occasion, by WHO and other UN agencies, the US government and other national governments, PPPs, and population control agencies, as well as by progressive anti-nuclear, environmental, and universal health care movements (Brown, Cueto, and Fee 2006; Garay, Harris, and Walsh 2013)—suggesting competing interests over its use. However, its resurrection has been greeted mostly uncritically (with some exceptions) or justified ex post facto either aspirationally, albeit with concerns regarding Western unilateral or hegemonic globalism, or as a theoretical and methodological challenge (Bozorghmehr 2010; Janes and Corbett 2009; Kickbusch 2002; Stuckler and McKee 2008). Others contend that global health primarily reflects HIC agendas, major donors, and priorities of wealthy elites (Ollila 2005; van der Rijt and Pang 2013).

For example, the US Institute of Medicine's (1997, p. 2) definition of global health as "health problems, issues, and concerns that transcend national boundaries, may be influenced by circumstances or experiences in other countries, and are best addressed by cooperative actions and solutions" remains mum on the directionality, nature, and causes of these influences and what is meant by cooperation. In a 2009 update, global health is characterized optimistically as "the goal of improving health for all people in all nations by promoting wellness and eliminating avoidable disease, disabilities, and deaths," and even calls for "an understanding of health determinants," before returning to the aim of "improv[ing] health in low and middle-incomes countries" through "basic and applied research on disease and disability" and their risk factors (Institute of Medicine 2009, p. 18).

Perhaps most widely cited of late is Koplan and colleagues' (2009, p. 3) "common definition of global health," as:

> an area for study, research, and practice that places a priority on improving health and achieving equity in health for all people worldwide. Global health emphasises transnational health issues, determinants, and solutions; involves many disciplines within and beyond the health sciences and promotes interdisciplinary collaboration; and is a synthesis of population-based prevention with individual-level clinical care.

This definition merits extensive analysis precisely because it sidesteps so many crucial issues. Remarkably, the definition excludes the political context of global health altogether. There is no mention of who the stakeholders are and who wields power in global health. Nor is there discussion of questions regarding who/what drives the global health agenda and to what ends. Moreover, the devised definition of Koplan et al. invokes globalization but ignores its documented negative effects on health, including the impact of: trade liberalization on inequality and economic insecurity; international financial institution conditionalities and privatization policies on access to social services; deregulation on environmental and occupational

Table 2-3 Continuities and Differences between International and Global Health Conceptualizations and Rationales

Continuities		Differences
Under international health[a] (Roughly 1900–1990)	***Under global health (Since 1990)***	***New or more pronounced under global health***
Charity/missionary work	Charity/missionary work	Human rights approaches
War and disaster relief	Humanitarianism (also linked to charity)	Renewed ethical imperatives Disaster capitalism
Philanthropy	Philanthropy/ Philanthrocapitalism	Philanthropies supporting the role of the private sector in global health
Colonial power/paternalism	Cooperation (typically North-South and asymmetrical)	Increasing South-South cooperation
Diplomacy and imperial power/foreign policy	Diplomacy and foreign policy	Global health diplomacy
"Dual mandate," "civilizing" development/dependency under capitalism; emphasis on economic growth	Globalization/ free markets/ investment under neoliberal capitalism; emphasis on economic growth; development goals	"Sustainable" development Development alternatives: degrowth
Commercial interests: extractive industries; pharmaceuticals, etc.; productivity and profits	Commercial interests: extractive industries; pharmaceuticals, food and agribusiness etc.; productivity and profits	Corporate interests directly involved in funding/decisionmaking; commodification of health
Technology transfer/ transnational training and experts/producing knowledge; mostly HIC research in LMICs	Technology diffusion/ transnational training/ and experts producing knowledge; brain drain	Expansion/recognition of LMIC research capacity
Paternalistic public health and medical experimentation, with limited or no ethical protocols	Medical research following more ethical but still sometimes fraught protocols	Stronger ethics committees, including in LMICs
Trade/ access to resources and markets	Trade/ investment/access to resources and markets	Broader penetration of corporate and financial interests in HICs and LMICs under neoliberal capitalism
Data collection/disease surveillance	Data collection/disease surveillance	More comprehensive, adaptable, flexible, technologies able to recognize/address new diseases more quickly
Security and national self-interest (fear of pandemics and "exotic/deadly" diseases; emerging bioterrorism concerns)	Security and national self-interest (fear of pandemics and "exotic/ deadly" diseases; bioterrorism)	Global health security

Table 2-3 Continued

Continuities		Differences
International agreements/IHR	International agreements/IHR	IHR requiring more global cooperation
South-South cooperation/G-77 and non-aligned movement, following NIEO principles	South-South cooperation (mostly not heeding NIEO principles, but some social justice-oriented)	More prominent role of larger LMIC actors, especially BRICS
Cold War rivalries—countering communism (1946–1991)	War on Terror	Proliferation of non-state actors
Alternative players (progressive social movements and groups, and "comrades in health") engaged in health internationalism	Alternative players engaged in social justice/solidarity efforts	Alternative players engaged in addressing health inequities within both HICs and LMICs
Nomenclature: Developing/underdeveloped countries vs. non-aligned movement/ Third World	HICs vs. LMICs Global North vs. Global South	Majority World vs. Minority World (see chapter 3)
Local institutions	NGOs-civil society	"Partners"
Bilateral/international/private	Bilateral/multilateral/private	"Multi-stakeholder" initiatives
Political stability; staving off unrest	Political stability; staving off unrest	Addressing challenges of global health in "fragile states"

[a] Many of these dimensions also formed part of colonial health and tropical medicine.

health (Labonté, Mohindra, and Schrecker 2011); and massive financial fraud on the lives of billions of people (Benatar, Gill, and Bakker 2009).

Additionally, the distinctions drawn by Koplan et al. between international and global (and public) health are inadequate. While global health is "meant to transcend past ideological guises of international health—as a 'handmaiden' of colonialism or a pawn of Cold War political rivalries" (Birn 2006a, p. 1), in reality these terms lie along a continuum. International health arose, backed by powerful nations and economic interests, for similar reasons as global health has surfaced—to address health issues that cross borders, and to pursue security and economic/commercial goals (the international dimensions of health and health dimensions of international political and economic relations) (PAHO 1992).

Though many have contested its appropriateness, the global health moniker has stuck. It remains in desperate need of interrogation—well beyond the proliferation of global health definitions—in order to explain why global health has dislodged international health. Gradually some voices from the South are proposing an alternative (anti-hegemonic) vision of global health for Latin America (and the Third World generally) based on justice, human rights, and a critical consciousness (Franco-Giraldo 2016). But more such voices are sorely needed.

To say that global health is primarily concerned with "achieving equity" and "emphasizes transnational health issues, determinants, and solutions" (Koplan et al. 2009, p. 1995) sounds promising, but there is little evidence that global health addresses equity in any profound or contextualized way (Rowson et al. 2012) or overcomes the patronizing and self-interested patterns of the past (Garay, Harris, and Walsh 2013). It certainly belies global health's profit-oriented present. A more useful analysis would seek to examine health in the context of the global order of political and economic power, either explaining why global health deserves to displace international health—or rejecting this proposition.

Amid this muddle, a characteristic feature of the new global health is undoubtedly the huge investment opportunity for private capital, previously kept under check by the exigencies of the Cold War and prior trade barriers (Birn 2011a). The medicalization, monetization, and profit-making prospects of global health have been implicitly sanctioned by the explosion over the last few decades of PPPs (see chapter 4) (Benatar and Upshur 2011; Qadeer and Baru 2016; Richter 2004), and a growing number of for-profit consulting firms. This has been fortified by the WHO's 2000–2002 Commission on Macroeconomics and Health, with its double entendre of "Investing in Health" (WHO 2001) (echoing the World Bank's identically titled report of 1993) as a means of enhancing economic productivity and amassing private profits (Waitzkin 2003). This trend is widely evidenced by the stated missions and activities of numerous food, insurance, and pharmaceutical corporations, global health agencies, foundations, and PPPs.

If anything, global health distinguishes itself not just as *business as usual*, but as *far more business than was usual* under the field's international health designation. Notwithstanding this reality, the dominant articulations of global health exclude discussions of the commodification of health and essentials such as water, private profit-making, and the role of market capitalism. Moreover, despite widespread, inspiring invocations of equity, "benefiting everyone," and "including southern voices," mainstream approaches are silent on why social inequalities in health have developed in the first place, why they persist, and how they might be fundamentally addressed (Birn 2009a; Hunsmann 2016).

These debates engender a series of dilemmas and contradictions: Is global health (or the globalization of health) simply a reflection of "capitalism without borders" or does it incorporate a dialectic of power involving imposition from above, resistance from below, and opportunistic gameplaying in both directions from mid-level players? Is it a slogan that is naïvely descriptive—in the sense of geographic simultaneities or problems and common solutions transcending physical and political boundaries? Is the arena of global health uncynically sanguine as it strives for equity and transnational human rights? Is it a fashionable renewal and bowdlerizing of the previously used term *international health* (Holmes, Greene, and Stonington 2014)? Or is it flagrantly ideological in the sense of putting forth a metropolitan Euro- or North-centric hegemonic universalism to promote the diffusion of goods, technologies, financial products, and values (Labonté and Gagnon 2010; Lakoff 2010) while maintaining domestic security (Macfarlane, Jacobs, and Kaaya 2008; Pogge 2002)?

These issues are taken up in the coming chapters as we explore the political economy of health and development and review a panorama of the current global health field's actors and activities.

[N.B. This book utilizes the terms *international health* and *global health* in their particular contexts, problematizing them as relevant but also taking them as general descriptors—with global health serving as the dominant term at present.]

CONCLUSION

Learning Points:

- World War II marked the beginning of a bumpy transition away from the imperial era, involving decolonization and liberation struggles across Asia, Africa, and the Caribbean, the rebuilding of Europe and Japan, and the Cold War rivalry between US-led and Soviet-led blocs.
- The new geopolitical order brought global legitimacy for international development cooperation and economic regulation via the UN and Bretton Woods institutions, with WHO at the helm of the international health agenda and activities.
- Shaped by the contemporary context, WHO's disease eradication approach—most notably its technology-based campaigns against yaws, malaria, and smallpox—also built on the legacy of earlier international health actors and activities.
- The logic of the Cold War and the accompanying impetus of economic development were also challenged by Third World aspirations to a New International Economic Order, entangling WHO in sharp disputes over how it should address health and development.
- As the non-aligned countries gained more voice and influence, WHO spearheaded

comprehensive PHC as a socially just, locally contextualized, integrated approach to enhancing health in contrast to more narrowly conceived top-down disease campaigns.
- The debt crises of the 1980s had devastating economic and social effects, with drastic repercussions for health and health services in LMICs. WHO was also faced with plummeting dues and deliberate US underfunding, stymying PHC's implementation and overshadowing it with SPHC-oriented efforts led by UNICEF and bilateral agencies.
- The waning of WHO as the fulcrum of international health activity coincided with the growing dominance of neoliberal globalization and the entry of new actors in the field that would be re-christened as global health.

The half century following World War II provides a crucial backdrop to understanding the institutions, activities, tenets, and challenges of global health today. Of course, the priorities and practices of international health played out differently in distinct settings, and the various actors and alliances were not uniform or static. Yet they remained indelibly shaped by the larger geopolitical concerns around the newly decolonized world, the Cold War, and how development would intersect with these contexts and processes.

Focusing on WHO as international health's one-time mid- and late-20th century beacon does not imply it was the only or most influential actor. Indeed, in many ways, the US government (including USAID's population control effort) and other bilateral and multilateral actors (especially the World Bank, as of the late 1980s) were far more powerful shapers of the international health agenda (see chapter 4 for a broad overview of players). Furthermore, although since its founding WHO was connected to a greater or lesser extent to a myriad of health issues, sometimes its involvement was minimal and belated, such as around aging, noncommunicable diseases, and HIV.

Even at its peak, WHO faced competition from and overlap with UNICEF, among other agencies, and was constrained in meeting its goals by the uneven enthusiasm of the United States and other donors. Still, some of its smaller initiatives, including, since the 1980s, health promotion and the healthy cities movement (see chapter 13), have engaged local and national governments and civil society in creative and forward-thinking ways.

But in the end, WHO—and the global health field writ large—have been most marked by disease control initiatives: the continued resonance of the now mythic eradication of smallpox, despite the shortcomings of this approach, is undeniable. The next chapter turns to a critical political economy of health framing to help explain and analyze the contemporary contours of the global health and development arena.

NOTES

1. The ILO was also intermittently influenced by progressive values, but its governance structure was more limited.
2. Yet more than 20 years later, at an October 1992 Ministerial Malaria Conference in Amsterdam, the inability to achieve eradication was attributed to a set of non-technical factors, including low education levels, low levels of community involvement, insufficient knowledge about malaria at the community level, and inadequate funding for and development of health services (Beigbeder 1995).
3. This approach was resurrected in 2006 through the Rockefeller and Gates Foundations' Alliance for a Green Revolution in Africa (AGRA), which, similar to predecessors, focuses on technological and market models for increased agricultural output. Ultimately aiming to integrate African food consumption and agricultural production into the (corporate cartel-controlled) global food chain, this emphasis comes at the expense of equitable, democratic, and sustainable approaches based on securing land rights for small producers and supporting local and regional food distribution networks (Morvaridi 2012).
4. This was diplomatically significant, given that the People's Republic of China only became a WHO member in 1972, replacing Taiwan.
5. At the time, Mahler's closest advisor, Joshua Cohen, recommended that the resolution call for polio to be *eliminated* rather than eradicated, due to the existence of wild poliovirus. However, the WHA's enthusiasm for a repeat success of eradication outvoted the cautionary approach (which has since proven prescient).

REFERENCES

Agostoni C. 2016. *Médicos, Campañas y Vacunas: La Viruela y la Cultura de su Prevención en México, 1870–1952*. México: Universidad Nacional Autónoma de México.

Ahmad OB, Lopez AD, and Inoue M. 2000. The decline in child mortality: a reappraisal. *Bulletin of the World Health Organization* 78:1175–1191.

Ajayi SI and Ndikumana L, Editors. 2015. *Capital Flight from Africa: Causes, Effects, and Policy Issues.* Oxford: Oxford University Press.

Allina-Pisano E. 2012. Imperialism and the colonial experience. In Haslam P, Schafer J, and Beaudet P, Editors. *Introduction to International Development: Approaches, Actors, and Issues (Second Edition)*. New York: Oxford University Press.

Altink H. 2014. 'Fight TB with BCG': Mass vaccination campaigns in the British Caribbean, 1951–6. *Medical History* 58(04):475–497.

Amrith S. 2006. *Decolonizing International Health: India and Southeast Asia, 1930-65.* Basingstoke, UK: Palgrave.

Anderson W. 2007. Immunization and hygiene in the colonial Philippines. *Journal of the History of Medicine and Allied Sciences* 62(1):1–20.

Anshan L. 2011. *Chinese Medical Cooperation in Africa: With Special Emphasis on the Medical Teams and Anti-Malaria Campaign.* Uppsala: Nordiska Afrikainstitutet.

Arita I, Wickett J, and Nakane M. 2004. Eradication of infectious diseases: Its concept, then and now. *Japanese Journal of Infectious Diseases* 57:1–6.

Asiedu K, Fitzpatrick C, and Jannin J. 2014. Eradication of yaws: Historical efforts and achieving WHO's 2020 target. *PLOS: Neglected Tropical Diseases* 8(9):e3016.

Atangana M-R. 2009. *French Investment in Colonial Cameroon: The FIDES Era (1946–1957).* Bern: Peter Lang.

Bair J. 2015. Corporations at the United Nations: Echoes of the New International Economic Order? *Humanity: An International Journal of Human Rights, Humanitarianism, and Development* 6(1):159–171.

Bandung Conference. 1955. Final Communiqué of the Asian-African Conference. Bandung.

Banerji D. 1999. A fundamental shift in the approach to international health by WHO, UNICEF, and the World Bank: Instances of the practice of 'Intellectual Fascism' and totalitarianism in some Asian countries. *International Journal of Health Services* 29(2):227–259.

Bashford A. 2014. *Global Population: History, Geopolitics, and Life on Earth.* New York: Columbia University Press.

Bassett MT. 2013. From Harlem to Harare: Lessons in how social movements and social policy change health. In Birn A-E and Brown TM, Editors. *Comrades in Health: U.S. Health Internationalists, Abroad and at Home.* New Brunswick, NJ: Rutgers University Press.

Beigbeder Y. 1995. *L'Organisation Mondiale de la Santé (Publications de L'Institut Universitaire de Hautes Etudes Internationales, Geneve).* Paris: Presses universitaires de France.

Beldarraín Chaple. E. 2006. Public health in Cuba and its international experience (1959-2005). *História, Ciências, Saúde – Manguinhos* 13(3):709–716.

Benatar S, Gill S, and Bakker I. 2009. Making progress in global health: The need for new paradigms. *International Affairs* 85(2):347–371.

Benatar S and Upshur R. 2011. What is global health? In Benatar S and Brock G, Editors. *Global Health and Global Health Ethics.* Cambridge: Cambridge University Press.

Bértola L and Ocampo JA. 2012. Turning back to the market. In *The Economic Development of Latin America since Independence.* Oxford: Oxford University Press.

Bhattacharya S. 2006. *Expunging Variola: The Control and Eradication of Smallpox in India, 1947–1977.* Hyderabad: Orient Longman.

———. 2013. International health and the limits of its global influence: Bhutan and the worldwide Smallpox Eradication Programme. *Medical History* 57(4):461–486.

Birn A-E. 2006a. Introduction: Canada, Latin America, and international health. *Canadian Journal of Public Health* 97(6):I–1.

———. 2006b. *Marriage of Convenience: Rockefeller International Health and Revolutionary Mexico.* Rochester, NY: University of Rochester Press.

———. 2009a. Making it politic(al): Closing the gap in a generation: Health equity through action on the social determinants of health. *Social Medicine* 4(3):166–182.

———. 2009b. The stages of international (global) health: Histories of success or successes of history? *Global Public Health* 4(1):50–68.

———. 2011a. Remaking international health: Refreshing perspectives from Latin America. *Pan American Journal of Public Health* 30(2):106–110.

———. 2011b. Small(pox) success? *Ciência & Saúde Coletiva* 16(2):591–597.

———. 2014. Backstage: The relationship between the Rockefeller Foundation and the World Health Organization, Part I: 1940s–1960s. *Public Health (Royal Society for Public Health)* 128(2):129–140.

Black M. 1996. *Children First: The Story of UNICEF, Past and Present.* New York: Oxford University Press.

Bond P. 2006. Resource extraction and African underdevelopment. *Capitalism Nature Socialism* 17(2):5–25.

Borowy I. 2008. Manoeuvering for space: International health work of the League of Nations during World War II. In Solomon SG, Murard L, and Zylberman P, Editors. *Shifting Boundaries of Public Health: Europe in the Twentieth Century.* Rochester, NY: University of Rochester Press.

———. 2016. Medical aid, repression, and international relations: The East German Hospital at Metema. *Journal of the History of Medicine and Allied Sciences* 71(1):64–92.

Bozorgmehr K. 2010. Rethinking the 'global' in global health: A dialectic approach. *Global Health* 6(19).

Brandt W. 1980. *North-South: A Program for Survival.* Cambridge, MA: MIT Press.

Brickman JP. 2013. Medical McCarthyism and the punishment of internationalist physicians in the United States. In Birn A-E and Brown TM, Editors. *Comrades in Health: U.S. Health Internationalists, Abroad and at Home.* New Brunswick, NJ: Rutgers University Press.

Brown TM and Birn A-E. 2013. The making of health internationalists. In Birn A-E and Brown TM, Editors. *Comrades in Health: U.S. Health Internationalists, Abroad and at Home.* New Brunswick, NJ: Rutgers University Press.

Brown TM, Cueto M, and Fee E. 2006. The World Health Organization and the transition from 'international' to 'global' public health. *American Journal of Public Health* 96(1):62–72.

Caprio ME and Sugita Y. 2007. *Democracy in Occupied Japan: the U.S. Occupation and Japanese Politics and Society.* Abingdon, UK: Routledge.

Centre Tricontinental, Gresea, and Editions Syllepse. 2007. Coalitions d'Etats du Sud: Retour de l'esprit de Bandung? Points de vue du Sud. *Alternatives du Sud.* 14(3).

Chakrabarty D. 2010. The legacies of Bandung: Decolonization and the politics of culture. In Lee CJ, Editor. *Making a World after Empire: The Bandung Moment and Its Political Afterlives.* Athens: Ohio University Press.

Chernomas R and Sepehri A. 2002. Is globalization a reality, a tendency or a rationale for neoliberal economic policies? *Globalization* 2(2):1–27.

Chetley A. 1986. *The Politics of Baby Foods: Successful Challenges to International Marketing Strategies.* Basingstoke, UK: Palgrave Macmillan.

Chorev N. 2012. *The World Health Organization between North and South.* Ithaca, NY: Cornell University Press.

Colombo Plan Secretariat. 2011. History. http://www.colombo-plan.org/index.php/about-cps/history/. Accessed April 27, 2016.

Connelly M. 2008. *Fatal Misconception: The Struggle to Control World Population.* Cambridge, MA: Belknap Press.

Cooper F. 1996. *Decolonization and African Society: The Labor Question in French and British Africa.* Cambridge: Cambridge University Press.

Cooper F and Packard RM, Editors. 1997. *International Development and the Social Sciences: Essays on the History and Politics of Knowledge.* Berkeley: University of California Press.

Cueto M. 2004. The origins of primary health care and selective primary health care. *American Journal of Public Health* 94(11):1864–1874.

———. 2007a. *Cold War, Deadly Fevers: Malaria Eradication in Mexico, 1955–1975.* Washington, DC: Woodrow Wilson Center Press.

———. 2007b. *The Value of Health: A History of the Pan American Health Organization.* Rochester, NY: University of Rochester Press.

———. 2008. International health, the early Cold War and Latin America. *Canadian Bulletin of Medical History* 25(1):17–41.

Cueto M, Brown T, and Fee E. 2011. El proceso de creación de la Organización Mundial de la Salud y la Guerra Fría. *Apuntes: Revista de Ciencias Sociales* 38(69):129–156.

Cueto M and Palmer S. 2014. Primary health care, neoliberal response, and global health in Latin America. In *Medicine and Public Health in Latin America: A History.* Cambridge: Cambridge University Press.

Cueto M and Zamora V. 2006. *Historia, salud y globalización.* Lima: Universidad Peruana Cayetano Heredia e Instituto de Estudios Peruanos.

Cullather N. 2010. *The Hungry World: America's Cold War Battle against Poverty in Asia.* Cambridge, MA: Harvard University Press.

Davis K. 1956. The amazing decline of mortality in underdeveloped areas. *The American Economic Review* 46(2):305–318.

Deutsch A. 1958. *The World Health Organization; its Global Battle against Disease.* New York: Public Affairs Committee.

Dobson MJ, Malowany M, and Snow RW. 2000. Malaria control in East Africa: The Kampala Conference and the Pare-Taveta Scheme: A meeting of common and high ground. *Parassitologia* 40(1-2):149–166.

Duara P. 2003. Introduction: The decolonization of Asia and Africa in the twentieth century. In Duara P, Editor. *Decolonization: Perspectives from Now and Then.* London: Routledge.

Ehrlich P. 1969. *The Population Bomb*. New York: Sierra Club.

Ekbladh D. 2015. Harry S. Truman, development aid, and American foreign policy. In Geselbracht RH, Editor. *Foreign Aid and the Legacy of Harry S. Truman*. Kirksville, MO: Truman State University Press.

Engerman DC. 2011. The Second World's Third World. *Kritika: Explorations in Russian and Eurasian History* 12(1):183–211.

Ermisch M-L. 2014. *Children, Youth and Humanitarian Assistance: How the British Red Cross Society and Oxfam Engaged Young People in Britain and its Empire with International Development Projects in the 1950s and 1960s*. Montreal: McGill University.

Escobar A. 2011. The problematization of poverty: The tale of three worlds and development. In *Encountering Development: The Making and Unmaking of the Third World*. Princeton, NJ: Princeton University Press.

Everill B and Kaplan J, Editors. 2013. *The History and Practice of Humanitarian Intervention and Aid in Africa*. Basingstoke, UK: Palgrave Macmillan.

Fabic MS, Choi Y, Bongaarts J, et al. 2015. Meeting demand for family planning within a generation: The post-2015 agenda. *Lancet* 385(9981):1928–1931.

Fang X. 2015. Reinterpreting the role of traditional Chinese medicine in public health in rural China in 1970s. In Medcalf A, Bhattacharya S, Momen H, et al, Editors. *Health for All: The Journey to Universal Health Coverage*. Hyderabad: Orient Blackswan.

Fanon F. 1963. Colonial war and mental disorders. In *The Wretched of the Earth: The Handbook for the Black Revolution that is Changing the Shape of the World* [Translated by Farrington C]. New York: Grove Press.

Farley J. 2008. *Brock Chisholm, the World Health Organization, and the Cold War*. Vancouver: UBC Press.

Federal Deposit Insurance Corporation (FDIC). 1997. The LDC debt crisis. In *History of the Eighties: Lessons for the Future*. FDIC: Washington, DC.

Feinsilver J. 2010. Fifty years of Cuba's medical diplomacy: From idealism to pragmatism. *Cuban Studies* 41:85–104.

Fenner F, Henderson DA, Arita I, et al. 1988. *Smallpox and its Eradication*. Geneva: WHO.

Ferguson J. 1999. *Expectations of Modernity: Myths and Meanings of Urban Life on the Zambian Copperbelt*. Berkeley: University of California Press.

Fitzgerald D. 1986. Exporting American agriculture: The Rockefeller Foundation in Mexico, 1943-53. *Social Studies of Science* 16(3):457–483.

Franco-Giraldo A. 2016. Salud global: Una visión latinoamericana. *Revista Panamericana de Salud Pública* 39(2):128–136.

Frank AG. 1972. The development of underdevelopment. In Cockroft J, Frank AG, and Johnson D, Editors. *Dependence and Underdevelopment: Latin America's Political Economy*. Garden City, NY: Anchor Books.

Frey M, Kunkel S, and Unger CR, Editors. 2014. Introduction: International organizations, global development, and the making of the contemporary world. In *International Organizations and Development, 1945–1990*. Basingstoke, UK: Palgrave Macmillan.

Fuhrer H. 1996. *A History of the Development Assistance Committee and the Development Co-operation Directorate in Dates, Names, and Figures*. Paris: OECD.

Fukuyama F. 1992. *The End of History and the Last Man*. New York: Free Press.

Garay J, Harris L, and Walsh J. 2013. Global health: Evolution of the definition, use and misuse of the term. *Face à face* 12 [online] http://faceaface.revues.org/745. Accessed May 26, 2016.

Gates B. 2005. Prepared Remarks to the 2005 World Health Assembly, May 16, 2005. http://www.gatesfoundation.org/speeches-commentary/Pages/bill-gates-2005-world-health-assembly.aspx. Accessed June 12, 2010.

Giles-Vernick T and Webb Jr. JLA, Editors. 2013. *Global Health in Africa: Historical Perspectives on Disease Control*. Athens: Ohio University Press.

Gillespie J. 2003. International organizations and the problem of child health, 1945-1960. *Dynamis* 23:115–142.

———. 2008. Europe, America, and the space of international health. In Solomon SG, Murard L, Zylberman P, Editors. *Shifting Boundaries of Public Health: Europe in the Twentieth Century*. Rochester, NY: University of Rochester Press.

Gilman N. 2015. The new international economic order: A reintroduction. *Humanity: An International Journal of Human Rights, Humanitarianism, and Development* 6(1):1–16.

Glendon MA. 2001. *A World Made New: Eleanor Roosevelt and the Universal Declaration of Human Rights*. New York: Random House.

Godlee F. 1994. WHO in retreat: Is it losing its influence? *BMJ* 309:1491–1495.

Goldman M. 2006. *Imperial Nature: The World Bank and Struggles for Social Justice in the Age of Globalization*. New Haven: Yale University Press.

Gómez-Dantés H and Birn A-E. 2000. Malaria and social movements in Mexico: The last 60 years. *Parassitologia* 42(1–2):69–85.

Gonzalez CL. 1965. *Mass Campaigns And General Health Services, Public Health Paper No. 29*. Geneva: WHO.

Goodman RA, Foster KL, Trowbridge FL, and Figueroa JP, Editors. 1998. Global disease elimination and eradication as public health strategies. *Bulletin of the World Health Organization* 76(Suppl 2):5–162.

Greene JA. 2010. When did medicines become essential? *Bulletin of the World Health Organization* 88:483–483.

Greenough P. 1995. Intimidation, coercion and resistance in the final stages of the South Asian Smallpox Eradication Campaign, 1973–1975. *Social Science and Medicine* 41(5):633–645.

———. 2011. "A wild and wondrous ride": CDC field epidemiologists in the East Pakistan smallpox and cholera epidemics of 1958. *Ciência & Saúde Coletiva* 16(2):491–500.

Gutiérrez JL. 1975. Health planning in Latin America. *American Journal of Public Health* 65(10):1047–1049.

Gutner T. 2016. *International Organizations in World Politics.* Thousand Oaks, CA: CQ Press.

Harrison M. 2015. A global perspective: Reframing the history of health, medicine, and disease. *Bulletin of the History of Medicine* 89(4):639–689.

Hartmann B. 1997. Population control I: Birth of an ideology; and Population control II: The population establishment today. *International Journal of Health Services* 27(3):523–557.

Harvey D. 2005. *A Brief History of Neoliberalism.* Oxford: Oxford University Press.

Helleiner E. 2014. *Forgotten Foundations of Bretton Woods: International Development and the Making of the Postwar Order.* Ithaca, NY: Cornell University Press.

Henderson DA. 2009. *Smallpox - the Death of a Disease: The Inside Story of Eradicating a Worldwide Killer.* Amherst, NY: Prometheus Books.

Hess GR. 2003. Waging the Cold War in the third world: The foundations and the challenges of development. In Friedman LD and McGarvie MD, Editors. *Charity, Philanthropy, and Civility in American History.* Cambridge: Cambridge University Press.

———. 2005. The role of American philanthropic foundations in India's road to globalization during the Cold War era. In Hewa S and Stapleton D, Editors. *Globalization, Philanthropy, and Civil Society: Toward a New Political Culture in the Twenty-First Century.* New York: Springer.

Hochman G. 2008. From autonomy to partial alignment: National malaria programs in the time of global eradication, Brazil, 1941–1961. *Canadian Bulletin of Medical History* 25(1):161–192.

———. 2009. Priority, invisibility and eradication: The history of smallpox and the Brazilian public health agenda. *Medical History* 53:229–252.

Hodge JM. 2016. Writing the history of development (part 2: longer, deeper, wider). *Humanity* 7(1):125–174.

Hodges S, Editor. 2006. *Reproductive Health in India: History, Politics, Controversies.* Delhi: Orient Longman.

Holmes SM, Greene JA, and Stonington SD. 2014. Locating global health in social medicine. *Global Public Health* 9(5):475–480.

Hong Y-S. 2015. *Cold War Germany, the Third World, and the Global Humanitarian Regime.* Cambridge: Cambridge University Press.

Howard-Jones N. 1981. The World Health Organization in historical perspective. *Perspectives in Biology and Medicine* 24(3):467–482.

Humphreys ME. 2001. *Malaria: Poverty, Race, and Public Health in the United States.* Baltimore: Johns Hopkins University Press.

Hunsmann M. 2016. Pushing 'global health'out of its comfort zone: Lessons from the depoliticization of AIDS control in Africa. *Development and Change* 47(4):798–817.

Immerwahr D. 2015. *Thinking Small: The United States and the Lure of Community Development.* Cambridge, MA: Harvard University Press.

Independent Commission on International Development Issues. 1983. *Common Crisis North-South: Co-Operation for World Recovery. The Brandt Commission.* Cambridge, MA: MIT Press.

Institute of Medicine. 1997. *America's Vital Interest in Global Health: Protecting Our People, Enhancing Our Economy, and Advancing Our International Interests.* Washington, DC: The National Academies Press.

———. 2009. *The U.S. Commitment to Global Health: Recommendations for the Public and Private Sectors.* Washington, DC: The National Academies Press.

Janes C and Corbett K. 2009. Anthropology and global health. *Annual Review of Anthropology* 38:167–183.

Johansson SR and Mosk C. 1987. Exposure, resistance and life expectancy: Disease and death during the economic development of Japan, 1900–1960. *Population Studies* 41(2):207–235.

Jones SG, Hilborne LH, Anthony CR, et al., Editors. 2006. Japan. In *Securing Health: Lessons from Nation-Building Missions.* Santa Monica: RAND Center for Domestic and International Health Security.

Kapur D, Lewis JP, and Webb R. 1997. *The World Bank: Its First Half Century.* Vol. 1. Washington, DC: The Brookings Institution.

Kassalow J. 2001. *Why Health is Important to U.S. Foreign Policy.* New York: Council on Foreign Relations and Milbank Memorial Fund.

Keller RC. 2006. Geographies of power, legacies of mistrust: Colonial medicine in the global present. *Historical Geography* 34:26–48.

Kerr RB. 2012. Lessons from the old Green Revolution for the new: Social, environmental and nutritional issues for agricultural change in Africa. *Progress in Development Studies* 12(2-3):213–229.

Kent G. 1991. *The Politics of Children's Survival*. New York: Praeger Publishers.

KFF [Kaiser Family Foundation]. 2015. *Fact Sheet: The U.S. Government and International Family Planning & Reproductive Health*. Menlo Park, CA: KFF.

Kickbusch I. 2002. Influence and opportunity: Reflections on the US role in global public health. *Health Affairs* 21:131–141.

Kinkela D. 2011. *DDT and the American Century: Global Health, Environmental Politics, and the Pesticide that Changed the World*. Chapel Hill: University of North Carolina Press.

Koplan JP, Bond TC, Merson MH, et al. 2009. Towards a common definition of global health. *Lancet* 373(9679):1993–1995.

Kumar R, Birn A-E, and McDonough P. 2016. International cooperation in women's health: Critical analysis of a quarter century of paradigm shifts. In Gideon J, Editor. *Handbook on Gender and Health* Cheltenham, UK: Edward Elgar Publishing.

Labonté R and Gagnon ML. 2010. Framing health and foreign policy: Lessons for global health diplomacy. *Globalization and Health* 6:14.

Labonté R, Mohindra K, and Schrecker T. 2011. The growing impact of globalization for health and public health practice. *Annual Review of Public Health* 32:263–283.

Lakoff A. 2010. Two regimes of global health. *Humanity: An International Journal of Human Rights, Humanitarianism, and Development* 1(1):59–79.

Lal P. 2015. African socialism and the limits of global familyhood: Tanzania and the new international economic order in sub-Saharan Africa. *Humanity: An International Journal of Human Rights, Humanitarianism, and Development* 6(1):17–31.

Latham ME. 2011. *The Right Kind of Revolution: Modernization, Development, and US Foreign Policy from the Cold War to the Present*. Ithaca, NY: Cornell University Press.

Liang W, Wang Y, Cao G, et al. 2014. China's Approach in the Blooming South-South Health Cooperation: Chances, Challenges and the Way Forward. http://www.uni-heidelberg.de/md/awi/ssdc_liang_wenjie.pdf. Accessed May 23, 2015.

Litsios S. 1997. Malaria control, the cold war, and the postwar reorganization of international assistance. *Medical Anthropology* 17(3):255–278.

———. 2002. The long and difficult road to Alma-Ata: A personal reflection. *International Journal of Health Services* 32(4):709–732.

Logan JA. 1955. Counteracting communism through foreign assistance programs in public health. *American Journal of Public Health and the Nation's Health* 45(8):1017–1021.

López, J. 1998. External financial fragility and capital flight in Mexico. *International Review of Applied Economics* 12(2):257–270.

Macfarlane SB, Jacobs M, and Kaaya EE. 2008. In the name of global health: Trends in academic institutions. *Journal of Public Health Policy* 29(4):383–401.

Magalhães RC da S. 2016. *A erradicação do Aedes aegypti: Febre amarela, Fred Soper e saúde pública nas Américas (1918–1968)*. Rio de Janeiro: Editora Fiocruz.

Mahler H. 1976a. A social revolution in public health. *WHO Chronicle* 30:475–480.

———. 1976b. Social perspective in health. World Health Organization [Offprint report; Rec 234].

Manela E. 2010. A pox on your narrative: Writing disease control into Cold War history. *Diplomatic History* 34(2):299–323.

———. 2014. Globalizing the Great Society: Lyndon Johnson and the pursuit of smallpox eradication. In Gavin FJ and Lawrence MA, Editors. *Beyond the Cold War: Lyndon Johnson and the New Global Challenges of the 1960s*. New York: Oxford University Press.

Mann Wall B. 2015. *Into Africa: A Transnational History of Catholic Medical Missions and Social Change*. New Brunswick, NJ: Rutgers University Press.

Manton J. 2003. Global and local contexts: The Northern Ogoja Leprosy Scheme, Nigeria, 1945-1960. *História, Ciências, Saúde-Manguinhos* 10(suppl 1):209–223.

Mazower M. 2009. *No Enchanted Palace: The End of Empire and the Ideological Origins of the United Nations*. Princeton, NJ: Princeton University Press.

McMillen CW and Brimnes N. 2009. Medical modernization and medical nationalism: Resistance to mass tuberculosis vaccination in postcolonial India, 1948–1955. *Comparative Studies in Society and History* 52(1):180–209.

Meier BM. 2013. Making health a human right: The World Health Organization and the United Nations Programme on Human Rights and Scientific and Technological Developments. *The Journal of the Historical Society* 13(2):195–229.

Mohamed D. 2016. "'No other help wins more friends': The Cold War, decolonization, and the WHO Global Yaws Control Programme, ." Annual Meeting of the American Association for the History of Medicine, April 28-May 1. Minneapolis.

Monson J. 2010. Working ahead of time: Labor and modernization during the construction of the TAZARA railway, 1968–86. In Lee CJ, Editor. *Making a World after Empire: The Bandung Moment and Its Political Afterlives*. Athens: Ohio University Press.

Morvaridi B. 2012. Capitalist philanthropy and the new Green Revolution for food security. *International Journal of Sociology of Agriculture and Food* 19(2):243–256.

Muniz ÉS. 2013. *Basta aplicar uma injeção?: Desafios e contradições de saúde pública nos tempo de JK (1956-1961).* Rio de Janeiro: Editora Fiocruz.

Nair R. 2011. The construction of a 'population problem' in colonial India 1919–1947. *Journal of Imperial and Commonwealth History* 39(2):227–247.

Nandy A. 1987. *'Towards A Third World Utopia,' in Traditions, Tyrannies, and Utopias: Essays in the Politics of Awareness.* New Delhi: Oxford University Press.

Nasser A. 2003. The tendency to privatize. *Monthly Review* 54(10):22–37.

Navarro V. 1984. A critique of the ideological and political position of the Brandt report and the Alma-Ata declaration. *International Journal of Health Services* 14(2):159–172.

Necochea López R. 2014. *A History of Family Planning in Twentieth-Century Peru.* Chapel Hill: University of North Carolina Press.

Neill DJ. 2012. *Networks in Tropical Medicine: Internationalism, Colonialism and the Rise of a Medical Specialty, 1890–1930.* Redwood City, CA: Stanford University Press.

Nishimura S. 2008. Promoting health during the American occupation of Japan the public health section, Kyoto Military Government Team, 1945-1949. *American Journal of Public Health* 98(3):424–434.

———. 2009. Promoting health during the American occupation of Japan: Resistance to Allied public health measures, 1945-1952. *American Journal of Public Health* 99(8):1364–1375.

Obadare E. 2005. A crisis of trust: history, politics, religion and the polio controversy in Northern Nigeria. *Patterns of Prejudice* 39(3):265–284.

Ollila E. 2005. Global health priorities — priorities of the wealthy? *Global Health* 1(6):1–5.

Packard RM. 1998. "No other logical choice": Global malaria eradication and the politics of international health in the postwar era. *Parassitologia* 40(1–2):217–230.

———. 2007. *The Making of a Tropical Disease: A Short History of Malaria.* Baltimore: Johns Hopkins University Press.

———. 2016. *A History of Global Health: Interventions into the Lives of Other Peoples.* Baltimore: Johns Hopkins University Press.

PAHO. 1992. *International Health: A North-South Debate.* Washington, DC: Pan American Health Organization.

PAI. 2005. *2005 Update: Trends in international development assistance for reproductive health and population.* Washington, DC: Population Action International.

———. 2015. *Organizations Urge Obama to Stop Blocking Abortion Access for Women Overseas.* Washington, DC: Population Action International.

Pearson-Patel J. 2015. Promoting health, protecting empire: Inter-colonial medical cooperation in postwar Africa. *Monde(s): histoire, espace, relations* 7:213–230.

PHM, Medact, and Global Equity Gauge Alliance. 2005. *Global Health Watch 2005-2006: An Alternative World Health Report.* London: Zed Books.

Pires-Alves FA and Maio MC. 2015. Health at the dawn of development: The thought of Abraham Horwitz. *História, Ciências, Saúde-Manguinhos* 22(1):69–93.

Pogge T. 2002. *World Poverty and Human Rights: Cosmopolitan Responsibilities and Reforms.* Cambridge: Polity Press.

Prashad V. 2007. *The Darker Nations: A People's History of the Third World.* New York: The New Press.

———. 2013. *The Poorer Nations: A Possible History of the Global South.* Brooklyn, NY: Verso Books.

Qadeer I and Baru R. 2016. Shrinking spaces for the 'public' in contemporary public health. *Development and Change* 47(4):760–781.

Reinhardt BH. 2015. *The End of a Global Pox: America and the Eradication of Smallpox in the Cold War Era.* Chapel Hill: University of North Carolina Press.

Reinisch J. 2013a. 'Auntie UNRRA' at the Crossroads. *Past & Present* 218(Suppl 8):70–97.

———. 2013b. *The Perils of Peace: The Public Health Crisis in Occupied Germany.* Oxford: Oxford University Press.

Rich B. 2013. *Mortgaging the Earth: The World Bank, Environmental Impoverishment, and the Crisis of Development.* Washington, DC: Island Press.

Richter J. 2004. Public–private partnerships for health: A trend with no alternatives? *Development* 47:43–48.

Ringen K. 1990. Karl Evang: A Giant in Public Health. *Journal of Public Health Policy* 11(3):360–367.

Rostow WW. 1960. *The Stages of Economic Growth: A Non-Communist Manifesto.* Cambridge: Cambridge University Press.

Rowson M, Willott C, Hughes R, et al. 2012. Conceptualising global health: Theoretical issues and their relevance for teaching. *Globalization and Health* 8(3 6).

Roy J. 2010. *Smallpox Zero: An Illustrated History of Smallpox and its Eradication.* Johannesburg: Nic Buchanan, Umlando Wezithombe, African Comic Production House.

Rupprecht T. 2015. *Soviet Internationalism after Stalin: Interaction and Exchange between the USSR and Latin America during the Cold War.* Cambridge: Cambridge University Press.

Sawyer WA. 1947. Achievements of UNRRA as an international health organization. *American Journal of Public Health* 37(1):41–58.

Schneider WH. 2009. Smallpox in Africa during Colonial Rule. *Medical History* 53(2):193–227.

Schuknecht R. 2010. *British Colonial Development Policy after the Second World War. The Case of Sukumaland, Tanganyika*. Berlin: Lit Verlag.

Shrestha N. 1995. Becoming a development category. In Crush J, Editor. *Power of Development*. Abingdon, UK: Routledge.

Siddiqi J. 1995. *World Health and World Politics: The World Health Organization and the UN System*. Columbia: University of South Carolina Press.

Sikkink K. 2014. Latin American countries as norm protagonists of the idea of international human rights. *Global Governance* 20(3):389–404.

Silva KT. 2014. *Decolonisation, Development and Disease: A Social History of Malaria in Sri Lanka*. New Delhi: Orient Blackswan Private Limited.

Sivaramakrishnan K. 2015. Global histories of health, disease, and medicine from a" zig-zag" perspective. *Bulletin of the History of Medicine* 89(4):700–704.

Smith I and Smith S. 2015. Universal health coverage and missionary medicine. In Medcalf A, Bhattacharya S, Momen H, et al, Editors. *Health for All: The Journey to Universal Health Coverage*. Hyderabad: Orient Blackswan.

Staples A. 2006. *The Birth of Development: How the World Bank, Food and Agriculture Organization, and World Health Organization Have Changed the World, 1945-1965*. Kent, OH: Kent State University Press.

Stapleton DH. 2004. Lessons of history? Anti-malaria strategies of the International Health Board and the Rockefeller Foundation from the 1920s to the era of DDT. *Public Health Reports* 119(2):206–215.

Starrels J. 1985. *The World Health Organization: Resisting third world ideological pressures*. Washington, DC: The Heritage Foundation.

Steil B. 2013. *The Battle of Bretton Woods: John Maynard Keynes, Harry Dexter White, and the Making of a New World Order*. Princeton, NJ: Princeton University Press.

Stepan N. 2011. *Eradication: Ridding the World of Diseases Forever?* Ithaca, NY: Cornell University Press.

Stuckler D and McKee M. 2008. Five metaphors about global-health policy. *Lancet* 372(9633):95–97.

Sze S. 1982. *The Origins of the World Health Organization: A Personal Memoir, 1945–1948*. Boca Raton, FL: L.I.S.Z. Publications.

Taffet JF. 2007. *Foreign Aid as Foreign Policy: The Alliance for Progress in Latin America*. New York: Routledge.

Thomas KJA. 2002. Development projects and involuntary population displacement: The World Bank's attempt to correct past failures. *Population Research and Policy Review* 21(4):339–349.

Truman HS. 1949. Truman's Inaugural Address, January 20, 1949. https://www.trumanlibrary.org/whistlestop/50yr_archive/inagural20jan1949.htm. Accessed May 4, 2016.

UN. 1948. *Universal Declaration of Human Rights*. New York: United Nations Department of Public Information.

Unger CR. 2014. India's Green Revolution: Towards a New Historical Perspective. *Südasien-Chronik -South Asia Chronicle* 4:254–270.

UNICEF. 1996. Fifty years for children. In *The State of the World's Children 1996*. New York: UN.

U.S. Congress, Senate Committee on Government Operations. 1959. *The United States and the World Health Organization*. Washington, DC: GPO.

U.S. Department of State. 1979. Foreign Relations of the US, 29 May 1953, Vol. III, 69. Washington, DC.

van der Rijt T and Pang T. 2013. How "global" is "global health?" Examining the geographical diversity of global health thinkers. *Global Health Governance* 6(2):1–20.

Vastag B. 2003. The siren song of disease eradication: Is it out of tune with the times? *JAMA* 289(9):1090–1091.

Venediktov D. 1998. Alma-Ata and after. *World Health Forum* 19(1):79–86.

Vicziany M. 1982. Coercion in a soft state: The family-planning program of India: Part I: The myth of voluntarism. *Pacific Affairs* 55(3):373–402.

Vojtech M. 2010. The Soviet Union's partnership with India. *Journal of Cold War Studies* 12(3):50–90.

Waitzkin H. 2003. Report of the WHO Commission on Macroeconomics and Health: A summary and critique. *Lancet* 361(9356):523–526.

Walsh JA and Warren KS. 1979. Selective primary health care: An interim strategy for disease control in developing countries. *New England Journal of Medicine* 301(18):967.

Warren K. 1988. The difficult art, science, and politics of setting health priorities. *Lancet* 332(8609):498–499.

Watt CA and Mann M, Editors. 2011. *Civilizing Missions in Colonial and Postcolonial South Asia: From Improvement to International Development*. London: Anthem Press.

Webb Jr. JLA. 2014. *The Long Struggle against Malaria in Tropical Africa*. Cambridge: Cambridge University Press.

Werner D and Sanders D. 1997. *Questioning the Solution: The Politics of Health Care and Child Survival*. Palo Alto: HealthWrights.

Westad OA. 2005. *The Global Cold War: Third World Interventions and the Making of Our Times*. Cambridge: Cambridge University Press.

Whelan DJ. 2015. "Under the aegis of man": The right to development and the origins of the new international economic order. *Humanity: An International Journal of Human Rights, Humanitarianism, and Development* 6(1):93–108.

WHO. 1978. *Declaration of Alma-Ata. International Conference on Primary Health Care*. Alma-Ata, USSR.

———. 1980a. *The Global Eradication of Smallpox. Final Report of the Global Commission for the Certification of Smallpox Eradication*. Geneva: WHO.

———. 1980b. *The Work of WHO 1978-1979: Biennial Report of the Director-General to the World Health Assembly and to the United Nation*. Geneva: WHO.

———. 2001. *Investing in Health: A Summary of the Findings of the Commission on Macroeconomics and Health*. Geneva: WHO.

———. 2008. *WHO in 60 years: A Chronology of Public Health Milestones*. Geneva: WHO.

World Bank. 2016. World Development Indicators. http://data.worldbank.org/data-catalog/world-development-indicators. Accessed April 5, 2016.

Wright-Carozza P. 2003. From conquest to constitutions: Retrieving a Latin American tradition of the idea of human rights. *Human Rights Quarterly* 25(2):281–313.

Yekutiel P. 1981. Lessons from the big eradication campaigns. *World Health Forum* 2(4):465–490.

Youde J. 2010. China's health diplomacy in Africa. *China: An International Journal* 8(1):151–163.

Zimmer T. 2014. In the name of world health and development: The World Health Organization and malaria eradication in India, 1949–1970. In Frey M, Kunkel S, and Unger CR, Editors. *International Organizations and Development, 1945-1990*. Basingstoke, UK: Palgrave Macmillan.

3

POLITICAL ECONOMY OF HEALTH AND DEVELOPMENT

Suppose you are a middle-aged minibus driver working for a medium-sized company in a highly populated city. Transport, like most industries in your country, is largely unregulated. Vehicle emissions contribute to dangerously high pollution levels throughout the year, and road collisions take an enormous toll on the lives of young adults. The pay is low and in order to earn enough to provide for your family, you work upwards of 12 hours per day, 6 days a week, in fierce competition with other minibus drivers. Throughout the day you barely get to rest or even take a toilet break. You buy food from street vendors, eating meals as you drive.

Despite your long work hours, you are chronically behind on bills and can only afford an apartment in a dilapidated building that you know is structurally unsound, and lacks potable water and reliable electricity. Your wages must also cover school fees for your children, as the government only partly subsidizes education. There is no labor union for transit workers, your employer offers no benefits, and the government offers meager social welfare provisions—a worthless pension and inadequate health insurance, requiring high out-of-pocket payments. Although business is booming throughout your country, with new buildings and companies appearing almost every month, you have not enjoyed the benefits of this economic growth.

One morning, while driving your bus, you experience a brief but frightening episode of shortness of breath and tightness in your chest. You try to ignore it but feel weak after finishing your route and decide to see a doctor on your way home. After conducting an ECG and other tests, the doctor diagnoses you with high blood pressure, symptoms of angina, and possible early coronary heart disease. She recommends blood tests to assess cholesterol levels, as these may be elevated given your sedentary and stressful occupation and excess weight. After advising you to make dietary and physical activity changes, and prescribing an expensive medication that might lower your risk of a heart attack, the doctor charges you the equivalent of a day's wages for the consultation.

How can we understand and address your (the driver's) health problems?

POLITICAL ECONOMY OF HEALTH (AND DEVELOPMENT)

Key Questions:

- What are the underlying causes of health and illness?
- Do, or how do, the main models of understanding health and disease incorporate these factors?
- How have political economy approaches developed over time?
- What do these approaches tell us about how good or ill health and particular patterns of disease and death are produced and how they might be addressed?

This chapter begins with three sets of explanations for health and disease patterns, comparing and contrasting the dominant biomedical and behavioral/lifestyle approaches with a political economy understanding, which is used as a framework for this textbook. We explore various historical dimensions of a critical political economy of health framing and apply it to case examples of tuberculosis in South Africa and the post-Soviet mortality crisis to illustrate how political economy differs from prevailing approaches to understanding health. In the second part of the chapter we focus on political economy of development as related to global health, covering mainstream development discourses and strategies—foreign policy, aid, and financing arrangements—and highlighting several current development approaches, including human capabilities and rights, and the Millennium and Sustainable Development Goals. We conclude with an analysis of global governance issues, discussing the constraints to global health governance under the contemporary political economy order.

Approaches to Understanding Health and Disease

Determining and addressing the factors that produce (or lead to) health and disease are central concerns of the global health arena, its institutions, ideologies, and practices. However, there is no universally accepted approach to understanding health and illness. Here we examine two dominant models (biomedical and behavioral/lifestyle) that are mostly taken for granted by global health actors and one alternative (a critical political economy approach). We present them separately, though in practice there is overlap among them. To be sure, these models are not exhaustive. For example, they do not encompass various Indigenous paradigms, such as Andean *Buen Vivir*, stressing the role of ecological harmony—the balance of community needs and preservation of the natural environment—in shaping health and the quality of life (see chapter 13).

Biomedical Approach

According to a biomedical approach, health and illness are viewed at an individual level and in predominantly biological terms, with the body conceptualized as a machine with constituent processes and parts (i.e., genes, organ systems, and so on) that can be manipulated or repaired through technical interventions (Clarke et al. 2003). Health is understood primarily in terms of the absence of disease, rather than as an integrated (social, psychological, cultural) sense of well-being. This reductionist understanding decontextualizes health, illness, and healing from the social and political environment and from subjective human experience (Fee and Krieger 1993).

While the biomedical approach is largely curative, it also rests on a preventive armamentarium (e.g., vaccines, diagnostic screening, and genetic testing) and incorporates the role of behavioral determinants of health insofar as they affect so-called "risk factors"—personal characteristics related to heredity, biology, and "lifestyle" that are believed to predispose individuals to disease (Krieger 1994; Pearce 1996; Susser 1998). Much of the appeal of a biomedical approach stems from the dramatic technological advances in medical treatment over the last century or two, as in surgery (anesthesia and asepsis) and pharmacotherapy (Bell and Figert 2015), but it is also closely connected to the commodification of health (i.e. treating health as a good or service that can be bought and sold), and, as we will discuss, biomedicine has become a massive business enterprise in itself.

The search for and application of so-called "magic bullets"—quick-fix tools including medical technologies, drugs, and devices—most vividly characterizes this model. For example, the biomedical model has helped spur technical approaches to addressing child malnutrition, such as "Ready-to-Use Therapeutic Foods" (RUTF)—energy-dense and enriched food products to treat severe acute malnutrition. RUTF and similar techno-fixes (e.g., food fortification and nutritional supplements to treat micronutrient deficiencies) are often linked to vested commercial interests, and they are typically implemented without addressing the root economic and social causes of chronic malnutrition (see chapter 7).

Although RUTF was developed as a short-term emergency response to severe malnutrition in crisis or conflict situations, UNICEF has promoted its use on a wider scale, even where not requested. In 2009, the Indian government asked UNICEF to take back a batch of RUTF, judging it an inappropriate form of assistance and of dealing with child malnutrition (PHM et al. 2011). Indeed, RUTF, especially when used beyond emergency scenarios, treats malnutrition as a bio-technical problem, divorced from malnutrition's underlying causes. In rural India these include farm and employment losses due to land-grabbing, costly farm inputs and prohibitive credits, inadequate government support for rural infrastructure, and high rates of poverty, among other factors (Desai et al. 2016).

In sum, though it is tempting (and convenient) to attribute health improvements largely or exclusively to narrow interventions, as examined ahead, without concomitant societal changes most biomedical developments have played a limited role in increasing life expectancy historically and to the present.

Per a biomedical approach, as the bus driver in the earlier example you need to take blood pressure and cholesterol-lowering prescription drugs, antiplatelet therapy, and continue to be monitored by a physician. You should also heed medical advice on lifestyle modification (see next model) for secondary prevention of coronary heart disease.

Behavioral/Lifestyle Approach

A behavioral/lifestyle approach views health and illness primarily as a consequence of individual or household comportment and beliefs (Kahan et al. 2014). This approach focuses on the regulation or modification of personal conduct and attitudes through education, counseling, and incentives aimed at achieving desirable health outcomes. Although the social environment and policy measures can be considered mediating factors, for the most part behavioral approaches deem the individual (and sometimes the household or community) to be responsible for health and typically ascribe poor health to poor decisions or lack of volition.

Behavioral approaches to health are often nested within medicalization, which has the effect of "pathologising normal behaviour, disempowering individuals when subject to control by medical professionals or models of care, decontextualising experience, and depoliticising social problems" (Clark 2014, p. 2). (Biomedicalization is discussed in chapter 11.)

Of course, healers have long proffered advice to the infirm on routines of sleep, work, and diet, commonly filtered through spiritual or supernatural beliefs. The moralizing dimensions of such approaches—with rewards for healthy living or punishment for the (inevitable) outcome of poor "lifestyle" choices and personal deficiencies—continue to the present.

In recent decades behavior has taken on renewed scientific pretense as a primary determinant of health. Its modern rebirth was most vividly articulated by Marc Lalonde, then Canada's Minister of National Health and Welfare, who issued a report arguing that the country's recently universalized health care system was "only one of many ways of maintaining and improving health" (Lalonde 1974, p. 5). Even more important, he proposed:

> [O]minous counter-forces have been at work to undo progress in raising the health status . . . They include environmental pollution, city living, habits of indolence, the abuse of alcohol, tobacco and drugs, and eating patterns which put the pleasing of the senses above the needs of the human body (ibid).

This official articulation of the "lifestyle model" brought legitimacy to the notion that health is a personal responsibility and that individuals (can) choose to be either healthy or unhealthy (Knowles 1977). The report helped ignite the health promotion movement (see chapter 13), which, though framed broadly in terms of societal influences on health, has been interpreted in an increasingly narrow behavioral fashion (Baum and Fisher 2014).

The key argument underpinning this model—applied in countless superficial studies and problematic public health policies—is that "human behavior is the single most important determinant of variations in health outcomes" (Satcher and Higginbotham 2008, p. 401). Accordingly, changing harmful behaviors is portrayed as essential to improving health, leading to victim blaming, that is, culpabilizing individuals for their unhealthy behavior (Crawford 1977). Despite abundant and consistent evidence that decisions are shaped by far more than individual will and that behavior alone cannot explain patterns of health and health inequities, the narrow behavioral model persists (Skalická, Ringdal, and Witvliet 2015), leaving the structural determinants that undergird health comportment virtually untouched (Baum and Fisher 2014).

Lifestyle approaches have particular resonance in mainstream policies and initiatives that place the onus on individuals to eat and exercise right, wear seatbelts, avoid alcohol, tobacco, or drug use, practice safe sex, and so on, without addressing the context and constraints in which behaviors unfold, or the many other (often more) important determinants of health (Carey et al. 2016). Moreover, behaviorally oriented programs deflect attention away from governmental responsibility for ensuring that public policies (including regulation of the private sector) enhance health and health equity. Such deflections are not innocent but politically-framed decisions and approaches.

According to a behavioral/lifestyle approach to health, you must make better choices regarding the food you eat, avoid stressful situations, take more breaks on the job, work fewer hours, and engage in exercise in order to improve your health status.

Political Economy Approach

A political economy approach to understanding health and disease integrates the political, social, cultural, historical, and economic contexts in which ill health arises. This text uses political economy of health as shorthand for *critical political economy of health*: the idea that health and disease are produced via societal structures (i.e., political and economic practices, policies, and institutions [systems of production, social protection, and governance], and class/gender/race interrelations). These structures and relations, in turn, interact with the particular conditions that lead to good or poor health.

A growing body of scientific knowledge shows that social interactions affect (human) biology in heretofore little recognized ways (Lewontin 2000), making context and life experiences central to producing good or ill health at individual and collective levels. The societal order sustaining the distribution of power and resources within and across societies (and the material conditions thereby experienced) is reflected in a range of linked factors that operate at multiple levels and junctures—individual, household, community, social relations, workplace, nation, and global political and economic conditions—to shape health. (Attempts to understand the environmental or ecological pathways through which such determinants operate are also termed *political ecology of health* approaches, explored further in chapter 10.)

Political economy of health perspectives consider the role of, for example, public policies around transportation and housing conditions, medical care and public health, environmental contamination and resource depletion, as well as social justice strategies (gender and racial equity, unionization), and social-class-mediated political involvement aimed at bettering redistribution and overall societal welfare across all social groups (see Box 3-1 for political economy definitions). These efforts include, but go far beyond, biomedical interventions and behavior/lifestyle change.

According to a political economy approach, your health reflects/derives from social, political, and economic structures and relations that constrain your control over stressful situations and the work environment, and limit your access to health care, recreation, decent housing, education, and good nutrition (Hervik and Thurston 2016). As such, notwithstanding awareness of the importance of making better choices around diet, exercise, and stress and heeding your doctor's advice, your actions and personal agency are limited by the power dynamics produced by the conditions described above. That said, mobilizing collectively for better living and working conditions together with other bus drivers, workers, and social movements—depending on conditions of oppression in your setting/country and political and economic pressures globally—may lead to partial or wholesale transformation of the circumstances that negatively affect your health.

While ideologically distinct, in practice the three models at times intersect. In a more conducive environment, bus drivers might be able to exercise greater control over some of the factors affecting health. This could take the form of establishing/joining a union and bargaining for higher wages and better working conditions, or participating in a political process that results in an improved welfare state. Stress levels would be lessened if housing quality were regulated and education provided free of charge, potentially enabling shorter work hours and improved health habits. Under a tax-payer-funded national health care system, medical practitioners could be consulted free of charge before the onset of severe symptoms; in less pressured work circumstances and a more favorable

Box 3-1 Key Political Economy Definitions

- *Capitalism* is an economic system in which: the means of production are predominantly privately owned; production is operated on a for-profit basis; and the "free market" (representing the sum of rational individual decisions) governs levels and patterns of wages, production, distribution, investment, and prices and availability of goods and services. For more on capitalism's emergence and phases, see chapters 1 and 9.
- *Social classes* are broad social groupings indicating societal stratification and hierarchies. Social class may be understood in terms of: one or more measures of socioeconomic status (education, occupation, income); a combination of wealth, power, and prestige (Max Weber's classification); relation to the means of production (as per Karl Marx)—either the class of owners (exploiters) or workers (the exploited) or in an intermediate (contradictory) position as both worker and owner (e.g., administrator, manager, overseer); or caste (social position and occupation determined through heredity and/or racial/ethnic heritage).
- *Redistribution policies* aim to even out the spread of wealth (income, property, assets) across a society. Redistribution can be realized through a mix of progressive taxation (higher taxes on the rich), minimum wages and maximum compensation levels, and targeted or universal social programs in a capitalist system or, in a socialist system, through collective ownership and equitable distribution of societal assets. Redistribution is just one element of battling oppression (see chapter 14).

physical environment, it would be easier to change behavior to exercise and eat more nutritious meals.

A political economy of health model is often associated with a critique of capitalism, yet it is not enough to assert that capitalism causes ill health or to demonstrate without elaboration that poverty is correlated with high rates of disease and premature death. As Lesley Doyal (1979) argues cogently, every form of societal organization has corresponding patterns of death and disease, and careful delineation of how the societal political and economic structure affects these patterns is needed in order to comprehend and tackle them.

Certainly communist bloc countries, which all but eradicated poverty, unemployment, and homelessness by the mid-20th century, nonetheless had high rates of heart disease, cancer, lung diseases, and other causes of premature death, albeit having experienced notable health and health equity improvements after World War II. This may be explained by the industrial model pursued by the Soviet bloc to compete against the capitalist bloc that led to enormous pollution and continued workplace stress, which, combined with varying levels of political repression, deeply influenced the prevalence of chronic diseases.

Another illustration of why the capitalism-induced-poverty-causes-disease formulation is insufficient arises from the conundrum of why HIV infection rates are higher among many urban, better-off sub-Saharan African populations than their rural counterparts. Part of the answer, as discussed in chapter 6, is differential exposure to HIV, even as urban, wealthier populations benefit more from prevention and have greater access to treatment (Doyal 2013). And of course, neither of these examples touches upon the complex array of other social factors, including race-ethnicity/racism and sex-gender/patriarchy, that shape health and disease processes. Without identifying and tracing the patterns and mechanisms (and causal pathways), truisms about the links among capitalism, poverty, and health offer little by way of understanding and addressing them, both in the short term, through specific policies, and in the longer transformative processes needed to create healthier, more equitable societies. We begin this endeavor ahead, and then build upon it in chapter 7, where we explore two additional lenses on health and disease patterns and health inequity: psychosocial and ecosocial models.

A further caveat: by no means does employing a critical political economy framing discount the role and place of public health and medical care in global, national, and local policies and efforts. To the contrary, they remain salient: integrated into a political economy approach, biomedical and behavior change measures can improve well-being and provide much-needed care and relief from suffering. However in isolation, even if efficacious in driving down certain disease rates, they do not in and of themselves produce health.

Case Study: Working Conditions, Poverty, and Tuberculosis in South African Mines and Beyond

The rate of pulmonary tuberculosis (TB)—a chronic lung ailment—is one of the most sensitive indicators of social and political conditions in a society. The relationship among working and living conditions, poverty, and TB in Black miners in South Africa in the 20th century was comparable to the situation of 19th-century British factory workers and coal miners (Packard 1989). In both countries and eras, TB epidemics surged in conjunction with industrialization. Migration to urban industrial centers in Britain and mining towns in South Africa brought many workers in contact with TB for the first time. In both settings, once workers and their families were exposed to TB, their immunological systems were ill-equipped to resist the disease due to crowded and unhygienic living conditions, deficient nutrition, long hours of exhausting and unsafe labor, inadequate wages to redress these circumstances, and for the miners, poorly ventilated mines filled with toxic mineral dust. The powerful economic and political interests of the state and industry in maximizing production relied on exploitation of the working class, in South Africa especially Black Africans: vested interests were opposed to social and labor reforms to improve social conditions.

> "... 200,000 subterranean heroes who, by day and by night, for a mere pittance, lay down their lives to the familiar "fall of rock" and who, at deep levels ranging from 1,000 to 3,000 feet in the bowels of the earth, sacrifice their lungs to the rock dust which develops miner's phthisis [tuberculosis] and pneumonia."
> —Solomon Tshekisho Plaatje, Journalist, Political Activist, and Linguist, 1916

In Europe, struggles to improve housing, working conditions, and nutrition (often met with violent repression) in conjunction with public health efforts to isolate the sick in sanatoria, had gradually enabled declines in TB rates starting in the late 19th century. But in mid-20th century South Africa under the brutal, racist apartheid regime, the African working class was unable to gain comparable broad-based improvements in labor or social conditions. To the contrary, white workers colluded with the political regime in order to preserve white settler privilege against an organized multiracial labor force.

As a result, while white South African miners experienced modest improvements in conditions, Black workers continued to live in abject poverty. To explain the high mortality rates of TB among the Black working class, white administrators and medical officers relied on biomedical and behavioral frames, attributing TB increases to poor hygiene, supposed racial susceptibility, and an inadequate diet. This sidestepped the underlying conditions that fueled the disease. Administration of effective antituberculosis drugs in the 1950s eventually led to a sharp drop in TB deaths among Black South Africans, but as new laborers continued to migrate to mining and industrial areas with poor working and living conditions, the incidence of TB cases remained extremely high (Packard 1989).

By the 1990s, after South Africa's apartheid regime was dismantled, the mining sector remained an important source of jobs for over half a million migrant workers. Under continued substandard social and working conditions, hundreds of thousands of miners have become sick not only with TB but also with HIV, partially via sex workers unknowingly exposed to and spreading the disease. Both TB and HIV rates have soared in mining areas over the past two decades, with the more than 40,000 cases of active TB in miners each year exacerbated by the HIV epidemic. Meanwhile, understaffed and poorly coordinated health services have dispensed TB drugs in an unregulated fashion (and until recently without HIV drugs), leading to the emergence of extensively drug-resistant TB strains (see chapter 6).

When miners have returned to their homes, their families, too, have become infected with TB and HIV, multiplying the crisis across the country and elsewhere in Southern Africa, given the large proportion of migrant workers (e.g., from Lesotho, Mozambique, and Swaziland) who have long been employed in the mines (Corno and de Walque 2012).

All told, the intractable legacy of apartheid-era labor practices and working conditions remains

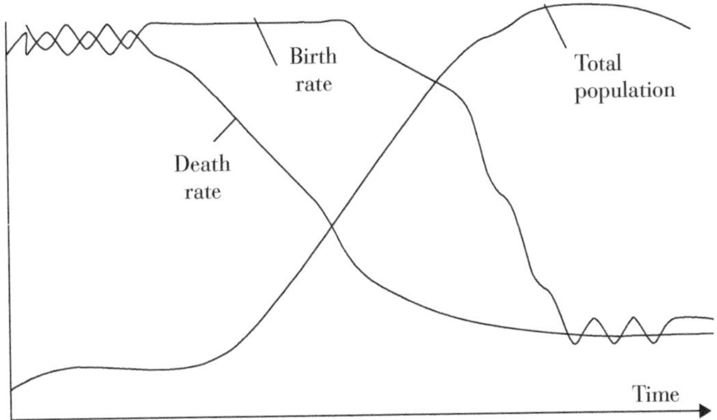

Figure 3-1: Demographic transition.
Source: Based on Notestein (1945).

difficult to resolve; even after legalized racial apartheid ended, a form of economic apartheid that goes beyond South Africa's borders persists.

Over the past few decades, a similar phenomenon has taken place in societies as diverse as Peru and the United States, where increased homelessness, malnutrition, marginalization, and problems of health care access have caused TB, once close to elimination, to reemerge as the leading global infectious disease killer, surpassing HIV (WHO 2015a). Inadequate health care is certainly part of the story, but TB's resurgence cannot be understood without considering larger structural issues, from poor housing and nutrition to unemployment and undemocratic governance, all framed by poverty and growing inequality (Neely 2015).

In sum, an ailment that by the late 19th century was largely preventable through improved housing, nutrition, and other infrastructural factors, and curable by the mid-20th century through antibiotics, has returned as a significant problem while its political economy dimensions have been largely disregarded.

Tying the Past to the Present

Transition Intransigencies

A background motif of global health is identifying historical patterns of mortality, fertility, and disease and gleaning what factors have driven these changes. This enables determination of past paths of progress, informs decisions on current actions and activities, and even helps predict future patterns. The "demographic transition" concept is credited to Princeton University professor F.W. Notestein (though parallel ideas were articulated by others). As illustrated in Figure 3-1, the concept outlines changes in birth and death rates that historically accompanied the shift from "traditional" to "modern" society based on the experience of Western European countries. In Notestein's classic description, a stage of high birth and death rates and little or no population growth gives way to a transitional stage of falling mortality, foremost infant mortality, during industrialization (as food supplies and living conditions improve), sustained high birth rates, and population growth. This is followed, after a lag, by a reduction in fertility, and then to a new stationary stage in which birth and death rates and population growth are relatively low. Such transitions can dramatically alter a population's age structure, featuring proportionately fewer children, more older people, and a substantial increase in median age and life expectancy.

Although this singular, unidirectional process of demographic transition is widely cited, it is a (highly problematic) characterization drawing from certain observed Eurocentric population patterns, rather than a generalizable theory. Not only have many countries, such as those in Latin America, followed patterns distinct from Notestein's account, demographic transition does not explain *how* changes take place or through what kinds of mechanisms. Despite extensive study, there are no universal explanations underpinning patterns of fertility decline in the past (Coale and Watkins 1986). The following hypotheses have been advanced (yet none of them convincingly fit even the well-documented English case [Szreter 2005]):

1. Shift from subsistence agriculture to factory work eventually requiring a smaller family size to maintain household revenues
2. Higher marginal cost of each additional child in urban settings (especially after child labor was prohibited)
3. Decline of multi-family/multi-generational households that facilitate child-raising
4. Larger numbers of women educated and working in the paid labor force, and delayed age at marriage
5. Social security beginning to replace family responsibility for elderly
6. Long workdays/shift work resulting in less time for child-rearing
7. Contraceptive technologies (e.g., condoms developed in 1840s)
8. Expanded use of fertility control methods, with women's networks relaying relevant knowledge
9. Infant mortality declines (and greater child survival) and increased birth spacing

Whether select high-income country (HIC) experiences offer a relevant template for low- and middle-income countries (LMICs) is debatable. Most observers consider this unlikely, given vast cultural, political, and contextual differences across settings. Moreover, even in Europe, transitions did not necessarily follow a smooth or universal pattern. Many rapidly industrializing cities of the early 19th century—for example Manchester, England and Liège, Belgium—saw mortality increase rather than decline due to miserable urban living and working conditions. As well, in various places mortality declines have not always been followed by fertility declines, due to cultural preferences, social necessity, or incentives for large family sizes.

The political context of demographic transition's emergence is key to understanding its endurance, despite these flaws. Although Notestein and colleagues originally held that high fertility was based on cultural preferences, not ignorance about contraception, by the early 1950s they reversed course, advocating concerted family planning efforts in the context of emerging Cold War population ideologies (Szreter 2005) (see chapter 2 for details). Around this time the US government began to view fertility declines in "developing countries" (via contraceptive campaigns) as both a precursor to economic development and a means of defusing population pressures perceived as a breeding ground for communism.

Preoccupation with hastening fertility declines through population control efforts motivated epidemiologist Abdel Omran's elaboration of "epidemiologic transition" (Weisz and Olszynko-Gryn 2010). According to Omran (1971), the major causes of death evolved from patterns of "pestilence and famine" to "receding pandemics," and then "degenerative and human-made diseases." In Western Europe and North America, he postulated, transition took approximately 100 years, whereas in Japan and Eastern Europe it started later and unfolded more rapidly ("the accelerated model"). In LMICs, transition was purportedly nearing completion in some settings, though not universally ("the contemporary delayed model"). With overarching, undemonstrated generalizations, epidemiologic transition is as wrongheaded as demographic transition. Detailed studies of Britain's population, for instance, show that although famine and plague ended by the 1670s, the rapid growth of England's population after 1750 was primarily due to rising fertility, not declining mortality. Moreover, both famine (Ireland 1840s) and infectious/epidemic mortality (soaring through much of the 19th century) resumed (Wrigley and Schofield 1989).

Indeed, the assumptions behind epidemiologic transition are so suspect it should arguably be discarded (Jones and Greene 2013). Notwithstanding Omran's eventual elaboration of new stages to take into account diseases of aging and emergent and resurgent diseases, he still did not cover the role of warfare and violence, the interaction of food insecurity with contagious diseases, or the emergence of occupational, environmental, and trade-related ailments, such as kidney disease, that also shape mortality patterns.

Despite these shortcomings, the ideological appeal of transition models triumphantly charting "progress" has led to their wide application as a policy-justification tool (Zijdema and Ribeiro de Silva 2014) and, even, combination into a single "health transition" that involves health care, socio-cultural, and behavioral responses (Frenk et al. 1991). This latter approach critiques but also seeks to rescue epidemiologic transition, arguing that its phases are plausible but may be overlapping, co-existing (especially where there is high social inequality) or reversible (leading to "countertransition") (Weisz and Olszynko-Gryn 2010). Yet life expectancy declines during the 1990s in the former Soviet Union amid a total breakdown of social welfare systems and in sub-Saharan Africa in the context of structural adjustment and AIDS and TB epidemics (see ahead for both) may not so much indicate transition reversals as question the validity of epidemiologic transition altogether.

Moreover, the notion of epidemiologic transition, even with modifications, overlooks social differences within populations and reinforces the presumption that people in LMICs die of infectious diseases whereas those in HICs die of noncommunicable diseases (NCDs) (this despite NCDs becoming the leading cause of death in a growing number of LMICs) and that the latter pattern is "more advanced" than the former. Given these multiple deficiencies (Santosa et al. 2014), it is puzzling that epidemiologic transition remains a touchstone for global health.

McKeown's Provocative (and Flawed) Thesis, and its Continuing Resonance

Alongside descriptions of the modern rise of population, the question of what factors have driven declines in mortality rates, including disease-specific trends, has gripped the worlds of health and development since the 1960s, with potentially enormous policy implications. Among the first to address this crucial question was a Canadian-English physician and social medicine professor, Thomas McKeown, who examined cause-of-death patterns in England and Wales from the late 18th to the mid-20th century. He postulated four possible avenues for mortality declines (McKeown 1976; McKeown and Record 1962):

1. Spontaneous change in the virulence of microorganisms
2. Medical measures
3. Public health measures
4. Economic growth and improvements in standard of living

In Sherlock Holmes style, McKeown discarded the first three options: (1) by discounting the possibility of spontaneous virulence declines except for scarlet fever; (2) by deeming modern medicine largely irrelevant based on his assessment that effective interventions appeared only after mortality rates had already fallen substantially, as illustrated by Figure 3-2's declining TB curve that preceded BCG and streptomycin (Worboys 2010); and (3) by arguing that public health (for McKeown equated with sanitation) had little relevance because it affected waterborne diseases and

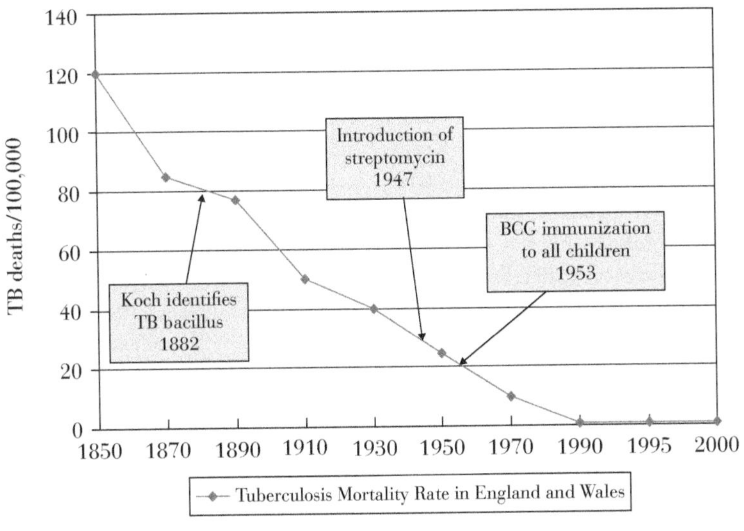

Figure 3-2: Tuberculosis mortality and medical interventions.
Source: Based on McKeown, Record, and Turner (1975).

most of the mortality decline was due to airborne diseases. By process of elimination, McKeown concluded that (4) economic growth and a rising standard of living—particularly shaping better nutrition (and thus immunological resistance)—were the key explanatory factors.

McKeown's provocative thesis was met with both praise and vitriol from distinct quarters. Skeptics of biomedicine, notably Austrian philosopher Ivan Illich (1976), applauded his findings for deflating technological triumphs (Colgrove 2002), as did advocates of lifestyle approaches. Demographers, meanwhile, soon discovered that McKeown had misread the data on Britain's mortality decline (Wrigley and Schofield 1989). McKeown's political bias and methodological misjudgments were most trenchantly exposed by historian Simon Szreter (2005), who found that because McKeown conflated TB with other respiratory deaths, his dismissal of the role of social policy and public health measures—such as sanitation, improved milk supplies, and housing improvements—was erroneous. McKeown's ideas also came under fire for privileging economic growth as the key influence on mortality patterns, without considering the role of political struggles for redistribution and social improvements (Burström 2003).

Still, the questions posed in McKeown's work have stimulated numerous national and local level mortality studies and ongoing debates around the enormous complexity of relevant factors and experiences (Corsini and Viazzo 1997; Cutler and Miller 2005; McGuire 2010; Wolleswinkel-van den Bosch et al. 2000; Woods 2000), including an "urban penalty" of increased mortality in northern Europe during the early phases of industrialization (Kearns 1988), and studies of mortality dynamics in Japan (Johansson and Mosk 1987) and the Americas (Birn, Cabella, and Pollero 2010).

Although McKeown's thesis, like Omran's, was discredited by historians, demographers, and other scholars, his interpretation is still invoked by economists and policymakers across the ideological spectrum. The World Bank, for example, took up certain aspects of McKeown's interpretation regarding the secondary importance of medicine and public health, arguing that economic growth, instead of health care, should be prioritized as the motor of improved standard of living, including better nutrition, to generate better health. Paradoxically, the same report portrayed the "dramatic health improvement" over the 20th century as a triumph of scientific knowledge and accompanying behavioral change (World Bank 1993, p. 6). Others hold that the effectiveness of HIV prevention and antiretrovirals in reducing mortality in recent decades significantly contests McKeown's thesis (Farmer et al. 2013).

While McKeown's work has been justifiably challenged, it is also important not to consider HIV therapeutics and their dissemination as separable from contextual factors—they are as much a political success as a medical one (Doyal 2013). Muddled as these various interpretations may be, they indicate the (global) health field's hunger for answers (often as oversimplified as McKeown's) on what are the best approaches to improving health.

Historical Factors Shaping Mortality Trends

Indeed, a recurring question in global health, if not *the* key question, is what are the elements and conditions that lead to improved health, health equity, and well-being (both within and across societies)? Historical patterns offer valuable evidence on this matter. As discussed in chapter 1, health conditions deteriorated across much of the colonized world in the context of warfare, disruption of livelihoods, and forced labor, although precise estimates are impossible because mortality statistics were not systematically collected. Mortality and mortality differentials between social groups also increased in Europe (Antonovsky 1967) (which has the most complete historical mortality records) during the first phase of industrialization starting in the late 18th century. Mortality increased among the poor majority especially, with peasants forced from communal pastoral life (itself far from idyllic) into urban settings, where from a young age they toiled long hours in dangerous factories. Cities at this time were deadlier than rural settings, plagued by crowding and filth, violence, infectious diseases, and pollution.

In the late 19th century, health conditions started to improve, albeit unevenly, as workers, supported by social reformers and some medical allies, struggled for better conditions. As a result, from roughly 1860 to 1950, Western European life expectancy increased from 35 years to over 65 years

(Gapminder 2009). An abundance of public health and demographic research demonstrates that the sustained (if uneven) mortality decline across Europe and beyond, particularly after 1900, was not due to market forces or income growth per se (Easterlin 1999; Preston 1975), but instead attributable to policies aimed at improving living and working environments.

But which policies and what drove them? The mix of factors propelling this increase in life expectancy (with interruptions from two world wars and the 1918–1919 influenza pandemic) has been traced to shorter working hours, prohibition of child labor, better access to and quality of nutrition, universal primary education, housing regulation, and urban upgrades (street paving, garbage collection), together with public health measures including sewage and sanitation systems, and maternal and child hygiene policies. However, it can be difficult to parse these factors (Riley 2001). Behavioral changes (such as hand washing and contraceptive use) were heavily mediated by education level, social class, location, and other features of the socio-political landscape. Fundamental was a secure and regular water supply for urban populations (separable from sewers and sanitation, which often came much later), a factor with continuing resonance (Bartram 2015).

Unfolding more gradually and slightly later than these broad social and political changes was a small but effective medical armamentarium. Early therapeutics included smallpox vaccine, which had a major impact initially in the late 18th century but took another century to be fully accepted and implemented; diphtheria antitoxin as of the late 1890s; Salvarsan (the first chemotherapy against syphilis) from 1909; and sulfonamides starting in the 1930s. Use of therapeutics accelerated after World War II, with the diffusion of antibiotics (e.g., streptomycin) and the proliferation of new vaccines.

Meanwhile, burgeoning welfare states covered a slew of social policies: unemployment compensation, old-age pensions, maternal benefits and family allowances, health care benefits, and other taxpayer-funded redistributive measures. These were undergirded by labor and other social movements (Brown and Fee 2014) together with ever greater public health improvements, including screened windows and doors preventing mosquito entry, indoor plumbing extended to rural areas, and occupational health protections.

So what ultimately caused mortality to decline? A political economy framework helps explain why the argument that "wealthier is healthier" (Steckel and Floud 1997) does not bear out—historically or contemporaneously—unless the distribution of increased wealth is taken into account. Indeed, despite soaring economic growth in 19th-century European cities, mortality rates stagnated or even increased (Schofield, Reher, and Bideau 1991). Why? Initially this was because the benefits of growth were not spread across social classes: industrial laborers faced atrocious living and working conditions while factory owners, suburban landowners, and urban landlords accumulated wealth.

Periods of extremely rapid capitalist expansion, as in China in the 1980s and the former Soviet bloc in the 1990s, suggest certain parallels with Britain's capitalist surge through the 19th century, when rapid economic growth was accompanied by disruption, deprivation, disease, and death (Szreter 2005). This seemingly counterintuitive idea—that wealth does not necessarily bring health—has now been demonstrated for 20th-century United States (Tapia Granados and Diez Roux 2009), contemporary China, Europe, and elsewhere (Deaton 2013). (Unsurprisingly, the financial sector has been reluctant to let go of the nostrum that GDP growth drives life expectancy improvements [Zijdema and Ribeiro de Silva 2014].)

What are the implications of all of these studies for LMICs? As discussed in chapter 2, some welfare state policies were implemented in the late colonial period (at least in urban areas), and adapted, as possible, by post-colonial governments navigating domestic claims on the state and Cold War exigencies. Leading economists and demographers attribute post-war mortality declines in LMICs to either the indirect by-products of economic development or the direct results of social policies. Demographer Samuel Preston (1980) estimates that only 20% of these life expectancy improvements are associated with increases in income, leaving deliberate policymaking (covering improved nutrition, education, sanitation, and diffusion of medical technologies, etc.) as a far more important explanatory factor. Nobelist Robert Fogel (2012) emphasized the importance of a "technophysio evolution"—that is, increased caloric intake due to technological advances in food production that has improved human physiology and thus increased longevity—across all settings. Others posit that in the decades following WWII, mortality improvements in LMICs derived largely from vaccines, antibiotics, vector control, oral rehydration therapy, and other technical and biomedical measures (Cutler Deaton, and Lleras-Muney 2006), as well as the institutional infrastructure required to enable these developments (Deaton 2013).

Arguments that mortality declines in LMICs resulted more from technical and medical interventions than was the case in Europe remain speculative, even as they have enormous implications for current global health policy (Jamison et al. 2013). Indeed, because LMIC mortality declines were coterminous with various enhancements in social and political conditions, including decolonization, education, and income, significant infrastructure support from both US-led and Soviet blocs, as well as medical and public health measures, it is nearly impossible to untangle the separate effects of each factor. As such, the *interaction* of scientific and technological gains *with* improvements in social conditions and the redistribution of economic, social, and political power remain as central to understanding past mortality dynamics as they are to analyzing the contemporary political economy of health. We return to the question of building healthy societies in "unexpected" LMIC settings (Riley 2007) in chapter 13.

Social Medicine Origins of Political Economy of Health Approaches

Healers and philosophers in societies as distinct as ancient China, Greece, medieval Europe, and the Middle East recognized that a range of local geographic and occupational factors influenced health beyond prevailing spiritual and comportment explanations. By the time of Europe's 19th century Industrial Revolution, the displacement, death, and distress experienced by the masses of workers stimulated new ideas linking political and social conditions to health. A pivotal moment was 1848, when an unprecedented wave of social uprisings unfurled across the world, demanding political representation and democratic governance and decrying horrendous workplaces, inhumane living conditions, and imperialist oppression (Krieger and Birn 1998) (see chapter 1).

Just before these revolutionary movements erupted, Rudolf Virchow, a brilliant young physician and founder of cellular pathology, was commissioned by the Prussian government (present-day Germany) to investigate a severe typhus outbreak among mostly Polish peasants in the impoverished Upper Silesia region. In his report to Prussian authorities, Virchow called the epidemic "artificial," and documented economic misery, poor housing, intense overcrowding, and government neglect during a famine as the critical reasons for widespread illness and death. Citing the epidemic's causes as political and economic, Virchow concluded that preventing future outbreaks required "full and unlimited democracy" (Virchow 1848a, p. 307).

Aware of the work of Engels (see chapter 1) tying harsh working and living circumstances of factory workers to specific health problems—including poor diet, chronic lung ailments, and musculoskeletal problems—Virchow was involved in the protest movements of his day (notably, he raced back to Berlin's barricades to participate in the short-lived 1848 Prussian revolution, then founded a medical politics weekly). His report recommended "radical" measures: improved working conditions, better housing, establishment of agricultural cooperatives, a more redistributive taxation system, and the decentralization of political authority, in addition to creation of public health services. Virchow's structural prevention approach—which astonished the report's commissioners, who expected recommendations geared toward medical intervention—served as a manifesto for the new field of *social medicine*, as it was soon dubbed by French physician Jules Guérin.

Virchow's contribution to political economy of health drew directly from his role as a researcher and physician. He understood the limits to scientific advances absent political and social equality, arguing: "medicine is a social science, and politics is nothing else but medicine on a large scale" (Virchow 1848c, p. 33). Further noting that disease was usually produced by conditions of deprivation, Virchow deemed physicians to be "the natural advocates of the poor" (Virchow 1848b, p. 4).

This work helped lay the foundation for a new approach to health and disease with a growing audience. Predictably, because it challenged the reigning economic model of factory-based capitalist production that exploited and immiserated workers, social medicine was rejected by Prussia's political and medical elites, and Virchow himself was forced out. After spending 7 years as a pioneering professor of pathological anatomy, he returned to politics, albeit with a less revolutionary agenda. But Virchow's earlier social medicine ideas spread throughout Europe, to the Americas, and beyond, where they were kept alive through generations of social medicine adherents and labor and political movements that systematically documented the social and political underpinnings of ill health and challenged the emerging (bio)medical model (Brown and Birn 2013).

One of the most important 20th century heirs to the social medicine approach was Salvador Allende, a physician and a founder of the Chilean Socialist Party. Allende's social medicine roots date from his days as a medical student activist. When the Popular Front coalition of leftist parties won the 1938 national elections, Allende became Health Minister. In his 1939 book *The Chilean Socio-Medical Reality* (*La realidad médico-social Chilena*), Allende outlined the relationship between poor social conditions and ill health; like Virchow's, his prescription included social reforms such as more equal income distribution and better housing (Waitzkin 2011). As Minister, and later Senator, Allende shepherded into law Chile's National Health Service, convinced it would help "prevent the tremendous injustices that arise due to the existence in this country of distinct social strata" (Allende 1951, p. 1525). Allende was elected President of Chile in 1970, committing suicide during a 1973 US-backed, right-wing military coup that aborted his government's policies against exploitation, imperialism, and other forms of oppression.

Latin American social medicine traditions extend both backward in time—to Ecuadorian physician Eugenio Espejo, who in the 18th century struggle against Spanish oppression identified the connection between epidemics and poverty (Breilh and Paz y Miño 2001), portending Virchow's more famous critique—and forward. Argentine physician Ernesto "Che" Guevara, who participated with Fidel Castro in the 1959 Cuban Revolution, came to see revolution as an extension of social medicine:

> integrating the doctor or any other health worker into the revolutionary movement [is crucial], because . . . the work of educating and feeding the children . . . and . . . of redistributing the land from its former absentee landlords to those who sweat every day on that very land without reaping its fruits—is the grandest social medicine effort that has been done in Cuba (Guevara 1960, p. 119).

We return to Latin American social medicine in chapter 13, and throughout the text refer to the work of many practitioner- and scholar-activists around the world who engage in political economy of health analyses and participate in social (medicine) movements.

Critical Political Economy of (Global) Health Framework

According to a political economy perspective, social structures (namely, observable, patterned relationships among groups, i.e., *relations of power*), and the asymmetries of power perpetuated through these structures, are largely (though not entirely) determined by political and economic forces. Economic power roughly correlates with social and political power and, in Karl Marx's term, relations to the means of production (i.e., whether one is an owner or a worker). As such, business owners have more power than workers, property owners more power than tenants, and so on.

As noted, a political economy analysis shows how political, social, and economic factors are intertwined at societal, community, and household levels to produce health or ill health in individuals. Economically, this approach assesses the ownership of national resources, the main engines of the economy, and what a country buys and sells on international markets. Socially, the approach examines the organization of society (its social arrangement and stratification), including by class, race, and gender divisions, and the extent to which certain social groups are marginalized. Politically, the approach assesses the organization and distribution of political power at local, national, and international levels, as well as the extent of human rights and political freedoms.

Some critics argue that, with its HIC provenance, political economy of health underplays the importance of various dimensions of power, such as race/ethnicity, gender, Indigeneity, subaltern and (neo-)colonial oppression, and biological embodiment of political and social processes (Jones 2013). As Boaventura de Sousa Santos (2014) argues, there is a fundamental need for "epistemologies of the South" to overcome the cognitive injustice created by the centuries-long Western dismissal of knowledge, practices, and existential meaning generated in the Global South. We return to these issues in subsequent chapters.

Incorporating a range of power dimensions and helping visualize the interplay of these factors, Figure 3-3 schematically represents a critical political economy of health framework. It delineates how the broad political, social, and economic order, relations, and interests affect and interact with health conditions in individual, household, community, local, national, and global (or micro, meso, and macro) contexts. This approach seeks to understand how power relations influence absolute and relative access to the medical, environmental, economic, and other societal determinants of health. As with any such visual scheme, the framework portrays relationships but cannot convey processes. Generally speaking, conditions and forces on the left shape those to the right, either directly or indirectly. Health and disease at the individual level, are thus shaped by and interconnect with all of these global, national, and community-level determinants.

Key factors that influence health directly and indirectly include: distribution of wealth and power; the larger political order; historical experiences of colonialism and militarism; class, racial/ethnic, and gendered social structures; and global trade and financial regimes. Trade agreements and treaties, for example, typically eliminate subsidies and protections for minor producers in LMICs, and encourage entry of agribusiness transnational corporations (TNCs) that displace small farmers, incentivize mono-cropping, and lead to environmental degradation, together resulting in declines in land tenure, food production for export rather than local consumption, and concomitant income declines and nutritional deficiencies, all affecting health. Of course, structural factors can also generate positive consequences: land redistribution and equitable trade policies can improve farmer livelihoods; and democratization of power can help meet the collective demands of those formerly excluded from decisionmaking.

As we explore these processes and seek to understand health and disease patterns within and between populations and countries, it is important to include the role of local agency (and variation across settings) in shaping public policies and consequent health outcomes. Of course at the "local" level there are many groups representing different ideological, political, and cultural stances that create internal clashes, compromise, and competition. Power differences between groups, as well as varying degrees of state corruption and adherence to democratic processes, shape whose interests are served and whose are ignored, whether in HICs, like the United States or Lichtenstein, or LMICs, such as Mongolia or Togo.

Although a political economy of health framework offers the most integrative approach to addressing health issues—involving biological, behavioral, and structural elements—it has been sidelined by most mainstream policymakers as overly ambitious and thus impossible to achieve in the short or medium term (Birdsall 1994). The World Bank has repeatedly asserted that "In the past 100 to 150 years, medical technologies have been effective at saving lives from a range of fatal diseases" (World Bank 2016a, p. 35). Indeed, World Bank-sponsored studies seek to highlight disease control priorities in terms of how best to roll out technologies (Frost and Reich 2009), giving little consideration to contextual and political economy factors. Technological measures are undoubtedly important, but as poignantly articulated by a malnourished person living with HIV in Mozambique, if "All I eat is ARVs" (Kalofonos 2010, p. 363), this means technology, not people, come first (Biehl and Petryna 2013).

Why is the seemingly obvious role of political economy left out of these analyses? The simplest explanation is that it challenges dominant political and economic forces: biomedical and behavioral approaches are compatible with and reinforce the status quo of the international distribution of power and resources. The behavioral approach seeks the answer to ill health through individual actions, and the biomedical approach through technical interventions, with overlap between the two. As such, most global health initiatives emphasize, many exclusively so, techno-behavioral solutions. For example, Roll Back Malaria provides therapies and insecticide-treated bednets to control malaria,

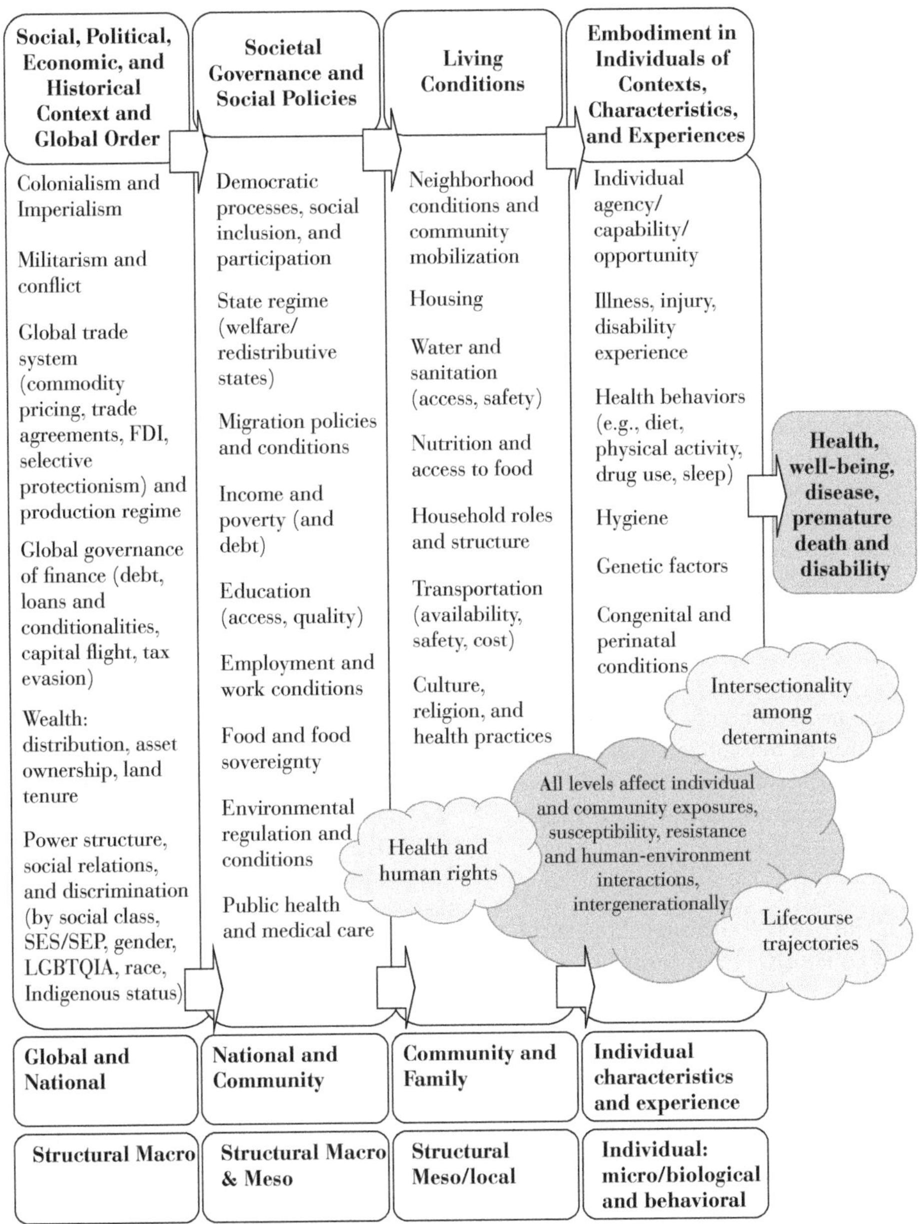

Figure 3-3: Political economy of global health framework.
Source: Extensively adapted with permission from Gloyd (1987).

instead of also integrating these with social and political measures around improved housing and clean water access as part of a larger strategy to address the underlying determinants and causes of malaria, including unfair distribution of societal resources.

Table 3-1 provides a summary of the central questions that run through political economy of health writings as articulated by Vicente Navarro, a Catalan doctor who in the 1960s fled Franco's dictatorship in Spain, becoming (as professor at Johns Hopkins University) one of the world's leading critics of

Table 3-1 Critical Political Economy Questions from the Writings of Vicente Navarro

Questions Relating to the Structure, Relations, and Organization of Society	Implications for Health
Economic structure: • Who owns and controls what? • What does a country produce? • What does it buy and sell on the international market?	• Social (by class, race, gender) patterns of population health inequities (see chapter 7) • Production and trade-related effects on health (see chapter 9)
Social structure: • Who works in what sector? • What are the class/race/gender structures of ownership and labor?	• Type and orientation of health care system (universal coverage vs. universal access; selective vs. comprehensive primary health care; public system vs. privatized services; health promotion vs. disease emphasis) (see chapter 11)
Political structure: • Who wields political power? • How is power distributed?	• Redistribution and building healthy societies (see chapter 13)

Source: Inspired by and adapted from Navarro (2009); Coburn (2015).

capitalism's effects on health. Navarro's questions are useful analytic tools, differing markedly from standard global health evaluations and analyses, which typically count interventions, health personnel and facilities, cost-effectiveness, and so on.

Using a Political Economy Approach to Analyze Health Problems

Life Expectancy Trends

A political economy of health approach remains as relevant today as it was in the 19th century, helping to explicate why overall global trends of life expectancy increases have seen extraordinary reversals in certain settings facing cataclysmic circumstances (Figure 3-4).

Perhaps the most well-known illustration of how contemporary life expectancy patterns remain highly sensitive to political, social, and economic conditions can be found in the case of life expectancy, which dropped dramatically in various African countries (by over 15 years in the case of Botswana and Zimbabwe) starting in the mid-1980s, only beginning to recuperate in the mid to late 2000s (Figure 3-5). While most global health agencies and analysts attribute this mortality pattern to HIV—and the behavioral/cultural dimensions of its sexual transmission (World Bank 2006)—a political economy of health approach offers a deeper explanation (Katz 2002). High rates of HIV and deaths from AIDS are but the visible epidermis of complex layers of historical events and relations that in turn shape present-day disease circumstances (Ichoku, Mooney, and Ataguba 2013; Parikh 2007). The effects of both colonial and current structures of favoritism, land dispossession, brutal authoritarian regimes (bolstered by Cold War rivalries and TNC interests), racial discrimination, environmental and human exploitation, debt, structural adjustment and austerity, gender oppression, and labor migration have coalesced to create ideal conditions for the spread of HIV via work and social survival patterns, extreme poverty, and social desperation (Doyal 2013; Fassin 2006; Hunter 2010). Premature death is further facilitated by crumbling health care systems, global patent protection regimes, and rapacious pharmaceutical prices, which together limit access to care and medication.

To be sure, civil society activism and government measures from South Africa to Brazil have played a key role in challenging the power of Big Pharma and the intransigence of national governments (see chapters 9 and 11). Also essential is the fact that the spread of HIV coincided with structural adjustment austerity across LMICs,

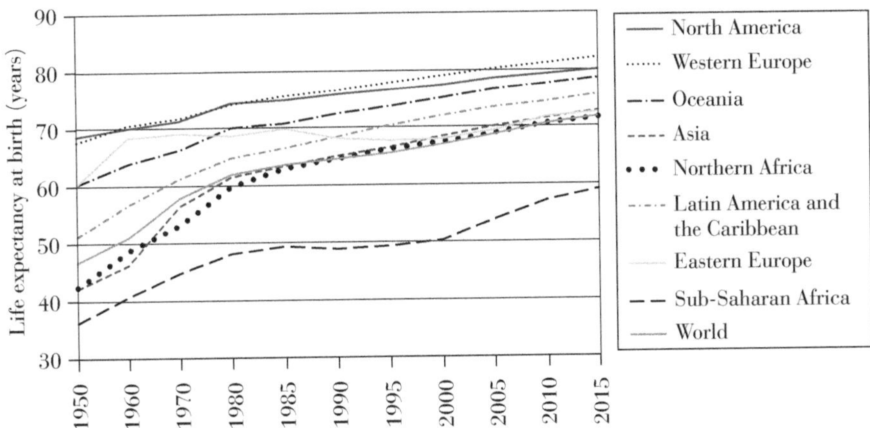

Figure 3-4: Trends in life expectancy by region (5-year averages), 1950–2015.
Data Source: UN (2015c).

both exacerbating AIDS and also provoking a far wider mortality crisis in Africa involving, inter alia, infant mortality and TB, due to much reduced public health funding for treatment and control (Bijlmakers, Bassett, and Sanders 1998; Maynard, Shircliff, and Restivo 2012).

In another part of the world, following the collapse of the Soviet Union, why did rates and deaths from infectious disease, violence, and chronic diseases increase, leading to an unprecedented 5-year drop in life expectancy in an industrialized setting? The explanations are linked to the severe social, economic, and political upheaval of the 1990s, including massive deindustrialization of the country (except for extractive sectors) and the dismantling of Soviet social protection and safety net systems. The effects of "shock therapy" capitalism in the early 1990s and the 1998 devaluation of the ruble and ensuing financial crisis were even more extreme in the Russian Federation than in other former Soviet republics, as seen in comparative life expectancy patterns (Figure 3-6).

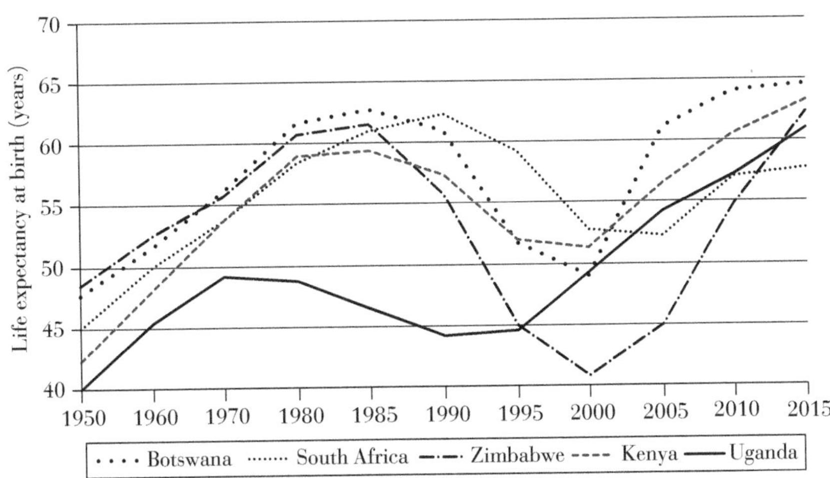

Figure 3-5: Trends in life expectancy in selected sub-Saharan African countries (5-year averages), 1950–2015.
Data Source: UN (2015c).

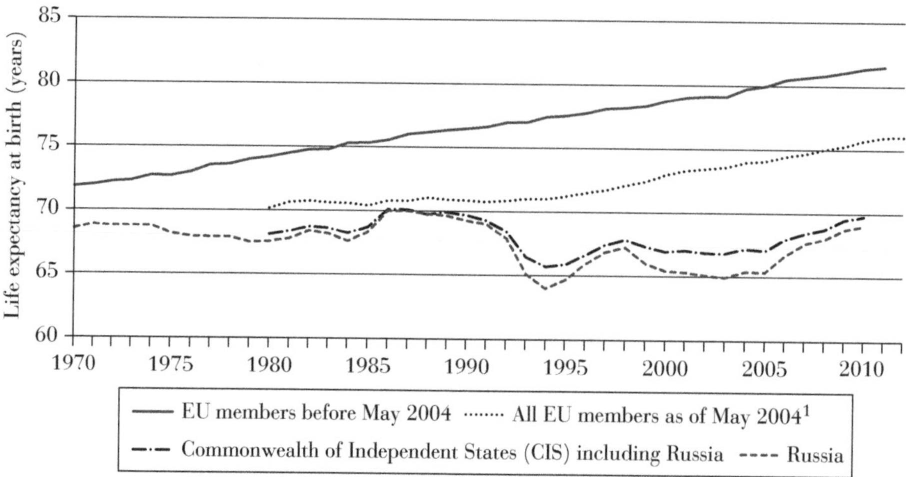

Figure 3-6: Life expectancy in EU member states and the Commonwealth of Independent States, 1970–2012.
Data Source: WHO EURO (2014).

Case Study: Life Expectancy in Russia Following the Dissolution of the USSR

When the Soviet Union dissolved in 1991, many believed that the establishment of a capitalist economy would rapidly generate untold improvements in health and well-being. The reality proved otherwise: rather than bettering quality of life, it worsened (Stuckler, King, and McKee 2009). The shift from socialism to market capitalism provoked social disruption, sharp declines in per capita income, unemployment, and deteriorating health conditions. Between 1987 and 1994 there was a 50% increase in premature death for Russian males, with a slight recovery until 1998 when the ruble collapsed, leading to economic chaos. At the lowest point in 1994, overall life expectancy was 64.5 years (males 57.6 years; females 71.7 years).

Underscoring these patterns were explosive increases in violent and occupational deaths, suicide, chronic diseases, and a resurgence of previously controlled infectious diseases (Men et al. 2003). For example, a diphtheria epidemic swept through Russia and former Soviet republics from 1991 to 1997, with 140,000 cases and 4,000 deaths (Vitek and Wharton 1998).

Russia's economy slowly recovered by the mid-2000s, yet in 2009 Russia's male life expectancy, at 62.8 years, was still barely higher than the 1960 figure of 62.1 years. This mostly reflected the situation of the working class population and marked the country's "protracted demographic crisis since the end of communist rule" (Eberstadt 2010).

By 2014, male life expectancy at birth rose to 65 years; female, to 76 years (World Bank 2016b). But HIV, drug-related deaths, and TB continue to ravage the lives of many young men. The rates of adult male mortality in Russia (as well as Kazakhstan and Turkmenistan) are currently similar to those in sub-Saharan Africa, and the countries of the former Soviet Union (with the exception of the Baltic states) have worse overall life expectancy than all world regions except South Asia and sub-Saharan Africa (ibid).

One view is that male mortality, in particular, is related to abuse of alcohol, especially vodka. Soviet restrictions on alcohol in 1985 resulted in a 25% decline in premature male deaths (under 55 years of age); however, with the collapse of the USSR, drinking rates increased sharply as did the number of premature deaths. By 2006, premature deaths started to decline again in part due to restrictions on alcohol production and sales, albeit with 37% of men continuing to die under the age of 55, compared with 7% in the UK (Zaridze et al. 2014).

Blaming alcohol use for high mortality in Russia is nothing new. A decade ago the World Bank proffered its own behavioral analysis, recommending that Russians "ease back on the bottle, cut down on smoking, watch their diet, and lead healthier lives" (Reuters, Moscow, Dec. 8, 2005 cited in [King, Stuckler, and Hamm 2006, p. 16]). The Bank's rationale for targeting specific factors rather than the changed economic and social context was based on gender differences in smoking and alcohol consumption, which, they argued, partially protected women and validated their findings in men (World Bank 2005).

While the male–female gap in life expectancy is almost twice as large as in most HICs, Russian women's life expectancy also trails behind European figures, with close to 1 million excess deaths per year beyond expected mortality rates, into the mid-2000s. Part of the explanation resides in widening educational and social class differentials in mortality. Russia's mortality increases mainly affected less educated (with less than high school completion) men and women, whose mortality differences with university-educated counterparts grew ten-fold over the crisis, concomitant with the loss of universal protections. Meanwhile gender differentials in life expectancy stayed constant among the university educated but grew among those with less education (Vandenheede et al. 2014). Larger male–female differences among less-educated groups may derive from women's greater flexibility in a changing economic environment and better collective coping mechanisms against stress.

Indeed, independent experts present a much more complex picture of differential mortality and morbidity rates that go far beyond alcohol and behavioral factors to include the collapse of public infrastructure and social safety nets, significant declines in the minimum wage, mounting class divergence in living standards, deregulation of ethanol (alcohol) production, and loss of employment protections. All of these stressors influenced smoking, drinking, and dietary patterns, among other pathways that have heightened exposure and susceptibility to disease, leading to premature death (Bessudnov et al. 2012; Shkolnikov et al. 2014). Also missing in the World Bank's analysis are the restructuring of, and sharp decline in funding for, public health and medical services in the 1991–2005 period, driven by market-oriented reforms (Aleksandrova et al. 2013), as well as huge increases in the cost of living, especially housing and food prices.

Comparing Bio-Behavioral and Political Economy Approaches

Comparative analyses of bio-behavioral and political economy approaches to particular health problems and to global health overall are illuminating. For instance, not only do causal explanations for high diarrheal rates diverge, the range and level of prevention and treatment responses are of an entirely different order (Table 3-2).

A similar analysis can be made for chronic kidney disease (CKD), laying out the causal explanations and therapeutics from medical and behavioral perspectives compared with a political economy counterpart. Between 1990 and 2013, the global age-standardized mortality rate from CKD increased from 11.6 to 15.8 deaths per 100,000 population and it went from being the 27th to the 13th leading cause of death (Naghavi et al. 2015). CKD is a soaring global problem arising from both chronic conditions, such as diabetes and hypertension, and infections—including HIV, TB, malaria, hepatitis B and C, and parasitic diseases—plus use of poor quality medicines and exposure to pesticides, heavy metals, and industrial waste. Even though most of these wide-ranging determinants stem from substandard living and working conditions, reflecting larger societal oppression, the major global health emphasis has been on early detection and management of hypertension and diabetes (which account for less than half of kidney disease cases). In focusing so narrowly on these factors, structural determinants are left out, and epidemiological research does not adequately examine environmental and work-related conditions and hazards.

To illustrate, in settings as distinct as Central America, Egypt, India, and Sri Lanka, an epidemic of CKD in agricultural workers has raised questions around "non-traditional" causes: growing evidence suggests exposure to toxic agents (especially pesticides and heavy metals) and strenuous work conditions in agribusiness plantations (causing severe dehydration and heat stress) are the principal factors (Hanson et al. 2014; Orantes Navarro et al. 2015; Ordunez et al. 2014), yet mainstream health agencies, in part pressured by the industries involved, have been slow to recognize CKD in agricultural workers as a problem, and when they have, the focus has been on genetic and behavioral approaches (Lenzer 2015; Ramirez-Rubio et al. 2013).

Table 3-2 Causes of and Therapeutics for Diarrhea According to Contrasting Approaches to Health

- Approximately 1.7 billion cases worldwide each year (WHO 2013)
- Second largest postneonatal killer of children globally—accounting for an estimated 550,000 deaths of children under 5 per year (UNICEF 2015)
- A leading cause of malnutrition in children under 5 (WHO 2013)

Approach to Health	Determinants/Causal Explanations	Prevention/Treatment
Biomedical	• Infectious agents enter the body and cause illness • Certain intestinal diseases or other illnesses or disorders • Allergic reaction to certain foods or medications • Death occurs primarily as a result of dehydration	• Vaccines against certain viruses and bacteria that cause diarrhea • Antibiotic/antiparasitic drugs • Oral rehydration therapy (ORT)
Behavioral	• Ingesting food or water contaminated with an infectious agent • Lack of knowledge/education about infectious agents and treatment • Lack of personal hygiene, such as hand-washing • Inadequate use of health services	• Avoiding untreated water and potentially infected food • Improving health education regarding causes and treatment of diarrhea • Improving personal hygiene, including hand-washing practices
Political economy	Biobehavioral explanations above nested within: • Lack of access to safe water • Poor basic sanitation • Lack of access to primary health care • Poverty/malnutrition • Crowded shelter • Water privatization • Austerity cutbacks/tax declines on wealthy • Revenue insufficiencies due to capital flight/tax evasion • Agribusiness misuse of water • Global economic and trade regime skewed against needs of poor	• Universal access to safe drinking water; water as a human right • Improving sanitation and living conditions, including housing and nutrition (also to stave off respiratory co-infection) • Universal access to health care • Social protections; fair wages • Redistribution of wealth and political power all shaping and interacting with biobehavioral measures specified above

In sum, that political economy approaches to global health are overlooked is itself a political economy issue. That is to say, naming the political, corporate, and other forces that shape health and disease is not in the interest of major power wielders within and across societies; thus, such perspectives are rarely articulated by mainstream global health scientists and other actors.

Not only does a critical political economy of health lens prompt us to broach such difficult questions, it also seeks to understand *why* inequities exist and explores what can and should be done about them.

This framework's interrogating of class, race and ethnic, and gender relations and the distribution of resources (skills, access to finance, wealth, etc.) is threatening both to those with significant political and economic power and to those comfortably oblivious to national and worldwide poverty and social inequalities.

Imagine you are a middle-aged minibus driver in a highly populated city. The government regulates emissions and traffic safety standards. You are a member of a union and receive benefits and inflation-linked wage increases negotiated by the union. You work 8 hours per day, 5 days a week, and earn paid holidays and sick days. According to national workplace regulations, you have the right, daily, to two 20-minute (toilet) breaks and an hour-long lunch period and are encouraged to participate in neighborhood-sponsored sporting events and physical activities. The transit depots for bus drivers offer a lunch program with nutritious food options. Your salary enables you to adequately meet living expenses for your family, including a home (located half an hour from your workplace) with consistent supplies of electricity, potable running water, and proper sanitation for all residents. Thanks to redistributive social policies and a progressive and efficient taxation system—with revenues assured by global rules against illicit financial flows—the state fully covers medical care and education through high school and subsidizes university tuition.

During one of your yearly medical check-ups, your doctor discusses the potential problems of high blood pressure, high cholesterol, and heart disease given your occupation and family history. She recommends that you take greater advantage of healthy meals and exercise programs at your workplace; reviews the possible need for medication should you develop high blood pressure; asks you about your work, community, and home environments in seeking to identify and reduce sources of stress and help prevent future illness; and encourages you to keep politically active.

What more might be done to understand and address your health problems?

Reimagining the life and health of this bus driver shows the relevance and importance of stretching beyond biomedical and behavioral models in order to understand how health is affected by global, societal, workplace, and municipal policies, intertwined with and influencing health status, as evidenced in a political economy of health framework (Figure 3-3). The bus driver could be 35 years old or 65, female or male, in Berlin, Bangkok, or Bogotá; the broad determinants of her/his health and illness do not change, although the social, political, and cultural contexts mediate particular responses to agents of disease. Earlier in the chapter we presented a case study of how poor working and social conditions—and concentration of political power among white elites—in South Africa led to high incidence of TB among Black miners. We also examined what happened when a broad system of social protection was dismantled with the dissolution of the Soviet Union. *Consider how the life of the bus driver might change under such conditions . . .*

Undoubtedly, there are limits to prevailing approaches to understanding and addressing national and international patterns of health and disease. Rather than looking to individual (biological and/or behavioral) characteristics, a critical political economy approach examines health and health equity in relation to a range of societal factors, in an effort to inform greater understanding and effective action. Now we turn to a critical political economy analysis of global development, exploring how contemporaneous strategies seek to address the challenges of social well-being and health through various economic, foreign aid, social, and governance approaches and what are their shortcomings.

POLITICAL ECONOMY OF DEVELOPMENT (AND HEALTH)

Key Questions:

- How is global health linked to development?
- Which development strategies have IFIs favored in recent years and what are the implications for LMICs?
- How are foreign policy, development, and health connected?
- What are the major sources of contention over development aid?

While global health is a large and complex domain, like its colonial medicine and international health predecessors, it is not set apart from social and geopolitical arenas but deeply embedded in them. In particular, the sphere of international development, which brings together economic, foreign policy, and a host of societal well-being issues, interacts closely with global health ideas and practices. We begin this section of the chapter by analyzing contemporary development discourses and practices through a political economy lens. We then pick up where chapter 2's discussion of neoliberalism and health ended, examining IFI development strategies since the mid-1990s, the foreign policy-development-health nexus, and aid effectiveness from donor and "recipient" sides, especially as applied to health aid. Next, we turn to the problem of aid in the context of debt burdens and the trade system, casting doubt on the overall development enterprise in the absence of a wholesale revamping of global economic relations. Subsequently, we review current development and health approaches including, "development as freedom," "sustainable development," human rights, the UN's development goals, global governance concerns as applied to health, and the dilemmas of growing TNC presence in these arenas.

What is *development*? A range of associations may come to mind: progress; economic expansion; productivity; industrialization; profitability; better health, education, and well-being; democracy; improved living and working conditions; loss of tradition; uneven growth and inequality; and economic globalization, among other concepts.

Despite extensive use, development and the term *developing countries* have no universal definitions (Rist 2007), even as both concepts are widely invoked to describe and justify an array of social and economic schemes (Box 3-2). Notwithstanding definitional ambiguities, development is a large domain involving multiple players: government

Box 3-2 What's in a Name?: Categorizing Countries by "Development" Level

In comparing different countries and their political and economic trajectories, politicians, researchers, and practitioners use certain social and economic labels and dichotomies as shorthand. Terms such as *developed* vs. *developing, Global North* vs. *Global South, industrialized* vs. *industrializing, wealthy* vs. *poor*, or the descriptors *low-income, middle-income*, and *high-income* are the most commonly used. Most of these are value-laden and rank countries according to a generalized hierarchy based on stage of "human development," colonial stereotypes, or social and economic "advancement" according to crude criteria (Box 2-3). These are often defined in terms of gross national income (GNI[a]) per capita but may include gender empowerment, school attendance, life expectancy, access to piped water and other factors linked to standard of living (see Human Development Index in Box 3-3).

These categorizations do not take into account fundamental social (and health) distinctions across the world, including the social class divide through which upper class elites in both HICs and LMICs (and transnationally) wield unequal power and advance their own interests over workers and marginalized populations, resulting in inequitable distribution of power and resources both among and within countries. Nor do they consider histories of colonialism, slavery, and ongoing imperialism in shaping power differentials. As discussed in chapter 7, class power interacts and intersects with other forms of power and oppression, especially racism and patriarchy. Global political and economic forces further influence the shape of domestic policies: power differentials and geopolitical struggles between larger and smaller economies, both historically and contemporaneously, shape class relations and constrain the ability of countries to redistribute resources and wealth.

During the Cold War, a categorization emerged that at least partially reflected political ideologies and realities but has largely fallen out of favor: First World (industrialized, capitalist countries); Second World (industrialized/ing communist countries); and Third World (mostly former colonies "held back" through unfair trade systems and political domination) (also see chapter 2) (Sauvy 1952). The contested terms *underdeveloped* countries (referring to development arrested by global capitalist forces) and the perhaps willfully naïve *resource-poor* countries (ironically, most countries designated as such have enormous resource wealth, if little control and/or minimal redistribution of it) also appeared in this period. Whereas Third World remains favored by some for its association with the non-aligned political movement for sovereignty among "poorer nations" (Prashad 2013), Global South is employed by others who prefer this geographic (perhaps evoking "tropical") as opposed to political designation, even as various Global South countries (e.g., so-called Western European offshoots, like Australia) do not fit the presumed categorization. Others use "World Systems" classifications of core, periphery, and semi-periphery. When possible we use the newer *Majority World*, coined by Bangladeshi photographer Shahidul Alam (2008), to avoid the disparaging stereotypes of poor communities and poor regions and re-center the debate around addressing development needs for the majority rather than the economic and political imperatives of the *Minority World*.

Yet because the current dominant classification of countries and collection of data is according to income per capita levels—per the World Bank's 2016-2017 classification high-income countries (HICs: \$12,476 or more GNI/capita), and low- and middle-income countries (LMICs: upper-middle: \$4,036 - \$12,475 GNI/capita; lower-middle: \$1,026 - \$4,035 GNI/capita; low-income \$1,025 or less GNI/capita) and various gradations therein—the textbook mostly relies on these for consistency. However, we recognize that these terms tell us very little about the nature of societies, their governments and other institutions, social structures, historical trajectories, cultures and values, and social policies, let alone how these factors manifest in health conditions and outcomes. Though these various classifications can be useful for grouping apparently similar countries and regions together, they risk oversimplifying differences among countries and obscure social and economic inequalities within each society. An alternative political-economy classification might incorporate both GNI/capita level and the structures and relations of political power in terms of redistribution and battling oppression, showcasing how societies that share power and allocate resources more equitably are healthier even without high per capita income levels. In chapters 7 and 13 we discuss different kinds of welfare states and their implications for health equity and building healthy societies across the world.

[a] GNI refers to income and taxes earned by the residents and government of a country from both domestic and international sources.

ministries, multilateral agencies, big and small business, technical experts, philanthropies, politicians, social movements, NGOs, and, most importantly, the population of places subject to development. Accordingly, as argued by the late Uruguayan novelist Eduardo Galeano, experts' designation of "developing countries" may most accurately depict places "trampled by someone else's development" (Galeano 2001, p. 36).

Although a detailed examination of development is beyond the scope of this book (there is a brief historical account in chapter 2), it is important to signal that various analysts recognize many of the contemporary crises facing the world (see chapter 8) as deriving from problematic forms of development: violent, oppressive, extractive, and discriminatory political arrangements, colonial planning and industrial practices, as well as ongoing prejudices, exploitation, and other features of the post-war development project as a whole (Hodge 2016b). The recurring theme that there is a moral responsibility for development by the "West for the rest" is linked to an ongoing set of dilemmas: a paradigm implemented by HICs is called upon to resolve the contradictions of uneven global development engendered by this very paradigm (Harvey 2006), with development ideologies and practices sustaining historical power asymmetries (Sumner 2006).

Still, the critique that "[d]evelopment was—and continues to be for the most part—a top-down, ethnocentric, and technocratic approach, which treated people and cultures as abstract concepts, statistical figures to be moved up and down in the charts of 'progress'" (Escobar 2011, p. 44) seems overly generalized and does not adequately reflect dynamics over time and place (Hodge 2016a). The questions of how and how much development efforts are shaped by larger power relations and societal structures at local, national, and transnational or imperial levels—and the diversity of experiences of contestation, albeit constrained by power structures (Sahle 2011)—remains a key tension of the development arena.

Recognizing greater primacy for human action as a way of reclaiming development may also overstate the agency of people living in circumstances of poverty and social and political oppression, past and present. Indeed, Johan Galtung's (1969) notion of structural violence, adapted to the health arena by medical anthropologists such as Paul Farmer (2004) and Didier Fassin (1996), points to how political-economy-framed structures and processes (discussed earlier in the chapter) are biologically embodied (see chapter 7)—creating a kind of biologized inequality. As such, material needs, the distribution of resources, and the possibilities of collective political change remain bound and constrained by the larger context (Sridhar 2008). Under such conditions, the bulk of global health and development "interventions into the lives of other peoples" (Packard 2016) are either complicit in maintaining structural imbalances of power or are unable to transcend them.

Among the many research insights of recent years are that the side effects of development projects may be far more consequential than the actual projects, themselves invariably unable to reach the stated objective of "helping poor people." In fact, the understandings of development actors may bear little resemblance to reality. One striking example is the World Bank's troubled 1970s–1980s agricultural scheme in Lesotho. There, "experts" erroneously characterized the majority of the population as farmers in need of education and technical inputs to increase agricultural productivity and income, all the while ignoring the historical legacy of Dutch land-encroachment policies that made land parcels so small that surplus production was near impossible. These experts also ignored ways to improve working conditions for migrant workers in South African mines, which was the source of most household income in Lesotho (Ferguson 1990).

Dominant development actors ought not simply be excused for failing to achieve program goals due to unforeseeable factors or local complexities and commended for inadvertent outcomes that may change circumstances for the better. As evidenced by the World Bank's 1980s–1990s nutrition project in Tamil Nadu, India, there was a mismatch between how "experts" measured and evaluated malnutrition and how it was understood on the ground. Contemptibly, the World Bank misleadingly touted the project as a success and deployed it as a blueprint across multiple settings (Sridhar 2008). Not only are these fraught claims tragic for the purported beneficiaries, the Bank's considerable control over development funding and approaches gives such manipulations of evidence enormous bearing on how development is and is not practiced.

> "I sit on a man's back, choking him and making him carry me, and yet assure myself and others that I am very sorry for him and wish to ease his lot by all possible means except by getting off his back."—Leo Tolstoy (1886).

To be sure, across distinct eras mainstream development analysts, whether from HICs or LMICs, have been critiqued for providing inconsistent and unfounded advice to LMIC governments. Paternalistic economic prescriptions—and even more "consensual" forms of development aid between HIC or BRICS (Brazil, Russia, India, China, South Africa) donors and LMIC "partners"—are often self-interested, damaging, serve as a disincentive for governments to act on their own, and prevent societies from choosing their own path (Deaton 2013; Easterly 2014). Yet a slew of books critical of development aid patterns—each with a scheme for change, whether calling for more aid, less aid, or better aid (Collier 2007; Banerjee and Duflo 2011; Easterly 2014; Moyo 2009; Ncayiyana 2007; Sachs 2015) reproduces the mentality of seeking to fix development without altering global and domestic structures of power, including in the contemporary era of neoliberal capitalism. Jeffrey Sachs, for example, argues that aid is a "practical bargain": a set of simple steps realizable "at a cost that would be nearly unnoticeable to the world's wealthiest nations" and that would "eas[e] the economic and environmental strains" imposed on impoverished nations (Sachs 2008, p. 36). At a multilateral level, much of the recent debate on development aid has been about how to improve its effectiveness without addressing larger power imbalances, as discussed ahead.

Furthermore, most development aid critiques do not take into sufficient account the role of colonial exploitation in enabling Western industrial development in the first place and of neocolonialism continuing today in creating vast inequalities between and within countries that are perpetuated by the current global order via foreign investment patterns, indebtedness, unfair terms of trade, capital flight, tax evasion, and aid (Kothari 2005) (see chapter 9).

Zambian economist Dambisa Moyo argues that the Western aid system is authoritarian, infantilizing, and damaging to the poor:

> Scarcely does one see Africa's (elected) officials or those African policymakers charged with a development portfolio offer an opinion on what should be done, or what might actually work to save the continent from its regression. This very important responsibility has, for all intents and purposes, and to the bewilderment of many an African, been left to musicians [e.g., Irish rockstar, Bono, who was instrumental in convincing US President George Bush to finance PEPFAR] who reside outside Africa (Moyo 2009, p. 27).

Moyo's remedy is African entrepreneurialism, hardly the stuff of equitable redistribution within societies. Counter to this, documented development successes have historically occurred where free trade or neoliberal nostrums have been defied (Currie-Alder et al. 2014) through protectionist and redistributional strategies. This holds whether in HICs starting in the 19th century or East Asian countries, which pursued import substitution industrialization since the 1950s and 1960s.

Yet mainstream criticisms of development have largely sidestepped these matters. A contemporary pairing of the discourse of development with more flexible qualifiers, such as "human," "social," and "sustainable," at least rhetorically seeks to create distance from neoliberal development orthodoxy (Rist 2007). As we shall see, it is highly debatable whether this new era of "millennial" development is in any way more equitable and transformative than the prior orthodoxy.

IFI Development Strategies since the SAPs Debacle: Debt Relief and Poverty Reduction

Starting in the 1980s, structural adjustment programs (SAPs) and other loan conditionalities, the hallmark of neoliberal ideology as applied to LMICs (see chapter 2), imposed tremendous hardship on dozens of countries, undermining social well-being by reducing public education, public health, and other social-sector spending, jeopardizing both health and future economic security (Pfeiffer and Chapman 2010; Rowden 2009). Rather than stabilizing economies, the policies wreaked havoc by abolishing controls on financial flows and encouraging reliance on a few commodities for export earnings, leaving economies vulnerable to overnight crashes as prices of copper, coffee, or cotton plummeted. Moreover, the combination of unfair lending practices and the IMF's inflation control measures locked countries into "debt bondage" which is near impossible to escape (Toussaint and Millet 2010).

Faced with mounting civil society activism and even critics from within (Stiglitz 2002), the IMF and World Bank were forced to respond to certain negative assessments of SAPs. In 1996, they jointly inaugurated the Heavily Indebted Poor Countries Initiative (HIPC) aimed at making the external debt of some of the world's poorest and most indebted countries "sustainable," and thus protecting creditors, the integrity of IFIs, and the larger global financial system. Indeed, HIPC does not cancel debt but provides "relief" for those countries complying with IMF economic conditions (for example around debt–export ratios). Though hailed for "constructively" addressing LMIC debt, HIPC has not included large countries (Brazil, Nigeria, India, Indonesia, China, Pakistan, Mexico, the Philippines, etc.) where most poor people live, instead covering just 11% of the LMIC population living in fewer than 40 countries. As well, debt servicing has actually increased, initially because HIPC countries had to take loans to pay off arrears to join the program (!), and later because IMF growth and export estimates (following implementation of IMF-recommended liberalization measures) were too "optimistic" and new loans had to be undertaken to meet HIPC conditions. Most importantly, HIPC governments, never creditors or IMF advisors, have been made responsible for debt even as the initiative augmented undemocratic, outside control over economic policies and continued exploitation of local resources (Katz 2005; Toussaint and Millet 2010).

Following further public-interest campaigning, the G8 countries (France, Germany, Italy, the United Kingdom, Japan, the United States, Canada, and Russia) agreed to a 2006 Multilateral Debt Relief Initiative (MDRI) fully "forgiving" the debts of countries satisfying at least 3 years of strict compliance with IFI criteria. Although debt relief was welcomed, the initiative resulted in similar terms as before, but with a slightly more human face. In 2015, the IMF determined that there was no longer outstanding MDRI-eligible debt. It terminated the MDRI and transferred remaining funding to a new Catastrophe Containment and Relief Trust launched in 2014 to provide loans and debt relief (with macroeconomic policy conditionalities) to countries hit by the Ebola epidemic and for future ecological and public health crises (IMF 2016d) (Table 3-3).

Meanwhile, the Poverty Reduction Strategy Papers (PRSPs; 1999–present) undergirding both HIPC and MDRI eligibility have offered a carrot of more "inclusive" approaches—whereby governments themselves design "pro-poor" efforts through greater country "ownership" and consultation with domestic and international development stakeholders—as well as a stick: needing to be endorsed by the IMF and World Bank boards before debt relief can be initiated. Thus, while more money has been designated to social sectors and reducing poverty, the IFIs have sought to guide this spending into particular sanctioned policies, such as conditional cash transfers. What is more, privatization, liberalization, and deregulation continued as terms of IFI agreements, with the added burden of micro-management through PRSPs (Dijkstra 2011; Rückert 2010).

Still, if the debt relief process imposes conditions on participating countries that are similarly onerous as under SAPs, it eventually frees up resources and decisionmaking latitude once debt servicing and IFI structures are terminated (Tan 2007). Cognizant of these new "policy spaces" for sovereign agenda-setting that potentially end the IMF's role in shaping LIC economic and social policies, the IMF has also developed Policy Support Instruments (PSIs) for countries that "graduate" from their loans yet wish to "voluntarily" receive advice and a credit rating, which is all but a prerequisite to participate in the global economy. As such, even the "enlightened" aim of poverty reduction and debt relief plays into the ongoing cycle of debt dependency and neoliberal globalization (Bretton Woods Project 2010).

In recent years, an alphabet soup of renewed loan facilities to replace SAPs has emerged under the umbrella of the IMF's Poverty Reduction and Growth Trust (PRGT), with concessional loans for low-income countries (LICs) (with lower interest rates and/or longer grace periods) and a range of non-concessional loans available to all IMF members. Responding to the global financial crisis of 2008, the PRGT offers three new credit facilities with different time frames (IMF 2016b) but requiring frequent monitoring and conditions, making LIC populations eternally indebted (literally, certainly not metaphorically!) to the financial elites of the global economy (PHM et al. 2014).

In sum, the IFIs are serving old wine—namely donor-driven priority setting and dominance over LMIC economies via new conditional loans drawing from the same market logic barrels as before (downsizing the state, deregulation, trade liberalization, etc.) (Toussaint and Millet 2010)—in new bottles, with labels touting more progressive rhetoric regardless of the similarity in content and effects.

Foreign Policy, Development, and Health

Global health cooperation is linked not only to development strategies but to foreign policy, with goals that go well beyond improving health conditions (see chapters 4 and 14 for discussion of health diplomacy). At the same time, given that global health "assistance" is usually accompanied by substantial matching donations at the country level, global health-related

Table 3-3 Selected IFI Development Strategies

	Heavily Indebted Poor Countries Initiative (HIPC)	Poverty Reduction Strategy Papers (PRSPs)	Multilateral Debt Relief Initiative (MDRI)	Policy Support Instruments (PSIs)	Poverty Reduction and Growth Trust (PRGT)
Main Actors	World Bank, IMF	World Bank (IDA), IMF (ECF)	IMF, World Bank (IDA), IDB, African Development Fund	IMF	IMF
Year Started	1996	1999	2006 (terminated in 2015)	2005	2010
Countries Involved	36 countries as of 2016, with 3 additional eligible countries	66 countries reporting PRSPs as of 2016; required from all countries seeking debt relief under HIPC	37 countries received debt relief by 2015	18 PSIs for 7 countries as of 2016	18 countries as of 2016
Main Features	Debt reduction for countries meeting the HIPC profile (and which have completed a PRSP); countries must adhere to certain policy conditions	Demonstrate how governments will achieve poverty reduction and macroeconomic growth through 3-year or longer programs, as "defined" by recipient countries with participation from domestic stakeholders, the IMF, and World Bank	Cancels 100% of debt from participating institutions for countries that have reached HIPC completion point (to help them achieve the MDGs)	Support to countries no longer getting IMF loans but seeking advice to "design effective economic programs that deliver clear signals to donors, multilateral development banks, and markets of the Fund's endorsement of the strength of a member's policies" (IMF 2016e).	Three concessional facilities for LICs with zero interest until end of 2016 (permanently zero rate for Rapid Credit Facility [RCF]): the Extended Credit Facility (ECF) for medium-long-term loans; the Standby Credit Facility (SCF) for short-term balance of payments needs; the RCF for urgent balance of payments needs (without conditionalities)

Sources: IMF (2015, 2016a, 2016b, 2016c, 2016e); World Bank (2011).

activities constitute a sizeable component of health-related spending across the world. Approximately US$180 billion in overall bilateral and multilateral development assistance in 2014 went to economic development and infrastructure, debt relief, disease control, and other sectors (OECD 2016b). Of this total, about US$20 billion was for health (with another US$16 billion coming from private foundations and partnerships) (IHME 2016), not counting military spending in health (the amounts are not public knowledge-see chapter 4).

The selected foreign policy statements examined here offer a window on the larger geopolitical context of development and health aid from the perspective of major donors. Generally, longtime foreign policy strategies of dominant capitalist countries, including the United States, the United Kingdom, and Canada, cover development, defense, market access, and diplomacy, reflecting economic priorities of safeguarding global capitalism with accompanying political and security concerns. Indeed, most HIC development agencies are located within or closely connected to foreign affairs, and increasingly trade, ministries (Hyman 2010).

Official US foreign policy goals include: "eliminating extreme poverty and promoting sustainable development," "[advancing] democracy and human rights," "[promoting] trade and investment to harness job-rich economic growth," and "improving global health security" (United States Government 2015). Yet these priorities are not evenly balanced. For example, in the 1980s and early 1990s, Israel and Egypt were the largest beneficiaries of US assistance, reflecting their strategic and political importance. Even today, Israel—categorized as an HIC—receives more US aid than some of the world's poorest countries—about US$360 per capita (Sharp 2015) compared with US$12 per capita received by Burkina Faso (OECD 2016b).

As during the Cold War, when combatting communism was a prime development rationale, the current context of the "war on terror" leads the US Agency for International Development (USAID) to conflate foreign policy goals with development objectives (Essex 2013). Unabashedly nesting development goals in this fashion is neither new nor masked. As USAID itself notes, "U.S. foreign assistance has always had the twofold purpose of furthering America's interests while improving lives in the developing world" (USAID 2016). Yet many health and development workers are surprisingly unaware of this reality.

Canada—like the United States—has national interests in mind when providing foreign assistance, with aid justified on the basis of: enhancing commerce and "stimulating sustainable economic growth"; responding to humanitarian needs; and promoting "Canadian values," outlined as "responsible business conduct" and human rights, on the international stage. Canada's foreign policy health goals also include supporting "evidence-based global efforts to improve the health of women, adolescents and children and to secure a better future for children and youth" (Government of Canada 2016), but which kind of evidence is not specified and economic and national security interests are emphasized over human rights and global public goods (Labonté, Runnels, and Gagnon 2012).

Most troubling is the flaunting of "Canadian values," hubristic indeed in a country with: (1) child poverty rates higher now than when Canada pledged to address this problem as an early signatory to the 1989 UN Convention on the Rights of the Child; and (2) a shameful track record on the well-being of Indigenous communities, hundreds of which suffer from inadequate housing (i.e., poor quality, overcrowded, unsafe), lack of safe drinking water and sanitation, substandard schools, and limited health care access (Reading and Halseth 2013), as well as child poverty rates up to 60%, more than three times the rates of non-Indigenous children (Macdonald and Wilson 2016) (see chapter 7). There are certainly legitimate reasons for countries with domestic problems of poverty, such as the United States, South Africa, the United Kingdom, Brazil, China, and others to furnish development aid, but to showcase human rights values and responsible business conduct as does Canada, seems hypocritical to say the least (see chapter 9 for discussion of Canada's mining sector).

Also illustrating how health fits in to the politics of foreign assistance, in recent years, the United Kingdom's cross-government strategy for global health explicitly focuses on three action areas: global health security, international development, and trade for better health, integrated into its goals of "achieving national and global security, creating economic wealth, supporting development in LICs and promoting human dignity through the protection of human rights and the delivery of humanitarian assistance" (Government of the United Kingdom 2011, pp. 3–4). Like its North American counterparts, this proposal has been primarily driven by security, and economic interests, as well as improving the UK's global reputation following its much critiqued role in the Iraq War (Gagnon and Labonté 2013). Meanwhile, the UK's 2016 vote to withdraw from the European Union (EU)—which occurred as this text was going to press—may well diminish its voice and influence in global health (Garrett 2016). Moreover, while the United Kingdom has a track record for providing effective, long-term development assistance and debt relief, it cannot escape the contradictions between promoting health and facilitating trade that harms health, most egregiously involving the sale of arms (the United States, France, Germany, Canada, among others, are also major arms exporters to LMICs) (Mahmudi-Azer 2011).

The stated goals of EU development aid are sustainable development and reducing poverty. With regard to health, the EU articulates "values of solidarity towards equitable and universal coverage of quality health services" as the basis for the EU role in global health (EU Council 2010) and generally promotes an intersectoral "health in all policies" (HiAP) approach (Amaya, Rollet, and Kingah 2015). Yet despite claims of impartiality and independence, EU aid remains politicized, linked to security concerns (Dany 2015), and self-interested. Lofty goals notwithstanding, the EU's internal security and economic priorities are evidenced in its fragmented and frankly un-humanitarian treatment of refugees from Syria and other countries (Smith and Daynes 2016) (see chapter 8) and in its failure to implement reparations for slavery and genocide as a just form of development (CARICOM 2014).

Within this larger foreign policy context, health aid is understood to confer a number of advantages on donor countries, which are often far greater than the benefits for "recipient" countries. In the case of the United States, these include: protecting the health security of its own citizens ("narrow self-interest"); promoting "political stability," "economic productivity," and growth ("enlightened self-interest"); and promoting research, partnerships, and debt relief ("global engagement") (Kassalow 2001).

Calls in the United States and beyond for global health to become a vital issue of national interest and of foreign policy (Bustreo and Doebbler 2010; Institute of Medicine 2009) are accompanied by a broad trend of health aid being increasingly shaped by commercial and industrial interests (PHM et al. 2014). There is also remarkable continuity with past economic and geopolitical aims (Table 2-3), though combatting communism has been replaced with counterterrorism and security concerns around "fragile" states, and prior humanitarian and charitable motivations have been recast as human rights concerns. All told, despite rhetoric to the contrary, foreign aid from the United States and other OECD countries benefits donor and recipient country political elites the most, while potentially harming the well-being of average LMIC residents—clearly at odds with stated humanitarian rationales motivating aid (de Mesquita and Smith 2009).

One effort that has sought to defy certain old patterns is the Foreign Policy and Global Health Initiative, established at a 2006 meeting of the Ministers of Foreign Affairs of Brazil, France, Indonesia, Norway, Senegal, South Africa, and Thailand. As per the 2007 Oslo Ministerial Declaration, these nations called for, inter alia, application of a "health lens" for evaluating foreign policy and development strategies on the basis of their impact on health, plus "respect for national sovereignty, a sense of shared responsibility, and . . . transparency, trust, accountability, and fairness" (Amorim et al. 2007, p. 1374). The absence of the three leading donors (US, Germany, and UK) enabled bold language on collaborative approaches (so as to better reflect the needs of recipient countries over charity or donor interests), fair trade, and health care systems as top priorities. Yet to date the initiative has had limited impact on these priorities or on making health central to foreign policy; much of its agenda for action remains framed around global health security (Fidler 2011).

Aid Effectiveness (and Financing for Development)

Longtime calls for reforming foreign assistance prompted a series of OECD co-sponsored international forums starting in the early 2000s to redress ineffective and donor-driven aid priorities. The initial meeting, held in Rome (2003) marked the first time (!) LMICs ("recipients") had been invited to discuss foreign assistance with donor countries. The next forum produced the Paris Declaration on Aid Effectiveness (2005), stressing the need for: "ownership" (recipient countries to "set their own strategies for poverty reduction, improve their institutions and tackle corruption"), alignment (between donors and local priorities and systems), harmonization (coordination, information sharing, and simplified procedures among donors to reduce duplication), focusing on achieving and measuring results, and "mutual accountability" (OECD 2015).

Adopted by 137 countries and 30 international organizations, the Paris Declaration set targets for 2010 for each component of the framework including, for example, that at least 25% of aid go to long-term programs instead of short-term projects and that 75% of aid be disbursed according to agreed-upon schedules. The 2008 Accra Agenda for Action built on these pledges, also promising to increase aid predictability, untie aid (from spending within donor countries), ensure that aid conditionalities are mutually decided, and boost civil society involvement (OECD 2015).

The 2011 Busan meeting shifted the language from "aid effectiveness" to "effective development cooperation," emphasizing "partnerships for development" that go beyond traditional North-South arrangements to incorporate South-South efforts, BRICS donors, civil society organizations, private funders, and "triangular cooperation" (among three countries) (OECD 2015).

Endorsed by over 160 governments and 50 international agencies, the Busan Partnership for Effective Development Co-operation has met with criticism for encouraging a strong private sector role in setting development policies and strategies. This approach will likely increase the level of inappropriate or ineffective aid and subsidize donor country companies through awarding of contracts, going against the principle of (recipient) country ownership (ActionAid 2014). Thus far, reports on Busan show limited alignment of donor aid with national priorities, slow and uneven country ownership of the aid management process, and limited progress on predictability and reducing "tied aid" (Global Partnership 2014).

Indeed, tied aid, which must be spent in the donor country (on personnel, equipment, products, and services) constitutes over 75% of all aid on average. Aid that is not formally tied but still goes back to donor countries has doubled between 2003 and 2010 to more than 50% of contracted aid; slightly more than one third goes to LMICs, with just 4% to the poorest countries. Some donors, such as the United Kingdom, United States, Austria, and Australia, grant more than 80% of the value of aid contracts to domestic companies (ActionAid 2014).

At the 2015 Financing for Development Summit in Addis Ababa, UN members agreed on a framework for financing the Sustainable Development Goals (SDGs), discussed ahead. As in Busan, attendees welcomed private sector financing for development, but the United States, United Kingdom, and France ensured that the proposal for a tax body to stop illicit financial flows was excised from the framework. Other issues evaded were the continuing debt burden and failure of development aid to fulfill the almost half-century commitment of HICs to provide 0.7% of GNI as official development assistance (ODA)[2], and 0.15% to 0.2% of GNI as ODA to the lowest-income countries (Eurodad 2015).

In the end, despite ambitious goals—and the commitment of certain well-meaning actors—donors, and many LMIC elites, have little interest in reforming the aid system. Even the OECD's internal evaluations find donor agencies extremely lagging in applying the Paris Declaration, with only a few recipient countries (gradually) implementing change. Although development aid levels have increased (including private donors' growing role), alignment with national priorities remains limited, with little improvement around aid management, aid predictability, and reduction of tied aid. Most importantly, with infrequent exceptions, the needs of the most vulnerable groups have not been prioritized (OECD 2011).

Donor–Recipient Dialectics

Sector-Wide Approaches

In the late 1990s, even before the Paris Declaration, dissatisfaction with the minimal impact of and the fragmentation, duplication, and disruption caused by development activities led the World Bank, together with WHO, donor agencies, and several African countries, to fashion a new sector-wide approach (SWAp) to aid. SWAps are an attempt to coordinate various actors on a particular issue (or within a region) in order to reduce overlapping service provision, pursue a coherent approach and goals, and lessen reporting burdens. Health has been at the forefront of this approach because of the urgency of problems and the large number of donor agencies and NGOs involved in this area.

SWAps herald various advantages, for instance increasing local say over agenda-setting, but few donors participate fully, precisely because they are unwilling to cede control over their contributions. Moreover, implementation of SWAps has been linked to a reduction in development assistance for health in 16 LICs because donors have pulled out rather than participate in SWAps (Sweeney, Mortimer, and Johnston 2014). Although some SWAp experiences have been positive—Ghana, the Solomon Islands, and Tanzania—elsewhere, as in Zambia, limited governance capacity amid political turmoil has proved an obstacle. Moreover, the HIV epidemic and vertical donor initiatives like PEPFAR (see chapters 4 and 12) have undermined SWAps in many sub-Saharan African countries (Peters, Paina, and Schleimann 2013).

"Recipient" Country Challenges with Health and Development Assistance

Aid, of course, is not a one-sided issue, and it is problematic to portray HIC donors as uniformly self-interested and LMIC recipients unwitting victims of such a system. Indeed, class alliances (especially elite interests) across countries of different income levels may be more relevant than the more typical distinctions between HICs and LMICs. Waste, self-interest, and inefficiencies, as well as corruption and favoritism, may occur on all fronts, with elites in all countries inevitably benefiting at the expense of vulnerable populations.

While there is enormous diversity among LMICs, there are certain shared characteristics—such as unpredictable revenue streams, multiple demands and priorities competing for attention, and sometimes insufficient governance capacity—that have great bearing on aid effectiveness from recipient country perspectives. Thus, part and parcel of a political economy analysis of donor aid, the structural factors influencing the incentives for and definition, practice, and obligations of cooperation on the part of participating countries should be carefully scrutinized. Analyses of particular instances and mechanisms of cooperation are scattered throughout the text; here we provide a set of common contextual factors that may shape the environment and reception of international cooperation in LMICs.

To be sure, each setting is unique, and has its own trajectory and experiences, and even the weakest states are not without agency. Moreover, distinct cultural approaches and bureaucratic idiosyncrasies mark every society. Still, the imbalance of power between "peripheral" and "core" countries (Box 2-3) limits the former's prospects for policy maneuvering domestically and for negotiation with donor agencies.

To begin, domestic governance capacity is essential to setting effective health agendas (Testa 2007). Nonetheless, as illustrated through analysis of policies around health care systems (also relevant to other dimensions of the health agenda), ministries of health in many LMICs face sizeable constraints in their stewardship of national health systems (Nervi 2014). This is especially the case where there is a large private sector role in health services delivery, and when significant health aid goes directly to NGOs. Moreover, as in the United States, many LMIC health care systems are heavily fragmented across insurance schemes/population coverage (i.e., social security systems, public health sector, private insurance, traditional healers), making regulation and monitoring challenging.

Health ministries are expected to fulfill aspirational agendas (e.g., building universal health systems) with grossly insufficient resources and little power to make key legislative changes. What may be perceived as lack of "capacity" from the outside is often linked to financial and other structural constraints. Moreover, health ministers do not typically participate in setting non-health sector government priorities, yet these may impinge on the realization and implementation of cooperative projects.

As well, although health ministers participate in the World Health Assembly (WHA) and other international summits, they usually have limited decisionmaking power over international cooperation. Particularly in the case of loans and the ability to repay them, these are central government decisions to be made based on credit repayment possibilities and the implications of indebtedness. This also means (too) many players are engaged in the governance of cooperation (ministries of health, foreign affairs, finance, economic development) creating competition among actors.

Ministries of health in recipient countries have to deal with a plethora of poorly coordinated initiatives and actors with several (sometimes contradictory) agendas and pressure to fulfill deadlines: bilateral agencies; multilateral organizations for technical cooperation (several from the UN, each with their owns goals and projects with the ministry of health); multilateral banks; universities and other research institutions; medical missions and brigades of all kinds (religious, training, etc.); diplomatic missions; global funds and global health initiatives; international NGOs; decentralized cooperation from donor countries (municipalities, regions, and communities); foundations and corporate philanthropy; and pharmaceutical and technology companies that make donations (just reading such a list is unwieldy). With so many moving parts, national health authorities may not even be aware of all cooperative activities at the local level (e.g., projects between sister municipalities, or efforts funded via NGOs or churches) (Nervi 2014).

As discussed, donor funding is unpredictable and usually short-term (long-term projects are the exception, not the norm), and fear of losing resources increases dependency. There is a pervasive "never-say-no" attitude to donor aid (though larger countries such as South Africa and Brazil have rejected certain aid offers in recent decades). Even so, if the ministry of health refuses an aid offer, donors may turn to other government officials to override the decision.

Particularly germane to smaller cooperation efforts are regulatory issues that put material donations (medicines, supplies, and medical equipment) and medical missions in limbo. Sometimes regulations exist but are not enforced when certain actors (including government officials) want to accept (and be recognized for) donations even if they are obsolete or unnecessary. Ministries of health may be compelled to accept all kinds of unapproved (and difficult to discard) donations of medical equipment, expired or off-list pharmaceuticals, and medical services, for the sole reason that they have been given at no cost.

Donors, especially those involved in disease campaigns or "global health initiatives" as opposed to more reciprocal primary health care collaborations, often fund a "one size fits all" set of interventions regardless of country and ministry of health priorities and needs (Batniji and Songane 2014). Further, there is growing evidence that (the resurgence of) narrowly technological, top-down global health initiatives are having negative consequences on health care systems in LMICs (Roalkvam and McNeill 2016).

Although most LMICs share a gamut of pressing issues around poverty, social infrastructure, and employment generation, they are not homogenous in their needs, capacity, or historical experience. Yet because donor aid requires national co-financing and the allocation of personnel and other in-kind resources, stock programs and global health initiatives can squeeze out or disrupt domestic priorities and redirect resources into unnecessary areas, consuming considerable portions of health budgets. Another challenge arises from tensions between lengthy negotiation periods for projects (at times longer than the projects themselves!) and recipient countries' urgency to implement their health policies before a political cycle ends (and there is staff turnover, etc.).

Other concerns derive from the conflict between creating separate project implementation units versus using national capacity. Historically, vertical disease campaigns (e.g., against smallpox and malaria) and multilateral banks created independent project implementation units that operated essentially as parallel ministries of health. This arrangement intensified in the early 2000s with an infusion of large-scale donor funding for HIV programs. But because "No health system in the world is actually built on 'vertical' programs" (Maciocco and Italian Global Health Watch 2008, p. 47), many national and international actors called for change (even as some donors have resisted). The Paris Declaration specified that donors use national procedures and mechanisms for project implementation in order to: (a) recognize recipient countries' capacities, and (b) strengthen their management systems. Yet few donors provide funds to strengthen these systems, all the while overestimating the capacities of national ministries to quickly process acquisitions and services. This leaves national procurement offices overwhelmed with work and unable to meet donor timeframe expectations.

A huge concern relating to international assistance is governmental obligation to manage different planning, monitoring, and project evaluation frameworks to satisfy each donor agency. These systems are oriented toward financial aspects and simplistic or uni-causal outcomes (to show results), rather than trying to improve the quality of cooperation by identifying problems. National teams have to manage dozens (if not hundreds) of different aid instruments that are not useful in monitoring the country's own health policy and may overlook what is actually happening for fear of presenting disappointing results. Echoing Rockefeller Foundation principles of ensuring a priori success and short-term, easy-to-count results, the accountability burdens on the part of donor agencies distort aid and health priorities in multiple ways (Holzapfel 2014) (Box 1-4). All of these problems might be addressed if donors adhered to SWAps and the Paris Declaration principles.

It is important to underscore that the impediments outlined here have been overcome in various notable LMIC health equity exemplars. As well, South–South cooperation (see chapters 4 and 14) is sometimes presented as an antidote to aid asymmetries and problems because LMICs are seen to share mutual governance and bureaucratic challenges and may, as does China, refrain from imposing conditionalities on aid (Information Office of the State Council 2014). However, South–South aid may differ little from North–South aid. Exceptionally, as in the case of Cuba's South–South cooperation, shared values around health equity may lead to long-term primary care and other collaborations (Walker and Kirk 2013).

The dilemmas linked to aid in political, bureaucratic, systemic, and cultural terms cannot be resolved facilely, as vividly analyzed in a 1980s study of Nepal's aid milieu that still resonates today. In this case, attempts to incorporate local perspectives and needs through consultation with Nepalese officials only perpetuated donor and elite self-interest because national officials, mostly Western-trained urban elites, knew little of the challenges of local policy implementation and on-the-ground conditions (Justice 1986). Moreover, aid is only one part of the political economy of development and health story.

The Paradox of ODA: Aid in Relation to Debt, Tax Evasion, (Unfair) Terms of Trade, Remittances, and Other Financial Flows and Subsidies

While donors consider ODA and other forms of development aid an important impetus for economic growth, in many LMICs debt, debt service, tax evasion, and profit sheltering, among other factors, far outstrip aid flows. Even as ODA has risen since 1970, the total stock of external debt has increased even more dramatically, as have capital flight and other

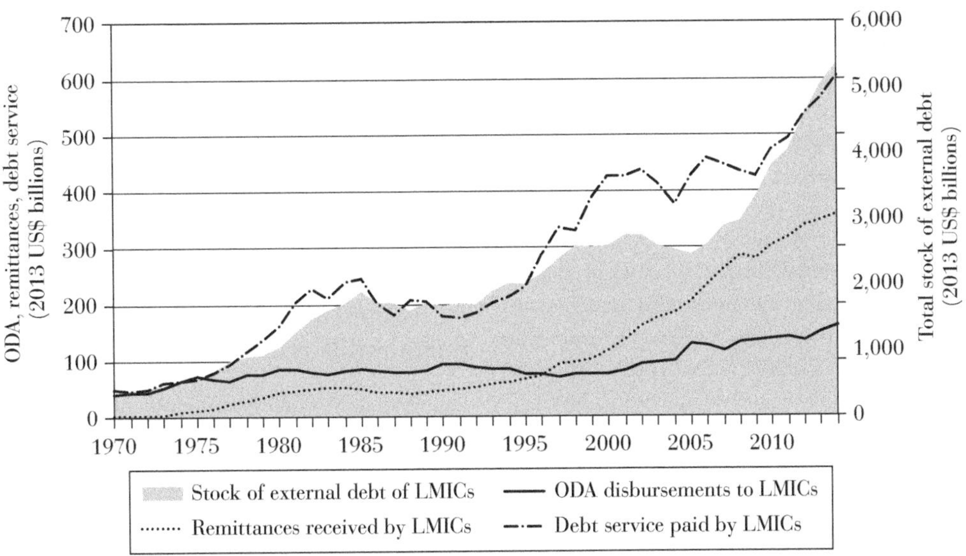

Figure 3-7: Long-term LMIC trends of ODA, remittances, debt service, and total stock of external debt (constant 2013 US$ billions[3]), 1970–2014.

Data Sources: OECD (2016b); World Bank (2016b).

illicit financial outflows. Also far overshadowing aid are migrant remittances to LMICs, reaching over twice the level of ODA in recent years (Figure 3-7).

The debt–aid paradox especially affects LICs. Aid disbursement to LICs has increased at only one quarter the rate of overall ODA. In 2014, LIC total external debt exceeded US$167 billion (collectively, LIC debt amounted to 27% of GNI and 100% of exports) (World Bank 2016b) compared with just US$47 billion in ODA received that year (OECD 2016b). For all LMICs combined, between 1985 and 2007, US$759 billion more was paid in debt service than received in new loans, locking in a self-perpetuating debt cycle (Toussaint and Millet 2010). To add insult to injury, the LIC debt cancellation programs of the 2006–2015 decade (Table 3-3) were typically counted as aid.

In addition to the stranglehold of debt, development aid is dwarfed by preferential treatment of donor country industries. In 2014, OECD countries reported spending US$239 billion on domestic farm subsidies (OECD 2016a), but just US$136 billion on development aid (OECD 2016b). It is estimated that each cow in the West is subsidized to the value of $2.50 per day compared with $0.90 cents per year for each child in LICs (Ware 2010).

Not only do HICs give themselves unfair trade advantages, they have done virtually nothing to improve the terms of trade or pricing policies for LMIC exports, which are a key source of revenue. In 2011, for example, coffee-producing countries earned US$23.5 billion of the US$70.86 billion generated from the global retail sale of coffee, with growers receiving only 7% to 10% of retail coffee prices in supermarkets (Fairtrade Foundation 2012). But the issue of fair commodity prices—which, if used for social distribution, could potentially help LMICs achieve far greater health and development gains than from foreign aid—has been eclipsed in recent decades by a different concern.

Globalized trade and investment under a neoliberal development model, more amply explored in chapter 9, have privileged TNC interests and displaced domestic development priorities in most LMICs. Yet many LMIC industries have the potential to generate employment, a secure tax base, and a diverse economy. Instead, in rural areas, farmers are increasingly dispossessed from their land and forced into debt by agribusiness and financial interests. Meanwhile, global investment-driven, export-oriented urban manufacturing and extractive industries condemn large swaths of LMIC populations to miserable work and living conditions and loss of state regulatory protections.

At the same time, many LMIC governments do not adequately enact or enforce tax laws and have insufficient regulations around capital flight, which—together with debt servicing and reigning macroeconomic policies of strict monetarism and fiscal austerity—impedes them from making needed social investments (Rowden 2012). All told, far more money flows out of than into LMICs: for every $1 entering LMICs from foreign direct investment, remittances, and aid, $2 to $6 leave in illicit financial flows, lending to wealthy countries, repatriated profits by foreign investors, and debt servicing (Griffiths 2014).

Accordingly, fundamental to improving global well-being is contesting the dominant development model that serves as recipe for continued immiseration.

RECENT DEVELOPMENT AND GLOBAL HEALTH APPROACHES

Key Questions:

- What new development ideas have emerged in recent decades? What are the implications for health?
- Why is reducing poverty an insufficient health and development strategy?
- How is health addressed in the SDGs compared with the MDGs? What is missing?
- What is global (health) governance and what is the role of TNC interests therein?

Development as Freedom, Sustainability, and Human Rights

Since the rise of the Washington consensus in the 1980s, "development" has been linked to policies around trade and investment liberalization, privatization, and deregulation. These policies, together with economic crises, have exacerbated poverty and inequality across much of the world (see chapter 2). As such, a continuing debate is whether development efforts should focus on reducing poverty or promoting economic growth (Brown 2012). Some argue that the poverty versus growth debate is a distraction in the sense that addressing poverty reduction as a development problem that is independent of, or isolated from, the political economy order completely misses the larger forces that create poverty in the first place (Rowden 2012).

Countering the neoliberal economic model espoused by many of his colleagues, Amartya Sen, 1998 Nobel Laureate in economics, has been hailed for bringing a humanistic approach to development economics. Building on a generation of economists who abandoned more orthodox paradigms of development to focus on poverty diminution instead of, or alongside, economic growth, Sen has proposed that human freedom is both the ultimate goal and the means of achieving development. Accordingly, "Development requires the removal of major sources of unfreedom: poverty as well as tyranny, poor economic opportunities as well as systematic social deprivation, neglect of public facilities as well as intolerance" (Sen 1999, p. 3).

Sen helped craft a "capabilities approach" to poverty that moves development away from exclusively economic concerns. Based on philosopher John Rawls' "theory of justice," which conceptualizes individual well-being as the possession of "social primary goods," Sen's "idea of capability is linked with substantive freedom . . . it gives a central role to a person's *actual* ability to do the different things that she values doing" (2009, p. 253).

Contrary to many policymakers, Sen places humans and human agency at the center of development, making material resources (e.g., income) primarily a means to realizing capabilities or freedoms rather than an end in itself (Klugman, Rodríguez, and Choi 2011). This approach renders the income per capita measure of well-being emphasized by orthodox economists grossly inadequate, inspiring the human development index as an alternative for measuring human well-being (Box 3-3).

Even with its acclaimed human development focus, Sen's approach has been critiqued for overemphasizing individual freedoms while underplaying the "social, and therefore political, nature of human wellbeing . . . This leads to an uneven account of the role of power, in all its forms, in its approach to the construction of human wellbeing" (Deneulin and McGregor 2010, p. 502). Sen also lacks an in-depth political economy and class analysis. For example, he does not focus on issues like unequal trade and the role of international financial instruments (O'Hearn 2009) and addresses political factors in a simplistic binary fashion, contrasting dictatorships with democracies, but overlooking who wields power and to what ends (Navarro 2004).

The related concept of "sustainable development," popularized via the 1987 Brundtland Commission report "*Our Common Future*," proposed that equity, economic growth, and environmental sustainability were not mutually exclusive but rather simultaneously possible goals (Du Pisani 2006). An accompanying "sustainable livelihoods" approach offers a framework for implementing interventions that address poverty and hunger, education, gender equality, and health as necessities of life, and thus core components of development, but there has been little attempt to assess whether this approach has made a "meaningful difference" to people's lives (Morse and McNamara 2013).

Moreover, "sustainable development" (as later embodied in the SDGs, discussed ahead) has not challenged the economic growth imperative, ignoring more radical approaches to ecological sustainability such as degrowth, or steady-state alternatives (see chapter 13). Indeed, a growing chorus argues that protecting the environment and promoting "development" are inherently incompatible, if not oxymoronic (Martínez Alier et al. 2010).

A human rights framework has brought yet another lens to development and health that departs from the standard health-development dyad (whether development leads to health or health to development). Building on the UN's Universal Declaration of Human Rights and subsequent international treaties around economic and social rights (see chapter 2), the 1986 Declaration on the Right to Development recognizes development as "an inalienable human right" and a "comprehensive economic, social, cultural and political process, which aims at the constant improvement of the well-being of the entire population and of all individuals on the basis of their active, free and meaningful participation in development and in the fair distribution of benefits resulting therefrom" (UN General Assembly 1986).

The "right to development" has notable implications for health-related social and economic rights,

Box 3-3 The Human Development Index

Sen's ideas animated creation of the Human Development Index (HDI), which employs the capabilities approach in an "applied measure" of human welfare. Developed in 1990 by Mahbub ul Haq, former Pakistani Finance Minister turned development specialist, the HDI is a composite index of education level, life expectancy, and GNI/capita in each country that has featured in the UNDP 's annual *Human Development Report* (HDR) since 1993. By incorporating measures of health, education, and material living standards, the HDI, which is used to rank countries in the HDR, represents an important first step toward establishing a more holistic evaluation of the human condition. More recently joined by a Multidimensional Poverty Index (MPI) and a Gender Inequality Index (GII), the use of the HDI has sought to shift development indicators from purely economic measures to assessing a range of human opportunities gauged via levels of literacy, health, access to sanitation, water, and other basic resources, and civil and political freedoms. Within this framework, health is considered a powerful means of gauging overall economic and social progress in society (Agarwala et al. 2014).

The HDI has been critiqued on methodological grounds, for the uneven quality of data used, its partial reflection of "reality," and for insufficiently measuring the effects of particular policies (Deb 2015; Hou, Walsh, and Zhang 2015). Crucially, the HDI is silent on who/what is responsible for inequality and low levels of development and on how to resolve these problems. Despite these deficiencies, the HDI remains the sole instrument that allows for an annual comparative snapshot of the world's social and economic conditions.

An HDI variant, the Social Progress Index (SPI), is composed of three parts: basic human needs (nutrition and basic medical care, water and sanitation, shelter, personal safety); foundations of well-being (literacy, school enrollment by age and gender, access to Internet and mobile phones, press freedoms and communications, health and wellness, ecosystem sustainability); and opportunity (personal rights, personal freedom and choice, tolerance and inclusion, access to advanced education) (Porter and Stern 2015). Importantly, while expanding the dialogue on well-being beyond economic growth, neither the HDI nor the SPI take on societal distribution of resources and power as the central determinants of well-being, instead focusing on symptoms.

helping inform a health and human rights approach (see Chapter 14), which synergistically links the right to health as both a goal of and a means to fulfilling the right to development. This framework also requires paying attention to the harms development projects may bring to health, the environment, and other areas. Moreover, rights-based approaches contend that economic constraints do not justify curtailment of human rights (Tarantola et al. 2013). For example, girls' education should be seen as its own good, not instrumentally in the name of economic development, and its realization should not be jeopardized by economic crisis.

In sum, these frameworks have extended the boundaries of poverty and health approaches to embrace, variously, human rights, social entitlements, capabilities, the natural environment, social relations, and vulnerability. Although these and other efforts transcend orthodox economic approaches to development by integrating social progress and well-being (Stiglitz, Sen, and Fitoussi 2009), they nonetheless refrain from challenging the larger world order.

Millennium Development Goals and Sustainable Development Goals

In 2000, world leaders gathered in New York to sign the UN Millennium Declaration, which called for "collective responsibility to uphold the principles of human dignity, equality and equity at the global level" and work toward eradicating poverty

Box 3-4 Health-Related Millennium Development Goals and Selected Targets

1. Eradicate extreme poverty and hunger
   Target: Halve the proportion of people living on less than $1 per day and who suffer from hunger
4. Reduce child mortality
   Target: Reduce by two-thirds the mortality rate among children under five
5. Improve maternal health
   Target: Reduce by three-quarters the maternal mortality ratio
   Target: Achieve universal access to reproductive health (added in 2007)
6. Combat HIV/AIDS, malaria, and other diseases
   Target: Halt and begin to reverse the spread and incidence of these diseases

and underdevelopment (UN 2000). The following year, 189 countries (nearly all UN member states) plus all major UN and other international agencies (including the World Bank and IMF) agreed to eight interdependent Millennium Development Goals (MDGs), and accompanying measurable targets to be met by 2015 (Box 3-4). Three of the eight MDGs, eight of the original 16 targets, and 18 of the original 48 indicators relate directly to health, and most others are linked to the underlying determinants of health (UN Millennium Project 2007).

While the Millennium Declaration and the setting of MDGs were widely lauded for demonstrating a shared global commitment to development and poverty reduction, many scholars and advocates have critiqued the MDGs' conflation of poverty reduction with development, their embeddedness in free market ideologies, and their failure to address unequal power relations (Cheru 2013). By contrast, LMICs that have been successful at lessening poverty have historically pursued comprehensive economic and social policies rather than poverty reduction programs (Gore 2013).

A key dispute surrounded the MDGs' extremely narrow definition of poverty, based on the World Bank indicator: people living on less than $1/day (1985 PPP[4]). Incredibly, the level was twice ratcheted downward (!!) ending at the equivalent of $0.69 1985 PPP (a more than 30% decline!) even though it looked like the level had been raised to $1.25/day (because the level was converted to 2005 PPP). This was an impressive feat of data gymnastics to make the global poverty trend appear more positive (Pogge and Sengupta 2015).

Of course, any universal poverty line is problematic. A PPP$1.25/day allotment is entirely insufficient for *daily survival* in most Latin American countries (and thus PPP$3/day—or considerably more in urban areas—is a better measure), whereas in some rural regions in sub-Saharan Africa, PPP $1.25/day may adequately gauge *extreme poverty*. The World Bank's approach to measuring poverty remains contentious, with many researchers arguing it substantially underestimates the magnitude of global poverty (Anand, Segal, and Stiglitz 2010).

Inadequate as they are, even these poverty lines show that in the lowest income region, sub-Saharan Africa, the proportion of the population living below PPP$1.25/day and PPP$3/day barely declined between 1990 and 2011. Moreover, if one were to count real poverty, the proportion of the population in LMICs living below PPP$10 per day, only declined from 94% to 88% in this time period (World Bank 2015) (Figure 3-8). Further, by artificially moving the MDG starting date to 1990 instead of 2000, the UN's clocking of poverty declines incorporated improvements in China, which lifted hundreds of millions of people out of poverty through domestic policies that predated and were entirely unrelated to the MDGs (Hickel 2016). Meanwhile, in Latin America, where poverty has fallen most dramatically, significant redistributive policies under leftist governments elected across the region in the early 2000s, rather than the MDGs, have played the major role (see chapter 13).

This points to a further, deep-seated deficiency of the MDG approach: it sidesteps the root causes of and long-term solutions to poverty. The Millennium campaign not only bowdlerized the "urgent struggle

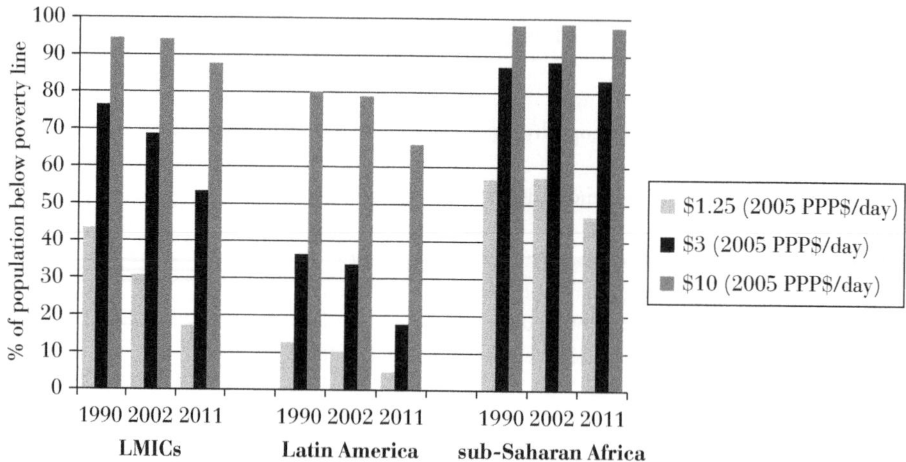

Figure 3-8: Percentage of population in LMICs living in poverty (2005 PPP$), 1990–2011.
Data Source: World Bank (2015). Note: PPP refers to purchasing power parity, a measure that seeks to adjust for national differences in the prices of goods and services.

to end exploitation" (by refraining from recognizing the role of dominant countries, business interests, and other elite actors in creating and perpetuating poverty and inequality), it excluded and was downright hostile to efforts emphasizing effective welfare state and other redistributive measures in either LMIC or HIC settings (Navarro 2007). Aside from renewed emphasis on the importance of economic growth (despite ample evidence, discussed previously, that growth alone does not lead to improvements in health and development), the MDGs proposed no real strategies to realize the shared goals within and across societies or on how to achieve and sustain improvements in human well-being into the future. In the end, this resulted in very uneven achievements both between and within countries (Fehling, Nelson, and Venkatapuram 2013).

At the designated 2015 endpoint, the UN took stock of the MDGs, finding that although all but one region met the target of halving the proportion of people living in extreme poverty (again, according to misleading measures), about 836 million people were still living in these conditions (a figure that might go as high as 3.5 billion people—half the world's population—if poverty were accurately gauged [Hickel 2016]). The highest level (41%) and slowest improvements were in sub-Saharan Africa, which did not meet the target. In Central Africa, the number of undernourished people doubled since 1990, part of 795 million undernourished people globally, including 161 million children (UN 2015b).

The largest health-related improvements were linked to diseases targeted by major global investments. HIV incidence fell from 3.5 million new cases in 2000 to 2.1 million in 2013. Additionally, an estimated 6.2 million malaria deaths and 37 million TB deaths were averted between 2000 and 2015 due to prevention and treatment efforts.

But the target for reducing child mortality by two thirds since 1990 was missed, and preventable causes of disease such as diarrhea, pneumonia, and malaria continued to kill about 16,000 children under-5 per day in 2015. Moreover, neonatal mortality saw virtually no reductions. Damningly, not a single LMIC region met the target of reducing maternal mortality by three quarters, and 13 countries with some of the highest maternal mortality in the world, including Côte D'Ivoire, Kenya, and Cameroon, saw extremely limited progress (UN 2015b).

Overall, those targets most closely tied to improved living conditions, requiring considerable socially redistributive investments, were especially disappointing. For example, in 2015, 663 million people still used unimproved drinking water sources (UN 2015b), and even those with "improved" drinking water did not necessarily have a household connection to make water accessible, nor did MDG measures assure affordability (see chapter 7).

Despite these shortcomings, UN Secretary General, Ban Ki-moon argued that the MDGs were the "most successful global anti-poverty push in history" (UN 2013, p. 3) and represented an unprecedented mobilization of resources for global health (WHO 2015b).

Seeking to build on the MDGs, 192 UN members adopted the Sustainable Development Goals (SDGs) for the 2015–2030 period. More extensive than the MDGs and involving a consultative process with "stakeholders," the SDGs comprise 17 goals and 169 targets. Goal 3, *Ensure Healthy Lives and Promote Well-Being for All at All Ages*, includes targets to, inter alia, reduce global maternal mortality, achieve universal access to sexual and reproductive health services, and reach universal health coverage (discussed in chapter 11), as well as targets relating to NCDs, mental health, injuries, exposure to hazardous chemicals and environmental pollution, and health repercussions from disasters and violence in conflict situations. However, only certain health care system components are mentioned, with important aspects such as access to medicines and health facilities excluded (Williams and Blaiklock 2015), and health inequity not sufficiently considered. Broader health-related SDGs include poverty and malnutrition eradication, equitable access to education, universal access to water and sanitation, full and decent employment, reducing social inequality, addressing climate change, and promoting peace and justice (UN 2015a).

The SDGs seek to avoid the uniform approach of the MDGs, encouraging a more ambitious scope and nationally determined targets. The SDGs recognize that HICs must also address poverty and pursue environmentally sustainable economic policies.

In contrast to the MDGs, which were significantly financed by development aid and debt "forgiveness," atop domestic spending, this time national governments have been enjoined to partner with the private sector, academia, and civil society to achieve the SDGs (UNIDO and UN Global Compact 2014). The Post-2015 Platform for Philanthropy, for example, invites funding from philanthropies (including corporate foundations) as partners with government and other non-state actors in the SDG agenda (Martens and Seitz 2015). With such private involvement there is the risk of diluted goals: already, a private initiative to re-package the SDGs as "Global Goals" eliminates important language around "sustainability" and "inclusivity" (Adams 2015). Either way, economist Jeffrey Sachs, among others, has equated sustainable development with sustainable economic growth—rehashing a troubled formula from the past (Wilson 2015).

Finally, while the SDGs repeatedly invoke human rights, they do not recognize health or any of the goals as human rights (Chapman 2015). Moreover, the same problematic metric for measuring poverty—income—is employed, again failing to capture the multidimensional conditions that shape poverty such as illiteracy, child labor, exposure to violence, and lack of safe drinking water (Pogge and Sengupta 2015).

All of these issues are ultimately connected to the fundamental problem: asymmetry of power in global policymaking and the larger world order.

Politics of Global (Health) Governance

Since the 1990s, and particularly since 2000, the array of players and policy mechanisms in international development and health have undergone a marked transformation. In the global health arena, powerful new multi-stakeholder partnerships (e.g., the Global Fund) private actors (e.g., foundations), and new or renewed bilateral players (e.g., BRICS countries) have upended prior decisionmaking forums, most notably the World Health Organization's (WHO's) Executive Board and WHA. Previously, WHO and its bodies were a hub of global health policymaking, based on quasi-democratic and representative structures. Today there are rising concerns not only that policymaking is occurring behind closed doors, sidelining shared governance principles, but that the entry of private actors and inadequate representation of LMICs is further skewing existing power imbalances (Buissonnière 2012).

Responding to these concerns, advocates of intergovernmental decisionmaking have called attention to the notion of "global health governance" as an effort to clarify the structures and norms of policymaking in the global health arena. This framing draws from overall global governance discussions in the post-Cold War era of deepening globalization, inequalities, and economic crises. Governance in this context refers, variously, to leadership, decisionmaking processes, mediating institutions and their rules, establishment of priorities and cooperative roles, and a chain of command for emergencies (Batniji and Songane 2014).

Espousing lofty goals around the need for collective global action based on human rights and for widening policymaking on such issues as development and trade beyond a few powerful players (OHCHR et al. 2013), the global governance agenda faces an uphill struggle.

Transposed into the health arena, there are similar salient concerns regarding concentrated decisionmaking. The United States and other powerful entities have emphasized a global health security paradigm in response to, for example, the HIV pandemic, the global economic crisis since 2008, the outbreak of H1N1 in 2009, and, increasingly, climate change, but these concerns are largely driven by self-interested priorities.

Moreover, though some non-state (mostly private sector) players such as the Bill and Melinda Gates Foundation (BMGF; see chapter 4)—and the organizations it has helped shape, including GAVI and the Global Fund—have been brought in, power-wielding structures have not been democratized, but rather privatized. In addition to marshalling (often by incentivizing large government contributions) significant amounts of new funding, these organizations are now in explicit, as well as more circuitous, decisionmaking roles that upstage the traditional policy processes of governments and multilateral agencies.

So what global health governance arrangement is needed to make the field responsive and accountable in a just and democratic fashion? Certain progressive voices call for a return to what WHO (2016) defines as the application of legally binding rules of engagement, including international law as it applies to public health as well as policymaking processes based on historic practices. This approach focuses particularly on multilateral institutions that play a role in global health (i.e., UN agencies), with reforming WHO (and returning it to its prior central position) a top priority (Velásquez and Alas 2016).

Another approach, championed by the Lancet-University of Oslo Commission on Global Governance for Health (Ottersen et al. 2014) acknowledges that global political arrangements continue to reproduce an unfair distribution of power and that "unacceptable health inequities within and between countries cannot simply be addressed within the health sector by technical measures" or solely at a national level (McNeill and Ottersen 2015, p. 834). Yet the Commission meekly recommends new "multi-stakeholder" advisory and monitoring bodies without addressing how skewed "structural and power relations have arisen and could be changed" or challenging "the dominating influence of large monopolistic and oligopolistic corporations" on the global health agenda and activities (Gill and Benatar 2016, p. 351). Clearly, pragmatism and treating the symptoms of the global health governance crisis are insufficient (McCoy 2014).

Corporatization of Governance and Aid

At the heart of governance concerns is the rise of corporate power in global governance, UN agencies, and international development writ large. The UN has become increasingly subject to corporate influence via two main pathways: the UN Foundation and the UN Global Compact (Adams and Martens 2015). In light of chronic underfunding to the UN system (spawned by US refusal to pay its regular contributions in the 1980s—see Chapter 2), the UN Foundation (launched in 1998) became an unprecedented channel for receiving and channeling private donations. Meanwhile, the UN's traditional operations via intergovernmental partnerships are being endangered by new cooperative relationships with multinational corporations and philanthropic foundations. This has transpired through the UN Global Compact (launched in 1999), a UN-corporate "social responsibility" initiative of 10,000 partners who agree to "align strategies and operations with universal principles on human rights, labour rights, environment and anti-corruption, and take actions that advance societal goals" (UN Global Compact 2016).

Promising as this sounds, corporations are not bound to abide by these principles, and many companies only adhere to them rhetorically. These approaches are known as "bluewashing" (blue being the UN's signature color), providing legitimacy to corporations through association with UN agencies. This is a profitable strategy for companies, enabling them to burnish their reputations *and* making them privy to internal UN discussions (even as they strategically shirk their Global Compact obligations by taking superficial measures and avoid more costly restructuring and monitoring of their human rights and environmental practices) (Berliner and Prakash 2015).

Moreover, although the financial contributions from corporations and private foundations constitute only a fraction of the UN budget, the leverage and influence garnered by such funding is much greater, as donations furnish access to decisionmaking and the shaping of UN strategies around global issues (Adams and Martens 2015). As such, in the current era of public-private partnerships (PPPs) (see chapter 4), private interests manage to present themselves as "part of the solution" and erase past malfeasance by closely interacting with the UN.

The Global Compact is but one element of a multistakeholder governance transformation. In 2009, the World Economic Forum's corporate-led Global Redesign Initiative set out to restructure the architecture of global decisionmaking so that UN agencies become just another "stakeholder" in polycentric, global, "multi-stakeholder governance" (Gleckman 2016). As discussed, key bilateral agencies have already enthusiastically embraced the idea that the private sector should be a full participant in setting foreign aid agendas (EU Council 2010; United States Government 2015).

Beyond private sector *funding*, health and development efforts increasingly involve *high financing*—high-level investment in global health business ventures. The Global Health Investment Fund (GHIF), designed by JP Morgan Chase & Co. and the BMGF, brings financing instruments to global health projects/products, treating them as "start-ups" with a financial return for investors when projects/products are successful. But unlike standard ventures, which run the risk of failure as per capitalist precepts, the GHIF protects investors, including by using public monies: the BMGF and the Swedish International Development Cooperation Agency guarantee up to 60% of losses through the GHIF! With the minimum investment set at US$250,000, not only is the GHIF limited to wealthy venture capitalists, but its very structure gives shareholders legal rights on the outcome of global health initiatives that trump the health needs of recipient populations (Erikson 2015).

Such new forms of financing mean more resources leveraged by nimble foundations and philanthrocapitalists—who infuse philanthropy with the principles and practices of for-profit enterprise *and* seek to demonstrate capitalism's altruistic potential through innovations that allegedly "benefit everyone, sooner or later, through new products, higher quality and lower prices" (Bishop and Green 2013). But this also means bypassing or coopting the UN system, trampling over public governance, inserting market models, and entrenching business interests, all funded by the public purse. Impact investing, as articulated by the Rockefeller Foundation, for instance, calls for turning a profit while addressing problems of poverty and other social and environmental issues (Dassel et al. 2015).

In the global health arena, it is important to recall that PPPs are not a surprising or unexpected development but a willful outgrowth of the neoliberal clawback of WHO and UN funding (and authority) starting in the 1980s, which has made the private sector appear as the only untapped source of funds. However, the insistence by donors for greater control over programs and policymaking means that private industry is "invited" as a full partner in decisionmaking processes concerning what are, in fact, public issues. This proliferation of private, less than democratic, health aid has diverted attention away from the corporate sector's role in, for example, maintaining inequitable trade arrangements that jeopardize the livelihoods of millions of LMIC country workers and farmers and allow the penetration of private interests in the public sphere (Rückert and Labonté 2014).

In sum, addressing global health governance is a useful exercise but only insofar as it returns us to a political economy understanding of who wields power in global health and development.

CONCLUSION: WHAT DOES A CRITICAL POLITICAL ECONOMY APPROACH BRING TO THE GLOBAL HEALTH ARENA?

Learning Points:

- A critical political economy approach to global health differs from bio-behavioral models by analyzing and addressing health and disease patterns in the context of social, political, and economic relations at local, national, and global levels, not solely in individual terms.
- Biomedical and behavioral models and interventions dominate the contemporary (global) health field because political economy-informed understandings and action represent a threat to the status quo of distribution of power and resources.

- Global health, like international health in the past, is linked to the international development arena and reflects its inherent tensions. A political economy lens shows how development strategies and donor aid are shaped by global political and ideological exigencies.
- A panoply of ideas and strategies—MDGs/SDGs, sustainability, aid effectiveness—seek to advance development and address poverty but do not ultimately challenge the reigning neoliberal capitalist model.
- Locally shaped ideas and plans aimed at improving equity are typically considered unwieldy and expensive; donor priorities dominate aid agendas, regardless of their (ir)relevance or possible negative impact on health and social justice.
- Discussions of global health governance offer the potential for understanding and addressing unfair power arrangements, but to date efforts toward a more democratic and equitable global health architecture have been thwarted by vested interests.

A critical political economy framework illustrates why global health efforts need to go beyond individual level interventions (technical quick fixes and changing the behavior of individuals) to changes in the distribution of power and resources. In an asymmetrical world, characterized by the historically powerful Minority World of HICs, the far larger but less powerful Majority World, and the growing influence of corporations and philanthropies on UN and other multilateral institutions (including WHO), it is especially important to understand how these forces and factors affect health equity and the health of nations that depend on aid.

While the "practical bargain" of mainstream aid is appealing to those comfortable with the status quo of power and resource distribution across the world and within countries, this approach of tinkering at the margins offers limited prospects for addressing the underlying determinants of global health problems. It contrasts markedly with bona fide social, political, and economic redistributional efforts within legitimate and representative political processes that are sustained by fair and equitable transnational economic and political rules, and involve social justice-oriented cooperation.

Although contested, if not ignored, in the international aid and development world—and addressed only rhetorically in global health—a critical political economy of health approach is invaluable to comprehending how complex political, economic, and social forces combine to produce health and ill health within and across societies and how these forces influence the global health actors and activities discussed in chapter 4. The approaches presented in this chapter—particularly critical political economy and the analytic questions regarding how the distribution of wealth and power influence patterns of health and its multilayered determinants—serve as a framework for the remainder of the book, both in terms of understanding the challenges of global health and in addressing them.

NOTES

1. On May 1, 2004 ten countries joined the EU: Cyprus, the Czech Republic, Estonia, Hungary, Latvia, Lithuania, Malta, Poland, Slovakia, and Slovenia. This was the largest single accession of new member states to the EU.
2. In 1969, Lester B. Pearson, who had just stepped down as Canada's Prime Minister, released a report for the World Bank calling for HICs to jointly agree to dedicating 0.7% of GNI for ODA to LMICs. In 1970, the UN General Assembly agreed to the target of 0.7% of GNI for ODA by 1975, but most countries did not reach this mark, with rare exceptions (typically a handful of Scandinavian countries and a few others). In recent years, ODA as a percentage of donor GNI has remained relatively steady at approximately 0.3% of GNI (Figure 4-1).
3. An OECD ODA deflator has been applied to the data in this figure to enable rough comparability over time (recognizing that the precise amounts are not accurate).
4. Purchasing power parity.

REFERENCES

ActionAid. 2014. *Aid to, with and through the Private Sector: Emerging Trends and Ways Forward.* London: ActionAid.

Adams B. 2015. Public SDGs or private GGs. *Social Watch*, September 25.

Adams B and Martens J. 2015. *Fit for Whose Purpose? Private Funding and Corporate Influence in the United Nations.* New York and Bonn: Global Policy Forum.

Agarwala M, Atkinson G, Fry BP, et al. 2014. Assessing the relationship between human well-being and ecosystem services: a review of frameworks. *Conservation and Society* 12(4):437–449.

Alam S. 2008. Majority World: Challenging the West's rhetoric of democracy. *Amerasia Journal* 34(1):87–98.

Aleksandrova OI, Gabueva LA, Gradoboev VV, et al. 2013. *Reformy systemy zdravookhraneniia v Rossii (2006-2012): Podkhody, problemy, perspektivy.* [Health Care Reform in Russia (2006-2012): Approaches, Problems and Prospects]. http://papers.ssrn.com/sol3/papers.cfm?abstract_id=2345880. Accessed July 13, 2015.

Allende S. 1951. *Sesión 33.a, en jueves 6 de septiembre de 1951. Diario de sesiones del senado.* Santiago: Biblioteca del Congreso Nacional de Chile.

Amaya AB, Rollet V, and Kingah S. 2015. What's in a word? The framing of health at the regional level: ASEAN, EU, SADC and UNASUR. *Global Social Policy* 15(3):229–260.

Amorim C, Douste-Blazy P, Wirayuda H, et al. 2007. Oslo Ministerial declaration—global health: A pressing foreign policy issue of our time. *Lancet* 396(9570):1373–1378.

Anand S, Segal P, and Stiglitz JE. 2010. *Debates on the Measurement of Global Poverty.* New York: Oxford University Press.

Antonovsky A. 1967. Social class, life expectancy, and overall mortality. *The Milbank Memorial Fund Quarterly* 45(2):31–73.

Banerjee AV and Duflo E. 2011. *Poor Economics: A Radical Rethinking of the Way to Fight Global Poverty.* New York: PublicAffairs.

Bartram J, Editor. 2015. *Routledge Handbook of Water and Health.* Abingdon, UK: Routledge.

Batniji R and Songane F. 2014. Contemporary global health governance: Origins, functions, and challenges. In Brown GW, Yamey G, and Wamala S, Editors. *The Handbook of Global Health Policy, First Edition.* Hoboken: John Wiley & Sons, Ltd.

Baum F and Fisher M. 2014. Why behavioural health promotion endures despite its failure to reduce health inequities. *Sociology of Health & Illness* 36(2):213–225.

Bell SE and Figert AE, Editors. 2015. *Reimagining (Bio) Medicalization, Pharmaceuticals and Genetics: Old Critiques and New Engagements.* New York: Routledge.

Berliner D and Prakash A. 2015. "Bluewashing" the firm? Voluntary regulations, program design, and member compliance with the United Nations global compact. *Policy Studies Journal* 43(1):115–138.

Bessudnov A, McKee M, and Stuckler D. 2012. Inequalities in male mortality by occupational class, perceived status and education in Russia, 1994–2006. *The European Journal of Public Health* 22(3):332–337.

Biehl J and Petryna A, Editors. 2013. *When People Come First: Critical Studies in Global Health.* Princeton, NJ: Princeton University Press.

Bijlmakers LA, Bassett MT, and Sanders D. 1998. *Socioeconomic Stress, Health And Child Nutritional Status In Zimbabwe At A Time Of Economic Structural Adjustment: A Three Year Longitudinal Study,* vol. 105. Uppsala: The Nordic Africa Institute.

Birdsall N. 1994. Pragmatism, Robin Hood, and other themes: Good government and social well-being in developing countries. In Chen LC, Kleinman A, and Ware NC, Editors. *Health and Social Change in International Perspective.* Cambridge, MA: Harvard University Press.

Birn A-E, Cabella W, and Pollero R. 2010. The infant mortality conundrum in Uruguay during the first half of the twentieth century: An analysis according to causes of death. *Continuity and Change* 25(3):435–461.

Bishop M and Green M. 2013. FAQ. http://philanthrocapitalism.net/about/faq/. Accessed April 23, 2016.

Breilh J and Paz y Miño J. 2001. *Eugenio Espejo: La otra memoria* [Nueva lectura de la historia de las ideas científicas]. Cuenca, EC: Universidad de Cuenca.

Bretton Woods Project. 2010. The IMF's framework for low-income countries. http://www.brettonwoodsproject.org/2010/06/art-566378/. Accessed April 20, 2016.

Brown S. 2012. National development agencies and bilateral aid. In Haslam PA, Schafer J, and Beaudet P, Editors. *Introduction to International Development: Approaches, Actors, and Issues,* Second Edition. New York: Oxford University Press.

Brown TM and Birn A-E. 2013. The making of health internationalists. In Birn A-E and Brown TM, Editors. *Comrades in Health: U.S. Health Internationalists, Abroad and at Home.* New Brunswick, NJ: Rutgers University Press.

Brown TM and Fee E. 2014. Social movements in health. *Annual Review of Public Health* 35: 385–398.

Buissonnière M. 2012. La nouvelle donne de la santé globale: dynamiques et écueils. *Revue internationale de politique de développement* 3.

Burström B. 2003. Social differentials in the decline of infant mortality in Sweden in the twentieth century: The impact of politics and policy. *International Journal of Health Services* 33:723–741.

Bustreo F and Doebbler CF. 2010. Making health an imperative of foreign policy: The value of a human rights approach. *Health and Human Rights* 12(1):47–59.

Carey G, Malbon E, Crammond B et al. 2016. Can the sociology of social problems help us to understand and manage 'lifestyle drift'? *Health Promotion International* [Epub ahead of print].

CARICOM. 2014. CARICOM Ten Point Plan for Reparatory Justice. http://caricom.org/caricom-ten-point-plan-for-reparatory-justice. Accessed July 16, 2016.

Chapman AR. 2015. SDG Series: Evaluating Universal Health Coverage as a Sustainable Development Goal. *Health and Human Rights Journal Blog*, September 2.

Cheru F. 2013. Goals, rights, and political economy: Daring to break out of the liberal ideological box! In Langford M, Sumner A, and Yamin AE, Editors. *The Millennium Development Goals and Human Rights: Past, Present and Future.* Cambridge: Cambridge University Press.

Clark J. 2014. Medicalization of global health 1: Has the global health agenda become too medicalized? *Global Health Action* 7.

Clarke AE, Shim JK, Mamo L, et al. 2003. Biomedicalization: Technoscientific transformations of health, illness, and U.S. biomedicine. *American Sociological Review* 68(2):161–194.

Coale AJ and Watkins SC, Editors. 1986. *The Decline of Fertility in Europe.* Princeton, NJ: Princeton University Press.

Coburn D. 2015. Vicente Navarro: Marxism, medical dominance, healthcare and health. In Collyer F, Editor. *The Palgrave Handbook of Social Theory in Health, Illness and Medicine.* London: Palgrave MacMillan.

Colgrove J. 2002. The McKeown thesis: A historical controversy and its enduring influence. *American Journal of Public Health* 92(5):725–729.

Collier P. 2007. *The Bottom Billion: Why the Poorest Countries are Failing and What Can Be Done About It.* New York: Oxford University Press.

Corno L and de Walque D. 2012. Mines, migration and HIV/AIDS in southern Africa. *Journal of African Economies* 21(3):465–498.

Corsini CA and Viazzo PP, Editors. 1997. *The Decline of Infant and Child Mortality: The European Experience: 1750–1990.* Cambridge: Kluwer Law International.

Crawford R. 1977. You are dangerous to your health: The ideology and politics of victim blaming. *International Journal of Health Services* 7(4):663–680.

Currie-Alder B, Kanbur R, Malone DM, and Medhora R. 2014. The state of development thought. In *International Development: Ideas, Experience, and Prospects.* Oxford: Oxford University Press.

Cutler DM, Deaton AS, and Lleras-Muney A. 2006. The determinants of mortality. *Journal of Economic Perspectives* 20(3):97–120.

Cutler D and Miller G. 2005. The role of public health improvements in health advances: The twentieth-century United States. *Demography* 42(1):1–22.

Dany C. 2015. Politicization of humanitarian aid in the European Union. *European Foreign Affairs Review* 20(3):419–437.

Dassel K, Saxena R, Funk B, and de Bruin C. 2015. *Accelerating Impact: Exploring Best Practices, Challenges, and Innovations in Impact Enterprise Acceleration.* New York: Monitor Deloitte and The Rockefeller Foundation.

Deaton A. 2013. *The Great Escape: Health, Wealth and the Origins of Inequality.* Princeton, NJ: Princeton University Press.

Deb S. 2015. The Human Development Index and its methodological refinements. *Social Change* 45(1):131–136.

de Mesquita BB and Smith A. 2009. A political economy of aid. *International Organization* 63(2):309–340.

Deneulin S and McGregor JA. 2010. The capability approach and the politics of a social conception of wellbeing. *European Journal of Social Theory* 13(4):501–519.

Desai S, Haddad L, Chopra D, and Thorat A, Editors. 2016. *Undernutrition and Public Policy in India: Investing in the future.* Abingdon, UK: Routledge.

de Sousa Santos B. 2014. *Epistemologies of the South: Justice against Epistemicide.* Boulder, CO: Paradigm Publishers.

Dijkstra G. 2011. The PRSP approach and the illusion of improved aid effectiveness: Lessons from Bolivia, Honduras and Nicaragua. *Development Policy Review* 29(s1):s110–s133.

Doyal L [with Pennell I]. 1979. *The Political Economy of Health.* New Brunswick, NJ: Rutgers University Press.

Doyal L [with Doyal L]. 2013. *Living with HIV and dying with AIDS: Diversity, Inequality and Human Rights in the Global Pandemic.* Farnham, UK: Ashgate Publishing, Ltd.

Du Pisani JA. 2006. Sustainable development–historical roots of the concept. *Environmental Sciences* 3(2):83–96.

Easterlin RA. 1999. How beneficent is the market? A look at the modern history of mortality. *European Review of Economic History* 3(3):257–294.

Easterly W. 2014. *The Tyranny of Experts: Economists, Dictators, and the Forgotten Rights of the Poor.* New York: Basic Books.

Eberstadt N. 2010. The demographic future: What population growth—and decline—means for the global economy. *Foreign Affairs*, November/December 2010.

Erikson SL. 2015. Secrets from whom? Following the money in global health finance. *Current Anthropology* 56(S12):S306–S316.

Escobar A. 2011. The problematization of poverty: The tale of three worlds and development. In *Encountering Development: The Making and Unmaking of the Third World.* Princeton, NJ: Princeton University Press.

Essex J. 2013. *Development, Security, and Aid: Geopolitics and Geoeconomics at the US Agency for International Development.* Athens: University of Georgia Press.

EU Council. 2010. *Council Conclusions on the EU Role in Global Health.* Brussels: Council of the European Union.

Eurodad. 2015. Addis Ababa summit falls short of addressing financing for development. http://www.eurodad.org/Entries/view/1546466/2015/07/24/Addis-Ababa-summit-falls-short-of-addressing-financing-for-development. Accessed February 20, 2016.

Fairtrade Foundation. 2012. *Fair Trade and Coffee: Commodity Briefing.* London.

Farmer P. 2004. An anthropology of structural violence. *Current Anthropology* 45(3):305–325.

Farmer P, Kim JY, Kleinman A, and Basilico M, Editors. 2013. *Reimagining Global Health: An Introduction.* Oakland: University of California Press.

Fassin D. 1996. *L'espace politique de la santé. Essai de généalogie.* Paris: Presses Universitaires de France.

———. 2006. *Quand les corps se souviennent. Expériences et politiques du sida en Afrique du Sud.* Paris: La Découverte.

Fee E and Krieger N. 1993. Understanding AIDS: Historical interpretations and the limits of biomedical individualism. *American Journal of Public Health* 83(10):1477–1486.

Fehling M, Nelson BD, and Venkatapuram S. 2013. Limitations of the Millennium Development Goals: A literature review. *Global Public Health* 8(10):1109–1122.

Ferguson J. 1990. *The Anti-politics Machine: "Development," Depoliticization, and Bureaucratic Power in Lesotho.* Cambridge: Cambridge University Press.

Fidler DP. 2011. *Assessing the Foreign Policy and Global Health Initiative: The Meaning of the Oslo Process.* London: Centre on Global Health Security at Chatham House.

Fogel R. 2012. *Explaining Long-Term Trends in Health and Longevity.* Cambridge, UK: Cambridge University Press.

Frenk J, Bobadilla JL, Stern C, et al. 1991. Elements for a theory of the health transition. *Health Transition Review* 1(1):21–38.

Frost LJ and Reich M. 2009. *Access: How Do Good Health Technologies Get to Poor People in Poor Countries?* Cambridge, MA: Harvard University Press.

Gagnon ML and Labonté R. 2013. Understanding how and why health is integrated into foreign policy - A case study of Health is Global, a UK government strategy 2008 -2013. *Globalization and Health* 9:24.

Galeano E. 2001. *Upside Down: A Primer for the Looking Glass World.* New York: Picador.

Galtung J. 1969. Violence, peace, and peace research. *Journal of Peace Research* 6(3):167–191.

Gapminder. 2009. 200 years that changed the world. http://www.gapminder.org/videos/200-years-that-changed-the-world/. Accessed April 12, 2016.

Garrett L. 2016. Brexit is a global health risk. *Foreign Policy*, July 13.

Gill S and Benatar S. 2016. Global health governance and global power: A critical commentary on the Lancet-University of Oslo Commission Report. *International Journal of Health Services* 46(2):346–365.

Gleckman H. 2016. *Multi-Stakeholderism: A Corporate Push for a New Form of Global Governance.* Amsterdam: The Transnational Institute.

Global Partnership [for Effective Development Co-operation]. 2014. *Progress since Busan: Country and Democratic Ownership.* Paris: Global Partnership.

Gloyd S. 1987. Child survival and resource scarcity. Paper presented at the International Congress of the World Federation of Public Health Associations, Mexico City. March 1987.

Gore C. 2013. Beyond the romantic violence of the MDGs: Development, aid, and human rights. In Langford M, Sumner A, and Yamin AE, Editors. *The Millennium Development Goals and Human Rights: Past, Present and Future.* Cambridge: Cambridge University Press.

Government of Canada. 2016. Global Affairs Canada. http://www.international.gc.ca/international/index.aspx?lang=eng. Accessed March 24, 2016.

Government of the United Kingdom. 2011. *Health is Global: An Outcomes Framework for Global Health 2011-2015.* London: Department of Health.

Griffiths J. 2014. *The State of Finance for Developing Countries, 2014: An Assessment of the Scale of all*

Sources of Finance Available to Developing Countries. Brussels: Eurodad.
Guevara E. 1960. Discurso a los estudiantes de medicina y trabajadores de la salud. In Ariet Garcia MdC and Deutschmann D, Editors. *Che Guevara Presente.* Melbourne: Ocean Press.
Hanson L, Haynes LK, and Turiano L. 2014. Chronic kidney disease in Central America: The big picture. *American Journal of Public Health* 104(7):e9.
Harvey D. 2006. Notes towards a theory of uneven geographical development. In *Spaces of Global Capitalism: Towards a Theory of Uneven Geographical Development.* Brooklyn, NY: Verso Books.
Hervik SEK and Thurston M. 2016. 'It's not the government's responsibility to get me out running 10 km four times a week'-Norwegian men's understandings of responsibility for health. *Critical Public Health* 26(3):333–342.
Hickel J. 2016. The true extent of global poverty and hunger: Questioning the good news narrative of the Millennium Development Goals. *Third World Quarterly* 37(5):749–767.
Hodge JM. 2016a. Writing the history of development (part 1: the first wave). *Humanity: An International Journal of Human Rights, Humanitarianism, and Development* 6(3):429–463.
———. 2016b. Writing the history of development (part 2: longer, deeper, wider). *Humanity: An International Journal of Human Rights, Humanitarianism, and Development* 7(1):125–174.
Holzapfel S. 2014. *Boosting or Hindering Aid Effectiveness? An Assessment of Systems for Measuring Agency results.* Bonn: German Development Institute.
Hou J, Walsh PP, and Zhang J. 2015. The dynamics of human development index. *The Social Science Journal* 52(3):331–347.
Hunter M. 2010. *Love in the Time of AIDS: Inequality, Gender, and Rights in South Africa.* Bloomington: Indiana University Press.
Hyman GF. 2010. *Foreign Policy and Development Structure, Process, Policy, and the Drip-by-Drip Erosion of USAID.* Washington, DC: Center for Strategic & International Studies.
Ichoku HE, Mooney G, and Ataguba JEO. 2013. Africanizing the social determinants of health: Embedded structural inequalities and current health outcomes in sub-Saharan Africa. *International Journal of Health Services* 43(4):745–759.
IHME [Institute for Health Metrics and Evaluation]. 2016. *Financing Global Health 2015: Development Assistance Steady on the Path to New Global Goals.* Seattle.
Illich I. 1976. *Medical Nemesis: The Expropriation of Health.* New York: Pantheon Books.
IMF. 2015. The Multilateral Debt Relief Initiative. https://www.imf.org/external/np/exr/facts/mdri.htm. Accessed April 21, 2016.
———. 2016a. Debt relief under the Heavily Indebted Poor Countries (HIPC) Initiative. https://www.imf.org/external/np/exr/facts/hipc.htm. Accessed April 21, 2016.
———. 2016b. IMF support for low-income countries. http://www.imf.org/external/np/exr/facts/poor.htm. Accessed April 21, 2016.
———. 2016c. Poverty Reduction Strategy in IMF-supported programs https://www.imf.org/external/np/exr/facts/prsp.htm. Accessed April 21, 2016.
———. 2016d. The Catastrophe Containment and Relief Trust. https://www.imf.org/external/np/exr/facts/ccr.htm. Accessed May 7, 2016.
———. 2016e. The Policy Support Instrument. https://www.imf.org/external/np/exr/facts/psi.htm. Accessed April 21, 2016.
Information Office of the State Council. 2014. *Preamble of White Paper on China's Foreign Aid.* Beijing: The State Council, The People's Republic of China.
Institute of Medicine. 2009. *The U.S. Commitment to Global Health: Recommendations for the Public and Private Sectors.* Washington, DC: The National Academies Press.
Jamison DT, Summers LH, Alleyne G, et al. 2013. Global health 2035: A world converging within a generation. *Lancet* 382(9908):1898–1955.
Johansson SR and Mosk C. 1987. Exposure, resistance and life expectancy: Disease and death during the economic development of Japan, 1900–1960. *Population Studies* 41(2):207–235.
Jones BG. 2013 Slavery, finance and international political economy: Postcolonial reflections. In Seth S, Editor. *Postcolonial Theory and International Relations: A Critical Introduction.* Abingdon, UK: Routledge.
Jones DS and Greene JA. 2013. The decline and rise of coronary heart disease: Understanding public health catastrophism. *American Journal of Public Health* 103(7):1207–1218.
Justice J. 1986. *Policies, Plans and People: Culture and Health Development in Nepal.* Berkeley: University of California Press.
Kahan S, Gielen AC, Fagan PJ, and Green LW, Editors. 2014. *Health Behavior Change in Populations.* Baltimore: Johns Hopkins University Press.

Kalofonos IA. 2010. "All I eat is ARVs": The paradox of AIDS treatment interventions in Central Mozambique. *Medical Anthropology Quarterly* 24(3):363–380.

Kassalow J. 2001. *Why Health is Important to US Foreign Policy*. New York: Council on Foreign Relations and Milbank Memorial Fund.

Katz A. 2002. AIDS, individual behaviour and the unexplained remaining variation. *African Journal of AIDS Research* 1(2):125–142.

———. 2005. The Sachs report: Investing in health for economic development—or increasing the size of the crumbs from the rich man's table? *International Journal of Health Services* 35(1):171–188.

Kearns G. 1988. The urban penalty and the population history of England. In Brändstrom A and Tedebrand LG, Editors. *Society, Health and Population during the Demographic Transition*. Stockholm: Almqvist and Wiksell International.

King L, Stuckler D, and Hamm P. 2006. Mass privatization and the postcommunist mortality crisis. Working Paper Series No. 118. Amherst: Political Economy Research Institute, University of Massachussetts Amherst.

Klugman J, Rodríguez F, and Choi H-J. 2011. *Human Development Research Paper 2011/01; The HDI 2010: New Controversies, Old Critiques*. New York: UNDP.

Knowles JH. 1977. The responsibility of the individual. *Daedalus* 106(1):57–80.

Kothari U, Editor. 2005. *A Radical History of Development Studies: Individuals, Institutions and Ideologies*. London: Zed Books.

Krieger N. 1994. Epidemiology and the web of causation: Has anyone seen the spider? *Social Science & Medicine* 39(7):887–903.

Krieger N and Birn A-E. 1998. A vision of social justice as the foundation of public health: Commemorating 150 years of the spirit of 1848. *American Journal of Public Health* 88(11):1603–1606.

Labonté R, Runnels V, and Gagnon M. 2012. Past fame, present frames and future flagship? An exploration of how health is positioned in Canadian foreign policy. *Administrative Sciences* 2(2):162–185.

Lalonde M. 1974. *A New Perspective on the Health of Canadians*. Ottawa: Government of Canada.

Lenzer J. 2015. Centers for Disease Control and Prevention: Protecting the private good? *BMJ* 350:h2362.

Lewontin RC. 2000. *The Triple Helix: Gene, Organism, and Environment*. Cambridge, MA: Harvard University Press.

Macdonald D and Wilson D. 2016. *Shameful Neglect: Indigenous Child Poverty in Canada*. Ottawa: Canadian Centre for Policy Alternatives.

Maciocco G and Italian Global Health Watch. 2008. From Alma Ata to the Global Fund: The history of international health policy. *Social Medicine* 3(1):36–48.

Mahmudi-Azer S. 2011. The international arms trade and global health. In Benatar S and Brock G, Editors. *Global Health and Global Health Ethics*. Cambridge: Cambridge University Press.

Martens J and Seitz K. 2015. *Philanthropic Power and Development. Who Shapes the Agenda?* Aachen/Berlin/Bonn/: Bischöfliches Hilfswerk MISEREOR, Evangelisches Werk für Diakonie und Entwicklung Brot für die Welt – Evangelischer Entwicklungsdienst, Global Policy Forum.

Martínez-Alier J, Pascual U, Vivien F, and Zaccai E. 2010. Sustainable de-growth: Mapping the context, criticisms and future prospects of an emergent paradigm. *Ecological Economics* 69(9):1741–1747.

Maynard G, Shircliff E, and Restivo M. 2012. IMF structural adjustment, public health spending, and tuberculosis: A longitudinal analysis of prevalence rates in poor countries. *International Journal of Sociology* 42(2):5–27.

McCoy D. 2014. The Lancet-UiO Commission on Global Governance For Health Commissioners should withdraw their recommendations and come up with better ones. http://www.medact.org/medact-blog/david-mccoy-lancet-commission/. Accessed June 26, 2015.

McGuire JW. 2010. Politics, policy, and mortality decline in Chile, 1960-1995. In Salvatore RD, Coatsworth JH, and Challú AE, Editors. *Living Standards in Latin American History: Height, Welfare, and Development, 1750–2000*. Cambridge, MA: David Rockefeller Center for Latin American Studies, Harvard University.

McKeown T. 1976. *The Modern Rise of Population*. London: Edward Arnold.

McKeown T and Record RG. 1962. Reasons for the decline of mortality in England and Wales during the nineteenth century. *Population Studies* 16(2):94–122.

McKeown T, Record R, and Turner R. 1975. An interpretation of the decline of mortality in England and Wales during the twentieth century. *Population Studies* 29(3):391–422.

McNeill D and Ottersen OP. 2015. Global governance for health: How to motivate political change? *Public Health* 129(7):833–837.

Men T, Brennan P, Boffetta P, and Zaridze D. 2003. Russian mortality trends for 1991–2001: Analysis by cause and region. *British Medical Journal* 327(7421):964–966.

Morse S and McNamara N. 2013. *Sustainable Livelihood Approach: A Critique of Theory and Practice.* London: Springer Science & Business Media.

Moyo D. 2009. *Dead Aid: Why Aid Is Not Working And How There Is A Better Way for Africa.* New York: Farrar, Straus and Giroux.

Naghavi M, Wang H, Lozano R, et al. 2015. Global, regional, and national age–sex specific all-cause and cause-specific mortality for 240 causes of death, 1990–2013: A systematic analysis for the global burden of disease study 2013. *Lancet* 385(9963):117–171.

Navarro V. 2004. Development and quality of life: A critique of Amartya Sen's *Development as Freedom.* In Navarro V and Muntaner C, Editors. *The Political and Economic Determinants of Population Health and Well-being.* Amityville, NY: Baywood Publishing Company.

———. 2007. A Note for the IAHP's History. http://www.healthp.org/node/255. Accessed September 22, 2007.

———. 2009. What we mean by social determinants of health. *International Journal of Health Services* 39(3):423–441.

Ncayiyana DJ. 2007. Combating poverty: The charade of development aid. *British Medical Journal* 335(7633):1272–1273.

Neely AH. 2015. Internal ecologies and the limits of local biologies: A political ecology of tuberculosis in the time of AIDS. *Annals of the Association of American Geographers* 105(4):791–805.

Nervi LL. 2014. Easier said than done (in global health): A glimpse at nonfinancial challenges in international cooperation. *Policies for Equitable Access to Health,* February 20. http://www.peah.it/2014/02/easier-said-than-done-in-global-health-a-glimpse-at-nonfinancial-challenges-in-international-cooperation/.

Notestein FW. 1945. Population—the long view. In Schultz T, Editor. *Food for the World.* Chicago: University of Chicago Press.

OECD. 2011. *Evaluation of the Implementation of the Paris Declaration.* Paris: OECD.

———. 2015. *Development Co-operation Report 2015: Making Partnerships Effective Coalitions for Action.* Paris.

———. 2016a. Agricultural support (indicator). https://data.oecd.org/agrpolicy/agricultural-support.htm. Accessed April 21, 2016.

———. 2016b. Query Wizard for International Development Statistics (QWIDS). http://stats.oecd.org/qwids/. Accessed February 27, 2016.

OHCHR, OHRLLS, UNDESA et al. 2013. *Global governance and governance of the global commons in the global partnership for development beyond 2015: Thematic Think Piece.* UN System Task Team on the Post-2015 UN Development Agenda.

O'Hearn D. 2009. Amartya Sen's development as freedom: Ten years later. *Policy & Practice: A Development Education Review* 8:9–15.

Omran AR. 1971. The epidemiologic transition: A theory of the epidemiology of population change. *Milbank Memorial Fund Quarterly* 49(4):509–538.

Orantes Navarro CM, Herrera Valdés R, Almaguer López M, et al. 2015. Epidemiological characteristics of chronic kidney disease of non-traditional causes in women of agricultural communities of El Salvador. *Clinical nephrology* 83(1):S24–S31.

Ordunez P, Martinez R, Reveiz L, et al. 2014. Chronic kidney disease epidemic in Central America: Urgent public health action is needed amid causal uncertainty. *PLoS Neglected Tropical Diseases* 8(8):e3019.

Ottersen OP, Dasgupta J, Blouin C, et al. 2014. *The Lancet*–University of Oslo Commission on Global Governance for Health: The political origins of health inequity: prospects for change. *Lancet* 383 (9917): 630–667.

Packard R. 1989. *White Plague, Black Labor: Tuberculosis and the Political Economy of Health and Disease in South Africa.* Berkeley: University of California Press.

———. 2016. *A History of Global Health: Interventions into the Lives of Other Peoples.* Baltimore: Johns Hopkins University Press.

Parikh SA. 2007. The political economy of marriage and HIV: The ABC approach,"safe" infidelity, and managing moral risk in Uganda. *American Journal of Public Health* 97(7):1198–1208.

Pearce N. 1996. Traditional epidemiology, modern epidemiology, and public health. *American Journal of Public Health* 86(5):678–683.

Peters DH, Paina L, and Schleimann F. 2013. Sector-wide approaches (SWAps) in health: What have we learned? *Health Policy and Planning* 28(8):884–890.

Pfeiffer J and Chapman R. 2010. Anthropological perspectives on structural adjustment and public health. *Annual Review of Anthropology* 39:149–165.

PHM, Medact, Health Action International, et al. 2011. *Global Health Watch 3: An Alternative World Health Report.* London: Zed Books.

PHM, Medact, Medico International, et al. 2014. *Global Health Watch 4: An Alternative World Health Report.* London: Zed Books Ltd.

Plaatje ST. 1916. *Native Life in South Africa, Before and Since the European War and the Boer Rebellion.* London: P.S. Kind and Son, Ltd

Pogge T and Sengupta M. 2015. The Sustainable Development Goals: A plan for building a better world? *Journal of Global Ethics* 11(1):56–64.

Porter ME and Stern S. 2015. *Social Progress Index 2015.* Washington, DC: Social Progress Imperative.

Prashad V. 2013. *The Poorer Nations: A Possible History of the Global South.* Brooklyn: Verso Books.

Preston SH. 1975. The changing relation between mortality and level of economic development. *Population Studies* 29(2):231–248.

———. 1980. Causes and consequences of mortality decline in less developed countries during the twentieth century. In Easterlin R, Editor. *Population and Economic Change in Developing Countries.* Chicago: University of Chicago Press.

Ramirez-Rubio O, Brooks DR, Amador JJ, et al. 2013. Chronic kidney disease in Nicaragua: A qualitative analysis of semi-structured interviews with physicians and pharmacists. *BMC Public Health* 13:350.

Reading J and Halseth R. 2013. *Pathways to Improving Well-Being for Indigenous Peoples: How Living Conditions Decide Health.* Prince George, BC: National Collaborating Centre for Aboriginal Health.

Riley JC. 2001. *Rising Life Expectancy: A Global History.* New York: Cambridge University Press.

———. 2007. *Low Income, Social Growth, and Good Health: A History of Twelve Countries.* Berkeley and Los Angeles: University of California Press.

Rist G. 2007. Development as a buzzword. *Development in Practice* 17(4-5):485–491.

Roalkvam S and McNeill D. 2016. What counts as progress? The contradictions of global health initiatives. *Forum for Development Studies* 43(1):69–88.

Rowden R. 2009. *The Deadly Ideas of Neoliberalism: How the IMF Has Undermined Public Health and the Fight against AIDS.* London: Zed Books.

———. 2012. Advocates for global health aid must call for a new development model. Schrecker T, Editor. *The Ashgate Research Companion to the Globalization of Health.* Abingdon, UK: Routledge.

Rückert A. 2010. The forgotten dimension of social reproduction: The World Bank and the poverty reduction strategy paradigm. *Review of International Political Economy* 17(5):816–839.

Rückert A and Labonté R. 2014. Public–private partnerships (PPPs) in global health: The good, the bad and the ugly. *Third World Quarterly* 35(9):1598–1614.

Sachs J. 2008. Primary health for all: Ten resolutions could globally ensure a basic human right at almost unnoticeable cost. *Scientific American,* December 16, 34–36.

———. 2015. *The Age of Sustainable Development.* New York: Columbia University Press.

Sahle EN. 2011. Interview with Professor Eunice N. Sahle: "Moving Beyond the Language of 'Help' ". *AfricAvenir,* March 1.

Santosa A, Wall S, Fottrell E, et al. 2014. The development and experience of epidemiological transition theory over four decades: A systematic review. *Global Health Action* 7.

Satcher D and Higginbotham EJ. 2008. Commentary: The public health approach to eliminating disparities in health. *American Journal of Public Health* 98(3):400–403.

Sauvy A. 1952. Trois mondes, une planète. *l'Observateur,* August 14.

Schofield R, Reher D, and Bideau A, Editors. 1991. *The Decline of Mortality in Europe.* Oxford: Clarendon Press.

Sen A. 1999. *Development as Freedom.* New York: Oxford University Press.

———. 2009. *The Idea of Justice.* Cambridge, MA: Harvard University Press.

Sharp JM. 2015. *U.S. Foreign Aid to Israel.* Washington, DC: Congressional Research Service.

Shkolnikov V, Andreev E, McKee M, and Leon DA. 2014. Rost prodolzhitel'nosti zhizni v Rossii 2000-kh godov. *Demograficheskoe obozrenie* 1(2):5–37.

Skalická V, Ringdal K, and Witvliet MI. 2015. Socioeconomic inequalities in mortality and repeated measurement of explanatory risk factors in a 25 years follow-up. *PLoS ONE* 10(4): e0124690.

Smith J and Daynes L. 2016. Borders and migration: an issue of global health importance. *Lancet Global Health* 4(2):e85–e86.

Sridhar D. 2008. *The Battle Against Hunger: Choice, Circumstance, and the World Bank.* New York: Oxford University Press.

Steckel R and Floud R, Editors. 1997. *Health and Welfare during Industrialization.* Chicago: University of Chicago Press.

Stiglitz J. 2002. *Globalization and its Discontents.* New York: W.W. Norton and Co.

Stiglitz JE, Sen A, and Fitoussi J-P. 2009. *Report by the Commission on the Measurement of Economic*

Performance and Social Progress. Paris: Institut national de la statistique et des études économiques.

Stuckler D, King L, and McKee M. 2009. Mass privatisation and the post-communist mortality crisis: A cross-national analysis. *Lancet* 373(9661):399–407.

Sumner A. 2006. What is development studies? *Development in Practice* 16(6):644–650.

Susser M. 1998. Does risk factor epidemiology put epidemiology at risk? Peering into the future. *Journal of Epidemiology and Community Health* 52(10):608–611.

Sweeney R, Mortimer D, and Johnston DW. 2014. Do Sector Wide Approaches for health aid delivery lead to 'donor-flight'? A comparison of 46 low-income countries. *Social Science & Medicine* 105:38–46.

Szreter S. 2005. *Health and Wealth: Studies in History and Policy*. Rochester, NY: University of Rochester Press.

Tan C. 2007. *Debt and Conditionality: Multilateral Debt Relief Initiative and Opportunities for Expanding Policy Space*. Penang, MY: Third World Network.

Tapia Granados JA and Diez Roux AV. 2009. Life and death during the Great Depression. *Proceedings of the National Academy of Sciences* 106(41):17290–17295.

Tarantola D, Byrnes A, Johnson M et al. 2013. Human rights, health and development. In Grodin MA, Tarantola D, Annas GJ, and Gruskin S, Editors. *Health and Human Rights in a Changing World*. New York: Routledge.

Testa M. 2007. Decidir en salud, ¿Quién?, ¿Cómo? y ¿Por qué? *Salud Colectiva* 3(3):247–257.

Tolstoy LN. 1886. *Writings on Civil Disobedience and Nonviolence* [published in 1967, New York: Bergman Publishers].

Toussaint É and Millet D. 2010. *Debt, the IMF, and the World Bank: Sixty Questions, Sixty answers*. New York: Monthly Review Press.

UN. 2000. *United Nations Millennium Declaration*. New York.

———. 2013. *The Millennium Development Goals Report, 2013*. New York.

———. 2015a. Sustainable Development Knowledge Platform: Sustainable Development Goals. https://sustainabledevelopment.un.org/sdgs. Accessed 15 December 2015.

———. 2015b. *The Millennium Development Goals Report 2015*. New York: UN.

——— [Department of Economic and Social Affairs, Population Division]. 2015c. *World Population Prospects: 2015 Revision, Volume I: Comprehensive Tables*. New York: UN Population Division.

UN General Assembly. 1986. Declaration on the Right to Development. A/RES/41/128.

UN Global Compact. 2016. What is UN Global Compact? https://www.unglobalcompact.org/what-is-gc. Accessed April 21, 2016.

UNICEF. 2015. *Committing to Child Survival: A Promise Renewed. Progress Report 2015*. New York: UNICEF.

UNIDO [UN Industrial Development Organization] and UN Global Compact. 2014. *Series of Dialogues on Means of Implementation of the Post-2015 Development Agenda Engaging with the Private Sector in the Post-2015 Agenda*. New York: UN.

UN Millennium Project. 2007. *Goals, targets and indicators*. http://www.unmillenniumproject.org/goals/gti.htm#goa11. Accessed March 23, 2007.

United States Government. 2015. *National Security Agenda: February 2015*. Washington, DC: The White House.

USAID. 2016. Who we are: Assistance to foreign countries. https://www.usaid.gov/who-we-are. Accessed April 21, 2016.

Vandenheede H, Vikhireva O, Pikhart H, et al. 2014. Socioeconomic inequalities in all-cause mortality in the Czech Republic, Russia, Poland and Lithuania in the 2000s: Findings from the HAPIEE Study. *Journal of Epidemiology and Community Health* 68:297–303.

Velásquez G and Alas M. 2016. The slow shipwreck of the World Health Organization? *Third World Network*, May 19.

Virchow R. 1848a. Report on the typhus epidemic in Upper Silesia. In Rather L, Translator and Editor. *Collected Essays on Public Health and Epidemiology (1985)*. Canton, MA: Science History Publications.

———. 1848b. The aims of the journal "Medical Reform." In Rather L, Translator and Editor. *Collected Essays on Public Health and Epidemiology (1985)*. Canton, MA: Science History Publications.

———. 1848c. The charity physician. In Rather L, Translator and Editor. *Collected Essays on Public Health and Epidemiology (1985)*. Canton, MA: Science History Publications.

Vitek C and Wharton M. 1998. Diphtheria in the former Soviet Union: Reemergence of a pandemic disease. *Emerging Infectious Diseases* 4(4):539–550.

Waitzkin H. 2011. *Medicine and Public Health at the End of Empire*. Boulder, CO: Paradigm Publishers.

Walker C and Kirk JM. 2013. From cooperation to capacitation: Cuban medical internationalism in the South Pacific. *International Journal of Cuban Studies* 5(1):10–25.

Ware E. 2010. After the crisis, is now the moment to cut Western farm subsidies? *Global Policy Forum*, March 30.

Weisz G and Olszynko-Gryn J. 2010. The theory of epidemiologic transition: The origins of a citation classic. *Journal of the History of Medicine and Allied Sciences* 65(3):287–326.

WHO. 2013. Diarrhoeal disease: Fact sheet. http://www.who.int/mediacentre/factsheets/fs330/en/. Accessed June 21, 2015.

———. 2015a. *Global Tuberculosis Report 2015*. Geneva: WHO.

———. 2015b. *Health in 2015: from MDGs, Millennium Development Goals to SDGs, Sustainable Development Goals*. Geneva: WHO.

———. 2016. Trade, foreign policy, diplomacy and health: Global governance. https://ideeaeuropeanaugal.files.wordpress.com/2016/01/who-_-global-governance.pdf. Accessed July 16, 2016.

WHO EURO. 2014. European health for all database. http://data.euro.who.int/hfadb/. Accessed July 17, 2015.

Williams C and Blaiklock A. 2015. SDG Series: With SDGs Now Adopted, Human Rights Must Inform Implementation and Accountability. *Health and Human Rights Journal Blog*, September 29.

Wilson J. 2015. Book review essay: The age of sustainable development by Jeffrey Sachs. *Human Geography* 8(2):103–110.

Wolleswinkel-van den Bosch JH, van Poppel FWA, Looman CWN, and Mackenbach JP. 2000. Determinants of infant and early childhood mortality levels and their decline in the Netherlands in the late nineteenth century. *International Journal of Epidemiology* 29(6):1031–1040.

Woods R. 2000. *The Demography of Victorian England and Wales*. Cambridge: Cambridge University Press.

Worboys M. 2010. Before McKeown: Explaining the decline of tuberculosis in Britain, 1880-1930. In Condrau F and Worboys M, Editors. *Tuberculosis Then and Now: Perspectives on the History of an Infectious Disease*. Montreal: McGill-Queen's University Press.

World Bank. 1993. *World Development Report 1993: Investing in Health*. New York: Oxford University Press.

———. 2005. *Dying Too Young: Addressing Premature Mortality and Ill Health due to Non-Communicable Diseases and Injuries in the Russian Federation*. Washington, DC: World Bank.

———. 2006. *World Development Report 2006: Equity and Development*. Washington, DC: World Bank.

———. 2011. What are PRSPs?. http://web.worldbank.org/WBSITE/EXTERNAL/TOPICS/EXTPOVERTY/EXTPRS/0,,contentMDK:22283891~menuPK:384209~pagePK:210058~piPK:210062~theSitePK:384201,00.html. Accessed September 21, 2014.

———. 2015. PovcalNet: an online analysis tool for global poverty monitoring http://iresearch.worldbank.org/PovcalNet/index.htm?0. Accessed February 20, 2016.

———. 2016a. *Live Long and Prosper: Aging in East Asia and Pacific*. Washington, DC: World Bank.

———. 2016b. World Development Indicators. http://data.worldbank.org/data-catalog/world-development-indicators. Accessed April 20, 2016.

Wrigley EA and Schofield RS. 1989. *The Population History of England 1541-1871: A Reconstruction*. Cambridge: Cambridge University Press.

Zaridze D, Lewington S, Boroda A, et al. 2014. Alcohol and mortality in Russia: Prospective observational study of 151 000 adults. *Lancet* 383(9927):1465–1473.

Zijdema RL and Ribeiro de Silva F. 2014. Life expectancy since 1820. In van Zanden JL, Baten J, d'Ercole MM, et al, Editors. *How Was Life?: Global Well-Being Since 1820*. Paris: OECD Publishing.

4

GLOBAL HEALTH ACTORS AND ACTIVITIES

There is a dizzying panorama of organizations and people operating in the global health arena, with new organizations appearing almost monthly. To be sure, the term *global health* (like international health) is a bit of a misnomer. The vast majority of work in this arena is not divvied up among relevant actors as though they had an equivalent voice or a unified vision. Instead, it reflects the prevailing political and economic order and its historical trajectory, whereby most health cooperation is "channeled" via high-income countries (HICs)—their bilateral organizations, corporations, non governmental organizations (NGOs), and philanthropies, as well as the multilateral agencies heavily influenced by these players—and "received" in low- and middle-income countries (LMICs). Why, we might ask, are there no LMIC foreigners interfering or "helping" HICs organize their public health systems; for example, where are the Madagascan agencies funding services for Swiss residents with disabilities in NGO-run clinics? Amid the enthusiasm that so many share in finding solutions and "making a difference," it is essential to remember that the global health field reflects contemporary geopolitical relations and reproduces dominant (im)balances of power and resources.

Still, large multilateral, bilateral, private, and nongovernmental entities (see Box 4-1 for definitions) are not the only global health actors. Many other health organizations, with far smaller budgets but often sizeable memberships, have emerged in recent decades. Active in HICs and LMICs, these include community action and public-interest NGOs, human rights organizations, and advocacy movements. Many of these groups agree on the importance of local priority-setting and advocate an integrated social, political, and technical approach to health in the context of economic redistribution, struggles against oppression, and bona fide democratic accountability. Unlike dominant global health players, social justice actors insist that the ultimate aim of global health is for sovereign states to be in a position—economically and politically—to meet their own people's needs (or, in the interim, to participate in cooperation based on solidarity principles, not outsider prescriptions).

In recent years, the term *global health diplomacy* has taken hold, referring both to the formal structures of global health decisionmaking in foreign affairs ministries and multilateral and summit organizations—such as the G20, African Union, and Organization of Islamic Cooperation, as well as United Nations (UN) agencies—and the interaction and negotiations among state (and non-state) actors around the dynamic factors that influence health (or the use of health to shape foreign policy and vice versa) (Kickbusch and Kökény 2013). Of course, as discussed in prior chapters, health has

Box 4-1 Definitions

Agency—an organization with a defined purpose, often administratively related to or subsumed under a larger governmental or intergovernmental structure

Bilateral—denoting the involvement of two nations (e.g., a bilateral agency)

Community-based organization (CBO)—public or private not-for-profit organization that represents members of a community and seeks to address issues related to that community

Foundation—a tax-exempt, nonprofit charitable organization, usually supported by a philanthropic endowment

Fund—a sum of money collected and set aside for a particular purpose, and/or the entity that administers it

Global health initiative—effort focused on particular diseases, interventions, products, or services, organized and operated by a PPP

Global health partnership—organization with multiple partners that seeks to address complex health challenges beyond what individual members of the partnership can achieve

INGO (International nongovernmental organization)—NGO that works internationally or transnationally

International—relating to activities or relations between/among two or more nations; like *global*, also connoting interaction that transcends national boundaries (see chapter 2 for further discussion of international and global health)

Multilateral—denoting the involvement of three or more nations (e.g., a multilateral agency)

NGO (Nongovernmental organization)—not-for-profit civic entity or network that is not directly related to government structures and focuses on a particular issue or purpose

Organization—a group or organized structure of people working together with the aim of achieving collective goals

Program—an umbrella structure (often overseen by an agency or organization) involving several related projects, generally with a particular purpose

Project—an endeavor with a defined time-frame and resources, designed to reach a specific goal

Product Development Partnership (PDP)—PPP aimed at innovating and commercializing drugs, vaccines, and other products for global health markets

Public-Private Partnership (PPP)—collaborative entity involving both public and private sector organizations

long been a foreign policy and diplomacy concern in relation to disease notification and cross-border transmission, as well as (asymmetrical) protection and promotion of national political, economic, and private interests.

The intertwining of health and foreign affairs agendas through "soft power" diplomacy, exemplified in China's and Brazil's growing involvement in health cooperation (Carrillo Roa and Silva 2015), raises the prospects of "horizontal" global health relationships based on mutual health equity aims (Buss and Faid 2013), even as uneven power dynamics persist (Labonté and Gagnon 2010). Such changed configurations have been afoot in the flourishing arena of South–South cooperation, involving an array of "emerging" powers and other LMICs. Operating outside the old nexus of imperial power, South–South interchange has opened the possibility of cooperation on a more equal and just basis, especially when partners share social and political values.

SNAPSHOT OF GLOBAL HEALTH ACTORS, AGENCIES, AND PROGRAMS

Key Questions:

- Who are the major players in global health and what are their roles?
- What political, economic, and ideological rationales guide their policies and activities?

This chapter presents a scan of organizations and activities in global health: those with a direct mandate for health; those that shape and provide public health and health care services through public and private channels; and those that influence the determinants of health, from international financial agencies to social justice organizations. This is not a comprehensive survey: we pay closest attention to those actors that have the greatest bearing on global health policymaking and practice or that illustrate particular kinds of actors.

Global health agencies and other actors may be characterized by their: sources of funding; influence over local, regional, and global agendas; relationship to other actors and priorities; accountability and breadth of membership; aims, approaches, motivations, and values; functions and activities; and impact on health, well-being, and the broader context. Other important features include technical and management capacity, political legitimacy, whether staff is voluntary or paid, and historical trajectory. Here we classify them according to funding source, mission, scope of activities, and their role and influence in the field, focusing on key examples in each category (Table 4-1). Importantly, the categories applied here are not mutually exclusive; some health actors cross categories. For example, Catholic Relief Services is both a religious agency and a humanitarian NGO; likewise, the Barcelona Institute for Global Health (ISGlobal) is a public-private partnership (PPP)/think tank hybrid that brings together academics, the public sector, and philanthropy to carry out scientific research and policy analysis, educational activities, and technical assistance.

Table 4-1 Typology of Global/International Health Actors and Programs

Type	Examples
UN (Multilateral) Agencies	WHO, UNICEF, UNAIDS, UNFPA, UNDP, UNEP, UN Women
International Financial and Economic Institutions	World Bank, International Monetary Fund (IMF), World Trade Organization (WTO)
Bilateral Aid and Development Agencies	United States Agency for International Development (USAID), Swedish International Development Agency (Sida), UK Department for International Development (DFID)
Military Actors	US Department of Defense, North Atlantic Treaty Organization (NATO), European Union Force (EUFOR)
South-South Cooperation	BRICS, China South-South Cooperation Fund, Ministerio de Relaciones Exteriores (Cuba)
Contract Providers and Consulting Firms	Management Sciences for Health, John Snow, Health Systems Trust, Abt Associates, FHI 360
Government Technical Agencies and Research Institutions	Centers for Disease Control and Prevention (CDC), Fundação Oswaldo Cruz (Fiocruz), European Centre for Disease Prevention and Control (ECDC), Medical Research Council MRC), icddr,b
Regional Organizations and Economic Unions	Organization for Economic Cooperation and Development (OECD), African Union, European Union (EU), CELAC

Table 4-1 **Continued**

Foundations	
The Old Guard	Rockefeller Foundation (RF), Ford Foundation, Wellcome Trust
The New Guard	Bill and Melinda Gates Foundation (BMGF), Clinton Foundation, Elton John AIDS Foundation
LMIC Foundations	Aga Khan Foundation, Carlos Slim Health Institute
Business Interests	
Private Health Insurance	Aetna
Big Pharma	Merck, Pfizer, GSK
Corporate Foundations and Alliances	Shell, ExxonMobil, Walmart
Public–Private Partnerships (PPPs)	Global Fund, GAVI, the Vaccine Alliance, Stop TB Partnership, Global Alliance for Improved Nutrition (GAIN), Global Polio Eradication Initiative
Emerging Global Financing Approaches	UNITAID
Missionaries and Religious Agencies and Charities	World Vision, Diakonia, Mennonite Central Committee, Islamic Relief Worldwide
Joint Health and Development Initiatives	IHP+, H8
NGOs	
Large Humanitarian NGOs	Save the Children, CARE, Concern Worldwide, Plan International
Relief Groups	National Societies of the Red Cross & Red Crescent, International Rescue Committee, Gift of the Givers
Social Rights-Oriented/ Service Provision NGOs	Oxfam, Médecins Sans Frontières (MSF), Partners In Health (PIH), Doctors for Global Health (DGH)
Human Rights and Health Groups	Physicians for Human Rights, Amnesty International, Dignitas International, Association for Women's Rights in Development (AWID)
LMIC NGOs	BRAC, Urmul Trust, Jamkhed Comprehensive Rural Health Project
Global Health and Development Think Tanks	Center for Global Development, Overseas Development Institute, CPATH
Advocacy Groups and Alliances	Global AIDS Alliance, NCD Alliance
Social Rights NGOs and Scholar-Activist Organizations	People's Health Movement (PHM), Treatment Action Campaign, Focus on the Global South, Equinet, ALAMES, Universities Allied for Essential Medicines
Social and Political Movements	International Labor Rights Forum, World Social Forum
University and Hospital Initiatives	Emory Global Health Institute, Instituto Nacional de Salud Pública (Mexico), AMPATH
Research Alliances	Council on Health Research for Development (COHRED), Global Forum for Health Research
Professional Membership Organizations	INCLEN, World Federation of Public Health Associations
Small-Scale and Consumer Driven Efforts	Kiva, GlobalGiving, (RED)

United Nations (Multilateral) Agencies

UN agencies, involving representation/membership of most countries, are aimed at aid, technical cooperation, and the setting of international norms and standards (see chapter 2 on the UN's origins). Traditionally funded through member state dues assessments (according to country size and wealth), via the UN directly, the World Bank, or in the case of the UN Children's Fund (UNICEF), voluntary contributions (from governments and millions of individuals), some agencies are governed through quasi-democratic decisionmaking processes. While high-income member states have long held more sway, greater funding from private and philanthropic donors gives these actors growing agenda-setting roles. Some UN agencies are focused exclusively on public health (most notably the World Health Organization [WHO] and the Joint United Nations Programme on HIV/AIDS [UNAIDS]), whereas others—such as the UN High Commissioner for Refugees (UNHCR), UN Environment Programme (UNEP), and UN Entity for Gender Equality and the Empowerment of Women (UN Women)—have different mandates, though their work bears significantly on health (Table 4-2).

Some autonomous specialized agencies are linked to the UN through specific agreements (Table 4-3). These organizations help set standards, formulate policies, and provide technical assistance in their areas of expertise.

While most UN agencies operate independently from one another, their in-country activities are meant to be complementary and they occasionally cooperate through large initiatives. Since the 1960s, every decade has had a designated UN theme. Among the most salient to health was the 1980s International Decade for Clean Drinking Water. Although 1.2 billion people gained access to water by 1990, the goal of universal access to safe water and sanitation was not met;

Table 4-2 Selected UN Organizations

Organization	Mission/Function
UN Development Programme (UNDP)	Addresses poverty and reducing inequities through three main foci: sustainable development; democratic governance and peace building; and climate and disaster resilience
UN Children's Fund (UNICEF)	Lead UN organization focused on survival, protection, and development of children Works on immunization, family planning, nutrition, maternal and child health, primary education, and child rights
UN Environment Programme (UNEP)	Encourages sound environmental practices and assesses global, regional, and national environmental conditions
UN High Commissioner for Refugees (UNHCR)	Protects rights and well-being of refugees, internally displaced persons, asylum-seekers, and stateless people
World Food Programme (WFP)	Largest international food aid organization for emergency relief
UN Population Fund (UNFPA)	Promotes sexual and reproductive health and rights of women and girls
UN Human Settlements Programme (UN-HABITAT)	Promotes socially and environmentally sustainable settlements for humans and adequate housing for all
UN Conference on Trade and Development (UNCTAD)	Promotes fair inclusion in the global economy, particularly addressing LMIC concerns
UNAIDS	Coordinates UN HIV and AIDS efforts
UN Office of the High Commissioner for Human Rights (OHCHR)	Promotes and protects the rights established in the UN Charter and in international human rights laws and treaties
UN Entity for Gender Equality and the Empowerment of Women (UN Women)	Promotes women's empowerment; supports development, implementation, and monitoring of global standards on gender equality

Table 4-3 Selected UN Autonomous Specialized Agencies

Agency	Mission/Function
World Health Organization (WHO)	Serves as directing and coordinating authority on health within the UN system
International Labour Organization (ILO)	Sets and monitors employment standards, promotes workplace rights, decent employment, and social protection
Food and Agriculture Organization (FAO)	Works to improve agricultural productivity and eliminate food insecurity, and better the conditions of rural populations
UN Educational, Scientific and Cultural Organization (UNESCO)	Promotes peace, universal education, intercultural understanding, scientific cooperation, protection of the world's natural and cultural heritage, and freedom of expression
International Fund for Agricultural Development (IFAD)	Mobilizes financial resources for poor rural producers in LMICs (including fishers, pastoralists, smallhold farmers, agricultural laborers, foresters, and small entrepreneurs) to help integrate them into national and global markets
UN Industrial Development Organization (UNIDO)	Promotes the "sustainable industrial development" of LMICs through technical cooperation, policy advisory services, research, and training

currently some 2.4 billion people lack access to safe water and basic sanitation (WWAP 2015).

The UN also sponsors large international gatherings directly or indirectly relating to health, such as a series of women's conferences and population and development conferences (see chapter 2). The Beijing Women's Conference of 1995, for example, produced a thorough declaration on women's rights—incorporating issues of poverty eradication, sexuality and reproduction, fair pay for work, the effects of armed conflict, racial and ethnic discrimination, natural resource management, and the special needs of girls.

Table 4-4 Major United Nations Meetings (with Health-Related Dimensions) since 2010

Subject/Short Title	Year	Site
Noncommunicable Diseases	2011	New York
Sustainable Development (Rio + 20 Summit)	2012	Rio de Janeiro
International Migration and Development	2013	New York
Ageing (6th)	2015	New York
Climate Change (21st)	2015	Paris
Convention to Combat Desertification (12th)	2015	Ankara
Financing for Development (3rd)	2015	Addis Ababa
Road Safety (2nd)	2015	Brasilia
Sustainable Development Summit (SDGs)	2015	New York
World Water Forum (7th)	2015	Daegu & Gyeongbuk (Rep. of Korea)
Disarmament (annually)	2016	Geneva
Framework Convention on Tobacco Control (7th)	2016	Noida
Permanent Forum on Indigenous Issues (15th)	2016	New York
Trade and Development (14th)	2016	Nairobi

However, progress around gender (and health) justice remains uneven (Esfandiari 2014). Indeed the UN has no power to implement or enforce resolutions, declarations, and programs of action generated by the conferences: even as these can have significant bearing on social and economic policy, compliance is a matter of domestic politics.

Various conferences since 2010 have focused on environmental sustainability concerns (Table 4-4), garnering attention but yielding limited results (see chapter 10). Two major development summits (in 2000 and 2015, on the heels of multiple development "decades") concretized agreed-upon sets of goals to drive UN activities as well as the global development agenda writ large (see chapter 3).

The World Health Organization

WHO is the flagship global health organization. Founded in 1948 as an independent technical agency within the UN (see chapter 2), it grew rapidly in the 1950s and 1960s as newly decolonized states joined. Today WHO's membership includes 194 countries (Palestine and the Vatican have observer status; Taiwan, which used to be a member, was replaced in the UN system by China in 1971; Taiwan's status remains contentious) (Herington and Lee 2014).

Mission and Functions

Spelled out in Article 1 of its Constitution, WHO's mission is: "the attainment by all peoples of the highest possible level of health." Its specific functions, listed in article 2, are no less ambitious. WHO is to:

- Act as the directing and coordinating authority on international health work
- Assist governments in strengthening health services and emergency aid
- Promote maternal and child health and welfare
- Foster activities in the mental health field
- Promote the improvement of nutrition, housing, sanitation, recreation; and of economic, working, and environmental conditions
- Study and report on public health and medical care
- Promote research and health training
- Advance work to eradicate epidemic, endemic, and other diseases, and to prevent injuries
- Propose conventions, agreements, and regulations, and make recommendations regarding international health matters
- Standardize diagnostic procedures and revise as necessary international nomenclatures of diseases, causes of death, and public health practices
- Develop, establish, and promote international standards with respect to food, biologicals, pharmaceuticals, and similar products

WHO's work is divided into two major categories: central technical services and technical assistance to governments. Central services include epidemiologic intelligence, development of international agreements concerned with health, standardization of vaccines and pharmaceuticals, and dissemination of knowledge through meetings of experts and technical reports. At the request of member countries, WHO provides technical assistance through its six regional offices (Table 4-5) and coordinates inter-regional and intraregional

Table 4-5 WHO Regional Offices

Region	Headquarters
Europe (EURO)	Copenhagen, Denmark
Eastern Mediterranean (EMRO)	Cairo, Egypt
Africa (AFRO)	Brazzaville, Republic of the Congo
Southeast Asia (SEARO)	New Delhi, India
Western Pacific (WPRO)	Manila, Philippines
Americas (PAHO)[a]	Washington D.C., United States

[a] Founded in 1902 as the International Sanitary Bureau, later the Pan American Sanitary Bureau (see chapter 1), it maintains more independence than the other regional offices for historical reasons and because it has a double system of governance (through WHO and the Organization of American States).

projects. WHO headquarters in Geneva also coordinates the work of hundreds of WHO collaborating centers, laboratories, and institutes across the world that provide expert advice and services. WHO has an international staff of over 7,000 people working at 150 country offices, its six regional offices, and headquarters. WHO also establishes commissions on specific health topics—such as the 2000–2001 Commission on Macroeconomics and Health (see chapter 12), the 2003–2006 Commission on Intellectual Property Rights, Innovation and Public Health, the 2005–2008 Commission on Social Determinants of Health (see chapter 7), and the 2014–2016 Commission on Ending Childhood Obesity.

Governance

The parliament-like World Health Assembly (WHA) meets each May to set policy priorities and approve WHO's program budget. It is attended by voting delegates of all member governments, plus observers from affiliated NGOs, intergovernmental organizations, and other agencies. A 34-member executive board (EB) also meets semi-annually, supporting the WHA and setting its agenda. EB members are health experts who represent national governments—balanced among WHO regions—and serve 3-year terms.

WHO is led by the Director-General, elected by the WHA for a 5-year term and subject to the authority of the EB. Director-General Dr. Margaret Chan from the People's Republic of China, first elected in 2006 (an accelerated election due to the death in office of her predecessor), was re-elected in 2012, serving until 2017.

It is important to note that WHO can only intervene in countries when requested and that all resolutions request or *urge* but never *oblige* member states to act. WHO members provide routine reports on domestic health conditions, and, according to the 2005 International Health Regulations (implemented in 2007), must notify WHO headquarters in the case of important epidemic outbreaks (see chapter 5 for details).

WHO country representatives are assigned to a specific country (or cover several small adjacent countries) and typically work closely with national health authorities and other international agencies and donors, assisting governments in reviewing health needs and resources, and supporting the planning, coordination, implementation, and evaluation of national health programs and policies.

Budget

WHO operates with a fixed budget comprised of required member state contributions (established on a sliding scale, based on national wealth and population size) as well as "extrabudgetary" funds—voluntary contributions that may be "flexible" (WHO can decide how to allocate the resources) but are predominantly earmarked (designated a priori for specific programs). Amid the economic crises and ideological conflicts of the 1980s and 1990s, WHO faced a stagnation in fixed dues, with some countries in arrears (the United States also cut back or withheld its assessed contribution during several years) (see chapter 2).

WHO's overwhelming reliance on voluntary, earmarked contributions not subject to regulation and priority-setting by the WHA has soared since the 1980s. The 2016–2017 biennial budget of US$4.43 billion (i.e., approximately US$2.2 billion/year, roughly the same as for the 2014–2015 biennium) includes US$929 million from assessed member contributions and US$3.5 billion from voluntary contributions. WHO's 2016–2017 budgetary structure provides a window on its key activities: communicable diseases (US$765 million); noncommunicable diseases (NCDs) (US$340 million); promoting health through the lifecourse (US$382 million); health care systems (US$595 million); preparedness, surveillance, and response (US$380 million); enabling functions/corporate services (leadership, evaluation and accountability, management, communications) (US$734 million); polio (US$895 million); outbreak and crisis response (US$205 million); and research (US$92 million) (WHO 2016).

Incredibly, polio eradication alone is allocated 20% of the 2016-2017 budget. This program, discussed ahead, is illustrative of the problem of donor-driven agenda-setting: eradicating polio, which threatens health in only a few isolated locales, is more a priority for a handful of donors than for most of WHO's member countries.

Meanwhile, funds allocated to outbreak and crisis response were cut by 50% to less than US$230 million from 2012–2013 to 2014–2015 (WHO 2014b), contributing to WHO's delayed and disjointed Ebola response (see chapter 6). Member countries also share the blame for starving the regular dues-based budget and thus impeding WHO's lead global health role (Kamradt-Scott 2016). Despite the evident shortcomings, assessed contributions were not raised for 2016–2017 (with flexible voluntary donations having risen slightly from the 7% 2014–2015 level). Moreover, even *after* the Ebola crisis, outbreak and crisis response funding was cut even further for 2016–2017, although preparedness and surveillance funding increased by roughly US$90 million.

A burgeoning concern is the influence of private donors (Shah 2016). Of late, the Bill and Melinda Gates Foundation (BMGF) has been the first or second largest single voluntary donor to WHO, alternating ranking with the US government. The US's 2016–2017 assessed contributions were US$227 million, with voluntary earmarked contributions of US$180 to 300 million annually since 2010. In recent years, the BMGF has donated US$200 to 300 million dollars per annum to specific programs, especially polio eradication, to which the BMGF has contributed over US$1.3 billion to WHO in total (BMGF 2016; WHO 2015a). Other private donors include large pharmaceutical companies, such as GlaxoSmithKline, Hoffmann-La Roche, and Novartis and their philanthropic arms, who collectively contributed some $40 million in earmarked contributions in 2014 (WHO 2015a), raising serious questions about corporate influence on WHO decisionmaking (Adams and Martens 2015).

WHO's Framework for Engagement with Non-State Actors (FENSA), adopted in 2016, sets guidelines for WHO's engagement with NGOs (a category covering public interest advocacy groups and networks, development NGOs, health professional associations, as well as PPPs), the private sector, philanthropic foundations, and academic institutions (Third World Network 2016). Alas, rather than protect WHO from undue private influence, FENSA deliberations succumbed to the pressure of a group of HICs seeking to protect the interests of corporations by legitimizing inclusion of big business and "venture philanthropies" on equal footing with public-interest actors in WHO decisionmaking. Additionally, FENSA discussions blurred the conflict of interest concept so that WHO's main institutional conflict of interest—between the aim of attracting more funds and its duty to fulfill and protect its mandate (Richter 2015b)—was masked. FENSA has been heavily criticized by public-interest NGOs, who call for ending the freeze on assessed member contributions that has made WHO so dependent on voluntary and private funding (IBFAN 2016).

In essence, the extrabudgetary arrangement gives both government and private donors the power to determine precisely how their contributions are allocated, leading to funding instability, coordination difficulties, and undemocratic policymaking and priority-setting processes. Today, between 70% and 80% of WHO's budget is earmarked by donors, a situation so dire that when Denmark offered US$11 million in fully flexible funding, this contribution was highlighted on the WHO web site as a pathbreaking strategy (WHO 2014a)!

Unlike from the 1950s to the 1970s, when approximately two thirds of total spending in international health passed through WHO (Kates, Morrison, and Lief 2006), today WHO is no longer the hub of global health activity. In recent years less than 10% of total development assistance for health has been channeled via WHO (IHME 2016), leaving it dwarfed by direct spending by bilaterals (foremost USAID) and philanthropies (led by the BMGF) and their indirect spending passing through PPPs, many NGOs, and the World Bank.

With most WHO activities funded jointly by WHO's regular budget, bilateral sources, and UN and private entities—as well as the country concerned—coordination, predictability, and governance are hampered. In recent years WHO has been pressed to undergo reform to make it more nimble and better managed (Clift 2014), but grave concerns persist about how such reforms will entrench corporate and philanthropic influence over WHO even further and prevent it from working in accordance with member state decisionmaking processes (Gupta and Lhotská 2015).

UNAIDS

The Joint United Nations Programme on HIV/AIDS (UNAIDS) was established in 1996 to lead the UN's efforts to prevent new HIV infections and improve treatment for people living with HIV to reduce the economic and social impact of the epidemic. Because HIV was deemed a problem beyond the scope of any one UN agency, UNAIDS coordinates activities among: the International Labour Organization (ILO), UN Office on Drugs and Crime (UNODC), WHO, UNICEF, UN Women, World Bank, UNHCR, World Food Programme (WFP), UN Development Programme (UNDP), UN Organization for Education, Science and Culture (UNESCO), and UN Population Fund (UNFPA). With a 2016–2017 US$485 million core budget, UNAIDS is based in Geneva and has offices in the countries most affected by HIV as well as in major donor countries. It is managed by an executive director and governed by a Programme Coordinating Board, which is composed of 22 UN member states, the co-sponsoring UN agencies as well as civil society representatives, including people living with HIV from various regions of the world.

UNICEF

UNICEF was established in 1946 in the aftermath of World War II to provide food and clothing for European children suffering from displacement and war devastation. In 1953 UNICEF became a permanent part of the UN and had its mandate extended to work globally. Headed by a US appointee since its founding, UNICEF is funded solely through voluntary donations. UNICEF focuses on all issues related to the well-being of the child—health, education, child protection, birth registration, and gender equality—coordinating, but also occasionally clashing with WHO, such as around primary health care (see chapter 2). UNICEF, which in recent years has had a budget roughly twice the size of WHO's, is headquartered in New York, with field offices in most UN member states.

International Financial and Economic Institutions

International financial and economic institutions (IFIs)—most notably, the World Bank Group (World Bank), the International Monetary Fund (IMF), and the World Trade Organization (WTO)—are involved in setting macroeconomic policy and establishing and overseeing trade rules, as well as providing sector-specific grants and loans (often employing incentives and "conditionalities"). These activities directly affect the delivery of health and other social services and indirectly influence health through policies relating to the labor market, employment, and living and social conditions.

In contrast to some other multilateral agencies, and though both the World Bank and the IMF are designated independent specialized UN agencies, IFIs have no pretense of democratic governance: wealthier countries, especially the United States through the US Treasury and the Federal Reserve, exert considerable power over decisionmaking processes and priority-setting (Table 4-6). IFI policies emphasize the primacy of free markets, financial liberalization, national and international deregulation of health and environmental protections, and privatization of public assets and services. Under the World Bank's aegis, global health policy has emphasized efficiency, private

Table 4-6 Voting Power as a Function of Shareholding

IFI	Country	Percent of Total Votes
World Bank	United States	16%
	Japan	7.4%
	China	4.8%
	Germany	4.3%
	United Kingdom	4.1%
	France	4.1%
	Top Six Country Total	**41%**
	Other countries with significant voting power: Saudi Arabia (3%), India (3%), Russia (2.8%), Italy (2.6%), Canada (2.6%)	
IMF	Similar pattern, with the United States holding 16.8% of votes	

Data Sources: World Bank (2016b); IMF (2016a).

investment, and market-based delivery of health services.

The World Bank

The World Bank Group includes two lending institutions for development and a tripartite investment arm, each with discrete roles:

- The International Bank for Reconstruction and Development (IBRD) provides 15- to 20-year loans to middle-income countries (MICs) (annual per capita income of US$1,026 to US$12,475) and "credit-worthy lower income countries," (below US$1,025 per capita) (World Bank 2015). Interest rates are below commercial bank levels but may still be burdensome.
- The International Development Association (IDA) provides low-interest or no-interest loans and grants to countries with annual income of less than US$1,215 per capita (in 2015). In 2015, IDA committed US$19 billion in loans and grants to eligible LMICs (IDA 2016). Since 1960, IDA has disbursed over US$312 billion to 112 countries. Typically, IDA credits mature in 25 to 38 years, with a 5- to 10-year grace period before repayment of the principal (World Bank 2012).
- The International Finance Corporation (IFC) promotes private investment in LMICs, with investments guaranteed by the Multilateral Investment Guarantee Agency and disputes resolved through the International Center for the Settlement of Investment Disputes (usually a win–win situation for investors; see chapter 9).

In the 1980s, the Bank became involved in questions of financing and organizing health care systems, to the chagrin of many public health advocates. The detailed studies it began to publish paved the way for its highly influential 1993 *World Development Report: Investing in Health,* which emphasized user fees, private sector competition, and cost-effectiveness as prime strategies and principles for the health sector (see chapter 12).

Meanwhile, beginning with a loan to Tunisia in 1981 for health care system development, the Bank has financed billions of dollars in projects across LMICs around health care system policies and financing, hospitals, pharmaceuticals, and nutrition, often in rural areas. These loans, together with Bank advice and involvement in structural adjustment programs (see ahead), are part of the Washington Consensus development agenda (see chapter 2), based on market principles and predominance and a downsizing of the state.

By the mid-1990s the World Bank became the world's largest external funder of health, securing US$2.4 billion in health-related loans annually (at least three times WHO's total spending at the time), over 10% of its overall commitments (Sridhar 2008). In this period, lending for all sectors was over US$22 billion annually, about US$16 billion of which were IBRD loans and US$6 billion IDA credits. The largest recipient of IBRD/IDA funding is India, which received US$3.8 billion in loans in 2016 for 12 projects, with about US$2 billion in health sector projects that were active or in the pipeline at the time of writing (World Bank 2016a).

Bank personnel are grouped into various practice areas, such as Health, Nutrition, and Population (HNP) and several around water, as well as networks—the Human Development Network; the Poverty Reduction and Economic Management Network; the Environment and Socially Sustainable Development Network; and the Finance, Private Sector, and Infrastructure Group—and six geographic regions: Africa, East Asia and the Pacific, Europe and Central Asia, Latin America and the Caribbean, the Middle East and North Africa, and South Asia. From 1970 through 2015 the HNP sector of the Bank lent US$47.2 billion to over 100 countries for over 1,200 projects (World Bank 2016c).

Since the 1990s, the World Bank's position as preeminent global health financier has been partially displaced—due to the appearance of new players and initiatives, most notably the Global Fund, the US President's Emergency Plan for AIDS Relief (PEPFAR), and the BMGF, but also owing to the failure of its prescriptions (Levine and Buse 2006). The HNP's current 10-year strategy highlights health care system strengthening, despite admissions that its prior efforts in this area were not systematically evaluated. Analysts have decried the HNP strategy, given the World Bank's ongoing role in promoting market-oriented policies that deteriorated access to care for the poor and reduced health care "to a set of tradeable commodities" (McCoy 2007, p. 1500). The IFC's ongoing Health in Africa private investment initiative appears to be validating this critique, given that private health sector expansion caters mainly to wealthier urban populations (Marriott and Hamer 2014).

One key concern relates to the World Bank's undemocratic voting structure, whereby decision-making and funding priorities are governed by a handful of major shareholders (Table 4-6). The Bank has always had a US President, but in 2012 the US nominee was challenged for the first time by candidates from LMICs. Shareholders ultimately selected an American, Jim Yong Kim, co-founder of Partners In Health (see ahead), but assurances were made that the next President would come from the Global South.

For some, the appointment of Kim as World Bank President heralded welcome change. In a 2013 speech to the WHA titled *Poverty, Health and the Human Future*, Kim focused on the need to end poverty, share prosperity, and make health care accessible through "universal health coverage" (see chapter 11). However, given the history of the Bank and the politics of its major shareholders, the extent to which Kim can refocus the Bank toward the "science of delivery" may be overstated (Horton 2013b).

Other Development Banks

In addition to the World Bank Group, regional level lending is conducted by the Inter-American Development Bank, the Asian Development Bank, the African Development Bank, the Islamic Development Bank, and the European Bank for Reconstruction and Development. As well, the Caribbean Development Bank, the East African Development Bank, the Development Bank of Southern Africa, the West African Development Bank, and the Central American Bank for Economic Integration are funded regionally and provide loans to member states. While these banks have less capital than the World Bank, they also reflect financial sector interests (and most have HIC representatives on their governing boards) in shaping loans and grants in various fields, including health, and in their regional training and research programs.

The International Monetary Fund

Established in 1945 alongside the World Bank, the IMF is charged with maintaining the stability of the international monetary system—the balance of payments (the financial flows relating to imports and exports, credit, and debit among countries) and the exchange rate system—to ensure economic growth and trade. It provides member countries with "advice" on how to avoid crises, technical assistance and training, and temporary financing when they are low on foreign exchange. With promises of protection, most countries became members of the IMF (the former Soviet bloc countries joined in the 1990s), and its current membership stands at 189 countries with loans outstanding to 74 members (IMF 2016b).

In recent decades especially, the IMF has played a significant role in restructuring LMIC economies in the context of financial and debt crises, with significant negative health and social sector (including health care) spending consequences (Stuckler et al. 2010). In accordance with its charter, the IMF swings into action to "help" indebted economies by providing short-term financing to restrain immediate balance-of-payment problems and minimize volatility for the international economy (as–problematically—the IMF, European Commission, and European Central Bank have done in Greece). In return for this financing, countries must commit to rescheduling debt repayments, government spending cuts and imposition of user fees for social services (and sometimes higher taxes), and overall economic restructuring. Since the 1980s, the World Bank has joined with the IMF in implementing structural adjustment loans (see chapter 2) and successor lending instruments that have come with a similarly heavy-handed quid pro quo. The details and effects of these policies are examined in chapters 3 and 9.

The World Trade Organization

The WTO was founded in 1995 to replace the post-war General Agreement on Tariffs and Trade (GATT), which lasted through the Cold War and sought to balance the goal of free trade against geopolitical concerns. More powerful than GATT, the WTO administers trade agreements and negotiations, monitors and enforces trade policies, and resolves trade disputes internally among its 164 members. Today, it governs approximately 96% of global commerce (WTO 2015) and ostensibly promotes laissez-faire free trade, open markets, global competition, and "nondiscrimination" (against foreign goods) by eliminating import tariffs, lowering subsidies, and homogenizing rules and trade concessions. Of course this official view is one-sided—over the past decade the WTO has forced open the economies of many LMICs, whereas HICs have retained many tariffs and subsidies. Indeed, as historically borne out, free trade overwhelmingly favors rich countries at the expense of poor countries and, within countries, the rich at the expense of the poor.

Proponents of the WTO (large financial and business interests and their government partners) claim that its policies have led to increased economic growth in LMICs, which according to the WTO is reducing poverty for hundreds of millions of people. Critics (including unions and many civil society organizations) denounce the WTO for being an unelected international authority and blame its trade rules for causing enormous losses to local industries and jobs, for privileging transnational corporations (TNCs) over human lives, and for challenging and/or overruling national laws, regulations, and political processes, among them public health regulations. In recent years, bilateral and regional trade and investment treaties and agreements have begun to usurp the WTO's primacy (see chapter 9 for further details).

Critiques of and Alternatives to International Financial Institutions

Over time, IFIs have played an increasingly active role in LMIC economies overall and in particular sectors, such as health. One set of critiques ties immiseration, exploitation, and dependency in LMICs to IFI policies that advocate deep domestic cuts in social sector spending, privatization, unfettered trade, deregulation, and the ratcheting down of social rights. Another decries the undemocratic decisionmaking structures at the World Bank and IMF, which give far greater voting power to large donors (and pro-business interests) than to other members, perpetuating neocolonialism via cycles of indebtedness, devaluation, tax evasion, and capital flight. For all of these reasons, a chorus of social movements, including Jubilee 2000 and 50 Years is Enough, have called for the immediate dismantling of these institutions (Global Social Justice 2013).

Since 2000, various Global South financing approaches to development have been pursued as IFI alternatives. Venezuela, with the support of Brazil, Argentina, Bolivia, Ecuador, Uruguay, and Paraguay, created a "Bank of the South" (Banco del Sur) in 2009, emphasizing social development and rejecting IFI privatization pressures. It has been slow to launch, however, given tensions around its focus and modus operandi as well as the region's recent financial turmoil (Garcia 2016).

The BRICS (Brazil, Russia, India, China, South Africa, from an acronym coined by an investment banker to characterize key "emerging" economies) began to associate formally in 2006. In 2015, the BRICS, which constitute 40% of the global population with an estimated combined US$16.8 trillion in gross national income (GNI) (about 22% of world GNI), launched the New Development Bank, motivated by desire to counter the World Bank's power and decisionmaking structure and the slow pace of IFI reforms. Still, the BRICS bank, which focuses on infrastructure and sustainable development in LMICs, is not a nonprofit credit cooperative, but rather a capitalist institution created by capitalist countries (Bond and Garcia 2015).

The Grameen Bank, based in Bangladesh, has provided microcredit for over 30 years, reaching over 8.8 million people (Grameen Bank 2016). By extending small loans, primarily to women, the Grameen Bank attempts to alleviate poverty through small-scale economic development. Founder Muhammad Yunus was awarded the Nobel Peace Prize in 2006, and his model of microfinance and microenterprise has been adopted throughout the world. Yet the complement to economic self-sufficiency—social services and infrastructure—remains unaddressed by this model.

Grameen has been critiqued for failing to reach the poorest populations, creating circuits of indebtedness and debt traps, and ultimately disempowering women (Karim 2011). It has also been accused of furthering capitalism on a large scale in Bangladesh through its commercial bank, private university, hotels, and real estate (Faraizi et al. 2011). In Latin America and elsewhere, not only has microcredit never been shown to eradicate poverty, it became captive to spectacular profiteering. Despite the wide adoption of microfinance approaches to development, even its proponents agree that its poverty-reduction ability is inadequate (Sinclair 2012). Meanwhile, critics cite the increasingly financialized forms of poverty and dispossession created by microfinance approaches (Mader 2015).

Bilateral Aid and Development Agencies

In addition to the programs and projects supported through multilateral organizations, most HICs maintain separate official development aid organizations to fund bilateral projects (i.e., those involving one donor and one recipient government). The greater part of official development assistance (ODA), which includes both bilateral and multilateral support, comes from the members of the Organization for Economic Cooperation and Development (OECD), made up of many HICs plus a smaller group of emerging economies. ODA is big business, with annual flows of almost US$180 billion in 2014 (OECD 2016). At the OECD's periodic Development Assistance Committee (DAC) meetings, representatives of the donors (28 countries plus the European Union) review and compare their respective national contributions to both bilateral and multilateral aid programs.

Bilateral donor agencies are official arms of the governments of many former (or current) colonial powers in Western Europe, North America, and the Pacific, although, as we shall see in subsequent sections, there is increasing involvement of bilateral agencies from the Global South. Typically subsidiary to or dependent on foreign affairs and trade ministries, bilateral agencies sponsor a range of health and development activities in LMICs through counterpart government channels. Collectively the largest source of development funding, these agencies are also often in charge of channeling national contributions to multilateral and international financial agencies. Countries are usually targeted for health assistance for strategic reasons, due to conflict and emergency situations, to address a particularly heavy burden of disease, and based upon historical and political ties (e.g., Australia has focused its aid in the Pacific region; half the countries receiving Spanish aid are in Latin America).

Bilateral agencies—most established after World War II—are diverse in scope and focus (Table 4-7). Some have a substantial personnel component actively involved in projects. Most sponsor, oversee, and assess rather than implement, usually operating through contracts with intermediary organizations including universities, humanitarian groups, for-profit companies, and NGOs. Donor country motivations and policies regarding ODA vary widely (see chapter 3). Bilateral ODA may be limited to certain sectors, or even to specific activities that would not have been the first priority of the recipient country's government and people. Various countries link their foreign aid even more directly to commercial and private investment interests. For instance, in 2013 the Canadian International Development Agency was collapsed into the Department of Foreign Affairs, Trade and Development (now Global Affairs Canada), which launched a controversial set of development projects partnering Canadian mining companies with international nongovernmental organizations (INGOs) in West Africa and Latin America (PHM et al. 2014).

Typically the procurement of goods and equipment (or the use of airlines and other services) is "tied aid" (also known as phantom aid), restricted to spending in the donor country. The same holds true for the hiring of technical personnel to design or implement projects. This practice is not only wasteful—procurement via tied aid raises the costs of projects by 15% to 30% (GPEDC 2014)—it makes aid more of a domestic subsidy to domestic private and nonprofit sectors than foreign assistance per se.

All told, more than half of aid from major donors like the United States, France, and Germany is estimated to be "substandard" (ActionAid 2011) because it: primarily serves donor interests (i.e., commercial, military, geopolitical); fails to support country priorities (i.e., is donor-driven); includes refugee expenditures within donor countries (permitted by OECD rules); double-counts debt cancellation as aid; is badly targeted (i.e., not reaching the poorest); and is tied to unsolicited, low-quality, and/or expensive technical assistance.

Some countries attribute expenditures never designed as ODA to foreign aid—the United Kingdom considers pensions paid to its former colonial officers, military training for African officials, and "English language and culture training" to foreign officials as bilateral aid expenditures (Provost 2014). Even more troubling, the United Kingdom, like the United States, Canada, and other donors, sells billions of dollars of military equipment to LMICs each

Table 4-7 Selected Bilateral Agency Budgets and Priorities

Agency	Budget	Agency-defined Priorities
UK Department for International Development (DFID)	£7.2 billion (2015–2016)	Poverty alleviation, job creation, projects directed at women and girls, humanitarian aid
Agence Française de Développement (AFD)	€8.3 billion (2015)	Poverty reduction, improving living conditions, economic growth, addressing climate change
German Society for International Cooperation (GIZ)	€2 billion (2015)	Works with the German Federal Ministry for Economic Cooperation and Development and private sector on sustainable development, trade, environmental, and other international cooperation projects
Japanese International Cooperation Agency (JICA)	US$1.3 billion (2015)	Poverty reduction through equitable growth, improving country governance, building capacity to deal with humanitarian threats (e.g., civil unrest, disasters, and poverty)
Swedish International Development Cooperation Agency (Sida)	SEK 30.2 billion (2016)	Rights-based approaches to poverty alleviation
US Agency for International Development (USAID)	US$27.1 billion (2015)	Economic growth, agriculture and trade, global health, democracy, conflict prevention, and humanitarian assistance.
Korea International Cooperation Agency (KOICA)	US$568 million (2015)	Improving access to quality education, increasing access to health services, supporting/consulting on industrial development, agriculture, forestry and fisheries projects
India Ministry of External Affairs (MEA)	US$830 million (for technical and economic cooperation 2015–2016)	Infrastructure for trade, investment, and "mutually beneficial" development; training; technical expertise; emergency aid after natural disasters
China (Ministry of Commerce, China Eximbank, and others)	US$7.1 billion (total aid and loans disbursed in 2013)	Grants, interest-free loans, and concessional loans prioritizing agriculture (including food security), rural development, and poverty reduction.
Brazil (mainly Brazilian Cooperation Agency [ABC])	US$52.5 million (ABC's budget for 2010[1]); US$160.3 million (total aid disbursed in 2010)	Coordinates both incoming assistance and outgoing technical cooperation projects based on South-South cooperation principles, responding to LMIC requests.

Sources: Agency web sites; AidData (2015b); Kitano and Harada (2014); Milani (2014).

[1] Most recent year available.

year, often as an implicit quid pro quo for aid (Whall, Ray, and Kirkham 2013).

United States Bilateral Assistance

The United States is the largest ODA donor in the world, providing almost US$33 billion in bilateral (27 billion) and multilateral (5.5 billion) aid in 2014, but it lags far behind most OECD countries in the percentage of GNI dedicated to ODA (Figure 4-1). Its flagship development office, the US Agency for International Development (USAID), and the State Department carry out and fund a variety of global health programs (US$8.5 billion in 2016) relating to HIV (55% of spending), tuberculosis (TB), maternal and child health, malaria, family planning, nutrition, and neglected tropical diseases (Wexler, Valentine, and Kates 2016).

USAID's formal mission is to "partner to end extreme poverty and to promote resilient, democratic societies while advancing [US] security and prosperity" (USAID 2014). With an annual budget of up to US$27 billion over the past few years, USAID characterizes itself as a "business-focused development agency focused on results" (USAID 2015b). Indeed, much of its work is aimed at opening LMICs to investment—for example helping create a US$50 billion annual market for private energy—and trade, in recent

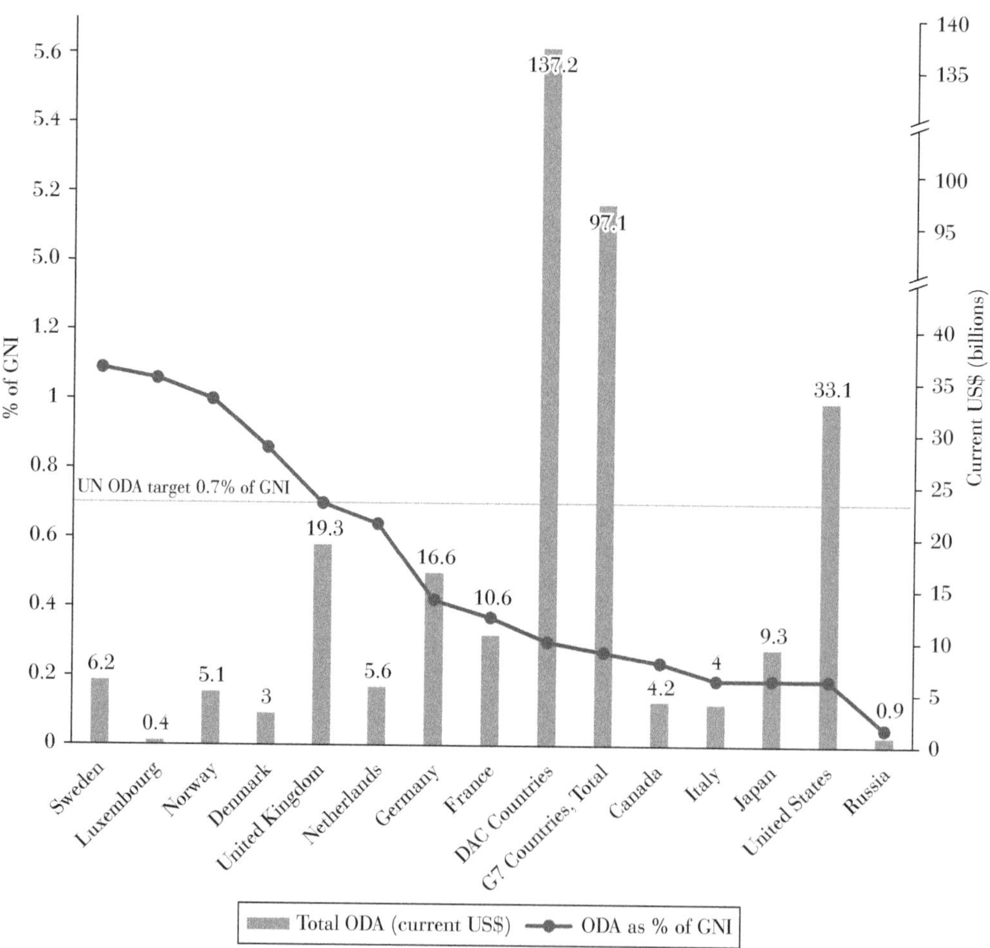

Figure 4-1: Total ODA and ODA as a percentage of GNI by country, 2014.
Data Source: Based on data from OECD, Query Wizard for International Development Statistics (QWIDS), http://stats.oecd.org/qwids/, Accessed February 27, 2016.

years helping Vietnam, Ukraine, and Cape Verde become WTO members (USAID 2015b).

In the health arena, USAID's longstanding focus on family planning (see chapter 2) has more recently been overshadowed by several large-scale global health programs that operate directly out of the US Department of State. These include PEPFAR (see just ahead); the President's Malaria Initiative (allocating over US$3.6 billion since 2005) (USAID 2015a) to increase funding for mosquito nets, indoor insecticide spraying, and antimalarial drugs; and the Millennium Challenge Corporation, founded in 2004 with a multibillion dollar budget to support "good governance, economic freedom" (providing grants that favor pro-growth private sector efforts in countries selected according to development, governance, and political criteria). An additional US$3.5 billion program, Feed the Future, addressing agricultural productivity, rural poverty, and hunger, was founded in the early 2010s (and has problematic ties to the private food industry).

The US government has also used its enhanced global health platform to push for multilateral efforts around health security. In 2014, US President Obama spearheaded the Global Health Security Agenda (GHSA)—a coalition of almost 50 member countries and various advisor organizations (such as WHO and FAO)—to boost global epidemic response capacity (e.g. against biowarfare).

PEPFAR

In 2003, then US President George W. Bush launched the US President's Emergency Plan for AIDS Relief, administered by the US Department of State with in-country involvement of USAID, the Centers for Disease Control and Prevention (CDC), the Department of Defense, and the Peace Corps, the highest profile bilateral health program in decades and the largest disease-specific initiative ever (IOM 2013). PEPFAR originally had 15 "focus countries," now expanded to 65 partner countries (OGAC 2016), selected based on a mix of factors including HIV burden, population size, "political stability," and strategic importance (Fan et al. 2013b).

Since 2004, US$66 billion has been committed through PEPFAR, making the US government the largest donor to the HIV epidemic global response. As of 2015, 9.5 million people were receiving antiretroviral drugs (ARVs) via PEPFAR. That fiscal year, 5.5 million orphans and vulnerable children received care and support, and 68.2 million people were tested and counseled, covering 14.7 million pregnant women, 831,500 of whom were administered ARVs to prevent mother-to-child HIV transmission (OGAC 2015).

PEPFAR initially purchased patented ARVs at "discounted" rates negotiated by the Clinton Foundation. However, annual per person treatment costs remained high (US$1,100 in 2004) until lower-cost generic ARVs manufactured in LMICs (US$315 in 2013 per year) were later adopted (Venkatesh et al. 2012).

PEPFAR's extraordinary reach has not been universally hailed. Early on, critics cited its vertical (siloed, narrowly-targeted, top-down) approach and hiring away (with better pay) of personnel from other needed health activities (Sepúlveda et al. 2007). While some health workers have been recruited back, the problem of internal migration away from primary care persists (IOM 2013).

Still, PEPFAR has attempted to shift toward health system strengthening, aiming to ensure sustainable transition to national government responsibility for the HIV epidemic response. Yet, this is unrealistic for countries with high levels of donor dependency (IOM 2013) or where the volume of patients receiving treatment exceeds current capacity, as in South Africa (Katz, Bassett, and Wright 2013).

Another set of controversies has surrounded PEPFAR's policies relating to abstinence (i.e., delayed onset of sexual debut) and "be faithful" (reduced number of concomitant partners) prevention programs as well as its original "anti-prostitution pledge" for sex workers, now overturned. PEPFAR currently employs biomedical (i.e., male and female condoms; male circumcision), behavioral (i.e., health education), and structural interventions (i.e., legal and policy reforms to address discrimination against gender-discriminated groups) (OGAC 2011), but remnants of earlier ideological approaches remain. Countries continue to be encouraged to report on abstinence and faithfulness spending (Santelli, Speizer, and Edelstein 2013), abstinence programs do not have to be integrated with other approaches, and condoms are only distributed to those older than 15 (Center for Health and Gender Equity 2011).

Remarkably, in over a decade of operations, PEPFAR has surpassed its own targets for expanding treatment access—a feat largely attributed to lower costs from the use of generic ARVs and improved health care system capacity.

OECD Donor Comparisons

In 2014, OECD members provided US$137.2 billion in ODA, a net increase of 260% in real dollars since 1960. Nonetheless, ODA, which covers both bilateral assistance and contributions to UN and multilateral agencies, began to decline in real terms since 2011 as a result of austerity measures following the 2008 financial crisis (UNCTAD 2014). Moreover, various countries disguise loans as aid (Crisp 2014). In 2014, the US spent US$33.1 billion in aid, of which US$357 million went to Iraq, US$1.9 billion to Afghanistan, and US$9.4 billion to countries in sub-Saharan Africa (OECD 2016).

For 2014, the only countries to meet or exceed the UN target of at least 0.7% of GNI in aid, and 0.15% to 0.2% of GNI to the poorest countries, were Sweden, Luxembourg, Norway, Denmark, and the United Kingdom (Figure 4-1). Finland and Ireland met the target of ODA directed to the poorest countries, but not the overall 0.7% target (OECD 2016).

Approximately 14% of DAC ODA is allocated to health (infrastructure and disease control), population policies and reproductive health, and water/sanitation projects, with another 10% for humanitarian efforts. The remainder goes to a range of economic sectors (including agriculture, industry, energy, transport, mining, communications), government and civil society, multi-sector programs, and debt relief (the latter garnering 0.5% of ODA) (OECD 2016).

Military Actors' Involvement in Global Health

Over the past few decades, the role of the military in global health has grown markedly, adding to long-standing activities of colonial and war-related military medicine (see chapters 1 and 2). The United States, with the largest military in the world, is also the principal military global health actor, involving at least US$580 million in US Department of Defense (DoD) global health spending in FY 2012. This conservative estimate covers: (1) "health protection" of Armed Forces (US$171.5 million); (2) medical stability operations and partnership engagement (US$149 million); and (3) biological "threat reduction," such as preparedness training in "partner countries" (US$259.5 million) (Michaud, Moss, and Kates 2012). But these are not actual DoD budget categories. DoD global health expenditures (including recent allocations of US$8 million to HIV and US$17.2 million to malaria) are not publicly released and may be managed under multiple DoD agencies (Licina 2012). Even if underestimated, DoD global health spending surpassed the FY 2012 global health budgets of the CDC and the National Institutes of Health (NIH) at US$348.9 million and US$511.5 million, respectively (Michaud, Moss, and Kates 2012).

The bulk of health protection efforts revolve around US Army and Navy overseas laboratories. Established in their contemporary form during World War II, today DoD laboratories in Egypt, Kenya, Peru, Singapore, Thailand, Cambodia, and Georgia conduct medical research and clinical trials for vaccines, medical devices, and prophylactics (Peake et al. 2011). These labs also support the Armed Forces Health Surveillance Center's Global Emerging Infectious Surveillance and Response System (AFHSC-GEIS), established in 1997, which operates in over 500 sites worldwide and plays an important public health role beyond Armed Forces protection (Russell et al. 2011). In 2009, for example, the first novel cases of influenza A/H1N1 in the United States, Nepal, Bhutan, Peru, and Kuwait were detected and subsequently monitored by AFHSC-GEIS-supported laboratories (Burke et al. 2011). Together, DoD overseas medical research laboratories including AFHSC-GEIS have an annual budget of about US$111 million (Peake et al. 2011).

The global health work of US combat forces focuses on medical stability operations (MSOs), covering both health care delivery for "warfighters" and technical assistance in conflict settings. Following a 2010 directive, MSOs were "given priority comparable to combat operations . . . [to] be explicitly addressed and integrated across all [Military Health Systems] activities" (US DoD 2010). Since 2003, MSOs have built health clinics and run public health campaigns in Iraq and Afghanistan as part of "counterinsurgency" efforts (Michaud, Moss, and Kates 2012).

After Haiti's 2010 earthquake, the US military delivered food, water, medical supplies, and medical care (Licina 2012), and in 2014–2015, the DoD provided US$474 million in the effort against Ebola in five African countries (Kates et al. 2015) through short-term medical assistance, training of 1,500 Liberian health care workers, a medical unit plus mobile labs and treatment units, vaccine research and disease surveillance, and procuring 1.4 million sets of personal protective equipment (US DoD 2015). They stopped short of transporting ill persons in and out of difficult terrain, however, and only transported US government staff into (but not out of) affected zones.

Other national armed forces involved in disaster relief include India's military, which provided humanitarian support to Sri Lanka and Indonesia after the 2004 Indian Ocean Tsunami, to the United States after Hurricane Katrina in 2005, and to Myanmar after Cyclone Nargis in 2008 (Mohan 2014). Regional military organizations, for example the North Atlantic Treaty Organization, the Sinai Peninsula-based Multinational Force and Observers, and the European Union Force also play a relief role, often in partnership with the UN.

An advantage of humanitarian relief delivered by the military is their ability to deploy resources quickly and efficiently (Licina 2011; Mohan 2014), but the ethics of their actual role is concerning to many. Increasingly, military forces work closely with national and international NGOs (US DoD 2010), skewing the non-military aims of humanitarian intervention (see chapter 8). Indeed, numerous NGOs have critiqued the use of military capacity for attending to basic needs in non-emergency contexts—such as the US military's health involvement in Afghanistan—due to fear that NGO neutrality will be compromised through direct collaboration or simply by virtue of military presence and the militarization of the US's image (Michaud, Moss, and Kates 2012; Serafino 2008). MSOs have also been faulted for their short-term design, neglect of needs assessments and evaluation, and lack of sustainability once the military leaves (Buhmann et al. 2010).

Still others argue that MSOs are inimical to the larger aims of global health because they are used to justify military intervention and militarism writ large, and because of potential ethical dilemmas for health care practice—an example is breach of patient confidentiality in favor of gaining national security information (Levy and Sidel 2008). To be sure, such an argument can also be made more broadly regarding the use of global health as a tool of commercial and foreign policy interests of powerful countries (Labonté and Gagnon 2010) (see chapter 3).

Regardless of how these debates play out in the long term, at present the military (especially that of the United States) plays an under-analyzed role in global health that warrants further research.

South–South Cooperation

A growing number of so-called "emerging countries" are engaged in government-to-government health cooperation among LMICs, from BRICS countries, the Gulf States, and other players. In recent years, ODA from 38 non-DAC countries has reached between US$11 and US$41.7 billion annually. This is undoubtedly a gross underestimate because most development assistance from non-DAC donors is not counted as ODA (AidData 2015a). While smaller than HIC ODA disbursements, aid to the poorest countries from non-DAC countries such as China and India increased three-fold between 2000 and 2012 (UNCTAD 2014) (though numbers are in flux because of volatile commodity prices).

The notion that "developing countries" should find ways to help one another is, of course, not new (see chapter 2). Historically, the Soviet Union and other Soviet bloc countries were deeply involved in building health infrastructure in LMICs; over 50 years, the USSR trained some 90,000 foreign doctors, the vast majority from the Third World. Most notably, since the early 1960s, Cuba has sent medical missions to over 100 countries in Asia, Africa, and Latin America to aid in disaster relief, provide medical services in under-resourced areas, support medical education, and offer health policy advice (Feinsilver 2010). Tens of thousands of Cuban health personnel serve overseas at any given time, more than all leading humanitarian NGOs together (Huish 2013). Cuba has also provided free medical education in Havana to thousands of students from socially excluded backgrounds, especially from the Americas (see chapter 11 for details). Unlike virtually all other donors, Cuba bases its cooperation on shared egalitarian principles of the right to health (Beldarrain 2006).

With rising economies (largely commodity-based) in a key group of "emerging" countries, South–South cooperation accelerated after 2000. In 2003, the IBSA trilateral agreement among Brazil, India, and South Africa was formed "to promote South–South dialogue, cooperation and common positions on issues of international importance" (IBSA 2013), including social development, information exchange, and economic cooperation. IBSA's working group on health focuses on epidemiological surveillance, sanitary regulations, traditional medicines, production of generic medicines, health technology and research, and intellectual property rights.

Venezuela has also undertaken social and development cooperation activities, primarily with other Latin American countries, in the form of debt relief, oil for doctor exchanges with Cuba (see chapter 13), and the provision of subsidized household heating oil, also covering low-income Americans. The Bolivarian Alternative (now Alliance) for the Americas (ALBA), created in 2004 and involving Bolivia, Venezuela, Cuba, Nicaragua, and several Caribbean islands, has pursued various cooperative financial, telecommunications, and educational efforts. Its own virtual currency, the *sucre*, is used instead of the US dollar (Mahud 2013). Another South–South modality is triangular cooperation, through which multilateral or bilateral agencies (e.g., Spain's AECID) partner with or help fund South–South cooperation, such as the Pan American Health Organization's (PAHO's) sponsorship of a group of Cuban health professionals who have assisted El Salvador's Ministry of Health develop and manage various public health programs in recent years.

A growing number of MICs are both aid donors and recipients: in 2014, Thailand received US$351 million and gave US$69 million; Turkey received US$3.4 billion, mostly from the EU, and gave US$3.6 billion, more than half of which went to Syria; with similar dual directionality of aid to/from Romania, Bulgaria, Saudi Arabia, and others. Brazil (receiving US$911 million), India (US$3 billion), and South Africa (US$1.1 billion) also both disburse and receive aid (OECD 2016). South Africa, for example, has paid for Cuban primary health care doctors to work in Mali and Sierra Leone and provided TB diagnostics to the Democratic Republic of Congo, while also welcoming aid via Tunisian ophthalmologists helping eliminate a backlog of cataract operations.

As per Table 4-7, the bilateral agencies of China, Brazil, and India have been particularly active. From the perspective of East and Southern African countries, mutual interests around health cooperation (e.g., access to medicines) with Brazil, India, and China are amplified in the context of aligned economic priorities (Brown et al. 2015).

China is currently the largest player in South–South development assistance, providing between US$4 and US$25 billion/year. It works mostly in Asia and Africa in areas of health, population, water, and sanitation—with the majority of projects focusing on infrastructure and human resource development—to the tune of hundreds of millions of dollars per year in Africa (Grépin et al. 2014). As well, the US$5 billion China–Africa Development Fund established in 2007 provides loans and credits to Africa, together with US$2.8 billion in cancelled debts. In 2015 China announced a new US$60 billion development and investment package to Africa for 2016–2018 (Agutamba 2015). In Latin America and the Caribbean, China has also become a key source of loans. In 2015, it surpassed lending to the region from the World Bank and the Inter-American Development Bank combined, reaching US$29 billion (plus almost US$35 billion in further credit), upwards of US$125 billion since 2005 (Gallagher and Myers 2015).

Critics have argued that China's development aid is not motivated by solidarity but linked to its quest for natural resources and to expand markets for its products (Liu et al. 2014), a charge that is just as applicable, past and present, to HICs (see chapters 1, 2, and 9). While these efforts certainly demand scrutiny, China also has a history of humanitarian solidarity with countries including Ethiopia, Tanzania, and Angola (Adem 2012; King 2014) (see chapter 2). In a further instance of the pot calling the kettle black, Western countries have charged China with overlooking human rights violations and governance concerns in, for example, Sudan, where EU and US companies are barred from working (see chapter 8 and Table 9-3 on human rights violations by mining and other interests). China counters that most of its aid and trade take place elsewhere (Brautigam 2011). Like other economic powerhouses, China is involved in a range of problematic extractive industry investments alongside its aid.

Other BRICS players are also active donors: India (purveying US$700 million to >US$ 2 billion per year), Russia (US$500 million), and South Africa (<US$150 million/year) (Dornsife 2013). Much smaller than Chinese assistance, Brazilian aid was estimated at US$160.3 million for 2010 (AidData 2015b) plus other forms of in-kind technical cooperation for agriculture, education, and health. Brazil's priority regions are Latin America, the Caribbean, and Africa, particularly focusing on African Countries of Portuguese Official Language. As in the case of China and most OECD donors, critical concerns have been raised about the connections between bilateral cooperation and corporate investments, such as in Mozambique, where Brazil's mining and construction sectors have major interests (Bond and Garcia 2015). Brazil's international cooperation in health is central to its South–South efforts and has been part of the Labor Party's National Health Plan. Activities include training, promoting universal health systems, and sharing expertise around achieving a unitary health system (Santos and Cerqueira 2015) (see chapter 14).

The new donor countries may appear to be pursuing a novel paradigm of mutual assistance via more progressive language around equality of development partners, but it remains to be seen whether there is a bona fide shift in approaches and aims of South–South cooperation (Harmer and Buse 2014). Presently, Cuba stands out—at times joined by Brazil, Venezuela, South Africa, and China—as moving beyond the rhetoric of solidarity to pursue truly social justice-oriented South–South cooperation (Birn, Muntaner, and Afzal 2017).

Contract Providers and Consulting Firms

Contractors and consulting firms play a growing role in global health project planning and implementation. Many, for example, Abt Associates and John Snow Inc. operate on a for-profit basis; others are mainline NGOs or have an NGO-like character, such as FHI 360. Large nonprofits include Management Sciences for Health, and JHPIEGO (initiated by Johns Hopkins University in 1974). Most are based in HICs—typically concentrated in and around Washington, DC, London, Geneva, Seattle, and other cities with large donor agencies, maintaining satellite offices in countries where they are working. Similar organizations implement projects in Africa and elsewhere, for instance the African Medical Research Foundation, based in Kenya, and South African-based Health Systems Trust. A large number of individual consultants in all areas of global health are employed on a subcontracted basis by such companies, which themselves receive contracts from bilateral and multilateral agencies.

Although contractors are intermediaries rather than agenda setters, per se, they often play an instrumental role in project evaluation and in determining which programs are deemed successful by donors. The accountability and transparency of these projects can be questionable when the financial stakes are high and oversight from donors is lacking.

The US "rebuilding" efforts in Iraq and Afghanistan offer a case in point. The Iraq war alone generated at least US$138 billion in contracts to consulting firms and private companies, many involved in health and development activities. Not only have these businesses engaged in gross profiteering and questionable spending, they have been linked to extensive environmental contamination (Hansia 2014).

Government Technical Agencies and Research Institutions

Some national disease-control agencies—notably the CDC, the Public Health Agency of Canada, the European Centre for Disease Prevention and Control, and various European surveillance networks (such as Euro TB)—provide technical assistance and capacity building support to government disease-control programs and emergency preparedness in a variety of settings. The CDC also supports PEPFAR, GHSA, international surveillance efforts, and outbreak investigations.

Other government-affiliated institutions and national research foundations involved in global health research, training, and funding include: the Fogarty International Center (part of NIH); Britain's Medical Research Council; and France's Institut Pasteur, together with its network of national affiliates in former French colonies. Canada's small International Development Research Centre (IDRC) has long supported collaborative eco-health research with LMIC researchers at the helm (Cole, Crissman, and Orozco 2006).

While public, some technical agencies have partnered with private donors to advance their work. Recent revelations about a project sponsored by the CDC Foundation (which has raised hundreds of millions of dollars from the corporate sector to support CDC's work) and funded by the sugar industry to investigate a chronic kidney disease outbreak that has killed 20,000 sugar plantation workers in Central America raises serious concerns about the credibility and impartiality of this research (Lenzer 2015).

There are also notable technical and research agencies in LMICs. Brazil's Fundação Oswaldo Cruz engages in global health research and domestic, regional, and South–South training, as well as producing vaccines and developing public health innovations. The International Centre for Diarrhoeal Disease Research, Bangladesh (icddr,b)—building on its predecessor, the Cholera Research Laboratory (founded in 1960)—was established by the Bangladesh government in 1978, and is supported by numerous bilateral and multilateral agencies and private foundations. In addition to carrying out community-based and hospital care and research—which has expanded to include child health and HIV prevention—icddr,b has trained over 25,000 health professionals from almost 80 countries.

Regional Organizations and Economic Unions

Regional and economic organizations have potentially powerful effects on health through specific trade rules, policy frameworks, and mutual priority-setting, as well as direct aid programs. The G8 (the United States, Canada, France, Germany, Italy, Japan, Russia, and the United Kingdom) (or G7, with Russia excluded) wields enormous influence on the global economy and global health priority-setting, although its formal interest in global health waxes and wanes (Kirton, Guebert, and Kulik 2014). G8 nations account for about half of the global economy (in terms of aggregate GNI), exercise significant shareholder control over the IMF and World Bank, have four of five permanent seats on the UN Security Council, and provide 55% of all annual ODA (Laub 2014; OECD 2016).

G8 countries also played a key role in setting the MDGs and in backing the Global Fund. Undoubtedly, the G8's commitment to a market-driven global economy has worsened health conditions for the world's poor and working class (Schrecker, Labonté, and Sanders 2007). For instance, the G8's New Alliance for Food Security and Nutrition, promising to "boost agriculture and relieve poverty" in Africa by easing investment restrictions on agribusiness, has been condemned for "ushering in a new era of colonialism" (Provost, Ford, and Tran 2014) and for threatening food sovereignty and likely driving small farmers out of business (Anderson and Bellows 2012).

The EU's 28 states (soon to be 27, with the United Kingdom's imminent departure) together contribute a substantial portion of global development aid (about 56% of public aid; and 30% of global humanitarian health funding) through its "Agenda for Change." The EU articulates a "unified" global health voice in multilateral organizations supporting health care equity, with over €3.2 billion in aid spent on health system strengthening and improving access to health services in recent years (European Commission 2016). The European Commission also sponsors overseas aid activities, for example through its Humanitarian Aid and Civil Protection Department, which funds disaster preparedness programs and emergency relief, implemented through the UN and NGOs (€1.27 billion in 2014) (European Commission 2015).

Trade and investment treaties also influence health and health care policy. NAFTA (the North American Free Trade Agreement, among Canada, Mexico, and the United States) and Mercosur (a common market covering Argentina, Brazil, Uruguay, Paraguay, Venezuela, and Bolivia, with several additional associate members) govern commercial policies among member countries, involving reductions in state subsidies and tariffs and openness to private foreign investors. Nefarious health-related outcomes of NAFTA, for example, have included the proliferation of factories in Mexico with scaled-down and little enforced occupational health protections and the squeezing out of small-scale agriculture (see chapters 7 and 9).

The Southern African Development Community (SADC) and the African Union, meanwhile, have designed a framework for mutual health assistance and guidelines for donors regarding health aid to Africa. Similarly, the Union of South American Nations (UNASUR) has a health council that enhances cooperation among the health ministries of the 12 member countries and an associated research institute aimed at health, health care systems, human resources policy, and knowledge exchange and coordination.

Foundations

Private philanthropies have long been active in international health work. Funded through the donations or bequests of wealthy individuals or of companies, these organizations operate according to missions specified by their founders. Unlike government agencies, which are subject to public scrutiny, philanthropies are accountable only to their self-selected boards, and decisionmaking is often in the hands of a few executives. In North America and various other settings, foundations enjoy tax-exempt status and thus are indirectly subsidized by the public, which has no role in how these monies are spent. The majority of global health philanthropies are based in the United States and to a smaller extent in Europe, but newer health philanthropies are appearing in India, Latin America, and elsewhere.

While many foundations state altruistic aims, the particular conceptions of how to meet those aims can be contested. The Rockefeller Foundation (RF) in the early 20th century, like the BMGF today, had an inordinate influence over the global health agenda, at least in part because it could mobilize resources quickly and allocate substantial sums to large or innovative efforts (Youde 2013). The boom in mega-foundations, dubbed "philanthrocapitalism," refers both to applying business approaches to philanthropy and to demonstrating the benevolent approach of private enterprise (Bishop and Green 2008). From a social justice perspective that sees health as a right rather than the object of charity, however, philanthropic actors have limited legitimacy and their growing direct and indirect purview over the field is worrisome indeed.

The Old Guard

As discussed in chapter 1, the RF was instrumental in molding the international health field's early priorities, paradigms, and activities through disease campaigns and public health activities in almost 100 countries, support for health ministries, the establishment of dozens of schools of public health, and extensive public health training efforts, as well as agricultural development technologies (the "Green Revolution"). At the same time, the RF gave substantial financial, material, and personnel support to core health agencies (including WHO), and helped institutionalize and shape the international health field as a whole (Birn 2014a).

Having made some US$2 billion (unadjusted) in grants since its 1913 founding, and with current assets of US$4.2 billion, today the RF focuses on "urban resilience," "inclusive markets," and environmental efforts, with global health a continuing interest. For instance, the RF was instrumental in developing the PPP arrangement for global health (examined ahead), launched a major health equity initiative in the 1990s, and is one of the forces backing "universal health coverage" (see chapter 11).

Other philanthropies established in the early 20th century with broad health and human welfare interests include the Wellcome Trust, the Ford Foundation, the Kellogg Foundation, and the smaller Milbank Memorial Fund (Table 4-8).

The New Guard

The Seattle, US-based Bill and Melinda Gates Foundation was established in 2000 by Bill Gates (Microsoft founder and for most of the last few decades the world's wealthiest individual) together with his wife Melinda. The largest global health philanthropy (also funding in areas of advocacy and policy, development, education, and regional US programs), its 2015 endowment of US$39.6 billion includes about US$17.3 billion in installments received from Berkshire Hathaway mega-investor Warren Buffet, who in 2006 pledged US$31 billion in stock paid over time (BMGF 2015b). Up to the end of 2015, the BMGF had cumulatively disbursed US$36.7 billion in grants.

With program spending reaching US$6.1 billion in 2015—US$5.3 billion going to a trio of global programs: global health (especially HIV, malaria, and TB); global development (covering polio, vaccine delivery, maternal and child health, family planning, and agricultural development); and global policy and advocacy (e.g. tobacco control)—the BMGF's budget for global health-related

Table 4-8 Endowments and Current Priorities of Selected Foundations

Foundation	Endowment/Total Spending, 2015	Selected Health-Related Priorities
Bill and Melinda Gates Foundation	US$39.6 billion/ $6.3 billion	• Infectious diseases, vaccines, HIV and AIDS, pneumonia, malaria, diarrheal diseases, TB • Reproductive and child health, nutrition
Wellcome Trust	£18.3 billion/£1.1 billion	• Fellowships; vaccines research in LMICs
Ford Foundation	US$11.9 billion/ $711 million	• LGBTQIA rights • Sexual/reproductive health and rights
William and Flora Hewlett Foundation	US$9 billion/ $438.3 million	• Population and reproductive health
W.K. Kellogg Foundation	US$8.4 billion/ $358.4 million	• Early child development • Educational programs in health, agriculture
John D. and Catherine T. MacArthur Foundation	US$6.5 billion/ $368.7 million	• Population and reproductive health
David and Lucile Packard Foundation	US$6.8 billion/ $339.4 million (2014)	• Population and reproductive health • Child health and education
Rockefeller Foundation	US$4.2 billion/ $163 million (2014)	• Universal health coverage • Equity in health
Aga Khan	N/A/US$600 million (2014)	• Health, education, information technology, and rural development
Clinton Foundation	US$55.7 million/ $249.5 million including via channeled funds (2014)	• HIV and AIDS • Human resources for health • Malaria • Access to medicines • Vaccines • Health care systems
Nuffield Foundation	£304 million/ £9.6 million	• Health care policy • Research, training, capacity building • Mental health • Neglected diseases
Carlos Slim Health Institute	US$3.5 billion endowment	• Maternal/infant health • Surgical procedures for the poor
Sir Dorabji Tata Trust and the Allied Trusts	US$295.3 million including trust fund/ $75 million	• Primary, secondary, and tertiary education • NCDs, disability, gender-based violence

Sources: Foundation web sites/annual reports.

activities has surpassed that of the WHO in some recent years. Its sheer size—and the renown of its founder—turned the BMGF into a leading global health player virtually overnight (Birn 2014b).

The BMGF's primary global health aim is "harnessing advances in science and technology to reduce health inequities" (BMGF 2011) through the innovation and application of health technologies, encompassing both treatment (via diagnostic tools and drug development partnerships) and prevention (through, for example, vaccines and topical microbicides). Its priorities include HIV prevention and treatment, malaria, TB, pneumonia, diarrheal diseases, and "neglected" diseases. Initially, the BMGF sought to avoid expanding its portfolio too quickly, focusing on a few disease-control programs mostly as a grant-making agency. This has changed lately, with efforts reaching over 100 countries, the establishment of offices in Africa, China, India, and the United Kingdom, and the growth of its staff to more than 1,300 people.

The BMGF's most prominent global health-related commitment involves support for vaccine development—in 2010 it committed US$10 billion over 10 years to vaccine research, development, and delivery. Leading donations include US$3.2 billion to GAVI, the Vaccine Alliance (which the BMGF was instrumental in launching, and still has a heavy hand in overseeing), over US$530 million in grants to Aeras (a nonprofit biotechnology organization developing TB vaccines), US$456 million to the PATH Malaria Vaccine Initiative, and over US$3.4 billion in grants for HIV and AIDS-related work. It has also supported the Global Polio Eradication Initiative with a cumulative total of almost US$2 billion, and the Alliance for a Green Revolution in Africa (AGRA) with US$264.5 million (BMGF 2015b). As of early 2016, three quarters of the total funds granted by the BMGF Global Health Program went to 60 organizations, 90% of which are located in the United States, United Kingdom, or Switzerland. Among the largest grantees is PATH and its Drug Solutions and Vaccine Solutions partners, which have together received over US$2.4 billion (BMGF 2016). In agriculture the BMGF backs use of expensive chemical inputs and patented seeds (including genetically modified seeds), ultimately enabling the penetration into Africa (and financing) of agribusiness and seed and chemical multinationals such as Monsanto, Cargill, Bayer, and Dupont (Curtis 2016).

Because the BMGF, like the RF before it, operates according to co-financing incentives (whereby other donors and governments match or surpass its funding), it has had enormous influence on the global health agenda in the space of just a few years. Following a technically oriented approach—with programs designed to achieve positive evaluations through narrowly defined goals—its business model emphasizes short-term achievements (Birn 2014b). Thus, many global health agencies are keen to join with the BMGF in order to be associated with a successful, high-profile activity: indeed, it has an extraordinary capacity to marshal other donors to its efforts, including bilateral donors, which collectively contribute 10 times more resources to global health each year than does the BMGF itself but with considerably less recognition (IHME 2016; McCoy and McGoey 2011).

The BMGF's connections to big business are palpable, if publicly downplayed, and involve close ties to pharmaceutical, agro-chemical, and biotechnology sectors (whence many of its executives hail) both directly and via the foundation's investment arm, BMGF Trust. Its past and present holdings in various corporations with long histories of causing harm to health include Coca-Cola, McDonald's, Barrick Gold, Monsanto, and Nestlé, as well as up to US$1.4 billion invested in fossil fuel companies in recent years (Curtis 2016).

In addition, the BMGF has channeled over US$230 million (mainly for health and agriculture projects) via the UN Foundation. Launched with a US$1 billion personal gift by US media mogul Ted Turner, the UN Foundation purports to support the UN's aims but serves as a gateway for corporate influence on the UN by channeling donations without consultation through its bodies (Adams and Martens 2015). At a far smaller scale, the BMGF has begun to fund "universal health coverage" through a US$2.2 million grant to the Results for Development Institute, which works to "Remov[e] barriers impeding efficiency in global markets for essential commodities (for instance, in health)" (Results for Development 2016).

PPPs, also going by the name multi-stakeholder initiatives, are among the key levers of BMGF influence at WHO and in global health generally (see ahead). The BMGF shapes the composition of boards of key PPPs, including that of GAVI, and BMGF executives and staff members are often members of, or even chair, these boards—particularly interim boards of new organizations that set broad policy directions.

In sum, even as it has infused resources and visibility to global health, the BMGF has been greatly criticized by public-interest civil society organizations for wielding broad public policymaking powers without democratic accountability (Bowman 2012; Curtis 2016).

Beyond the BMGF, the global health activities of the Clinton Foundation, founded by former US President Bill Clinton in 2001, focus on HIV and AIDS and the Clinton Health Access Initiative. The foundation, also involving Clinton's family, acts as a "hub" for other health and development actors, which channel funds through it. It has also worked to convince pharmaceutical companies to reduce the prices of some medications, notably ARVs (Clinton Foundation 2014). Due to its founder's high profile, the foundation has convened major figures and marshaled considerable media attention. Clinton and his foundation walk a fine line between negotiating lower (but still profitable) prices for Big Pharma drugs sold to LMICs and threatening trade sanctions against LMICs that produce and sell generics. The foundation has also been scrutinized for financial mismanagement and on ethical grounds for receiving donations from foreign governments while Bill Clinton's wife, Hillary Clinton, was US Secretary of State between 2009 and 2013 (Grimaldi and Ballhaus 2015).

A number of other global health philanthropies have been established by wealthy and/or well-known individuals. Investor and currency speculator George Soros started the Open Society Foundations (OSF) in 1979. Engaged in a range of human rights issues, OSF have invested US$737 million in public health issues such as HIV and AIDS, TB, palliative care, harm reduction, and patients' rights. Their much larger human rights and educational efforts also have global health relevance (Open Society Foundations 2016). Singer and songwriter Elton John founded his eponymous AIDS Foundation (EJAF) in 1992 with offices in New York and London. EJAF has raised over US$350 million to support projects on HIV prevention, testing, and treatment around the world. Founded in 2003, the Stephen Lewis Foundation, started by a former Canadian politician and ambassador to the UN, funds community-based organizations (CBOs) seeking to mitigate the impact of HIV and AIDS at the grassroots level, with to-date over CAD$89 million in funding going to over 300 CBOs in 15 sub-Saharan African countries.

LMIC Foundations

The Aga Khan Foundation (AKF) is among the earliest international philanthropies focused on health originating in the Majority World. Established in 1967 by H.H. the Aga Khan, 49th Imam (spiritual leader) of the Shia Imami Ismaili Muslims, this non-denominational agency works in Pakistan, India, Bangladesh, Kenya, and elsewhere in Africa and South Asia. AKF has supported hundreds of educational and health institutions, international workshops, and conferences.

The recent proliferation of billionaires in LMICs is sparking a host of new foundations. Mexican telecom billionaire Carlos Slim (who ping-pongs with Bill Gates as the world's richest person) founded the Carlos Slim Health Institute in 2007 to support activities in Latin America. Endowed with US$3.5 billion, the institute's priority health issues include child and maternal health, renal health and kidney transplants, addiction rehabilitation services, palliative care, and genomic medicine research (the latter in Mexico).

The multinational Tata conglomerate in India (annual revenues exceeding US$100 billion), funds health programs through the Sir Dorabji Tata Trust and the Allied Trusts. These philanthropic trusts provide grants to NGOs working on community-based health interventions, NCDs, violence against women, and disability. In 2013–2014, about US$ 8 million (23% of all NGO grants) went to health initiatives (Sir Dorabji Tata Trust et al. 2014).

In South Africa, the Motsepe Foundation, launched by mining billionaire Patrice Motsepe, supports projects related to poverty alleviation and education. Another new entrant is Saudi Arabian billionaire investor Prince Alwaleed bin Talal, who, inspired by Bill Gates, has pledged his US$32 billion dollar fortune to Alwaleed Philanthropies, which goes to women's empowerment, disaster relief, and "cultural understanding."

For-Profit Business Interests in Global Health

The private sector's concerns with international health date back to the colonial period, centered around increasing labor force productivity, preventing the interruption of commerce due to epidemics, and establishing international markets for health-related goods and services (see chapter 1). Past and present, business interests benefit from bilateral and multilateral agency spending on health and development aid both through procurement, subsidies, and distribution of products and services (e.g., US government food aid purchased from US agribusiness; GAVI funding for vaccine distribution, underwriting Pharma profits), and through overall government support for expanding markets for private health insurance, pharmaceuticals, medical devices, and services (e.g., through trade agreements). Private interests are increasingly directly involved in agenda-setting and particular policies via PPPs (see ahead).

TNCs also have direct and indirect bearing on health through: environmental contamination; poor workplace conditions and low wages in the manufacturing, service, and agricultural sectors; marketing of food, tobacco, and other goods; regulatory incompliance; and through influence over global agreements and trade treaties affecting these industries and practices (Baum and Anaf 2015) (see chapter 9). For example, certain industries, such as the US Sugar Association, have sought to prevent WHO from issuing guidelines recommending that consumption of their products be limited due to the harms posed to health (Owens 2014).

Global health often takes center stage at the World Economic Forum (an annual meeting held in the Swiss resort of Davos that gives the world's wealthiest and most powerful a platform for shaping "inclusive" globalization and development agendas while preserving a world order that sustains their riches and power [Prashad 2016]), and similar meetings, where discussions abound around investment prospects in such areas as digital health, and charitable pledges are made for cost-effective interventions to "help" the "global poor." In conjunction with these events, the private sector is also invited to donate to the Global Fund and other PPPs and to sit on their boards (World Economic Forum 2014), helping shape global health policies and enhance private sector involvement. Though portrayed as humanitarian philanthropy, business participation in these partnerships remains consistent with the fiduciary responsibilities of corporations to maximize profits for shareholders. For instance, a 2016 Davos report signals the potential returns on investments in preventing NCDs and mental ill-health, as generating "opportunities across all industries, not just typical healthcare players" (World Economic Forum 2016, p. 3).

Private Health Insurance and Other Global Health "Business Opportunities"

The private health insurance industry has been expanding its reach in both HICs and LMICs, as more countries have privatized parts of their health care systems and extended coverage via private sector delivery. Over the past quarter century, the World Bank has actively encouraged private insurance expansion, arguing that this will increase access to health services where public systems are inadequate (Preker, Zweifel, and Schellekens 2010). The BMGF, too, is involved as the largest funder of the UK-managed HANSEP initiative to "improve the performance" of private health care delivery for low-income populations in the Global South (Curtis 2016). Ironically, the turn to the private sector and the deterioration of public sector health systems is linked to the very loan conditionalities imposed by IFIs (Waitzkin, Jasso-Aguilar, and Iriart 2007) (see chapter 9). In the 1990s, US private health insurance company penetration soared in Latin America (Iriart, Merhy, and Waitzkin 2001); in Colombia, a 1994 regulated health insurance market reform involving both domestic and US insurance companies has increased obstacles to access and exacerbated inequities (Vargas et al. 2010). Today largely US-based health insurance companies, together with corporate diagnostics, device, and health management industries, continue to pursue new overseas markets (Murphy et al. 2015) such as the efforts by insurance giant Aetna to expand its coverage in the Middle East.

Big Pharma

The trillion-dollar pharmaceutical sector is among the most powerful and profitable industries in the world and a major global health player, with emerging markets constituting a growing proportion of revenues. The top ten pharmaceutical companies, with combined 2014 revenues of US$454 billion and profits of US$82 billion (*Fortune* 2015), enjoy about a third of their sales in emerging economies (Buente et al. 2013). Represented by the International Federation of Pharmaceutical Manufacturers & Associations in Geneva, Big Pharma has enormous influence over global access, and inequity thereof, to medicines. Its drug development practices, marketing and pricing policies, and stance on patents and generic production often pit Big Pharma against what WHO and civil society campaigns articulate as the right to "essential medicines," especially since the passage of the WTO's 1996 TRIPS agreement (see chapter 9), which globalizes patent protections (Forman and Kohler 2012).

Big Pharma also has a direct and indirect role in shaping global health policy and particular initiatives (and in turn having its products purchased) through donations to WHO and other agencies, through influence on bilateral spending and procurement, and via PPPs such as GAVI and the Global Fund (see ahead), where it has board representation. As such, Big Pharma's involvement in assuring that (patented) drugs for LMIC populations are purchased via global health financing entities gives it an increasing say in the overall global health agenda. Growing attention to NCDs in LMICs also represents a boon for Big Pharma (among other business interests), with the prospect of expanded global health financing for NCD therapeutics (PHM et al. 2014).

The profit-making drivers and nefarious practices of the pharmaceutical industry are best understood from a political economy perspective: Big Pharma's lack of interest in unprofitable diseases (viz. low-income populations)—that is, its motivation to participate in global health is directly linked to profit-making—has impelled the proliferation of multiple organizations, initiatives, partnerships, and financing mechanisms to entice Big Pharma and ensure development of and access to drugs for major ailments, including HIV, TB, and malaria, as well as so-called "neglected diseases."

Though their main aim is to sell products at the maximum price possible, certain pharmaceutical companies garner attention for making donations or offering discount drug stocks in disaster situations. Sometimes these drugs are near or past expiry or have been replaced with better alternatives. Other times, an outright donation is made, for instance through the International Trachoma Initiative, started by Pfizer and the Edna McConnell Clark Foundation in 1998 to integrate treatment with community and personal hygiene. Since then Pfizer has donated hundreds of millions of doses of the antibiotic azithromycin to prevent and treat this eye infection that leads to blindness in many LICs. While such donations may seem admirable, it is important to note that companies receive tax deductions and good publicity in return: fair pricing, generic production, and a just patent regime would do far more for global health than the occasional donation.

Most famously, since 1987, Merck has donated Mectizan© to treat onchocerciasis (river blindness) free of charge to hundreds of millions of people exposed to the disease (and, later, donated to treat lymphatic filariasis). But the story of Merck's self-proclaimed generosity is less inspiring than meets the eye. When Mectizan© was developed from Merck's existing veterinary de-worming drug, the company initially intended to sell the drug but realized they could not make money from it given the extreme poverty of the affected populations; then it sought to strong-arm the WHO and US Congress into purchasing and distributing it. Only after these strategies failed did Merck consider a donation (Collins 2004)—as a last resort, not as a model of philanthropy. Elsewhere, Merck has used donations as a segue into sales. In Botswana, Merck joined with the BMGF to donate ARVs in 2000, subsequently "systematically transitioning" the program to the government of Botswana and eliminating funding (Merck & Co. Inc. 2014). In China and the United States, where the Merck Foundation also supports HIV programs, it has not donated ARVs (which must be purchased), instead funding accompanying prevention and care management efforts.

Corporate Foundations and Alliances

Various corporations also run foundations, invariably as public relations and marketing efforts, or as a means of distributing their own products. Among the largest are the Bristol Myers Squibb Foundation, which reports US$47 million in 2014 spending, and the Merck Company Foundation with US$819 million in spending since 1957, focused on vaccines and HIV treatment. Examples of "corporate philanthropy" include: the ExxonMobil Foundation working in malaria control; the Walmart Foundation, involved in nutrition, environmental sustainability, and disaster relief; the Shell Foundation, working on sustainable transportation; and the Nestlé Foundation, which since 1968 has funded public health and nutrition activities in LMICs—even as Nestlé is linked to unethical marketing of baby formula (see Box 9-3). Meanwhile Coca-Cola's international philanthropic arm reports spending approximately US$820 million during the course of 30 years on empowering women, water access, and "active healthy living" (Coca-Cola Company 2015). Other companies, including agricultural feed supplier Cargill, agribusiness multinational Louis Dreyfus, and fruit giant Dole, have formed partnerships with development NGOs such as CARE (Cargill 2012) to create an image of corporate social responsibility, notwithstanding their infinitely larger for-profit endeavors that carry on business as usual. Indeed, corporate foundations are often active in areas in which their workers, factories, and markets are located.

In 2008 ten of the largest food and beverage multinationals, including Coca-Cola, PepsiCo, Unilever, Nestlé and General Mills, joined the International Food and Beverage Alliance (IFBA), committing their support to WHO's *Global Strategy on Diet, Physical Activity and Health*, involving responsible marketing and healthier (re-)formulation of products (Yach et al. 2010). Needless to say, these activities are self-governing, self-regulating, and non-binding and have not demonstrated effectiveness (Moodie et al. 2013). IFBA has lobbied aggressively to influence WHO's standard-setting and policymaking activities around diet-related NCDs. As such, a healthy degree of skepticism is warranted about the motives of commercial enterprises that purport to be concerned about the nutrition of the public when the products they purvey are unhealthy (and knowledge of this may limit their profits) (Richter 2015a).

Public–Private Partnerships

Philanthropic and business interests have long had ties to international health organizations, but it was not until the mid-1990s that PPPs were formalized as a central modality of global health (Buse and Walt 2000). The proliferation of global health PPPs coincided with plunging base budget (dues-based) funding for the WHO and increased bilateral and private sector funding—including substantial grants from the BMGF—to targeted initiatives. Typically portrayed in a positive light, these now pervasive "collaborations" between the private sector and public agencies (both multilateral and national) have given the business sector a major role in public health policymaking, consciously drawing on profit-making principles as a driver of policies, product development, and other activities (Velásquez 2014).

There are now many large-scale global PPPs in existence, with WHO involved in dozens of them. PPP budgets range from millions to many billions of dollars. Among the most prominent are the Stop TB Partnership, Roll Back Malaria, the International AIDS Vaccine Initiative, and the Global Alliance for Improved Nutrition. Many were launched by the BMGF or receive(d) funding from it. While some global health PPPs have spurred research and facilitated the supply of medicines, on the whole they bring most of the same problems as health donors writ large: imposition of outside agendas, and poor harmonization with national governments and other actors (Buse and Harmer 2007).

Almost by definition, narrowly-targeted PPPs entrench vertical and technically-focused programs (there is no PPP for primary health care!), jeopardizing health systems development and impeding integrated approaches. WHO's mandated responsibility for global health is superseded in some PPPs, which relegate it to the margins. In others, there are so many partners (e.g., Roll Back Malaria has nearly 200) that management and governance problems are insuperable, especially when the organizational members of PPPs have divergent interests. Furthermore, when their governing Secretariats are too small and under-resourced to manage the growing number of operations, PPPs are more likely to take a "one size fits all" approach that lacks local relevance (Buse and Tanaka 2011). Illustrating this concern, NGOs working with PPPs often find it challenging to incorporate complex social determinants of health, such as gender and race, that do not fit PPPs' formulaic approaches (Gideon and Porter 2016).

One of the most longstanding PPPs is the Global Polio Eradication Initiative—launched in 1988 with participation of WHO, Rotary International, CDC, UNICEF, and national governments. Nearly 3 billion children have been immunized since 2000 leading WHO to estimate that administering the oral polio vaccine has prevented more than 13 million cases of childhood paralysis (WHO 2015b).

Yet more than a quarter century into the campaign, over US$14 billion has been invested in it, with polio recently accounting for a staggering onefifth of WHO's budget. Increasingly, critics decry the campaign's top-down approach, contentious scientific decisions, and its role in squeezing out many other health priorities (Muraskin 2012). Problems persist: wild poliovirus or polio resurgence (including vaccine-derived poliovirus) in Afghanistan, Nigeria, Pakistan, and up to 10 other "vulnerable" countries have led to considerable re-evaluation of existing approaches. Even Bill Gates, one of the largest proponents of and donors to technical approaches to global health (including over US$3 billion for tackling polio) belatedly recognized that targeted eradication needs to be integrated with broader health infrastructural approaches (Guth 2010).

Another PPP is Salud Mesoamérica, a regional health initiative, established in 2010 by the Inter-American Development Bank, the Carlos Slim Health Institute, the Government of Spain, and the BMGF. Its aim is to improve the health conditions of 1.8 million women and children in the Mesoamerican region. Donor and country partner contributions have totaled US$155 million since its initiation (Salud Mesoamerica 2015).

With far less funding but tackling a key issue, the WHO-based Global Health Workforce Alliance brings together governments, the private sector, foundations, UN agencies, NGOs, academics, and professional associations to address the health personnel shortage across low-income regions.

A particular genre of PPPs, product development partnerships (PDPs), harness donations from public and private actors to develop medicines and other health technologies for specific problems. PDPs are themselves largely nonprofit, but the patents they generate are usually retained by partnering companies or academic institutions. PDPs include the International AIDS Vaccine Initiative, the Medicines for Malaria Venture, Aeras (focused on new and accessible/affordable TB vaccines); and DNDi (the Drugs for Neglected Diseases Initiative), created in 2003 to jumpstart neglected disease therapeutics. A quasi-PDP is PATH (formerly Program for Appropriate Technology in Health), a "global health innovation" nonprofit, funded primarily by philanthropies (especially the BMGF), the US government, and other public agencies. With over US$300 million in annual spending, it focuses on the development of vaccines, drugs, diagnostics and other health technologies, and service delivery. In 2011, PATH absorbed the US's first nonprofit pharmaceutical company, the Institute for One World Health, which had aimed to develop and ensure affordability and access to needed medicines in LMICs. PDPs have arguably helped spur research and development (R&D), enabled better diffusion of pharmaceuticals, and raised hundreds of millions of dollars for medicines for "neglected diseases." For the most part, however, PDPs have had relatively little impact on health because they focus on incremental innovations and products developed by partner organizations, stifling overall R&D for "neglected diseases" (Grace 2010). Moreover equitable access to their products, particularly for poor populations, remains problematic (Pratt and Loff 2013).

The largest PPP and one of global health's biggest financing channels (about 10% of total global health spending [IHME 2016]), the Global Fund to Fight AIDS, Tuberculosis and Malaria (now the Global Fund), was established as an independent Swiss foundation in 2002, becoming fully autonomous in 2009. Inaugurated with a US$100 million grant from the BMGF, it raises money, reviews proposals, and disburses grants aimed at combating the three diseases to government ministries, CBOs, private sector entities, and other organizations. Designed to bypass the bureaucratic "encumbrances" of UN agencies, the Global Fund's governing board is split between donors and "implementers," including HICs and LMICs, NGOs, people living with the three diseases, and the private sector. Remarkably, WHO and UNAIDS are board members but have no vote, whereas both the BMGF (representing private foundations) and pharmaceutical company Merck (representing the private sector) are voting members.

Although bilateral aid constitutes 95% of the Fund's budget, with the private sector contributing just 5%, the latter has an ample voice not only on the board but also in country coordinating groups. As of early 2016, the Global Fund had disbursed US$33 billion to fund programs in 140 countries (Global Fund 2016). Its disbursements, currently US$4 billion per year, focus on vertical programs to deliver therapeutics, with 54% spent on HIV prevention and treatment (funding, for example, the distribution of 300 million condoms and the initiation of 7.3 million people on ARVs), 27% on malaria, 16% on TB, and 1%

on HIV and TB together, constituting most donor spending on these diseases.

The Global Fund's Debt2Health initiative arranges for debtor and creditor nations to, respectively, forgive and divert debt repayment to Global Fund-approved programs in the debtor ("beneficiary") country, but thus far entails small sums. Long critiqued by both activists and governments for ignoring health care system needs (Patel, Cummings, and Roberts 2015), the Global Fund has sought to increase cross-cutting health systems spending to 40% of spending yet most is still channeled through disease programs, with just 12% going to building and strengthening policymaking, service delivery, financial management, health worker training, and procurement (Global Fund 2015).

The Global Fund has also come under scrutiny over corruption and misuse of up to two thirds of funds (Boseley 2011). Part of the problem is that the Global Fund puts oversight in the hands of private accounting and auditing firms with little expertise in public health. Concerns around conflicts of interest also stem from the frequent rotation of personnel among grant recipients, the Global Fund, and the oversight agents (PHM et al. 2014). The Global Fund's performance-based funding mechanism allots limited negotiating leverage for countries, including on the types of health interventions and targets that should be pursued, creating power asymmetries (Barnes, Brown, and Harman 2015). Additionally, the grant rating process has been found to be highly discretionary and non-replicable, creating accountability concerns both for the public and recipients (Fan et al. 2013a). Furthermore, the reporting system is expensive and cumbersome for LICs (Biesma et al. 2012). Not only has the Global Fund's creation further debilitated WHO, like many PPPs it offers "business opportunities"—lucrative contracts—as a prime feature of its work, elucidating how global health is being captured by business interests both in agenda shaping and as a source of profit-making.

The model for most PPPs is the highly visible GAVI, the Vaccine Alliance (formerly the Global Alliance for Vaccines and Immunization), founded by the BMGF in 1999 and based in Geneva. GAVI focuses on increasing children's access to vaccines in over 60 countries (currently eligible) through support for R&D and distribution of existing vaccines at subsidized prices. Bringing together foundations, UNICEF, WHO, the World Bank, private businesses, and NGOs, GAVI maintains a vertical focus on global immunization coverage financed by national governments (77%) and the BMGF (22%). GAVI has been critiqued for being heavily "top-down," and paying scant attention to local needs and conditions (Muraskin 2004).

Critics have also faulted GAVI for the hefty representation of industry on its board and for directly subsidizing the profits of already mega-profitable Big Pharma through dubious contracts and incentives, not doing enough to reduce the prices of new vaccines, and not supporting production and registration of vaccines by new manufacturers in LMICs, all in the name of "saving children's lives" (Birn and Lexchin 2011). Indeed, GAVI has subsidized Merck, among other companies, for already profitable products such as pneumococcal vaccine, whereas countries that "graduate" from GAVI price eligibility lose direct subsidies and access to lower negotiated vaccine prices (MSF 2015b). Moreover, GAVI's discounted products remain prohibitive for many countries, even as they assure sales to Big Pharma: although GAVI's price for Pfizer's pneumonia vaccine Prevnar 13 (the world's biggest-selling vaccine) is discounted from US$170 to US$10 per child, Pfizer's patent is being contested in India, where generic production at US$6 would make it more affordable for use in India and other LMICs (Siddiqui 2016).

Another PPP, Family Planning 2020, launched in 2012, partners with UNFPA, DFID, USAID, and the BMGF and collaborates with LMIC governments and private sector actors especially Big Pharma (e.g., Merck, Pfizer and Bayer) in a bid to expand access to, and profit-making from, family planning services (FP2020 2015).

Despite these problems, UN agencies and governments favor the PPP model. At the 2011 UN high-level meeting on the prevention and control of NCDs, there was a special call for collaboration among the public sector, the private sector, and civil society. It is thus not surprising that public-interest groups question whether partnerships with companies that produce unhealthy goods are the right response to reducing the global rise in chronic disease, given the opportunities for corporate cooptation of disease prevention efforts (Katz 2013).

The concerns outlined here are compounded by the contradictions between the profit-making mandates of corporations (and their philanthropic spinoffs) and WHO's commitment to health as a human right. PPPs have marshaled billions of dollars to global health, resulting in unprecedented commercialization and extensive private sector influence on global health policymaking without quid pro quo accountability (Lawson 2013), such that most PPPs channel public money into the private sector, not the other way around (Ollila 2005; Richter 2015a).

In sum, PPPs—whether in health or other domains—are narrowly focused, duplicative of existing efforts and one another, lack transparency, and are insufficiently subject to public safeguards that would prevent conflicts of interest between corporate and public objectives (Buse and Tanaka 2011; Ruckert and Labonté 2014; Utting and Zammit 2006).

Emerging Global Financing Approaches

An "innovative financing mechanism for global health" was introduced with the establishment of UNITAID by Brazil, Chile, France, Norway, and the United Kingdom in 2006 (now also partnered with the Gates and Clinton foundations). UNITAID raises funds for the purchase of medicines and diagnostic technologies for HIV, malaria, and TB (including drug-resistant TB) to increase treatment access in LICs. Over 60% of funding comes from a levy on airline tickets in ten countries, including several LICs, which brought in almost US$1.5 billion by the end of 2014 (Silverman 2013).

Through "market interventions" such as bulk purchasing and developing better-adapted products, UNITAID is able to lower prices and improve access to therapies and diagnostics. Its focus on pediatric HIV detection and medicines is especially important given that, until recently, three fourths of children with HIV were not on ARVs (UNITAID 2015). UNITAID has also supported a Medicines Patent Pool, which negotiates "with patent holders to share their intellectual property with the Pool" and licenses producers to make low-cost generics for people with HIV living in LMICs (Medicines Patent Pool 2014). The concerns raised by civil society organizations around product selection (PHM 2009), potential market segmentation, and maintenance of TRIPS flexibilities seem to be allayed through the Pool's contractual provisions, transparency policy, and collaboration with a range of "stakeholders" (Medicines Patent Pool 2015).

Missionaries and Religious Agencies and Charities

Religious missions have sponsored health-related activities for hundreds of years, building and operating leprosaria, hospitals, and orphanages in Asia, Africa, and Latin America (Hardiman 2006). Historically, Christian medical missions were often associated with repressive colonial regimes and used health activities to proselytize religious beliefs. Today some missionary groups oppose contraception and family planning, termination of pregnancy, and artificial insemination, others, immunization and blood transfusions, and many faith-based institutions discriminate against LGBTQIA populations (Tomkins et al. 2015). Yet faith-based organizations do not only proselytize, and serve far more than believers. Though barely visible in mainstream global health, faith-based groups provide health care to 30%–70% of the world's poorest populations (noting that information is limited and these may be overestimates) (Olivier et al. 2015). Moreover, much global health involvement today continues to be motivated by a mix of humanitarian, social-justice oriented, ethical, and deeply personal beliefs that intersect in complex ways with religious missions (Holman 2015) (Table 2-3).

Sub-Saharan Africa is the region perhaps most marked by religious medical humanitarianism, with some missions broadening to include community development, agricultural work, primary health care efforts, and struggles around gender and health rights (Mann Wall 2015). Religious missions are funded primarily through contributions from members/congregations/headquarters in Europe and North America, also receiving support from development agencies.

Most contemporary religious health aid is centralized in multimillion dollar charitable and relief agencies—World Vision, American Friends Service Committee, Adventist Development and Relief

Agency, France's Comité Catholique contre la Faim et pour le Développement, Samaritan's Purse—and so on (Table 4-9). Catholic Relief Services, for example, was founded in 1943 by the US Catholic Bishops and now supports low-income communities in almost 100 countries.

While Christian charity predominates, Jewish, Islamic, Hindu, and other religious agencies also sponsor global health and relief work, typically aimed at people of the same faith. Among the largest are Islamic Relief Worldwide and American Jewish World Service. Khalsa Aid, established in 1999 and largely funded by the diaspora community, is based on Sikh principles of selfless service and universal love.

For some groups, religion (and religious conversion) may serve more as background inspiration than an overt goal. Christian Aid, Diakonia (made up of five Swedish churches), and Norwegian Church Aid espouse economic justice and human rights in their work, the latter as part of the Scandinavian tradition of anti-imperialist missions. Combined efforts include Caritas Internationalis, a confederation of over 160 Catholic development, social service, and relief agencies that work in 200 countries; ACT (Action by Churches Together) Alliance, made up of over 140 churches; the Lutheran World Federation, providing emergency relief in over 140 countries; the Church World Service, which encompasses 35 Protestant, Anglican, and Orthodox denominations; and Coopération Internationale pour le Développement et la Solidarité, an alliance of 17 European and North American Catholic development organizations. Global health alliances also form across religions. The Global AIDS Interfaith Alliance provides community-based HIV services in LICs through partnerships with religious organizations.

There are also many small Christian missions with explicitly religious aims operating today. Over 100 organizations belong to the Mission Exchange. The Mission Doctors Association sends Catholic doctors from the United States to serve at mission hospitals and clinics overseas, and the Aloha Medical Mission is active in Asia. The Fellowship of Associates of Medical Evangelism sees medical aid as a path to evangelism. Some "faith-based" organizations, such as Christian Connections for International Health, have been criticized for infusing fundamentalist values (sexual abstinence, prohibition on abortion) into their work, for refusing to hire gay men and lesbians, and for blocking the implementation of harm reduction initiatives.

Pentecostal and other evangelical churches are spreading across Latin America, Africa, the former Soviet Union, and Asia. In some settings church healing is replacing the role of traditional healers, whose rising fees and sometime connection with global health players is viewed with suspicion (Pfeiffer 2005).

Joint Health and Development Initiatives and Partnerships

In 2007, a group of 8 international organizations working in the health field began to meet informally to "stimulate a global sense of urgency for reaching the health-related MDGs" and to focus "on better ways to speed up efforts to bring lifesaving health improvements to people worldwide" (UNAIDS 2011). Dubbing themselves the Health 8 (H8), echoing the G8 political grouping, H8 is comprised of WHO, UNICEF, UNFPA, UNAIDS, the World Bank, the BMGF, GAVI, and the Global Fund—the world's leading global health institutions. The H8 holds meetings, like the G8, at which the mainstream global health agenda is shaped behind closed doors, and organizations considerably influenced by Gates and the BMGF constitute a majority (Horton 2013a).

The International Health Partnership (IHP+), also formed in 2007, aims to accelerate progress on the health-related SDGs, particularly universal health coverage. IHP+ members include a range of "development partners:" all H8 members, plus many HICs and their bilateral aid agencies, the African Development Bank, ILO, UNDP, and European Commission, and three dozen low-income "partner countries," mostly in Africa. However, no BRICS, MICs, or civil society organizations participate (IHP+ 2015). Members sign the IHP+ Global Compact, committing to the principles of the Paris Declaration (see chapter 3): national ownership of projects; alignment with national development priorities; harmonization between agencies; managing for results; and mutual accountability. Despite these pledges, IHP+'s future remains uncertain (McCoy et al. 2011).

Table 4-9 Selected Religious Agencies—Spending and Activities

Religious Agency	Total Spending, 2015	Health-Related Activities
World Vision International	US$2.3 billion	• Works in 95 countries • Emergency relief, nutrition and community-based health projects (treating acute malnutrition, HIV testing, training health workers)
Catholic Relief Services	US$733.3 million (11% to health)	• 134 health projects in 43 countries • Early child development, immunizations, maternal and newborn care, malnutrition
Samaritan's Purse	US$517.8 million	• Works in 150 countries • Disaster relief, child nutrition, clean water projects
Islamic Relief Worldwide	£78.1 million (8% access to health care and water) (2014)	• Works in over 30 countries • Install water wells/water pumps, childhood cancer treatment, drug addiction services
Mennonite Central Committee	US$90.6 million	• Works in 48 countries • HIV prevention and support to people living with HIV and AIDS; support to health clinics
American Jewish World Service	US$61.6 million	• Supports grassroots efforts to end violence, poverty, and inequality
Adventist Development and Relief Agency	US$56.1 million (2014)	• 140 health projects (e.g., family planning and reproductive health); 84 water, hygiene, and sanitation projects; 87 food security projects
Comité Catholique contre la Faim et pour le Développement	€38.5 million	• 442 projects in ~60 countries • Food sovereignty, natural resource protection, rights of women, children, and the poor
Muslim Aid	£31.3 million (4.6% on health care programs) (2014)	• Health care, child nutrition, emergency relief, water and sanitation, poverty alleviation
American Friends Service Committee	US$36.1 million	• Works in 15 countries for peace, economic and social justice, humanitarian assistance, human rights

Source: Agency web sites/annual reports.

NGOs

NGOs are enormously diverse, ranging from local grassroots efforts to small or large INGOs that work transnationally purveying resources and personnel from one (usually high-income) to another (usually low or middle-income) country. NGOs are involved in expert consultation, training, direct service delivery, advocacy, contract work, and many other activities. Networks of NGOs, such as the US alliance InterAction or the International Council of Voluntary Agencies, are formidable advocacy groups.

It is important to note that NGOs and civil society groups—understood to be separate from the state and private sector, even as there can be conflation—are a pervasive feature of modern societies. The proliferation of NGOs since the 1980s—estimated in the tens of thousands, though there are no official counts—has been viewed as a sign of vibrant civil society. Yet in many settings, they have arisen to meet social well-being, neighborhood, and larger collective needs no longer addressed by government in the context of the shrinking public provision of services. NGOs may be fostered or coopted by business interests to help fulfill particular agendas or operate in parallel or competition with public agencies. Others have succumbed to survival-by-any-means strategies to ensure revenue streams for the NGO.

But many other NGOs play a far more progressive role, especially at the local or domestic level. Under repressive or unresponsive regimes, or in countries emerging from dictatorships as was the case in Latin America in the 1980s, countless public-interest NGOs have pursued social justice concerns and made claims on the state to improve social conditions, democratic decisionmaking, and human rights. As such, the umbrella term NGO is extremely broad and should be used with qualification.

Within the international "aid community," NGOs, foundations, and bilateral agencies may work in conjunction or, more typically, compete unproductively. Some groups receive contributions from foundations and government agencies and are bound by the funder's mandate. In the field of population and family planning activities, for example, USAID has allocated hundreds of millions of dollars to NGOs such as the International Planned Parenthood Federation, Pathfinder International, and EngenderHealth. Other NGOs directly appeal to the public for resources. Still others (like BRAC in Bangladesh) generate income from the sale of products or services.

Increasingly, INGOs are contracted by their home government's bilateral development agencies to implement particular projects or provide humanitarian relief. Such contracting can facilitate work in the field where the funding agency lacks experience, personnel, and equipment. Contractors may also permit a more rapid, flexible, and informal response, can circumvent government bureaucracies, and present a more acceptable face to the public and to donor countries. Some 95% of USAID global health funding directed to NGOs "is channeled through US-based NGOs" (Moss 2014). Yet INGOs are not necessarily more knowledgeable than governments and often poach local staff from health ministries (at a higher pay rate), denuding domestic health services. INGOs also frequently subcontract to local NGOs, creating bureaucratic burdens and displacing grassroots efforts, particularly as they must respond and report more to donors than to beneficiaries (Adams, Craig, and Samen 2015; Chahim and Prakash 2014).

NGOs, especially INGOs, do not necessarily offer a neutral "third way" that transcends the public and private sectors. They may be unaccountable, undemocratic, and—to the extent to which they exist because appropriate, democratically-determined structures for public service have been destroyed—may be a dangerous development. INGOs can fragment health care systems and other social services, cause chaos and undercut local decisionmaking, exacerbate inequality, drain resources and staff from health systems, and generate unproductive hierarchies among health workers and between outsiders and nationals (Pfeiffer 2013; Mussa et al. 2013).

As Indian novelist-activist Arundhati Roy (2012) provocatively argues:

> In the NGO universe, which has evolved a strange anodyne language of its own, everything has become a "subject", a separate, professionalised, special-interest issue. Community development, leadership development, human rights, health, education, reproductive rights, AIDS, orphans with AIDS—have all been hermetically sealed into their own silos with their own elaborate and precise funding brief. Funding has fragmented solidarity in ways that repression never could. Poverty too, like feminism, is often framed as an identity problem. As though the poor have not been created by injustice but are a lost tribe who just happen to exist, and can be rescued in the short term by a system of

grievance redressal (administered by NGOs on an individual, person to person basis), and whose long-term resurrection will come from Good Governance.

Thus, even as NGOs can be crucial to bringing cooperative health efforts to fruition, their place in the donor assistance organizational arrangement risks depoliticizing, isolating, and disempowering the very struggles that civil society and social rights efforts helped bring to the fore.

In sum, at their best, committed NGOs can deliver imaginative, appropriate, and meaningful grassroots or solidarity assistance. At their worst, NGOs can become, or are created as, inefficient, unresponsive contract service providers with little innovation or dedication to the public welfare, dislodging and discrediting the public provision of services.

Here we present a sample of NGOs according to size, aim, and mode of operation. Most of the organizations in this overview have a primary, but not exclusive, focus on health; arguably all of their activities affect health in some dimension.

Large Humanitarian NGOs

Large humanitarian agencies, many with national donor or operating affiliates, work in multiple settings, on multiple issues, with enormous budgets. The International Committee of the Red Cross (ICRC), the first such entity, was established in 1863 by Swissman Jean-Henri Dunant with the aim of assisting people wounded and displaced by warfare while heeding a principle of neutrality (see chapters 1 and 8). Operating with an annual budget of almost US$1.8 billion, ICRC is engaged in health and economic issues in some 80 countries, involving war-related relief, post-war infrastructural redevelopment, promotion of international law and human rights, and protection of people affected by conflict and detention (ICRC 2016).

Save the Children, comprised of Save the Children International and 30 member organizations, was founded by English children's rights advocate Eglantyne Jebb in 1919 to help starving children in Eastern Europe in the wake of World War I. Today it operates in 120 countries around the world with annual program spending of about US$1 billion in areas such as emergency relief, nutrition and sanitation, HIV prevention, reproductive health, education, and children's rights (Save the Children International 2015).

CARE International, started in 1945 to provide relief to World War II survivors, operates humanitarian projects aimed primarily at helping women via education, sanitation, health programs, and economic support. It operates in 90 countries, spending €477 million on programs and emergency relief in 2014 (CARE International 2015).

Founded in 1937, Plan International is one of the oldest child development NGOs. It focuses on meeting basic needs and promoting child rights in over 50 countries. In 2015, Plan reported spending €810 million on programs with over 85,000 communities. Core project areas include health, education, water and sanitation, sexual health, and economic security (Plan International 2016).

Relief Groups

As witnessed in the public and institutional response to 2013's Typhoon Haiyan in the Philippines, the 2015 Nepal earthquake, and many other "ecologic disasters" (see chapter 8), relief aid is among the most active and publicly supported aspects of global health. The 190 national societies affiliated with the International Federation of Red Cross and Red Crescent Societies constitute by far the largest of these efforts, and are active in emergency relief and the provision of medical services in the countries in which they are based as well as abroad. In conflict situations, the Red Cross typically takes on the role of caring for and protecting people within the conflict zone, whereas protection and care of war refugees is largely left to the UNHCR.

The International Rescue Committee (IRC), whose founding was urged by Albert Einstein in 1933, began by rescuing people suffering under German fascism. Today, with annual spending of almost US$670 million, the IRC provides emergency relief and support to refugees in Africa, Central and South Asia, and other settings where people are uprooted by war and ethnic persecution. More modestly sized NGOs, for example, Merlin, based in the United Kingdom; Project Hope, Mercy Corps, and International Relief Teams, of the United States; and Gift of the Givers, the largest African-originated disaster relief NGO (based in South Africa) provide emergency medical care, training, and health and sanitation infrastructure support. Although these efforts sometimes support long-term rebuilding and conflict/disaster prevention, short-term and immediate relief take priority.

Social Rights-Oriented Service Provision NGOs

These agencies, some large, others with more limited budgets, operate in similar arenas as humanitarian and relief agencies but have explicitly political and social rights missions. Oxfam International, one of the largest such organizations, with 2014-2015 spending of €1 billion, funds small-scale development projects, emergency relief, and campaigns for social/economic justice (Oxfam International 2015).

Médecins Sans Frontières (MSF), with 2015 expenditures of approximately €1.3 billion, is a humanitarian medical aid agency that operates in some of the most crisis-ridden places in the world (MSF 2015a) (see chapter 8). MSF has made the witnessing and reporting of atrocities—particularly those conveniently ignored by dominant political actors—central to its mission, as recognized by the Nobel Prize committee in 1999. MSF also carries out policy and advocacy work, for example in its Essential Drugs Campaign and DNDi. Somewhat smaller, Médecins du Monde (Doctors of the World) carries out similar activities.

Partners In Health (PIH) co-founded by Paul Farmer and current World Bank president Jim Yong Kim, has drawn attention to the possibility—and indeed the human right—of providing first-rate medical care to people with multidrug-resistant TB, HIV, and other ailments deemed "untreatable" in marginalized settings in Peru, Russia, Rwanda, and Haiti (Farmer and Weigel 2013). PIH was among the organizations that successfully demonstrated that highly active antiretroviral therapy can be delivered in resource-poor circumstances. These efforts have also helped drive down the cost of ARVs worldwide (see chapter 6).

There are also various groups with clear political, social justice, and health aims, such as Doctors for Global Health, working in a small number of places where their projects can be locally sustained. Similarly, Health Alliance International explicitly links its efforts towards increasing access to quality health care among disadvantaged populations to underlying structural and policy changes, most notably in Mozambique (see chapter 14 for more on both). Other groups, for instance Physicians for Peace, focus on international peace-building through medical education, clinical care, or medical donations.

Human Rights and Health Groups

This diverse group of NGOs puts human rights at the forefront of their approach to global health. They include professionally-based groups that operate health cooperation projects, small think tanks and advocacy NGOs that carry out research on health and human rights, such as the Center for Social and Economic Rights, and large human rights organizations. For example, both Amnesty International and Human Rights Watch have established health programs as part of their larger mandate. Most of these groups are experienced in using media outlets to raise awareness and provoke political responses.

Only a small sampling of groups active in this area are showcased here. Dignitas International, which provides services to people living with HIV, puts human rights at the center of its activities. Physicians for Social Responsibility, founded to prevent the use and spread of nuclear weapons, now also focuses on environmental conditions, and Physicians for Human Rights, drawing attention to the role of US policies in impeding the realization of health of peoples around the world, has effectively used physicians as advocates. AWID (the Association for Women's Rights in Development) is a membership organization led by Majority World women and comprises feminist activists working globally on diverse women's rights issues: economic justice, environmental sustainability, and challenging religious fundamentalism. Wemos is a Netherlands-based advocacy organization that works toward attainment of the right to health for all. It emphasizes the role of government policies in improving and protecting public health across the globe.

Health and human rights efforts are also advanced by the Hesperian Foundation, a nonprofit community health and advocacy publisher. Its many handbooks, including *Where There is No Doctor,* first issued in 1977, and others covering midwifery, community health activism, among many subjects, have been translated into dozens of languages and used all over the world as health activist and primary health care "bibles."

LMIC NGOs

There are literally hundreds of thousands of NGOs working locally in diverse settings across the world. Here we highlight a few in South Asia (other regions are featured in different chapters) that are linked to global health as service deliverers, grantees, and contributors to the larger policy agenda. The largest and most well-known of these is the Bangladesh Rehabilitation Assistance Committee, better known as BRAC, which began as a donor-funded war relief effort following the Bangladesh independence struggle in the early 1970s and has been transformed into a self-funded development effort. Today, it reaches 135 million people in 12 countries through poverty alleviation, employment generation, and maternal and child health programs. BRAC's total annual spending in Bangladesh for 2014 was US$537 million, with another US$65 million spent through BRAC International. BRAC has been widely praised for its numerous health and anti-poverty projects, and for investing in research and higher education (Chowdhury et al. 2013). However, BRAC has also come under attack for its corporate approach and limited impact on poverty alleviation (Muhammad 2015).

On a much smaller scale, the Urmul Trust, founded in 1972 in Rajasthan, India, is a group of organizations "guided by the spirit and trust placed in people's capabilities to bring about the much-needed social change with their own efforts" (Urmul Trust 2015). It began as a milk cooperative that went from producing 200 L/day to 1 million L/day and soon expanded into health and education outreach to women and girls. Following a 1987 drought, the Urmul Trust's participants collectively adapted themselves into a weaving cooperative that has followed in the successful footsteps of its predecessor. Urmul Trust, now in over 500 villages in rural Rajasthan, works on training community health workers, drought and disaster mitigation, women's empowerment, and child rights. Also remarkable is the Comprehensive Rural Health Project (CRHP), founded in 1970 in Ahmednagar, Maharashtra, India. It provides community-based primary health care in rural areas, with a special focus on training women village health workers. Considered a model by WHO and UNICEF, its approach has been emulated across the world (CRHP 2016).

Alliances of grassroots organizations to create a broader powerbase and influence local action across multiple countries are also important. One example is the South Asian Alliance of Grassroots NGOs, formed after the World Social Forum in 2004. It links grassroots organizations in Afghanistan, Bangladesh, India, Nepal, and Sri Lanka and focuses on child rights and the provision of services to children and families.

Global Health and Development Think Tanks

Think tanks engage in wide-ranging research and advocacy activities in an effort to improve access to health services and push for the effectiveness and accountability of donor development aid, including health aid. These organizations, for example the Center for Global Development in Washington and the Overseas Development Institute in London, often have close connections to multilateral and bilateral agencies and to politicians, and can have significant influence on decisionmaking. The US-based Treatment Action Group is a research and policy think tank fighting for better treatment, a vaccine, and a cure for HIV and TB. The modestly-sized yet highly effective CPATH (Center for Policy Analysis on Trade and Health) addresses public health concerns in international trade agreements and engages in transnational advocacy (see chapter 9).

Advocacy Groups and Alliances

There is a broad array of global health advocacy groups and alliances, some focused on diseases, for instance the Global AIDS Alliance, others regionally-based (e.g., the Washington Global Health Alliance, which fosters PPPs). Many are aimed at leveraging private sector agenda-setting over global health. For example, the expanding NCD Alliance is comprised of NGOs, foundations, and private sector players (including Big Pharma) that advocate for attention to NCDs as a global health emergency, thereby expanding support for treatment (and new product markets) for controversial conditions such as "pre-hypertension" (PHM et al. 2014). Meanwhile, the US-based Global Health Council (GHC) is a 40-year-old advocacy group that brings together individual and organizational members to advocate for global health research and spending. However, like a growing number of hybrid entities, the GHC is not a public-interest organization, given the significant presence of corporate, contractor, and foundation members in addition to universities, NGOs, and individuals (Subramaniam 2015).

Social Rights NGOs and Scholar-Activist Organizations

The People's Health Movement (PHM), founded in 2000 in Bangladesh, is an international network of health workers and activists who carry out research and advocacy work, host conferences, and undertake political action. With a presence in 70 countries, PHM played an instrumental role in the establishment of the WHO's Commission on Social Determinants of Health in 2005. PHM also hosts courses for activists around the world through its International People's Health University, helps coordinate WHO Watch and PAHO Watch, and helps prepare the noteworthy triannual publication, *Global Health Watch* (see chapter 14).

Among the most effective social rights NGOs is South Africa's Treatment Action Campaign (TAC), which has had a crucial impact on policy by pressuring the South African government, in alliance with Global North groups such as Treatment Action Group, to provide HIV therapeutics. The All India Drug Action Network similarly fights for access to medicines as part of a larger struggle against poverty and social injustice.

Various social rights alliances, for example Malaysia-based Third World Network and Focus on the Global South (headquartered in Thailand) embrace activist, advocacy, and research activities. Solidarity social rights NGOs based in the Global North include CETIM (Centre Europe-Tiers Monde) and the South Centre (which promotes learning, cooperation, and coordination among Global South countries to advance equity and justice-oriented interests in international fora), both located in Geneva, and Belgian-based Third World Health Aid, which focuses on the right to health and sovereign development. Some issue-based, public-interest NGOs, notably the International Baby Food Action Network (IBFAN—see Box 9-3), also engage in public-interest advocacy around democratic governance in global health.

Scholar-activist organizations include the Latin American Social Medicine Association (ALAMES, see chapter 13), Equinet (the Regional Network on Equity in Health in Southern Africa), and the European-based International Association of Health Policy. These networks of academics, health workers, scientists, and activists carry out rigorous analysis of public health issues and offer a forum for international and regional political debate on global health issues, also engaging in research and advocacy from the perspective of health as a social and political right.

Like PHM, all of these groups are guided by the principle of political solidarity with allies across the world and work hand-in-hand with social movements to redress the unequal distribution of political power and resources.

Student Activism

A growing number of student groups work as effective global health advocates and activists. The International Federation of Medical Students Associations (IFMSA) is an alliance of 127 medical student organizations from 119 countries—the largest of its kind. IFMSA advocates for public health, sexual and reproductive health, medical education, human rights and peace, and organizes medical exchanges among its members. Another student organization, Universities Allied for Essential Medicines (UAEM), has chapters in 46 research universities across 15 countries, with student members from medicine, the sciences, public health, economics, and other disciplines. UAEM advocates for LMIC access to the benefits of biomedical and other university research. These and other groups also participate in activities such as WHO Watch, which seeks to increase the public accountability of multilateral health agencies.

Social and Political Movements

While not global health players in the strictest sense, grassroots and transnational movements, also involving anti-WTO, anti-G20, and anti-G7/8 activism, draw attention to the untoward health and social consequences of global economic policies. Their efforts have been instrumental in raising awareness and resistance to international financial and trade policy.

The first World Social Forum (WSF) took place in 2001 in Porto Alegre, Brazil to counterbalance the annual closed Davos forum held by corporate and government elites (see above). Under the slogan "Another World is Possible," the WSF convenes open meeting spaces for "groups and movements of civil society that are opposed to neoliberalism and to domination of the world by capital and any form of imperialism, and are committed to building a planetary society directed towards fruitful relationships among Humankind and between it and the Earth" (World Social Forum 2001). Recent gatherings (Dakar 2011, Tunis 2013 and 2015, and Montréal 2016, also sometimes taking place in multiple sites simultaneously) have attracted up to 100,000 people from over 130 countries, mostly representing grassroots movements, who relay experiences of activism and resistance, spurring further mobilization.

Innumerable networks, such as Shack/Slum Dwellers International, solidarity groups, trade unions, and people's movements of all kinds have enormous bearing on health locally, but also have considerable international resonance in that their ideas and actions are shared from place to place. Their explicitly political activities—for land reform (e.g., Brazil's MST [Movimento dos Trabalhadores Rurais Sem Terra], with over 1.5 million landless members); for keeping water in public hands (e.g., Bolivia's Coalition in Defense of Water and Life); for labor rights (e.g., International Labor Rights Forum)—do more for health by fighting for water, land, workplace, and other rights than dozens of global health programs (see chapters 9, 10, and 14).

Another notable grassroots movement is the India-based Bachpan Bachao Andolan (Save the Childhood) Movement. Founded in 1980 by activist and 2014 Nobel Peace Prize laureate, Kailash Satyarthi, the movement has advocated for children's rights and legislation to protect against trafficking and child labor in India and across South Asia. It has also led the Global March Against Child Labour, a network of child rights activists that began with a massive march across 103 countries in 1998.

University and Hospital Initiatives

In recent decades, university-based researchers and hospitals have become increasingly involved in global health, carrying out donor-funded research, establishing collaborations between researchers in HICs and LMICs (e.g., AMPATH, a consortium among Indiana University, Moi University, and the Kenyan government), and establishing "subsidiaries" (such as Cornell-Weill Medical College's counterpart in Qatar, and Harvard's in the United Arab Emirates). Hospital exchanges furnish equipment, short-term in-country training programs, and intensive "donation" of medical services, for instance cataract operations and surgery for children.

Some LMICs also have extensive scholarship programs. The Latin American School of Medicine (ELAM), based in Havana, provides free medical education for thousands of students from LMICs, with the understanding that those students will practice in underserved areas in their home countries (see chapter 11). In 2007 a sister school—the Alejandro Prospero Reverend School of Medicine—opened in Venezuela.

In HICs there is a proliferating number of academic enterprises in global health. Columbia University's International Center for AIDS Care and Treatment Programs (ICAP, founded in 2004) delivers HIV services and is now one of the larger PEPFAR partners in various countries. The Harvard Initiative for Global Health participates in global health research, training, and cooperation. The François-Xavier Bagnoud Center for Health and Human Rights, also at Harvard, was the first academic unit with an explicit focus on health and human rights. Johns Hopkins University also has a Center for Health and Human Rights and its Center for Global Health offers training courses and fellowships, and collaborates on research projects with public health schools in LMICs. Similar initiatives are based at Duke Emory, Universities of Washington, Iowa, Toronto, Copenhagen, Maastricht, and elsewhere. European countries, for example Portugal (Instituto de Higiene e Medicina Tropical in Lisbon), the United Kingdom (London School of Hygiene and Tropical Medicine; Liverpool School of Tropical Medicine), Belgium (Antwerp's Institute of Tropical Medicine), and Germany (Hamburg's Bernhard Nocht Institute for

Tropical Medicine), also retain tropical medicine institutes founded during the colonial period.

The Aga Khan University, based in Pakistan, trains medical and public health practitioners and maintains hospitals in Karachi and Nairobi. In the Americas, Mexico's Instituto Nacional de Salud Pública co-hosts the International Association of National Public Health Institutes, undertakes research on local and global health issues, and offers postgraduate training in public health for students from across Latin America. Thailand's Thammasat University, Ecuador's Universidad Andina Simón Bolívar, Peru's Universidad Peruana Cayetano Heredia, the Public Health Foundation of India, the University of Chile, and Makerere University in Kampala, among others, also carry out global health training and research.

Research Alliances

Members of the Switzerland-based Council on Health Research for Development (COHRED)—established in 1993—undertake global health research with an explicit focus on equity and social justice issues and giving voice to partners from the Global South. COHRED's annual global health research forums seek to strengthen global research capacity and coherence.

The Global Forum for Health Research—also based in Switzerland—has since its founding in 1998 used research and advocacy to draw attention to global health issues, including the "10/90 gap" whereby only 10% of health sciences research dollars address the health problems of 90% of the world's population (see Box 14-1). Each year, the Global Forum hosts a global health research conference with attendance of many key players in global health.

The WHO-hosted Alliance for Health Policy and Systems Research was established in 1999 with a mandate to generate, capacity-build for, and disseminate health policy research to strengthen health care systems in LMICs. A topically related but separate membership organization, Health Systems Global, holds a biennial research symposium.

University College London's Institute for Global Health hosts the Global Alliance for Chronic Diseases. The Alliance's aim is to build scientific evidence for chronic NCDs to assist policymaking in LMICs. It raises funds for research and prioritizes research in cardiovascular diseases, cancers, chronic respiratory conditions, Type II diabetes, and mental illness.

The Berlin-based M8 Alliance, founded in 2009, is a network of universities, academic health centers, and national academies that develop "science-based solutions" to global health problems. Its annual World Health Summit seeks to influence the global health agenda via dialogue with global governance organizations, commerce and industry leaders, and government representatives.

The One Health Initiative is a global movement to galvanize collaboration in research, training, communication, and practice among professionals and government agencies focused on human, animal, and environmental public health (especially related to zoonoses).

Professional Membership Organizations

Many people who work with global health agencies also belong to professional organizations, whose members include public health and medical personnel, academics, policy actors, field workers, and activists who are involved in research, advocacy, running programs, and communication with the public. One example is the Canadian Society for International Health, which also carries out cooperative projects.

Various professional public health and medical associations are engaged in global health work. Two international associations that partner with the WHO are the World Federation of Public Health Associations and the International Association of National Public Health Institutes. The formerly Philadelphia-based, now New Delhi-headquartered International Clinical Epidemiology Network (INCLEN) of over 100 universities, medical faculties, and research centers in 34 countries with almost 2,000 member-professionals aims to improve "health for all" through multidisciplinary research and training.

Many countries also have national public health associations. The oldest, the American Public Health Association, founded in 1872, early on served as a regional public health association for US, Canadian, Mexican, and Cuban health professionals, but since the 1950s its international involvement has mainly been channeled through collaboration with USAID, CDC, and various NGOs. Others include the Bangladesh Public Health Association, the Ethiopian Public Health Association, the Afghanistan National

Public Health Association, the Brazilian Association of Collective Health, the China Preventive Medicine Association, the Public Health Association of Georgia, the Indonesian Public Health Association, the Public Health Association of South Africa, and the Turkish Public Health Association. The African Federation of Public Health Associations is an important regional group.

Small-Scale and Consumer Driven Efforts

Numerous doctor and nurse groups and civic organizations are involved in global health cooperation on a small scale, sometimes as "flying doctors," whose commitment is minimal. Medical Expeditions International and International Health Service organize such volunteer stints.

Other charitable models operate via direct donations. Microcredit networks such as Kiva and the crowd funding initiative Global Giving, connect individuals in HICs with LMIC residents seeking loans or donations. Likewise, GiveDirectly conducts cash transfers directly from small donors to poor households in Kenya and Uganda. It forgoes partnerships with NGOs to increase effectiveness, transparency, and accountability of donor funds' use. As of 2014 it had committed over US$10 million in cash transfers (GiveDirectly 2015). Meanwhile, Giving What We Can operates on a tithing model, whereby individual donors set aside a percent of their salary to international charities that have been evaluated to maximize impact (Giving What We Can 2015).

The high-income public has also been drawn into "marketized philanthropy," whereby some profits from consumer purchases, for example through Irish rock star Bono's Product (RED), are channeled to the Global Fund. (In a companion "celebrity humanitarianism" effort, Bono's ONE campaign raises awareness about—and persuades governments to invest in reducing—poverty and ill health in Africa [Kapoor 2012].)

POLITICAL ECONOMY OF GLOBAL HEALTH ACTORS AND ACTIVITIES

Key Questions:

- How are decisions made and who wields power in global health?
- What arrangements might lead to greater health equity and social justice?

The panorama of institutions and activities presented in this chapter suggests that the field is marked by a flurry of energy, resources, and goodwill. In 2004 approximately US$18 billion (in 2014 US$) was spent in the global health arena—within a decade this had doubled to US$36 billion (IHME 2016).

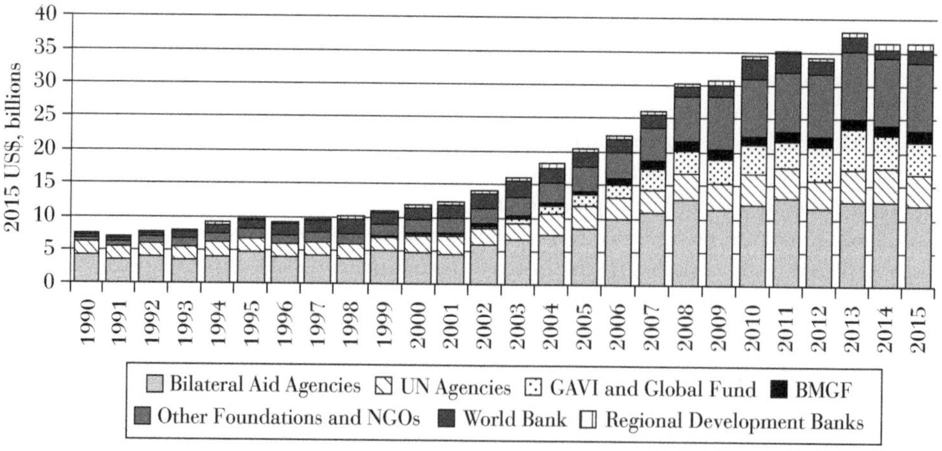

Figure 4-2: Development assistance for health by source, 1990–2015.
Data Source: Adapted from Institute for Health Metrics and Evaluation (2016).

Despite the slowdown in the rate of increase of development assistance for health since 2010 (Figure 4-2), the current level of resources for global health is unprecedented (IHME 2016). Alongside this interest come a series of dilemmas around who and what drives (and should drive) the global health agenda. The varied players and activities that we have covered—from grassroots movements to bilateral and multilateral agencies, philanthropies, and pharmaceutical multinationals—have competing, overlapping, and only rarely shared, approaches to global health even as the field has experienced explosive growth. Another reading of this situation, then, is that the global health scene is chaotic and requires a new governance system.

Global health governance (see chapter 3) analysts rightly point out that there is: much duplication and inefficiency in health cooperation; greed, self-interest, arrogance, and lack of transparency on the part of donors (Birdsall 2004; Youde 2012); insufficient management, technical capacity, decisionmaking power, resources (or control of resources in the health arena) and regulatory weaknesses, clientelism, and other problems at the country level (Nervi 2014); and little coordination between country needs and the allocation of aid (Sridhar 2010). Various strategies to address these problems have emerged in recent years, from calls for greater capacity-building at the national level to reforming the very terms of aid through pledges of donors to better align with country needs (Fidler 2010). While not lacking merit, these efforts have borne few fruits, in large measure because they do not take into account either the evolution or nature of the global health arena in recent years or the larger contemporary political-economic context.

As per chapter 2 and evidenced here, the last few decades have seen a return of global health initiatives, typically involving top-down, technological approaches to health. This followed a period in the 1970s and early 1980s when progressive efforts sought to rescript international health as participatory, locally defined, equity-oriented, and harnessing the technical aspects of health and medicine to the political goal of health as a human right, all within the context of WHO's democratization to reflect the interests of the majority of member countries and the goal of Health for All. The backlash against this initiative was directly realized through defunding of WHO. But it also unfolded indirectly through Washington Consensus favoring of financial liberalization and free trade, among other factors, generating or exacerbating enormous human misery and health inequity.

Given such circumstances, the large infusion of money into global health since 2000 has been widely welcomed. But the money has come, so to speak, at a very steep price—channeled via private sector actors and the bilateral and multilateral aid they influence. These efforts have largely bypassed WHO and public sector decisionmaking, either by earmarking WHO contributions or operating through PPPs or bilateral programs, themselves increasingly shaped by private interests, outside WHO's ambit. They also have resurrected the prior flawed vertical model, offering reductionist technical solutions to political problems, but this time with the heavy hand of unaccountable private actors, commercial interests and attendant conflicts of interest, and profiteering. Any semblance of democratic health governance is being lost through this process.

The BMGF offers a case in point. It appeared on the scene precisely at the apex of neoliberalism—a moment when overall spending for global health was stagnant, suspicion of ODA was at an all-time high, and many LMICs were floundering under the multiple burdens of HIV, re-emerging infectious diseases, violence, and soaring chronic ailments (including both undernutrition and obesity), compounded by decades of World Bank and IMF-imposed policies, such as social expenditure cuts. Today, virtually all key global health actors have received BMGF funding (McCoy et al. 2009).

Yet, emblematic of elite interests in contemporary society, the BMGF disregards the underlying causes of ill health, overlooks what role the enormous accumulation of wealth in the hands of a few has played therein, and stakes a moral high ground regarding its generosity and narrow technically-oriented savoir-faire, all the while remaining generally under-scrutinized by scientists and unaccountable to the wider public (Birn 2014b).

The BMGF has been, largely uncritically, hailed as a savior of global health (McGoey 2015), but this assessment excludes the question of what could be achieved through combined social, political, and public health measures such as investing in peace, improved living and working conditions, creating a fair global system of finance and trade, ensuring food sovereignty, building redistributive welfare states and strong public and universal health care systems, or even abolishing the military.

To be sure, this is not simply a global health problem but a profound problem of the marked asymmetry of power in the global economy—not only in terms of who controls the purse strings and decisionmaking, but who decides the rules of the game. In addition to the undue influence of private actors *within* the global health field, the corporate sector and its government partners have a crucial *indirect* effect on global health via exploitative trade relations, dismantling of decades of hard-won workplace protections and improvements in social conditions, and the stripping away of already insufficient and inequitable health, education, and other social services, jeopardizing the lives and livelihoods of literally billions of people across the world in LMICs, especially, but also in HICs (see chapter 9).

These ideas can be difficult to grasp, particularly for those new to the global health field and who are attracted to the aspirational language of many global health actors and initiatives. As discussed throughout the book, such rhetoric can distract

Table 4-10 Largest Current Global Health Actors

Organization	Donors	Funds Pledged/Spent/Committed to Health
President's Emergency Plan for AIDS Relief (PEPFAR)	US Government	US$ 6.8 billion committed for 2016 US$66 billion committed between 2004 and 2016 (3% to bilateral TB programs, 19% to Global Fund, 78% to bilateral HIV and AIDS programs)
Global Fund	Governments, foundations, corporations	US$33 billion committed and spent between 2002–2015 US$4 billion per year pledged for 2014–2016
Bill and Melinda Gates Foundation	Bill and Melinda Gates, Warren Buffett	US1.1 billion spent in global health in 2014
World Health Organization	Governments, non-state actors (e.g., PPPs, corporations, foundations, academic institutions)	US$4.4 billion budget (2016–2017)
GAVI, the Vaccine Alliance	Gates Foundation, governments, NGOs, private businesses, multilateral agencies, other philanthropies	US$11.7 billion committed between 2000–2015 US$9.5 billion pledged for 2016–2020
World Bank	Governments	US$2.6 billion budget (2015)
OECD ODA	28 DAC countries	US$8.8 billion to family planning and reproductive health; US$5.3 billion to general health; US$4.5 billion to water supply and sanitation (2014)
European Union	Member countries[1]	US$2.9 billion to family planning and reproductive health; US$2.8 billion to water supply and sanitation; US$1.8 billion to general health (2014)

[1] As of 2016 the EU had 28 member countries, but that year the United Kingdom voted to leave the EU, with a timetable and repercussions unclear when the book went to press.

Sources: Agency web sites; OECD (2016).

from, or even coopt, progressive social justice goals that are widely shared by the majority of the world's population. This rhetoric may also mask deeper tensions around the extent to which global health serves as a strategic issue of security and commercial interests.

If global health efforts were to serve as stopgap measures on the way to a world in which all countries had the (control over their) resources and sovereignty to make their own decisions about health and its determination in pursuit of equity, global health initiatives might well play a legitimate—and vital—role (Farmer et al. 2013). But the proliferation of global actors and technical quick fixes appears to be more a reflection (or even reinforcement) of the increasing inequalities within and between countries than an indication of the forging of sustainable health approaches in the context of locally responsive and representative policymaking.

Indeed, a handful of large bilateral agencies, multilateral financial agencies, and foundations finance most global health cooperation (Figure 4-2 and Table 4-10). These agencies not only have an inordinate role in shaping the major global approaches and practices to health—oriented to magic bullet-based, vertical disease-control interventions over short timelines—they also reinforce dominant ideological paradigms that view health as a function largely of individual and medical factors. Moreover, because of aid stipulations that require recipient governments to allocate substantial matching funds to donor programs, national needs and decisionmaking, including around health system strengthening, frequently become subsidiary to the priorities of donors (Chilundo et al. 2015; Chima and Homedes 2015).

Of course, the direct work of global health actors has far less impact on health status across the world than do the combination of international economics and domestic politics (i.e., how redistributive each country is in terms of providing access to health, education, and other social services, in ensuring fair working and living conditions, and in addressing oppression). Health is subject to the enormous structural influence of global economic institutions, ideologies, and practices (commodity prices, terms of trade, capital flight, trade agreements, role of TNCs) and IFI loans and policies (and those of private banks) on national production patterns, wage levels, social infrastructure, redistributive policies, health care system characteristics, and politics writ large.

In sum, global health governance and donor assistance have been critiqued on a number of grounds:

- Political and economic interests—rather than health needs—drive health aid.
- Underlying determinants of health are rarely addressed by donor assistance.
- Private interests have largely hijacked global health agenda-setting.
- Bureaucratic institutions act to preserve and expand their power; smaller organizations to ensure their survival.
- Annual project cycles mean narrow objectives.
- Political interests upstage health outcomes.
- Ideologically driven policies promote a market ethos.
- Threats to commerce and HICs (e.g., Avian influenza), strategic interests, and fears of bioterrorism shape global health donor assistance more than needs-based rationales.
- Little aid reaches the neediest—and up to half of aid is spent in HICs.
- Most cooperation is more accountable to donors than "beneficiaries."
- Substantial co-financing expectations on the part of national governments means that donor projects significantly influence national health agendas.
- Health "cooperation" is rarely fully cooperative, in both conception and implementation, instead reflecting donor agendas and assessment of priorities.
- "Aid" tends to exacerbate inequalities in already profoundly unequal societies.
- Poverty alleviation and social justice principles are much touted but little practiced.

CONCLUSION

Learning Points:

- There has been a proliferation of new global health actors in recent years, including philanthropies, PPPs, and large and small NGOs, as well as renewed spending by bilateral organizations.

- These new organizations, and above all, the power of private interests, have led to undemocratic agenda-setting, investment of large sums of public (bilateral) monies in commercial products and activities, and a focus on short-term, technology based approaches to health that ignore or downplay the socio-political context and the societal determinants of health.
- A small, but important, set of efforts are challenging global (health) hegemony: South–South cooperation, particularly that long purveyed by Cuba's solidarity efforts around the right to health and the training of health personnel; and a variety of civil society-based public interest organizations that mobilize for representation of collective grassroots voices and push for global health accountability on multiple fronts.

The organization of global health today is marked by both historical legacies and new developments. The way aid is organized, who provides the funds, on what terms, and its effectiveness remain issues of great importance. Without a better alignment of global health priorities and the underlying determinants of premature death and disability, global health initiatives—no matter how well funded—are unlikely to achieve truly sustainable health improvement. But this diverts attention from the main issue: underpinning such an alignment are the larger arrangements around who and what wield power and resources in the contemporary global political order. This reality cannot be sidestepped.

Before contemplating what might be done to improve global health, we must first deepen our knowledge and understanding of the patterns of health across the world and their social, political, and economic determinants.

REFERENCES

ActionAid. 2011. *Real Aid 3*. London: ActionAid.

AidData. 2015a. Track Emerging Donors. http://aiddata.org/track-emerging-donors#nondac_donors. Accessed August 8, 2015.

———. 2015b. AidData Dashboard. http://aiddata.org/dashboard. Accessed August 1, 2015.

Adams B and Martens J. 2015. *Fit for Whose Purpose? Private Funding and Corporate Influence in the United Nations*. New York and Bonn: Global Policy Forum.

Adams V, Craig SR, and Samen A. 2015. Alternative accounting in maternal and infant global health. *Global Public Health* 11(3):276–294.

Adem S. 2012. China in Ethiopia: Diplomacy and economics of sino-optimism. *African Studies Review* 55(1):143–160.

Agutamba K. 2015. Africa: How will Rwanda benefit from China's $60bn aid to Africa? *Forum on China-Africa Cooperation*, December 22.

Anderson MD and Bellows AC. 2012. Introduction to symposium on food sovereignty: Expanding the analysis and application. *Agriculture and Human Values* 29(2):177–184.

Barnes A, Brown GW, and Harman S. 2015. Locating health diplomacy through African negotiations on performance-based funding in global health. *Journal of Health Diplomacy* 1(3):1–19.

Baum FE and Anaf JM. 2015. Transnational corporations and health: A research agenda. *International Journal of Health Services* 45(2):353–362.

Biesma RG, Makoa E, Mpemi R, et al. 2012. The implementation of a global fund grant in Lesotho: Applying a framework on knowledge absorptive capacity. *Social Science and Medicine* 74(3):381–389.

Birdsall N. 2004. *Seven Deadly Sins: Reflections on Donor Failings. Working Paper 50*. Washington, DC: Center for Global Development.

Birn A-E. 2014a. Backstage: The relationship between the Rockefeller Foundation and the World Health Organization, Part I: 1940s–1960s. *Public Health* 128(2):129–140.

———. 2014b. Philanthrocapitalism, past and present: The Rockefeller Foundation, the Gates Foundation, and the setting(s) of the international/ global health agenda. *Hypothesis* 12(1):e8.

Birn A-E and Lexchin J. 2011. Beyond patents: The GAVI Alliance, AMCs, and improving immunization coverage through public sector vaccine production in the Global South. *Human Vaccines* 7(3):291–292.

Birn A-E, Muntaner C, and Afzal Z. 2017. Social justice oriented South-South cooperation in health: Theorizing (and politicizing) the debate. *Cadernos de Saúde Pública*, forthcoming.

Bishop M and Green M. 2008. *Philanthrocapitalism: How the Rich Can Save the World*. New York: Bloomsbury Press.

BMGF [Bill and Melinda Gates Foundation]. 2011. *Global Health Data Access Principles*. Seattle: BMGF.

———. 2015a. *2015 Gates Annual Letter: Our Big Bet for the Future.* Seattle: BMGF.

———. 2015b. Who we are: Foundation fact sheet. http://www.gatesfoundation.org/who-we-are/general-information/foundation-factsheet. Accessed March 5, 2016.

———. 2016. Grantmaking: Awarded grants. http://www.gatesfoundation.org/How-We-Work/Quick-Links/Grants-Database#. Accessed March 3, 2016.

Bond P and Garcia A, Editors. 2015. *The BRICS: An Anti-Capitalist Critique.* London: Pluto Press.

Boseley S. 2011. Can the Global Fund weather the corruption storm? *The Guardian*, January 28.

Bowman A. 2012. The flip side to Bill Gates's charity billions. *New Internationalist*, April 1.

Brautigam D. 2011. Chinese development aid in Africa: What, where, why, and how much? In Golley J and Song L, Editors. *Rising China: Global Challenges and Opportunities.* Canberra: ANU E Press.

Brown GW, Loewenson R, Modisenyane M, et al. 2015. Business as usual? The role of BRICS co-operation in addressing health system priorities in East and Southern Africa. *Journal of Health Diplomacy* 1(3):1–23.

Buente M, Danner S, Weissbäcker S, and Rammé C. 2013. *Pharma emerging markets 2.0: How emerging markets are driving the transformation of the pharmaceutical industry.* New York: Strategy.

Buhmann C, Santa Barbara J, Arya N, and Melf K. 2010. The roles of the health sector and health workers before, during and after violent conflict. *Medicine, Conflict and Survival* 26(1):4–23.

Burke RL, Vest KG, Eick AA, et al. 2011. Department of defense influenza and other respiratory disease surveillance during the 2009 pandemic. *BMC Public Health* 11(2):S6.

Buse K and Harmer A. 2007. Seven habits of highly effective global public-private health partnerships: Practice and potential. *Social Science and Medicine* 64(2):259–271.

Buse K and Tanaka S. 2011. Global public-private health partnerships: Lessons learned from ten years of experience and evaluation. *International Dental Journal* 61(Suppl. 2):2–10.

Buse K and Walt G. 2000. Global public-private partnerships: Part I—A new development in health? *Bulletin of the World Health Organisation* 78(4):549–561.

Buss P and Faid M. 2013. Power shifts in global health diplomacy. In Kickbusch I, Lister G, Told M, and Drager N, Editors. *Global Health Diplomacy.* New York: Springer.

CARE International. 2015. *CARE International Annual Report 2014: Fighting Poverty by Empowering Women and Girls in the Poorest Communities Around the World.* Geneva: CARE International.

Cargill. 2012. *Cargill's Nutrition and Health Partnerships.* Minneapolis: Cargill.

Carrillo Roa A and Silva FRP. 2015. Fiocruz as an actor in Brazilian foreign relations in the context of the Community of Portuguese-Speaking Countries: An untold story. *História, Ciências, Saúde-Manguinhos* 22(1):153–169.

Center for Health and Gender Equity. 2011. *Female Condoms and US Foreign Assistance: An Unfinished Imperative for Women's Health.* Washington, DC: Center for Health and Gender Equity.

Chahim D and Prakash A. 2014. NGOization, foreign funding, and Nicaraguan civil society. *VOLUNTAS: International Journal of Voluntary and Nonprofit Organizations* 25(2):487–513.

Chilundo B, Madede T, Cliff J, et al. 2015. Implicações de suporte de iniciativas de saúde globais no Sistema de Saúde de Moçambique. *Revista Científica da UEM: Série Ciências Biomédicas e Saúde Pública* 1(1):41–56.

Chima CC and Homedes N. 2015. Impact of global health governance on country health systems: the case of HIV initiatives in Nigeria. *Journal of Global Health* 5(1):1–13.

Chowdhury AMR, Bhuiya A, Chowdhury ME, et al. 2013. The Bangladesh paradox: Exceptional health achievement despite economic poverty. *Lancet* 382(9906):1734–1745.

Clift C. 2014. *What's the World Health Organization For? Final Report from the Centre on Global Health Security Working Group on Health Governance.* London: Chatham House.

Clinton Foundation. 2014. *Unlocking Human Potential: Clinton Foundation 2013-2014 Annual Report.* New York: Clinton Foundation.

Coca-Cola Company. 2015. The Coca-Cola Foundation. http://www.coca-colacompany.com/our-company/the-coca-cola-foundation. Accessed July 17, 2015.

Cole DC, Crissman CC, and Orozco AF. 2006. Canada's International Development Research Centre's eco-health projects with Latin Americans: Origins, development and challenges. *Canadian Journal of Public Health* 97(6):I8.

Collins KL. 2004. Profitable gifts: A history of the Merck Mectizan donation program and its implications for international health. *Perspectives in Biology and Medicine* 47(1):100–109.

CRHP. 2016. About Us. http://www.jamkhed.org/about_us/comprehensive_rural_health_project. Accessed March 15, 2016.

Crisp J. 2014. Growing share of European development aid disguised as loans. *EurActiv.com*, December 12.

Curtis M. 2016. *Gated Development Is the Gates Foundation Always a Force for Good?* London: Global Justice Now.

Dornsife C. 2013. BRICS countries emerging as major aid donors. *Asia Pathways*, October 25.

Esfandiari H. 2014. Revisiting the Beijing Declaration. In Heideman K, Nietsche C, Romano JC, et al. *Beijing +20: Looking Back and the Road Ahead: Reflections on Milestones in Women's Leadership in the 21st Century*. Washington, DC: Woodrow Wilson International Center for Scholars.

European Commission. 2015. *Echo Factsheet – Humanitarian Aid*. Brussels: European Commission.

———. 2016. Global health. http://ec.europa.eu/health/eu_world/global_health/. Accessed January 26, 2016.

Fan VY, Duran D, Silverman R, and Glassman A. 2013a. Performance-based financing at the Global Fund to Fight AIDS, Tuberculosis and Malaria: An analysis of grant ratings and funding, 2003–12. *Lancet Global Health* 1(3):e161–e168.

Fan V, Silverman R, Duran D, and Glassman A. 2013b. *The Financial Flows of PEPFAR: A Profile*. Washington, DC: Center for Global Development.

Faraizi A, Rahman T, and McAllister J. 2011. *Microcredit and Women's Empowerment: A Case Study of Bangladesh*. New York: Routledge.

Farmer P, Kim JY, Kleinman A, and Basilico M, Editors. 2013. *Reimagining Global Health: An Introduction*. Los Angeles: University of California Press.

Farmer P and Weigel J. 2013. *To Repair the World: Paul Farmer Speaks to the Next Generation*. Berkeley: University of California Press.

Feinsilver JM. 2010. Fifty years of Cuba's medical diplomacy: From idealism to pragmatism. *Cuban Studies* 41(1):85–104.

Fidler DP. 2010. *The Challenges of Global Health Governance*. New York: Council on Foreign Relations.

Forman L and Kohler JC, Editors. 2012. *Access to Medicines as a Human Right: What are the Implications for Pharmaceutical Industry?* Toronto: University of Toronto Press.

Fortune. 2015. Global 500. http://fortune.com/global500/?iid=G500_sp_. Accessed July 24, 2015.

FP2020. 2015. *Commitment to Action 2014-2015*. FP2020.

Gallagher KP and Myers M. 2015. *China-Latin America Finance Database*. Washington: Inter-American Dialogue.

Garcia G. 2016. The rise of the Global South, the IMF and the future of law and development. *Third World Quarterly* 37(2):191–208.

Gideon J and Porter F. 2016. Challenging gendered inequalities in global health: Dilemmas for NGOs. *Development and Change* 47(4):782–797.

GiveDirectly. 2015. *2014 Annual Report*. New York: GiveDirectly.

Giving What We Can. 2015. Political change. https://www.givingwhatwecan.org/research/charities-area/political-change. Accessed May 12, 2015.

Global Fund. 2015. *Building Resilient and Sustainable Systems for Health*. Geneva: Global Fund.

———. 2016. Financials. http://www.theglobalfund.org/en/financials/. Accessed February 25, 2016.

Global Social Justice. 2013. BRICS challenge IFIs. *Global Social Justice*, April 9.

GPEDC [Global Partnership for Effective Development and Cooperation]. 2014. *Progress since Busan: Country and Democratic Ownership*. Paris and New York: GPEDC.

Grace C. 2010. *Product Development Partnerships (PDPs): Lessons from PDPs Established to develop New Health Technologies for Neglected Diseases*. London: DFID.

Grameen Bank. 2016. About us: Introduction. http://www.grameen.com/index.php?option=com_content&task=view&id=16&Itemid=112. Accessed July 13, 2016.

Grépin KA, Fan VY, Shen GC and Chen L. 2014. China's role as a global health donor in Africa: What can we learn from studying under reported resource flows? *Globalization and Health* 10:84.

Grimaldi JV and Ballhaus R. 2015. Foreign government gifts to Clinton Foundation on the rise. *The Wall Street Journal*, February 17.

Gupta A and Lhotská L. 2015. A fox building a chicken coop? - World Health Organization reform: Health for All, or more corporate influence? *Asia & the Pacific Policy Society*, December 5.

Guth RA. Gates rethinks his war on polio. *Wall Street Journal*, April 23.

Hansia F. 2014. KBR and Halliburton can be sued for Iraq toxic burn pits, court rules. *CorpWatch Blog*, April 17.

Hardiman D, Editor. 2006. *Healing Bodies, Saving Souls: Medical Missions in Asia and Africa*. Amsterdam: Rodopi.

Harmer A and Buse K. 2014. The BRICS: A paradigm shift in global health? *Contemporary Politics* 2:127–145.

Herington J and Lee K. 2014. The limits of global health diplomacy: Taiwan's observer status at the world health assembly. *Globalization and health* 10(1):1–9.

Holman SR. 2015. *Beholden: Religion, Global Health, and Human Rights*. New York: Oxford University Press.

Horton R. 2013a. Offline: Challenging America's hegemony in global health. *Lancet* 382(9890):382.

———. 2013b. Offline: The capture, incarceration, and release of Jim Kim. *Lancet* 381(9881):1888.

Huish R. 2013. *Where No Doctor Has Gone Before*. Waterloo, ON: Wilfrid Laurier University Press.

IBFAN. 2016. Press Release: Trade vs Health – WHO opens the door to big business while trying to protect babies. http://www.babymilkaction.org/archives/9786. Accessed July 18, 2016.

IBSA. 2013. About IBSA – introduction. http://www.ibsa-trilateral.org/. Accessed July 16, 2015.

ICRC. 2016. *Annual Report 2015*. Geneva: ICRC.

IDA. 2016. IDA at work in the poorest countries. https://ida.worldbank.org/content/infographic-ida-work-poorest-countries. Accessed July 19, 2015.

IHME. 2016. *Financing Global Health 2015: Development assistance steady on the path to new Global Goals.* Seattle: IHME.

IHP+. 2015. IHP+ partners. http://www.internationalhealthpartnership.net/en/ihp-partners/. Accessed July 4, 2015.

IMF. 2016a. IMF Members' Quotas and Voting Power, and IMF Board of Governors. http://www.imf.org/external/np/sec/memdir/members.aspx#I. Accessed February 27, 2016.

———. 2016b. Total IMF Credit Outstanding. http://www.imf.org/external/np/fin/tad/balmov2.aspx?type=TOTAL. Accessed July 13, 2016.

IOM [Institute of Medicine]. 2013. *Evaluation of PEPFAR*. Washington, DC: The National Academies Press.

Iriart C, Merhy EE, and Waitzkin H. 2001. Managed care in Latin America: The new common sense in health policy reform. *Social Science and Medicine* 52:1243–1253.

Kamradt-Scott A. 2016. WHO's to blame? The World Health Organization and the 2014 Ebola outbreak in West Africa. *Third World Quarterly* 37(3):401–418.

Kapoor I. 2012. *Celebrity Humanitarianism: The Ideology of Global Charity*. New York: Routledge.

Karim L. 2011. *Microfinance and its Discontents: Women in Debt in Bangladesh*. Minneapolis: University of Minnesota Press.

Kates J, Morrison JS, and Lief E. 2006. Global health funding: A glass half full? *Lancet* 368(9531):187–188.

Kates J, Michaud J, Wexler A, and Valentine A. 2015. *The US Response to Ebola: Status of the FY2015 Emergency Ebola Appropriation*. Menlo Park, CA: Kaiser Family Foundation.

Katz AR. 2013. Noncommunicable diseases: Global health priority or market opportunity? An illustration of the World Health Organization at its worst and at its best. *International Journal of Health Services* 43(3):437–458.

Katz IT, Bassett IV, and Wright AA. 2013. PEPFAR in transition—implications for HIV care in South Africa. *NEJM* 369(15):1385–1387.

Kickbusch I and Kökény M. 2013. Global health diplomacy: Five years on. *Bulletin of the World Health Organization* 91(3):157–236.

King K. 2014. China's higher education engagement with Africa: A different partnership and cooperation model? *International Development* Policy 5(1): 151–173.

Kirton JJ, Guebert J, and Kulik J. 2014. G8 health governance for Africa. In Besada H, Cooper AF, Kirton JJ, and Lisk F, Editors. 2014. *Moving Health Sovereignty in Africa: Disease, Governance, Climate Change*. Surrey, UK: Ashgate Publishing Ltd.

Kitano N and Harada Y. 2014. *Estimating China's Foreign Aid 2001-2013. JICA-RI Working Paper No. 78*. Tokyo: JICA Research Institute.

Labonté R and Gagnon M. 2010. Framing health and foreign policy: Lessons for global health diplomacy. *Globalization and Health* 6(14):1–22.

Laub Z. 2014. The Group of Eight (G8) industrialized nations. *Council on Foreign Relations*, March 3.

Lawson ML. 2013. *Foreign Assistance: Public-Private Partnerships (PPPs)*. Washington, DC: Congressional Research Service.

Lenzer J. 2015. Centers for Disease Control and Prevention: Protecting the private good? *BMJ* 350:h2362.

Levine R and Buse K. 2006. The World Bank's new health sector strategy: Building on key assets. *Journal of the Royal Society of Medicine* 99:569–572.

Levy BS and Sidel VW. 2008. The roles and ethical dilemmas for military medical care workers. In Levy BS and Sidel VW, Editors. *War and Public Health, Second Edition*. New York: Oxford University Press.

Licina D. 2011. Disaster preparedness—formalizing a comparative advantage for the Department of Defense in US global health and foreign policy. *Military Medicine* 176(11):1207–1211.

———. 2012. The military sector's role in global health: Historical context and future direction. *Global Health Governance* 6(1):1–30.

Liu P, Guo Y, Qian X, et al. 2014. China's distinctive engagement in global health. *Lancet* 384(9945):793–804.

Mader P. 2015. *The Political Economy of Microfinance: Financializing Poverty*. Basingstoke: Palgrave Macmillan.

Mahud M. 2013. Explainer: What is ALBA? http://www.as-coa.org/articles/explainer-what-alba. Accessed May 11, 2015.

Mann Wall B. 2015. *Into Africa: A Transnational History of Catholic Medical Missions and Social Change.* New Brunswick, NJ: Rutgers University Press.

Marriott A and Hamer J. 2014. *Investing for the Few: The IFC's Health in Africa Initiative.* Oxford: Oxfam International.

McCoy D. 2007. The World Bank's new health strategy: Reason for alarm? *Lancet* 369(9572):1499–1501.

McCoy D, Kembhavi G, Patel J, and Luintel A. 2009. The Bill & Melinda Gates Foundation's grant-making programme for global health. *Lancet* 373(9675):1645–1653.

McCoy D and McGoey L. 2011. Global health and the Gates Foundation—in perspective. In Williams EO and Rushton S, Editors. *Health Partnerships and Private Foundations: New Frontiers in Health and Health Governance.* Basingstoke, UK: Palgrave MacMillan.

McGoey L. 2015. *No Such Thing as a Free Gift: The Gates Foundation and the Price of Philanthropy.* New York: Verso Books.

Medicines Patent Pool. 2014. About the MPP. http://www.medicinespatentpool.org/about/. Accessed October 11, 2014.

———. 2015. Licenses in the MPP. http://www.medicinespatentpool.org/licensing/current-licences/. Accessed July 4, 2015.

Merck & Co. Inc. 2014. ACHAP. http://www.merckresponsibility.com/access-to-health/key-initiatives/achap/. Accessed May 13, 2015.

Michaud J, Moss K, and Kates J. 2012. *US Global Health Policy: The US Department of Defense and Global Health.* Menlo Park, CA: Kaiser Family Foundation.

Milani C. 2014. *Brazil's South-South Co-operation Strategies: From Foreign Policy to Public Policy. Occasional Paper No. 179.* Johannesburg: South African Institute of International Affairs.

Mohan CR. 2014. *Indian Military Diplomacy: Humanitarian Assistance and Disaster Relief.* Singapore: National University of Singapore/Institute of South Asian Studies.

Moodie R, Stuckler D, Monteiro C, et al. 2013. Profits and pandemics: Prevention of harmful effects of tobacco, alcohol, and ultra-processed food and drink industries. *Lancet* 381(9867):670–679.

Moss K. 2014. *NGO Engagement in US Global Health Efforts: U.S.-Based NGOs Receiving USG Support through USAID.* Menlo Park, CA: Kaiser Family Foundation.

MSF. 2015a. *Médecins Sans Frontières Financial Report 2015: Key Figures.* Geneva: MSF.

———. 2015b. *The Right Shot: Bringing Down Barriers to Affordable and Adapted Vaccines.* Geneva: MSF Access Campaign.

Muhammad A. 2015. Bangladesh—A model of neoliberalism: The case of microfinance and NGOs. *Monthly Review* 66(10):35.

Muraskin W. 2004. The Global Alliance for Vaccines and Immunization: Is it a new model for effective public-private cooperation in international public health? *American Journal of Public Health* 94(11):1922–1925.

———. 2012. *Polio Eradication and its Discontents: An Historian's Journey Through an International Public Health (Un)Civil War.* New Delhi: Orient Blackswan.

Murphy K, Weisbrod J, Jain N, et al. 2015. *Global Healthcare Private Equity Report 2015.* Boston: Bain and Company.

Mussa AH, Pfeiffer J, Gloyd SS, and Sherr K. 2013. Vertical funding, non-governmental organizations, and health system strengthening: Perspectives of public sector health workers in Mozambique. *Human Resources for Health* 11(1):26.

Nervi LL. 2014. Easier said than done (in global health): A glimpse at nonfinancial challenges in international cooperation. *PEAH – Policies for Equitable Access to Health,* February 20.

OECD. 2016. Query Wizard for International Development Statistics (QWIDS). http://stats.oecd.org/qwids/, Accessed February 27, 2016.

OGAC [Office of US Global AIDS Coordinator]. 2011. *The US President's Emergency Plan for AIDS Relief: Guidance for the Prevention of Sexually Transmitted HIV Infections.* Washington, DC: US State Department.

———. 2015. *2015 PEPFAR Latest Result: Fact Sheet.* Washington, DC: OGAC.

———. 2016. PEPFAR bilateral countries. http://www.pepfar.gov/countries/bilateral/index.htm. Accessed July 8, 2016.

Olivier J, Tsimpo C, Gemignani R, et al. 2015. Understanding the roles of faith-based health-care providers in Africa: Review of the evidence with a focus on magnitude, reach, cost, and satisfaction. *Lancet* 386(10005):1765–1775.

Ollila E. 2005. Restructuring global health policy making: The role of global public-private partnerships. In Mackintosh M and Koivusalo M, Editors. *Commercialization of Health Care: Global and Local Dynamics and Policy Responses.* Basingstoke, UK: Palgrave Macmillan.

Open Society Foundations. 2016. About us: Expenditure. http://www.opensocietyfoundations.org/about/expenditures. Accessed July 14, 2016.

Owens B. 2014. Storm brewing over WHO sugar proposal. *Nature* 507(7491):150–150.

Oxfam International. 2015. *Oxfam Annual Report 2014-2015.* Oxford: Oxfam International.

Patel P, Cummings R, and Roberts B. 2015. Exploring the influence of the Global Fund and the GAVI Alliance on health systems in conflict-affected countries. *Conflict and Health* 9:7.

Peake JB, Morrison JS, Ledgerwood MM, and Gannon SE. *The Defense Department's Enduring Contributions to Global Health: The Future of the US Army and Navy Overseas Medical Research Laboratories.* Washington, DC: Center for Strategic and International Studies.

PHM. 2009. PHM letter to UNITAID board on Patent Pool plan. http://www.phmovement.org/en/node/2720. Accessed July 14, 2015.

PHM, Medact, Medico International, et al. 2014. *Global Health Watch 4: An Alternative World Health Report.* London: Zed Books Ltd.

Pfeiffer J. 2005. Commodity fetichismo, the Holy Spirit, and the turn to Pentecostal and African Independent Churches in central Mozambique. *Culture, Medicine and Psychiatry* 29:255–283.

———. 2013. The struggle for a public sector: PEPFAR in Mozambique. In Biehl J and Petryna A, Editors. *When People Come First: Critical Studies in Global Health.* Princeton, NJ: Princeton University Press.

Pratt B and Loff B. 2013. Linking research to global health equity: The contribution of product development partnerships to access to medicines and research capacity building. *American Journal of Public Health* 103(11):1968–1978.

Plan International. 2016. *Plan International: Worldwide Annual Review 2015.* Surrey: Plan International.

Prashad V. 2016. The Davos Club: Meet the people who gave us a world in which 62 people own as much as 3.6 Billion. *AlterNet*, January 21.

Preker AS, Zweifel P, and Schellekens OP. 2010. *Global Marketplace for Private Health Insurance: Strength in Numbers.* Washington, DC: World Bank.

Provost C. 2014. Millions of pounds of overseas aid money spent in Britain. *The Guardian*, February 13.

Provost C, Ford L, and Tran M. 2014. G8 New Alliance condemned as new wave of colonialism in Africa. *The Guardian*, February 18.

Results for Development. 2016. Our approach. http://www.resultsfordevelopment.org/about-us/our-approach. Accessed March 5, 2016.

Richter J. 2015a. Conflicts of interest and global health and nutrition governance - the illusion of robust principles. *BMJ* 349:g5457 [response].

———. 2015b. Time to debate WHO's understanding of conflicts of interest. *BMJ* 348:g3351.

Roy A. 2012. Capitalism: A ghost story. *Outlook India*, March 26.

Ruckert A and Labonté R. 2014. Public–private partnerships (PPPs) in global health: The good, the bad and the ugly. *Third World Quarterly* 35(9):1598–1614.

Russell KL, Rubenstein J, Burke RL, et al. 2011. The Global Emerging Infection Surveillance and Response System (GEIS), a US government tool for improved global biosurveillance: A review of 2009. *BMC Public Health* 11(Suppl 2):S2.

Salud Mesoamerica. 2015. Resources. http://www.iadb.org/en/salud-mesoamerica-2015/sm2015/resources,6585.html. Accessed July 5, 2015.

Santelli JS, Speizer IS, and Edelstein ZR. 2013. Abstinence promotion under PEPFAR: The shifting focus of HIV prevention for youth. *Global Public Health* 8(1):1–12.

Santos RdF and Cerqueira MR. 2015. South-South Cooperation: Brazilian experiences in South America and Africa. *História, Ciências, Saúde-Manguinhos* 22(1):23–47.

Save the Children International. 2015. *Trustees' report, strategic report and financial statements for 2014.* London: Save the Children International.

Schrecker T, Labonte R, and Sanders D. 2007. Breaking faith with Africa: The G8 and population health after Gleneagles. In Cooper A, Kirton J, and Schrecker T, Editors. *Governing Global Health.* Burlington, VT: Ashgate Publishing.

Sepúlveda J, Carpenter C, Curran J, et al., Editors. 2007. *PEPFAR Implementation: Progress and Promise.* Washington, DC: Institute of Medicine.

Serafino NM. 2008. *The Department of Defense Role in Foreign Assistance: Background, Major Issues, and Options for Congress.* Washington, DC: Congressional Research Service.

Shah S. 2016. From Zika to Antibiotic-Resistant Superbugs: Welcome to the New Age of Contagions Today's deadly new pathogens aren't just a scientific challenge, they're a political one. *The Nation*, June 16.

Siddiqui Z. 2016. Médecins Sans Frontières files to block Pfizer patent on pneumonia vaccine in India. *Thomson Reuters*, March 11.

Silverman R. 2013. *UNITAID: Background Paper Prepared for the Working Group on Value for Money: An Agenda for Global Health Funding Agencies.* Washington, DC: Center for Global Development.

Sinclair H. 2012. *Confessions of a Microfinance Heretic: How Microlending Lost its Way and Betrayed the Poor.* San Francisco: Berrett-Koehler Publishers, Inc.

Sir Dorabji Tata Trust and the Allied Trusts. 2014. *Annual Report 2013-2014.* Mumbai.

Sridhar D. 2008. *The Battle Against Hunger: Choice, Circumstance, and the World Bank: Choice, Circumstance, and the World Bank.* New York: Oxford University Press.

———. 2010. Seven challenges in international development assistance for health and ways forward. *Journal of Law, Medicine and Ethics* 38(3):459–469.

Stuckler D, Basu S, Gilmore A, et al. 2010. An evaluation of the International Monetary Fund's claims about public health. *International Journal of Health Services* 40(2):327–332.

Subramaniam C. 2015. Did the WHO just invite corporates to set health policy? *The News Minute*, May 19.

Third World Network. 2016. WHO: Health Assembly adopts framework for non-State actor engagement. May 31, *Third World Network*.

Tomkins A, Duff J, Fitzgibbon A, et al. 2015. Controversies in faith and health care. *Lancet* 386(10005):1776–1785.

UNAIDS. 2011. Health 8 group meet to discuss maximizing health outcomes with available resources and getting "more health for the money." http://www.unaids.org/en/resources/presscentre/featurestories/2011/february/20110223bh8. Accessed July 4, 2015.

UNCTAD. 2014. *The Least Developed Countries Report 2014: Growth with structural transformation: A post-2015 development agenda*. Geneva: UNCTAD.

UNITAID. 2015. About UNITAID. http://www.unitaid.eu/en/who/about-unitaid. Accessed May 12, 2015.

Urmul Trust. 2015. About Urmul. http://www.urmul.org/?page_id=5. Accessed June 27, 2015.

USAID. 2014. USAID: Mission, vision and values. http://www.usaid.gov/who-we-are/mission-vision-values. Accessed October 4, 2014.

———. 2015a. *The President's Malaria Initiative: Ninth Annual Report to Congress April 2015*. Washington, DC: USAID.

———. 2015b. Results and data. http://www.usaid.gov/results-and-data. Accessed June 25, 2015.

US DoD [Department of Defense]. 2010. Department of Defense Instruction Number 6000.16: May 17, 2010.

———. 2015. DoD helps fight Ebola in Liberia and West Africa. http://www.defense.gov/News/Article/604184. Accessed July 7, 2015.

Utting P and Zammit A. 2006. *Beyond Pragmatism. Appraising UN-Business Partnerships. Markets, Business and Regulation Programme Paper Number 1*. Geneva: United Nations Research Institute for Social Development.

Vargas I, Vázquez ML, Mogollón-Pérez AS, and Unger JP. 2010. Barriers of access to care in a managed competition model: Lessons from Colombia. *BMC Health Services Research* 10(1):297.

Velásquez G. 2014. *Public-Private Partnerships in Global Health: Putting Business Before Health? Research Paper No 49*. Geneva: South Centre.

Venkatesh KK, Mayer KH, and Carpenter CCJ. 2012. Low-cost generic drugs under the president's emergency plan for AIDS relief drove down treatment cost; more are needed. *Health Affairs* 31(7):1429–1438.

Waitzkin H, Jasso-Aguilar R, and Iriart C. 2007. Privatization of health services in less developed countries: An empirical response to the proposals of the World Bank and Wharton School. *International Journal of Health Services* 37(2): 205–227.

Wexler A, Valentine A, and Kates J. 2016. *The US Global Health Budget: Analysis of Appropriations for Fiscal Year 2016*. Menlo Park, CA: Kaiser Family Foundation.

Whall H, Ray DB, and Kirkham E. 2013. *Getting it Right: The Pieces that Matter for the Arms Trade Treaty*. Oxford: Oxfam International.

WHO. 2014a. Denmark delivers. http://www.who.int/about/funding/denmark-new-strategy/en/. Accessed July 5, 2015.

———. 2014b. *Programme Budget 2014–2015*. Geneva: WHO.

———. 2015a. *Annex to the Financial Report for the Year Ended 31 December 2014*. Geneva: WHO.

———. 2015b. What is vaccine-derived polio?: Online Q&A. http://www.who.int/features/qa/64/en/. Accessed July 18, 2016.

———. 2016. *Programme Budget 2016–2017*. Geneva: WHO.

World Bank. 2012. IDA Financing. http://www.worldbank.org/ida/financing.html. Accessed May 8, 2015.

———. 2015. International Bank for Reconstruction and Development. http://www.worldbank.org/en/about/what-we-do/brief/ibrd. Accessed July 19, 2016.

———. 2016a. India Projects & Programs. http://www.worldbank.org/en/country/india/projects. Accessed July 15, 2016.

———. 2016b. *International Bank for Reconstruction and Development, Subscriptions and Voting Power of Member Countries. Data as of: February 24, 2016*. Washington, DC: World Bank.

———. 2016c. World Bank HNP Lending. http://datatopics.worldbank.org/hnp/worldbanklending. Accessed July 15, 2016.

World Economic Forum. 2014. *Global Agenda: World Economic Forum Annual Meeting 2014 Programme*. Davos: World Economic Forum.

———. 2016. *Future of Healthy: How to Realize Returns on Health*. Cologny/Geneva: World Economic Forum.

World Social Forum. 2001. *Charter of Principles*. São Paulo: WSF.

WTO. 2015. *Handbook on Accession to the WTO: Introduction and Summary*. Geneva: WTO.

WWAP (United Nations World Water Assessment Programme). 2015. *The United Nations World Water Development Report 2015: Water for a Sustainable World*. Paris: UNESCO.

Yach D, Khan M, Bradley D, et al. 2010. The role and challenges of the food industry in addressing chronic disease. *Globalization and Health* 6:10.

Youde J. 2012. *Global Health Governance*. Cambridge: Polity Press.

———. 2013. The Rockefeller and Gates Foundations in global health governance. *Global Society* 27(2):139–158.

5

DATA ON HEALTH

What Do We Know, What Do We Need to Know, and Why Does it Matter

A political economy approach to global health provides a theoretical framing of the factors underpinning the distribution of health and sickness within and across countries. Identifying these disease patterns, in turn, depends on the existence of health data—both data about the people who are ill or who have died (the numerators of health rates) and data about the people who comprise the population in which the cases of illness and death have occurred (the denominators). Health-related information, and knowing how to obtain and analyze it, is thus essential to taking action to improve health. Although the policies that affect health—both inside and outside the health sector—are ultimately determined in the political arena, health data play a vital role in helping to recognize needs and shape solutions (Table 5-1).

This chapter discusses the nature, strengths, and limitations of health-related data collection and analysis at local, national, and global scales, and examines the various types of health data that are currently used. At issue are the completeness and accuracy of the data, their ability to detect and monitor health inequities, and their utility for evaluating adequacy of health policies and services.

WHY HEALTH DATA MATTER

Key Questions:

- Why are the collection, analysis, and interpretation of health data important?
- What can health data tell us about health inequities?
- What is at stake, politically and technically, in generating health data that can be used to promote accountability and health equity?

The health and mortality data we come across in official documents, scholarly work, and the media—such as life expectancy and infant mortality rates (Table 5-2 for definitions)—appear impressively precise and objective. For instance, according to a recent WHO report, global life expectancy has increased considerably in the last few decades. A baby girl born in 2015 has a life expectancy on average of 73.8 years and a baby boy 69.1 years; a child born in 2015 has a life expectancy 6 years longer than one born in 1990 (WHO 2016). These data, tabulated at national and international levels, are believed to be the unequivocal baseline for public health decisionmaking. But not all lives are equally recorded: one third of births and two thirds of the estimated 56 million global annual deaths, including almost 50% of child deaths, are not registered (WHO 2014a).

Table 5-1 Some Uses and Limitations of Population Health Data

Uses of Population Health Data	*Explanations*
1. Gauge trends and identify emerging problems and needs	Follow population health patterns in relation to changes in the economy, the environment, and demographics; recognize health issues and identify the social characteristics and geographic areas in which they occur
2. Priority-setting, planning, legislation, and budgeting	Identify types and distribution of health problems to anticipate future needs and set public health priorities and budgets; collect data for planners and legislators including the number of people who must be reached, their characteristics and location
3. Serve information needs of governments, multilateral organizations, business, and nonprofit sectors	Produce statistics for education campaigns and for presentation to voters, workers, schoolchildren, experts, and officials; and guide health-related programs and activities in other sectors
4. Policy and program monitoring and evaluation, including on equity	Monitor progress and assess policies and programs, including their impact on particular social groups, and reconfigure them if necessary
5. International sharing, comparison, and reporting	Carry out surveillance (ongoing data collection, analysis and reporting) of public health emergencies; monitor and report health statistics to global health agencies
6. Health impact assessment	Assess the health implications of a range of decisions in order to inform policymaking
Limitations:	
7. The very collection and analysis of health data are not neutral processes	Health data do not exist in a vacuum and how they are collected and analyzed cannot be assumed: political and institutional decisionmaking processes affect what data are collected in the first place and how these data are analyzed
8. Health data cannot determine on their own the policies that affect health	Once data are collected and analyzed, they enter into political and institutional decisionmaking processes as one of a variety of factors to be considered
9. Health data cannot give causal explanations	Mortality and morbidity data alone do not provide causal pathways, nor do they explain how and why health and disease rates follow particular patterns

Source: Points 1–4 adapted from Woolsey (1979).

Table 5-2 Commonly Used Health Indicators

Life expectancy

Not a prediction or a rate, but a calculation of how long people are expected to live given current age-specific mortality rates. Life expectancy can also be calculated at specific age points. The life expectancy indicator is a hypothetical measure based upon current health and mortality conditions.

Annual crude[a] live birth rate (= birth rate)

$$\frac{\text{Number of births occurring in a defined population during a year}}{\text{Number in that population at midyear of the same year}} \times 1{,}000$$

Annual fertility rate

$$\frac{\text{Number of live births in an area during a year}}{\text{Midyear female population age 15-44 in same area in same year}} \times 1{,}000$$

Annual crude[a] death rate (= mortality rate, death rate)

$$\frac{\text{Number of deaths occurring in a defined population during a year}}{\text{Number in that population at midyear of the same year}} \times 1{,}000$$

Annual specific death rate (by age, sex/gender, cause or a combination)

$$\frac{\text{Number of deaths of a specified age, sex, or cause occurring in a defined population during a year}}{\text{Number of the specified age group in that population at midyear of the same year}} \times 1{,}000$$

Annual infant mortality rate (= infant mortality rate or IMR)

$$\frac{\text{Number of deaths under 1 year of age in a defined population during a year}}{\text{Number of live births occurring in that population during the same year}} \times 1{,}000$$

Annual neonatal mortality rate

$$\frac{\text{Number of deaths under 28 days of age in a defined population during a year}}{\text{Number of live births occurring in that population during the same year}} \times 1{,}000$$

Annual post-neonatal mortality rate

$$\frac{\text{Number of deaths between 28 days and 1 year of age in a defined population during a year}}{\text{Number of live births occurring in that population during the same year}} \times 1{,}000$$

Annual fetal death rate (stillbirth rate)

$$\frac{\text{Number of deaths at } 20^{b} \text{ or more weeks gestational age in a defined population during a year}}{\text{Number of live births occurring in that population during the same year}} \times 1{,}000$$

Annual maternal mortality rate

$$\frac{\text{Number of deaths from materal causes in a defined population during a year}}{\text{Number of women of childbearing age in that population during the same year}} \times 100{,}000$$

Annual maternal mortality ratio

$$\frac{\text{Number of deaths from materal causes in a defined population during a year}}{\text{Number of live births in that population during the same year}} \times 100{,}000$$

Table 5-2 Continued

Proportionate mortality

$$\frac{\text{Number of deaths in a specified category in a defined population during a year}}{\text{Total number of deaths occurring in that population during the same year}} \times 100$$

Annual incidence rate for occurrence of a specified condition

$$\frac{\text{Number of new cases of the condition occurring in a defined population in a year}}{\text{Number of people in that population at midyear in the same year}} \times 10^{n c}$$

(Point) prevalence of a specified condition

$$\frac{\text{Number of cases of the specified condition existing in a defined population at a particular point in time}}{\text{Number of people in that population at the same point in time}} \times 10^{n c}$$

Morbidity rate (crude[a] or specific by age, sex/gender, occupation, etc.)

$$\frac{\text{Number of cases of a specified condition occurring in a specified population during a specific time period}}{\text{Average population in that category during the year}} \times 10^{n c}$$

[a]Crude measures refer to entire populations, without adjusting for age, sex or any other population characteristic. They are the raw count of cases divided by the overall population, often used when there are incomplete census data to qualify the denominator and numerator.

[b]Varies somewhat in different jurisdictions.

[c]Multiplier n varies depending on frequency of the condition.

Also see Table 6-1.

Source: Adapted from prior editions of this text and Porta et al. (2014).

This means that much of the available data are estimations, extrapolations from other settings, or "guesstimations," because over half the world's population is excluded from data collection. When priority-setting in public health is derived from flawed or weak data, interpreting the findings and making decisions based on those data is highly problematic and may even jeopardize health. A top priority in public health research, then, must be to secure reliable health statistics collection. But gathering data costs money, and the higher the quality, the greater the cost. In many low- and middle-income countries (LMICs) there are significant resource constraints around the collection and analysis of population health data.

Moreover, summary statistics—aggregate health indicators describing population-wide health—do not reflect variations by social class, geographic location, occupation, sex/gender, race/ethnicity, and other important factors. For example, while average global life expectancy has increased, regional differences in mortality rates remain stark: children born in sub-Saharan Africa are, on average, seven times more likely to die before the age of 5 than those born in Europe, and in 2015 life expectancy ranged from 53 years in Côte d'Ivoire, Central African Republic, and Chad to 83 years for Australia, Italy, and Switzerland (WHO 2016).

There is wide variation within countries, too. Residents of the city center of Glasgow, Scotland live to 73.4 years (men) and 78.7 years (women), whereas those living in the bordering affluent East Dunbartonshire area have a life expectancy of 80.7 years and 83.9 years respectively (National Records of Scotland 2015). Even more dramatically, in the United States the gap between counties with the highest and lowest life expectancy is 12 years for women and 18 years for men (Wang et al. 2013). When race and class are taken into account, there is a staggering 35-year life expectancy difference between the wealthiest white neighborhood and the poorest African-American neighborhood within a single county in Missouri, USA (Ferguson Commission 2015).

Understanding the patterns of health and mortality in a population—considering who is included in and excluded from this population and why—and being able to act on this information also requires knowledge of the social distribution of these patterns and of the constellation of factors that affect health (Krieger 2012). Despite increasing recognition of the influence of social, political, and economic factors on health, in most settings these variables are insufficiently captured by routine data collection. As well, many variables that directly affect health—such as pollution, housing quality, and poverty—are not typically considered *health* statistics, although they may be central to uncovering and addressing the root causes of ill health and premature death. For these reasons, a strict reliance on disease-specific health data may not accurately incorporate valuable areas of policy-relevant information.

Differences in the health of individuals and populations reflect intrinsic features of the societies in which they live (Marmot 2004). Some countries, such as Cuba, Denmark, and the Czech Republic, use a comprehensive array of data, including on economic, educational, occupational, and housing conditions, to inform health policy. Indeed, gauging health data according to these factors is an essential first step to addressing health inequities (explored in chapter 7), which are defined as "avoidable disparities in health or its key determinants that are systematically observed between groups of people with different levels of underlying social privilege, i.e. wealth, power, or advantage" (Braveman and Tarimo 2002, p. 1624).

The importance of documenting health inequities has been recognized for centuries. Among the earliest studies was by Frenchman Louis-René Villermé, a military physician turned researcher who investigated mortality patterns in different neighborhoods of Paris in the 1820s. In his pioneering work, he discovered that, in contrast to prevailing beliefs that disease was divinely ordained or influenced by topographic and climatic features, mortality rates in the city's dozen *arrondissements* (neighborhoods) were closely correlated with poverty levels: where there was a higher proportion of poor people, death rates were higher and vice versa. Pathbreaking as Villermé's framing and identification of poverty's link to mortality was, he did not advocate for public policies to address poverty, with the exception of championing France's 1841 prohibition on child labor. Instead, he attributed his findings to the moral shortcomings of the poor and called for—in addition to schooling children to enhance their sobriety and physical fitness for later employment—individual uplift and continuation of laissez-faire capitalism, which he held would lead to both higher wages and moral improvement.

In 1840s Britain, Edwin Chadwick and Friedrich Engels (see chapter 1) documented similar population patterns of health. Both provided empirical evidence of what many knew or suspected to be true about the effects, if not measurable per se, of social relations: typically, health status was worst among those sectors of the population most subjected to economic exploitation and oppression, and best among those sectors of the population who gained from exploiting and oppressing others. Groups in between experienced intermediate mortality levels. But these findings generated radically different prescriptions: Chadwick advocated meliorative public health and environmental cleanup without improvements in wages or working conditions, whereas Engels called for revolution to end the capitalist and class exploitation that produced poverty and elevated death rates (Birn 2009). In sum, documenting health inequities does not automatically result in addressing them (or doing so in a particular way), but it is an indispensable precursor to action.

In recent years, WHO's Commission on Social Determinants of Health (2008) has called for incorporating measures of health inequity into planning, policy, and technical work, including data collection, at WHO and in member countries (Figure 5-1). Not only are these data used to gauge health inequities, they can drive policies and practice.

In the absence of relevant data on societal variables, complex approaches and techniques are required. Without routine collection of social class data, for example, researchers must engage in various extra steps to understand the factors shaping location-based inequalities, employing such techniques as census tract or neighborhood-based coding, and indices of extreme concentrations of affluence and poverty (Carpiano, Lloyd, and Hertzman 2009; Krieger et al. 2005). The data problems around health inequities are best documented in high-income countries (HICs), which have the resources to do so. But these issues are just as salient elsewhere—the situation in most LMICs and various HICs only underscores the difficulty of gauging (health) inequities in countries lacking the requisite data (Speybroeck et al. 2012).

For instance, the Swedish government, which has historically taken important strides to redress health inequities (Linell, Richardson, and Wamala 2013), does not routinely collect socioeconomic data in death registries and must carry out particular studies that link mortality data to individual records from the

Health Inequities

Include information on:
Health-related variables (all cause, age-specific and cause-specific mortality; mental health; early childhood development; morbidity and disability; self-assessed health) disaggregated by:
- ☐ at least two socioeconomic stratifiers (education, income/wealth, occupational class);
- ☐ age;
- ☐ sex/gender;
- ☐ ethnic group/race/Indigeneity;
- ☐ other contextually relevant social stratifiers;
- ☐ place of residence (rural/urban and province or other relevant geographical unit)

The distribution of the population across these sub-groups

Consequences of Ill Health

Economic consequences; Social and psychological consequences; Somatic consequences; Familial consequences

Determinants of Health

Living/working conditions and social policies

Physical environment:
- water and sanitation;
- housing conditions;
- land and natural resource use and abuse;
- infrastructure, transport, and urban design;
- air and soil quality;
- global climate change

Social context:
- social support and networks;
- neighborhood characteristics, such as community institutions, parks, safety;
- quality and accessibility of nutritious food/food sovereignty

Family context:
- intimate partner relations;
- familial roles, relations, and responsibilities

Working conditions:
- workplace hazards and protections;
- stress and job control;
- job precariousness

Personal health characteristics:
- smoking, alcohol, and other psychoactive substance use;
- physical activity;
- diet and nutrition;
- sexual health;
- amount of sleep

Health care:
- comprehensiveness/universality/accessibility/equity;
- administration and infrastructure

Social protection:
- populations served/access/equity;
- level of solidarity/fragmentation/generosity

Structural forces underlying health inequities

Gender and sexuality factors:
- norms and values;
- economic participation;
- sexual and reproductive health

Race, ethnicity, Indigeneity, religion, immigrant status factors:
- level of tolerance/discrimination/ (de jure and de facto); and
- oppression, norms, values, and rights;
- effects of historical settler colonialism and redressing (i.e., via Indigenous rights recognition)

Socioeconomic factors:
- social exclusion;
- income and wealth distribution;
- land tenancy and property;
- education/literacy

Sociopolitical context:
- participation in community, regional, national, global decisionmaking;
- distribution of political power;
- civil, social, and other human rights;
- level of violence/militarism/oppression
- employment conditions;
- governance and public spending priorities;
- macroeconomic conditions;
- global political economy/trade treaties;
- labor force participation;
- unionization and social movement participation

Figure 5-1: Additional information to be included in routine data collection to enable measurement of health inequities and societal determinants of health.

Source: Adapted (with permission) from Box 16.3 of WHO Commission on Social Determinants of Health (2008, p. 182); WHO (2015e).

population census in order to track changes over time (Groenewold, van Ginneken, and Masseria 2008). In Canada, where routine health data are not collected on "visible minorities" (Khan et al. 2015), and Indigenous identification for birth and death registration remains inconsistent across provinces (Smylie, Fell, and Ohlosson 2010), it has been inordinately difficult to track the mortality effects of the Canadian government's racially motivated public policies. For example, starting in the 1890s and for almost a century, more than 150,000 Indigenous children were removed from their homes and compelled by Canadian government policy to attend Church-run residential schools. These children experienced notoriously high rates of tuberculosis, violent treatment, and atrocious living and nutritional conditions (Kelm 1999; Milloy 1999), with death rates up to five times higher than the overall school-aged population (for more details see chapter 7). The Truth and Reconciliation Commission of Canada (2015) compiled death registers verifying over 3,200 deaths at these schools (but representing just 10%–20% of the likely total due to incomplete burial records).

To recapitulate, population health data matter a great deal for knowledge and action. But they are not a "given" despite the word *data's* Latin etymological provenance. How data are compiled, collected, synthesized, presented, analyzed, and interpreted is not neutral. The importance of addressing the implicit assumptions and values regarding health data is incisively encapsulated by social epidemiologist Nancy Krieger. She notes that virtually every term and concept employed, from *population, rate,* and *disease* to "*geographic variation*" and "*differences in disease rates by social group*" must be problematized because:

> None of these ideas are intuitively obvious. . . . Also of note is who and what is omitted, not simply who and what is included . . . In other words, data are not simply "observed": there is active thinking behind the act of data acquisition. . . . [and] active thinking that guides data analysis, display, and interpretation (Krieger 2011, p. 17).

TYPES OF HEALTH DATA

Key Questions:

- What are the major kinds of health-related data?
- What are the challenges involved in collecting and using health data?
- How do these challenges, including gaps in the data, affect our understanding of, and actions to address, population health and health inequities?

A key issue, core to a political economy of health analysis, is: who counts? And, related: who is not counted? This means that for all types of health data, decisions around which and how data are collected, analyzed, and interpreted can help, ignore, or harm the prospect of more equitable population health.

But first we must know what the basic categories of health-related data are:

- *Population data*: The number of people in a population, who comprise the population at risk for disease, disability, and death. Important characteristics include the age structure of the population, its sex/gender composition, and the distribution of such social characteristics as occupation, race/ethnicity, nativity, social class, religion, and geographic location.
- *Vital statistics*: Live births; deaths by sex/gender, age, and cause; and marriages. In some countries, migration, adoptions, divorce, and other categories are also recorded by vital statistics agencies.
- *Morbidity statistics*: Morbidity by type, severity, and outcome (e.g., illness, injury, physical or mental disability), including data on notifiable diseases (whose reporting is mandated by law) and data obtained from registries for cancer and other diseases.
- *Health services statistics*: Numbers and types of facilities and services available; distribution, qualifications, and functions of personnel; nature of services, diagnostic and treatment modalities and their utilization rates; hospital and health center operations; organization of government and private health care systems; costs, payment mechanisms, and related information.
- *Data on social determinants of health inequities*: Societal factors that lead to inequities in health—rates of absolute and relative poverty, levels of education, and occupational exposures, among others; population groups categorized by social class, race/ethnicity, nativity, religion, location, and sex/gender in order to identify how equally or unequally health (and health care services) are distributed in a population.

Societal variables—including those that capture social protection and distribution of power and resources—are increasingly considered vital to health-related decisionmaking, although they are not collected to the same extent as other, more discrete indicators.

The compilation, analysis, interpretation, and issuance of health data on a continuing basis entails a great deal of governmental effort and expense. Politicians, analysts, and advocates employ health data to monitor and compare populations within and across countries, set policy agendas, evaluate the effects of particular programs and policies, and potentially adapt successful experiences from elsewhere (Siddiqi et al. 2012) (Table 5-1). Health improvements (e.g., lowering infant mortality) can serve to legitimize political decisions, and deterioration in health status may be attributed to failed public health efforts or economic and social policies.

Interpreting health-related data can be challenging, as it is difficult to define the metrics and get the numbers right, and governments may be reluctant to declare disease outbreaks as was the case with China during the 2003 SARS outbreak (Transparency Policy Project 2015). Administrators may be tempted, for example, to overestimate the number of inoculations given or to minimize reported disease or death rates to reach specified targets (Birn 1999). Concern with international trade or tourism may prompt cases of cholera to be reported as gastroenteritis (Hamlin 2009), and impending elections may entice politicians into downplaying or exaggeration. Children may be inappropriately labeled "autistic" to obtain needed school services or insurance coverage (Silverman 2011), and reporting of diseases may be used to justify physician reimbursement or hospital stays. As well, those in charge of data collection and monitoring may be simultaneously responsible for running programs that are expected to reach particular health goals, generating serious conflicts of interest (AbouZahr, Adjei, and Kanchanachitra 2007). Such distortions, arising from varied incentives and influences, need not be overemphasized but should be kept in mind when reviewing health-related data.

Deciding which variables to use in health data collection is a complex and sometimes ideologically fraught endeavor. Authorities may ignore essential information linked to health inequities, leading to flawed causal connections between existing variables, in lieu of searching for missing data. Accordingly, a focus on individual risk factors and behavioral variables (such as diet and exercise) when measuring health status and determinants (without examining, for instance, food production and accessibility, neighborhood conditions, and air quality) may generate data interpretations that "blame the victim" without going beyond "lifestyle factors" (see chapters 3 and 7).

Health data may also enter into hotly contested political and economic debates. Epidemiological findings associating cigarette smoking with lung cancer, firearms with homicides, and transfats with coronary heart disease, for example, have been cited as grounds for restrictive legislation. Past and present, proponents and opponents of everything from nuclear power plants to lead paint have identified and interpreted data to support their positions, with industrial interests particularly prone to concealing and denying the deleterious effects of their products and manufacturing processes (Markowitz and Rosner 2013). Additionally, advocates of a particular cause or disease may release selective health statistics to garner disproportionate funding, whereas others languish for lack of organized proponents (Martin and Mallela 2015).

In more propitious circumstances, health data are a key input to policymaking. One emergent tool is health impact assessment (HIA), which explicitly considers the health effects of both public and private sector actions in diverse arenas including zoning, transportation, environmental hazards, labor, energy, and education. The HIA approach also calls for action and accountability on the part of decisionmakers for the promotion of health and reduction of health inequities (Krieger et al. 2003; Pennington et al. 2015). HIA has been institutionalized in Finland to ensure healthy and sustainable development (National Institute for Health and Welfare 2013) and has been useful in shaping public policy in Australia and New Zealand (Haigh et al. 2013), among other countries.

From a political economy of health perspective, it is not surprising that political as well as technical considerations influence every element of health data, numerators and denominators alike.

Population Health Data

Two types of data are required to calculate a rate of disease, disability, or death: the number of cases (the numerators) and the number of persons from whom these cases arise (the denominators) (Table 5-2). The data on health outcomes are the product of health-related databases; the data on the number of persons in the population at risk come from either the census or other population-based data. Understanding population health data thus requires attention to data about the population as well as data about the health outcomes.

Population health data for a country or defined geographical area are usually obtained in two ways: enumeration and registration; a third approach is to obtain a representative population sample for use in health surveys, as will be discussed later. Enumeration is done by means of a census of the population, ideally every 10 years, also supplemented by more frequent data collection on nationally representative samples. Registration involves the routine collection of vital statistics such as births, marriages, and deaths.

To be sure, neither enumeration nor registration is done primarily for the purpose of compiling health statistics. Census data have been used for millennia to determine taxation, labor and production capacity, inheritance, and conscription. Among the earliest surviving census information is from the Han Dynasty in China (2nd century CE), when data were recorded on approximately 11 million households, including the heads of families and the name, sex, age, and birthplace of over 50 million people (von Glahn 2012).

The figures derived from the census serve as denominators for the mortality and morbidity rates defined in Table 5-2. Census data of adequate quality make possible more meaningful comparisons of the measures than can be obtained from crude (whole population) figures, largely because the risks of so many different kinds of morbidity and mortality vary enormously by age. Box 5-1 reviews how to make different populations comparable despite different age structures.

As an illustration of why the age distribution matters so much, the age and sex (noting that gender, discussed in chapter 7, is implicitly included) distributions of the population of three different countries are compared in Figure 5-2. These are known as age pyramids. The shape of each pyramid is affected by birth rates at particular periods in time and death rates for each age group (by sex). The age pyramids portray the childhood and old-age dependency ratios within each population: persons under 14 years of age and over 65 are generally considered to be dependent on the population segment aged 15 to 65. We see that the bulk of Botswana's population is under 30, and Spain's population bulges from ages 30 to 60, suggesting a forthcoming wave of old-age dependency. While China's population concentrates in a 15 to 60 age band, there is a significant dip in the 30 to 40 age range corresponding

Box 5-1 Age Adjustment

The varied age structure of different populations is evidenced in Figure 5-2: Botswana has more than twice the proportion of people under 15 and roughly one fourth the proportion of people over 65 as does Spain. It would be inappropriate and misleading to compare crude overall or cause-specific mortality rates between two such groups because their mortality experience differs on the basis of age structure alone. To increase the validity of international comparisons, the crude death rate of one population is apportioned into a set of age-specific death rates, which are then applied to the proportionate age distribution of a second population. In practice when many populations are compared, all are adjusted against a standard population, which may be real or a computer model generated for the purpose of the analysis. This process allows comparison of mortality experience between two or more populations as if they had the same age structure.[1] It is important to note that this is not only a technical issue but a political one. The choice of age-standard (whether the standard population is more heavily weighted towards younger or older ages) makes a difference: health inequities will look larger with a younger age standard compared with an older age standard, as most health inequities are greater at younger ages because eventually everyone dies (Krieger and Williams 2001).

[1]For further explanation and concrete examples of age standardization, see: Anderson RN and Rosenberg HM. 1998. Age standardization of death rates: Implementation of the year 2000 standard. *National Vital Statistics Reports* 47(3):1–17.

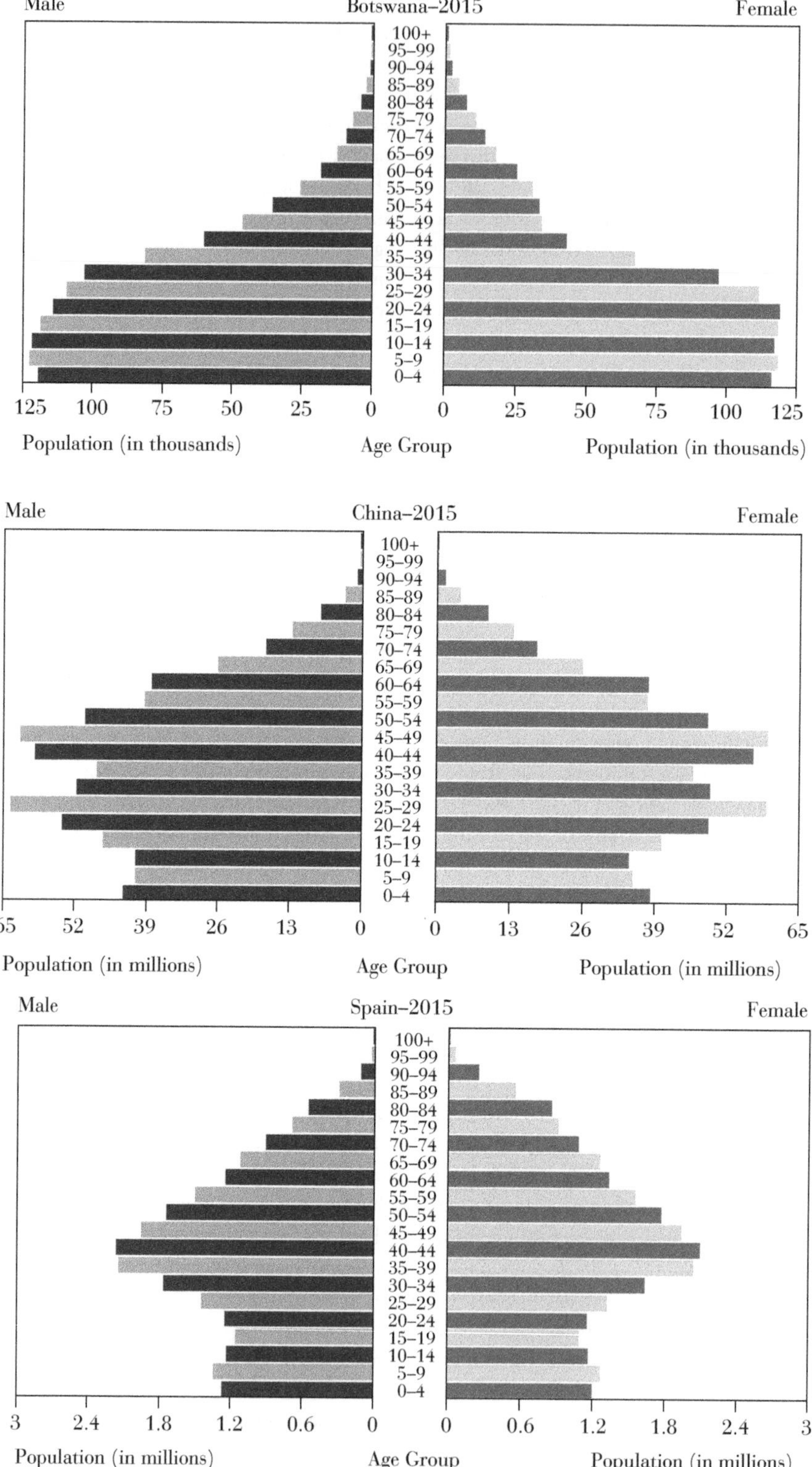

Figure 5-2: Age pyramids for populations of three countries, 2015.

Source: US Census Bureau (2015).

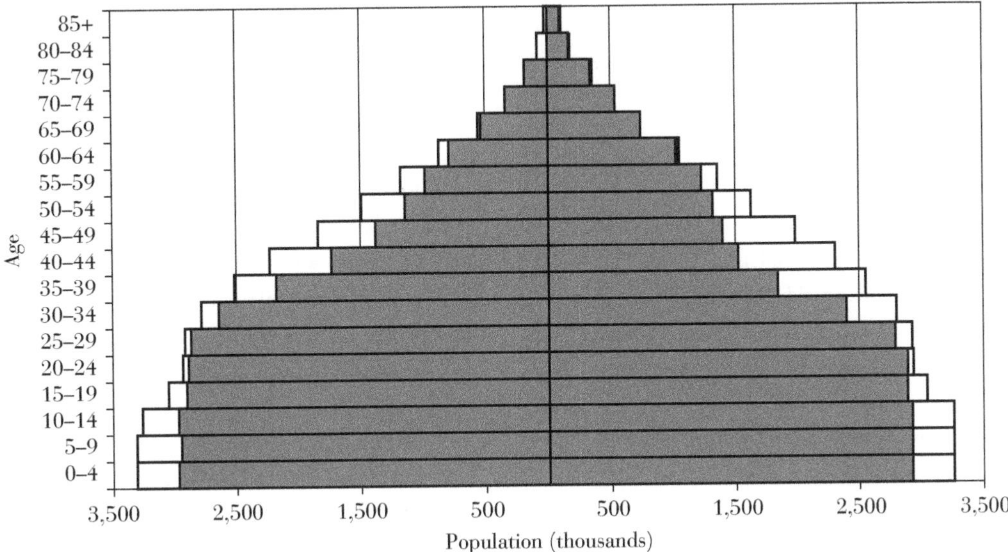

Figure 5-3: Population size estimates with and without the effect of AIDS, Southern Africa, 2015. Outer blocks estimate population size without the effect of AIDS.

Source: From *World Population Prospects: The 2010 Revision, Volume I*, p. 23, by UN Department of Economic and Social Affairs (Population Division), © (2011). Reprinted with the permission of the United Nations.

to the one-child policy in force from 1979 until 2015, designed to help steer the country from agrarian to market socialism. High mortality rates can drastically alter the age pyramid, as seen in the projected effect of HIV and AIDS in Southern Africa (Figure 5-3).

Census Procedures and Cost

During a census, information is collected on a variety of topics (Table 5-3). The information obtained from census data permit a population to be characterized by a range of classifiers, including age, sex/gender, education, literacy status, occupation, and ethnic group, among other features. Political considerations shape what data are and are not collected. For example, Brazil recently expanded its census to be more inclusive in enumerating its diverse Indigenous populations and has likewise experienced new debates over collection of racial/ethnic data pertaining to its population of African origin (Bailey and Telles 2006; Coimbra et al. 2013). Of late, the US Census has begun more accurately reporting data on same-sex couple households (Lofquist 2011), in contrast to prior policy as per the 1990 census, which "corrected" data from same-sex couple households to make them "opposite-sex" by randomly changing the sex of one of the members of the couple (Black et al. 2007). Awareness of political controversies about collecting information on different societal groups is vital for critical understanding and use of census data.

The essential features of a national population census are as follows (UN Department of Economic and Social Affairs Statistics Division 2008):

- Individual enumeration (each individual and each household should be counted and recorded separately);
- Universality within a defined territory (the entire country should be part of the census);
- Simultaneity (data should be collected at the same point in time for everyone);
- Defined periodicity (a census should be conducted at regular intervals, usually every 10 years)

An accompanying objective of the census is compilation, which requires that the data collected in the census be put in a useful form so that they are accessible, timely, coherent, interpretable, accurate, and relevant.

Table 5-3 Some Topics Recommended by the UN World Population and Housing Census Programme and Various National Census Agencies for Inclusion in a National Population Census

Priority Items	Other Useful Items
Place of usual residence	Housing conditions
Place at time of the census	Food security status
Place/country of birth	Access to health care services
Duration of current residence	Disability status
Place of previous residence	Sector(s) of employment
Place of residence in [year]	Years worked in each sector
Total population	Income
Locality	Language
Relationship to household head or other reference member	National/ethnic origin
Sex	Year of arrival (for migrants/refugees)
Age	Indigenous identity
Marital status	Educational qualifications
Citizenship	Live births in preceding 12 months
Number of children born alive	Infants born and died within last 12 months
Number of children living	Age of mother at birth of first child
Duration of marriage	Household deaths in the past 12 months
Educational attainment	Maternal orphanhood (loss of mother)
Literacy	Religion
School attendance	
Economic activity status	
Occupation	
Industry	
Status in employment/occupation	

Source: Adapted from UN Department of Economic and Social Affairs (2008).

Census-Taking around the Globe

Since 1950, the proportion of the world's estimated population that derives from total census enumeration has risen substantially. Almost all LMICs have had some experience in census-taking in recent decades. The UN's 2010 World Programme on Population and Housing Censuses recommended that all member states carry out a population census during the 2005–2014 period (United Nations 2016).

A census is a complex undertaking in any setting. In India, with the second largest population in the world, each decennial census requires the recruitment and training of 2.7 million enumerators to survey 240 million households within 25 days in an extensive and highly organized operation. During this exercise, information on the inhabitants of each dwelling is collected and the quality of housing assessed, allowing for measurement of changing living conditions (Chandramouli 2011). Nigeria's 2006 census required 6 years of preparation and 7 days to carry out. As the most populous country in Africa, with an estimated 120 to 150 million people and over 300 different ethnic groups, Nigeria faced a gargantuan organizational challenge. To ensure the most credible data collection, government authorities imposed a weeklong national stay-at-home order, and for the first time, digital processing of forms and satellite positioning were used to identify census areas. More than 1 million census workers were trained and went door to door across the country. In Myanmar, 120,000 school teachers were trained as enumerators to conduct the country's 2014 census—its first in over 30 years (UNFPA 2014b). After decades of military rule, census questions about ethnic identity and religious affiliation sparked civil protest (International Crisis Group 2014).

Elsewhere, the increasing use of Geographic Information System (GIS) and Global Positioning System (GPS) tools has enabled more countries to carry out censuses: in 2010 all but seven UN member states participated, compared with 25 abstaining in 2000 due to civil war or inadequate resources. Still, effective collection (and harnessing) of census data for policymaking remains a challenging and politicized endeavor (UNFPA 2003; 2014a). In 2011, Canada's Conservative administration cancelled the mandatory detailed "long form" census covering a range of social and economic questions. Critiqued as a deliberate move to minimize information on the country's growing inequalities (Scoffield 2011), the long form census was reinstated after the Conservatives were voted out of office in 2015.

Limitations of Census Data

After a national census is budgeted for and planned, enumerators trained, and data processing materials prepared, the rest may seem a simple matter. In actuality, appraising the completeness of census data calls for careful checks and sophisticated techniques. Errors and inaccuracies can tarnish the raw data, particularly when questions are asked of people who are suspicious of intent and confidentiality. Coverage of large populations is never perfect. Concerns around potential undercounts have been raised in various countries because these can result in lower government subsidies for education and other services based on population size; overcounts are similarly problematic. A common US practice considers short-term incarcerated individuals as residents of prison jurisdictions, artificially deflating the populations of their often minority and poorer home communities (Wood 2014).

A country's prior experience with census-taking, available equipment and human resource capacity, and existing infrastructure greatly affect census counts and compliance. The diversity within a country—including languages spoken, education levels, and presence of nomadic populations—is another factor that makes a population census count a formidable task. Where censuses have historically been utilized for repressive purposes, such as compulsory military service, there may be considerable resistance to participation. Regardless of available financial and human resources, complete enumeration of an entire population is nearly impossible. Even in HICs, millions of refugees, migrants, and homeless persons are likely to be missed by census counts. The extent to which these deficiencies are addressed through special surveys and adjustments is variable and highly politicized.

Challenges in Classification

The question of age may be taken as an example of the uncertainty inherent in census taking. Many people do not know their age and some may deliberately misstate it. Asking a person for his or her year of birth rather than age is considered more accurate, because the former figure remains constant (and is more likely to be recalled correctly) whereas the latter changes every year. Important local events may also be used as a reference. Local customs in reckoning age vary; in some cultures a child may not be counted until reaching 1 year of age.

The use of racial and ethnic classification on census counts may be both divisive and purposive in that how people are classified predetermines the types of conclusions that can be drawn, in turn affecting policies. While typologies of humans relating to climatic and geographic features have ancient roots, the contemporary system of classifying people according to such groupings originated with 19th century political authorities. They held (erroneously) that humans were composed of distinct, biologically determined races that needed to be distinguished for administrative and political purposes. These racialized classifications were used to determine domestic social and industrial policies and to justify imperial expansion and domination (Krieger 2005).

The most notable recent example of the deliberately racist use of such categorizations comes from the apartheid government in South Africa (1948–1994). The apartheid bureaucracy collected census and vital information according to the following categories: Black (of African descent), White (European), Asian (Indian and Pakistani), and Colored ("mixed race"). Every public agency in the country used these data to enforce differential treatment under the law, unequal distribution of education and welfare funds, and so on, further reifying these constructed racial categories. Even though the apartheid system was dismantled in the early 1990s, the South African Department of Health decided to retain these same racial categories in health statistics and census counts, in part to gauge the effect of post-apartheid policies on closing the equity gap between racial groups.

In the United States, census data are also collected by race and ethnicity, reflecting the country's legacy of slavery, segregation, and discrimination. For the 2000 census and continuing with the 2010 census, the US government adopted a larger array of racial and ethnic classifications and allowed respondents to self-identify in more than one category, recognizing the growing diversity of the population (US Census Bureau 2014).

How people are classified shapes to a great extent the types of policies undertaken to tackle health and other social problems. The decontextualized focus on race and ethnicity in the United States, whereby race/ethnicity is conflated with biological and cultural characteristics—and absent collection of data on racism—has greatly diverted attention from the interconnected societal factors that need to be modified to address health inequities (e.g., racial discrimination, skewed wealth distribution, inadequate environmental and occupational health protection). This does not mean that collection of data on race should end—to the contrary, retaining this variable in the census and other population health data, and including social class, enables the realities of *both* racial oppression and economic deprivation—and their effects on health—to be studied, understood, and addressed. Indeed, some countries that used to collect statistics by social class but not race/ethnicity (e.g., the United Kingdom) now collect data by both. These data clearly show that both variables, among others, matter greatly for understanding health inequities and population health (Iqbal et al. 2015).

Vital Statistics

Vital statistics are data collected through civil registration of major life events such as birth, adoption, marriage, divorce, and death. The UN deems "the critical act of recording important events in people's lives . . . [essential to provision of] official recognition and documentation necessary to establish legal identity, family relationships and civil status," (UNESCAP 2015) with full coverage crucial to achieving gender equity (WHO

Table 5-4 Some Personal/Social and Administrative Uses of Vital Records

Personal/Social	Administrative
Birth Certificate	
1. Establish date of birth and identity: enter school and access social services; obtain work permit/ identification/ passport/proof of citizenship or residency; qualify for voting, marriage, running for office, retirement pension	1. Provide basis for child health and immunization, education planning, etc.; evaluate family planning programs and prenatal clinics; oblige military service; serve as a basis for taxation (together with census data)
2. Establish family relationship: trace descent, prove parentage, birth order; prove legal dependency and inheritance benefits; qualify for insurance	2. Contribute to inter-censal estimate of population size
3. Protect against child labor and military inscription, child trafficking, and incarceration	3. Aid in family reunification efforts and in delivery of humanitarian assistance during times of war, conflict or disaster
Marriage and Civil Union Certificates[a]	
1. Qualify for housing allocation, inheritance, pension, insurance, tax deduction	1. Prove establishment of household for benefit programs
2. Prove legal responsibility of spouse, legitimacy of offspring, and citizenship	2. Predict population trends

Table 5-4 Continued

3. Child custody	
4. Medical decisionmaking for spouse/partner	
Divorce Certificate	
1. Establish right to alimony or other benefits	1. Determine right to remarry
Death Certificate	
1. Establish fact and cause of death: claim pension, insurance, inheritance	1. Provide basis for cause-of-death analysis and specific prevention or control programs, particularly for infant and maternal mortality 2. Clear files (e.g., electoral rolls, tax or social security registers, disease-case registers)
Identity Cards	
1. Many countries and jurisdictions require identity cards to be carried at all times, for access to virtually any public service	1. Historically, identity cards have also been used for racially-motivated oppressive purposes (e.g., in South Africa and Nazi-occupied countries), a potential problem that should be considered
2. In some settings, identity cards for minority, Indigenous, and Afro-descendant populations certifying lineage are critical for eligibility to land claims, reparations, and treaty rights based on Indigenous identity	

[a]In countries and jurisdictions in which marriage between same sex couples is not legally recognized, marriage certificates and the accompanying eligibility for services are limited to heterosexual marriages. To mid-2016, 23 countries, including many in Europe, Canada, the United States, New Zealand, Greenland, South Africa, and various countries (and municipalities) in Latin America legally recognize same sex marriages. Many other jurisdictions recognize same sex civil unions or domestic partnerships, usually providing more limited entitlements.

Sources: Based in part on Swaroop (1960); UN Department of Economic and Social Affairs (1973); WHO (2013a).

2011). Depending on local laws and practice, registration may take place at a police post, courthouse, municipal or district office, special civil registry agency, school, or other locale. Compilation of records by administrative/geographic divisions (towns/provinces/states/regions) provides a comprehensive picture of vital events feeding into the planning and allocation of government, including health services (Table 5-4).

Where effective registration systems exist, the availability of good quality data is often taken for granted, but in most settings civil registration is lacking or inadequate. Under the best circumstances, vital statistics provide approximately 95% coverage, with gaps due to non-registration of temporary or undocumented workers, technical errors, and poor coverage of marginalized populations, including in HICs. Under the worst scenario, such as in roughly 40 countries (mainly in Africa, South and Southeast Asia), fewer than 25% of deaths are registered (Mikkelsen et al. 2015).

Periodic surveys have been used in many countries to bridge the gap between the need for accurate data on health and deficient vital statistics coverage. In fact, most available health data in many LMICs do not come from vital statistics systems but from such surveys.

Since 1984, the US Agency for International Development has supported the demographic and health survey (DHS) program in over 90 LMICs. The program funds and provides technical assistance to collect and make available data on fertility, family planning, and maternal and child health, as well as infant mortality, HIV and AIDS, malaria, and nutrition. The data collected through DHSs are considered nationally representative and are used not only to underpin national health policy and public health programming but also to draw comparisons across countries. UNICEF-supported Multiple Indicator Cluster Surveys also focus on maternal and child health. The overwhelming majority of these surveys offer snapshots rather than cohort analyses that can track health status over time (Victora and Barros 2012). Moreover, they are far less effective at estimating youth and adult mortality, and in some countries they impede the development of full-fledged vital statistics systems. In addition, they rarely provide subnational data and therefore cannot be used to track regional variations in health status.

History of Birth, Marriage, and Death Records

Registry systems of births, marriages, and deaths existed (unevenly) across East and South Asia, Europe, and the Mediterranean over a millennium ago, serving taxation and ritual purposes (Breckenridge and Szreter 2012). In Europe, records were collected and maintained by local parishes, which combined religious and civic-administrative functions. As such, baptisms and burials (and marriages) were recorded rather than births and deaths. Perhaps the earliest and best-known national registry system was founded in England and Wales in 1538, initially as a means of ensuring property rights; other European countries, such as Sweden, soon followed suit. Circa 1600, England established its Poor Law system, which provided locally funded short-term "relief of the poor" in the case of unemployment or destitution. The Poor Laws relied on the parish record system, ensuring high levels of compliance even among uneducated and poor populations. This system remained in place for centuries (Szreter 2012).

In the 19th century, state-run birth and death registries began to be established across Europe, the Americas, and in many colonial settings—in conjunction with census enumeration—for explicit economic and political planning purposes. In an era of rapid industrial growth and inter-imperial rivalries, population size, migration and death patterns, and marriage and birth rates all had considerable bearing on economic output and expansion, military strength, and settlement policies. Today, vital records remain important not only to demographers, epidemiologists, and health planners but also to social and economic policymakers. These data contribute to decisions around public transport and social welfare transfers, how many schools are needed, and which regions merit priority, among countless other issues.

Birth Registration

The right to be registered at birth is recognized under the 1976 *International Covenant on Civil and Political Rights*, the 1989 *Convention on the Rights of the Child*, and other human rights charters. UNICEF refers to birth registration as "the first right, the right to an official identity" (Dow 1998), one that is key to fulfillment of other fundamental rights and that is essential to population health data. Infant mortality rates, an important indicator of health status, rely on accurate birth records as a denominator.

Yet almost one third (230 million) of children under five years of age are not registered—mostly in sub-Saharan Africa and Asia, with just 36% of births registered in Eastern and Southern Africa (World Bank and WHO 2014). Within countries, there are up to five-fold urban-rural differences in registration (UNICEF 2015b). As noted by former UNICEF director Carol Bellamy, these children "are in essence non-existent in the eyes of states. . . . Not having a birth certificate is the functional equivalent of not having been born" (Crossette 1998). Hence, from childhood and throughout life people who are unregistered lack the entitlements listed in Table 5-4.

Conversely, inclusion in statistical records can enable access to equity-enhancing services. In Brazil's flagship program to reduce child poverty through family benefits (see chapter 13), participants require birth certificates to establish eligibility, meet program obligations, and enter other programs (Hunter and Sugiyama 2014). Absent certificates, child benefits may not go to those who are most in need, in turn exacerbating inequities.

Mortality

Along with the expectation that governments collect population data as denominators, effective use of population health data rests on two assumptions:

first, that death and major diseases are certified by trained medical practitioners and publicly recorded, tabulated, and monitored over time; second, that there is an agreed-upon nosology—a disease classification that can be universally applied through common diagnostic procedures.

In the mid-17th century, there was a veritable revolution in social and medical thinking that led to the "scientific" study of societal health and disease and served as precursor to systematic mortality data collection and analysis. Based on his sustained observations of fevers in both privileged and impoverished patients, English physician Thomas Sydenham challenged the Hippocratic notion of disease being the result of humoral imbalances residing within the individual moral and physical being (in conjunction with both the divine and local environment). Instead he held that diseases were specific and distinct pathological entities, and thus could be counted as such.

This insight combined with the work of various contemporaries, starting with fellow physician-anatomist William Petty, who recognized the possibility of studying society systematically and objectively (just as one could anatomy) through what he held was neutral evidence. Petty in turn inspired and assisted London cloth merchant John Graunt in studying the bills (records) of mortality during the final years of the Black Death. The tabulations revealed remarkable findings about patterns of high child mortality and short lives for those surviving (Krieger 2011). Given the utility of this information to government and business, and bolstered by Sydenham's etiologic reasoning—which marked a stunning departure from prior understandings of disease in terms of human moral failings and divine will—the eclectic and ad hoc collection of parish mortality records gradually became systematized. Increasingly the records were studied for political, demographic, and economic purposes amid accelerating industrial and imperial demands.

It would take two centuries for these ideas to be transformed into a uniform disease nomenclature applicable cross-nationally. The need for international comparability of cause-of-death data, fueled by a wave of cholera pandemics and yellow fever outbreaks in the context of soaring trade and migration (see chapter 1), was a prime subject of discussion at the International Statistical Congresses that were first held in the 1850s. At the 1855 congress, William Farr of England and Marc d'Espine of Switzerland proposed tabulations that were later merged into a single list of 139 causes applicable to all countries. That list, officially adopted by the congress, formed the basis for subsequent classifications. At the 1893 meeting of the International Statistical Institute, Frenchman Jacques Bertillon proposed a classification system now known as the International Statistical Classification of Diseases and Related Health Problems or *International Classification of Diseases* (ICD). In 1900, the First International Conference for the Revision of the ICD was convened in Paris, and since then, revisions have appeared at approximately 10-year intervals.

The transition from one ICD revision to another always involves changes in the coding of certain categories: some diagnoses are reassigned, resulting in sudden increases or decreases in reported occurrences of affected categories and breaks in the comparability of statistics. Identification of new ailments and changes in medical knowledge and diagnostic and therapeutic technology contribute to new ways of defining and distinguishing among the many possible causes of death.

The ICD was substantially modified at the sixth revision in 1948, with the addition of coding rubrics for morbidity as well as for causes of death. The latest version, ICD-10, adopted in 1994 and used by 117 countries, has more than 2,036 categories, 12,159 subcategories, and 12,420 codes (Table 5-5). The extensive changes in ICD-10 required training programs to ensure uniformity and gave governments an opportunity to review and improve the entire flow of health-related statistics, reformulate data processing systems, and even redesign death certificates.

According to ICD procedures, when a death occurs, a death certificate should be completed (Figure 5-4). Medical certification of cause of death is typically the responsibility of the attending physician, when there is one. In cases of sudden, violent, or suspicious death, a coroner or other medico-legal officer may be the certifier. Certifiers may also include midwives, nurses, police officers, village chiefs, teachers, or lay persons. Many countries include social and economic information on death certificates; however, according to the ICD, only immediate physical and biological factors are considered causes of death.

Generally, a national statistical office receives the individual records and collates the data for administrative purposes, sending summaries to WHO for compilation. In some countries, multiple and/or

Table 5-5 Major Subdivisions of the International Classification of Diseases, Tenth Revision, 1994

Chapter	Subjects	Range of Codes
I	Certain infectious and parasitic diseases	A00–B99
II	Neoplasms	C00–D48
III	Diseases of the blood and blood-forming organs and certain disorders involving the immune mechanism	D50–D89
IV	Endocrine, nutritional, and metabolic diseases	E00–E90
V	Mental and behavioral disorders	F00–F99
VI	Diseases of the nervous system	G00–G99
VII	Diseases of the eye and adnexa	H00–H59
VIII	Diseases of the ear and mastoid process	H60–H95
IX	Diseases of the circulatory system	I00–I99
X	Diseases of the respiratory system	J00–J99
XI	Diseases of the digestive system	K00–K93
XII	Diseases of the skin and subcutaneous tissue	L00–L99
XIII	Diseases of the musculoskeletal system and connective tissue	M00–M99
XIV	Diseases of the genitourinary system	N00–N99
XV	Pregnancy, childbirth, and the puerperium	O00–O99
XVI	Certain conditions originating in the perinatal period	P00–P96
XVII	Congenital malformations, deformations, and chromosomal abnormalities	Q00–Q99
XVIII	Symptoms, signs, and abnormal clinical and laboratory findings not elsewhere classified	R00–R99
XIX	Injury, poisoning, and certain other consequences of external causes	S00–T98
XX	External causes of morbidity and mortality	V01–Y98
XXI	Factors influencing health status and contact with health services	Z00–Z99
XXII	Codes for special purposes	U00–U85

Source: WHO (2015c). Note: The ICD-10 has been updated every year since 1996 with the next full revision (ICD-11) scheduled for release in 2017.

contributory causes of death are tabulated but usually only the underlying cause of death is coded. It is under this rubric that the data finally appear in WHO's *World Health Statistics* annual update and other venues.

In the many countries in which traditional healers practice in parallel to Western allopaths, use of the ICD may be hindered due to local understandings of disease categories that do not coincide with biomedical nosology. Economic and political factors such as the cost of implementing classification changes and limited access to health and government services also help explain why more than 75 countries do not employ the ICD.

Albeit beset by such deficiencies, mortality statistics are the leading global health measure. Two categories of mortality rates are of particular significance: the infant mortality rate (IMR) and maternal mortality ratio/rate.

Infant Mortality Rate (and Child Mortality)

The IMR—defined as deaths that occur among liveborn infants in the interval between birth and 1 year—differs from other annual age-specific death rates in several important respects. First, both numerator and denominator are derived directly from registration data, whereas the denominator for other age-specific mortality rates generally comes from census-based estimates. More importantly, the denominator of the IMR is not the number of persons in that age group at midyear but the number of live births occurring in a

Cause of death		**Approximate interval between onset and death**
I Disease or condition directly leading to death*	(a)..	....
	due to (or as a consequence of)	
Antecedent causes Morbid conditions, if any, giving rise to the above cause, stating the underlying condition last	(b)..	....
	due to (or as a consequence of)	
	(c)..	....
	due to (or as a consequence of)	
	(d)..	....
II Other significant conditions contributing to the death, but not related to the disease or condition causing it	....	....
	....	....
*This does not mean the mode of dying, e.g. heart failure, respiratory failure. It means the disease, injury, or complication that caused death.		

Figure 5-4: International form of medical certificate of cause of death.
Source: WHO (1993).

defined population during the entire year (Table 5-2). Additionally, infant deaths are not uniformly distributed throughout the year, but are highest in the first day and weeks of life (neonatal mortality, or death before 28 days). While infant mortality rates have dropped markedly across the world over the past century, the almost 60-fold difference between Angola's IMR (from overwhelmingly preventable causes) and that of Iceland (Table 5-6) demonstrate one of the world's most pernicious dimensions of health inequity.

Although the global IMR has steadily declined over recent decades, since 1990 under-5 child mortality has risen in five countries (four in Africa) (WHO 2015a). Globally, an estimated 5.9 million children under five died in 2015, down from 12.7 million in 1990, mostly from preventable causes, and almost all in low-income countries (LICs). Five countries account for 50% of worldwide deaths in children under age 5, with India and Nigeria alone accounting for more than one third. About 50% of child deaths occur in sub-Saharan Africa and another 32% in South Asia (UNICEF 2015a), but there is considerable variation within countries by social class (Figure 7-1) and region (Figure 5-5 and Table 5-7).

Though reported infant mortality was almost halved from 8.9 million deaths in 1990 to 4.5 million deaths in 2015 (UNICEF 2015a), neonatal mortality as a proportion of infant mortality has risen (Victora and Barros 2012). Likewise, neonatal mortality as a proportion of under-5 mortality increased from 40% in 1990 to 45% in 2015 (UNICEF 2015a).

The question of statistical artifacts—that is, whether reported rates are correct—always arises when considering infant deaths. Where births are seldom registered and medical attention is lacking, many infant and child deaths are never recorded and are permanently lost to the statistical system. Yet the number of population-based studies to fill these gaps has been declining, even as epidemiological techniques are improving (Bryce, Victora, and Black 2013). According to the Partnership for Maternal, Neonatal, and Child Health (PMNCH), most neonatal deaths are not registered, resulting in an undercounting of both IMR and the under-5 mortality rate (PMNCH

Table 5-6 Countries with Highest and Lowest Infant Mortality Rates (IMR) and Corresponding Neonatal Mortality Rates (NMR), 2015

Highest IMR Countries	IMR	NMR
Angola	96	48.7
Central African Republic	91.5	42.6
Sierra Leone	87.1	34.9
Somalia	85	39.7
Chad	85	39.3
Democratic Republic of Congo	74.5	30.1
Mali	74.5	37.8
Nigeria	69.4	34.3
Lesotho	69.2	32.7
Equatorial Guinea	68.2	33.1
Côte d'Ivoire	66.6	37.9
Afghanistan	66.3	35.5
Pakistan	65.8	45.5
Lowest IMR Countries	**IMR**	**NMR**
Luxembourg	1.5	0.9
Iceland	1.6	0.9
Finland	1.9	1.3
Norway	2	1.5
Japan	2	0.9
Slovenia	2.1	1.4
Andorra	2.1	1.4
Singapore	2.1	1
Estonia	2.3	1.5
Sweden	2.4	1.6

Data Source: UNICEF (2015a).

2011). Such discrepancies are greater in settings with limited vital statistics systems, especially rural areas. There may be little parental or community incentive for reporting infant deaths, particularly in areas of economic deprivation in which the death toll is higher than elsewhere. Fatalism and tradition may render the subject of deceased infants and children unsuitable for discussion, especially with strangers. Likewise, fetal deaths, stillbirths (estimated at 2.6 million annually [Lawn et al. 2016]), and induced abortions are rarely reported, though they help in understanding infant mortality determinants, for example, to ascertain the harmful prenatal effects of toxic chemicals, other environmental hazards, and lack of access to effective contraceptives.

Maternal Mortality

A maternal death is defined in the ICD-10 as "the death of a woman while pregnant or within 42 days of termination of pregnancy, irrespective of the duration and the site of the pregnancy, from any cause related to or aggravated by the pregnancy or its management but not from accidental or incidental causes" (WHO 1992). The newer "pregnancy-related death" definition covers any cause of death in this period, in order to account for absence of medical certification and also for deaths due to intimate partner violence that are triggered by the pregnancy or the birth of the child and having a new infant in the home. A late maternal death is the death of a woman from direct or indirect obstetric causes between

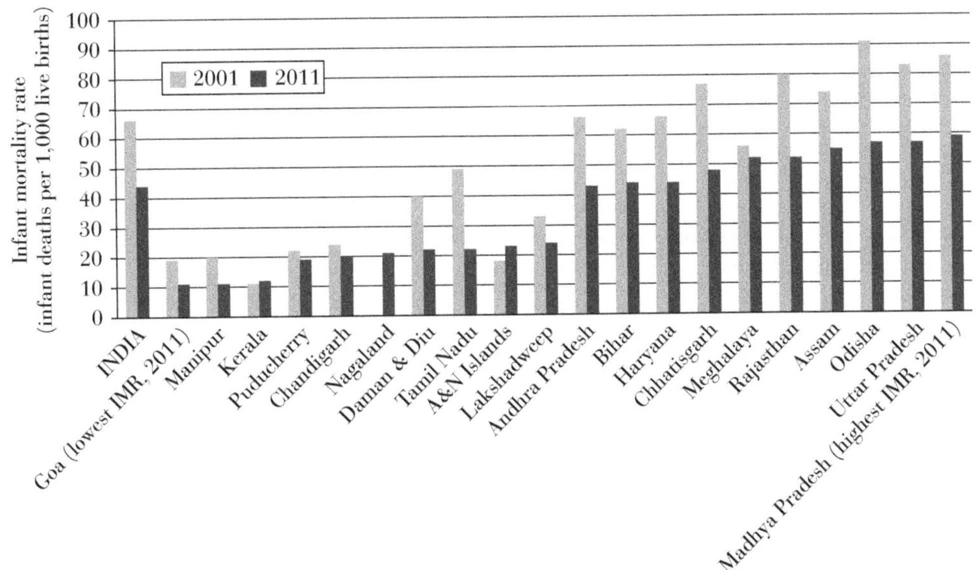

Figure 5-5: Infant mortality in India by state and union territory (highest and lowest IMR states), 2001 and 2011.
Data Source: Government of India (2014).

42 days and 1 year after termination of pregnancy (WHO 2015d).

Maternal mortality is calculated in two ways. The Maternal Mortality Rate indicates the number of deaths from maternal causes per 100,000 women of reproductive age range in a given year and requires reliable census estimates for the denominator (Table 5-2). The Maternal Mortality Ratio (MMR), usually a more accurate estimate, refers to the number of deaths in a given year from maternal causes per 100,000 live births the same year, thus measuring the obstetric risk per pregnancy. Sierra Leone and Central African Republic have two of the highest MMRs in the world at 1,360 and 882 deaths per 100,000 live births, respectively (WHO et al. 2015). Worldwide there were 216 maternal deaths per 100,000 births in 2015. Regional differences in the MMR are striking—in HICs it is 12 per 100,000, whereas in LMICs it is 239 per 100,000—spanning from a low of 27/100,000 in Eastern Asia to a high of 546/100,000 in sub-Saharan Africa (ibid).

Lifetime risk of maternal death takes into account both the probability of becoming pregnant and the probability of dying as a result of that pregnancy cumulated across a woman's reproductive years. Lifetime risk of maternal death is highest in LMICs, with as many as 1 woman in 150 likely

Table 5-7 Infant Mortality Rate by Region, Brazil, 2010

Brazil (National Rate)	**15.6 deaths/1,000 live births**
North	18.1/1,000
Northeast	18.5/1,000
Southeast	13.1/1,000
South	12.6/1,000
Central-West	14.2/1,000

Data Source: Instituto Brasileiro de Geografia e Estatística (2012).

to die from maternal causes in the course of her lifetime, compared with 1 in 3,300 in HICs (World Bank 2016).

Challenges Surrounding Mortality Data Collection

During recent decades there has been almost no progress in civil registration of deaths: in the early 1980s 36.2% of deaths were recorded globally, rising slightly to 38.6% for 2005–2009 (Mikkelsen et al. 2015). In Kenya, 45.6% of deaths were registered in 2013 but with huge regional variations: rural Mandera county registered only 3.1% of deaths versus 80.1% registered in Nairobi (Kenya National Bureau of Statistics 2015). Hand-in-hand with the registration problem is lack of medical certification, with just one third of 56 million annual deaths certified (Figure 5-6). There are exceptions, such as Australia, where a medical certificate is required to register a death, resulting in high certification (WHO 2013a), but this is not the predominant model elsewhere.

Even the death registration data that are available for 119 WHO member states (WHO 2014a) remain limited by coding problems—particularly due to the large percentage of causes labeled "ill-defined." The proportion of ill-defined deaths ranges from 3% in New Zealand to nearly 50% in Morocco (WHO 2015a). Overall, of the 194 WHO member states, only 34 provide high-quality cause-of-death statistics using ICD-9 or ICD-10, and covering at least 90% of all deaths (WHO 2014b).

The underlying cause of death is considered to be the disease or injury initiating the chain of events leading directly to death, or the circumstances producing fatal injury. But this causal chain does not extend to broader societal determinants discussed in chapter 7. The capability of the certifying physician and the presence of technical facilities (diagnostic laboratory support, pathology reports, and autopsy facilities) affect the reliability of certified cause of death. Most medical schools provide little or no training on coding: coronary artery disease is often the default diagnosis written on the death certificate.

As people become older and accumulate more chronic illnesses, the specific underlying cause of death (if there is one) becomes more difficult to determine. An elderly person may die *with* heart failure (and various other serious conditions), but that does not necessarily mean that the person died *due to* heart failure. Errors can also occur when coding and transcribing the cause of death, particularly if it relates to a socially sensitive or stigmatized condition. Some HIV-related deaths, for example, may be coded as pneumonia or tuberculosis.

WHO has sought to improve international comparability, and deal with differences in medical practice and rules for coding through distribution of visual displays of standardized classification of atherosclerotic lesions, hypertension, coronary heart disease, and tumors. Underreporting of certain mortality causes may also be driven by political factors. For example, although there exists an ICD cause of death "due to legal intervention," that is, caused by the actions of law enforcement officers (Krieger et al. 2015), there is likely significant underreporting because of the power and interest of the police to mask this information.

In an effort to capture cause-of-death data in LMICs lacking death certification and where most deaths occur outside a clinical setting, there is increasing use of verbal autopsy (VA) mortality surveillance (Box 5-2). In this technique, specific signs and symptoms of the deceased person, elicited from relatives or others who knew them, are compared with carefully constructed pre-coded algorithms based on well-defined diagnostic criteria (Murray et al. 2011). However, the approach raises vexing ethical and interpretive issues. The sensitive nature of the questions asked may take an emotional toll on the family of the deceased, and ensuring informed consent may be complicated (Fottrell and Byass 2010).

Despite standardization improvements, VA is less accurate at discerning cause of death when there are coexisting conditions leading to death, a common occurrence in old age, and when symptoms are non-specific or variable (Kay 2014; Thatte 2009). Moreover, VA is not a surrogate for medical certification because, among other reasons, not all causes of death can be assessed with VA, and some illnesses are not distinguishable through distinct symptoms, such as AIDS in children (Fottrell 2009; Garenne and Fauveau 2006). These limitations suggest potential for misleading results and highlight why VA is not an adequate replacement for vital statistics collection.

Problems with Vital Statistics

Over 100 countries lack a functional civil registration system (World Bank and WHO 2014), stemming

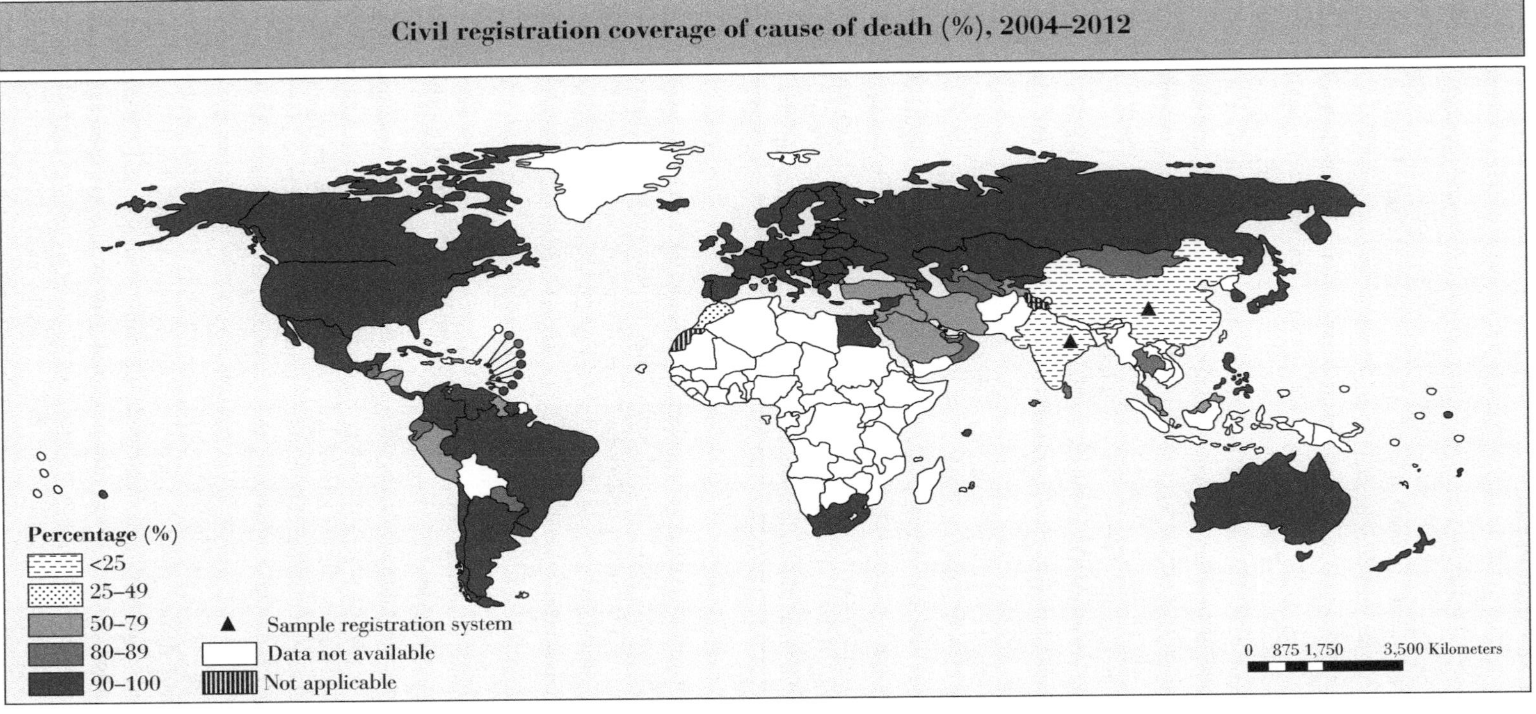

Figure 5-6: Coverage of vital registration of deaths (%), World, 2004–2012.
Source: WHO (2014c). Reprinted from Global Health Observatory, World Health Organization, Copyright (2014).

Box 5-2 Million Death Study in India

An example of the use—and drawbacks—of VA-based household survey data to gauge mortality patterns is the Million Death Study (MDS), carried out in collaboration with the Registrar General of India and a number of academic institutions in India and in HICs (Centre for Global Health Research 2016). With more than three quarters of deaths in India occurring at home, and over half of these lacking a certified cause, the MDS was set up to track a sample of 14 million people across 2.4 million households starting in 1998 (through 2014) to identify causes of and underlying factors in child and adult deaths. Cause of death is documented through VA, with ongoing household monitoring for occurrence of vital events. MDS researchers hope that this model for estimating cause-specific mortality in the absence of routine, comprehensive, sustainable, and reliable measurement of vital statistics may be replicable in other settings and help inform health priorities. Preliminary MDS results for deaths between 2001 and 2003 identified cardiovascular diseases, chronic respiratory diseases, and diarrheal diseases as leading causes (Jha and Laxminarayan 2009). Subsequent analyses have used MDS samples to estimate national mortality rates for other causes of death such as suicide (Patel et al. 2012), road traffic injury (Hsiao et al. 2013), and measles in children (Morris et al. 2013).

While an improvement over the prior paucity of data (Jha 2014), these studies face limitations inherent to all VA studies. The MDS has attributed 200,000 "unattended febrile deaths" to malaria in the absence of standard diagnosis, a 15-fold difference with WHO figures (Westly 2013). MDS could be grossly overestimating malaria deaths, given that fever can signal multiple other diseases. However, because the full data have yet to be released, other scientists are unable to verify these findings (Kay 2014). A further crucial concern is whether sample and VA-based systems may delay the expansion and implementation of full vital statistics capacity.

from many reasons. Vital statistics collection requires a sustained and steady budget allocation and well-trained personnel but is too frequently undervalued and underfunded. The absence of a clear administrative mandate is an impediment in some countries because responsibility for parts of this work may be divided among several government departments or ministries: health, finance, planning, census, social security, central statistics, or others.

Difficulties in data collection include the isolation of rural populations or inaccessibility of registry offices, prohibitive fees, insufficient knowledge about registration and its potential benefits, incompatibility with cultural and religious customs, and suspicion by the public that records may not be kept confidential or that they may be used by the government for taxation, enforced military service, or other undesirable purposes. Squatters, undocumented migrants, persons without identity cards, nomads without a fixed residence, persons engaged in illegal activities, and others may have strong disincentives toward registration.

Finally, the collection, dissemination, and use of vital statistics are far from neutral activities. A population group or national government may, for various reasons, wish population size to be either overstated or understated or may not wish to identify particular causes of death.

Morbidity Statistics and Data Sources

Illness statistics are sometimes more useful to health analysts than are data on deaths, but reliable figures are not always available. Global estimates comparing 2013 to 1990 figures indicate that morbidity (from disease and injury) has increased in accordance with population growth and aging, with a minuscule overall decline in morbidity rates after age standardization. However, years lived with disability from neonatal disorders have almost doubled (Vos et al. 2015), even as infant mortality has declined by almost 50% (WHO 2015a).

Ideally, morbidity statistics describe ill health by diagnosis, severity, duration, distribution in place and time, as well as characteristics of the persons affected, such as age, sex/gender, occupation, social class, and place of residence. In 2002, the WHO issued an International Classification of Functioning, Disability, and Health, complementing the ICD, but to date it has had limited implementation.

Morbidity statistics may be used for the following purposes:

- Control of communicable diseases
- Planning preventive, treatment, and rehabilitation services
- Research on social, environmental, and occupational factors and health
- Estimation of economic importance of sickness
- Research into etiology and pathogenesis
- Research on efficacy of preventive and therapeutic measures
- National and international studies of distribution of disease and disability

There are three general categories of sources for morbidity data: records routinely compiled (often from medical practitioners) and accumulated by various agencies; special surveys that obtain information on particular issues; and disease registries.

Many practitioners and organizations collect data on illness and disability. These include: health and statistics ministries, health centers, hospitals, public health departments, special clinics (e.g., sexually transmitted infection clinics and maternal and child health clinics); schools; workplaces; NGOs, aid agencies, visiting nurses, midwives, physicians' and dentists' offices; military and veterans' services; workers' compensation programs; census bureaus; police; traffic safety organizations; health insurance and life insurance companies; and disease-specific registries. Persons legally responsible for morbidity notification include physicians and other health workers, school and workplace authorities, directors of laboratories in which positive diagnoses are made, and heads of families.

To ensure consistent reporting of particular diseases, a strict case definition is needed. For example, a case of measles can be clinically defined as: a generalized rash of three or more days duration, a fever of 101°F (38.3°C) or more, and a cough, coryza, or conjunctivitis (Murphy, Xu, and Kochanek 2013). This clinical case definition distinguishes measles from other similar illnesses, but it is not always easy to identify a case. Applying the measles case definition involves observation, the use of a thermometer, and inquiring about duration of illness. Identifying other diseases, such as tuberculosis, requires laboratory studies. These can be costly and impractical in remote areas. The level of diagnostic services needed depends on the purpose and design of the investigation. A relatively straightforward and inexpensive ("quick-and-dirty") clinical survey, with some laboratory backup, may provide sufficient basis for a policy decision.

Compulsory reporting of disease occurrence in any country/jurisdiction is limited to certain ailments, plus those mandated by WHO (see next section: The International Health Regulations). In most countries, obligatory notification laws cover highly contagious diseases that pose an immediate threat to the community, and also include such diseases as botulism, caused by contaminated canned foods. Prompt notification may result in recalls of affected production lots and thus avert additional cases. Epilepsy may be a notifiable disease when a driver's license is involved. AIDS is widely reportable, but due to the complexity of diagnosis and a tangle of other factors, case reporting is incomplete. Occupational diseases and work-related injuries are legally notifiable in many countries, in part to gather data for control purposes, and in part for validation of workmen's compensation claims.

Some countries require immediate reporting of suspected cases, others only after laboratory confirmation. Often, notification focuses on institutions, such as schools, prisons, nursing homes, or resorts. Special regulations may govern outbreaks in particular facilities, including on dairy farms or in hospitals, requiring that healthy carriers be reported and registered.

Routine and continuous monitoring of health data is essential to the prompt detection of disease outbreaks, determining their cause, and minimizing hazards before larger groups are exposed. For example, starting in the late 1950s, reports of limb malformations in newborns led to the discovery that thalidomide, prescribed to pregnant women to combat morning sickness, was responsible. In the 1960s a syndrome of eye, ear, and heart damage was described in children whose mothers contracted rubella during pregnancy. Both discoveries resulted in worldwide awareness and control efforts. Similarly, the first cases of what became known as AIDS were detected in the early 1980s through physician reports and CDC epidemiological investigations of an unusual number of cases of Kaposi's sarcoma and *Pneumocystis* pneumonia among young gay men in Los Angeles. Other similar instances include ongoing surveillance efforts for avian influenza.

Population-based surveys, which typically rely on census data for the sampling frame, are employed to determine the prevalence of particular diseases, often, but not only, when resources for routine morbidity data are limited. Parasitological surveys for hookworm disease, for example, use stool samples to identify the characteristic worm ova; population surveys for malaria and filariasis use microscopic examination of blood films. Prevalence estimates of sexually transmitted infections (such as HIV), childhood diarrhea, hypertension, and nutritional deficiencies also rely on large survey methods.

Disease registries have been formed in various countries to monitor the distribution, incidence, and prevalence of certain diseases occurring in populations within a specified geographic area or institution. Frequently administered at the regional level, subnational registries then feed into national counterparts. Registries require considerable resources to ensure accurate and complete compilation of data on diagnostics, therapies, and specific outcomes and are useful to evaluate the effectiveness of interventions, calculate survival, and track trends. Most common are cancer registries, but there are also special registries for blindness, childhood disabilities, congenital conditions, and diseases of local importance.

The International Health Regulations

Under WHO's Constitution, member countries have a national responsibility to report annually on the actions taken and progress achieved in improving health. They must also keep WHO informed of important laws, regulations, official reports, and health statistics, in addition to providing statistical and epidemiological information as determined by the World Health Assembly. These responsibilities extend to the health problems encountered by migrants and travelers.

To ensure mutual reporting and collaboration, the *International Health Regulations* (IHR)—a legally binding agreement on disease notification—mandate that national governments notify WHO of cases or outbreaks of certain diseases, and of measures taken to prevent their spread. The IHR's precursor, the *International Sanitary Regulations,* was adopted by WHO in 1951 as a legal instrument to protect against the international spread of diseases. Originally, diseases subject to international reporting included cholera, plague, yellow fever (these three motivating international sanitary treaties starting in the 19th century), smallpox, relapsing fever, and louse-borne typhus. When the IHR were created in 1969, the latter two diseases were dropped, and other diseases "under surveillance" were added, including malaria and poliomyelitis. In 1981, after it was declared eradicated, smallpox was removed from the list, only to be re-added 25 years later as a possible bioterrorist threat. Accurate figures on cases of diseases near eradication, such as polio, are crucial for monitoring progress.

Starting in the 1980s the (re)appearance of old and new ailments, including plague in India, cholera in the Americas, and Ebola hemorrhagic fever in Africa, and the 2003 SARS outbreak concentrated in Asia and Canada (see chapter 6) motivated WHO to review and adapt the scope of the IHR. These emerging diseases, plus emergencies provoked by noninfectious diseases, made apparent the need for improvements in international surveillance of, and coordinated responses to, public health emergencies (Davies, Kamradt-Scott, and Rushton 2015).

In 2007, a revision of the IHR came into effect requiring that 196 country signatories, including all WHO members plus several observer states, notify WHO of all events that constitute a public health emergency. According to the revised IHR, a public health emergency is of international concern if it: (a) constitutes a public health risk to other states through the international spread of disease; and (b) potentially requires a coordinated international response. The IHR's legal framework requires signatories to notify WHO within 24 hours of the first official case of a listed disease, respond to public health emergencies, and ensure a mechanism for seeking technical assistance from WHO. If a particular event constitutes a public health emergency of international concern, the IHR require WHO to make "a 'real-time' response to the emergency" through immediate action (WHO 2007).

The Ebola outbreak in West Africa in 2013–2015 illustrates the importance of morbidity statistics and the IHR. Critical to the IHR's implementation is having the capacity to: conduct surveillance, ensure real-time reporting, and take urgent action to address the causes and consequences of the outbreak. All of these require a strong health system, lacking in the three countries most affected by the Ebola outbreak (WHO 2015b). But many other countries remain unprepared: only 78 signatories completed the self-assessment of their capacity to implement the IHR provisions (WHO 2015b). WHO also came under fire: its delayed response to the Ebola outbreak put its own IHR compliance under the microscope, potentially challenging its legitimacy (Gostin and Friedman 2015; Horton 2015).

Challenges of Gathering and Measuring Morbidity Statistics

The quality and completeness of morbidity records vary greatly, as does their accessibility. Many diseases exhibit a wide spectrum of severity from subclinical to extreme. Moreover, many infections go undetected and undiagnosed by those carrying them. Even for illnesses detected, few people can document their own complete health history over the lifecourse. Morbidity information may be considered confidential or privileged, particularly when the information forms the basis of legal claims for insurance or compensation. Many countries have laws protecting the privacy of personal data concerning mental illness or other conditions.

A high degree of coordination between regional and international reporting agencies is seldom achieved, even in HICs, because information is collected differently, for different purposes, and at different intervals. One opportunity to strengthen the quality of morbidity data is through implementation of electronic health records (EHR). Such longitudinal patient health information records are "generated by one or more encounters in any care delivery setting . . . [and include] . . . patient demographics, progress notes, problems, medications, vital signs, past medical history, immunizations, laboratory data, and radiology reports" (WHO 2012, p. 11). While potentially advantageous, EHR implementation requires extensive computerization, coordination, steady Internet access, privacy safeguards, and substantial resources. The UK's EHR project, for example, squandered £12.7 billion over 9 years (Currie 2014), an important cautionary for other settings.

Morbidity and Mortality Metrics

In addition to counts of occurrence of disease and death, there are also various metrics that seek to gauge the significance of ill health and premature death for individuals, communities, and nations. Examples include: years of potential life lost (YPLL), years lived with disability (YLD), quality-adjusted life years (QALY), and healthy life years (HeaLY). WHO's cross-cultural WHOQOL instrument assesses 26 quality-of-life facets covering physical and psychological health, environmental conditions, and social relationships.

Because these measures entail assessment of what constitutes a norm and assumptions regarding quality of life, they can be heavily value laden and fraught with controversy. People with disabilities, for example, may take umbrage at having quality of life assessed without accounting for societal lack of accommodation in influencing integration into work and school (see chapter 6).

Turning to YPLL, causes of death that typically strike young people, such as malaria and diarrhea, are weighted differently from the diseases characteristic of the elderly. The rationale is that a person who dies in infancy or early childhood loses almost all of his or her life expectancy, whereas an elderly person who dies loses only a few years. For this metric, the age at death must be known, as well as the expected age at which that person would otherwise have died (not always simple to determine). There is also a strong equity concern here: health inequities involving premature mortality are enormous. Calculating life expectancy of, for instance, people in the lowest income quintile compared with the highest quintile and framing YPLL differentially by income groups incorporates assumptions about who should and can experience both the benefits and the problems of longer life expectancy.

The potential life lost in a population can be a powerful incentive for policy changes by governments but also de-emphasizes certain chronic diseases among adults. Diabetes, the ninth leading

Table 5-8 The 12 Leading Causes of Death in the World, 2013 (and rank order in 2000)

No.	Cause	Estimated Number of Deaths (in Millions)	% of all Deaths
1	Coronary heart disease (1)	8.1	14.8
2	Cerebrovascular disease (2)	6.4	11.8
3	COPD (4)	2.9	5.3
4	Lower respiratory infections (3)	2.7	4.8
5	Alzheimer's disease and other dementias	1.7	3.0
6	Tracheal, bronchus, lung cancers (9)	1.6	2.9
7	Road injury (12)	1.4	2.5
8	HIV and AIDS (6)	1.3	2.4
9	Diabetes mellitus (10)	1.3	2.4
10	Tuberculosis (7)	1.3	2.4
11	Diarrheal diseases (5)	1.3	2.3
12	Cirrhosis of the liver (13)	1.2	2.2

Data Sources: Naghavi et al. (2015); WHO (2014d).

cause of death in 2013 (Table 5-8), rarely appears on YPLL "top ten" lists because death tends to strike later in life even if diabetes is now diagnosed at younger ages.

Global Burden of Disease

A large-scale effort to quantify the "global burden of disease" (GBD) was commissioned in the early 1990s by the World Bank and carried out jointly by WHO and Harvard School of Public Health researchers. Nowadays, the ongoing GBD studies are overseen by the University of Washington-based Institute for Health Metrics and Evaluation (IHME) with funding from the Bill and Melinda Gates Foundation and World Bank. The GBD's modeling approach estimates both mortality *and* morbidity (calculated via disability-adjusted life years [DALYs, see ahead]), combining them in a single measure. Diseases are grouped into three major classifications: Group I includes communicable diseases, perinatal conditions, and nutritional deficiencies; Group II comprises noncommunicable diseases (NCDs); and Group III all injuries. These groups are further subdivided into categories, and then into 240 separate causes of death according to ICD-10 (107 causes for ICD-9).

The GBD studies have also sought to estimate the burden of disease due to a series of "risk factors." High blood pressure, diet, high body mass index, child and maternal malnutrition, tobacco smoking, and air pollution were identified as the most harmful risk factors for death and DALYs for 2013 (Forouzanfar et al. 2015). It is important to note, as explored further in chapters 3 and 7, that risk factors focus on individual and behavioral matters without considering the social and political context in which they are generated (i.e., poverty, poor housing, and lack of energy alternatives leading to use of indoor cookstoves, creating household air pollution [and differential gendered exposures]; and the role of societal stress and transnational trade and marketing in influencing, respectively, blood pressure and tobacco use). This highlights that the very ways that data are parsed, analyzed, and presented have enormous bearing on how problems are defined and thus how policies and strategies are crafted and adopted to address these problems.

The GBD studies have catalogued significant shifts in mortality patterns over time. For 1990, 55% of all deaths worldwide were found to be due to NCDs; 35% to communicable diseases; and 10% to injuries (Murray and Lopez 1996). The comprehensive IHME update for 2013 found that 70% of deaths were due to NCDs; 21% to communicable diseases; and 9% to injuries (Naghavi et al. 2015). Table 5-8 shows that eight of the twelve leading causes of death worldwide are NCDs and that the three top causes—coronary heart disease, stroke, and chronic obstructive pulmonary disease (COPD)—account for nearly a third of all deaths. After stratification by country income-level, the LIC picture changes markedly, with communicable diseases constituting the bulk of leading causes of death (Table 5-9).

It is imperative to underscore that GBD figures are *estimates* derived from *modeling* techniques applied to the limited (and often non-comparable) data furnished by national governments, epidemiological studies, the UN, and WHO. Data sources include vital statistics, VAs, cancer registries, police reports, and demographic and health surveys (Lozano et al. 2012). Not only can such estimates be specious, they "can have unintended adverse effects, diminish country ownership, mislead users to think that empirical data are available, reduce pressures on governments to fix broken information systems, and discourage development partners from support to strengthen statistical systems, including CRVS [civil registration and vital statistics systems]" (AbouZahr et al. 2015a, p. 4). Moreover, although estimation methods are increasingly sophisticated, they may skew global results and, therefore, health policies. Ultimately "they cannot replace or replicate the policy value of high-quality, detailed, and timely vital statistics generated subnationally and nationally" (ibid).

Table 5-9 The 10 Leading Causes of Death by Country Income Level, 2012*

Low-Income Countries			High-Income Countries		
Cause	**Deaths (Thousands)**	**% of Total Deaths**	**Cause**	**Deaths (Thousands)**	**% of Total Deaths**
Lower respiratory infections	774	10.4	Coronary heart disease	2046	17.5
HIV and AIDS	549	7.4	Cerebrovascular disease	1226	10.5
Diarrheal diseases	446	6.0	Trachea, bronchus, lung cancers	630	5.4
Cerebrovascular disease	438	5.9	Alzheimer's disease and other dementia	549	4.7
Coronary heart disease	326	4.4	COPD	401	3.4
Malaria	296	4.0	Lower respiratory infections	395	3.4
Preterm birth complications	279	3,8	Colon and rectum cancers	352	3.0
Tuberculosis	263	3.5	Diabetes mellitus	254	2.2
Birth asphyxia and birth trauma	245	3.3	Hypertensive heart disease	253	2.2
Protein-energy malnutrition	225	3.0	Breast cancer	204	1.7

*Compared with 2000, there were several differences. In LICs, coronary heart disease went from 11th to 5th place and measles dropped far off the list. In HICs, Alzheimer's disease climbed from 8th to 4th place, and hypertensive heart disease went from 13th to 9th place.

Data Source: WHO (2014d)

Table 5-10 Leading Causes of Disease Burden (in DALYs) for Males and Females, Worldwide, 2012

Males	% of DALYs	Females	% of DALYs
Coronary heart disease	6.6	Cerebrovascular disease	5.4
Lower respiratory infections	5.4	Coronary heart disease	5.3
Cerebrovascular disease	4.9	Lower respiratory infections	5.3
Preterm birth complications	4.0	Diarrheal diseases	4.1
Road injury	3.9	Preterm birth complications	3.8
COPD	3.5	Unipolar depressive disorders	3.8
Diarrheal diseases	3.3	HIV and AIDS	3.5
HIV and AIDS	3.2	COPD	3.2
Birth asphyxia and birth trauma	2.9	Birth asphyxia and birth trauma	2.5
Unipolar depressive disorders	2.0	Diabetes mellitus	2.4

Data Source: WHO (2014d).

Disability-Adjusted Life Years

In the 1993 *World Development Report: Investing in Health*, the World Bank proposed a new composite measure called the DALY (rhymes with rally) as a generic indicator to help set health policy priorities, facilitate comparisons between countries, and standardize health sector decisionmaking. Its principal contribution is the incorporation of both mortality and morbidity (in terms of disability) into a single summary statistic. The DALY is defined as "the present value of the future years of disability-free life that are lost as the result of the premature deaths or cases of disability occurring in a particular year" (World Bank 1993, p. x). As originally formulated, it combines four elements: (1) levels of mortality by age, (2) levels of morbidity/disability by age, (3) the value of a healthy year of life at specific ages, and (4) a discount rate of 3%.

DALYs are calculated by adding premature death (years of life lost based on a "standard life" expectancy by sex, and adjusted for the extremes of young and old age, so that youth and adult deaths "count" more) and years living with a disability (weighted by the severity of the disability and adjusted for age of onset, making the lives of people with disabilities "valued" less), all discounted by 3% per year. The underlying assumption is that priority should be given to those health problems that cause a large disease burden and for which generally accepted cost-effective interventions (assessed by DALYs "saved") are available (Lopez et al. 2006).

The top 10 causes of death and of disease burden for males and females (Table 5-10) overlap but are not identical. For men and boys, preterm birth complications, birth trauma, and unipolar depression are leading causes of disease burden but not of death. Meanwhile, trachea, bronchus, and lung cancers, diabetes, and cirrhosis of the liver are leading causes of death (which tend to kill at older ages), but not of disease burden (because older age deaths are weighted less by the GBD). For women and girls, unipolar depressive disorders and birth trauma appear as leading causes of disease burden but are not leading causes of death, whereas breast cancer and hypertensive heart disease are main causes of death but not disease burden. This collapsing of morbidity and mortality into a single metric muddles decisionmaking by presuming universal priority-setting approaches, obscuring some diseases that are important to specific societies, and underplaying the role of intersectoral approaches for chronic diseases.

The 2012 GBD suggests that regional disparities in burden of disease are increasing. Sub-Saharan Africa's disease burden is 756 DALYs per 1,000 people, compared with 264 DALYs per 1,000 people in East Asia, 322 DALYs per 1,000 people in Europe and North America, and 388 DALYs per 1,000 people globally (WHO 2014d). An analysis of country income level-specific DALYs (Figure 5-7) shows the

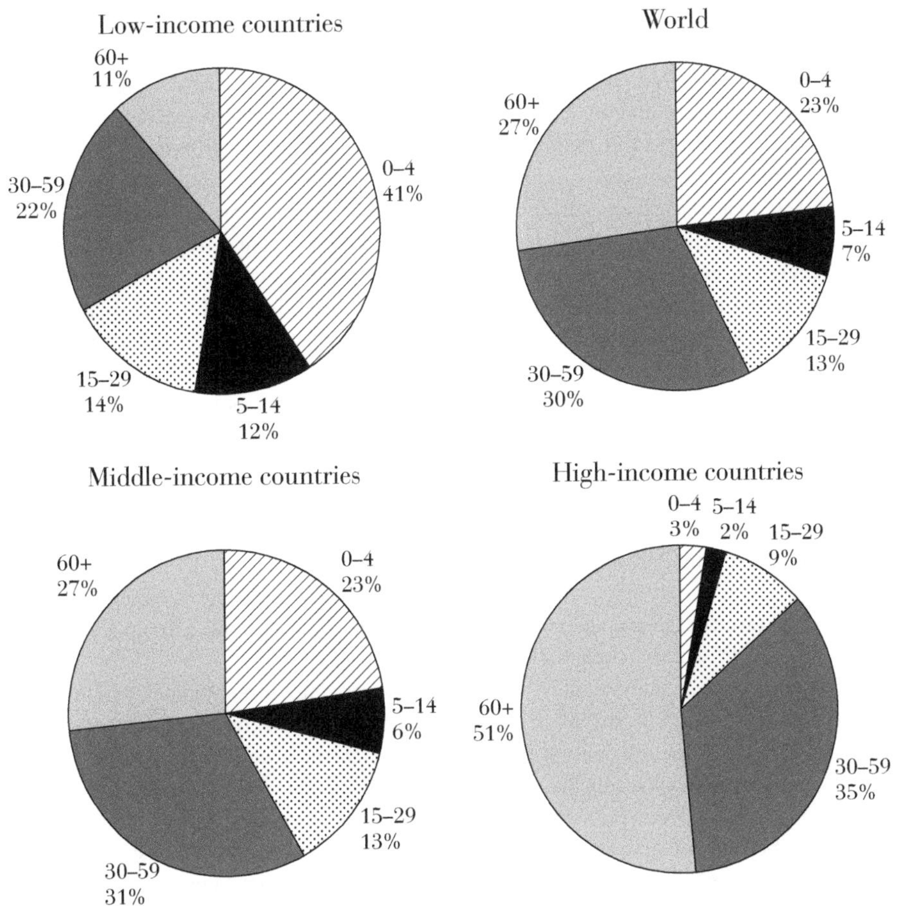

Figure 5-7: Distribution of disease burden (in DALYs) by age group and income group, 2012.
Data Source: WHO (2014d).

different contribution to DALYs according to age group, with LICs having a much higher proportion of DALYs at the youngest ages, HICs at the oldest ages, and MICs in between.

There have been few attempts to compare GBD estimates of number (and causes) of deaths to those based on other surveys or vital statistics (Victora 2015). Figure 6-4 shows the top 10 causes of death for Kenya according to the latest estimates from IHME and Kenya's vital statistics registry for 2013. In large part due to different disease classifications, only 4 of the top 10 causes are the same, so it can be near impossible to make a systematic comparison. But there are also striking differences in the *number* of deaths: Kenya's civil registration system estimated over 426,000 deaths for 2013, whereas IHME calculated some 295,000 deaths—a 30% difference!

To be sure, each source has its limitations. IHME's modeled estimates are based on a number of assumptions, extrapolations, and complex algorithms, and it is near impossible to know whether these truly reflect reality (Horton 2013). At the same time, with less than half of deaths registered and huge within-country variations, Kenya's vital statistics are severely lacking (Kenya National Bureau of Statistics 2015); it is unknown whether these death estimates would change significantly if the data were more complete. Which data are more useful or accurate?

This is difficult to answer with certainty, but "any estimate is only as good as the underlying data on which it is based" (AbouZahr et al. 2015a, p. 4). Though limited, Kenya's vital statistics reflect actual registered deaths (albeit those of more urban and less impoverished populations), whereas IHME's aggregated estimates derive from modeling based on multiple sources and methods. A key issue is which data collection and analysis approach can be strengthened by and at the country level. By building on existing vital registration and data compilation systems, Kenyan policymakers can discern where civil registration is weakest and correct these deficiencies. Moreover, only disaggregated data can help identify geographic and other social inequities in both data collection and health status, making local efforts crucial to addressing health inequity overall.

Critiques of DALYs

Soon after their appearance, DALYs came under fire on technical, philosophical, and political/social grounds. The main lines of criticism are (Anand and Hanson 2004; Bobadilla 1996; Parks 2014):

- DALYs reflect the (average) social values of a small group of "experts" who assume certain norms without taking social, cultural, and environmental contexts into account. The discount rate, age weights, and disability scores are arbitrary and were developed with little involvement of health care workers or the public.
- Valuing people's lives according to current and future productivity is ethically dubious and contradicts the notion of health as a human right.
- Valuing future years of life below present levels justifies activities that result in current environmental degradation at the expense of future generations.
- DALYs' disability weights are ethically troubling, devaluing the lives of people with disabilities and failing to contextualize how disabilities are experienced culturally and economically (i.e., via support systems that facilitate participation in the workforce and enhance quality of life). Revision of DALYs to "account" for culture by "averaging" the social situation of persons with disabilities remains inappropriate and inequitable (Reidpath et al. 2003).
- DALYs discriminate against the very young, persons who are sick and who have disabilities, and the elderly in part because death during youth and middle age corresponds to a higher DALY value than death in early or later years. The DALY is also insensitive to variations in how each life-year is lost. The value of 30 years lost by one individual's premature death may be equated to 1 year lost by 30 different individuals.
- DALYs are biased in favor of societies that use life-prolonging technologies.
- DALYs conflate measurement of need and resource allocation in the same universal metric.
- DALYs favor narrow, disease-specific interventions that can be used in cost-effectiveness analyses, overlooking long-term efforts that affect health, such as housing improvements and social security measures.
- DALYs do not account for inequity, for example differences by class and other social variables or distribution of wealth and resources within and across societies.
- Calculating DALYs is expensive because they require large quantities of data that are not readily available.
- Estimates for countries with limited data are based on questionable extrapolations from other settings.
- Maximizing the number of DALYs gained (akin to improving aggregate health status) via cost-effective interventions may not be the sole or most desirable means of deciding societal or health sector goals for health. Policymaking is guided better by comprehensive, rights-based approaches to improving health equity rather than increasing average health.

Despite more recent flexibility on whether age weighting and discounting are incorporated, DALYs' problematic social valuing of disability, ignoring of equity issues, and other flaws remain. Yet DALYs and the GBD approach have achieved ever more widespread application, especially as global health power and resources have become increasingly concentrated (Parks 2014). The use of average mortality rates as targets for the UN's development goals (United Nations 2015) are the subject of ongoing controversies around the inadequacies of aggregate summary statistics for addressing health inequities (Gibbons 2015).

Given the GBD's ubiquitous presence in WHO and other global health statistical repositories, this textbook perforce relies on GBD-generated death rates; however, because of the cited weaknesses of DALYs and the GBD, we minimize their use whenever possible. Crucial in this regard is Krieger's astute reminder that data do not:

> . . . tell stories. People do. An important caveat, however, is that the stories that people who are scientists tell are not simply or simple "stories": they are (or are supposed to be) transparent accounts, informed by theory, and premised on the public testing of ideas and explanations, using explicitly defined concepts and methods (Krieger 2011, p. 17).

Health Services Statistics

Information about the organization of health services is another element of health data useful to government agencies, insurance companies, health organizations, and researchers. Health services statistics refer not only to resources (facilities, personnel, financing, supplies, equipment) but also to activities and utilization patterns.

The main reasons for collecting health services statistics are to (WHO 2000):

- Support the administration, management, and coordination of local, regional, and national health services
- Develop short-, medium-, and long-term plans/policies
- Assess whether health services are equitable, effective, efficient, and responsive
- Keep track of expenditures
- Provide data on accountability to oversight bodies both locally and globally

Ideally, these data are compiled at a national level and forwarded to Geneva, and become accessible through WHO's Statistical Information System (WHOSIS), which is now integrated with the Global Health Observatory data repository. WHOSIS provides a set of core health system and health status indicators plus a national health accounts system, which includes information on health spending, system coverage, and epidemiological and demographic indicators. WHO's Global Health Expenditure Database is a separate repository for other data on specific health expenditure indicators.

Large-scale disease campaigns and initiatives, such as WHO's global TB control strategy (see chapter 6), also seek to gather standard data in an attempt to record activities and gauge their impact. However, data from program evaluations are not compiled consistently, making it difficult to draw conclusions or comparisons. Moreover, programs of this type are often organized and administered separately from the other activities of health ministries, impeding the routine and uniform collection of health services data.

The comparison of data on health services in different countries is generally challenging, as each society has a unique mosaic of formal and nonformal health services (chapter 11 returns to some of these issues). While important, health services statistics provide just one window on patterns of health within and across populations.

CONCLUSION

Learning Points:

- Reliable health data are the lifeblood of national and international health policies and decisionmaking, but there are major gaps in health and vital statistics collection across the world, especially in LMICs.
- Health data collection and analysis are simultaneously technical, political, cultural, and ideological activities.
- Availability of health data alone will not improve health status or equity, but they are necessary, if insufficient, for the making of effective and just policies affecting health.

As the old adage goes, "If you don't ask, you don't know, and if you don't know, you can't act" (Krieger 1992, p. 412). Though far less palpable than treating illness, the routine collection of population data, morbidity and vital statistics, health services statistics, and data on health inequities is essential to understanding local, national, and global patterns of disease and death and to formulating effective actions for health improvement (Phillips et al. 2015). What's at stake is no less than who gets counted and who counts in terms of policies, resource distribution, and health and well-being.

Global health actors have paid inadequate attention to the problem of civil registration and vital statistics, perhaps because these activities are perceived as less important or effective than disease-control efforts

(AbouZahr et al. 2015b). Although internationally sponsored health surveys and programs periodically collect key health data where they are not institutionalized, and IHME provides estimates of aggregate data based on models and extrapolations, these are no substitute for routine, inclusive, and comprehensive population health data collected by government agencies (AbouZahr et al. 2015a).

A further challenge is that where data are routinely collected and analyzed, they typically measure average levels of health and disease and do not reflect inequities in access to services within a population, nor do they expose how health is distributed according to different population characteristics. Failure to include socioeconomic indicators in the collection and analysis of health data (and failure to provide disaggregated data) severely impedes efforts to understand, routinely monitor and detect, and address health inequities through public policies (Krieger et al. 2005).

Indeed, as global attention to poverty and health inequities has grown—and given the post-2015 Sustainable Development Goals and the monitoring of their progress—the need for far more accurate and comprehensive health data and analysis that takes equity concerns into account is even more pressing. WHO and the World Bank's "Global Civil Registration and Vital Statistics Scaling Up Investment Plan 2015–2024" is a start (World Bank 2015), but this toolkit requires US$200 million and does not cover the far higher operational costs of maintaining these systems. Compiling and assessing health data, including data on health inequities, in an ongoing and permanent fashion—especially in the many countries that lack functional vital statistics systems—should be a global and national health priority (WHO 2013c).

REFERENCES

AbouZahr C, Adjei S, and Kanchanachitra C. 2007. From data to policy: Good practices and cautionary tales. *Lancet* 369(9566):1039–1046.

AbouZahr C, de Savigny D, Mikkelsen L, et al. 2015a. Towards universal civil registration and vital statistics systems: The time is now. *Lancet* 386(10001):1407–1418.

AbouZahr C, de Savigny D, Mikkelsen L, et al. 2015b. Civil registration and vital statistics: Progress in the data revolution for counting and accountability. *Lancet* 386(10001):1373–1385.

Anand S and Hanson K. 2004. Disability-adjusted life years: A critical review. In Anand S, Peter F, and Sen A, Editors. *Public Health, Ethics, and Equity.* Oxford: Oxford University Press.

Bailey SR and Telles EE. 2006. Multiracial versus collective black categories examining census classification debates in Brazil. *Ethnicities* 6(1):74–101.

Birn AE. 1999. Federalist flirtations: The politics and execution of health services decentralization for the uninsured population in Mexico, 1985–1995. *Journal of Public Health Policy* 20(1):81–108.

———. 2009. Making it politic(al): Closing the gap in a generation: Health equity through action on the social determinants of health. *Social Medicine/ Medicina Social* 4(3):166–182.

Black D, Gates G, Sanders S, and Taylor L. 2007. *The Measurement of Same-Sex Unmarried Partner Couples in the 2000 US Census.* Los Angeles: California Center for Population Research.

Bobadilla JL. 1996. Priority setting and cost effectiveness. In Janovsky K, Editor. *Health Policy and Systems Development: An Agenda for Research.* Geneva: WHO.

Braveman P and Tarimo E. 2002. Social inequalities in health within countries: Not only an issue for affluent nations. *Social Science and Medicine* 54(11):1621–1635.

Breckenridge K and Szreter S, Editors. 2012. *Registration and Recognition: Documenting the Person in World History.* Oxford: Oxford University Press.

Bryce J, Victora CG, and Black RE. 2013. The unfinished agenda in child survival. *Lancet* 382(9897):1049–1059.

Carpiano RM, Lloyd JEV, and Hertzman C. 2009. Concentrated affluence, concentrated disadvantage, and children's readiness for school: A population-based, multi-level investigation. *Social Science and Medicine* 69(3):420–432.

Centre for Global Health Research. 2016. Million Death Study. www.cghr.org/projects/million-death-study-project/. Accessed May 30, 2016.

Chandramouli C. 2011. Census of India 2011 – A Story of Innovations. http://pib.nic.in/newsite/efeatures.aspx?relid=74556. Accessed May 30, 2015.

Coimbra CEA, Santos RV, Welch JR, et al. 2013. The first national survey of Indigenous people's health and nutrition in Brazil: Rationale, methodology, and overview of results. *BMC Public Health* 13(1):52.

Crossette B. 1998. Third of births aren't registered, UNICEF says. *New York Times,* July 8.

Currie WL. 2014. Translating health IT policy into practice in the UK NHS. *Scandinavian Journal of Information Systems* 26(2):3–26.

Davies SE, Kamradt-Scott A, and Rushton S. 2015. *Disease Diplomacy: International Norms and Global*

Health Security. Baltimore: Johns Hopkins University Press.

Dow U. 1998. Birth registration: The "First" right. In Way C, Editor. *The Progress of Nations 1998*. New York: UNICEF.

Ferguson Commission. 2015. *Forward Through Ferguson: A Path Toward Racial Equity*. Ferguson, MO.

Forouzanfar MH, Alexander L, Anderson HR, et al. 2015. Global, regional, and national comparative risk assessment of 79 behavioural, environmental and occupational, and metabolic risks or clusters of risks in 188 countries, 1990–2013: A systematic analysis for the Global Burden of Disease Study 2013. *Lancet* 386(10010):2287–2323.

Fottrell E. 2009. Dying to count: Mortality surveillance in resource-poor settings. *Global Health Action* 2(1).

Fottrell E and Byass P. 2010. Verbal autopsy: Methods in transition. *Epidemiologic Reviews* 32(1):38–55.

Garenne M and Fauveau V. 2006. Potential and limits of verbal autopsies. *Bulletin of the World Health Organization* 84(3):164.

Gibbons ED. 2015. SDG Series: The Slippery Target for Child Survival in the 2030 Agenda for Sustainable Development. *Health and Human Rights Journal Blog*, September 3.

Gostin LO and Friedman EA. 2015. A retrospective and prospective analysis of the West African Ebola virus disease epidemic: Robust national health systems at the foundation and an empowered WHO at the apex. *Lancet* 385(9980):1902–1909.

Government of India. 2014. State-wise Infant Mortality Rate. *Data Portal India*. https://data.gov.in/catalog/state-wise-infant-mortality-rate. Accessed February 12, 2014.

Groenewold G, van Ginneken J, and Masseria C. 2008. *Towards Comparable Statistics on Mortality by Socio-economic Status in EU Member States*. Brussels: European Commission.

Haigh F, Baum F, Dannenberg AL, et al. 2013. The effectiveness of health impact assessment in influencing decision-making in Australia and New Zealand 2005–2009. *BMC Public Health* 13(1):1188.

Hamlin C. 2009. "Cholera Forcing" The myth of the good epidemic and the coming of good water. *American Journal of Public Health* 99(11):1946–1954.

Horton R. 2013. Metrics for what? *Lancet* 381:S1–S2.

———. 2015. Offline: An irreversible change in global health governance. *Lancet* 385(9983):2136.

Hunter W and Sugiyama NB. 2014. Transforming subjects into citizens: Insights from Brazil's Bolsa Família. *Perspectives on Politics* 12(4):808–828.

Hsiao M, Malhotra A, Thakur JS, et al. 2013. Road traffic injury mortality and its mechanisms in India: Nationally representative mortality survey of 1.1 million homes. *BMJ Open* 3:e002621.

Instituto Brasileiro de Geografia e Estatística. 2012. Censo Demográfico 2010 Resultados gerais da amostra. http://www.ibge.gov.br/home/presidencia/noticias/imprensa/ppts/0000000847310412201231572748398 5.pdf. Accessed April 21, 2014.

International Crisis Group. 2014. *Counting the Costs: Myanmar's Problematic Census. Asia Briefing N°144*. Yangon/Brussels: International Crisis Group.

Iqbal G, Gumber A, Johnson MRD, et al. 2009. Improving ethnicity data collection for health statistics in the UK. *Diversity in Health and Care* 6(4):267–285.

Jha P. 2014. Reliable direct measurement of causes of death in low-and middle-income countries. *BMC Medicine* 12(1):19.

Jha P and Laxminarayan R. 2009.*Choosing Health: An Entitlement for all Indians*. Toronto: Centre for Global Health Research, University of Toronto.

Kay M. 2014. Coding a million deaths in India, one interview at a time. *BMJ* 349:g5800.

Kelm M-E. 1999. *Colonizing Bodies: Aboriginal Health and Healing in British Columbia, 1900-50*. Vancouver: UBC Press.

Kenya National Bureau of Statistics. 2015. *Economic Survey 2015*. Nairobi.

Khan M, Kobayashi K, Lee SM, and Vang Z. 2015. (In) visible minorities in Canadian health data and research. *Population Change and Lifecourse Strategic Knowledge Cluster Discussion Paper Series* 3(1):5.

Krieger N. 1992. The making of public health data: Paradigms, politics, and policy. *Journal of Public Health Policy* 13(4):412–427.

———. 2005. Stormy weather: Race, gene expression, and the science of health disparities. *American Journal of Public Health* 95(12):2155–2160.

———. 2011. *Epidemiology and the People's Health: Theory and Context*. New York: Oxford University Press.

———. 2012. Who and what is a "population?" Historical debates, current controversies, and implications for understanding "population health" and rectifying health inequities. *Milbank Quarterly* 90:634–681.

Krieger N, Chen JT, Waterman PD, et al. 2005. Painting a truer picture of US socioeconomic and racial/ethnic health inequalities: The public health disparities geocoding project. *American Journal of Public Health* 95(2):312–323.

———. 2015. Police killings and police deaths are public health data and can be counted. *PLoS Medicine* 12(12):e1001915.

Krieger N, Northridge M, Gruskin S, et al. 2003. Assessing health impact assessment: Multidisciplinary and international perspectives. *Journal of Epidemiology and Community Health* 57(9):659–662.

Krieger N and Williams DR. 2001. Changing to the 2000 standard million: Are declining racial/ethnic and socioeconomic inequalities in health real progress or statistical illusion? *American Journal of Public Health* 91(8):1209–1213.

Lawn JE, Blencowe H, Waiswa P, et al. 2016. Stillbirths: Rates, risk factors, and acceleration towards 2030. *Lancet* 387(10018):587–603.

Linell A, Richardson MX, and Wamala S. 2013. The Swedish national public health policy report 2010. *Scandinavian Journal of Public Health* 41(10 suppl):3–56.

Lofquist D. 2011. *Same-Sex Couple Households: American Community Survey Briefs*. Washington, DC: US Census Bureau.

Lopez AD, Mathers CD, Ezzati M, et al., Editors. 2006. *Global Burden of Disease and Risk Factors*. Washington, DC: Oxford University Press and World Bank.

Lozano R, Naghavi M, Foreman K, et al. 2012. Global and regional mortality from 235 causes of death for 20 age groups in 1990 and 2010: A systematic analysis for the global burden of disease study 2010. *Lancet* 380(9859):2095–2128.

Markowitz G and Rosner D. 2013. *Lead Wars: The Politics of Science and the Fate of America's Children*. Berkeley: University of California Press.

Marmot M. 2004. Social causes of social inequalities in health. In Anand S, Peter F, and Sen A, Editors. *Public Health, Ethics and Equity*. Oxford: Oxford University Press.

Martin IG and Mallela S. 2015. Funding of cancer research: Do levels match incidence and mortality rates? *Therapeutic Innovation & Regulatory Science* 49(1):33–35.

Mikkelsen L, Phillips DE, AbouZahr C, et al. 2015. A global assessment of civil registration and vital statistics systems: Monitoring data quality and progress. *Lancet* 386(10001):1395–1406.

Milloy JS. 1999. *A National Crime: The Canadian Government and the Residential School System, 1879 to 1986*. Winnipeg: University of Manitoba Press.

Morris SK, Awasthi S, Kumar R, et al. 2013. Measles mortality in high and low burden districts of India: Estimates from a nationally representative study of over 12,000 child deaths. *Vaccine* 31(41):4655–4661.

Murphy SL, Xu J, and Kochanek KD. 2013. Deaths: Final data for 2010. Centers for Disease Control and Prevention. *National Vital Statistics Report* 61(4):1–117.

Murray CJL and Lopez AD, Editors. 1996. *The Global Burden of Disease: A Comprehensive Assessment of Mortality and Disability from Diseases, Injuries and Risk Factors in 1990 and Projected to 2020*. Cambridge: Harvard School of Public Health/Harvard University Press.

Murray CJ, Lopez AD, Black R, et al. 2011. Population Health Metrics Research Consortium gold standard verbal autopsy validation study: Design, implementation, and development of analysis datasets. *Population Health Metrics* 9(1):27.

Naghavi M, Wang H, Lozano R, et al. 2015. Global, regional, and national age–sex specific all-cause and cause-specific mortality for 240 causes of death, 1990–2013: A systematic analysis for the global burden of disease study 2013. *Lancet* 385(9963):117–171.

National Institute for Health and Welfare. 2013. Human Impact Assessment. https://www.thl.fi/en/web/thlfi-en/research-and-expertwork/tools/human-impact-assessment. Accessed May 10, 2015.

National Records of Scotland. 2015. *Life Expectancy for Areas within Scotland: 2012-2014*. Edinburgh: National Records of Scotland.

Parks R. 2014. The rise, critique and persistence of the DALY in global health. *The Journal of Global Health*, August 10.

Partnership for Maternal, Neonatal and Child Health. 2011. Newborn death and illness. http://www.who.int/pmnch/media/press_materials/fs/fs_newborndealth_illness/en/. Accessed April 27, 2015.

Patel V, Ramasundarahettige C, Vijayakumar L, et al. 2012. Suicide mortality in India: A nationally representative survey. *Lancet* 379(9834):2343–2351.

Pennington A, Dreaves H, Scott-Samuel A, et al. 2015. Development of an Urban Health Impact Assessment methodology: Indicating the health equity impacts of urban policies. *The European Journal of Public Health* [Epub ahead of print].

Phillips DE, AbouZahr C, Lopez AD, et al. 2015. Are well functioning civil registration and vital statistics systems associated with better health outcomes? *Lancet* 386(10001):1386–1394.

Porta MS, Greenland S, Hernán M, et al. 2014. *A Dictionary of Epidemiology*. New York: Oxford University Press.

Reidpath D, Allotey P, Kouame A, and Cummins R. 2003. Measuring health in a vacuum: Examining the disability weight of the DALY. *Health Policy and Planning* 18(4):351–356.

Scoffield H. 2011. Ex-chief statistician picks apart cancellation of long census. *Toronto Star*, September 20.

Siddiqi A, Kawachi I, Berkman LF, et al. 2012. Education determines a nation's health, but what determines educational outcomes? A cross-national comparative analysis. *Journal of Public Health Policy* 33:1–15.

Silverman C. 2011. *Understanding Autism: Parents, Doctors, and the History of a Disorder*. Princeton: Princeton University Press.

Smylie J, Fell D, and Ohlsson A. 2010. A review of Aboriginal infant mortality rates in Canada: Striking and persistent Aboriginal/non-Aboriginal inequities. *Canadian Journal of Public Health* 101(2):143–148.

Speybroeck N, Harper S, de Savigny D, and Victora C. 2012. Inequalities of health indicators for policy makers: Six hints. *International Journal of Public Health* 57(5):855–858.

Swaroop S. 1960. *Introduction to Health Statistics for the Use of Health Officers, Students, Public Health and Social Workers*. Edinburgh: Livingstone.

Szreter S. 2012. Registration of identities in early modern English parishes and among the English overseas. In Breckenridge K and Szreter S, Editors. *Registration and Recognition: Documenting the Person in World History*. Oxford: Oxford University Press.

Thatte N, Kalter HD, Baqui AH, et al. 2009. Ascertaining causes of neonatal deaths using verbal autopsy: Current methods and challenges. *Journal of Perinatology* 29(3):187–194.

Transparency Policy Project. 2015. Disclosing International Infectious Disease Outbreaks to Protect Public Health. http://www.transparencypolicy.net/infectious-diseases-.php. Accessed August 22, 2015.

Truth and Reconciliation Commission of Canada. 2015. *Honouring the Truth, Reconciling for the Future: Summary of the Final Report of the Truth and Reconciliation Commission of Canada*. Winnipeg: TRC.

UN Department of Economic and Social Affairs. 1973. *The Determinants and Consequences of Population Trends: New Summary of Findings of Interaction of Demographic, Economic and Social Factors*. New York: UN.

———. 2008. *Principles and Recommendations for Population and Housing Censuses, Revision 2*. New York: UN.

———. 2011. *World Population Prospects: The 2010 Revision, Volume I*. New York: UN.

UNESCAP. 2015. Civil registration and vital statistics. http://www.unescap.org/our-work/statistics/civil-registration-and-vital-statistics/about. Accessed May 14, 2015.

UNFPA. 2003. *Counting the People: Constraining Census Costs and Assessing Alternative Approaches: Population and Development Strategies Series, Number 7*. New York: UNFPA.

———. 2014a. *ICPD Beyond 2014 Global Report* [Unedited Version]. New York: UNFPA.

———. 2014b. *Making Sense of Myanmar's Census*. New York: UNFPA.

UNICEF. 2013. *Levels & Trends in Child Mortality: Report 2013 Estimates Developed by the UN Inter-agency Group for Child Mortality Estimation*. New York: UNICEF.

———. 2015a. *Levels and Trends in Child Mortality: Report 2015, Estimates Developed by the UN Inter-agency Group for Child Mortality Estimation*. New York: UNICEF.

———. 2015b. The births of nearly one third of the global population of children under five have never been registered. http://data.unicef.org/child-protection/birth-registration#sthash.nSNLGgSp.dpuf. Accessed April 27, 2015.

United Nations. 2015. Transforming our world: the 2030 Agenda for Sustainable Development. https://sustainabledevelopment.un.org/post2015/transformingourworld. Accessed September 10, 2015.

———. 2016. 2020 World Population and Housing Census Programme: Q & A. http://unstats.un.org/unsd/demographic/sources/census/wphc/QA.htm. Accessed June 30, 2016.

US Census Bureau. 2014. *2020 Census: Race and Hispanic Origin Research Working Group. National Advisory Committee on Racial, Ethnic and Other Populations*. Washington, DC: U.S. Census Bureau.

———. 2015. International Data Base. http://www.census.gov/population/international/data/idb/. Accessed June 22, 2016.

Victora CG. 2015. Causes of child deaths: Looking to the future. *Lancet* 385(9966):398–399.

Victora CG and Barros FC. 2012. Cohorts in low- and middle-income countries: From still photographs to full-length movies. *Journal of Adolescent Health* 51(6):S3.

von Glahn R. 2012. Household registration, property rights, and social obligations in imperial China: Principles and practices. In Breckenridge K and Szreter S, Editors. *Registration and Recognition: Documenting the Person in World History*. Oxford: Oxford University Press.

Vos T, Barber RM, Bell B, et al. 2015. Global, regional, and national incidence, prevalence, and years lived with disability for 301 acute and chronic diseases and injuries in 188 countries, 1990–2013: A systematic analysis for the Global Burden of Disease Study 2013. *Lancet* 386(9995):743–800.

Wang H, Schumacher AE, Levitz CE, et al. 2013. Left behind: Widening disparities for males and females in US county life expectancy, 1985–2010. *Population Health Metrics* 11(1):1–8.

Westly E. 2013. One million deaths: What researchers are learning from an unprecedented survey of mortality in India. *Nature* 504:22–23.

WHO. 1992. *ICD-10: International Statistical Classification of Diseases and Related Health Problems, Tenth Revision and updated version for 2007*. Geneva: WHO.

———. 1993. *International Statistical Classification of Diseases and Related Health Problems, Tenth Revision.* Vol. 2. Geneva: WHO.

———. 2000. *World Health Report 2000. Health Systems: Improving Performance.* Geneva: WHO.

———. 2007. Frequently asked questions about the International Health Regulations (2005). http://www.who.int/csr/ihr/howtheywork/faq/en/index.html#whatis. Accessed June 16, 2007.

———. 2011. Commission on information and accountability for women's and children's health. http://www.who.int/woman_child_accountability/about/coia/en/. Accessed June 8, 2015.

———. 2012. Management of patient information: Trends and challenges in Member States. *Global Observatory for eHealth Series, Volume 6.* Geneva: WHO.

———. 2013a. *Civil Registration and Vital Statistics 2013: Challenges, Best Practice and Design Principles for Modern Systems.* Geneva: WHO.

———. 2013b. Disease and injury regional estimates for 2000-2011. Geneva: WHO. http://www.who.int/healthinfo/global_burden_disease/estimates_regional_2000_2011/en/. Accessed February 11, 2014.

———. 2013c. *Strengthening Civil Registration and Vital Statistics for Births, Deaths and Causes of Death: Resource Kit.* Geneva: WHO.

———. 2014a. Civil registration: Why counting births and deaths is important. Fact sheet No. 324. Updated May 2014. http://www.who.int/mediacentre/factsheets/fs324/en/. Accessed 10 May 10, 2015.

———. 2014b. Civil registration of deaths. http://www.who.int/gho/mortality_burden_disease/registered_deaths/text/en/. Accessed April 24, 2014.

———. 2014c. Civil registration of deaths: coverage of registration. http://www.who.int/gho/mortality_burden_disease/registered_deaths/en/. Accessed June 26, 2015.

———. 2014d. Global health estimates. http://www.who.int/healthinfo/global_burden_disease/en/. Accessed February 9, 2016.

———. 2015a. Global Health Observatory data repository. http://www.who.int/gho/database/en/. Accessed June 1, 2015.

———. 2015b. Implementation of the International Health Regulations (2005): Responding to public health emergencies. http://reliefweb.int/sites/reliefweb.int/files/resources/B136_22-en.pdf Accessed May 2, 2015.

———. 2015c. International Statistical Classification of Diseases and Related Health Problems 10th Revision (ICD-10). http://apps.who.int/classifications/icd10/browse/2015/en#/XXII. Accessed May 14, 2015.

———. 2015d. Maternal mortality ratio (per 100 000 live births). http://www.who.int/healthinfo/statistics/indmaternalmortality/en/. Accessed February 9, 2016.

———. 2015e. *State of Inequality: Reproductive, Maternal, Newborn and Child Health.* Geneva: WHO.

———. 2016. *World Health Statistics 2016: Monitoring Health for the SDGs.* Geneva: WHO.

WHO Commission on Social Determinants of Health. 2008. *Closing the Gap in a Generation: Health Equity Through Action on the Social Determinants of Health. Final Report of the Commission on Social Determinants of Health.* Geneva: WHO.

WHO, UNICEF, UNFPA, et al. 2015. *Trends in Maternal Mortality: 1990 to 2015.* Geneva: WHO.

Wood E. 2014. *Implementing Reform: How Maryland & New York Ended Prison Gerrymandering.* New York: Dēmos.

Woolsey TD. 1979. *Needed Development Research for Measuring the Health of Populations in the Less Developed Countries. International Health Planning Methods Series,* Volume 10. Washington, DC: Agency for International Development.

World Bank. 1993. *World Development Report 1993: Investing in Health.* New York: Oxford University Press for the World Bank.

———. 2015. Global civil registration and vital statistics scaling up investment plan 2015-2024. http://www.worldbank.org/en/topic/health/publication/global-civil-registration-vital-statistics-scaling-up-investment. Accessed May 2, 2015.

———. 2016. World Development Indicators. http://databank.worldbank.org/data. Accessed June 30, 2016.

World Bank and WHO. 2014. *Global Civil Registration and Vital Statistics: Scaling up Investment Plan 2015–2024.* Washington, DC: World Bank.

6

EPIDEMIOLOGIC PROFILES OF GLOBAL HEALTH AND DISEASE

Having discussed the importance of—and challenges to—health data collection (see chapter 5), we now examine global health and disease patterns from several perspectives. While all causes of mortality and morbidity have "natural" histories and pathogenic processes, these are not inevitable and are shaped by larger political, economic, social, and demographic factors. Here, we start with a broad analysis of mortality profiles by country income level, age group, and other key aspects, including dimensions of gender and health, disability, Indigenous health, oral health, and the health of people who inject drugs. We continue with a detailed exploration of the major causes of illness and death based upon a political economy typology that categorizes diseases by the general societal conditions of marginalization, deprivation, and modernization in which they typically occur. Undoubtedly, there are significant challenges regarding the validity of global health data. Here we cite the most accurate data available, albeit cognizant of their deficiencies.

To begin, we review some basic epidemiologic terms that are essential to understanding public health epidemiology (Table 6-1).

LEADING CAUSES OF MORBIDITY AND MORTALITY ACROSS SOCIETIES AND THE LIFE CYCLE

Key Questions:

- How do patterns of mortality compare across countries?
- What are the structural factors shaping these patterns?
- How do the underlying causes of death change across the lifecourse?

Patterns of disease and death vary across and within countries, depending on political, economic, environmental, and social contexts, as well as biological susceptibility. We have chosen three countries with different levels of income and redistribution to demonstrate the range in causes of death.

1. High-income/redistributive: Italy
2. Middle-income/partially redistributive: Indonesia
3. Low-income/marginally redistributive: Kenya

Table 6-1 Public Health Epidemiologic Terms	
Acute disease	A disease of sudden onset, often brief, intense, or short-term.
Association	Statistical dependence between two or more events, characteristics, or other variables. It is present if the probability of occurrence of an event or characteristic, or the quantity of a variable, varies with the occurrence of one or more other events, the presence of one or more other characteristics, or the quantity of one or more other variables.
Case fatality rate	The proportion of cases of a specified condition that are fatal within a specified time. Defined as: $\frac{\text{Number of deaths from a disease (in a given period)}}{\text{Number of diagnosed cases of that disease (in the same period)}} \times 100$
Chronic disease	A disease that lasts from several weeks to many years. Often used interchangeably with NCD.
Communicable disease	An illness due to a specific infectious agent or its toxic products, arising through transmission of that agent or its products from an infected person, animal, or reservoir to a susceptible host, either directly or indirectly. Also known as infectious diseases. Contagious diseases refer to those transmissible via direct contact and through droplet transmission.
Death rate (crude)	An estimate of the portion of a population that dies during a specified period. See chapter 5 for full definition and formula.
Endemic disease	The constant occurrence and/or high prevalence of a disease, disorder, or noxious infectious agent in a geographic area or population group.
Epidemic	The occurrence in a community or region of cases of an illness, specific health-related behavior, or other health-related events clearly in excess of normal expectancy.
Exposure	Proximity or contact with a source of a disease agent in such a manner that effective transmission of the agent or harmful effects of the agent may occur.
Incidence	The number of new health-related events in a defined population within a specified period of time, a rate.
Infant mortality rate (IMR)	A measure of the yearly rate of deaths in children less than 1 year old.
Maternal death	Death of a woman while pregnant or within 42 days of termination of a pregnancy.
Noncommunicable disease (NCD)	A disease due to a non-infectious cause that is: non-transmissible between persons; not equivalent to the natural process of aging; arises through pathogenic processes within the human body, or as a result of toxic exposure; can be influenced by societal and environmental conditions.
Pandemic	An epidemic occurring worldwide, or over a very wide area, crossing international boundaries and affecting a large number of people.
Prevalence	The total number of individuals who have a health condition at a particular time (or during a particular period) divided by the population at risk of having the attribute or disease at this point in time or midway through the period. A ratio.
Stratification	The process or result of separating a group into several subgroups according to specified criteria, such as age or socioeconomic status.
Surveillance	Systematic ongoing collection, collation, and analysis of data and the timely dissemination of information to those who need to know so that action can be taken.

Sources: Last (2001) and Porta (2014) by permission of Oxford University Press, Inc.

Note: Other health indicators (such as MMR) and details on definitions may be found in Table 5-2.

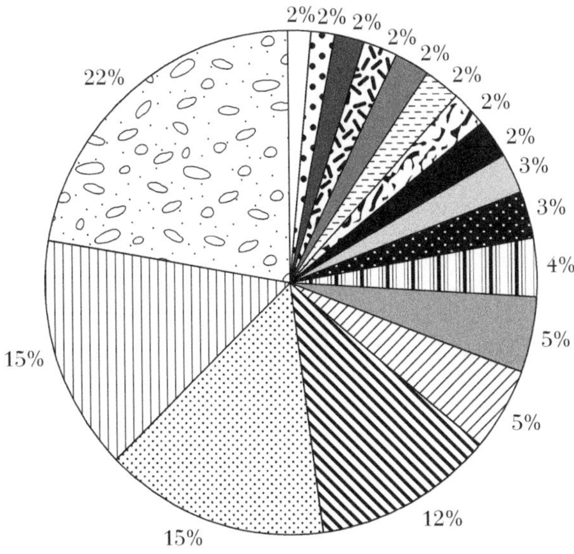

Self-harm (842,000)
Malaria (855,000)
Hypertensive heart disease (1.1 million)
Cirrhosis of the liver (1.2 million)
Diarrheal diseases (1.3 million)
Tuberculosis (1.3 million)
Diabetes (1.3 million)
HIV/AIDS (1.3 million)
Road injuries (1.4 million)
Alzheimer's disease and other dementias (1.7 million)
Neonatal disorders (2 million)
Respiratory infections (2.7 million)
COPD (2.9 million)
Stroke (6.4 million)
Coronary heart disease (8.1 million)
Cancers (8.2 million)
Other (12.2 million)

Top specific causes for broader cause of death categories
***Cancers*:** tracheal, bronchus and lung cancer; stomach cancer; liver cancer; colon and rectum cancer.
Neonatal disorders: preterm birth complications; birth asphyxia and trauma; neonatal sepsis and other infections.
Respiratory infections: upper and lower respiratory infections.
Stroke: ischemic stroke and hemmorhagic stroke.

Figure 6-1: Leading causes of death in the world, 2013.
Data Source: Naghavi et al. (2015).

Figure 6-1 shows the leading causes of death in the world (without any income stratification) reported by the Institute for Health Metrics and Evaluation's (IHME) Global Burden of Disease (GBD) project (discussed in chapter 5). Globally, the three leading causes of death are noncommunicable (chronic) conditions: coronary heart disease (CHD) (also known as ischemic heart disease), cancer, and cerebrovascular disease (stroke) (combined, 42% of all deaths).

Italy, a high-income country (HIC), has more income inequality and child poverty than many of its European neighbors. Although in the past decade Italy has significantly increased its social welfare spending, much of it has gone to pensions (OECD 2014). Life expectancy in Italy is high (83 years) and (under-5) child mortality rates are below 5 deaths per 1,000 live births (among the lowest 20 in the world). The maternal mortality ratio is also low, at 4 deaths/100,000 live births. Figure 6-2 shows the leading causes of death in the country: CHD, cerebrovascular disease, other cardiovascular diseases, and trachea, bronchus, and lung cancers.

Indonesia is a partially redistributive middle-income country (MIC). Life expectancy in Indonesia is considerably lower than in Europe: 69 years. The infant and child mortality rates are 22.8 and 27.2 deaths per 1,000 live births, respectively, over 5 times higher than Italy. Maternal mortality is over 30 times higher than in Italy, at 126 deaths per 100,000 live births. Figure 6-3 shows the leading causes of death in Indonesia: cerebrovascular disease, CHD, and tuberculosis (TB). Closely behind are diabetes, lower respiratory infections, and asthma.

Kenya is a marginally redistributive low-income country (LIC) with very poor health indices. Life expectancy in Kenya is only 63 years. The infant mortality rate (IMR) is 35.5 deaths per 1,000 live births, and the child mortality rate is 49.4 deaths per 1,000

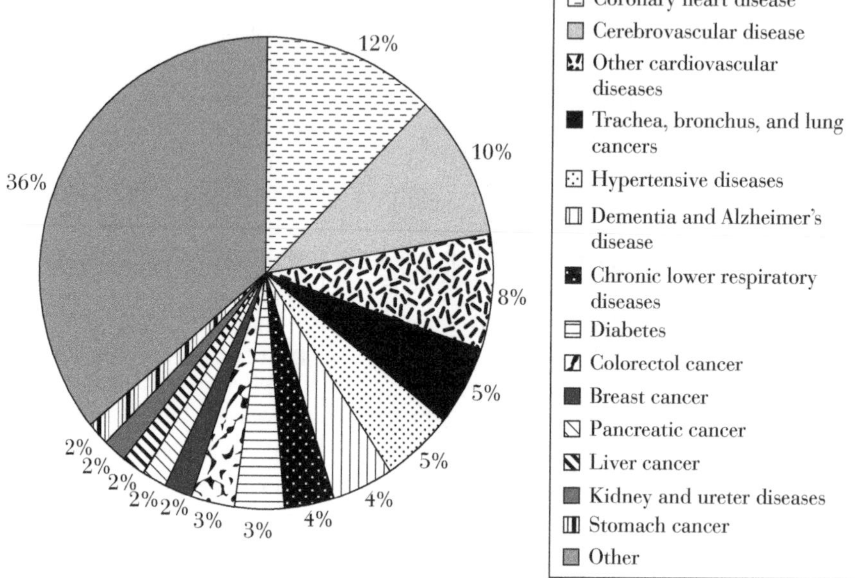

Figure 6-2: Leading causes of death in Italy, 2012.
Data Source: Istituto Nazionale di Statistica (2014).

live births. Maternal mortality is extremely high, at 510 deaths per 100,000 live births, more than 125 times Italy's level. Figure 6-4 shows the leading killers in Kenya, with malaria, pneumonia, and cancers topping the list of major causes according to registered deaths in Kenya's civil registration system, and AIDS, lower respiratory infections, and diarrheal diseases at the top of the list according to IHME's estimates. Chapter 5

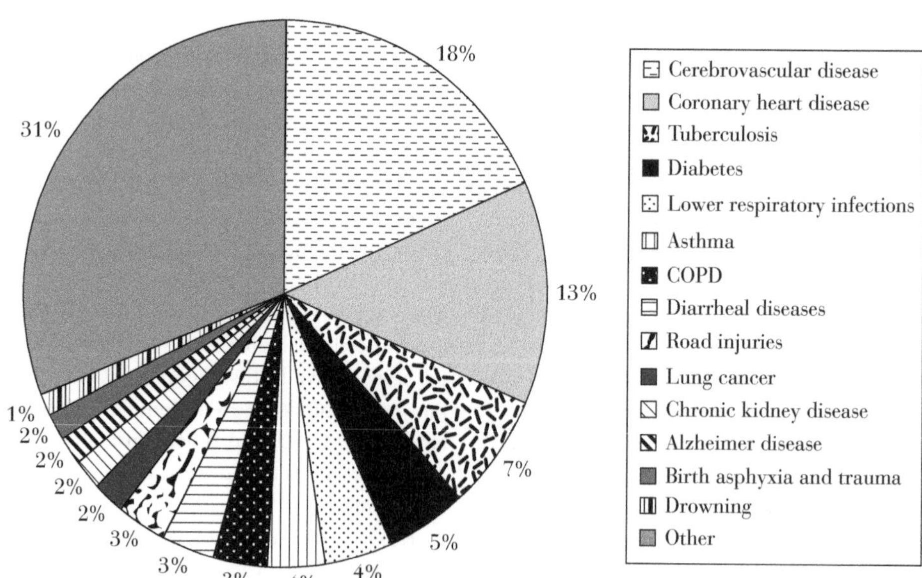

Figure 6-3: Leading causes of death in Indonesia, 2013.
Data Source: IHME (2013a).

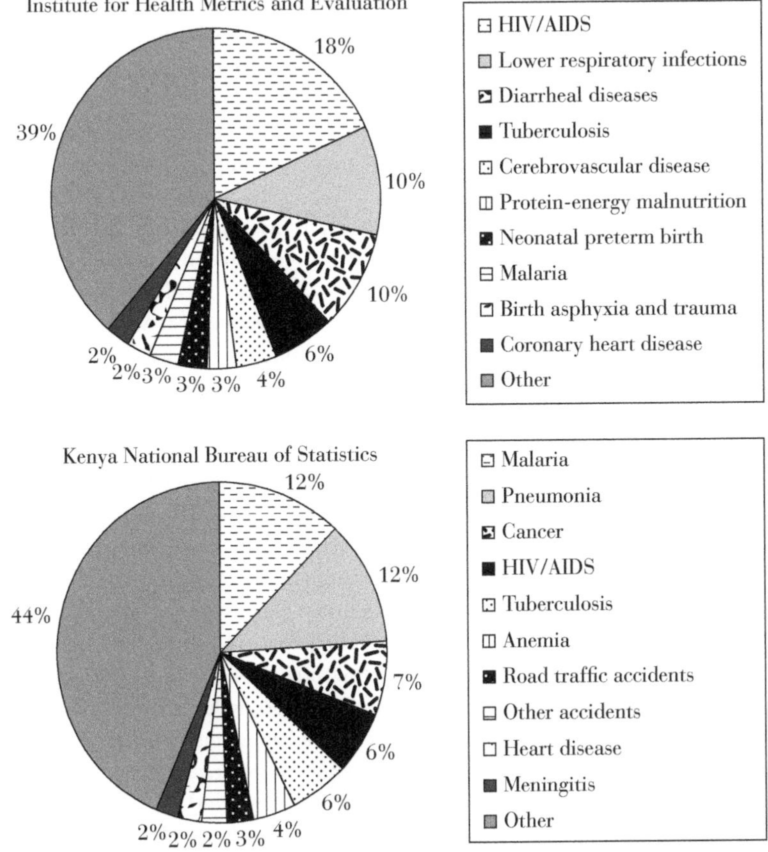

Figure 6-4: Leading causes of death in Kenya according to IHME and the Kenya National Bureau of Statistics, 2013.
Data Sources: IHME (2013a); Kenya National Bureau of Statistics (2015).

discusses the differences in leading causes of death between these sources.

Figure 6-5 shows a selection of countries in order from highest GDP per capita (Denmark) to lowest GDP per capita (Ethiopia). There is a tendency for LICs to have a higher age-standardized mortality rate from communicable, perinatal, nutritional, and injury-related causes. The trend is less clear for

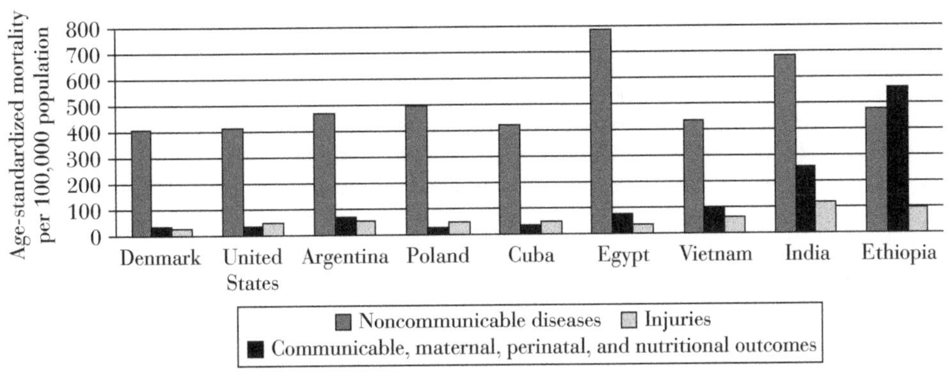

Figure 6-5: Age-standardized mortality rate among selected countries, 2012.
Data Source: WHO (2015f).

noncommunicable diseases (NCDs): lower-middle income countries Egypt and India have much higher NCD mortality rates than Denmark and the United States.

The Present Plagues: Noncommunicable Diseases

While these examples show a greater proportion of infectious disease deaths in low- and middle-income countries (LMICs) than HICs, the oft-repeated dichotomy between HICs experiencing principally chronic disease mortality and LMICs having mostly infectious mortality does not hold. At present another trend is indisputable: all countries face a growing burden of NCDs as well as the threat of health problems linked to climate change (see chapter 10).

NCDs—especially CHD, chronic lung diseases, cancer, and diabetes—now cause over two thirds of all deaths, with an estimated 74% of global NCD deaths in LMICs (WHO 2015o). In 2011 the UN General Assembly held a high level meeting to discuss the rising incidence of NCDs, adopting a political declaration on the need to reduce "risk factors," strengthen national capacity for prevention, promote research on prevention and control, and increase international cooperation (UN General Assembly 2012) (Box 6-1). Previously these diseases were regarded as "diseases of the affluent," often attributed to poor "lifestyle" choices such as unhealthy diets. In reality, NCDs are present in all countries, as demonstrated in Figures 6-2 to 6-5, and are closely linked to societal and global patterns of work, stress, trade, production, aging, marketing, and consumption (PHM et al. 2014).

To be sure, many HICs have seen dramatic decreases in heart disease and stroke in part due to medical (e.g., blood pressure-lowering drugs) and behavioral (e.g., smoking cessation and increased exercise) interventions. As per chapters 3 and 7, however, modifying personal risk factors through behavioral and medical approaches are only one part of the story.

Increasing rates of NCDs can be partially traced to a dietary shift from whole grains, pulses, and fresh fruits and vegetables to more processed diets high in sugar, transfats, and animal-source food (Popkin, Adair, and Ng 2012). Neoliberal capitalist globalization (see chapter 9) has played an important part in altering local production, access, cost, and availability of nutritious food in LMICs through deregulation of food markets, industrialized food production, global food marketing, displacement of small farmers, and penetration of transnational agribusiness corporations (Hawkes 2006).

Paradoxically, in HICs and LMICs alike, poor and socially excluded children are vulnerable to

Box 6-1 Approaches to Prevention and Control of NCDs

Control of NCDs resides at the confluence of politics, public health, business, and medicine. Public health campaigns often focus on primary prevention strategies of improving diet, promoting physical activity, and creating healthy environments to help reduce NCDs. Biomedical approaches (supported by Big Pharma, among other forces) usually promote interventions and medications at the level of individuals and specific diseases (see chapter 3).

Prevention measures are classified as primary, secondary, and tertiary. Primary prevention is undertaken to prevent infection or exposure, avoid the development of disease, and promote overall health. Secondary prevention is aimed at early detection (and treatment) of disease to prevent its further development, such as colonoscopy screening programs to detect colorectal cancer and remove polyps. Tertiary prevention is similar to disease management and attempts to mitigate the negative effects of, or any complications or disability arising from, an illness once a person is diagnosed.

While there is clearly a role for these forms of prevention, they neglect societal interventions that could prevent NCDs, including reducing carbon emissions through regulation of industry, regulating and taxing soft drinks, providing strong welfare state protections, and regulating food transnationals so that local healthy produce is not outpriced by processed foods. Chapters 3, 7, and 9 discuss in greater depth how social factors and political systems affect health.

both hunger and obesity (and diabetes), due to the low cost of energy-dense foods; moreover a dual burden of undernutrition and overnutrition may exist within the same household in Indonesia, Ecuador, and elsewhere (Tzioumis and Adair 2014).

Health of Infants and Children

One of the greatest achievements in international health over the past half century has been the dramatic reduction of overall infant and child mortality. In 1960 there were 20 million deaths of children under the age of 5; by 2015 this had been reduced to 5.9 million (2.9 million in sub-Saharan Africa alone). This greater than 75% decline (from 198 deaths per 1,000 live births to 43) was accomplished through improved sanitation, maternal and infant nutrition, vaccination, and primary health care interventions (UNICEF 2015a). In recent decades, countries as distinct as Cuba, South Korea, and Rwanda (post-genocide) have seen remarkable declines in under-5 mortality. Notwithstanding this progress, the numbers remain appallingly high—equivalent to 16,000 children dying every day, nearly all preventable, and many without access to care. Approximately 45% of under-5 deaths occur within the first month of life. Currently, most deaths in children under 5 result from treatable or preventable causes such as pneumonia, malaria, measles, diarrhea, and AIDS. Of the 60 countries with the highest rates of child mortality, only 14 met the 2015 Millennium Development Goal (MDG) of reducing under-5 mortality by two thirds (UN IGME 2015).

The IMR is often cited as the most sensitive indicator of a general level of "development" and the state of health of a population. High IMRs reflect underlying inadequacies in socioeconomic and sanitary conditions. Many of the leading causes of infant and child mortality are preventable through structural and redistributive policy approaches.

Despite declines in global childhood mortality, these are not equitably distributed. Advances have been made in many MICs but in LICs, especially in sub-Saharan Africa, reducing neonatal mortality and stillbirth rates has been slower than childhood mortality improvements overall (Darmstadt et al. 2014) (Figure 6-6). At present rates of decline, it will take over a century before survival prospects of African newborns match the current situation in North America and Europe (Lawn et al. 2014). Moreover, *within* many countries, a child from the poorest population group is almost twice as likely to die before his or her fifth birthday as a child from the wealthiest, and this gap is widening (UNICEF 2015a).

Potential causes of infant mortality begin in utero. Most importantly, poor maternal nutrition

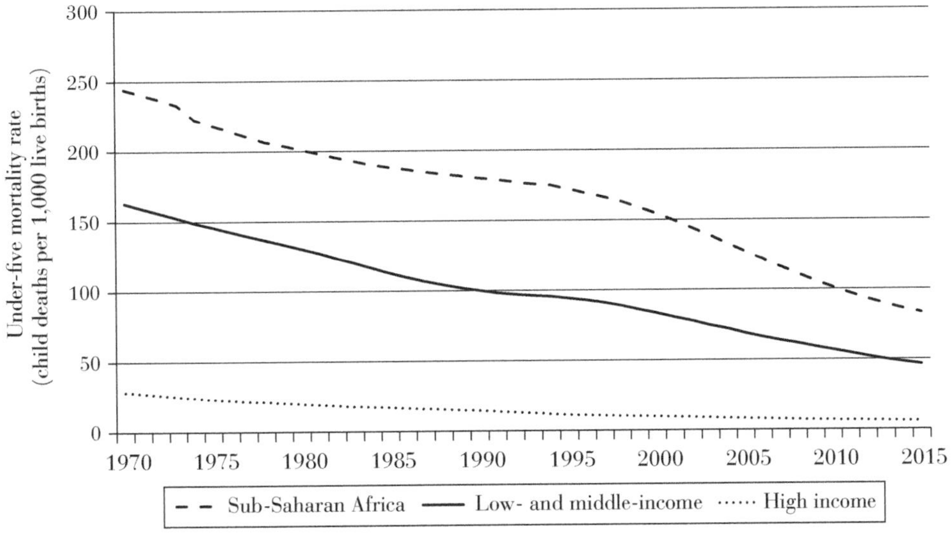

Figure 6-6: Trends in under-5 child mortality, 1970–2015.
Data Source: IGME (2015).

can lead to low birthweight, affecting, for example, cognitive and respiratory development. Infections transmitted perinatally include tetanus, syphilis, and HIV (Partnership for Maternal, Newborn and Child Health 2011). Hepatitis B virus—infecting more than 2 billion people—is primarily transmitted in utero and during birth, increasing likelihood of chronic liver conditions later in life (WHO 2015i).

Malnutrition is a key determinant of both respiratory illnesses and diarrhea, linked to just under half of child deaths (Black et al. 2013) (Figure 6-7). Chronic undernutrition into early childhood has serious consequences: vitamin A deficiency is linked to blindness; iodine deficiency to growth failure and intellectual disability, and iron deficiency to learning disabilities, all with lifelong effects. Early exposure to environmental contaminants, like air pollution, can also generate chronic problems, including lung disease, asthma, and cancer.

Although nearly half of under-5 mortality occurs in the neonatal period, only 4% of global maternal and child health funding goes to newborn health (Darmstadt et al. 2014). Yet wide implementation of existing interventions for maternal and child well-being—including skilled birth attendants at delivery, immunization and antibiotic treatment for pregnant women and newborns, hygienic practices during delivery, and exclusive breastfeeding for the first 6 months of life—could prevent most neonatal deaths (Bhutta et al. 2014). Still, these important interventions focus on the immediate determinants of child (and maternal) health but fall short of considering underlying factors. For example, breastfeeding has a crucial protective role against malnutrition, diarrhea, and other early childhood ailments. However, exclusive breastfeeding is often impeded by maternal–infant separation for work reasons, maternal illness, or weaning and mixed feeding practices promoted by infant formula companies (see Box 9-3 for details).

Toddlers (aged 12–36 months) are subject to a variety of respiratory illnesses (e.g., influenza virus and rhinovirus), diseases related to immature immunological systems (e.g., diarrhea), and environmental dangers (e.g., indoor pollution, malaria).

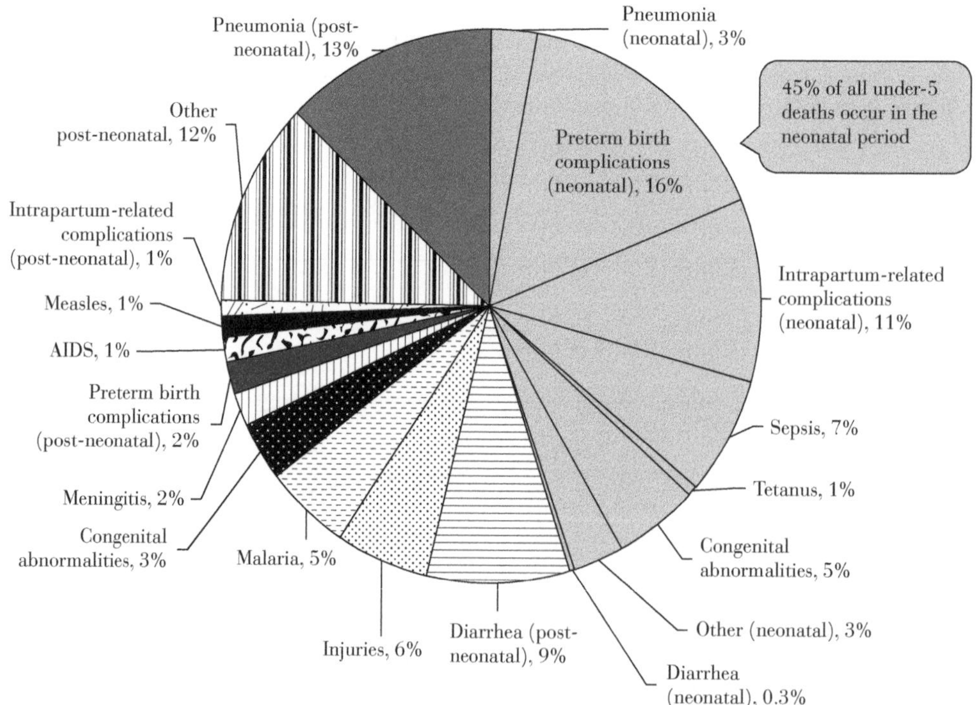

Figure 6-7: Global distribution of deaths among children under 5 by cause, 2015.
Source: WHO and Maternal and Child Epidemiology Estimation Group 2015.

Interventions to improve survival of young children overlap with those for infants and include providing potable water, improving cooking facilities, oral rehydration therapy for diarrhea, as well as malaria prevention and treatment (UNICEF 2015a).

The Health of Children Five and Older and of Young Adults: Unique Realities and Issues

Over 40% of the world's population is under 25 years old, representing the largest youth generation in history (US Census Bureau 2015). Childhood and youth may be the healthiest time of life, but 5 to 25 year olds face among the highest rates of death due to road injuries (WHO 2015q), poisonings (WHO 2013a), drownings (WHO 2014d) and other "accidental" causes of death, as well as suicide and homicide (WHO 2014f). Mental health disorders, and particularly depression, are a principal cause of disability in youth worldwide (WHO 2016a). Gender-based violence is a leading cause of death for young women in many countries. Asthma and other respiratory problems are common in childhood, and have significant effects on schooling, family life, and daily activities, especially in LMICs.

Societal factors in childhood are particularly important in shaping health across the lifecourse. Early education has great consequences for health and quality of life, yet as many as 58 million 5- to 12-year-olds do not attend school. Although girls have experienced a global increase in school attendance at all levels (UNICEF 2015b), there remains a sharp decline in female attendance following primary school. Almost one fourth of the world's youth live in extreme poverty, and in many LICs more than half of students must work to support their families instead of attending secondary school. Furthermore, an estimated 85 million children aged 5 to 17 years work in hazardous conditions (ILO 2015), and coerced work/human trafficking (related to sex work and indentured labor) is a major health problem.

Because many youth lack the ability or social support to delay the age of sexual debut, negotiate safer sex, or protect themselves against unintended pregnancy and sexually transmitted infections, globally 50% of HIV infections occur in people aged 15 to 24, and 1 in 7 new infections occur in adolescence, wherein it is the second leading cause of death (UNFPA 2014). Young women have twice the infection rate as young men (UNAIDS 2012), in large part due to inadequate or nonexistent sexual health education programs and health services, and laws that prohibit dispensing contraception to youth or unmarried women.

Health through the Lifecourse

The health of adults (defined by WHO as persons aged 25 to 60 years) is distinct from that of children and the elderly because adults typically have greater immunity and recover more readily from acute communicable illnesses. Conversely, adults face more chronic health problems. Rates of many noncommunicable (and some communicable) conditions are much higher in adults than among children.

Adults form the economic backbone of all countries, but their health, with exceptions in the area of reproduction and HIV, typically elicits little attention from policymakers and planners. Yet adult deaths, illnesses, injuries, and disabilities reduce productivity and family income and well-being. Moreover, the chronicity of many adult illnesses places heavy social and financial burdens on health services and caregivers.

Mental Health

Mental health is a long under-emphasized aspect of global health, framed by discrimination, concentration of mental illness in poor and socially excluded populations, and challenges in measurement and treatment (Becker and Kleinman 2013). One in four people are estimated to experience a mental health problem during their lifetime (Kessler et al. 2009). Worldwide, 350 million people are estimated to suffer from depression, 21 million from schizophrenia (WHO 2016e), over 40 million from alcohol use disorders, and over 29 million from drug use disorders (UNODC 2016). Accompanying and potentially contributing to this distress, "[a]n overwhelming majority of people with mental and psychosocial disabilities are living in poverty, poor physical health, and are subject to human rights violations" (WHO 2015m). These numbers are also framed by changes in the clinical definition of depression: people enduring suffering due to economic insecurity and other adverse circumstances are increasingly classified as depressed (Prins et al. 2015).

Mental health problems—especially suicide—often accompany other illnesses, particularly NCDs. Over 800,000 people commit suicide each year, three quarters taking place in LMICs. Even though women attempt suicide more than men, men's completed suicide rates are three times higher in HICs, and one and a half times higher in LMICs (WHO 2014g). Mental health disorders are often intertwined with substance abuse, as some may turn to addictive drugs like alcohol, cocaine, prescription painkillers, and heroin to relieve their symptoms. Few countries provide substance abuse counseling and treatment together with mental health services, despite high need. In the United States and countries with growing incarceration rates (especially linked to narcotics possession and minor infractions), up to one third of inmates suffer from mental illness, reflecting its increasing criminalization (Ford 2015).

Across the world, mental illness, especially schizophrenia, is disproportionately borne by the poor and oppressed. Accumulated lifelong stressors such as precarious living and working conditions, social isolation, exploitation and mistreatment, and lack of health care and social support, also lead to symptoms of distress consistent with what is characterized as depression. Higher rates of mental disorders among women and sexual minorities reflect discrimination, disenfranchisement, gender oppression, and poverty in HICs and LMICs alike (WHO 2010).

It is estimated that over three fourths of persons with serious mental illness in LMICs do not receive treatment, with as little as US$0.20 per capita spent on care in LICs compared with US$45 in HICs. In many LMICs only institutionally based services are available, and social support for family and caregivers is inadequate (WHO 2013b).

These deficiencies have garnered increasing attention, with experts calling for better integration of mental health services within health systems, expansion of a global research agenda, and greater drug availability (Lancet GMHG 2007; Patel and Prince 2010). In response, WHO established the Mental Health Gap Action Programme (mhGAP) in 2013 and has endorsed a mental health action plan (WHO 2013b).

While there are clearly unmet mental health needs in LMICs, the predominantly biomedical approach of the global mental health movement and its emphasis on the scaling-up of treatment interventions, notwithstanding vast contextual, cultural, and ideological differences among populations, has met with criticism (Timimi 2011). Accused of cultural and medical imperialism, the movement may inappropriately impose Western models of psychiatry in LMICs (Watters 2010), and ignore local and Indigenous understandings of mental health, emotional responses, and ways of coping (Das and Rao 2012; Fernando, 2014; Summerfield 2013). This is compounded by the powerful influence of the pharmaceutical industry on biomedical psychiatry (see chapter 11): in their endless pursuit of new markets and profits, pharmaceutical companies have been accused of participating in the medicalization of psycho-social distress (Mills 2014) and charged with illegally promoting their products (Moncrieff 2009; Whitaker and Cosgrove 2015).

Disability

An estimated 15% of the world's population, roughly 1 billion people, live with a disability (WHO 2015e). Because definitions of disability are shaped by cultural and societal factors, the term *impairment* is also used, defined as the point at which a person faces "problems in body function or structure," which may be physical, mental, and/or intellectual in nature. Whereas disability results from a confluence of factors—medical, physical, economic, and environmental, primarily determined by societal discrimination and exclusion from work, education, and other activities that could enable self-sufficiency—impairment is more discrete (WHO 2007b; ILO 2002). For example, a person may be impaired by the loss of a limb, but the impairment only becomes a disability if the person cannot fully participate in society. Technologies and medical interventions, such as hearing aids, may alleviate impairment, but disabilities are only countered through social change (Durham 2002).

Poverty both underlies and results from disability; 80% of people with disabilities live in LICs, often in isolated settings, and an estimated 20% of the world's poorest people live with disabilities. Throughout the world, persons with disabilities face social exclusion and disadvantages in accessing education, health, and social services (particularly in rural areas) and are more likely to be unemployed (Mitra, Posarac, and Vick 2013).

People living with disabilities often require specialized rehabilitation programs and therapy, which can alleviate some economic and social difficulties. But many countries do not provide such care. In LMICs, only 5% to 15% of persons in need of assistive devices (e.g., wheelchairs, prosthetics) have access to them. Furthermore, the devices that are available are frequently of poor quality and prohibitively expensive (WHO Kobe Centre 2013). In HICs, too, people with disabilities face significantly higher unemployment rates, and hard-won disability benefits have been slashed in financial crisis-justified austerity programs.

In 2006, following years of persistent civil society advocacy, the UN passed the *Convention on the Rights of Persons with Disabilities* "to promote, protect and ensure the full and equal enjoyment of all human rights and fundamental freedoms by all persons with disabilities, and to promote respect for their inherent dignity." Although many countries have ratified the convention, ableism—discrimination against people with disabilities—remains pervasive and disability issues still receive inadequate attention globally and in domestic policies, especially due to "lack of access to dignified living conditions, employment, housing, and health care services" (Fiorati and Elui 2015).

Sexually Transmitted Infections

Sexually transmitted infections (STIs), also referred to as sexually transmitted diseases (STDs), include viral, bacterial, and parasitic infections transmitted through sex. Some of the most common STIs are chlamydia, gonorrhea, syphilis, herpes simplex virus, human papillomavirus (HPV), pubic lice, and HIV.

Each year, there are over 350 million new STI infections. STIs are a main preventable cause of infertility among women, due to chronic, undiagnosed infection. Mother-to-child transmission of STIs can lead to stillbirth, neonatal death, pneumonia, and congenital deformities (WHO 2015r).

STIs are largely preventable through barrier methods of protection (e.g., condoms) during sexual activity. However, these methods are not always available or appropriate. The spread of STIs is largely determined by other factors, including transactional sex, forced sex, migrant labor, gender disparities, and inaccessible health services.

Most bacterial STIs are curable through short-course antibiotic therapy, and many viral STIs can be managed through medication and improvements in immunologic status. Factors such as stigma, cost, and availability of medical and laboratory services often inhibit people from seeking diagnosis and/or treatment.

People Who Inject Drugs

Substance use and abuse can have acute and long-term detrimental effects on health among people who inject drugs, including reduced memory and cognitive function, and increased injury rates resulting from impaired perceptive capabilities and reflexes. People who inject drugs are at increased risk of other conditions, such as dermatologic, pulmonary, cardiovascular, genitourinary problems, and diabetes and hypertension. They may face unemployment and associated impoverishment and homelessness, violence, mental illness, and family estrangement (Nambiar, Stoove, and Dietze 2014). There are an estimated 12 million people who inject drugs globally (UNODC 2016). Many viral infections are spread through injection drug use. Outside of sub-Saharan Africa, 30% of new HIV infections are attributed to injecting, and in some regions it is up to 80% (AVERT 2015). Currently, an estimated 130 to 150 million people are infected with hepatitis C virus (HCV), which is transmitted largely through injection drug use and non-sterile medical injections, and can lead to liver failure and cancer (WHO 2015j). Some HCV transmission may also occur through sex, in utero, and from blood transfusions. HCV can now be cured, but treatment costs US$84,000 per 12-week course, which few can afford. Hepatitis B virus is another liver infection that is commonly spread via unsterilized, reused needles and syringes, and also transmitted congenitally and in health care settings. Although the highly effective hepatitis B vaccine is increasingly administered at birth or early childhood in many countries, this will not affect rates of liver cancer or end-stage liver disease for another generation (WHO 2015i).

Addressing drug use and related health effects among people who inject drugs is complex. Some countries (Switzerland, Holland) and cities

(Vancouver, Berlin) have provided safe injection sites, clean needles and disposal facilities, opiate substitution therapy, and nursing and addiction counseling staff. These practices—known as harm reduction strategies—have reduced the spread of disease and other adverse health effects. However, many people still oppose needle-exchange programs, whose federal funding is banned in the United States.

Oral Health

Oral diseases are a major public health concern in most of the world's LMICs (Sheiham et al. 2011). Common problems include dental caries, periodontal disease, tooth loss, oral mucosal lesions and oropharyngeal cancers, HIV-related diseases, and trauma to the teeth as a result of violence, road collisions, unsafe sports, and falls. In HICs and LMICs alike, most adults and up to 90% of school-aged children, some 5 billion people, are affected by dental caries. In LICs over 90% of caries are untreated. Untreated dental caries are the world's most common health problem. Globally, up to one in five middle-aged adults suffers from severe periodontal (gum) disease. Almost half of people living with HIV suffer from oral fungal, bacterial, or viral infections (WHO 2012).

Throughout the world, oral health problems are common among poor populations (Sheiham et al. 2011). Increased consumption of soft drinks and prepackaged foods containing refined sugars, insufficient exposure to fluorides, and the expense of toothbrushes and, especially, of oral health care all contribute to this.

Despite increasing need, the density of dentists in LMICs is abysmal, with an average of 1 dentist per 10,000 people in Southeast Asia and 0.5 per 10,000 in Africa, compared with 5.7 dentists per 10,000 people in Europe (WHO 2015u). In Brazil dental care is covered by the national health system, but almost two thirds of the population, especially poor and rural populations, have no access to a dentist (Neumann and Quiñonez 2014). In HICs, too, oral health care is financially prohibitive for many. In Canada, poorer groups are more likely to suffer from oral pain, tooth decay, and missing teeth: because routine dental care is not included in provincial health plans, those without private insurance have less access to preventive dental services than wealthier counterparts (Ravaghi, Quiñonez, and Allison 2013).

Gender, Sex, and Health

Various health issues are related to a person's sex and/or gender. As discussed in chapter 7, gender is a social category relating to social roles, whereas sex is a biological category, distinguished by physical and genetic characteristics. Here we explore health determinants and status of men and women, which are expressions of both biological and gender differences (also see LGBTQIA section).

Women's Health

Women's health includes, but is not limited to, reproductive and sexual health: even health concerns linked to biology and reproductive roles are shaped by gender concerns. Although the leading cause of death in women worldwide is cardiovascular disease (CVD) (12.4% of deaths), there are marked differences by income (WHO 2015a). Women generally have a longer life expectancy but tend to experience more illness and disability than men.

In many societies, women have limited economic and social power, attain lower levels of education than men, and lack legal autonomy. These factors reproduce women's disadvantaged social position and result in gender-specific health problems. Violations of girls' and women's health and human rights include early and coerced onset of sexual activity, early marriage, gender-based violence (in particular intimate partner violence), humiliation, bride-burning and dowry deaths, inadequate nutrition, high rates of STIs, sexual trafficking, entrapment through sexual violence and coercion, among many others, all reflecting unequal power relations in the home, workplace, and community (UNICEF 2014). Such violations play a crucial role in women's emotional suffering, and generate high rates of depression and other mental health problems (Astbury 2010).

Where women are in the paid workforce, they may experience a similar range of occupational health problems as men, such as cancers linked to toxic exposures, deaths and injuries from unsafe workplaces, and CHD from job-related stress. In places with poor quality housing and inadequate ventilation, women working at home—together with children and the elderly—are exposed to high levels of indoor air pollution and associated respiratory disease.

Women's Reproductive Health

For reproductive-age women in LMICs, almost one fifth of illnesses and deaths are pregnancy related. Some 830 women die every day (303,000/year) due to maternal causes (primarily hemorrhage, infection, eclampsia [seizures], obstructed labor, complications from abortion, and ectopic pregnancy) (WHO et al. 2015). Maternal sepsis alone causes approximately 75,000 maternal deaths every year, primarily in LICs (van Dillen 2010).

Of all the health statistics monitored by the WHO, maternal mortality shows the largest discrepancy between HICs and LICs (Figure 6-8). Lack of proper infrastructure for prenatal care, poor resource allocation, and a low priority given to women's health result in enormous deficiencies in maternal health care and low presence of skilled birth attendants for delivery and postpartum care in LICs. In sub-Saharan Africa, women have a lifetime risk of 1 in 36 of dying from pregnancy-related causes, whereas in East Asian LMICs it is 1 in 860 and in HICs 1 in 3,300 (World Bank 2015b). India alone has more maternal deaths each week than all EU countries combined (with roughly 40% of India's population) have in an entire year (ibid).

Barriers to obtaining prenatal and obstetric services include distance from health services, cost (direct fees for medical services as well as the cost of transportation, drugs, and supplies), and women's lack of decisionmaking power within the family. Three main types of care are essential for pregnant women:

- *Antenatal care*: The percentage of women who access care during their pregnancies at least once is 78% in sub-Saharan Africa, 69% in South Asia, and 96% in Latin America and the Caribbean, but less than two-thirds of women worldwide receive the recommended minimum four visits (UNICEF 2016).
- *Perinatal care* (during childbirth): About one third of all births in LMICs take place without the assistance of a skilled birth attendant, such as a doctor or midwife (Figure 6-8). A leading cause of maternal death is preventable infections

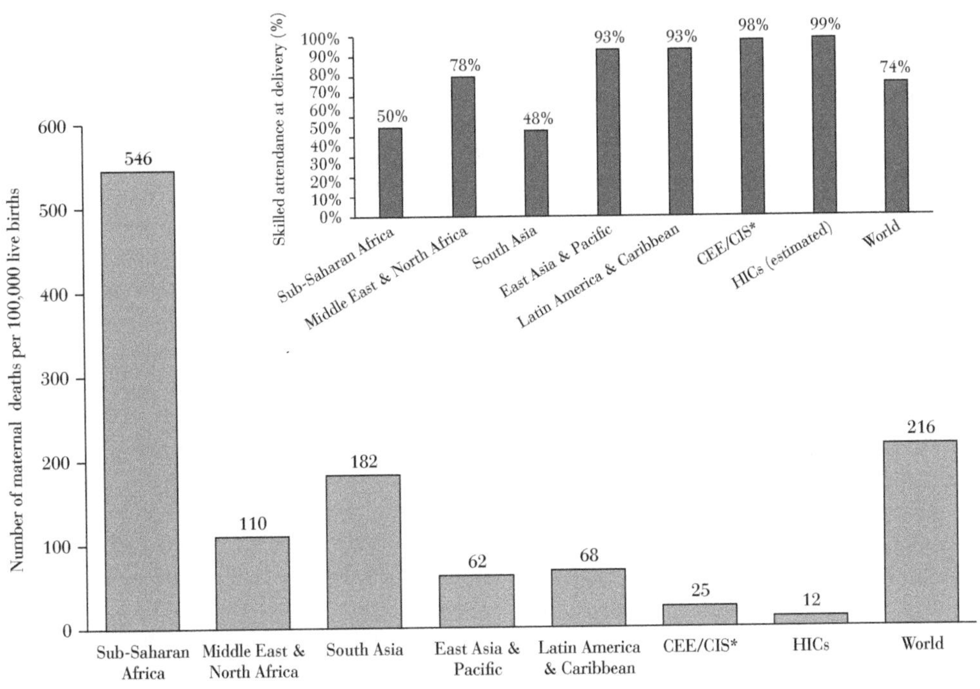

Figure 6-8: Maternal mortality ratios and percentage of births attended by skilled health personnel, 2015.
Data Sources: UNICEF (2016); WHO et al. (2015).

resulting from poor hygiene and contamination during childbirth. Skilled birth attendants can address these issues and have a major impact on reducing maternal mortality (Wilson et al. 2011).
- *Postpartum care*: Care after delivery can prevent life-threatening infections and provide support around issues such as breastfeeding and birth spacing. The majority of women in LMICs receive no postpartum care.

Poorly performed abortions are an important cause of maternal mortality. About half of all abortions are performed in an unsafe manner, nearly all in low-income settings. Unsafe abortions can result in long-term health problems including hemorrhage, genital damage, and necrotic bowels. Abortion is legal in 63 countries "without restriction as to reason" and legal in another 71 countries to preserve health and sometimes allowable on socioeconomic grounds (e.g., UK, India, Japan). However many of these countries restrict abortion based on weeks of gestation or only permit abortion under certain circumstances, such as rape, incest, and fetal impairment. In 60 countries—including Nigeria, the Philippines, Brazil, Venezuela, Ireland, and Iran—abortion is entirely prohibited or tightly restricted, such as only being permitted to save the woman's life (Center for Reproductive Rights 2016).

Men's Health

The principal health problems of men have been well studied, reflecting male dominance in most societies and among researchers and policymakers. Men experience higher rates of mortality and have higher rates of CVD, HIV (except in Africa), and physical injury, though women are "catching up" in many of these areas.

While some illnesses can be attributed to (biological) sex (e.g., only men can have prostate cancer), many differences are related to gender. Men's roles as primary breadwinners in numerous societies may lead them to travel and work in dangerous and/or stressful settings, and result in illness and/or injury. Most occupational mortality occurs in men (ILO 2009). Men drink alcohol and engage in armed conflict more than women and experience more deaths related to these activities. Of the nearly 6 million deaths linked to tobacco use each year, about 4.5 million occur in men (WHO 2015s).

Lesbian, Gay, Bisexual, Transgender, Queer, Intersex, and Asexual Health Issues

The health needs of lesbian, gay, bisexual, transgender, queer, intersex, and asexual[1] (LGBTQIA, also referred to as LGBT—the terminology is both dynamic and debated) people are often overlooked at the community, national, and global levels. In countless settings LGBTQIA individuals fear being publicly identified because this often leads to discrimination, violence, abuse, or death despite the UN's affirmation that these are human rights violations that states are obliged to combat (OHCHR 2015). Currently 75 countries have "anti-homosexuality" or "anti-sodomy" laws (Caroll and Itaborahy 2015). Until 1990, the WHO listed homosexuality as a mental disorder! In many Muslim societies, both civil and Shari'a (Islamic) law criminalize homosexual activity (including 10 countries in which it is punishable through the death penalty [HRC Foundation 2015]). Fundamentalist Christian countries and communities likewise criminalize or otherwise condemn homosexual activity.

Transgender (trans), non-binary, two-spirit, and intersex persons are subject to similar criminalization, though a dearth of information impedes precise documentation. Yet many faith-based, including Muslim, communities are supportive of LGBTQIA persons. Regardless of the legal or religious context, police abuse of LGBTQIA people, especially, trans, non-binary, and people of color (and the ignoring of anti-LGBTQIA violence by judicial systems) is common across the world, even as data are not systematically collected (another form of discrimination). In response, there are now 69 countries and 85 entities that prohibit discrimination on sexual orientation and, increasingly, gender identity/affirmation grounds (ILGA 2015). Yet these measures are not always effective.

Conventionally, LGBTQIA health issues have been framed narrowly in relation to STIs (beyond the issue of pathologizing the very existence of these groups) and, more recently, gender transitioning, involving hormones, surgery, and/or mental health services. Yet discrimination and abuse (sexual, emotional, physical) affects many other health behaviors and outcomes for LGBTQIA persons. Certainly HIV has disproportionately affected men who have sex with men, and trans persons (who may not identify as gay or queer), partly because contracting HIV is 18 to 20 times more likely via unprotected anal sex than vaginal sex (Patel et al. 2014). However, HIV is *not* an exclusively LGBTQIA concern: women, men, non-binary, LGBTQIA, and straight persons alike, may experience high HIV rates, especially where there is widespread racial, social, and economic oppression.

Devastating as the HIV epidemic has been for many LGBTQIA persons, far more is at stake. Societal homophobia (prejudice toward persons based on sexual orientation), transphobia, and heterosexism (favoring of heterosexual and heteronormative persons and behaviors) jeopardize LGBTQIA health through: discrimination in housing, education, and employment; denial of social security benefits (limiting financial security, access to health insurance, other social services); harassment, stress, social isolation, and community and family rejection; sexual assault/abuse, rape, psychological and physical harm, and extreme violence; imprisonment; and health provider ignorance, assumptions, and refusal to accept LGBTQIA patients. This discrimination and violence, in turn, may provoke depression, anxiety, and other mental health and/or substance abuse problems (Fish and Karban 2015).

On a more positive note, growing awareness, acceptance, and policy changes over recent decades are enabling more LGBTQIA persons to live with dignity, thanks to activism, education, monitoring, and solidarity, including around HIV (Biehl 2006; Fee and Brown 2001). Not only are changing societal norms and gender affirmation among LGBTQIA individuals improving health, they are ushering in new understandings: emerging research suggests care-taking roles in same-sex couples are more reciprocal than in heterosexual couples, casting new light on how heteronormative relations and practices may limit or harm health (Reczek and Umberson 2012).

Health and the Elderly/Aging

A "demographic shift" is underway as many populations live longer and often healthier lives. In 2000, 600 million people were aged 60 or older, and by 2050, this number will likely grow to 2 billion, with over 80% residing in LMICs. This shift results from factors such as improvements in health and its determinants throughout the lifecourse, and decreased fertility rates (WHO 2014c).

As we age, our physical and sometimes mental health capacity gradually deteriorates, but these changes do not necessarily precipitate ill health. Still, both physical and mental impairments are more common among the elderly, and many older people have long-term care problems that necessitate continual management. The major health conditions of older people include (WHO 2014c):

- Cardiovascular (coronary heart/cerebrovascular) disease
- Hypertension
- Diabetes
- Cancer
- Chronic obstructive pulmonary disease
- Musculoskeletal conditions (arthritis and osteoporosis)
- Mental health conditions (dementia and depression)
- Blindness and visual impairment
- Hospital infections, such as pneumonia, and medical errors

Deaths from preventable harm in health care facilities account for significant mortality in many countries, estimated to be the third-leading cause of death in the United States, with about 250,000 annual deaths (Makary and Daniel 2016). Medical errors, overdiagnosis and excessive medical interventions, and intra-hospital infections are among the principal underlying causes. A significant proportion of hospital errors are linked to hospital-acquired infections, including sepsis. This is also a grave concern in LMICs, although rarely captured by official statistics. Public, universal health systems tend to have lower iatrogenic (medical care-induced) deaths than where private services have a larger role (James 2013).

Older persons have higher rates of morbidity owing largely to accumulated exposure to environmental toxins, occupational stresses, and poor nutrition. Physical and social environments not supportive of aging contribute to increased health problems, including falls due to poor lighting and depression among isolated individuals. In some societies, the elderly experience widespread ageism—discrimination based on age.

The extent to which adults are able to age with health and dignity largely depends on the same societal and cultural factors that determine lifelong health trajectories and influence the level of care and social support received. These include family structure, retirement age and benefits, accessibility of transit systems and infrastructure, and opportunities to engage in mentally and physically stimulating activities (HelpAge International 2014). But end-of-life care decisions are not always discussed, and when debilitating illness strikes, life-sustaining interventions are often employed even when the quality of life is much diminished. In HICs and MICs, a high share of hospital expenditures occur at the end of life (frequently in the last month), even as there is inadequate access to palliative hospice care (Langton et al. 2014).

Health of Indigenous Populations

Over 370 million people living in 90 countries (approximately 5% of the global population) identify as Indigenous (UN 2009): persons who, according to J. Martinez Cobo, have a "historical continuity with pre-invasion and pre-colonial societies that developed on their territories, consider themselves distinct from other sectors of the societies now prevailing in those territories, or parts of them" (UNESCO 2006, p. 10).

Across the world, Indigenous groups consistently experience higher mortality rates and worse health than non-Indigenous populations (Table 6-2). In Canada, for example, First Nations communities have higher CVD mortality rates, 30% higher for men, 76% higher for women (Tjepkema et al. 2012), and rates of TB 32 times higher (Public Health Agency of Canada 2014) and diabetes 3–5 times greater than the general population (Health Canada 2013). For Inuit people, the incidence of TB is 400 times higher than for non-Indigenous people (Public Health Agency of Canada 2014). In the United States, TB rates are 5 to 13 times greater for Indigenous peoples and mortality rates from diabetes 1.6 times greater than in the general population (Bloss et al. 2011; Department of

Table 6-2 Selected Indigenous Populations and Related Health Indicators

Country	Estimated Numbers of Indigenous People[a]; as % of National Population (year)	Selected Health Disparities
China	113.8 million; 8.5% (2010)[b,c]	*IMR*: Yunnan province Han Chinese average: 53.64/1,000 Yunnan province ethnic minority[b]: 78/1,000 (Li, Luo, and De Klerk 2008)
India	84.3 million; 8.2%[c]	*Adult underweight prevalence, Kerala State*: Non-Indigenous: 24% Paniyas: 46% (Haddad et al. 2012)
Mexico[d]	16.9 million; 15.1% (2010)	*IMR*: National average: 14/1,000 Indigenous population: 20/1,000
Bolivia[d]	6.2 million; 62.2.% (2010)	*IMR*: National average: 35/1,000 Indigenous population: 65/1,000
Guatemala[d]	5.9 million; 41% (2010)	*IMR*: National average: 28/1,000 Indigenous population: 40/1,000
United States	5.2 million; 1.7% (2010) (US Census Bureau 2012)	*IMR*: National average: 6/1,000 American Indians & Alaska Natives: 7.6/1,000 (Mathews, MacDorman, and Thoma 2015)

Table 6-2 Continued

Canada	1.4 million; 4.3% (2011) (Statistics Canada 2015a)	*Projected life expectancy, males (2017):* National average: 79 First Nations: 73–74 Inuit: 64 *Projected life expectancy, females (2017):* National average: 83 First Nations: 78–80 Inuit: 73 (Statistics Canada 2015b)
Brazil[d]	900,000; 0.5% (2010)	*IMR:* National average: 15/1,000 Indigenous population: 22/1,000
Cameroon[c]	*Bagyeli, Baka, Bedzan*: 65,500; 0.4% *Mbororo*: 1,000,000; 12%[c]	N/A
Uganda[b,c]	*Benet, Batwa*: 26,700; 0.07% *Ik, Karamojong*: 990,029; 2.6%	*Life expectancy (2003–2008):* National average: 53 Batwa: 28 (Berrang-Ford et al. 2012)
New Zealand	712,000; 15.5% (2015) (Statistics New Zealand 2016)	*Life expectancy, females (2012–2014):* National average: 83.2 Maori: 77.1 (Statistics New Zealand 2015)
Australia	669,900; 3% (2011) (Australian Bureau of Statistics 2013)	*Life expectancy, females (2010–2012):* National average: 83.1 Indigenous: 73.7 (Australian Government 2014)
Democratic Republic of Congo	600,000-2 million; 1–3%[c]	N/A
Russia	260,000; 0.2%[c]	*Life expectancy, females (2004):* National average: 74 Northern Indigenous population: 55 (Ellsworth and O'Keeffe 2013)
Cambodia	150,000-300,000; 1–2%[b,c]	N/A
Burundi	*Batwa*: 78,000; 1% (2008)[c]	N/A
Greenland	*Inuit*: 50,000; 89%[c]	*Life expectancy, males (2014):* National average: 69 (Statistics Greenland 2016)
Denmark (to be compared with Greenland)	*Inuit*: 8,000; 0.15% (Bjerregaard et al. 2004)	*Life expectancy, males (2014)* National average: 78 (Ministry of Foreign Affairs Denmark 2015)

[a]Counts of Indigenous populations may be inaccurate due to censuses that do not distinguish among ethnic groups and differences in identification of Indigenous populations. For example, although some populations are classified as Indigenous based on language, others rely on self-identification. As well, various ethnic groups fall under the term *Indigenous* within a country. In Canada, the official term *Aboriginal Peoples* historically encompassed Inuit, First Nations, and Métis (people of mixed Indigenous and European ancestry) though the term *Indigenous* is increasingly preferred, whereas in Ecuador, Indigenous groups are distinguished from the mestizo population (who are descendants of mixed Indigenous and European heritage).

[b]Historically, these national governments have denied the presence of Indigenous groups. This estimate includes all ethnic minorities, as it is unclear which minorities are considered Indigenous.

[c]Estimates from IWGIA (2016); exact data years are not always provided.

[d]CEPAL (2014).

Health and Human Services 2012). Most telling is the enormous life expectancy differential: in Australia there is a 10-year gap between Indigenous and non-Indigenous life expectancy (Australian Institute of Health and Welfare 2014).

Health inequities between Indigenous peoples and dominant groups are related to historic colonization processes (see chapter 1) and to the ongoing practices of social, economic, political, and cultural oppression. While other groups (e.g., working class, women, and LGBTQIA groups) share certain aspects of this oppression, among Indigenous populations, as well as slave descendants, the effects are compounded over time owing to the profound and disruptive effects of colonization on spiritual and material ways of life and cultural history (see chapter 7).

Mainstream public health authorities and researchers typically seek biomedical and behavioral explanations for the health inequities between Indigenous and non-Indigenous groups, citing genetic differences, and supposed proclivities to substance abuse and violence. For example, the high rate of Type II diabetes among Indigenous people has been spuriously argued to result from a "thrifty gene" that enabled hunter-gatherer populations to conserve energy for later use (Krieger 2011). More recent research suggests that response to famine and deprivation at residential schools, together with economic and livelihood shifts, has shaped current diabetes-linked consumption patterns among Indigenous populations.

It is important that discourses around intergenerational trauma strike a careful balance between understanding the impact of past and ongoing oppression and not pathologizing the effects of these experiences at an individual level (Maxwell 2014).

EPIDEMIOLOGY AND THE POLITICAL ECONOMY OF DISEASE

Key Questions:

- What are the limits of traditional disease categories, such as communicable versus noncommunicable disease?
- What are the underlying causes of diarrheal diseases and Type II diabetes worldwide?
- How might we understand the mix of biologic, social, and economic factors linked to the transmission of HIV?
- What biologic and structural factors allow some emerging global diseases to spread rapidly, whereas others take years to spread?

While dichotomies of HICs/LMICs and communicable/noncommunicable disease, (supplemented by the GBD with an injuries category—see chapter 5) offer a useful snapshot of different disease patterns across the world, these fail to fully explain the complexity of the factors influencing and underpinning the health–disease process in a global context.

The now discredited epidemiological transition (see chapter 3) assumes a one-way path of mortality "progress." However, as evidenced in settings as varied as Russia in the 1990s and the US state of Mississippi more recently—where life expectancy and infant mortality rates, respectively, worsened notably amid deteriorating social protections—patterns of health and disease and their determinants follow complex pathways. Some diseases on the rise globally have different underlying processes in HICs and LICs. Sepsis, a serious systemic immune response to infection (Becker et al. 2009), may be exacerbated by water and sanitation problems and malnutrition in LICs (Tupchong, Koyfman, and Foran 2015), while in HICs is linked to a rise in chronic diseases. In all settings, attention to hygiene and handwashing plays an important part in reducing hospital-acquired sepsis (Ellingson et al. 2014). The emergence of new infectious diseases (e.g., Ebola, MERS) or re-emergence of old ones (e.g., chikungunya, cholera, Zika) and new patterns of mortality (e.g., soaring road deaths in LMICs) also demonstrate the fallacy of a unidirectional trajectory of improvement of health patterns.

Here we have developed the following typology to describe global patterns of disease and mortality, one that differs from the standard communicable/noncommunicable disease dichotomy:

- Diseases of marginalization and deprivation (MD)
  - Examples: diarrhea, neglected tropical diseases, malaria, acute respiratory infections
- Diseases of modernization and work (MW)
  - Examples: CVD, cancer, road traffic injury and death

- Diseases of marginalization and modernization (MM)
  - Examples: diabetes, chronic obstructive pulmonary disease, TB, HIV and AIDS
- Diseases of emerging (global) social and economic patterns (EG)
  - Examples: SARS, new strains of influenza, Ebola, and effects of substandard drugs

Each disease classification relates to the larger political economy order and cuts across high and low-income dichotomies. This means that Cuba, though long a LIC, has had a disease distribution that fits more into the MW category than the (expected) MD or MM, largely because it has addressed the diseases of extreme marginalization. Of course many countries do not fit neatly into one category—significant portions of the US population experience MD and MM even though MW dominate. Moreover, particular diseases that are both chronic and infectious and occur in varied contexts, such as HIV, may fit in all categories. Likewise, road traffic fatalities and CVD may traverse several categories.

Because the quality of much international morbidity data is poor, this chapter focuses more on mortality patterns, albeit recognizing the importance of morbidity to population health.

Figure 6-9 depicts the relative importance of the first three disease types in terms of their contribution to mortality in LMICs and HICs. Only the major MD, MW, and MM diseases listed on pp. 248–249 are calculated into each category. Together, these MD, MW, and MM diseases account for 72% of all causes of death worldwide (the remainder being EG, unknown, or diseases not easily classified by the typology, such as cirrhosis and suicide). LMICs, with 80% of the world population, account for 91% of deaths from MD diseases, 68% from MW diseases, and 87% from MM diseases. In spite of their economic importance and local priority at times of epidemics (frequently sensationalized in media reports), EG are not the chief contributors of mortality.

Diseases of Marginalization and Deprivation

Many diseases occur primarily as a result of marginalization and deprivation—that is, poverty, substandard living conditions, geographic isolation, discrimination, and political oppression. Many, if not all, MD ailments have been nearly eliminated in HICs and among elites everywhere. For example, it is rare for a rich person to fall ill from cholera, Chagas disease, or even TB, whether in Mali or Luxembourg. Yet a broad swath of people face a range of diseases that are largely preventable and controlled in societies with universal social welfare provisions, including some LICs. MD diseases often result from exposure to pathogens and toxins in contaminated water, air, food, and physical environments. Populations living in chronic poverty—who lack social benefits and healthy environments—are more susceptible and less resistant to illness due to compromised immune systems from conditions such as malnutrition, making them more likely to become ill or acquire disabilities, remain sick longer, and die earlier than wealthier groups.

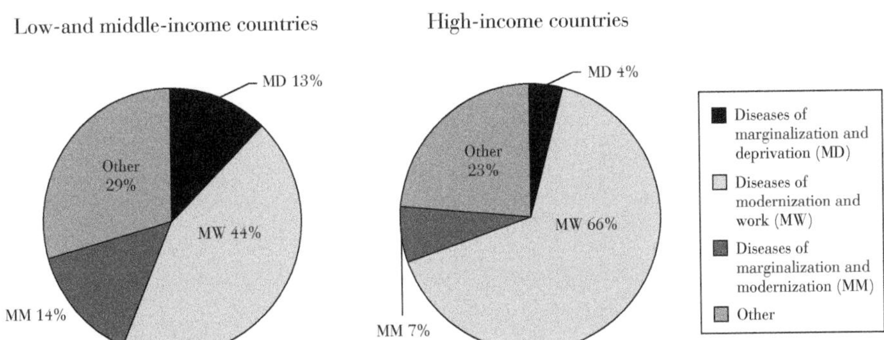

Figure 6-9: Deaths by typology as a proportion of all deaths in LMICs and HICs, 2013.
Data Source: Original calculations and figure based on data from IHME (2013c).

Diarrhea and Gastrointestinal Infections

Diarrheal disease can result from multiple causes of gastrointestinal infection, or from the effects of a pathogen's toxin on the body. There are approximately 1.7 billion cases of diarrhea throughout the world annually, causing 1.5 million deaths (3% of all deaths) (WHO 2014h). Globally, it is one of the leading causes of death among children. Although deaths from diarrhea have fallen dramatically over the past 40 years, the number of cases has remained constant (and high), at over three episodes per year for children living in LICs (Walker et al. 2013).

Epidemic diarrheal infection, including cholera (Box 6-2), often results from contamination of a common water source. The lack of adequate facilities to dispose of and treat human waste increases the likelihood of widespread infection, as does using contaminated water to prepare food and consuming raw foods that have not been peeled. Bottle-feeding with powdered milk or formula mixed with bacteria-laden water may lead to the death of infants very quickly. Leading diarrhea-causing agents are listed in Table 6-3.

The main determinants of diarrhea are structural factors such as water quality and level of sanitation, as well as overall health-promoting factors, including sufficient food of good quality and health status since birth. Thus, persons with suppressed or weakened immune systems, particularly those infected with HIV, are more susceptible.

Because the agents of diarrhea are generally found in food and drink (Box 6-3), it is possible to prevent many diarrheal diseases. Prevention can be undertaken by: changing biology (immunization) or behavior (education and training); improving community conditions (water supply, food regulation); and, at the political level, decreasing poverty. Improved access to clean water and sanitary disposal

Box 6-2 Cholera

Cholera occurs in pandemic waves, often related to conflict, displacement, trade, and weather changes, and underpinned by inadequate access to potable water and sanitation, in turn exacerbated by poor maintenance and privatization of these services in recent decades driven by neoliberal reforms. The current (eighth) pandemic of cholera began in Southeast Asia in the early 1990s and spread to Latin America through the discharged ballast of a ship, killing tens of thousands of people (Figure 6-10). In 2014, over 190,000 cholera cases and 2,200 deaths were reported to the WHO (WHO 2015f). However, these are underestimates, given the difficulty in accurately diagnosing each episode of diarrhea and the fear of trade- and travel-related sanctions. WHO estimates true numbers to be in the range of 3 to 5 million cases and 100,000 to 120,000 deaths per year (WHO 2014b). In 2010, cholera was imported into Haiti after 150 years, of absence, via UN peacekeeping forces from Nepal. Into mid-2016, there had been approximately 776,000 infections, with over 9,100 deaths (PAHO 2016), likely an underestimate.

Table 6-3 Some Enteric Agents that Can Cause Acute or Chronic Diarrhea

Viruses: Rotaviruses, noroviruses

Bacteria: *Campylobacter jejuni, Clostridium difficile, Escherichia coli, Salmonella, Shigella, V. cholerae, V. parahemolyticus*

Protozoa: *Entamoeba histolytica, Cryptosporidium parvum, Cyclospora* species, *Giardia lamblia, Balantinium coli*

Helminths (worms): *Ascaris lumbricoides* (roundworm), *Strongyloides stercoralis, Taenia solium* (pork tapeworm), *Trichuris trichiuria* (whipworm)

Box 6-3 Food-Related Morbidity and Mortality

More than 200 diseases can develop from consumption of foods that contain harmful bacteria, viruses, parasites, and chemicals, with an estimated 600 million foodborne illnesses and 420,000 deaths occurring from 31 leading hazards (WHO 2015t). Worldwide increases in reported foodborne problems have raised concerns that regulation and inspection are severely deficient. The food supply may be threatened by entry of the following substances (Friis 2012):

Microbiological hazards:

- Bacteria (including drug resistant strains), parasites, fungi, viruses, prions, worms

Chemical hazards:

- Heavy metals (e.g., mercury), pesticides, chemical preservatives and additives (used to increase the shelf-life of goods), antibiotic residues (used to keep penned animals, such as chickens, from getting sick)
- Packaging, including waxes, plastic, and other materials that leach into food
- Debris, cleaning chemicals

Physical hazards:

- Foreign objects such as glass, metal, stones, bones, radioactive materials

Nutritional hazards:

- Foods with excess or deficiency of nutrients

The most important sources of infectious foodborne illness are *E. coli, Campylobacter, Salmonella, Shigella, and norovirus,* all prime causes of diarrheal death among children living in poverty. While food contamination often occurs in the household, particularly where clean water is deficient, it is also common at other points in the food chain due to business cost-cutting measures, such as use of contaminated water, inadequate refrigeration, substandard working conditions, and poor hygienic facilities.

Raising commercial livestock also poses health risks, as animals in overcrowded pens spread diseases to one another and to humans (zoonoses). Several well-known (and preventable) zoonoses can be transmitted to humans through food (brucellosis, *M. bovis*) and food contamination (*Echinococcosis*). These problems go hand in hand with excess antibiotic use and inadequate inspections of farms, food plants, stores, restaurants, and street vendors.

The *Codex Alimentarius* was jointly developed by the WHO and FAO in 1963 to set nonbinding international foods standards, with the (sometimes contradictory) purposes of protecting health and facilitating trade. However, it has no enforcement capacity, leaving underfunded national and local surveillance systems responsible for food safety.

of waste are the cornerstones of disease control by environmental means. Rotavirus vaccine is highly effective for preventing up to 40% of diarrheal deaths (Munos, Walker, and Black 2010) but is underutilized due to cost. Exclusive breastfeeding for the first 6 months of an infant's life is also key to reducing diarrheal illness and many other childhood diseases and to boosting children's immune systems.

Oral rehydration therapy (ORT) is an effective treatment that has saved the lives of many, perhaps millions, of children in LMICs since WHO approved its use in 1969. ORT replaces lost fluids orally rather than intravenously. It is cheap, relatively simple, requires only basic training, can be employed at home by parents or even older siblings, and involves little time delay if ingredients are readily available. But

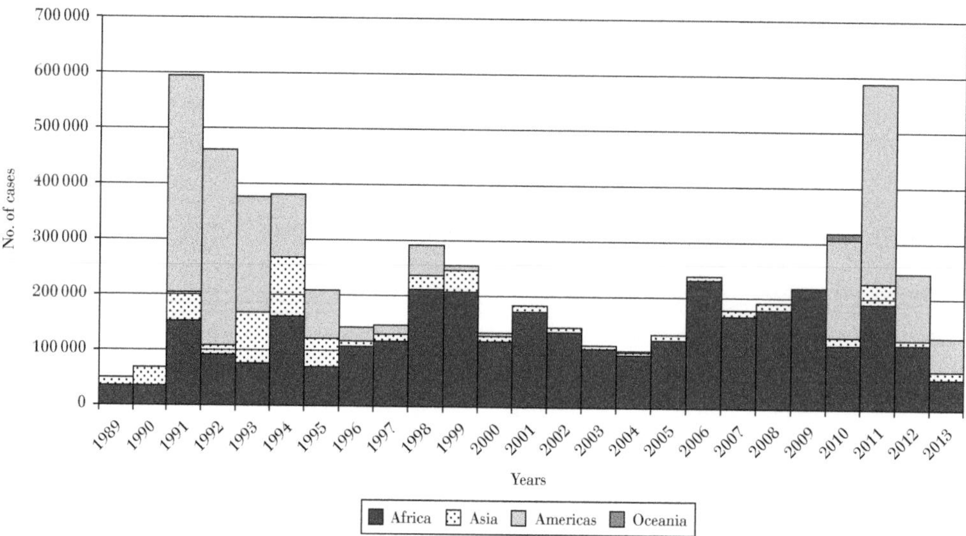

Figure 6-10: Cholera cases reported to WHO by year and by continent (1989–2013).
Source: WHO (2014a). Reprinted from *Weekly epidemiological record: Cholera*, 2013, 89, World Health Organization, p. 351, Copyright (2014).

ORT requires clean water, a major problem in areas with high diarrhea rates.

Measures such as ORT, education regarding sanitary practices, and newly developed vaccines for a few pathogens such as rotaviruses and cholera have contributed to control of diarrheal diseases. However, serious reductions in illness and death are likely to occur only after there have been substantial improvements in social and economic conditions and betterment of the living standards of disadvantaged populations. A prime illustration is Cuba, where acute diarrheal disease mortality in infants fell from 12.9 deaths per 1,000 live births in 1962 to 0.3 per 1,000 in 1993 concomitant with improvements in housing, nutrition, education, and public health (Riverón Corteguera 1995).

"Neglected" Tropical Diseases

Some diseases no longer attract world headlines, although they still pose an enormous burden on people living in poverty, mainly in tropical and subtropical areas of the world (Lancet 2014). Due to strong lobbying by MSF (Médecins Sans Frontières), WHO, CDC, and infectious disease experts, 18 diseases are now referred to as "neglected tropical diseases," or NTDs (WHO 2016h). The "neglected" is used because they are not global priority diseases and usually occur among the most marginalized, rural communities in the poorest parts of the world. The term *neglected* designation is itself problematic: it fails to indicate *who* has done the neglecting. At least 1 billion people suffer from at least one NTD (Table 6-4). Given that the main determinants of NTDs are unclean water, poor sanitation and hygiene, and lack of access to health care services, it is not surprising that they are among the most common infections in the over 2.1 billion people who live on less than US$3.10 per day (World Bank 2015a). Because those affected are also the most discriminated against—rural poor, minority populations, Indigenous groups, migrant workers, and slum dwellers—some argue that it is people, rather than diseases that are neglected.

NTDs lead to approximately 152,000 deaths annually, a relatively low toll, yet various NTDs have lifelong and intergenerational consequences including chronic illness, disability, and/or disfigurement. These, in turn, negatively affect education and work productivity, pregnancy, and fetal and child development (Hotez et al. 2014).

There are effective drugs for prevention and control of some NTDs. Filariasis, onchocerciasis, schistosomiasis, and soil-transmitted nematode infections can be controlled through regular chemotherapy against intestinal worms, reducing mortality and morbidity, enhancing the nutritional status and academic performance of schoolchildren, and improving the health and well-being of pregnant women and their babies. However, for-profit pharmaceutical

Table 6-4 Selected "Neglected Tropical Diseases"

Neglected Tropical Disease and Global Prevalence/New Cases Per Year	Description
Buruli ulcer ND/5,000-6,000	• Caused by bacterial infection • Most frequent near waterways • Leads to destruction of skin and soft tissue and long-term aesthetic and functional disability • 50% of affected people in Africa are under 15 years of age
Chagas disease 7–8 million/ND	• Caused by infection via Triatominae (kissing bug) insects, also via transfusion of infected blood, and mother-to-child transmission • 10,300 deaths/year • Leads to lymphatic and organ infection, especially fatal heart infection • Endemic in 21 Latin American countries
Dengue/dengue hemorrhagic fever ND/2.4 million	• Viral infection transmitted through mosquito bites • 14,700 deaths/year • Leads to flu-like symptoms, hemorrhage, convulsions • 2.5 billion people at risk
Dracunculiasis (guinea worm) ND/22	• Parasitic infection by ingesting water containing guinea worm larvae • 76% of 2013 cases occurred in South Sudan • Leads to intestinal and skin infection
African trypanosomiasis (sleeping sickness) ND/37,000	• Protozoa infection via bite of a tsetse fly • Found only in sub-Saharan Africa • 9,100 deaths/year • Leads to fatigue, damage to lymphatic, neurological, and endocrine systems • 70 million people at risk
Human leishmaniasis 10 million/1.3 million	• Parasitic infection through sandfly bites • 51,600 deaths/year • Leads to skin lesions, soft tissue deterioration, and organ inflammation
Leprosy 190,000/230,000	• Bacteria transmitted through human-to-human contact • Causes infection of skin, nerves, and mucous membranes, leads to loss of sensitivity, atrophy, and severe disfiguration
Lymphatic filariasis 120 million/36 million	• Parasitic infection transmitted through bites from infected mosquitoes • Causes damage to the lymphatic system and kidneys; causes extreme enlargement of limbs • Almost 1 billion at risk, requiring preventive chemotherapy • 40 million disfigured and incapacitated by the disease

Table 6-4 Continued

Onchocerciasis 30 million/ND	• Parasitic worm transmitted through blackfly bites • Second leading cause of blindness globally • 99% of infected live in sub-Saharan Africa • Leads to lesions, visual impairment • 123 million people at risk
Schistosomiasis ND/252 million (total)	• Infection via contact with freshwater parasites • More than 80% of infected people live in sub-Saharan Africa • 11,700 deaths/year • Causes bladder cancer, damage to the intestines, spleen, and kidneys
Soil-transmitted helminthiasis >1.5 billion/ND	• General term for worms that cause gastrointestinal and liver infections • Transmitted by ingesting food contaminated with helminth eggs, or by direct infection through contact with contaminated soil • Together with schistosomiasis, cause 1 billion infections worldwide

Data Sources: CDC (2013); Hotez et al. (2014); WHO (2015n; 2016g; 2016h)

Note: ND = No Data.

companies have little interest in manufacturing drugs for many NTDs since the market is not lucrative.

Some NTDs have received more attention than others. Since 1985, multidrug therapy has cured 14.5 million patients of leprosy; fewer than 1 million people currently have the disease. More recently, preventive chemotherapeutic treatment of almost 1 billion people for lymphatic filariasis has led to considerable reduction in its transmission (WHO 2015l). The Guinea worm disease eradication program, supported by the Carter Center in Atlanta, USA has reduced global prevalence from 3.5 million in 1986 to 22 individuals in 2015, with complete eradication possible soon (WHO 2016g). To take the "neglected" out of NTDs, the London Declaration of 2012 called for the control, elimination, or eradication by 2020 of ten NTDs. To that end, 1.35 billion treatments were donated in 2013, a 35% increase from 2011, and 70 countries have NTD plans (Lancet 2014). Ultimately, permanent control will rest on improvements in water, housing, sanitation, and environmental conditions to reduce exposure to the parasites and vectors that carry NTDs, as well as increased access to health care.

Other significant NTD-related problems include snake bites and viral rabies infection. Venomous snake bites, causing tissue damage, blood clotting, shock, neurotoxicity, and renal damage, result in up to 125,000 deaths per year; hundreds of thousands more people end up with disabilities, mostly in subsistence farming regions in South Asia, Southeast Asia, and sub-Saharan Africa. Anti-venom is available in some countries (though one of the most effective treatments has been discontinued); even so, anti-venom is typically only stocked in central repositories, making it inaccessible to the poor populations most likely to be bitten by snakes (Lancet 2015). Also acquired through animal bites or scratches, the rabies virus kills over 25,000 people per year. Rabies causes progressive damage to the central nervous system, particularly hydrophobia (fear of water), eventually resulting in death. Fifteen million persons per year receive post-exposure vaccine to prevent disease and death.

Malaria

Malaria is the most important vector-transmitted disease in the world. Caused by a parasite (most often *Plasmodium falciparum*) and producing fever and flu-like symptoms, it is transmitted to humans by female *Anopheles* mosquitoes found worldwide in tropical climates. An estimated 214 million malaria cases occur each year, primarily among young children, pregnant women, and immune-compromised adults, with 438,000 malaria deaths.[2] An estimated 306,000 of these deaths are in children under 5, equivalent to one child dying every two minutes (WHO 2015v). Malaria's biological features interact with environmental, social, and economic conditions, creating challenging health problems.

As far back as records extend, malaria has been endemic in much of Asia, Africa, and Latin America—but also in more temperate climates such as central Russia, Canada, and Northern Europe. Malaria's role as an obstacle to colonial conquest, the productivity of colonized peoples, and, more recently, to economic development, has kept the disease on the international health agenda for well over a century.

After the folding of WHO's Global Malaria Eradication Programme in the late 1960s (see chapter 2), malaria rates began to rise, reaching crisis proportions of well over 1 million annual deaths by the 1990s and peaking in 2004. With renewed support from global donors in recent years, and coordinated efforts through the Roll Back Malaria Partnership and WHO's Global Malaria Programme, there has been major growth in coverage and annual financing of malaria programs, rising from US$100 million in 2000 to US$2.5 billion in international and domestic funding in 2014. Technical support for battling malaria mortality has been particularly boosted by the billions committed since 2005 through the US President's Malaria Initiative, which accounts for over 20% of malaria funding (WHO 2015v).

Calls for the elimination of malaria, country by country, have been getting stronger. Since 2000, estimated malaria mortality rates have fallen 48% overall, and 58% in children under 5 years of age (WHO 2015v). Accounting for 90% of malaria deaths, sub-Saharan Africa remains disproportionately affected: 34.3% of the African population lives in moderate to intense transmission areas (Noor et al. 2014).

In addition to its mortality burden, malaria's high morbidity results in significant economic effects. These include direct costs for treatment and prevention, as well as indirect costs from lost work, time spent seeking treatment, and diversion of household resources. The cost to reach malaria control is currently estimated to be over US$6 billion per year (WHO 2015v).

Notwithstanding longtime investments in vector control, the *Anopheles* mosquito has proven resilient. Contemporary malaria control, drawing on certain prior approaches (such as screens and bednets; see chapters 1 and 2), centers on vector control through larval source management of obvious breeding sites (i.e., areas of stagnant water), interruption of transmission through use of insecticidal bednets (ITNs) and indoor residual spraying (IRS), prevention of malaria in pregnancy, and rapid diagnostic tests.

Long-lasting ITNs help reduce transmission within that household, also benefiting residents of adjacent houses, and lead to overall mortality reductions. UNICEF, among other organizations, includes ITNs as part of basic child intervention packages (covering free prenatal care and childhood vaccines), because the nets often cost the equivalent of a family's full week's wages.

Between 2004 and 2010, the number of ITNs delivered to endemic countries jumped from 6 million to 145 million, and over 150 million ITNs were delivered to sub-Saharan Africa in 2015. As a result, the proportion of the population sleeping under an ITN in sub-Saharan Africa rose from less than 2% in 2000 to an estimated 55% in 2015 (WHO 2015v). With growing use of insecticides, however, more than 60 countries in Africa have reported increases in mosquito resistance to pyrethroids, the class of insecticides used in ITNs.

Antimalarial drugs are used for both prevention and treatment, but coverage for the 28 million pregnant women in sub-Saharan Africa at risk is sorely lacking, with only 17% receiving the desired three doses during antenatal care (WHO 2015v).

At the end of the 1990s, a new antimalarial was introduced: the artemisinin group of compounds, derived from a plant native to China. Because these drugs are cleared from the blood quickly, they must be given in concert with longer acting drugs, so-called artemisinin-based combination therapy (ACT), which is now the standard worldwide treatment for *P. falciparum* malaria. A major impediment to use of artemisinins is cost; at their cheapest, they cost at least 10 times as much as the prior standard, chloroquine. Additionally, because monotherapy—artemisinin-based single course drugs (missing the combined therapy)—is cheaper and thus widely available in pharmacies, artemisinin resistance is rising.

Indeed, drug resistance has increased much faster than the ability of pharmaceutical chemists to produce and test new compounds. The reduced effectiveness of chloroquine in treating malignant *falciparum* malaria was reported independently in Colombia and in Thailand in 1960 and has since become widespread. All subsequent drugs have faced the same fate. Since resistance to artemisinins was detected in Cambodia, Myanmar, Thailand, and Vietnam, strains of *Plasmodium* have become resistant to virtually every drug, including quinine. This has led to a shift in strategy: rapid diagnostic tests enable ACT treatment to be used only for confirmed cases, helping limit resistance.

Substandard or fake artemisinin drugs are a further problem linked to hundreds of thousands of deaths each year. With demand far outstripping supplies, poor quality drugs are readily available in marketplaces in malaria-endemic regions. In 2013, poor quality malaria medications were responsible for the deaths of over 120,000 children in 39 sub-Saharan African countries (Renschler et al. 2015).

It is estimated that between 2000 and 2015, three malaria control interventions—IRS, ITN, and ACT—averted 663 million new cases in sub-Saharan Africa, over two thirds attributed to ITNs (Bhatt et al. 2015). However, progress in malaria control will only be incremental as long as the focus remains on residual spraying and therapeutics, without attention to underlying social conditions. These include inadequate housing and poor environmental conditions (Tusting et al. 2015). With the problems of drug and insecticide resistance mounting, scientists are revisiting prior approaches based on upgraded housing that were enormously effective in eliminating malaria in Europe and North America in the first half of the 20th century. A 2015 review found a dramatic 45% to 65% reduction in malaria among people living in houses with screened doors and windows and enclosed ceilings, also protective against a range of vector-borne diseases. The role of other environmental and infrastructural approaches, such as road paving and piped water supply to reduce breeding sites (including those due to household storage of water), would be a welcome next step in a (return to a) political economy approach to addressing malaria and a host of childhood diseases. Such improvements were all critical to eliminating malaria in settings as varied as the United States, Sri Lanka, Southern Europe, and Cuba.

Acute Respiratory Infections

Acute respiratory tract infections (ARIs) comprise a broad mix of illnesses, all affecting the lungs and respiratory tract through viral or bacterial infection. Measles can cause subsequent pneumonia in young children and thus is included in this category (Box 6-4). Although virtually everyone experiences mild upper respiratory tract (throat) infections, ARI death rates from lower respiratory tract infections overwhelmingly affect the most socially excluded populations.

There are an estimated 150 million episodes of childhood pneumonia in LMICs annually. Pneumonia claims the lives of nearly 1 million children under the age of 5 each year, accounting for about 16% of child deaths (UNICEF 2015a) (Figure 6-7). The majority of these deaths are in sub-Saharan Africa, Southeast Asia, and the Eastern Mediterranean, where vaccination rates remain low.

The consequences of respiratory tract infections are wide-ranging. In people with strong immune systems, viral infections usually clear up on their own or with minimal medical intervention. Bacterial infections are much more serious, and generally require antibiotic treatment. For the many children in LMICs who lack access to proper housing, medical care, food, and water, these infections are often fatal. Moreover, respiratory tract infections are a leading cause of missed work and wage losses.

Pediatric pneumonia can be prevented through immunization (with the *Haemophilus influenzae* type b, measles, and pneumococcal vaccines), adequate nutrition (e.g., through exclusive breastfeeding and zinc intake), and reduction of indoor air pollution

Box 6-4 Measles

Despite the existence of a vaccine, measles causes about 325,000 cases annually, most of which occur in LMICs (WHO 2016d). Due to underreporting, the true number of cases and deaths could be 10 to 20 times greater (Strebel et al. 2011). Measles most severely affects children in the poorest communities with the least financial and human resources, reflecting inequitable measles vaccination coverage. For example, in Cameroon, the vaccine is given to 52% of children from the poorest quintile but to 86% from the wealthiest quintile (WHO 2015f). The WHO estimates that measles is responsible for more child deaths than any other cause due to the ensuing complications of pneumonia, diarrhea, and malnutrition. Measles is also one of the main causes of preventable blindness (WHO 2016d).

There is only one effective vaccine for lifelong protection from measles infection. Global efforts to expand vaccine use since 2000 have resulted in remarkable under-5 mortality reduction, with annual deaths reduced by 79% from 546,800 in 2000 to 114,900 in 2014 (WHO 2016d). Most children in HICs receive the vaccine, but this is not the case in many parts of the world, including Nigeria, where measles is the fifth leading cause of death. In 2014–2015 there was a resurgence of measles in North America and Europe, largely due to parents refusing to vaccinate their children (CDC 2015). Currently, aerosolized vaccines are being tested to replace the traditional syringe method. Of course, as with other health interventions, improved nutrition could help prevent the development of disease and aid in speeding up recovery time.

(Wardlaw et al. 2006). Prompt antibiotic treatment can be lifesaving (because most severe cases are bacterial), yet poor access to antimicrobials results in hundreds of thousands of preventable pneumonia deaths each year (Das and Horton 2015).

Diseases of Modernization and Work

As most societies shift from rural, agriculturally based economies to urban, service and industrially based economies, their populations face ailments related to work, transport, stress, toxic exposures, and consumption patterns. Yet largely agrarian societies are not shielded from such problems: use of toxic chemicals and dangerous machinery and work methods have multiplied in recent years as countries have been pressured to reduce health and safety measures in order to compete on the global market. As such, NCDs and injuries are on the rise in rural areas.

Cardiovascular Disease

Cardiovascular disease refers to both CHD and cerebrovascular disease (stroke). Although CVD caused fewer than 10% of all deaths in the early 20th century, since 1990 it has been the leading cause of death globally. And while death rates have declined in many HICs, they are increasing in LMICs, where death rates from CVD are higher than in HICs (Yusuf et al. 2014). An estimated 17.5 million people die of CVD each year (7.4 million due to CHD and 6.7 million due to stroke); 80% of these deaths occur in LMICs (WHO 2015b). CHD occurs when there is a limitation of blood flow to parts of the heart due to either clots or blockages to coronary arteries. CHD is often a leading cause of mortality even in countries with a high prevalence of infectious diseases.

A stroke occurs when there is a lack of oxygen to parts of the brain, causing damage to brain tissue. Major strokes have severe consequences, including paralysis, disability, and death. Caring for a patient after a stroke can be expensive, time consuming, and difficult, putting an enormous onus on caregivers where rehabilitative services are not accessible. Prevalence of stroke is highest in HICs, where it is the third leading cause of death, but incidence and stroke mortality rates are higher in LMICs, particularly in younger populations (Feigin et al. 2014).

The main biological determinants of CVD are high blood pressure and high cholesterol levels, typically attributed to low levels of physical activity, significant tobacco use, and consumption of foods high in saturated fats. These biological and behavioral determinants are, in turn, influenced by societal factors, including affordability and availability of nutritious food, time and safe spaces for exercise, and high stress levels related to employment and income. These factors help explain why lower-income groups experience disproportionately high rates of CVD mortality (see chapter 7). CVD is mostly seen in older populations, owing to the cumulative effects of lifetime exposures, but the disease can manifest even before age 50. The existence of other ailments, such as diabetes, also increases the likelihood of stroke.

CVD interventions usually emphasize smoking cessation, exercise, and dietary changes, such as increasing consumption of fruits and vegetables. Medications to reduce blood pressure and cholesterol levels are common, and surgical interventions may be performed to clear arterial blockage and keep damaged arteries open. These mainstream approaches focus on individual behavior (often termed lifestyle issues) and medical interventions without adequately addressing the societal factors outlined above, plus racial and other forms of discrimination, political disempowerment, and sexual harassment, among others, which helps explain why lower-income groups experience higher rates of CVD fatality than the wealthy.

Cancer

Cancer is the overarching term used for over 100 different conditions characterized by an abnormal division of cells. In 2013, cancer caused 15% of all deaths (8.2 million); 60% to 70% of cancer deaths occur in LMICs. Overall, five cancers account for the majority of cancer deaths (Naghavi et al. 2015):

- Lung (1.6 million deaths/year)
- Stomach (841,000 deaths/year)
- Liver (818,000 deaths/year)
- Colon (771,000 deaths/year)
- Breast (471,000 deaths/year)

The causes of cancer range from workplace exposure to chemicals and other substances, environmental toxins, inherited genes that are activated by viral infections, and infectious diseases. Unlocking the key to cancer causation and treatment is one of the most challenging problems of modern epidemiology and medicine. Tobacco use is believed to be the leading preventable cause of cancer and is related not only to lung cancer but also to cancers of the mouth, esophagus, stomach, kidney, bladder, and cervix, as well as heart disease and stroke, with mortality rates higher in lower-income groups.

Important environmental hazards linked to cancer (also see chapter 10) include radiation, chemical and material pathogens (such as asbestos and vinyl chloride), air pollution (IARC 2013), prolonged exposure to electromagnetic fields, and contaminated food (causing liver and stomach cancers). Infectious agents leading to cancer include hepatitis B and C virus to liver cancer, HPV to cervical cancer, *H. pylori* bacteria to stomach cancer, schistosomiasis to bladder cancer, and HIV to Kaposi's sarcoma and lymphomas. More than 20% of cancers are thought to be due to chronic infections, which occur more commonly among the working class and people living in poverty.

Just as there are many different forms of cancer, so too are there differing methods of prevention and treatment and rates of survival. The WHO estimates that over 40% of cancers are preventable, and many curable if detected early. Cancers may be categorized into three groups. The first group—liver, esophageal, lung, and pancreatic cancers—are extremely difficult to treat and have high case fatality rates. Interventions often focus on primary prevention, such as environmental measures, smoking cessation, reduction in toxic exposures like asbestos, and immunization against infectious agents. The second group includes cancers for which effective screening and secondary prevention are available, including early detection and treatment for breast, bowel, and cervical cancers. Screening for cervical cancer through regular Papanicolaou testing followed by treatment can be effective in lowering rates, but inadequate detection and treatment programs mean 80% of cervical cancer deaths occur in LMICs (Soliman and Boffetta 2013). The third group includes cancers for which treatment is more involved and expensive, such as leukemia and lymphoma. These are treated through high-cost and highly technological interventions. Inadequate and inequitable access to cancer treatment is a major global health issue: in 2015, WHO added 16 cancer drugs to the List of Essential Medicines to promote their availability, affordability, and equitable access (Shulman, Torode, and Wagner 2015).

The HPV vaccine was first introduced in 2006 and now exists in three different versions that can prevent between 70% and 90% of cervical cancers related to HPV, as well a variety of other HPV-associated cancers (vulvar, vaginal, anal, penile, oropharyngeal cancers) (Wailoo et al. 2010). The vaccine is administered to adolescent girls and, in some settings, adolescent boys. As of early 2015, 80 national HPV vaccination programs and several dozen pilot programs had been implemented in over 100 countries with licensed HPV vaccines (Wigle, Fontenot, and Zimet 2016). To date widespread HPV vaccine implementation has mostly occurred in HICs: the vaccine remains contentious in LMICs due to its high cost—US$120 per dose (with three needed)—and where adopting the vaccine perforce squeezes out other public health priorities.

Efforts to lower the cost for LMICs include PAHO's Revolving Fund, which has negotiated prices of US$10 to US$15 per dose for MICs in Latin America (Levin 2013). Meanwhile, GAVI, the Vaccine Alliance is supporting national introduction of HPV vaccine at local prices as low as US$0.20 per dose (with a government co-payment of US$4.50 per dose), but this is limited to fewer than 50 countries whose GNI per capita is US$1,580 or less.

Road Traffic Injury and Death

Road traffic crashes cause considerable injury and death and are the leading cause of death in persons aged 10 to 24. Men and low-income groups generally have a higher likelihood of death or injury from road collisions, the latter linked to significant long-term consequences including physical and mental disability, chronic pain, and job and income loss. Over the past three decades, traffic fatality and injury rates have dramatically declined in HICs, primarily owing to regulations regarding seatbelt and car seat use, speeding, punitive measures for alcohol use before or while driving, rest periods for long haul drivers, vehicle safety laws, helmet laws for bicycles and motorcycles, and road design improvements. Improved public transit has also helped reduce vehicle fatalities. At the same time, road injuries and deaths have soared in LICs and MICs, which have fatality rates, respectively, three times and two times higher than the rates in HICs. Rising LMIC fatalities, with up to 40% of deaths occurring among pedestrians (Haagsma et al. 2016), are linked both to growth in vehicle ownership (Figure 10-3) and inadequate safety regulations. Road traffic incidents cause 1.3 million deaths per year, with 90% of deaths in LMICs (WHO 2015g). Thailand, an upper-middle income country, has the third highest death rate from traffic collisions in the world (38/100,000 persons), and China alone experiences an estimated 200,000 road deaths per year due to a recent surge in car ownership (Schwartlander 2015).

Diseases of Marginalization and Modernization

This section discusses a set of globally prevalent causes of death that are present in settings in which modernization and marginalization coexist. Although the diseases of marginalization and deprivation are typically associated with the lowest-income countries, they are also present in MICs and among socially excluded populations within HICs whose social welfare systems are patchy or have been undermined by spending and coverage clawbacks. Similarly, given rapid industrialization and urbanization across LICs, diseases of modernization have proliferated amid widespread marginalization.

As such, in most of the world, modernization and marginalization and their corresponding ailments coexist to varying degrees. Those socially excluded not only experience diarrhea and respiratory mortality, but also have increasing rates of CVD, cancer, and road deaths, as well as diseases at the intersection of marginalization and modernization, such as diabetes, TB, and HIV. The pie charts at the beginning of the chapter showing causes of death for Indonesia and Kenya illustrate the point that diseases associated with marginalization and with modernization can overlap in the same place. For example, China is nowhere near eliminating diseases of marginalization yet experiences high rates of diabetes, cancer, and respiratory diseases related to industrialization. Indeed, environmental toxins and air pollution disproportionately affect socially marginalized populations throughout the world.

Diabetes Mellitus

Sharing features of MW, MD, and EG, diabetes has become a global menace in less than a generation. Diabetes is a noncommunicable, chronic disease characterized by disturbances in blood sugar regulation and metabolism. Type I diabetes occurs when the pancreas produces little or no insulin (it typically has childhood onset). Type II is diagnosed when a person cannot effectively use the insulin that the pancreas produces; 90% of diabetics have Type II diabetes. In HICs diabetes is among the top 10 causes of death, but its ranking is likely higher because it often goes unrecorded on death certificates. The rate of diabetes in HICs and LMICs alike is skyrocketing, having increased by over 45% since 1990, although much diabetes in LICs remains undiagnosed. About 415 million people (projected to increase to 642 million by 2040) have diabetes globally, with adult prevalence exceeding 20% in Saudi Arabia and other Gulf states and in various South Pacific islands (International Diabetes Federation 2015). Diabetes directly causes an estimated 1.5 million deaths per year (many more deaths are indirectly related, especially chronic kidney disease). Of diabetes deaths, 80% occur in LMICs (WHO 2015d); China, India, Russia, and the United States have the highest number of diabetes deaths.

The main biological and behavioral determinants of diabetes are low physical exercise levels and diets high in processed sugars and fats, together with overweight and obesity. As countries have modernized, populations have faced increasing challenges in maintaining physical activity levels and healthy eating traditions of the past due to the industrialization of agriculture, corporatization of food production (with local production shifted to export crops), global marketing of foods high in sugar and saturated fats, built environments designed for motorized vehicles, and the shift from agriculture to factory and service sector work plus soaring precarious employment (with the attendant time constraints around exercise and food preparation) (see chapters 7 and 9 for further discussion of these issues). These trends, which particularly affect low-income populations, who have limited food options, will likely worsen as TNCs selling low-cost mass-produced food further expand into LMICs. Rates of diabetes are especially high in populations whose ways of living—including market penetration of imported foodstuffs—have undergone rapid change (such as in Samoa). Low birthweight and early stunting followed by rapid weight gain in childhood, especially common in low-income populations, also increases likelihood of future diabetes (WHO 2016c).

Type II diabetes is largely preventable and many of its consequences can be delayed, if not avoided altogether. Diabetes interventions may be categorized into three broad approaches: behavioral-educational, medical, and social policy related (WHO 2016c). Behavioral-educational measures include individual counseling for self-care practices and health education to promote modifications in diet and exercise (WHO 2016c). Medical approaches include surgery (e.g., bariatric surgery for weight loss and procedures to stop complications from organ damage) and pharmacologic management. Recent evidence suggests that older persons with diabetes are being over-treated with hypoglycemic drugs, with harms likely exceeding the benefits for older patients with complex or poor health status. Of course the greater than US$40 billion dollar diabetes drug industry has a strong financial incentive in widespread drug treatment (Lipska 2015).

While these behavioral and medical interventions may help manage diabetes, sustainable prevention and societal management require addressing the structural factors associated with the rise of diabetes in HICs and LMICs alike, including corporate food and beverage production and their global marketing; safe, convenient, and affordable spaces for physical activity; the high cost and inaccessibility of healthy food and clean water; work schedules that do not provide time for exercise and food preparation; and poverty.

Chronic Obstructive Pulmonary Disease

Chronic obstructive pulmonary disease (COPD) is an umbrella term for several diseases (e.g., chronic bronchitis and emphysema) characterized by decreased airflow in the lungs. Sixty-four million people worldwide have COPD, and about 3 million people die of it annually; 90% of these deaths occur in LMICs (Naghavi et al. 2015; WHO 2015c). It is the fifth leading cause of death in HICs, accounting for 5% of total deaths, and in MICs it is the third leading cause of death, accounting for 6% of deaths (WHO 2014h).

In HICs, most COPD mortality is related to tobacco smoke (with outdoor air pollution also important), whereas in LMICs indoor air pollution from stoves (which causes about one third of annual COPD deaths—see chapter 10) and outdoor air contamination are both important. Other factors that increase or exacerbate COPD include crowding, poor nutrition, inadequate access to health care, early-age respiratory infections, and occupationally related dust and vapors.

As the global population ages and smoking rates rise in LMICs (with tobacco companies marketing aggressively [Savell et al. 2015]), COPD rates will likely increase. China's rapid development without adequate controls on industrial pollution has already led to soaring COPD rates (Hughes 2012). All told, industrial and vehicle emissions controls, occupational and safety standards, tobacco regulations, and improvements in housing quality (involving cookstoves and ventilation) are all important to preventing COPD and its disproportional impact on people working and living in precarious conditions.

Tuberculosis

Tuberculosis is an infectious disease that commonly affects one or both lungs, causing pneumonia and slow destruction of lung cells. A healthy and strong immune system can prevent an infected person from becoming sick for many years. Conversely, those with weakened or compromised immune systems fall ill sooner. Without treatment, TB is fatal in most patients, though a diseased person may live for many years before dying.

TB, in its various forms, is estimated to have killed more people in the history of the world (≈2 billion) than any other infectious disease (Ryan 1992). Tuberculosis prevalence in Europe increased after 1700 as the population rapidly urbanized, facing crowded living and miserable working conditions. By the early 19th century, TB was responsible for one quarter of all European deaths. TB accompanied European colonialism to Africa and Asia, and in India and China, TB rates reached epidemic levels circa 1900 (Stead et al. 1995). These two countries, joined by Indonesia, still have the highest numbers of new cases in the world per year, with 23% in India, 10% in China, and another 10% in Indonesia—4.1 million cases in 2014 combined (WHO 2015h).

As discussed in chapter 1, TB's decline in Europe was aided by improvements in social (such as housing and nutritional) conditions, with antibiotics available after World War II yielding further declines. By 1990, however, rising racial and socioeconomic inequalities, along with increased homelessness and deteriorating housing, all contributed to an increase in TB rates globally, including in various HICs. Where resources were available, sometimes intrusive TB control efforts enabled a marked decline in rates, but in other parts of the world TB rates were soaring by the late 1990s.

One of the primary causes of the resurgence in TB globally is the increase in HIV infection, including in rural areas. HIV suppresses the body's immune system, which promotes progression to active tuberculosis in people with TB infection. Between 1990 and 1999, the incidence of TB in sub-Saharan Africa increased by over 250% (WHO 2005), with an estimated one third of all new TB cases among HIV-infected people, part of a growing syndemic (presence of several diseases that are mutually exacerbating).

Early in the 21st century, TB remains the number one infectious disease killer in the world, with an estimated 9.6 million new cases of TB in 2014, and 1.5 million deaths. The incidence and mortality rates vary widely by region (Figure 6-11): LMICs bear the brunt of the epidemic, with 95% of cases and 98% of TB deaths worldwide.

Despite the availability of antibiotics, TB resists effective control in many regions, chiefly owing to the inadequacy of public health services, the spread of HIV, and the emergence of drug resistance. TB is not only a matter of infection, it is also the preeminent disease of poverty, a telling indicator of a country's level of wealth and inequality (Kim et al. 2005). The emerging worldwide epidemic of multidrug-resistant tuberculosis (MDR-TB) is a human-made problem—an entirely treatable problem became untreatable due to government inaction and apathy and the political disempowerment of the billions of people living in poverty (Citro et al. 2016). Moreover, treatment of MDR-TB fell victim to cost-effectiveness exigencies. From 1993-2002, WHO advice to donors, NGOs, and governments called for persons with MDR-TB to be left out of treatment programs due to cost concerns, despite evidence from HICs that case-finding and treatment had effectively controlled MDR-TB (Nicholson et al. 2016).

Drug-resistant strains appear where treatment is inconsistent or interrupted, when the wrong drugs are prescribed for the wrong amount of time, when drugs of inferior quality are given, or when the drug

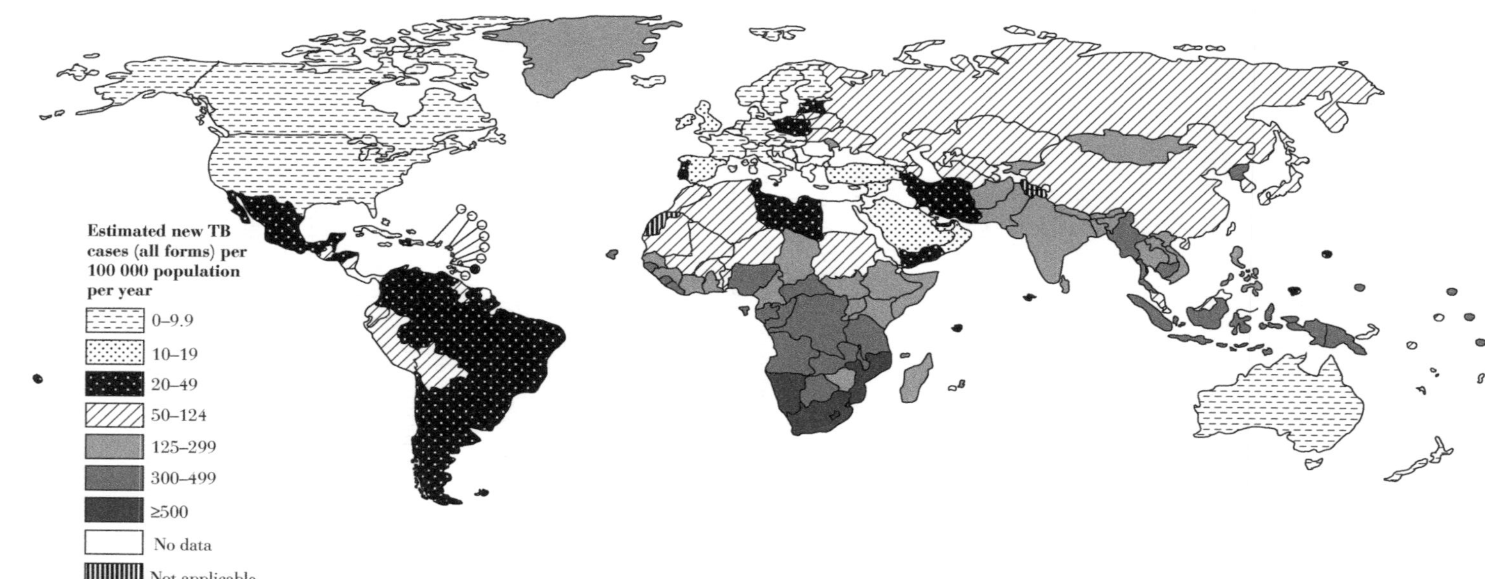

Figure 6-11: Estimated TB incidence rate, by country, 2014.

Source: Reprinted from *Global Tuberculosis Report 2015*, World Health Organization, Disease burden and 2015 targets assessment, Figure 2.6, p. 18, Copyright (2015).

supply is unreliable. Globally, approximately 3.3% (about 300,000) of all new TB cases and 20% of previously treated cases are MDR-TB, over half occurring in India, China, and Russia (WHO 2015h). The CDC described extensively drug-resistant tuberculosis (XDR-TB) in 2005 as MDR-TB that is also resistant to any fluoroquinolone and to one of the three second-line injectable drugs (almost one tenth of MDR-TB cases) (CDC 2006). XDR-TB is now found in at least 105 countries. Even the most effective treatment efforts are estimated to cure only 30% to 40% of XDR-TB cases (Leimane et al. 2010).

In the face of rising TB rates, the WHO declared TB a "global emergency" in 1994 and launched a five-component program called Directly Observed Therapy, Short-course (DOTS): standardizing funding, screening, treatment, pharmaceutical management, and evaluation. In 2001 the Stop TB PPP was established, and WHO became host to the "Global Drug Facility" to ensure access to and public funding for anti-TB drugs. In 2006 the Stop TB Global Strategy widened the scope to include: addressing TB/HIV and drug-resistant TB; contributing to health system strengthening; engaging all public and private providers in TB control; empowering people with TB and their communities; and promoting research into new drugs, vaccines, and diagnostic methods (Stop TB Partnership 2006). Since 2015, the End TB Strategy includes three pillars: integrated, patient-centered care and prevention; bold policies and supportive systems; and intensified research and innovation (Uplekar et al. 2015). With prior approaches critiqued for being coercive, excluding "low priority" patients, under-emphasizing the need for new diagnostics and drugs, and ignoring those needing re-treatment (Hakokongas 2005), the new strategy is more flexible though still biomedically focused.

WHO estimated in 2014 that global incidence rates had been slowly falling (1.5% per year) for a decade, in part due to international control programs. With overall TB mortality declines of 47% since 1990, the MDG target of halving TB deaths by 2015 was almost reached. However, the African and European regions did not achieve this target, owing to the large caseload of HIV-infected incident TB in sub-Saharan Africa (870,000 cases), and drug-resistant TB in countries of the former Soviet bloc (WHO 2015h). In the long run, global tuberculosis control will require integration of technical approaches with equitable improvements in socioeconomic conditions, which has long proven effective in settings with strong welfare states.

HIV and AIDS

Of all the health problems that have emerged in recent decades, none better illustrates the challenges, prospects, and ongoing problems for global health than the human immunodeficiency virus (HIV) and acquired immunodeficiency syndrome (AIDS). This reflects the way HIV and AIDS are intertwined with poverty, oppression, disability, modernization, neoliberal globalization, inequality, the commitment of health workers and activists, scientific advances and technological innovation, corporate greed, health and social welfare deficiencies, personal desires, and a host of other matters from the cellular to the secular.

At the biological level, HIV is a retrovirus (i.e., it can use a host's DNA to self-replicate) and is the viral infectious agent that causes AIDS. HIV targets the body's infection-fighting CD4 cells and slowly disables the immune system, which normally wards off common infections. AIDS is the term given to a collection of conditions found in persons with advanced HIV. There is frequently a long time lapse—as much as 5 to 10 years (or even longer, with treatment)—between initial HIV infection and progression to AIDS. Because most people do not get tested routinely, they may infect others in this period.

HIV is spread through blood, semen, breastmilk, and other bodily fluids (but not saliva). Transmission can occur through: unprotected sex; sharing of injection equipment by people who inject drugs; medical injection with a contaminated needle or syringe; organ or tissue transplantation of infected body parts; semen donation; and mother-to-child transmission (MTCT) during childbirth or breastfeeding. STIs also increase exposure to HIV via open sores or abrasions.

There were an estimated 1.1 million deaths due to AIDS in 2015 (UNAIDS 2016), with a cumulative total of 39 million deaths since the epidemic was recognized (WHO 2015k). In 2014 there were approximately 2.1 million people newly infected (5,750 every day), including 150,000 children (7% of the total). Overall, an estimated 36.7 million people are living with HIV

(UNAIDS 2016). Notwithstanding these large numbers, the epidemic may have reached its peak in 2005: child deaths have more than halved since 2000, and overall annual AIDS-related deaths have declined by 45% since 2004 (ibid). As well, annual new infections are down by over one third globally, although the number of people living with HIV is still rising (Figure 6-12).

HIV gradually emerged into public vision during the late 1970s and was first labeled a distinct clinical entity in 1981. The epidemic was characterized by media hysteria and severe discrimination (which persists in many places) against people infected or suspected of being susceptible to the disease, at the time primarily gay men, hemophiliacs, people who inject drugs, and Haitians.

Public health prevention and control measures adopted in some settings during the 1980s, such as mandatory HIV testing especially in so-called "risk groups," quarantine of HIV-infected people and their exclusion from schools and workplaces, exacerbated prejudice and discrimination (Fee and Fox 1988; Mann 1999). Meanwhile, many governments failed to adequately screen blood products even after the development of sensitive ELISA testing, leading to tens of thousands of avoidable infections and associated deaths. The extent of human rights violations led Jonathan Mann, founding director of WHO's Global Programme on AIDS, to declare human rights as central to the global AIDS challenge as the disease itself.

AIDS was recognized as an epidemic across affluent countries in the early 1980s, but a decade passed before the situation in LMICs elicited a global response. Today sub-Saharan Africa bears the brunt: only 10% of the world's population lives in this region, but it is home to almost 70%—25.5 million people—of the global HIV-infected population and nearly 85% of children with HIV (UNAIDS 2016). In 2015, 1.4 million Africans were newly infected and 800,000 died from AIDS. HIV seroprevalence (proportion with disease verified by blood specimens) varies across the continent, ranging from less than 1% in Mauritania to 29% in Swaziland. The impact on mortality and well-being in sub-Saharan Africa has been immense (ibid) (Box 6-5). In five African countries, life expectancy is lower than it was 20 years ago (African Health Observatory 2014). Yet there is also reason for guarded

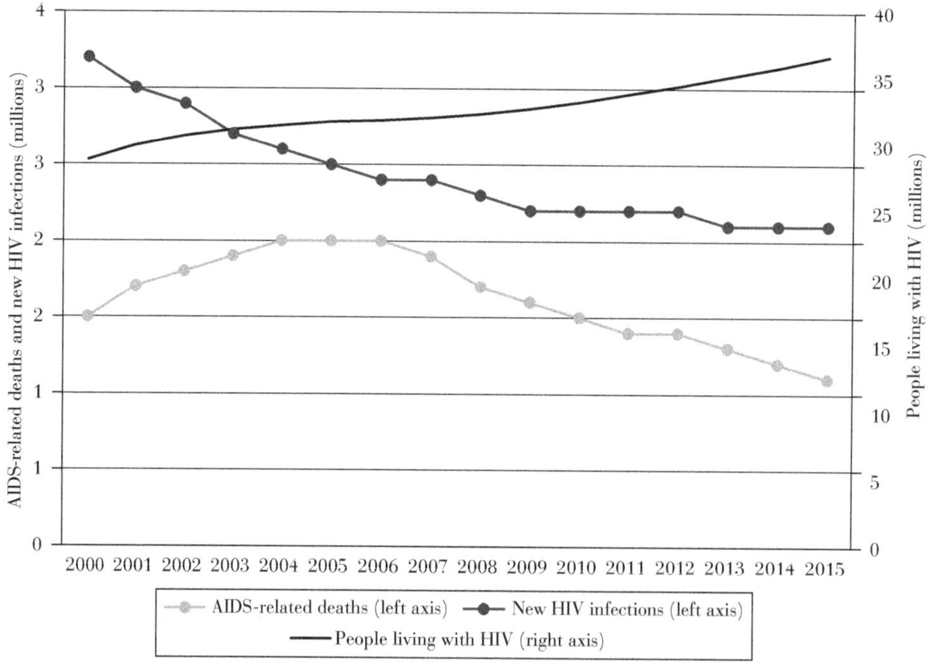

Figure 6-12: Annual estimates on the number of AIDS-related deaths, new HIV infections, and people living with HIV globally (2000–2015).
Data Source: UNAIDS (2016).

optimism: among young people (15–24 years) in sub-Saharan Africa, HIV prevalence fell by 42% between 2001 and 2012, with concomitant life expectancy gains (e.g., South African life expectancy increased from 57 years in 2009 to 62 years in 2013) (Dorrington et al. 2014). Of course it is important to remember that those who live longer are not cured, remaining HIV-infected with associated care needs.

Epidemiologic explanations of HIV typically focus on individual "risk behaviors" (e.g., unprotected sex and drug use) without considering the societal-level factors that shape and limit individuals' choices and options. The underlying assumption of the biomedical approach is that individuals make autonomous and informed decisions that are not constrained by the broader context of their lives (Hunter 2010). Yet in much of the world, HIV has become a disease of marginalization: poverty is both cause and consequence of the disease. People with long-term nutritional deficiencies and untreated infections are more biologically vulnerable to HIV, and low-income women, for example, may feel forced into transactional or unprotected sex. Once ill, persons of low socioeconomic status have less access to health and social services, and if they are unable to work, they and their households will be further impoverished (Doyal with Doyal 2013). Indeed, a 2001 UN General Assembly Special Session recognized that "poverty, underdevelopment, and illiteracy are among the principal contributing factors to the spread of HIV/AIDS" (UN 2001).

At a global level, the distribution of infection reflects regional economic and political inequities; the majority of people infected live in the poorest regions of LMICs. Within countries, the most socially excluded groups are typically the most affected by the disease, such as homeless individuals in North America, low-income Black women in South Africa, and people who inject drugs imprisoned in Russia. Yet HIV also poses certain paradoxes: in much of Africa, higher HIV seroprevalence is linked to people who have more education and income, live in urban areas (where prevalence is higher), and have more transactional sex and multipartner concurrency, resulting in increased exposure to HIV (Gould 2009; Mishra et al. 2007). At the same time, more educated groups have a greater likelihood of benefiting from HIV prevention and treatment (Doyal with Doyal 2013).

Box 6-5 Social Impact of HIV and AIDS in sub-Saharan Africa

The disruptions caused by HIV and AIDS to social and family life in parts of sub-Saharan Africa are extreme. There are an estimated 13.4 million children worldwide orphaned, of whom some 81% were living in sub-Saharan Africa (UNAIDS 2016). In countries with the highest prevalence—Botswana, Lesotho, Swaziland, and Zimbabwe—more than 1 in 5 children are orphans, and other children are made vulnerable by AIDS. Orphans are often cared for in female-headed households—typically grandmothers and aunts looking after several children—and many face poverty, malnutrition, and exploitation. This in turn may lead to increased vulnerability to subsequent HIV infection. Many orphans experience interrupted schooling and can be forced into lives of early labor, crime, violence, and exploitative sex. Orphans must not only cope with the severe emotional consequences of losing a parent but also with discrimination, at the same time as they face an uncertain future (Iliffe 2006).

The effects of HIV and AIDS range from profound personal harm, including pain and distress, to loss of livelihood, increases in inequality within countries, and global injustices writ large (Doyal with Doyal 2013). The growing number of people with HIV-related disabilities has an enormous impact on family caregivers, especially in the context of inadequate rehabilitation and social support services (Hanass-Hancock et al. 2015). A decade ago it was estimated that AIDS would lead to the loss of 20% of the agricultural workforce in Africa and a high proportion of teachers and health care workers (UNAIDS 2004). While the introduction of large-scale HIV treatment has diminished the magnitude of these estimates, the dire consequences of the AIDS crisis will continue to be felt in generations to come.

Preventing and Treating HIV

Initially the sole means of controlling the spread of HIV involved strategies to prevent individuals from engaging in unprotected sex and avoid blood-borne transmission both in health care settings and in the context of injecting drug use. Condoms do serve as an effective, if imperfect, barrier against possible infection through sexual intercourse, as demonstrated by Thailand's successful nationwide condom campaign. However, condom promotion faces multiple obstacles including cost (especially for female condoms, developed only recently), access, and public resistance due to cultural and religious values and desire for children. In some settings, use of condoms has become synonymous with infidelity and/or HIV infection (Bauman and Berman 2005). But promotion of the controversial alternative of abstinence from sex is unrealistic and ineffective. Still, consistent condom use makes childbearing difficult, and for many a choice they are unwilling to make. Needle exchange for people who inject drugs, too, has been opposed in many communities across the world because it is viewed as an encouragement to drug use (Lurie and Drucker 1997).

In the early 1990s, researchers found highly active antiretroviral therapy to be the most effective intervention for reducing morbidity and mortality in persons with HIV. For those already infected, antiretroviral therapy (ART) can dramatically slow the progression of HIV to AIDS and reduce transmission to others due to a low viral load maintained in the bloodstream. Starting in the mid-1990s antiretrovirals (ARVs) were widely prescribed in most HICs and covered by national health insurance, but the thousands of dollars in annual medication costs made ART prohibitive in LMICs, with certain exceptions (Box 6-6). Unwilling to accept this

Box 6-6 Case Study: Brazil's National AIDS Program

Brazil's National AIDS Program is widely recognized as a leading example of integrated HIV prevention and AIDS care and treatment based on the principle of health as a human right. The program has provided an important model for other countries in Latin America and Africa through AIDS control cooperation projects.

Brazil's epidemic has primarily affected men who have sex with men and people who inject drugs. In the early 1990s, the World Bank estimated that 1.2 million Brazilians would have HIV by 2000. Due to its aggressive HIV prevention activities and universal access to free treatment, Brazil cut that projected number nearly in half by the early 2000s (UNAIDS 2016). In 1996 the government of Brazil began offering universal and free access to ARVs, reaching 458,000 persons in 2015 (UNAIDS 2016). In 1992, during negotiations for a loan to support its national AIDS program, Brazil effectively refused World Bank demands that it abandon free distribution of the drug AZT (which it had begun several years earlier) as a condition to the loan agreement (Berkman et al. 2005). Brazil has also resisted US challenges to its generic manufacture of some ARVs (see chapter 9).

Brazil's success is based on widespread distribution of condoms, needle exchange and harm reduction programs, and HIV testing, as well as treatment, all within the context of its public and universal health care system. Prevention programs have addressed issues around sexual practices and increasing condom use, while also combating homophobia and discrimination, and supporting sexual diversity. The government has promoted community-based prevention programs that work with men who have sex with men, sex workers, and youth (Berkman et al. 2005). In 2005, the Brazilian government refused the remaining US$40 million in a 5-year grant from USAID to protest restrictions on funding that required all recipient organizations to agree to a declaration condemning prostitution.

None of these efforts would have been possible without an engaged civil society, activist NGOs, and organizations led by people living with HIV, who have pushed for effective government policies and helped reduce discrimination, educated the public, and provided care and support for other people living with HIV (Biehl 2006).

situation, a range of advocacy organizations and activists engaged in protracted negotiations and concerted pressure and protest against the pharmaceutical industry (Chan 2015).

Meantime, two nonprofits ignored arguments that ARVs were too complicated and expensive to administer in Africa. MSF launched several small-scale initiatives in South Africa and Malawi, and now runs projects in 25 countries. Partners In Health set up community-based treatment programs in Haiti, Rwanda, Malawi, and low-income areas of the United States (Mukherjee et al. 2006).

After 2000, the goal of "universal treatment" obtained greater support. WHO's campaign to get 3 million people on ART by 2005 (3 by 5) was not reached but it played an important role in pressuring companies to drive down the price of first-line ARVs from US$2,500 per year to US$300 per year by 2004, and further down to US$115 by 2013 (AVERT 2014). South Africa, with the world's largest number of people living with HIV, has also been the site of tireless social mobilization and transnational solidarity on this issue. In the early 2000s, the Treatment Action Campaign vociferously pressed the South African government, whose then President denied the link between HIV and AIDS, to provide ARVs to pregnant women, while a human rights lawsuit accused international pharmaceutical companies of gross profiteering. Its out-of-court settlement resulted in substantial price drops (Singh, Govender, and Mills 2007). South Africa's recent willingness to confront AIDS denialism and its surge in treatment volume have led it to use its purchasing power to press for the lowest ARV prices in the world (Simelela et al. 2015).

International progress in the scale-up of ART over the past decade has been notable, although many challenges remain. In South Africa, for example, women are substantially more likely to be on treatment than men, and prevalence has declined among youth. However, despite optimistic projections otherwise, there is consistently high HIV prevalence and incidence among adults aged 25 to 49 even with ARV availability (Eaton et al. 2015).

As of June 2016, it was estimated that 17 million people living with HIV were receiving ART, a thirty-fold increase from 2001 and up from 15 million in 2014 (UNAIDS 2016) (Figure 6-13). Where treatment has become available, more people have sought to be tested, though many others have not. Today, the largest funders for ART worldwide are the Global Fund and PEPFAR (see chapter 4 for details). From 1995 to 2013, ARV treatment averted an estimated 7.6 million AIDS-related deaths

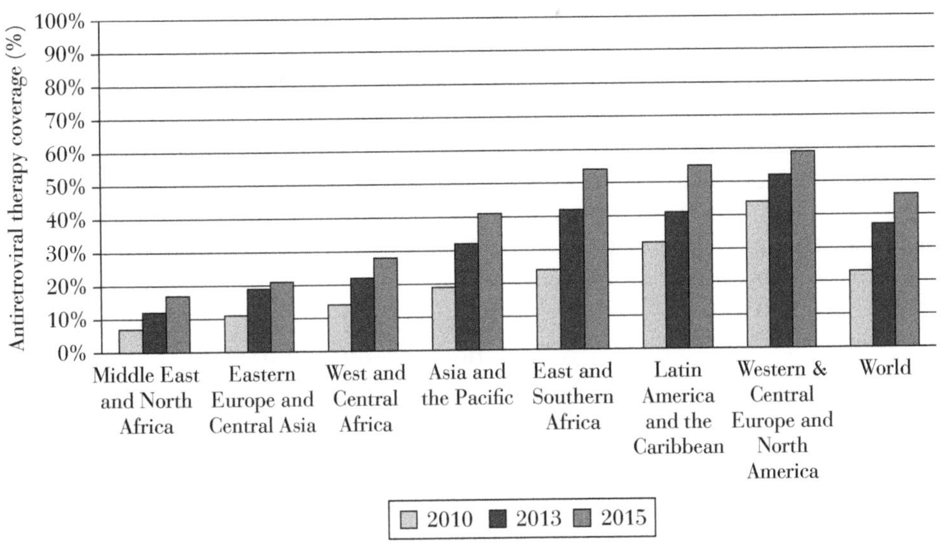

Figure 6-13: Percentage of adults and children receiving antiretroviral therapy among all people living with HIV, by region (2010–2015).

Data Source: UNAIDS (2016).

worldwide (UNAIDS 2014b). However, almost 20 million people worldwide (three of five people living with HIV), still lacked access to ART in 2015, most in LMICs. An estimated 46% of adults, and 50% of eligible children were receiving ARV treatment in 2015 (UNAIDS 2016).

Since 2002, MTCT of HIV in utero (5%–10% risk), intrapartum (10%–20%), and during breastfeeding (5%–20%) has been reduced dramatically through a worldwide initiative to administer nevirapine at delivery (noting that exclusive breastfeeding for the first 6 months nevertheless protects against diarrheal and respiratory illnesses) (Barron et al. 2013). In 2015 Cuba became the first country in the world to eliminate MTCT of HIV and congenital syphilis, portending the possibility for global elimination of all new perinatal HIV infections (Kamb et al. 2015).

Preventing MTCT has been more of a priority than long-term treatment for infected mothers, however. The Option B+ program (started in 2011) aims to provide lifetime ARV treatment to all HIV-infected pregnant and breastfeeding women, though there remain concerns about pursuing this approach without overall strengthening of health and social services (Coutsoudis et al. 2013).

ARVs can be used for HIV prevention in several ways: as treatment to reduce the viral load of HIV infected persons, as oral chemoprophylaxis after a high risk exposure, or orally or vaginally as daily pre-exposure prophylaxis in "high-risk persons" with repeated exposures. The "Treatment as Prevention" approach, universal HIV testing and immediate initiation of ART, also known as "Test and Start," reduces transmission to others by over 90% (Cohen 2013). Other prevention methods include voluntary medical male circumcision, found to be 60% efficacious in preventing HIV infection in men, leading to 9.1 million men being circumcised between 2008 and 2014 (UNAIDS 2015; WHO 2014i).

The public health response to the global HIV epidemic now focuses on 12 key populations deemed to be most vulnerable to infection and disease: people living with HIV, adolescent girls and women, prisoners, migrants, people who inject drugs, sex workers, men who have sex with men, transgender persons, children living with HIV, displaced persons, persons with disabilities, and people over 50 (UNAIDS 2014b). The latest round of UNAIDS targets for epidemic control by 2020 are: (1) 90% of all people living with HIV knowing their HIV status; (2) 90% of people with HIV on ARVs; and (3) 90% of those on ART having viral suppression—all therapeutically oriented (UNAIDS 2014a).

However, for HIV to be addressed more equitably and, arguably, more quickly, the social and political dimensions of the epidemic must also be tackled. Structural interventions dealing with, for example, gender and power inequities and livelihood security are relevant not only for prevention but for access and adherence to treatment (Seeley et al. 2012).

Notwithstanding the global response to the epidemic in the last decade, involving a wide array of partnerships and initiatives showing extraordinary persistence and dedication (Quigley 2009), HIV is on the increase in some settings. In India and parts of Southeast Asia for example, it has been fueled by a lack of political commitment to early prevention, compounded by poverty, illiteracy, population mobility, discrimination, and gender inequality. In the former Soviet bloc, HIV infections and deaths have increased by 40% since 2000. Globally there is rising prevalence among people who inject drugs, and HIV prevalence exceeds 25% among men who have sex with men in some areas (Beyrer et al. 2012).

Moreover, advances in treatment and prevention have not been accompanied by concomitant attention to the complex personal and societal circumstances that generate and exacerbate the epidemic. Indeed, in a bitter paradox, the privileging of therapeutics over social context means that although there has been a massive scale-up of ARV treatment in Mozambique, for example, adequate nutrition, essential to keeping people living with HIV healthy, remains out of reach and forces people to compete for scarce food resources, undermining community-based solidarity efforts that address AIDS (Kalofonos 2010).

Diseases of Emerging (Global) Social and Economic Patterns

Over recent decades, new and renewed infectious diseases, from HIV to SARS, have emerged alongside globalization, with increased surveillance improving the ability to detect them. Especially in the Global South, the rise in agribusiness and low-wage factory labor have pushed people and production into urban areas, generating new disease patterns. For example, across Asia, as in Africa and Latin America, rural residents increasingly seek work in cities—expensive high-stress contexts with low levels of worker protection and crowded housing, enabling easy pathogen transmission. Workers who become infected with TB or HIV may then bring infection home to their villages. With social and work conditions jeopardized by deregulation and the collapse of public services, old diseases have resurged and new ones have materialized, often defying public health efforts to control them. These changes, in turn are linked to the neoliberal phase in global capitalism, shaping production, finance, trade, and consumption patterns, as well as labor and social policies (see chapter 9), ergo the EG nomenclature.

In a rash of misplaced optimism, some scientists in the 1960s suggested that infectious diseases were a thing of the past. Nobel laureate Sir Frank MacFarlane Burnet, for example, noted that the mid-20th century marked "the end of one of the most important social revolutions in history—the virtual elimination of the infectious disease as a significant factor in social life" (Burnet and White 1962, p. iii).

Yet the threat of infectious diseases is perhaps higher now than ever. Many common ailments, such as pertussis, TB, and cholera, never really disappeared. Instead, HIC authorities lost interest in them and only perceived their "re-emergence" when they began to threaten high-income settings (Farmer 1996). New and re-emerging zoonoses linked to ecological shifts in the habitats of mosquitoes and others that cross species barriers, for example in the context of factory farms, have raised particular alarm.

Another emerging problem has to do with indiscriminate use of antibiotics (up to 50% unnecessary) in humans plus widespread use in the commercial livestock industry. These practices have led to increasing antimicrobial resistance (to penicillin and other commonly used antibiotics), with at least 700,000 associated deaths each year (Review on Antimicrobial Resistance 2016). Still, a predominant concern around antibiotics remains inadequate access, especially in LMICs (Das and Horton 2015).

Concern with emerging infectious diseases (EIDs), what we call EG diseases, motivated establishment in 2001 of the Global Outbreak Alert and Response Network, coordinated by WHO and involving UN and government technical agencies (e.g., CDC), as well as MSF, the International Committee of the Red Cross, and other organizations involved in outbreak alert and responses. The US government's Global Health Security Agenda involves a similar multi-entity collaboration (Frieden et al. 2014). But it has been accused of focusing too narrowly on diseases without considering their social determinants, and of closely paralleling US national security interests (Gostin and Phelan 2014).

Arguably, various MM ailments, such as diabetes, are as much a part of EG as infectious diseases. Here we have decided to retain the EID focus, but consciously employ EG as a political economy categorization.

EG diseases (Table 6-5) fall into one of three groups:

1. Truly new diseases, including HIV and Ebola in the 1970s, and SARS in 2003.
2. Newly recognized entities, such as amebic infection of the sinuses and brain, which existed previously but were only recently identified.
3. Diseases on the rise where they were previously absent or infrequent, such as cholera in Africa and Latin America, or XDR-TB in sub-Saharan Africa and Eastern Europe.

Most emerging infections are caused by organisms already present in the environment, which become prominent through some change in societal conditions (Table 6-6).

SARS and MERS

Demonstrating the rapid global spread of infectious disease and its connection to massive economic shifts in Asia was SARS (severe acute respiratory syndrome), the first emergent disease of the new millennium. Although it likely started in late 2002, Chinese officials only reported the first signs of SARS in February 2003: in Guangdong Province over 100 persons died from a mysterious atypical pneumonia. A physician who had treated some of the patients became infected and subsequently traveled to Hong Kong, where he infected at least 13 other people in his hotel. These individuals then traveled and inadvertently seeded large outbreaks in Vietnam, Singapore, and Toronto. The virus spread quickly to six other countries in Asia and several Canadian cities. Thousands of people were quarantined for weeks in order to stop the spread of SARS.

Table 6-5 Some (Re-) Emerging Infections and Probable Factors in their Emergence and Spread

Disease (or Agent Causing Disease)	Factors Contributing to Emergence and Spread
Bovine spongiform encephalopathy (cattle)	Agricultural practices (changes in rendering processes; human cases of variant Creutzfeldt-Jakob disease (vCJD) believed to be linked to consuming infected cattle products)
Viral Syndromes/Diseases	
Argentine, Bolivian hemorrhagic fever	Changes in agricultural practices favoring rodent hosts
Chikungunya, dengue hemorrhagic fever, Zika	Travel, commerce migration, urbanization, housing and sanitation deficiencies (i.e., stagnant water); spreading worldwide, especially in the Americas
Ebola, Marburg	Initial cases through contact with infected natural host (probably bats, whose habitats shifted due to deforestation); human contact may be linked to increased foraging, shaped by livelihood pressures; subsequent cases through close contact with patient's body fluids by family and caregivers, exacerbated by extreme health care system deficiencies due to war, structural adjustment, illicit financial outflows
Hantavirus	Ecological or environmental changes increasing contact with rodent hosts
Lassa fever	Human settlement patterns (e.g., near diamond mines), favoring rodent exposure in homes
Rift Valley fever	Dam building, agriculture, irrigation
SARS (Severe Acute Respiratory Syndrome)	Food animal agricultural practices (from handling infected food animals that acquired virus from other species in live animal markets); contact with infected bodily fluids or respiratory droplets, especially in health care settings; international travel
West Nile fever	Bird migratory patterns enabling introduction of virus into area with suitable indigenous mosquito vectors
Bacterial Syndromes/Diseases	
Helicobacter pylori	Most common chronic bacterial infection in world, but largely unrecognized. Linked to urbanization, contaminated water, and inadequate sanitation.
Hemolytic uremic syndrome	Mass food processing technology allowing *E. coli* 0157:H7 contamination of meat, or contamination of other products with infected cattle manure
Legionella (Legionnaire's disease)	Cooling and plumbing systems
Lyme borreliosis (*Borrelia burgdorferi*)	Deforestation around homes and other conditions favoring tick vector with deer (a secondary reservoir host)
Streptococcus, group A (invasive, necrotizing, "flesh-eating")	Unknown
Toxic shock syndrome (*Staphylococcus aureus*)	Ultra-absorbent tampons
Parasitic Diseases/Agents	
Cryptosporidium, *Cyclospora*, other waterborne pathogens	Transnational trade in food and produce, contaminated surface water, faulty water purification
Schistosomiasis	Dam building

Source: Adapted and updated from Morse (1995).

Table 6-6 Some Factors in the (Re-)Emergence and Spread of Infectious Diseases

Category	Factors	Examples of Disease
Ecological changes	Agriculture, dams, changes in water ecosystems, deforestation and reforestation, flood and drought, famine, climate change	Schistosomiasis, Hantavirus pulmonary syndrome, Rift Valley fever, dengue, Zika, chikungunya, malaria
Demographic shifts, political and economic factors, human behavior	Population growth and migration, urbanization, war and civil conflict, urban decay, sexual behavior changes, injection drug use, vaccine refusal	Introduction of HIV, spread of dengue fever, sexually transmitted infections, hepatitis, measles
International travel and commerce	Worldwide movement of goods and people, transcontinental air travel	MERS, introduction of cholera to South America, SARS
Technology and industry	Globalization of food supplies, changes in food processing and packaging, organ and tissue transplantation, drugs causing immune suppression, widespread use of antibiotics, intensified food animal production	Hemolytic uremic syndrome (*E. coli* O157:H7), bovine spongiform encephalopathy, transfusion-associated hepatitis B and C, opportunistic infections in immunosuppressed patients, SARS, H5N1 avian influenza
Microbial adaptation and change	Response to health care-related and human-related selection factors, microbial evolution	Antibiotic-resistant bacteria (MDR- and XDR-TB), "antigenic drift" in influenza virus
Breakdown in public health measures	Curtailment or reduction in prevention programs, inadequate sanitation and vector control measures, lack of infection control measures	Resurgence of TB and MDR/XDR-TB in Eastern Europe and Africa, cholera and yellow fever in Africa, resurgence of diphtheria in the former Soviet Union, dengue, Zika, and chikungunya in the Americas

Source: Adapted and extensively updated from Morse (1995).

By the time the outbreak was declared contained in July 2003, there had been 8,098 cases of probable or confirmed SARS—over 5,000 in China—with 774 deaths reported in 29 countries.

The causative agent was a new pathogen, the SARS-coronavirus, almost identical to a virus found in civet cats, raccoon dogs, and bats sold in animal markets in southern China—the fastest urbanizing setting in the world. With farm and wild animals in close proximity and increased demand for meat, amid unregulated slaughtering, Chinese markets proved a fertile ground for transmission to humans. The rapid spread was facilitated by air travel of some infected individuals, and respiratory droplet spread of the virus. With health facilities an extremely conducive environment for transmission, health care workers, exposed through intubation and close contact, accounted for one fifth of all SARS cases. The overall case fatality rate was 9.6%.

The pathogen was identified and laboratory diagnostics developed extremely rapidly, but without drugs or a vaccine, strict infection control measures were vital. These traditional approaches included identifying and managing contacts and quarantining those potentially exposed. Fear and panic led to travel bans, scapegoating in some settings, such as shunning of Chinese restaurants in Toronto, and travel and investment losses of up to US$100 billion. SARS clearly showed that inadequate surveillance and response capacity in one country can have global implications (Heymann 2004). The outbreak tested disease notification systems and WHO's response capability, motivating the development of new International Health Regulations (see chapter 5).

Mirroring the nature and spread of SARS in 2003, a new coronavirus emerged in 2012 in Saudi Arabia, baptized the Middle East Respiratory Syndrome coronavirus (MERS-CoV). As of mid-2016, 1,769 cases (with at least 630 deaths) had been reported in 27 countries including Saudi Arabia, Malaysia, Jordan, Qatar, United Arab Emirates, Tunisia, Philippines, South Korea, Taiwan, and the United States (WHO 2016f). Although the origins are still unclear, the epidemiology points to multiple zoonotic transmission channels from common unknown sources, possibly dromedaries (Hui, Perlman, and Zumla 2015). MERS has raised particular concern around the Hajj—the annual pilgrimage of millions of Muslims to Mecca—but as of 2015, there were no associated cases, perhaps due to precautionary measures (Lessler et al. 2014). A 2015 outbreak in South Korea saw the fastest spread of the virus to date, revealing weaknesses in the Health Ministry's preparedness. Transmitted by a businessman returning from the Middle East, it was exacerbated by inadequate infection control, consultation of specialists at multiple facilities, and crowded hospital quarters with overnight visitors (WHO 2015w).

Ebola in West Africa

Ebola virus disease (EVD) was first detected in West Africa in late 2013, traveling slowly between villages in rural eastern Guinea. Some epidemiologists thought that, like outbreaks elsewhere, it would be short-lived. However, within a few months, EVD spread to neighboring Liberia and Sierra Leone, with rapidly increasing case counts and fatalities, and has since become the largest EVD outbreak ever: Sierra Leone experienced 14,124 cases and 3,956 deaths; Liberia 10,675 cases and 4,809 deaths; and Guinea 3,811 cases and 2,543 deaths (WHO 2016b). On 14 January 2016, WHO declared that Ebola transmission had ended in West Africa.

Ebola first emerged in 1976 in the Democratic Republic of Congo, with over 20 outbreaks since then, each causing a few hundred deaths before being contained. The Congo strain of Ebola likely spread to West Africa through bat migration, resulting from reduced habitats in central Africa due to deforestation. Extreme poverty and thinning forests in West Africa led rural populations into ever more remote forests foraging for game, wood, and minerals, and exposing them to zoonotic pathogens.

Dire economic conditions also shaped the health system response—long-neglected health facilities lacking staff, supplies (including syringes, disinfectants, and gloves), and hospital beds—and further exacerbated the spread of disease throughout the health system and into the community. The governments of the three hardest hit countries had limited ability to contain EVD within the region (Bausch and Schwarz 2014). Once established in the community, EVD quickly spread through close contact, and funerals and burials caused massive transmission to those who touched and bathed the body.

As with many other illnesses to afflict the global poor, there is a complex interwoven political ecology framing Ebola. Reminiscent of HIV in the early 1980s, EVD was accompanied by distrust, discrimination, and fear, leading to difficulties in tracking down infected individuals (Gonsalves and Staley 2014). These sentiments were aggravated by the legacy of slavery—shifting alliances determined capture versus survival—the colonial period, when punitive actions were taken to enforce quarantines (and in the case of Liberia, the powerful role of US interests, including the rapacious Firestone rubber company [Mitman 2014]), as well as the more recent history of authoritarian and corrupt regimes backed by the international community, unspeakably brutal civil wars and population displacement (Benton and Dionne 2015), and the impact of structural adjustment programs and their long aftermath on health and social services infrastructure (Leach 2015). The political economy context of EVD is discussed further in chapter 11.

The affected countries had fragile health care systems to begin with, which broke under the strain of the crisis (Pieterse and Lodge 2015). Infection control was a major problem (including due to shortage of rubber gloves, despite Liberia being the site of the largest rubber plantation in the world!). Diversion of support for Ebola control and the death of over 500 health workers resulted in closing of medical and nursing schools, secondment of health care workers away from TB and malaria control programs, closing of HIV clinics, and so on, with associated untreated disease and likely increased mortality. In Guinea, a 31% decline in overall outpatient visits during the epidemic especially affected children, with lowered vaccination rates and treatment of diarrhea and acute respiratory infections (Barden-O'Fallen et al. 2015). EVD's devastating indirect impact in Sierra Leone included a 30% increase in maternal deaths and 24% increase in newborn deaths (Jones and Ameh 2015), levels not experienced since the 1990s civil war.

There were multiple missed opportunities to stem the outbreak early on. Both CDC and WHO scientists admitted to letting down their guard when they thought the virus was contained (Bausch 2015). WHO arrived late to the response, and when the wider humanitarian system mobilized, the response was fragmented rather than being coordinated under WHO's lead. Indeed, WHO lacked the funding, global health emergency workforce, and organizational capacity to mount a full-scale emergency response to an epidemic like Ebola (WHO 2015p). From a public health practice perspective, a trained and agile workforce was critical to EVD's eventual control. A centralized "Incident Command Structure" in Liberia and Sierra Leone included case management, surveillance, safe burial teams, epidemiology, family support, water and sanitation teams, quarantine, and most importantly, social mobilization.

Portrayal of Ebola as a security crisis for the West was enormously problematic (Benton and Dionne 2015). Travel bans and quarantine were threatened and administered in North America and elsewhere based on prejudice, stereotypes, and ignorance. Racism was also manifest in the differential medical care (experimental medicines and serum from survivors) given to foreign versus African health workers who got sick with Ebola, and the relentless media dichotomy between "superstitious" locals and heroic foreign health personnel.

Influenza

There are approximately 1 billion cases of influenza (the flu) each year, with 3 to 5 million severe cases and 250,000 to 500,000 deaths annually, the vast majority in the elderly (WHO 2014e). Health authorities plan for the most likely strain of influenza and create yearly vaccines (of varying efficacy, due to challenges in identifying the right strains given the time lag in vaccine development) accordingly. WHO targets pregnant women as the highest priority group for vaccination, given the risk of complications and death, as well as the elderly, immunocompromised persons, health care workers, and children under 2 years of age (WHO SAGE 2012). Some HICs, such as the United States, have universal vaccine recommendations for all persons over 6 months old (Grohskopf et al. 2012).

New strains of influenza viruses can be transmitted to humans from other animal species, most often poultry and swine. An influenza pandemic occurs when one of these novel strains of influenza is introduced and adapts to become easily transmissible from human to human. A global epidemic could potentially kill millions more than seasonal influenza because no one would have immunity to the novel strain (WHO 2014e).

There were three influenza pandemics in the 20th century: the so-called Spanish flu (H1N1, 1918), the Asian flu (H2N2, 1957), and the Hong Kong flu (H3N2, 1968). Whereas the latter two were relatively mild, the 1918 epidemic struck young, healthy adults. Between 20% and 40% of the worldwide population became ill, exacerbated by WWI's massive troop movements and the crowded conditions of trench warfare. Seasonal flu mortality is normally less than 0.1%, but the Spanish flu killed 2% to 20% of those infected—some 50 to 100 million people over 10 months, including likely 20 to 25 million people in colonial India who were already facing famine (Patterson and Pyle 1991).

Avian influenza (H5N1) poses another potential public health concern. This highly pathogenic subtype of influenza virus was first documented in 1996 and crossed the species barrier to infect persons living and working with birds in Southeast Asia. In 2004, the first case of probable human-to-human transmission occurred in Thailand (WHO 2007a). Countries in Eastern Europe and Central Asia began detecting avian influenza in local flocks starting in 2005, and WHO (erroneously, as it turned out) forecasted up to 150 million fatalities and mobilized the enormously wasteful stocking of over 100 million doses of the antiviral drug Tamiflu,* which has since proven inefficacious and generated drug resistance (Velásquez 2012). As of mid-2015, WHO had confirmed 844 human cases of H5N1 and 449 deaths in 15 dozen countries, with presence in bird populations in 60 countries. Due to the potential consequences of large-scale, sustained transmission, more than 400 million birds were culled worldwide (1.6 million in Nigeria) (Donis and Cox 2013), although there has been little attention to the extreme conditions of the expanding livestock industry from North America to Asia and well beyond (Wallace 2016), as well as human crowding and poor nutrition.

While vaccine development is another potential approach, it would take 6 months to respond to an emerging pandemic, and efficacy would be limited depending on viral mutations. Another challenge is that some countries are refusing to share viral samples collected from patients, fearing (with apparently good reason, in the case of Indonesia) that viral strains will be passed on to pharmaceutical companies, which could produce a vaccine for profit rather than for public health, drastically limiting access to the vaccine in LMICs.

In April 2009, a novel influenza A(H1N1)pdm09 strain emerged in Mexico (likely through pigs imported from Asia) and caused a wave of illness in otherwise healthy people. Originally labeled an outbreak, WHO upgraded it to a pandemic as it spread worldwide. Through aggressive and targeted immunization by involved countries, as well as social isolation efforts, the pandemic tapered off in late 2009 and was declared over in August 2010. All told, there were 18,500 laboratory-confirmed deaths worldwide; an estimated excess 200,000 respiratory deaths and 83,000 cardiovascular deaths were attributed to H1N1, most among nonelderly persons (Dawood 2012). H5N1 pandemic planning had improved both preparedness for seasonal influenza A(H1N1) and, based on WHO guidelines, for future pandemics via sustained surveillance of flu viruses.

However, WHO came under fire after both the 2005 and 2009 pandemics, because the declaration of global epidemics, seemingly unsubstantiated, mobilized countries to stockpile billions of dollars worth of vaccines and antivirals (Cohen and Carter 2010). Not only did most of these go to waste, but the stockpiling recommendation itself represented a conflict of interest for some of WHO's expert advisors, who were also on the payroll of the pharmaceutical industry. These episodes represent a troubling development: the pharmaceutical industry, which profits handsomely from pandemic declarations, together with other private sector actors, has increasing sway over WHO's public health decisionmaking role (Velásquez 2012).

Substandard Drugs/Adverse Drug Reactions/Drug Overdoses

The global trade in substandard drugs is a mounting problem in HICs and LMICs alike (see chapter 11) and is estimated to result in US$75 billion annually in illegal revenues (Nayyar, Breman, and Herrington 2015). Spurred by access problems due to prohibitive "Big Pharma" prices (and lack of public financing for medicines), as well as an inadequate governance framework to guide regulations and policymaking pertaining to drug safety in many settings, the quest for affordable medicines has generated lucrative production and transnational distribution of substandard drugs (due to inadequate regulation or deteriorating quality, safety, and efficacy measures) via Internet sales, dubious companies, and market channels. Upwards of 700,000 deaths a year may be caused by poor quality or adulterated drugs, including 200,000 to 300,000 annual deaths in China and over 100,000 deaths per year in sub-Saharan Africa (Sambira 2013). In one Nigerian city, poor quality and inactive ingredients were found in over 15% of antimalarials (Kaur et al. 2015).

An accompanying problem is adverse drug reactions (ADRs, dangerous drug effects), which often go unreported, even more so in LMICs. In the United States alone, ADRs contribute to an estimated 2 to 4 million serious, disabling, or fatal injuries annually (Moscou, Kohler, and Lexchin 2013); they are considered one of the top 10 causes of death in the world. In addition, fatal poisonings from prescription painkillers are a growing problem: in the United States more than 47,000 people died in 2014 from overdoses, over half due to prescription drugs, especially opioids) (Rudd et al. 2016); at the global level, though precise data are lacking, deaths from painkillers are a fast-growing epidemic that may rival the 200,000 overdose deaths due to illegal narcotics (Martins et al. 2015).

CONCLUSION

Learning Points:

- Patterns of disease are shaped by social, political, and economic factors as well as biological and medical ones.
- Diseases are typically categorized by their communicability, but this approach is inadequate because (1) various diseases are both infectious and chronic (e.g., TB, HIV, and many NTDs); (2) so-called NCDs may be "socially communicable," that is, spread by social processes (marketing, societally-mediated consumption patterns, etc.); (3) the standard association of LMICs with communicable diseases and HICs with NCDs does not hold—all societies are affected by both kinds of disease; and (4) these categories do not take into account the larger context of disease.
- Global disease patterns can be categorized according to macro-structural causes as: (a) diseases of marginalization and deprivation; (b) diseases of modernization and work; and (c) diseases of marginalization and modernization; as well as (d) diseases of emerging (global) social and economic patterns.
- Treatment and preventive measures are available for many of the world's leading causes of morbidity and mortality, but there are myriad structural barriers to implementation.

This chapter began with a snapshot of disease profiles from selected countries. All populations experience morbidity and mortality due to both communicable diseases *and* CHD, chronic lung diseases, diabetes, and cancer. The relative weight of these causes is linked to the economic structure and socio-political features of different societies (e.g., level of urbanization, class/gender/race relations, and governance arrangements) as well as to biological factors.

For most childhood diseases, there are simple and effective interventions. There have been great strides in child health in the past 50 years, with millions of lives saved. Yet up to six million children continue to die each year from preventable causes, with large inequalities in infant and child morbidity/mortality, as well as maternal mortality, both *between* HICs and LMICs and *within* these settings. The inability to prevent child deaths and maternal mortality is as much a failure of politics as of health measures.

Malaria, measles, NTDs, and diarrhea plague many LMICs. The immediate determinants, such as nonpotable water, poor sanitation and hygiene, and lack of access to health care services, are influenced by larger structural factors. Distributing simple interventions for these ailments should not obscure the need for larger change. Most tellingly, although diseases of marginalization and deprivation are especially associated with LICs, they may also be present among socially excluded populations of HICs, where inequalities have worsened and social welfare systems have eroded under austerity policies.

Modernization has raised standards of living but has also exacerbated chronic NCDs and, particularly through the burning of fossil fuels, generated the looming effects of climate change (see chapter 10). Again, biological factors are intertwined with societal patterns of consumption and production, the affordability and availability of nutritious food, employment patterns (including job security and levels of occupational stress), and exposure to toxins, pollution, and violence, which all relate to the politics and distribution of power and wealth.

At the confluence of marginalization and modernization, there are increased rates of diabetes, lung disease, TB, and HIV. Claiming the lives of millions, these diseases fall along the fault lines of poverty and discrimination, with social and economic dynamics fueling the HIV pandemic. Meanwhile, diseases of emerging (global) social and economic patterns garner significant and sometimes unwarranted attention, which nonetheless typically overlooks the role of neoliberal globalization in directly and indirectly generating these diseases.

While smallpox and the cattle plague rinderpest have been eradicated, and polio and guinea worm are nearing eradication, addressing the underlying determinants of multiple causes of death is ultimately a far more effective and equitable approach than disease-by-disease eradication. The next chapter explores how the societal determinants of health, operating simultaneously at global, national, community, and household levels, shape the patterns of life expectancy, disease, and premature death presented here.

NOTES

1. Queer is an umbrella term that offers a fluid alternative to more rigid gender and/or sexuality labels. The Q in the abbreviation also refers to anyone questioning their gender and/or sexual identity or not conforming to standard categories. Transgender refers to people whose gender identity does not align with the one they were assigned at birth. Under the transgender umbrella, nonbinary refers to people whose gender identity does not fit within the gender binary (of male or female). Asexual refers to persons who do not experience sexual attraction (aromantics do not experience romantic attraction). These identities are on a spectrum. Intersex people may have (been born with) chromosomes, reproductive organs, and/or genitals that are not exclusively "male" or "female" sex traits.
2. See map showing the global distribution of malaria deaths at http://www.viewsoftheworld.net/?p=1541.

REFERENCES

African Health Observatory. 2014. Life expectancy. http://www.aho.afro.who.int/profiles_information/index.php/AFRO:Life_expectancy. Accessed June 16, 2015.

Astbury J. 2010. The social causes of women's depression: A question of rights violated. In Jack DC and Ali A, Editors. *Silencing the Self across Cultures: Depression and Gender in the Social World.* New York: Oxford University Press.

Australian Bureau of Statistics. 2013. Estimates of Aboriginal and Torres Strait Islander Australians, June 2011. www.abs.gov.au/ausstats/abs@.nsf/mf/3238.0.55.001. Accessed June 25, 2016.

Australian Government. 2014. *Aboriginal and Torres Strait Islander: Health Performance Framework 2014 Report.* Canberra: Australian Government.

Australian Institute of Health and Welfare. 2014. *Mortality and life expectancy of Indigenous Australians: 2008 to 2012. Cat. no. IHW 140.* Canberra: AIHW.

AVERT. 2014. Antiretroviral drug prices. http://www.avert.org/antiretroviral-drug-prices.htm. Accessed March 18, 2015.

———. 2015. People who inject drugs (PWID) and HIV/AIDS. http://www.avert.org/people-inject-drugs-hiv-aids.htm#footnote1_kpmw4uq. Accessed January 24, 2016.

Barden-O'Fallon J, Barry MA, Brodish P, and Hazerjian J. 2015. Rapid assessment of ebola-related implications for reproductive, maternal, newborn and child health service delivery and utilization in Guinea. *PLoS Currents Outbreaks* 7.

Barron P, Pillay Y, Doherty T, et al. 2013. Eliminating mother-to-child HIV transmission in South Africa. *Bulletin of the World Health Organization* 91:70–74.

Bauman LJ and Berman R. 2005. Adolescent relationships and condom use: Trust, love and commitment. *AIDS and Behavior* 9(2):211–222.

Bausch D and Schwarz L. 2014. Outbreak of Ebola virus in Guinea: Where ecology meets economy. *PLOS Neglected Tropical Diseases* 8(7):1–5.

Bausch DG. 2015. The year that Ebola virus took over West Africa: Missed opportunities for prevention. *The American Journal of Tropical Medicine and Hygiene* 92(2):229–232.

Becker AE and Kleinman A. 2013. Mental health and the global agenda. *NEJM* 369(1):66–73.

Becker JU, Theodosis C, Jacob ST, et al. 2009. Surviving sepsis in low-income and middle-income countries: New directions for care and research. *Lancet Infectious Diseases* 9(9):577–582.

Benton A and Dionne KY. 2015. International political economy and the 2014 West African Ebola outbreak. *African Studies Review* 58(01):223–236.

Berkman A, Garcia J, Muñoz-Laboy M, et al. 2005. A critical analysis of the Brazilian response to HIV/AIDS: Lessons learned for controlling and mitigating the epidemic in developing countries. *American Journal of Public Health* 95(7):1162–1172.

Berrang-Ford L, Dingle K, Ford JD, et al. 2012. Vulnerability of Indigenous health to climate change: A case study of Uganda's Batwa pygmies. *Social Science and Medicine* 75(6):1067–1077.

Beyrer C, Baral SD, van Griensven F, et al. 2012. Global epidemiology of HIV infection in men who have sex with men. *Lancet* 380(9839):367–377.

Bhatt S, Weiss DJ, Cameron E, et al. 2015. The effect of malaria control on Plasmodium falciparum in Africa between 2000 and 2015. *Nature* 526:207–211.

Bhutta ZA, Das JK, Bahl R, et al. 2014. Can available interventions end preventable deaths in mothers, newborn babies, and stillbirths, and at what cost? *Lancet* 384(9940):347–370.

Biehl J. 2006. Pharmaceutical governance. In Petryna A, Lakoff A, and Kleinman A, Editors. *Global pharmaceuticals: Ethics, Markets, Practices.* Durham, NC: Duke University Press.

Bjerregaard P, Kue Young T, Dewailly E, and Ebbesson S. 2004. Review article: Indigenous health in the arctic: An overview of the circumpolar Inuit population. *Scandinavian Journal of Public Health* 32(5):390–395.

Black RE, Victora CG, Walker SP, et al. 2013. Maternal and child undernutrition and overweight in low-income and middle-income countries. *Lancet* 382(9890):427–451.

Bloss E, Holtz TH, Jereb J, et al. 2011. Tuberculosis in Indigenous peoples in the U.S., 2003–2008. *Public Health Reports* 126(5):677–689.

Burnet FM and White DO. 1962. *Natural History of Infectious Disease*, Third Edition. Cambridge: Cambridge University Press.

Caroll A and Itaborahy LP. 2015. *State-Sponsored Homophobia 2015: A World Survey of Laws: Criminalisation, Protection and Recognition of Same-Sex Love*. Geneva: ILGA.

CDC [Centers for Disease Control and Prevention]. 2006. Notice to readers: Revised definition of XDR-TB. *Morbidity and Mortality Weekly Report* 55(43):1176.

———. 2013. Parasites – onchocerciasis (also known as river blindness). http://www.cdc.gov/parasites/onchocerciasis/epi.html. Accessed January 27, 2015.

Center for Reproductive Rights. 2016. The World's Abortion Laws 2016. http://worldabortionlaws.com/map/. Accessed July 1, 2016.

CEPAL. 2014. *Los Pueblos Indígenas en América Latina: Avances en el Último Decenio y Retos Pendientes para la Garantía de Sus Derechos*. Santiago: United Nations.

Chan J. 2015. *Politics in the Corridor of Dying: AIDS Activism and Global Health Governance*. Baltimore: Johns Hopkins University Press.

Citro B, Lyon E, Mankad M, et al. 2016. Editorial: Developing a human rights-based approach to tuberculosis. *Health and Human Rights Journal* 18(1):1–7.

Cohen D and Carter P. 2010. WHO and the pandemic flu "conspiracies." *BMJ* 340(2912):1274–1279.

Cohen MS, Smith MK, Muessig KE, et al. 2013. Antiretroviral treatment of HIV-1 prevents transmission of HIV-1: Where do we go from here? *Lancet* 382(9903):1515–1524.

Cohen SA. 2009. Facts and consequences: Legality, incidence and safety of abortion worldwide. *Guttmacher Policy Review* 12(4):2–6.

Coutsoudis A, Goga A, Desmond C, et al. 2013. Is Option B+ the best choice? – Authors' reply. *Lancet* 381(9874):1273–1274.

Darmstadt GL, Kinney MV, Chopra M, et al. 2014. Who has been caring for the baby? *Lancet* 384(9938):174–188.

Das P and Horton R. 2015. Antibiotics: Achieving the balance between access and excess. *Lancet* 387(10014):102–104.

Das A and Rao M. 2012. Universal mental health: Re-evaluating the call for global mental health. *Critical Public Health* 22(4):383–389.

Dawood FS, Iuliano D, Reed C, et al. 2012. Estimated global mortality associated with the first 12 months of 2009 pandemic influenza A H1N1 virus circulation: A modelling study. *Lancet Infectious Diseases* 12(9):687–695.

Department of Health and Human Services. 2012. *Diabetes in American Indians and Alaska Natives Facts At-a-Glance*. Rockville: Department of Health and Human Services, Indian Health Service Division of Diabetes Treatment and Prevention.

Donis RO and Cox NJ. 2013. So many questions, so little time. *Journal of Infectious Diseases* 207(2):208–210.

Dorrington RE, Bradshaw D, Laubscher R, and Nannan N. 2014. *Rapid Mortality Surveillance Report 2013*. Cape Town: South African Medical Research Council.

Doyal L with Doyal L. 2013. *Living with HIV and Dying with AIDS: Diversity, Inequality and Human Rights in the Global Pandemic*. Farnham, UK: Ashgate Publishing, Ltd.

Durham M. 2002. *Poverty, Disability and Impairment in the Developing World*. London: DFID and KAR.

Eaton JW, Bacaër N, Bershteyn A, et al. 2015. Assessment of epidemic projections using recent HIV survey data in South Africa: A validation analysis of ten mathematical models of HIV epidemiology in the antiretroviral therapy era. *Lancet Global Health* 3(10):e598–e608.

Ellingson K, Haas JP, Aiello AE, et al. 2014. Strategies to prevent healthcare-associated infections through hand hygiene. *Infection Control* 35(08):937–960.

Ellsworth L and O'Keeffe A. 2013. Circumpolar Inuit health systems. *International Journal of Circumpolar Health Supplement* (72):937–945.

Farmer PE. 1996. Social inequalities and emerging infectious diseases. *Emerging Infectious Diseases* 2(4):259–269.

Fee E and Brown TM. 2001. Walter J. Lear. *American Journal of Public Health* 91(6):902.

Fee E and Fox DM. 1988. *AIDS: The Burdens of History*. Berkeley: University of California Press.

Feigin VL, Forouzanfar MH, Krishnamurthi R, et al. 2014. Global and regional burden of stroke during 1990–2010: Findings from the global burden of disease study 2010. *Lancet* 383(9913):245–255.

Fernando S. 2014. *Mental Health Worldwide: Culture, Globalization and Development*. New York: Palgrave Macmillan.

Fiorati RC and Elui VMC. 2015. Social determinants of health, inequality and social inclusion among people with disabilities. *Revista Latino-Americana de Enfermagem* 23(2):329–336.

Fish J and Karban K, Editors. 2015. *Lesbian, Gay, Bisexual and Trans Health Inequalities: International Perspectives in Social Work*. Bristol, UK: Policy Press.

Ford M. 2015. America's largest mental hospital is a jail. *The Atlantic*, June 8.

Frieden TR, Tappero JW, Dowell SF, et al. 2014. Safer countries through global health security. *Lancet* 383(9919):764–766.

Gonsalves G and Staley P. 2014. Panic, paranoia, and public health—the AIDS epidemic's lessons for Ebola. *NEJM* 371(25):2348–2349.

Gostin LO and Phelan A. 2014. The Global Health Security Agenda in an age of biosecurity. *JAMA* 312(1):27–28.

Gould B. 2009. Exploring the anomalous positive relationship between AIDS and poverty in Africa. *Geography Compass* 3(4):1449–1464.

Grohskopf L, Uyeki T, Bresee J, et al. Prevention and control of influenza with vaccines: Recommendations of the Advisory Committee on Immunization Practices (ACIP) — United States, 2012–13 Influenza Season. *CDC Morbidity and Mortality Weekly Report* 61(32):613–618.

Haagsma JA, Graetz N, Bolliger I, et al. 2016. The global burden of injury: Incidence, mortality, disability-adjusted life years and time trends from the Global Burden of Disease study 2013. *Injury prevention* 22:3–18.

Haddad S, Mohindra KS, Siekmans K, et al. 2012. "Health divide" between Indigenous and non-Indigenous populations in Kerala, India: Population based study. *BMC Public Health* 12(390).

Hakokongas L. 2005. *Running Out of Breath? TB Care in the 21st Century.* Geneva: Médecins Sans Frontières.

Hanass-Hancock J, Myezwa H, Nixon SA, and Gibbs A. 2015. "When I was no longer able to see and walk, that is when I was affected most": Experiences of disability in people living with HIV in South Africa. *Disability Rehabilitation* 37(22):2051–2060.

Hawkes C. 2006. Uneven dietary development: Linking the policies and processes of globalization with the nutrition transition, obesity and diet-related chronic diseases. *Globalization and Health* 2(1):4.

Health Canada. 2013. First Nations & Inuit Health: Diabetes. http://www.hc-sc.gc.ca/fniah-spnia/diseases-maladies/diabete/index-eng.php. Accessed July 2, 2016.

HelpAge International. 2014. *Global AgeWatch Index 2014.* London.

Heymann DL. 2004. The international response to the outbreak of SARS in 2003. *Philosophical Transactions of the Royal Society of London Series B: Biological Sciences* 359(1447):1127–1129.

Hotez PJ, Alvarado M, Basáñez M-G, et al. 2014. The global burden of disease study 2010: Interpretation and implications for the neglected tropical diseases. *PLoS Neglected Tropical Diseases* 8(7):e2865.

HRC Foundation. 2015. Criminalization around the world. http://hrc-assets.s3-website-us-east-1.amazonaws.com//files/assets/resources/Criminalization-Map-042315.pdf. Accessed November 25, 2015.

Hughes V. 2012. Public health: Where there's smoke. *Nature* 489(7417):S18–S20.

Hui DS, Perlman S, and Zumla A. 2015. Spread of MERS to South Korea and China. *Lancet Respiratory Medicine* 3(7):509–510.

Hunter M. 2010. *Love in the Time of AIDS: Inequality, Gender, and Rights in South Africa.* Bloomington: Indiana University Press.

IARC [International Agency for Research on Cancer]. 2013. *Air Pollution and Cancer.* Geneva: WHO.

IHME. 2013a. GBD Arrow Diagram. http://vizhub.healthdata.org/gbd-compare/arrow. Accessed January 21, 2015.

———. 2013b. Global Burden of Disease (GBD). http://www.healthdata.org/gbd. Accessed February 1, 2015.

ILGA [International Lesbian, Gay, Bisexual, Trans and Intersex Association]. 2015. *The Lesbian, Gay and Bisexual Map of World Laws: May 2015.* Geneva: ILGA.

Iliffe J. 2006. *The African AIDS Epidemic: A History.* Athens, OH: Ohio University Press.

ILO. 2002. *Managing Disability in the Workplace: ILO Code of Practice.* Geneva: ILO.

———. 2009. *Providing Safe and Healthy Workplaces for Both Women and Men.* Geneva: ILO.

———. 2015. *World Report on Child Labour: Paving the Way to Decent Work for Young People 2015.* Geneva: ILO.

International Diabetes Federation. 2015. *IDF Diabetes Atlas, Seventh Edition 2015.* Brussels: IDF.

Istituto Nazionale di Statistica. 2014. Anno 2012: Le principali cause di morte in Italia. http://www.istat.it/it/archivio/140871. Accessed May 21, 2015.

IWGIA [International Work Group for Indigenous Affairs]. 2014. *The Indigenous World 2014.* Copenhagen: IWGIA.

James JT. 2013. A new, evidence-based estimate of patient harms associated with hospital care. *Journal of Patient Safety* 9(3):122–128.

Jones S and Ameh C. 2015. *Exploring the Impact of the Ebola Outbreak on Routine Maternal Health Services in Sierra Leone.* London: VSO.

Kalofonos IA. 2010. "All I Eat Is ARVs." *Medical Anthropology Quarterly* 24(3):363–380.

Kamb ML, Caffé S, Perez F, et al. Cuba eliminates mother-to-child transmission of HIV and congenital syphilis: A call to action for the Americas Region. *Jornal Brasileiro de Doenças Sexualmente Transmissiveis* 27(1-2):3–5.

Kaur H, Allan EL, Mamadu I, et al. 2015. Quality of artemisinin-based combination formulations for malaria treatment: Prevalence and risk factors for poor quality medicines in public facilities and private sector drug outlets in Enugu, Nigeria. *PLoS ONE* 10(5):e0125577.

Kenya National Bureau of Statistics. 2015. *Economic Survey 2015*. Nairobi: Kenya National Bureau of Statistics.

Kessler RC, Aguilar-Gaxiola S, Alonso J, et al. 2009. The global burden of mental disorders: An update from the WHO World Mental Health (WMH) surveys. *Epidemiologia e Psichiatria Sociale* 18(01):23–33.

Kim JY, Shakow A, Mate K, et al. 2005. Limited good and limited vision: Multidrug resistant tuberculosis and global health policy. *Social Science and Medicine* 61(4):847–859.

Krieger N. 2011. *Epidemiology and the People's Health: Theory and Context*. New York: Oxford University Press.

Lancet [Editorial]. 2014. Neglected tropical diseases: Becoming less neglected. *Lancet* 383(9925):1269.

———. 2015. Snake bite—the neglected tropical disease. *Lancet* 386(9999):1110.

Lancet GMHG. 2007. Scale up services for mental disorders: A call for action. *Lancet* 370(9594):1241–1252.

Langton JM, Blanch B, Drew AK, et al. 2014. Retrospective studies of end-of-life resource utilization and costs in cancer care using health administrative data: A systematic review. *Palliative Medicine* 28(10):1167–1196.

Last JM. 2001. *A Dictionary of Epidemiology*, Fourth Edition. New York: Oxford University Press.

Lawn JE, Blencowe H, Oza S, et al. 2014. Every newborn: Progress, priorities, and potential beyond survival. *Lancet* 384(9938):189–205.

Leach M. 2015. The Ebola crisis and post-2015 development. *Journal of International Development* 27(6):816–834.

Leimane V, Dravniece G, Riekstina V, et al. 2010. Treatment outcome of multidrug/extensively drug-resistant tuberculosis in Latvia, 2000–2004. *European Respiratory Journal* 36:584-593.

Lessler J, Rodriguez-Barraquer I, Cummings DA, et al. 2014. Estimating potential incidence of MERS-CoV associated with Hajj pilgrims to Saudi Arabia, 2014. *PLOS Currents Outbreaks* 6.

Levin C, Van Minh H, Odaga J, et al. 2013. Delivery cost of human papiloomavirus vaccination of young adolescent girls in Peru, Uganda and Viet Nam. *Bulletin World Health Organization* 91(8):585–592.

Li J, Luo C, and De Klerk N. 2008. Trends in infant/child mortality and life expectancy in indigenous populations in Yunnan province, China. *Australian and New Zealand Journal of Public Health* 32(3):216–223.

Lipska KJ. 2015. When diabetes treatment goes too far. *NY Times, January 12*.

Lurie P and Drucker E. 1997. An opportunity lost: HIV infections associated with lack of a national needle-exchange programme in the USA. *Lancet* 349(9052):604–608.

Makary MA and Daniel M. 2016. Medical error—the third leading cause of death in the US. *BMJ* 353:i2139.

Mann J. 1999. The transformative potential of the HIV/AIDS pandemic. *Reproductive Health Matters* 7(14):164–172.

Martins SS, Sampson L, Cerdá M, and Galea S. 2015. Worldwide prevalence and trends in unintentional drug overdose: A systematic review of the literature. *American Journal of Public Health* 105(11):e29–e49.

Mathews TJ, MacDorman MF, and Thoma ME. 2015. Infant mortality statistics from the 2013 period linked birth/infant death data set. *National Vital Statistics Reports* 64(9):1–30.

Maxwell K. 2014. Historicizing historical trauma theory: Troubling the trans-generational transmission paradigm. *Transcultural Psychiatry* 51(3):406–434.

Mills C. 2014. *Decolonizing Global Mental Health: the Psychiatrization of the Majority World*. Hove, UK: Routledge.

Ministry of Foreign Affairs Denmark. 2015. Facts and statistics. http://denmark.dk/en/quick-facts/facts/. Accessed January 30, 2015.

Mishra V, Bignami-Van Assche S, Greener R, et al. 2007. HIV infection does not disproportionately affect the poorer in sub-Saharan Africa. *AIDS* 21(7):S17–S28.

Mitman G. 2014. Ebola in a stew of fear. *NEJM* 371(19):1763–1765.

Mitra S, Posarac A, and Vick B. 2013. Disability and poverty in developing countries: A multidimensional study. *World Development* 41:1–18.

Moncrieff J. 2009. *The Myth of the Chemical Cure. A Critique of Psychiatric Drug Treatment*. Basingstoke, UK: Palgrave Macmillan.

Morse SS. 1995. Factors in the emergence of infectious diseases. *Emerging Infectious Diseases* 1(1):7–15.

Moscou K, Kohler JC, and Lexchin J. 2013. Drug safety and corporate governance. *Global Health Governance* 7(1):56–79.

Mukherjee JS, Louise I, Fernet L, et al. 2006. Antiretroviral therapy in resource-poor settings: Decreasing barriers to access and promoting adherence. *Journal of Acquired Immune Deficiency Syndrome* 43(Suppl 1):S123–S126.

Munos MK, Walker CLF, and Black RE. 2010. The effect of rotavirus vaccine on diarrhoea mortality. *International Journal of Epidemiology* 39(suppl 1):i56–i62.

Naghavi M, Wang H, Lozano R, et al. 2015. Global, regional, and national age–sex specific all-cause and cause-specific mortality for 240 causes of death, 1990–2013: A systematic analysis for the global burden of disease study 2013. *Lancet* 385(9963):117–171.

Nambiar D, Stoové M, and Dietze P. 2014. A cross-sectional study describing factors associated with utilisation of GP services by a cohort of people who inject drugs. *BMC Health Services Research* 14(1):308.

Nayyar GM, Breman JG, and Herrington J. 2015. The global pandemic of falsified medicines: Laboratory and field innovations and policy perspectives: Summary. *American Journal of Tropical Medicine and Hygiene* 92(6 Suppl):2–7.

Neumann DG and Quiñonez C. 2014. A comparative analysis of oral health care systems in the United States, United Kingdom, France, Canada, and Brazil. *NCOHR Working Papers Series* 1(2).

Nicholson T, Admay C, Shakow A, and Keshavjee S. 2016. Double standards in global health: Medicine, human rights law and multidrug-resistant TB treatment policy. *Health and Human Rights Journal* 18(1):85–101.

Noor AM, Kinyoki DK, Mundia CW, et al. 2014. The changing risk of plasmodium falciparum malaria infection in Africa: 2000–10: A spatial and temporal analysis of transmission intensity. *Lancet* 383(9930):1739–1747.

OECD. 2014. *Social Spending Is Falling in Some Countries, But in Many Others It Remains at Historically High Levels.* Paris: OECD.

OHCHR [Office of the High Commissioner for Human Rights]. 2015. Combatting discrimination based on sexual orientation and gender identity. http://www.ohchr.org/EN/Issues/Discrimination/Pages/LGBT.aspx. Accessed November 5, 2015.

PAHO. 2016. *Epidemiological Update, Cholera: 21 July 2016. Cholera in the Americas—Situation Summary. Epidemiological Alerts.* Washington, DC: PAHO.

Partnership for Maternal, Newborn and Child Health. 2011. Newborn death and illness. http://www.who.int/pmnch/media/press_materials/fs/fs_newborndealth_illness/en/. Accessed July 3, 2015.

Patel P, Borkowf CB, Brooks JT, et al. 2014. Estimated per-act transmission risk: A systematic review. *AIDS* 28(10):1509–1519.

Patel V and Prince M. 2010. Global mental health: A new global health field comes of age. *JAMA* 303(19):1976–1977.

Patterson KD and Pyle GF. 1991. The geography and mortality of the 1918 influenza pandemic. *Bulletin of the History of Medicine* 65(1):4–21.

PHM, Medact, Medico International, et al. 2014. *Global Health Watch 4: An Alternative World Health Report.* London: Zed Books Ltd.

Pieterse P and Lodge T. 2015. When free healthcare is not free. Corruption and mistrust in Sierra Leone's primary healthcare system immediately prior to the Ebola outbreak. *International health* 7(6):400–404.

Popkin BM, Adair LS, and Ng SW. 2012. Global nutrition transition and the pandemic of obesity in developing countries. *Nutrition Reviews* 70(1):3–21.

Porta MS, Greenland S, Hernán M, et al. 2014. *A Dictionary of Epidemiology.* New York: Oxford University Press.

Prins SJ, Bates LM, Keyes KM, and Muntaner C. 2015. Anxious? Depressed? You might be suffering from capitalism: Contradictory class locations and the prevalence of depression and anxiety in the USA. *Sociology of Health & Illness* 37(8):1352–1372.

Public Health Agency of Canada. 2014. Tuberculosis Prevention and Control in Canada. http://www.phac-aspc.gc.ca/tbpc-latb/pubs/tpc-pct/index-eng.php. Accessed January 19, 2015.

Quigley F. 2009. *Walking Together, Walking Far. How a U.S. and African Medical School Partnership is Winning the Fight against HIV/AIDS.* Bloomington: Indiana University Press.

Ravaghi V, Quiñonez C, and Allison PJ. 2013. The magnitude of oral health inequalities in Canada: Findings of the Canadian health measures survey. *Community Dentistry and Oral Epidemiology* 41(6):490–498.

Reczek C and Umberson D. 2012. Gender, health behavior, and intimate relationships: Lesbian, gay, and straight contexts. *Social Science & Medicine* 74(11):1783–1790.

Renschler JP, Walters K, Newton PN, and Laxminarayan R. 2015. Estimated under-five deaths associated with poor-quality antimalarials in sub-Saharan Africa. *American Journal of Tropical Medicine and Hygiene* 92(6 Suppl):119–126.

Review on Antimicrobial Resistance. 2016. *Tackling Drug-Resistant Infections Globally: An Overview of Our Work.* London: Review on Antimicrobial Resistance.

Riverón Corteguera RL. 1995. Strategies and causes of reduced infant and young child diarrheal disease mortality in Cuba, 1962–1993. *Bulletin of the Pan American Health Organization* 29(1):70–80.

Rudd RA, Aleshire N, Zibbell JE, and Gladden M. 2016. Increases in drug and opioid overdose deaths — United States, 2000–2014. *CDC Morbidity and Mortality Weekly Report* 64(50):1378–1382.

Ryan F. 1992. *Tuberculosis: The Greatest Story Never Told.* Worcestershire, UK: Swift Publishers.

Sambira J. 2013. Counterfeit drugs raise Africa's temperature. http://www.un.org/africarenewal/magazine/may-2013/counterfeit-drugs-raise-africa%E2%80%99s-temperature. Accessed June 28, 2015.

Savell E, Gilmore AB, Sims M, et al. 2015. The environmental profile of a community's health: A cross-sectional study on tobacco marketing in 16 countries. *Bulletin of the World Health Organization* 93(12):851–861.

Schwartlander B. 2015. Motorization not at the cost of kids' lives. *China Daily USA, May 6.*

Seeley J, Watts CH, Kippax S, Russell S, et al. 2012. Addressing the structural drivers of HIV: A luxury or necessity for programmes? *Journal of the International AIDS Society* 15(Suppl 1):1–4.

Sheiham A, Alexander D, Cohen L, et al. 2011. Global oral health inequalities: Task group-Implementation and delivery of oral health strategies. *Advances in Dental Research* 23(2):259–267.

Shulman LN, Torode J, and Wagner CM. 2015. Improving global access to cancer care and treatment. *Global Health NOW*, June 8.

Simelela N, Venter WF, Pillay Y, and Barron P. 2015. A political and social history of HIV in South Africa. *Current HIV/AIDS Reports* 12(2):256–261.

Soliman A and Boffetta P. 2013. *Cancer Epidemiology: Low- and Middle-Income Countries and Special Populations.* New York: Oxford University Press.

Statistics Canada. 2015a. Aboriginal peoples in Canada: First Nations people, Métis and Inuit. http://www12.statcan.gc.ca/nhs-enm/2011/as-sa/99-011-x/99-011-x2011001-eng.cfm#a1. Accessed June 25, 2016.

———. 2015b. Life expectancy. http://www.statcan.gc.ca/pub/89-645-x/2010001/life-expectancy-esperance-vie-eng.htm. Accessed June 25, 2016.

Statistics Greenland. 2016. *Greenland in Figures 2016.* Nuuk: Statistics Greenland.

Statistics New Zealand. 2015. New Zealand Period Life Tables: 2012–14. http://www.stats.govt.nz/browse_for_stats/health/life_expectancy/NZLifeTables_HOTP12-14/Commentary.aspx. Accessed June 25, 2016.

———. 2016. Māori Population Estimates: Mean Year ended 31 December 2015 – tables. http://www.stats.govt.nz/browse_for_stats/population/estimates_and_projections/MaoriPopulationEstimates_HOTPMYeDec15.aspx. Accessed June 25, 2016.

Stead WW, Eisenach KD, Cave MD, et al. 1995. When did Mycobacterium tuberculosis infection first occur in the New World? An important question with public health implications. *American Journal of Respiratory and Critical Care Medicine* 151(4):1267–1268.

Stop TB Partnership. 2006. *The Global Plan to Stop TB, 2006–2015.* Geneva: WHO.

Strebel PM, Cochi SL, Hoekstra E, et al. 2011. A world without measles. *Journal of Infectious Diseases* 204(Suppl 1):S1–S3.

Summerfield D. 2013. "Global mental health" is an oxymoron and medical imperialism. *BMJ* 346:f3509.

Timimi S. 2011. Globalising mental health: A neo-liberal project. *Ethnicity and Inequalities in Health and Social Care* 4(3):155–160.

Tjepkema M, Wilkins R, Goedhuis N, and Pennock J. 2012. Cardiovascular disease mortality among First Nations people in Canada, 1991-2001. *Chronic diseases and injuries in Canada* 32(4):200–207.

Tupchong K, Koyfman A, and Foran M. 2015. Sepsis, severe sepsis, and septic shock: A review of the literature. *African Journal of Emergency Medicine* 5(3):127–135.

Tusting LS, Ippolito MM, Willey BA, et al. 2015. The evidence for improving housing to reduce malaria: A systematic review and meta-analysis. *Malaria journal* 14(1):209.

Tzioumis E and Adair LS. 2014. Childhood dual burden of under-and over-nutrition in low-and middle-income countries: A critical review. *Food and Nutrition Bulletin* 35(2):230.

UN. 2001. Declaration of commitment to HIV/AIDS. Paper read at United Nations General Assembly, at New York.

———. 2009. *State of the World's Indigenous Peoples.* New York: UN.

UNAIDS. 2004. *2004 Report on the Global AIDS Epidemic.* Geneva: UNAIDS.

———. 2012. Fact sheet: Adolescents, young people and HIV. http://www.unaids.org/sites/default/files/en/media/unaids/contentassets/documents/factsheet/2012/20120417_FS_adolescentsyoungpeoplehiv_en.pdf. Accessed April 19, 2015.

———. 2014a. *90-90-90: An Ambitious Treatment Target to Help End the AIDS Epidemic.* Geneva: UNAIDS.

———. 2014b. *The Gap Report.* Geneva: UNAIDS.

———. 2015. *How AIDS Changed Everything--MDG 6: 15 Years, 15 Lessons of Hope from the AIDS Response.* Geneva: UNAIDS.

———. 2016. AIDSinfo Online Database. http://aidsinfo.unaids.org/. Accessed June 22, 2016.

UNESCO. 2006. *UNESCO and Indigenous Peoples: Partnership to Promote Cultural Diversity.* New York: UNESCO.

UNFPA. 2014. *Annual Report 2014: A Year of Renewal.* New York: UNFPA.

UN General Assembly. 2012. *Political Declaration of the High-level Meeting of the General Assembly on the Prevention and Control of Non-communicable Diseases,* U.N. Doc A/RES/66/2 January 24.

UNICEF. 2014. *Hidden in Plain Sight: A Statistical Analysis of Violence Against Children.* New York: UNICEF.

———. 2015a. *Committing to Child Survival: A Promise Renewed. Progress Report 2015.* New York: UNICEF.

———. 2015b. Girls' education and gender equality. http://www.unicef.org/education/bege_70640.html. Accessed June 8, 2015.

———. 2016. UNICEF Data: Monitoring the Situation of Children and Women. http://data.unicef.org/. Accessed June 22, 2016.

UN IGME [UN Inter-agency Group for Child Mortality Estimation]. 2015. *Levels & Trends in Child Mortality: Report 2015*. New York: UNICEF.

UNODC. 2016. *World Drug Report 2016*. Vienna: UNODC.

Uplekar M, Weil D, Lonnroth K, et al. 2015. WHO's new end TB strategy. *Lancet* 385(9979):1799–1801.

U.S. Census Bureau. 2012. *The American Indian and Alaska Native Population: 2010*. Washington, DC: U.S. Census Bureau.

———. 2015. International Data Base: World Population by Age and Sex. https://www.census.gov/population/international/data/idb/worldpop.php. Accessed December 23, 2015.

van Dillen J, Zwart J, Schutte J, and van Roosmalen J. 2010. Maternal sepsis: Epidemiology, etiology and outcome. *Current Opinion in Infectious Diseases* 23(3):249–254.

Velásquez G. 2012. The management of a (H1N1) pandemic: An alternative view. *Journal of Health Law* 13(2):108–122.

Wailoo K, Livingston J, Epstein S, and Aronowitz R, Editors. 2010. *Three Shots at Prevention: The HPV Vaccine and the Politics of Medicine's Simple Solutions*. Baltimore: Johns Hopkins University Press.

Walker CLF, Rudan I, Liu L, et al. 2013. Global burden of childhood pneumonia and diarrhoea. *Lancet* 381(9875):1405–1416.

Wallace R. 2016. *Big Farms Make Big Flu: Dispatches on Infectious Disease, Agribusiness, and the Nature of Science*. New York: Monthly Review Press.

Wardlaw T, Salama P, Johansson EW, and Mason E. 2006. Pneumonia: The leading killer of children. *Lancet* 368(9541):1048–1050.

Watters E. 2010. *Crazy Like Us: The Globalization of the American Psyche*. New York: Simon and Schuster.

Whitaker R and Cosgrove L. 2015. *Psychiatry Under the Influence: Institutional Corruption, Social Injury, and Prescriptions for Reform*. New York: Palgrave Macmillan.

WHO. 2005. *Global Tuberculosis Control: Surveillance, Planning, Financing*. Geneva: WHO.

———. 2007a. Cumulative number of confirmed human cases of Avian influenza A/(H5N1) Reported to WHO. http://www.who.int/csr/disease/avian_influenza/country/cases_table_2007_05_31/en/index.html. Updated 31 May 2007. Accessed July 16, 2007.

———. 2007b. International classification of functioning, disability, and health. http://www.who.int/classifications/icf/site/intros/ICF-Eng-Intro.pdf. Accessed July 15, 2007.

———. 2010. *Mental Health and Development: Targeting People with Mental Health Conditions as a Vulnerable Group*. Geneva: WHO.

———. 2012. Oral health: Fact sheet. http://www.who.int/mediacentre/factsheets/fs318/en/. Accessed January 17, 2014.

———. 2013a. Animal bites: Fact sheet. http://www.who.int/mediacentre/factsheets/fs373/en/. Accessed June 8, 2015.

———. 2013b. *Mental Health Action Plan 2013-2020*. Geneva: WHO.

———. 2014a. Cholera, 2013. *Weekly Epidemiological Record* 31(89):345–356.

———. 2014b. Cholera: Fact sheet. http://www.who.int/mediacentre/factsheets/fs107/en/. Accessed January 20, 2015.

———. 2014c. Facts about ageing. http://www.who.int/ageing/about/facts/en/. Accessed January 17, 2015.

———. 2014d. *Global Report on Drowning: Preventing a Leading Killer*. Geneva: WHO.

———. 2014e. Influenza (seasonal): Fact sheet. http://www.who.int/mediacentre/factsheets/fs211/en/. Accessed April 19, 2015.

———. 2014f. *Injuries and Violence: The Facts*. Geneva: WHO.

———. 2014g. *Preventing Suicide: A Global Imperative*. Geneva: WHO.

———. 2014h. The top 10 causes of death. http://www.who.int/mediacentre/factsheets/fs310/en/. Accessed January 20, 2014.

———. 2014i. Voluntary medical male circumcision for HIV prevention in priority countries of East and Southern Africa. http://www.who.int/hiv/topics/malecircumcision/male-circumcision-info-2014/en/. Accessed December 18, 2014.

———. 2015a. 10 leading causes of death in females. http://www.who.int/gho/women_and_health/mortality/situation_trends_causes_death/en/. Accessed June 15, 2015.

———. 2015b. Cardiovascular diseases. http://www.who.int/mediacentre/factsheets/fs317/en/. Accessed June 8, 2015.

———. 2015c. Chronic obstructive pulmonary disease: Fact sheet. http://www.who.int/mediacentre/factsheets/fs315/en/. Accessed January 21, 2016.

———. 2015d. Diabetes: Fact sheet. http://www.who.int/mediacentre/factsheets/fs312/en/. Accessed January 21, 2015.

———. 2015e. Disability and health: Fact sheet. http://www.who.int/mediacentre/factsheets/fs352/en/. Accessed June 29, 2016.

———. 2015f. Global Health Observatory data repository. http://www.who.int/gho/database/en/. Accessed June 9, 2015.

———. 2015g. *Global Status Report on Road Safety 2015*. Geneva: WHO.

———. 2015h. *Global Tuberculosis Report 2015*. Geneva: WHO.

———. 2015i. Hepatitis B: Fact sheet. http://www.who.int/mediacentre/factsheets/fs204/en/. Accessed June 29. 2016.

———. 2015j. Hepatitis C: Fact sheet. http://www.who.int/mediacentre/factsheets/fs164/en/. Accessed June 29, 2016.

———. 2015k. HIV/AIDS. http://www.who.int/gho/hiv/en/. Accessed May 29, 2015.

———. 2015l. Lymphatic filariasis. http://www.who.int/mediacentre/factsheets/fs102/en/. Accessed September 23, 2015.

———. 2015m. Mental health, poverty and development. http://www.who.int/mental_health/policy/development/en/. Accessed December 23, 2015.

———. 2015n. Neglected tropical diseases: Fact sheets. http://www.who.int/topics/tropical_diseases/factsheets/neglected/en/. Accessed June 27, 2015.

———. 2015o. Noncommunicable diseases: Fact sheet. http://www.who.int/mediacentre/factsheets/fs355/en/. Accessed June 30, 2015.

———. 2015p. *Report of the Ebola Interim Assessment Panel.* Geneva: WHO.

———. 2015q. Road traffic injuries: Fact sheet. http://www.who.int/mediacentre/factsheets/fs358/en/. Accessed June 8, 2015.

———. 2015r. Sexually transmitted infections (STIs): Fact sheet. http://www.who.int/mediacentre/factsheets/fs110/en/. Accessed June 29, 2016.

———. 2015s. Tobacco: Fact sheet. http://www.who.int/mediacentre/factsheets/fs339/en/. Accessed June 8, 2015.

———. 2015t. *WHO Estimates of the Global Burden of Foodborne Diseases.* Geneva: WHO.

———. 2015u. *World Health Statistics 2015.* Geneva: WHO.

———. 2015v. *World Malaria Report 2015.* Geneva: WHO.

———. 2015w. WHO statement on the ninth meeting of the IHR Emergency Committee regarding MERS-CoV. http://www.who.int/mediacentre/news/statements/2015/ihr-ec-mers/en/. Accessed July 2, 2015.

———. 2016a. Adolescents: health risks and solutions: Fact sheet. http://www.who.int/mediacentre/factsheets/fs345/en/. Accessed June 29, 2016.

———. 2016b. *Ebola Situation Report—30 March 2016.* Geneva: WHO.

———. 2016c. *Global Report on Diabetes.* Geneva: WHO.

———. 2016d. Measles: Factsheet. http://www.who.int/mediacentre/factsheets/fs286/en/. Accessed July 2, 2016.

———. 2016e. Mental disorders: Fact sheet. http://www.who.int/mediacentre/factsheets/fs396/en/. June 29, 2016.

———. 2016f. Middle East respiratory syndrome coronavirus (MERS-CoV) – Qatar: Disease outbreak news 29 June 2016. http://www.who.int/csr/don/29-june-2016-mers-qatar/en/. Accessed July 1, 2016.

———. 2016g. Monthly report on dracunculiasis cases, January–March 2016. *Weekly epidemiological record* 18(91):247-248.

———. 2016h. Neglected tropical diseases. http://www.who.int/neglected_diseases/diseases/en/. Accessed July 2, 2016.

WHO Kobe Centre. 2013. *Summary Report: Consultation on Advancing Technological Innovation for Older Persons in Asia.* Kobe: WHO Centre for Health Development.

WHO SAGE [Strategic Advisory Group of Experts on immunization]. 2012. *Background Paper on Influenza Vaccines and Immunization.* Geneva: WHO.

WHO, UNICEF, UNFPA, et al. 2015. *Trends in Maternal Mortality: 1990 to 2015.* Geneva: WHO.

Wigle J, Fontenot HB, and Zimet GD. 2016. Global delivery of the human papillomavirus vaccine. *Pediatric Clinics of North America* 63(1):81–95.

Wilson A, Gallos ID, Plana N, et al. 2011. Effectiveness of strategies incorporating training and support of traditional birth attendants on perinatal and maternal mortality: Meta-analysis. *BMJ* 343:d7102.

World Bank. 2015a. Poverty overview. http://www.worldbank.org/en/topic/poverty/overview. Accessed July 10, 2015.

———. 2015b. *World Development Indicators 2015.* Washington, DC: World Bank.

Yusuf S, Rangarajan S, Teo K, et al. 2014. Cardiovascular risk and events in 17 low-, middle-, and high-income countries. *NEJM* 371(9):818–827.

7

HEALTH EQUITY AND THE SOCIETAL DETERMINANTS OF HEALTH

Key Questions:

- Why do different social groups have differing health profiles?
- How does the society in which people live shape the health and ill health of social groups and their members?
- What are health inequities and how might they be addressed?

In 2013, Costa Ricans lived, on average, to the age of 79—the same as in the United States. Yet US per capita income was about five times that of Costa Rica (World Bank 2015). Even more striking, in 2011, inhabitants of the southern Indian state of Kerala, earning, on average, less than US$1,500 per year, had a life expectancy of 75 (Susuman, Lougue, and Battala 2014), identical to that of residents of Mississippi (United States), whose annual income was approximately 10 times larger at US$21,000 (Lewis and Burd-Sharps 2013). What makes Costa Ricans and Keralites live as long as those in significantly richer places?

Before addressing this question, we consider another remarkable set of comparisons that takes place *within* countries. In Australia, Indigenous persons live on average 10 years less than non-Indigenous counterparts (AIHW 2014). Meanwhile, life expectancy in China varies markedly by region, from 71 years in Qinghai province to 82 years in Shanghai (Zhou et al. 2015). In Colombia, too, Bogotá residents have an average life expectancy of 75 years, whereas those in Chocó department live to only 64 years (Eslava-Schmalbachet al. 2013). Why is there such variation within countries?

The answer to these questions has far less to do with the *specific individuals* living in these settings than with the *structure of their societies* and their corresponding position in the global economy. Recognizing that the health differences just described are neither inevitable nor natural, this chapter focuses on health inequities—that is, health status differences between socially defined groups that are unjust, unfair, and avoidable—and their underlying and interacting societal determinants (for further definitions see Box 7-1). These concepts enable us to link the ideas around political economy of health introduced in chapter 3 to the broad outline of global disease patterns based on conditions of marginalization, deprivation, modernization, and work presented in chapter 6.

Insights about the influence of social factors on health and the existence of mortality inequities by social group are not new (see chapters 3 and 5), but in recent decades theory and research in these areas have yielded increasingly systematic understandings of how health inequities are generated and how to diminish them. Here, we begin with an explanation of the societal determinants of health and show how they can be operationalized. We also examine several theories that posit pathways between societal determinants and health inequities. Then, we work

Box 7-1 SDOH and Health Equity Definitions

- *Population health,* broadly speaking, investigates three components and their interactions: "1) health outcomes and distribution in a population, 2) patterns of health determinants over the lifecourse, and 3) policies and interventions at the individual and social levels," (Kindig 2007, p. 141) aiming to "maximize overall health outcomes and minimize health inequities at the population level" (ibid, p. 158)
- *Social determinants of health* are "conditions in the environments in which people are born, live, learn, work, play, worship, and age that affect a wide range of health, functioning, and quality-of-life outcomes and risks . . . In addition to the more material attributes of 'place,' the patterns of social engagement and sense of security and well-being are also affected by where people live" (Office of Disease Prevention and Health Promotion 2016).
- *Societal determinants of health* are the political, economic, social, and cultural structures (institutions, rules, and social relationships between groups) that shape health and health patterns across key societal categories including social class, race/ethnicity, sex/gender, and geographic setting.
- *Social/societal determination of health* refers to social processes "directly shaping the modes or ways of living of communities within the broader context that in turn influence styles of living at the micro individual/family scale. . . [and] the processes whereby those who are affected also respond to these circumstances, within and across scales" (Spiegel, Breilh, and Yassi 2015, p. 4).
- *Health inequities*[a] are the differences in health profiles within and across countries by social group, geography, and other factors that "are unnecessary and avoidable but, in addition, are also considered unfair and unjust," giving "a moral and ethical dimension" (Whitehead 1992, p. 5) to the term *inequity.*

[a]The term "health disparities" (almost exclusively employed in the United States) may refer to health inequities, racial/ethnic health differences, or both.

through the structures and determinants in our political economy of global health framework, showing how, level by level, individually and synergistically, a range of societal factors influence both health and health equity. Finally, we touch upon various policies and practices that address the societal determinants of health and lead to sustained reduction of health inequities, a discussion that will be further explored in chapter 13.

HOW IS HEALTH SOCIETALLY DETERMINED AND WHAT EXPLAINS HEALTH INEQUITIES: PATHWAYS AND POSSIBILITIES

Key Questions:

- What makes the underlying determinants of health societal as opposed to individual?
- How does a political economy of health perspective help operationalize societal determinants of health?
- How do different theoretical and conceptual lenses explain health inequities?

Each case of illness occurs in individuals, and each of us experiences ill health individually. Yet virtually every bout of ill health or injury can also be understood in societal terms. Different groups in each population are exposed, susceptible, and resistant to different diseases in particular ways: pesticide plant workers or people residing near toxic waste dumps are more likely to get cancers linked to their exposure to dangerous chemicals; homicides are higher in populations wracked by poverty and state-sanctioned violence; narcotic drug use, while certainly personally addictive, is heavily mediated by economic insecurity, social exclusion, and organized crime; and infants living in dwellings without running water are more likely to get diarrhea, and their susceptibility and resistance to diarrhea are further influenced by their own and their mother's nutritional status.

Who works in dangerous occupations and who lives in hazardous conditions is not randomly decided, but rather reflects societal arrangements according to different axes of power, including wealth, social class, race and ethnicity, gender, location, political structure, and so on. Likewise, the quality and accessibility of medical treatment for these ailments and the social policies that mitigate exposure also vary considerably based on a variety of contextual factors. That is to say, diseases are distributed via chance variation (not everyone is exposed and not everyone exposed becomes ill), but at the same time, at a population level, these chances are "structured" by "historically contingent causal processes" that shape a hierarchy and range of existing, albeit dynamic, societal factors (Krieger 2014a, p. 660). This is what we mean by the *societal determinants of health.*

As such, the individual risk of becoming ill tells us little about who gets sick or dies of what, at which age, and why. More salient is who lives under what conditions, from neighborhood characteristics to the work environment, availability of and access to social services, such as education and transport, and overall economic and political system. Accordingly, though the term *social determinants of health* is widely used, here we employ *societal determinants of health* (SDOH) to refer more emphatically to the structural forces (e.g., institutional and political) that affect health. What is more, these factors are not static but can be influenced and changed by human agency and specific policies that unfold within (and across) societies. Strictly speaking, the *social* determinants of health refer to concrete factors related to resources and interactions among people and communities, whereas *societal* determinants emphasize a broader array of structural factors and processes that, in effect, determine the rules regarding access to resources and relationships between and among societal groups.

A further conceptual dimension relates to the mechanisms of power through which SDOH operate. The concept of social (or societal) *determination* of health was developed by Ecuadorian epidemiologist Jaime Breilh and others to shift emphasis from *what* (factors) to *who* (i.e., which groups and political and economic forces) is determining the factors and processes that produce and reproduce health (also known as the social production of health). Societal determination—understanding society as beyond the sum of individual experiences—is gaining traction as a more political and dialectical framing of SDOH (Morales-Borrero et al. 2013; Spiegel, Breilh, and Yassi 2015).

It is important to underscore that societal determination seeks to characterize the dynamics of the process—that is, determinants are not disembodied or separate from larger political forces but rather embedded in them, with actors and more proximate factors shaping how the SDOH play out in context and as circumstances change. Thus, instead of simply identifying housing as a key determinant of health, a societal determination approach examines how real estate and other business interests and government actors drive land costs, land use policies, housing markets, maintenance of housing stock (free from vermin, mildew, indoor air pollution, etc.), tenant and ownership policies (e.g., by gender), municipal services, neighborhood quality (parks, transport access, schools, food stores, recreation, etc.), water and sanitary conditions, waste and pollution, as well as zoning, class and racial discrimination, and so on. So housing is not a static category that independently shapes health, but one that is influenced by and interacts with a host of historical and contextual political, economic, environmental, geographic, and social factors.

Further explicating these relations, in many societies wealthier people historically had higher smoking rates than poorer counterparts, reflecting greater disposable income and leisure time. As smoking's harmful effects were revealed and social acceptability diminished, its prevalence followed a downward social class trend, also indicating fewer stress-release and addiction-controlling possibilities for working class people. In sum, the societal determination of health approach enables translation of political economy theory into mechanisms and pathways influencing health at multiple levels.

In other words, if social determinants of health are the "causes of the causes" of health and disease (Marmot 2005), societal determinants are "the causes of the causes of the causes" (that is, political economy forces driving the determinants) (Birn 2009), and societal determination of health reflects the dynamic production of health and disease as a process (Breilh 2003), with perpetrating and nameable forces that lead to the physical embodiment (experiences, behaviors, exposures expressed on human bodies) of health, illness, and premature death. The following section explores, and presents an illustration of, societal determinants/determination of health from each level of chapter 3's political economy of global health framework.

Operationalizing Political Economy of Health through SDOH

An SDOH approach serves to operationalize political economy of health understandings of how health and ill health are produced and reproduced at multiple levels even as all levels and factors coexist and interact, and societal determination takes place on each level simultaneously.

As per Figure 3-3 (p. 103), we begin our discussion at the broadest level, reviewing the underlying global and national forces (e.g., resource and wealth distribution, social structure, economic system) that influence health through various pathways. We then move to health determinants at the national or regional level, reflecting governance and social policies (e.g., affecting work and environmental conditions, social well-being, public health, and education). Next we examine living conditions and the array of factors (e.g., housing, water/sanitation, nutrition) operating at the neighborhood and household levels—factors that are concurrently shaped by larger policies and structural forces.

Individual exposure, susceptibility, resistance to, and recovery from, illness literally represent the embodiment of all of these determinants, drawing from personal and collective life experiences, health behaviors, congenital factors, and prior illness and injury, which in turn reflect community-level conditions, societal policies, and the global political order. It is important to note that various determinants, such as poverty and discrimination, operate at multiple levels, influencing neighborhood contexts and influenced by the larger politics of, for example, redistribution and land tenure.

Applying a societal determination lens to a concrete case, imagine Lee—a migrant laborer working in construction in a rapidly growing metropolis, who falls 10 stories from a scaffolding and dies. To understand the causes of his death we draw from four distinct but inter-connected perspectives. Although our first instinct may be to start at the individual level, in order to truly understand how SDOH are operationalized, we begin our analysis with the larger political and economic context.

At the **broadest (macro) level**, we may understand the fall to be linked to the free-market economic system whereby profits come before worker safety and well-being. A building boom driven by global financial interests and facilitated by trade treaties that are signed by governments—many under pressure and/or representing elite interests—gives investors and transnational corporations (TNCs) enormous power to evade taxes and flout labor laws. As such, working class efforts to organize for social security benefits and workplace safety are constrained by threats of job loss and government repression. At an **intermediate (macro-meso) level** linked to government policies, Lee's low earnings derive from minimum wage levels that are inadequate and poorly enforced; because his position as a foreign worker is precarious, he has little recourse. Moreover, the company's meager safety training and low-grade scaffolding materials are enabled by scant employment regulations and oversight. At the **individual level**, Lee may have been inattentive and insufficiently conscious of safety, or just unlucky (as the word *accident* implies), and thus slipped to his death. But if we examine Lee's living and home conditions **(meso-local level)**, we learn that he is chronically sleep-deprived due to his long and stressful commute to work—he can only afford to reside in a distant slum. Moreover, the flimsy walls of his dwelling cannot keep out biting and disease-bearing insects and rodents (whose colonies proliferate in the absence of garbage collection) causing an unpleasant skin rash. Perhaps in his exhaustion, he scratched his arm, inopportunely letting go of the scaffolding. Lee's fall—whether in Dubai or Dublin—may be construed as one person's misfortune, but viewed through a lens of societal determinants, it may be understood as the result of an interdependent set of political, economic, and social forces that involve global and individual determinants, and a range of factors in between.

Understanding Health Inequities

SDOH approaches offer essential ingredients for explaining the existence of health inequities, but in seeking to analyze health inequities and explain *how* they come about (and how to prevent or address them), we need theoretical frameworks that link ideas of society to human biology (recognizing that health takes place in actual bodies, even as people interact with one another and with the larger society). Three ways of understanding health and disease patterns were introduced in chapter 3—two mainstream models: biomedical and behavioral/lifestyle—and a critical political economy of health approach. Here we offer some additional theories and concepts to help us think about biology in context and flesh out how population health and health equity happens, quite literally, in the flesh (Table 7-1).

As a brief reminder, the biomedical model argues that health derives from a combination of one's genetic heritage and individual biology and lifelong health and disease experiences (and behavior). Health differences among individuals and groups thus result from natural variation, inherent differences that have evolved over time, individual risk factors, and different opportunities accorded by genetics and biology.

Following a behavioral/lifestyle model, health and health differences are a function of personal choices around how one lives in terms of diet, exercise, occupation, place of residence, and aspects of personal behavior, from abusing alcohol and drugs to practicing safe sex. Both of these models are based on individualized and decontextualized understandings of how health and health inequity are produced.

Just as the biomedical model sidesteps that every occurrence of disease, death, or injury is societally influenced (including genetic conditions, whose expression is environmentally-mediated and whose outcomes are societally-mediated,[1] via who and what gets detected and treated, what medical research, care, and funding policies exist, etc.), the lifestyle model often overlooks the day-to-day constraints of, for example, what foods are affordable and accessible, the presence/absence of parks and safe spaces, job possibilities, daily and long-term family responsibilities, stress, or how much political influence their communities have on people's behavior and decisions regarding how they live their lives.

A critical political economy approach, by contrast, sees society as more than the sum of individuals and their actions. In particular, it focuses on the role of power and control over resources—that is, political and economic systems and key actors, and their accompanying values and priorities—in structuring patterns of health and health inequity. These structural forces shape but do not negate human agency and biology, although political economy may not elaborate the exact mechanisms that connect the political to the biological.

Political economy is not the only alternative to mainstream theories. We now turn to two other theories: psychosocial and ecosocial, which will help concretize ideas around how societal determinants shape health and health inequities.

Psychosocial Theory

Psychosocial understandings emphasize the health impact of individual perceptions and responses to the social environment: family, community, school, workplace, and the wider society. These contexts and social interactions, combined with one's social status, shape experiences of psychological stress and associated emotions (responses such as depression, anger, anxiety), mediated by coping skills, social support, self-esteem, and sense of control. Stress, and adverse reactions to it, synergistically affect health through physiological and psychological responses, including harmful health behaviors (e.g., overeating, alcohol abuse, smoking) (Kubzansky, Winning, and Kawachi 2014).

Both exposure to stressors and forms of coping or buffering stress are socially patterned, with one's position or rank in the social hierarchy serving as the prime psychological stressor/buffer. Not only are working class persons exposed to greater stress than higher class individuals, the former experience similar situations in more stressful ways because they have fewer personal and social resources to manage stressful circumstances.

Among the postulated mechanisms regulating these processes are physiologic responses of distress and resentment which, especially when chronic, create endocrinologic, nervous system, and other regulatory imbalances due to cumulative over- and under-use of these systems from repeated or chronic stress over the lifecourse, also called allostatic load (Berkman and Kawachi 2014). These imbalances raise blood pressure and depress the immunological and central nervous systems, in turn negatively affecting cardiovascular, metabolic, and mental health, among other health consequences.

Table 7-1 Theories Explaining Health and Disease Patterns (and their Contribution to Understanding Societal Determinants and Health Inequities)

	Theory	Main arguments on health and disease determinants/health inequities
Mainstream	Biomedical	• Health derives largely from genetic heritage and other individual biological factors. • Age, chance, and prior health and disease experience and exposure explain health differences.
	Behavioral/Lifestyle	• Individual choices, behaviors, practices, and beliefs are key determinants of health outcomes. • Health differences arise from freely chosen lifestyles.
Alternative	Critical Political Economy	• Societal political structures and class relations are central to explaining health outcomes. • Explains the causes of health inequities as manifested through various power mechanisms (e.g., material conditions, distribution of power and resources through the political system and workplace).
	Psychosocial	• Individuals' perceptions of their social conditions, location within social hierarchies, and interactions—particularly via stress responses (and mitigators)—have psychological, behavioral, and physiological consequences. • Seeks to understand how responses to socially-structured environments affect health and health inequities.
	Ecosocial	• Health/disease is the embodiment of social and living conditions, political, economic, and ecologic context, and power relations—experienced inter-generationally and over the lifecourse. • Examines how the interplay over time of exposure, susceptibility, and resistance in individuals and social groups forms patterns of population health that result in greater or lesser health equity.

Source: Adapted extensively from Krieger (2011).

Exacerbating the physiological response are various coping mechanisms adopted to relieve stress—such as excessive eating, sleep disruption, and use of psychoactive substances—which have further negative effects on physical and mental health (Krieger 2011). According to psychosocial understandings, the *perception* of precarious, unfair, or inferior status may count as much as the *reality* of unequal resources, power differentials, and limited decisionmaking latitude (Matthews and Gallo 2011).

Unlike lifestyle and biomedical explanations, psychosocial theory does not focus solely on individual behavior and biology or overlook the role of social context. Indeed, it accepts the importance of social causes, stressing that psychological and physiological exposures (stressors) affect health. However, it de-emphasizes *who* and *what* cause the differential exposures and capacities of resistance to stress in the first place and how political, social, and economic agendas, values, power, and practices shape societal hierarchies and the nature and distribution of stress exposures.

Ecosocial Theory

An ecosocial model, developed by social epidemiologist Nancy Krieger, seeks to integrate political, social, and biological understandings of the determinants of health, reconciling the limits to political economy (which underplays biological mechanisms) and to psychosocial theory (which underplays the role of politics and power in shaping material and social conditions). Health outcomes in ecosocial terms are the biological expression of living conditions, social relations, and structures of power over the lifecourse and across generations. Ecosocial theory pays particular heed to:

> interrelationships between diverse forms of social inequality, including racism, class, and gender. A central focus is on "embodiment," referring to how we literally embody, biologically, our lived experience, in societal and ecological context, thereby creating population patterns of health and disease... (Krieger 2014b, p. 48).

Elucidating the notion of embodiment, ecosocial theory employs two key concepts: the "cumulative interplay of exposure, susceptibility, and resistance"—whereby past and ongoing biological incorporation of social relations of power are integrated into present health and disease experience—and "accountability and agency, historically and dynamically," which, like a political economy approach, incorporates relations of power not simply in the abstract, but through actors, institutions, actions and their inter-relations, past and present.

As such, ecosocial theory accounts for who and what is responsible for power asymmetries and uncovers how channels of resistance (agency) are able to upend power structures. Ecosocial theory also helps to bridge the (false) distance between so-called "upstream and downstream" approaches by showing how unequal power manifests at all levels—from the body to the body politic—shaping overall population health (Krieger 2008).

Thus, the ecosocial model builds upon a political economy approach to health by specifying not just macro- but also micro-level mechanisms through which social inequalities, societal conditions, and biological processes interact to produce health or ill health (Krieger 2011).

In sum, this roster of societal determination frameworks helps make concrete how injustice is embodied in health outcomes and inequity and lays out the dimensions of injustice that need to be considered, at what level and timescale, in order to address health inequity.

Three additional cross-cutting frames can help link society and biology: intersectionality, lifecourse approaches, and health and human rights.

Intersectionality

Intersectionality (coined by Kimberlé Crenshaw 1989) argues that simultaneous forms of identity and social position (race, class, gender, sex, and other categories) interact dynamically, making their separate, directly additive, or hierarchical analysis problematic. Applied to health research, the concept of intersectionality seeks to explain "how multiple social [factors] . . . reflect interlocking systems of privilege and oppression (i.e., racism, sexism, heterosexism, classism)" (Bowleg 2012, p. 1267). While this chapter retains a determinant-by-determinant organization for purposes of clarity, it recognizes the health effects of concurrent and synergistic forms of oppression and privilege posited by intersectionality (Kapilashrami, Hill, and Meer 2015) in several ways: through discussion of intersectionality and synergistic effects under many determinants, through use of embodiment theory (incorporating an understanding of concomitant experiences of oppression and the importance of historical and policy dimensions of exposure, susceptibility, and resistance that mediate how these factors operate), and through examples and illustrations of intersecting and interacting SDOH.

Lifecourse Approaches

Influences on health cannot be gleaned from a onetime snapshot; studying them across the lifetime offers more illuminating explanations. Lifecourse approaches consider: (1) important early-life experiences that shape development (especially brain development) and vulnerability or resistance to future disease into adulthood) (Walker et al. 2011); (2) the impact of early-life exposures on adult social conditions, in turn affecting adult health, as per a "social trajectory model"; and (3) accumulation over the lifetime of advantages and disadvantages—though not prenatal or early childhood exposure per se—marking adult health and disease (Berkman and Kawachi 2014, p. 10). A variety of theories (including those just discussed) employ lifecourse perspectives, because they offer a dynamic understanding of how determinants of health (and their interaction) operate within and across individuals and generations, and in population health writ large, relating past experience to current health status and possible future health directions (Lynch and Smith 2005).

Health and Human Rights

A third shared frame for understanding how societal determinants affect health and health equity is a health and human rights approach (see Box 14-2). Respecting, protecting, and fulfilling human, including health-related, rights—inter alia, racial and gender-based discrimination, substandard living and working conditions, and exclusion from democratic processes—are a government's responsibility in any society (Tarantola and Gruskin 2013). Consequently, government (in)actions and (absence of) policies related to multiple SDOH have a huge bearing on health and human rights. Because most (but not all) current SDOH are also in the legal purview of governments (as is addressing the harms of historical determinants), we can think of respecting, fulfilling, and enforcing health-related rights as being infused across SDOH.

The ideas presented thus far frame the next task at hand: identifying the constellation and intersection of factors and structures influencing health and health inequity.

The following pages flesh out, in rough order, the different components of Figure 3-3. While many of these societal determinants are discussed in greater depth in other chapters, our aim here is to present a comprehensive and structured, if condensed, array of the factors that influence health, paying particular attention to *how* societal determinants are translated into health inequities that unjustly and avoidably cut short millions of lives and cause enormous suffering.

At the level of population health, knowing how the presence, absence, and interaction of particular societal factors or policies affect health equity and outcomes—and to what extent—offers key insights as to their origins and the forces driving them, as well as their policy importance (Krieger 2014a) (bearing in mind the contingencies of time and space, since factors may operate differently in distinct settings or time periods).

In order to see how societal determinants unfold at different levels and culminate in people's (ill) health and lived experiences, throughout the chapter we provide a fictional but all too real account of two working mothers, in Bangladesh and the United States, and the range of influences shaping their—and their children's—lives and health.

FROM POLITICAL, ECONOMIC, SOCIAL, AND HISTORICAL CONTEXT TO POPULATION HEALTH AND HEALTH INEQUITIES

Key Questions:

- How do past patterns of political, economic, and social relations affect SDOH?
- What makes the uneven distribution of power and wealth a SDOH?
- How do global trade and financial regimes influence health?

At the broadest level, SDOH can be understood in relation to social, political, economic, and historical forces that play out in national and global arenas. At the global level, these forces include trade and financial governance systems, patterns of wealth and ownership, production processes, imperialism, and militarism (Ng and Muntaner 2014). At the national level (also reflecting global historical forces), a key factor is how power is exercised in terms of class, race, and gender relations through the structure, capacity, and accountability of political systems.

Although few colonies remain, the current global political structure reflects geopolitical relations that have been in place for centuries and which affect the SDOH (Czyzewski 2011). Systems of trade and commodity pricing, debt and global finance regimes, and international organizations for the most part maintain historical asymmetries between colonizer (high-income, powerful, dominant) and colonized (low-income, less powerful) countries (see chapters 1, 2, and 9 for further details).

Colonialism, Imperialism, Militarism, and Violence

The legacies of colonialism, imperialism, and ongoing militarism have enormous bearing on SDOH. Current power configurations, including the global financial system, discriminatory social structures and divisions, and the uneven distribution of wealth, derive from long historical processes of accumulation and exploitation under pre-feudal and feudalistic societies, processes that accelerated under imperialism and capitalism (see chapter 1), and now neoliberal globalization (see chapter 9). The rules and social arrangements under these systems—from slavery to tithing of peasant agricultural output; colonial military occupation, oppression, and uncompensated resource extraction; imperial domination; and current national and international governance mechanisms that protect corporate profit-making over virtually all other social values—all influence health across varied pathways and mechanisms that involve infringement of sovereignty and political self-determination, limited control over resources, repressive social policy, further conflict, and so on.

To explore just one avenue, the continued use of war to consolidate power and ensure access to resources is a contemporary manifestation of neo-imperial global capitalism. War, although justified under some circumstances, is indisputably bad for health. It leads to death, disease, rape, environmental contamination, and destruction of infrastructure, generating a host of other physical and mental health problems. During the 20th century, almost 200 million people lost their lives directly or indirectly as a result of wars, with civilians constituting over half of those killed. There were 69 armed conflicts in the 2000–2010 period alone (Levy and Sidel 2013). Use of weapons (e.g., machetes, landmines, guns, and bombs) can cause acute physical trauma followed by long-term disability (e.g., loss of limbs, reduction in sensory abilities, fistulae), as well as psychological trauma. Conflicts also decrease access to adequate nutrition and potable water, linked to elevated infant mortality rates (Gates et al. 2012), and generate millions of refugees and internally displaced persons (IDPs) (see chapter 8).

Militarism escalates all forms of violence within and between countries, with extremely damaging consequences to soldiers and civilians alike. Globally, about 1.3 million people die each year as a result of violence (WHO 2014). Military spending also channels resources away from social and infrastructural endeavors—parks, schools, quality housing, investing in safe employment, and so on.

Trade, Finance and Governance, and Production Regimes under Contemporary Global Capitalism

A range of global arrangements, including rule-making bodies, international financial institutions (IFIs), and trade treaties have direct and indirect health effects (Koivusalo 2011; Rudin and Sanders 2011) (see chapter 9 for details).

Succinctly, the market-driven capitalist world order is motored by growth, consumption, and a profit motive that trump values of equity, communitarianism, and social and environmental protection. That said, during capitalism's periodic crises—and when union and other social movements have struggled to challenge its dominance—there have been significant, if uneven, improvements in well-being (e.g., through the building of welfare states). Such challenges were particularly effective from the 1930s Great Depression through the height of the Cold War, when a possible socialist alternative to the capitalist world order existed.

Since the 1980s, however, the ideological sweep of neoliberal globalization has stifled labor and social movements and ushered in a renewed intensity in capital accumulation on a worldwide scale, featuring a massive surge in quantities, flows, and rapidity of trade and foreign direct investment (FDI), hand-in-hand with an even greater upsurge in speculation, financialization, public and private debt, and currency circulation (Panitch and

Gindin 2012). These changes have been bolstered by national governments that are increasingly at the service of transnational capital and capitalist classes, together integrated as a corporate and political force (Robinson 2014).

Under neoliberal globalization, the power, capacity, and accountability of democratically elected governments are ever more subsumed under trade and investment rules favoring financial interests and TNCs. These hegemonic processes accelerated during the 1980s debt crisis in low- and middle-income countries (LMICs), when IFI loans and accompanying conditionalities denuded government capacity, and reoriented regulation to favor capitalist interests over public need. Already financially fragile states were stripped of resources to invest in social policies and well-being, in turn provoking unemployment, malnutrition, hazardous exposures, and increased poverty. These consequences disproportionately affected the health of the most vulnerable populations (including children, women, Indigenous groups, and small-scale farmers).

Atop financial gouging, the global trade system, governed by the World Trade Organization (WTO) and separate trade and investment agreements, illustrates how unequal power is created and maintained and manifests in inequitable health outcomes. With limits on FDI and foreign ownership lifted, TNCs have relocated primary resource extraction and labor-intensive production to LMICs, where the cost of business is minimized through low wages, low taxes, inadequate and lax enforcement of environmental and occupational standards, tax evasion, and capital flight. Producer country gains are limited (although corrupt politicians, local elites, and intermediaries often benefit enormously), given paltry control over commodity pricing or power to retain/reinvest profits domestically. Moreover, in many countries a combination of subsistence living and political repression can make it difficult for workers to unionize and social movements to mobilize for accountable governance and equitable social policies.

In addition to undermining worker rights and environmental protection policies, trade and investment agreements affect health by promoting privatization of—and circumscribing access to—water provision, health care, and education, and by reducing tariffs and taxes, thereby lowering state income that could have been spent on social services (Friel, Hattersley, and Townsend 2015). These agreements also protect big businesses from "impediments to competition," such as subsidies for local industries and regulations, at the expense of small-scale producers and laborers in high-income countries (HICs) and LMICs alike.

Exemplifying the concentration of power enabled by contemporary global trade arrangements, world food production and trade is now controlled by a small number of mega-companies. The 10 largest food and beverage corporations have revenues of over US$1.1 billion/day, part of an industry worth US$7 trillion (10% of global GDP). Furthermore, one third of global grocery sales are in the hands of 30 food retailers, and just four TNCs—ADM, Bunge, Cargill, and Dreyfus—control 90% of world grain trade (Hoffman 2013). This powerful sector affects multiple SDOH, including food sovereignty, nutrition, water access, environmental contamination, and poverty.

Wealth and Health: Distribution, Assets, and Land Tenure

Wealth and Ownership/Income Distribution

Wealth and its distribution shape and are shaped by access to power and resources across countries and institutions, in many ways determining the basic political, economic, and social institutions and rules that govern society. For much of the 20th century, wealth extremes were declining due to growing demands of workers, peasants, and other social groups for improved living conditions, as well as decolonization struggles, all leading to deconcentration of assets and power and enabling fairer health, education, land, and employment policies. But since the 1970s, wealth inequalities have increased markedly within settings and across the world, alongside a decline in working class (and union) power (Jaumotte and Buitron 2015). Globally, in 2015 the world's 62 wealthiest individuals owned as much as the world's "bottom half"—3.6 billion people! Even more starkly, 1% of the world's population owns more than the remaining 99% (Hardoon, Ayele, and Fuentes-Nieva 2016).

Wealth (and its distribution) influences health *both* by determining the material circumstances that affect health in concrete terms—including via livelihoods and social conditions—*and* through its relation to societal power structures that shape broader social relations and policies, from economic security and social protections via welfare/redistributive states, to employment and workplace conditions, to political social justice struggles affecting those relations and structures (de Andrade et al. 2015). These will be explored ahead.

At the international level, skewed wealth distribution has translated into countries and regions with differing per capita wealth (as per Box 3-2: HICs, middle-income countries [MICs], and low-income countries [LICs]; previously stratified as developed and developing countries, roughly based on colonizer versus colonized societies). Overall GDP per capita levels roughly correspond to life expectancy (see chapter 12), as well as a society's degree of political power (or ability to manoeuver without threat of economic or military repercussions) on the international stage. But aggregate GDP per capita tells us little about wealth distribution and consequent health outcomes and health (in)equity within countries, or how various societies with relatively low GDP per capita are nonetheless able to achieve favorable health (equity).

Wealth levels within countries are consistently correlated with health (Figure 7-1), though patterns are not identical. For instance, in Indonesia and Jordan infant mortality is over three times higher in the lowest wealth quintile than the highest. But in the Philippines, the top and middle quintiles have almost identical infant mortality, less than half the rate of the bottom quintile. Across LMICs, infant mortality rates vary widely, with some settings (such as Cuba) clocking lower rates than the United States, as does Jordan's wealthiest quintile (WHO 2016a).

> "If the rich could hire others to die for them, we, the poor, would all make a nice living."—Mordcha, the innkeeper, *Fiddler on the Roof*

It is important to underscore that inequality is a symptom of wealth concentration (and the societal structures that undergird it) rather than a driver independent of power arrangements, as popularly portrayed. Moreover, wealth inequality is mostly studied in terms of income inequality (since income data are more readily available), meaning that wealth's far greater non-income components, including property, stocks, inheritance, investments, and

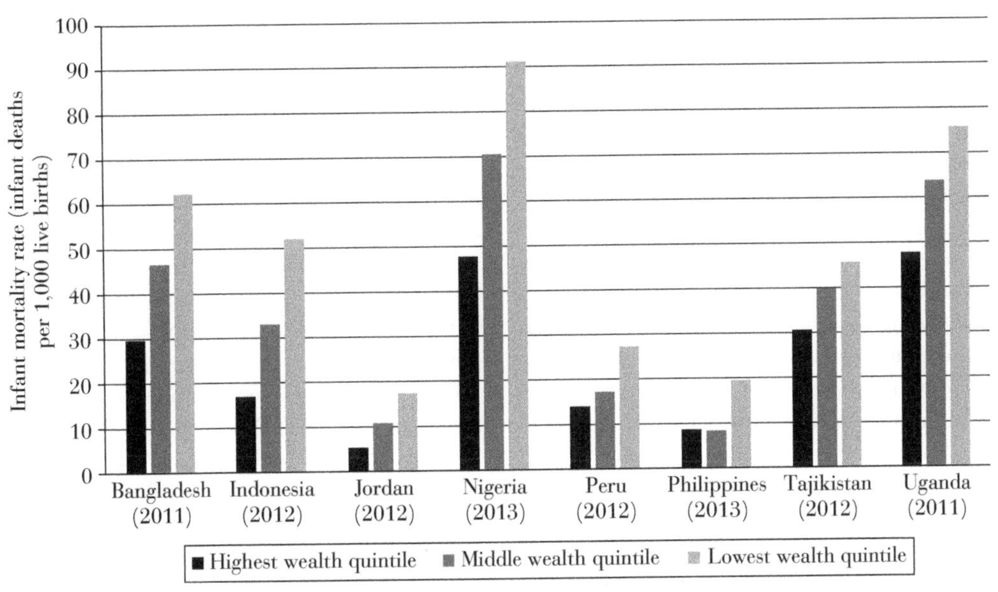

Figure 7-1: Infant mortality rate by wealth quintile, selected countries.
Data Source: WHO (2016a).

other assets, are not captured. As such, wealth inequality is far larger than income inequality, and thus decreases in income inequality may leave maldistribution of wealth (for example between men and women), and corresponding political influence/power, largely intact (Thrasher 2015).

Some point to income inequality as key to understanding population health patterns, arguing that for HICs, relative income inequality is more important than GDP per capita, poverty, or other social differences in determining shorter life expectancy (Wilkinson and Pickett 2009). This avenue relates to the psychosocial effects of inequality on individuals whose negative (or positive) perceptions of their hierarchical status influence their health, as psychosocial models assert. Accordingly, societies with greater income inequalities are less cohesive and have greater social distance between groups. As distrust and suspicion mount, support for society-wide institutions and infrastructure—such as public education, youth and social programs, public parks, and universal health care—decreases, thereby deteriorating quality of life for all but society's wealthiest.

Further postulated by psychosocial framings, even those at the top end of the income scale experience worse health than do people living in more egalitarian societies, because they fear losing their position or assets and may be isolated from other groups (Wilkinson and Pickett 2009). Meanwhile, those at the bottom end of the income distribution may be socially excluded, disrespected, and may themselves lose self-respect, with dire health consequences. In other words, "more unequal societies generate more anxiety, shame, depression, and other negative emotions" (Kawachi and Subramanian 2014, p. 135).

However, whether income inequality is associated with population health over and above levels of wealth and poverty—and, if so, why—is debated (Kawachi and Subramanian 2014; Mackenbach 2015; Wilkinson and Pickett 2015). While most agree that health inequities exist within societies, many contest whether income inequality at the societal level is associated with aggregate population health (e.g., gauged by infant mortality) (Beckfield, Olafsdottir, and Bakhtiari 2013). A central issue is how much poverty matters separately from inequality, even in HICs. Moreover, income inequality has a negative impact on life expectancy largely in countries with high poverty levels: other than in the United States, among HICs income inequality does not appear to be a major determinant of population health differences within or between countries, making inequality but one feature of the distribution of wealth and power (Rambotti 2015).

Ultimately, income, or even wealth, inequality alone, does not explain the effects of racial, gender, and other forms of discrimination or how unequal power structures and relations manifest in the workplace and the polis and affect patterns of health and health equity (Coburn 2011).

Land Tenure and Property Ownership

Property ownership and land tenure are a fundamental dimension of wealth and economic security in both rural and urban settings. Holding and farming the land is the prime rural livelihood source, involving 400 million subsistence or small-scale farms that support approximately one third of the world's population. In the mid-20th century, land reform was a key feature of social movements from Bolivia to Taiwan, improving the lot of millions of smallholders. In more recent decades, productive land has become increasingly concentrated in the hands not just of domestic elites, but of large agribusinesses, now operating massive soy, sugar, and palm oil plantations across the world, enabled by deregulation, trade agreements, and the penetration of TNCs. Not only do agribusiness interests monopolize use of water and other resources, they benefit from extensive credit and infrastructure support that displaced smallholders cannot access (Hoffman 2013). Demonstrating the connections between land tenure and multiple SDOH, an incredible 30% to 50% of all food produced is wasted (never eaten) due to both pre- and post-harvest losses, leading to untold volumes of wasted water and billions of tons of greenhouse gas emissions, while almost 1 billion people (or by some estimates over 2 billion) still experience hunger (Whitmee et al. 2015).

Small landholders have been squeezed out through various mechanisms. In India, for example, 1960s Green Revolution policies introduced pricey technologies and inputs that benefited the richer peasantry and saddled marginal farmers with growing debt. Over time, widespread use of fertilizers and pesticides, and hybrid and genetically modified seeds sold by TNCs, exacerbated these trends at the same time as neoliberal reforms privatized seed distribution, reduced access to public credit, and channeled irrigation systems to favor larger farms (Reddy and Mishra 2010). In India alone, millions of small farmers have lost their livelihoods in recent decades, unable to survive against large competitors, and hundreds of thousands of farmers have committed suicide in the context of bankruptcy, indebtedness, and crop failure (Radhakrishnan and Andrade 2012).

Worldwide, agribusiness takeovers by Monsanto and other multinationals have had drastic effects on local producers, in Argentina provoking a 25% reduction in the number of small farms from 1988 to 2002, affecting the livelihoods of small farmers and pushing the country into virtual monoculture: more than half of its fertile land is used for soybean cultivation almost entirely for export (Gras 2009). Some governments, such as Ethiopia's, serve as (reprehensible) intermediaries by nationalizing large swaths of land only to resell to private interests, simultaneously forcing local farmers and pastoralists onto unproductive land (Human Rights Watch 2012).

Loss of land tenure usually affects the poorest and women/girls first, causing lower nutritional intake, increased partner violence, and migration to urban factory jobs with dangerous working (and living) conditions. Landless farmers across the Majority World are among the world's most disenfranchised populations, even as in recent years they have organized politically, demanding food sovereignty (see ahead) through La Via Campesina and Brazil's Landless Workers' Movement.

Meanwhile, in cities, where 54% of the world's population now lives (UN-DESA 2014), inequitable property ownership influences health and well-being via the effects of real estate speculation, gentrification, and redevelopment policies. Past and present, urban poor and working classes (joined by rural populations dispossessed of their land) have experienced intense struggles over public space and private property (Harvey 2006). Urbanization was historically tied to industrialization, turning center cities into dangerous and deadly sites of production and reproduction of factory workers and more marginal groups. Elites escaped to outlying districts, with many retaining rural estates.

More recently, shifting urban economies have reversed this trend. From Manhattan to Mumbai, large-scale resettlement policies combined with rising land values and speculation have displaced low-income populations (Corburn 2015). Affordable urban housing markets have drastically diminished, compelling millions to move farther and farther from workplaces and vastly increasing commuting times, with attendant stress and time constraints and exposures to (and generation of) air pollution.

A nefarious accompanying trend is predatory lending, whereby bankers encourage working class—often racial and ethnic minority—populations to purchase property beyond their means, a move that strangles them with debt and eventual bankruptcy in a context of economic precariousness, aggravated by economic downturn (viz. the Great Recession of 2008–2012). In the worst hit places, a geography of foreclosure, home abandonment, and bank repossession marks urban landscapes amid further speculation (Dorling 2015). Even more repressive, slum clearance policies, euphemized as urban renewal, have forced the poorest (usually racialized) groups out of central urban locations, breaking up communities and jeopardizing social ties, livelihoods, and access to social services, all with negative health effects including rising mortality in informal urban settlements (Doshi 2013; Van de Poel, O'Donnell, and Van Doorslaer 2007).

Power Structure, Social Relations, and Discrimination

Social Class, Socioeconomic Status, and Socioeconomic Position

Important as income appears as a direct and indirect determinant of health, it does not tell the full story. Nor, as we have seen, can income inequalities completely explain health and mortality patterns within and across societies. Crucial is social class, theorized by Karl Marx as people's relation to ownership of assets and the production process—that is, whether one is an owner or a worker—or, in neo-Marxist terms, a manager/administrator (in a contradictory class location) (Wright 1998). Social class explains health outcomes above and beyond income via mechanisms of structure and agency: class relations are mediated by class structure (the balance of political power favoring capital or labor), reflecting the extent of effective class struggle against class oppression—that is, the deprivation, exclusion from control, and appropriation of the exploited group's productivity and assets. Capital-dominated class structures tend to produce less generous social welfare policies, affecting health by generating varying degrees of social inequalities across virtually all health determinants (Coburn 2015). Social class is thus a vital determinant of health inequities, and operates synergistically with other forms of oppression, including racism and patriarchy/gender oppression.

Although social class is well theorized, using it systematically poses a significant challenge, as most governments do not routinely collect data by class (at least partly reflecting ideological resistance to generation of information that portends social change) (see chapter 5). The United Kingdom is an exception in this regard,[2] making possible the landmark 1980 "Black Report," which tracked mortality and life expectancy differentials by five occupational classes from the 1930s through the 1970s (and visible to the present—Figure 7-2). Not only did mortality differences not diminish, they widened, even long after the UK's National Health Service was established in 1948 (see chapter 11). The Black Report argued that these inequalities in health result from inequities in living and working conditions, not in health care access and utilization, concluding that class-based mortality differences are "socially or economically determined" and therefore amenable to change through social and economic policies (Black et al. 1980).

With data gaps around social class, most health research refers to socioeconomic status (SES). Deriving from the ideas of Max Weber, SES refers to individuals' position in society in terms of three main categories: income or wealth, education, and status (prestige or power). In socially stratified contexts, and evidenced by numerous studies in HICs, SES helps explain how assets and characteristics intertwine to create social differences, impeding or enabling people to achieve health or other desired goals thanks to money, knowledge, and connections, including intergenerationally (Braveman et al. 2005; Glymour, Avendano, and Kawachi 2014). Social epidemiology research often employs continuous indicators such as wealth or education (plus

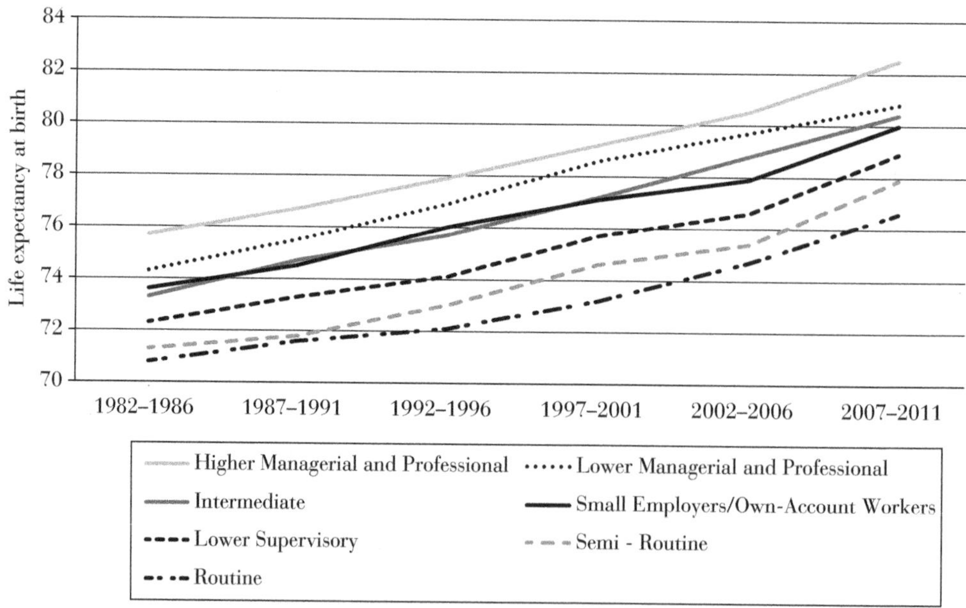

Figure 7-2: Life expectancy at birth by socioeconomic/occupational classification for men in England and Wales since the Black Report.

Data Source: Office for National Statistics (2015).

occupation); other studies seek to control for SES so as to exclude these effects and focus on other factors.

The UK's Whitehall Studies of tens of thousands of civil servants starting in the late 1960s employed occupational grade as a measure of SES, uncovering a "social gradient in health" even in the absence of poverty or material deprivation. Men in the lowest of four occupational grades were found to have the highest death rate from coronary heart disease (CHD), with mortality decreasing stepwise from the lowest to the highest occupational class (Rose and Marmot 1981). Subsequent studies including women replicated social gradient findings for CHD and other health indicators (Marmot and Brunner 2005) and linked the gradient to the work environment via job insecurity and imbalance between job demands and control (and between effort and rewards) (Bell et al. 2004). Study lead Michael Marmot, who went on to chair the World Health Organization's (WHO) Commission on Social Determinants of Health (see ahead), argues that social status and one's place in the employment hierarchy pattern health inequities through psychosocial mechanisms that condition health behaviors and shape stress pathways (Marmot 2004). Others explaining the social gradient put greater emphasis on employment power differentials, such as control over work process, workplace democracy, and social protections (Muntaner et al. 2010). As discussed ahead, physical working conditions, more than psychosocial environment, continue to play a major role in explaining occupational inequalities in health in post-industrial societies (Toch et al. 2014).

Many countries use SES as an indicator of health, together with household and community indicators (which can be easier to collect). For example, across LMICs, women with higher SES are more likely than those with lower SES to have a skilled health worker present at childbirth (Say and Raine 2007). SES has also been associated with contradictory patterns shaping childhood obesity in LMICs versus HICs: lower child obesity in higher SES groups in HICs is linked to education, safe recreation areas, and the higher cost of healthier foods, among other factors, whereas the opposite trend in LMICs links obesity to higher incomes, greater access to transnational food products, and less reliance on active transport (Gupta et al. 2012).

From a societal determination of health perspective, SES's reliance on income and social assets at the individual level sidesteps work and ownership relations—the major feature of power and power differences in capitalist societies. Consequently, a growing tendency is to discuss socioeconomic position (SEP), understood as being structured by social class *relations*, not just differences in material possessions and personal characteristics and networks (Krieger, Williams, and Moss 1997; Shaw et al. 2007). This means that via SEP income differences between, for instance, a CEO and a factory worker are understood as a function of their respective class positions (while SES would simply note the differences, not explain how they arose) (Glymour, Avendano, and Kawachi 2014). The past two decades have also witnessed efforts to employ a neo-Marxist approach to measure social class and transcend the focus on individual attributes, with an aim at better understanding the causal mechanism through which class affects health and the SDOH (Muntaner et al. 2015). The differences among these concepts—social class, SES, and SEP—are not only semantic but have enormous implications for the types of data collected (as per chapter 5) and policies employed to address inequalities in health.

Gender Inequality, Patriarchy, and Sexuality

Gender inequality and discrimination influence health in various ways, separately and in conjunction with other determinants. Gender refers to social conceptions, roles, and identities rather than biology. In other words, differing health outcomes due to sex-based differences in biology are not gendered per se, whereas health differences among persons who identify as women, men, or transgender (regardless of sexuality, "biological sex," or gender presentation) due to their differing household responsibilities, decisionmaking power in public and private spaces, occupational roles, or legal rights, are gendered. Gender-based differences in health status vary across time and place, just as gender roles differ according to era, society, and stage in life. That said, in most societies, women, transgender, and non-binary people bear the brunt of gender oppression and prejudice and their health consequences (Doyal and Payne 2011).

As discussed in chapter 6, gender and sexual identity constitute an important determinant of health worldwide, with particular concerns stemming from societal mistreatment. This occurs through institutionalized oppression via law, policing, health provider ignorance, or inadequate services (Math and Seshadri 2013). Other forms of discrimination, homophobia, transphobia, and heteronormativity—magnified by classism and racism—are manifest through social policies around housing, schooling, and employment, as well as threats, bullying, and violence, which cause physical harm or death as well as mental health problems and related substance abuse (Logie 2012).

The most egregious health manifestations of gender inequality relate to gender-based violence (GBV). Globally, over 35% of adolescent girls and adult women (over 15 years) have experienced physical and/or sexual violence, mostly perpetrated by sexual partners. Intimate partner violence is overwhelmingly directed by men toward women. It includes violence during pregnancy, which in addition to physically and psychologically harming women, can lead to premature labor, stillbirths, and neonatal mortality (UNICEF 2014c).

Notwithstanding incomplete data and considerable underreporting due to stigma, one pattern holds: the level of violence against women is unconscionably high across all world regions, reaching up to 60% of women in the Western Pacific, 46% in Africa, 40% in Southeast Asia, 36% in LMICs in the Americas and the Eastern Mediterranean, 33% in HICs, and 27% in LMICs in Europe (WHO 2013a).

Women may experience violence as adolescents or even earlier, with nearly 25% of girls aged 15 to 19 globally having been subject to physical violence and 10% of girls to sexual violence, and rates twice as high in conflict zones such as the Democratic Republic of Congo (see chapter 8). GBV can have lifelong consequences, from organ damage, disability, and mental illness to negative effects on other determinants of health including school attendance, mobility, and employment (UNICEF 2014c).

Certain societal factors shape the prevalence of GBV, particularly patriarchy (social systems defined by male power and predominance) and associated norms around male authority: tolerance of wife-beating, laws and practices limiting women's access to land, property, and other economic resources, as well as limits on female education and wage-earning. Greater educational access for girls and women's increased entry into the paid workforce appear particularly relevant for reducing GBV, moreso than higher GDP per capita (Heise and Kotsadam 2015).

Gender also matters for health outcomes that involve "sex"-linked biology, including reproductive health. For example, although only people with uteruses experience childbirth, the lifelong effects of nutrition, previous illness, and social support, as well as access to health care, are all influenced by gender roles and in turn affect the health of women during pregnancy and childbirth.

In addition to the abortion restrictions outlined in chapter 6, four countries (plus the Holy See) explicitly prohibit abortions under any circumstances: Malta, El Salvador, Nicaragua, and Chile (whose ban was under debate in 2016). Under El Salvador's extreme ban, illegal abortion carries a 2- to 8-year penalty, and dozens of women who have experienced miscarriages following rape or due to obstetric complications have been sentenced to prison for up to 50 years for "aggravated homicide" (often turned over to police by hospitals). This multiplies the violence women experience through: rape; violation of physician–patient confidentiality; the institutional violence of imprisonment; the societal violation of women's human rights; and the devastating impact on families (Center for Reproductive Rights 2014). Most are low-income women with poor heath care and contraceptive access; many are teenagers. The death rate due to clandestine abortions exceeds 10%. El Salvador also has the highest child and teen pregnancy rate in Latin America, with almost 60% of pregnancy-related deaths from suicide (Amnesty International 2014). Worldwide, bans or limited access to abortion result in 22 million unsafe abortions per year—causing over 5 million complications and 47,000 deaths—making unsafe abortion a leading cause of maternal mortality (WHO 2016b).

The connections between gender and health are complex. The gendered division of labor leads to differential health outcomes, with men more likely to work in dangerous or high-stress jobs outside of the home, and women, children, and the elderly—especially in LMICs—more exposed to strenuous and potentially hazardous household activities such as field work, water collection, and cooking with inadequate ventilation, which puts them at risk for cardiovascular and respiratory illnesses (Sehgal and Krishnan 2013). However, these roles are changing, with women's increased responsibility for income generation (e.g., through factory work) and growing male unemployment in many countries.

In most countries, women experience lower levels of mortality and longer life expectancy (but higher morbidity) than men, in large measure due to reductions in childbirth-related deaths over the past century and differential workplace exposures. Yet in some LICs, women's life expectancy is shortened by extremely high maternal mortality. Life expectancy at birth in 2013 in Afghanistan was 62 years for women (61 for men) and maternal mortality was 396 deaths/100,000 live births (WHO 2015a) (though WHO numbers are contested and may significantly underestimate maternal mortality [Carvalho et al. 2015]). This is not merely a question of low GDP per capita or war conditions. In neighboring Iraq, which also experienced over a decade of war, life expectancy was 74 years for women (67 for men) with 50 maternal deaths/100,000 live births (WHO 2015a). These indicators are considerably worse than those of HICs (e.g., Dutch women's life expectancy is 83 and maternal mortality 7/100,000 births), but far better than Afghanistan's levels. This at least partially reflects Iraq's greater gender equality among other structural factors, such as decades of foreign occupation and impoverishment in Afghanistan, outmigration of doctors and elites, and deterioration of social services.

Child marriage, defined as marriage before the age of 18, disproportionately affects girls, who may have limited ability to negotiate household roles and safer sex (leading to STI and HIV exposure). Child brides are also more likely to experience early pregnancy with less access to prenatal care. Currently, more than 700 million women worldwide were married before they turned 18 and 250 million before they turned 15 (UNICEF 2014b).

Also linked to gender discrimination is female genital mutilation (FGM), involving cutting, manipulation, or excision of part or all of the external genitalia and/or narrowing of the vaginal opening. FGM is linked to short- and long-term risks including, pain, hemorrhage, infections, urinary incontinence, discomfort during vaginal intercourse, birth and labor complications, and death (WHO 2016c). An estimated 200 million girls and women currently alive have undergone FGM (approximately 3 million per year), which is practiced in 30 countries in Africa and the Middle East and among immigrants in other countries (UNICEF 2016). Historical explanations for the practice include hygiene, coming-of-age (akin to male circumcision), female purity and chastity, religious tradition, and as a form of resisting rape during colonialism (Boddy 2002). Today, growing international consensus deems FGM a violation of human rights: 24 countries have banned it (some only criminalize FGM of minors, others also adult women), amid various efforts to eliminate or retain the ritual only symbolically; however, criminalization is not necessarily the best approach and may itself be harmful because it pushes the practice underground (Berer 2015).

While girls and women are more subject to both physical and sexual violence, boys and men are more likely to die from homicide—partly explained by higher male participation in crime-related activities such as gangs and street fighting (UNICEF 2014c)—linked to poverty and drug trafficking, as shaped by gendered norms. Globally, an estimated 475,000 homicides occur annually, 82% (389,500) among males, more than half of whom are 10- to 29-year-old youths (WHO 2014). Eight of the 10 countries with the highest homicide rates in the world are in Latin America and the Caribbean; in 7 of the region's countries, homicide is the leading cause of death among 10- to 19-year-old boys (UNICEF 2014c).

Gendered norms affect men's health in other ways. In Vietnam, women's life expectancy is 80 years whereas men's is 71, the latter shaped by higher smoking rates (48% of men versus 2% of women) (World Bank 2015), as well as greater en masse exposure to violence during the 1960s–1970s war as combatants, which jeopardized long-term physical and mental health (Teerawichitchainan 2014).

Gender interacts and intersects with class, race, and other categories of difference and discrimination in determining access to education, employment, health care, and social services (Connell 2012). Across the globe, women are poorer than men, earning on average just 75% of men's wages. In low-income settings, girls' school attendance may be deprioritized due to their household roles and lower family expectations around education-to-employment pathways (plus impediments including fees, lack of toilets, and unsafe conditions). Poverty increases morbidity and mortality for both men and women, but women typically have less control over the material and social conditions of life that foster good health. For example, women own only half as much land as men in Latin America (Deere, Alvarado, and Twyman 2012).

In places such as Kerala state, India, where girls' education and women's participation in civil and political life have been longtime priorities, health equity and overall population health have improved markedly (see chapter 13). Still, women's education alone—though important for employment, independence, and well-being—is insufficient to ensure gender equity and political inclusion (Joshi 2015), which are also affected by sexism and discrimination based on class and caste in the workplace and community.

Race and Racism

Race, like gender, is a social construction developed to classify groups based on arbitrary, usually visible, characteristics (e.g., skin color, shape of eyes). Historically, dominant societal groups have elaborated racial distinctions in order to establish or maintain power and privilege at the expense of "the other" group (e.g., to justify plantation economies using Black African slaves). The ongoing repercussions of these historical and contemporary patterns of power generate worse health profiles of oppressed groups compared with dominant groups.

Global data reveal a consistent pattern: groups subject(ed) to racial discrimination—tied to racial ideologies involving conquest of Indigenous populations, slavery, and subjugation—have the worst health status. Racism—distinguished from race—is the enactment of structural and systematic forms of oppression and discrimination against particular racial groups by institutions and individuals, with racial definitions themselves arising from oppressive systems of race relations. Here *institutions* refer to both state and non-state actors (i.e., private sector, civil society, and religious organizations), but from a human rights perspective, the state plays a critical legal and enforcement role that either permits or prohibits racism. Even so, dominance and oppression is institutionalized in multifarious extralegal ways through practices that maintain the privilege enjoyed by dominant groups (Krieger 2014a).

Descendants of African slaves in North America, Brazil, the Caribbean, and elsewhere have experienced unspeakable loss of freedom, social disruption, death, illness, disability, and physical and psychological abuse. Yet the legacy is not uniform across regions (Bergad 2007): slave descendants comprise the majority population in some countries and have realized important socio-political gains (e.g., in Barbados), whereas in other settings (e.g., the United States), there is ongoing racial discrimination and persistent "embodied" oppression, as among Indigenous populations (discussed in the next section). By no means are racism and its health effects exclusive to the Americas: former European colonial powers involved in the slave trade and more recently experiencing high immigration from the Middle East, Africa, Latin America, and other regions experience similar, if less studied, patterns (Gil-González et al. 2014).

Racism negatively affects health through simultaneous pathways, with historical context determining their relative significance (Box 7-2). An additional persistent feature of the impact of racism relates to how scientists investigate racism, race/ethnicity, and health. Only since the 1990s has a robust body of empirical work investigated how racism harms health. This research has refuted longstanding beliefs that observed differences in health status both among discriminated populations and in relation to dominant populations are due only to genetics (Krieger 2014a).

The embodied manifestations of discrimination are evidenced by health inequities and negative health outcomes in somatic health, mental health, health behaviors including substance use, self-rated health, blood pressure, preterm delivery, obesity, and use of health care services (Paradies et al. 2015). As well, life-course and intergenerational effects mean that adults who were materially and socially deprived as children may continue to experience the effects of deprivation even if their life circumstances improve (Krieger 2011).

These differences also go beyond SES explanations: in New Zealand racism experienced by Māori-descended populations is associated with adverse health outcomes irrespective of economic deprivation levels (Harris et al. 2012). Similar findings elsewhere show that racial discrimination and its attendant health effects occur across all socioeconomic strata, exacerbating class and other economic effects. For example, despite Brazil's national health insurance system, Black women are less likely than others to receive adequate prenatal care (Domingues et al. 2015).

In sum, *both* social class *and* racism, among other societal factors, explain the existence and persistence of racial inequalities in health. In the context of police violence in the United States, race/ethnicity remains far more predictive of health-harming, if not lethal, encounters than does socioeconomic position, but the two interact. Gender/sexism often

Box 7-2 Main Pathways Linking Racism to Health Effects

1. Economic and social deprivation, which restricts ability to obtain quality education and well-paying, safe, and secure employment
2. Greater exposure to toxic substances, pathogens, and hazardous conditions, often experienced as a result of segregated living and working conditions
3. Socially inflicted trauma, such as verbal, sexual, physical, and emotional abuse and the resulting psychological stress, anxiety, and injury
4. Targeted marketing of substances and activities that are harmful to health
5. Lower access to appropriate and quality health care, leading to inadequate and degrading medical treatment
6. Exclusion from political power and decisionmaking
7. Unequal treatment, including unjustified killings, via law and order (police and justice) systems
8. State oppression, including inadequate state responses to unfair treatment
9. Health-harming responses to discrimination
10. Environmental degradation and alienation from the land (especially affecting, but not limited to, Indigenous peoples and low-income ethnic and racial minority groups)

Sources: Adapted from Krieger (2014a); Williams and Mohammed (2013).

adds to this intersectional mix, as in the case of low-income Afro-Brazilian women with little education, who are disproportionately employed as domestic workers and in other informal sector jobs without social security (Daniel and Graf 2015).

Clearly policies matter in addressing the health effects of racism. In the United States, the 1964 US Civil Rights Act's overturning of Jim Crow laws (legalized segregation and racial discrimination enforced across a band of Southern states) resulted in a convergence of infant mortality rates between the Black population in states with and without Jim Crow laws. Abolition of these laws had significant consequences for population health and for the embodied histories shaping African-Americans' long-term mortality trends (Krieger et al. 2013). Even as political enfranchisement reduced certain health inequities, however, others have persisted, such as infant mortality rates 1.5 to 2.5 times higher for Black versus white Americans (Mathews, MacDorman, and Thoma 2015).

Racial and ethnic discrimination has likewise worsened health in other settings. In South Africa, the legacy of the racist apartheid system of state-sanctioned segregation and discrimination—which endured into the 1990s, even longer than in the United States—is evidenced in unequal health conditions, with under-5 mortality rates fives times higher among African children than among whites, lower than under apartheid and at the height of the HIV epidemic (with a peak eight-fold difference in 2002), but enormous nonetheless (Bradshaw et al. 2015). In Europe, the Roma ethnic minority, disenfranchised across the region, has a life expectancy up to 20 years lower than non-Roma populations (European Commission 2014).

Indigenous Status

Across the world, Indigenous status is associated with oppression and worse health relative to non-Indigenous populations (see chapter 6). These inequalities result from historical subjugation that has denigrated traditional ways of life, kinship structures, and spiritual beliefs—generating near universal patterns of racial and cultural discrimination (and government paternalism) damaging the health and well-being of Indigenous groups (Walters et al. 2011).

In a sign of persistent and deep-rooted prejudice, Australia, Canada, New Zealand, and the United States (all with Indigenous populations) voted against the UN's 2007 Declaration on the Rights of Indigenous Peoples, with 11 other countries abstaining. Indeed, the colonization process and ongoing discrimination against Indigenous peoples—including violence, forcible removal from ancestral lands, denial of heritage, loss of livelihood, government neglect, and absence of social protections—continues to reverberate through the lives of Indigenous peoples and to harm their health. This is illustrated by Australian and Canadian experiences, where for almost a century, the national government forcibly removed thousands of Indigenous children from their families and communities into residential schools, where they faced violence, overcrowding, poor nutrition, and forced labor.

Documenting the present as well as past harms generated by these policies, Canada's Truth and Reconciliation Commission's 2015 report on the more than century-long residential school system linked it to a "cultural genocide" policy that sought to "eliminate Aboriginal governments; ignore Aboriginal rights; terminate the Treaties; and, through a process of assimilation, cause Aboriginal peoples to cease to exist as distinct legal, social, cultural, religious, and racial entities in Canada" (TRC of Canada 2015, p. 1). The schools' dilapidated, unsanitary, and hazardous conditions led to up to 30,000 deaths due to tuberculosis (TB), influenza, pneumonia, and fires.[3] School staff tormented students with rampant physical and sexual abuse, which also created the conditions for student-to-student abuse. Adding to this mistreatment, in the 1960s large numbers of Indigenous children were removed without cause from their families and placed into foster care. These experiences have affected not only the health and well-being of survivors but also of their families, children, and broader communities, many of whom suffer mental health, narcotics addictions, and abuse problems.

Historical and contemporary oppression of Indigenous populations worldwide is reflected in alarmingly high poverty rates, limited access to potable water, poor quality housing stock, inadequate health care access, disproportionate incarceration and foster care rates, and high levels of exposure to environmental toxins, all jeopardizing health (UN-DESA 2015). Across the Americas, Indigenous populations experience extreme poverty rates of up to 90%, more than twice the rates of non-Indigenous groups, as well as high rates of suicide, and both chronic and infectious disease. In Mato Grosso do Sul, Brazil, for example, Indigenous people account for 3% of the population but 20% of suicide deaths, and in several Latin American countries, Indigenous children have twice the rate of chronic undernutrition as non-Indigenous counterparts (ECLAC 2014).

Some countries have begun to develop initiatives to promote health equity for Indigenous populations. In the 1980s in New Zealand, Māori activists reinvigorated efforts to improve their well-being, including health, by invoking the 1840 Treaty of Waitangi, long disregarded by colonial settlers because it officially recognized Māori sovereignty and outlined reparations and agreements. As a result of this advocacy, Māori perspectives on health and illness have begun to be incorporated into national and regional health plans. The New Zealand government has also prioritized housing and infrastructural needs of the Māori people—providing potable water, affordable housing, and an Indigenous justice system on Māori lands (Friel et al. 2012). While these policies have not eliminated inequalities in New Zealand, they demonstrate the role

T-shirt Travels

Dolores, a working mother of two school-aged children in Los Angeles, USA, spots brightly-colored T-shirts in a discount chain store in her neighborhood. Noticing the two for US$4.99 deal, she picks one for each child, depleting the remainder of her week's pay from her exhausting kitchen prep job at a fast-food restaurant. Fourteen time zones away, Disha, a pregnant mother of three outside Dhaka, Bangladesh, takes her foot off the pedal of her sewing machine to fan her face in a sweltering garment factory. A few weeks earlier, she made the T-shirts bought by Dolores; at Disha's current 21 taka hourly wage (less than US$0.50), the cost of her labor for these T-shirts was less than US$0.20. Ironically, Dolores's mother and aunts used to toil in a maquiladora (export-oriented sweatshop) in Guatemala, before factories closed and jobs moved to Southeast Asia when Dolores was a young girl. This prompted Dolores's family to enter the United States as undocumented migrants.

Meanwhile, Disha, originally from a rural village, was forced to seek employment in the city because farming could no longer sustain her family. She barely scrapes by, living in a poorly ventilated shack with a makeshift stove where her pregnant sister-in-law cares for Disha's children and elderly parents. The children are undernourished and asthmatic, and the grandparents have chronic obstructive pulmonary disease. Dolores's children are also malnourished—overweight for their age, primarily subsisting on inexpensive energy-dense foods. Both women are struggling to make ends meet within their own realities, their partners working far from home, respectively, as a migrant laborer in a California lettuce field and a construction worker for a Qatari building company.

What are the political, economic, social, and historical contexts shaping these scenarios of poor working and living conditions from both production and consumption ends? Both women live in countries that have actively participated in trade liberalization in the neoliberal phase of globalization. Domestic policies around export-processing zones, together with WTO and other trade and investment agreements, have enabled TNCs to outsource manufacturing and service industries and jobs to ever lower-wage settings. TNCs such as Walmart, Nike, and countless others subcontract to the most competitive suppliers who drive down wages, provide no benefits, and overlook occupational safety and health. The women's realities are framed by their gender, race/ethnicity, and social class, in turn shaping family responsibilities, migrant status, precarious work, and almost nonexistent social protections, all undergirded by the global economic order. The women are connected not only by the fabric of the T-shirts but the fabric of their lives.

of deliberate policymaking in improving the health of Indigenous populations, especially compared with neighboring Australia's failure to effectively address entrenched inequalities between Indigenous and non-Indigenous groups (Gracey 2014).

SOCIETAL GOVERNANCE AND SOCIAL POLICIES

Key Questions:

- How and why does the type of regime influence the kinds of social policies adopted?
- What are the most crucial health determinants that government policies and regulations can affect?

Governments employ a range of more or less protective and redistributive policies and entitlements that shape health via levels of poverty, inequality, and discrimination; access to and quality of education; employment and work conditions; food sovereignty; environmental conditions and industrial regulations; public health and medical care; and social security benefits (for families, persons with disabilities, the elderly, and unemployed). It is important to recall that societal measures are often constrained and intertwined with determinants at the global level, including via trade agreements, debt and financing obligations, and the enduring effects of colonialism, which, inter alia, created artificial political boundaries between peoples in many countries, to this day threatening democratic governance and social inclusion. Other SDOH-relevant state-level factors consist of democratic processes; transparency/corruption; social inclusion/exclusion; migration policies and conditions; and policing and justice systems. These policies are inherently linked to the ways (and extent to which) governments respect, protect, and fulfill human rights obligations.

Democratic Processes, Social Inclusion, and Participation

The relationship between democracy and health outcomes, such as infant mortality, has been widely studied (Grassi and Luppi 2014; McGuire 2010). But what is it about democracy that leads to better health? Social justice-oriented political values, solidarity, and representative institutions and power structures constitute critical elements of decision-making around improving health and health equity (Crammond and Carey 2016).

(Un)accountable and (un)representative governments (fail to) protect their citizens' economic, social, cultural, political, and civil human rights through (or because they lack) anti-poverty strategies, quality education, progressive taxation, decent employment, and effective regulation of the environment and the workplace. For example, countries that respect individual and collective rights and have fair legal and governance systems, including by controlling corruption, appear to have better health outcomes (Pinzon-Rondon et al. 2015). By contrast, authoritarian and militaristic societies have excessively harsh judicial systems and are more prone to violence and repression, generating death, disability, fear, and destruction, while restricting day-to-day activities and destroying dreams for the future.

The ability to participate fully in community and political life also appears to confer well-being. Social inclusion/exclusion describes the ability/inability of certain groups (e.g., people who are homeless, poor, racial and ethnic minorities, persons with disabilities or undocumented workers) to fully participate in civic life. Social exclusion may be the result of structural inequalities, lack of access to resources (economic, social, political, and/or cultural), prejudice, and stigma (Ruckert and Labonté 2014). In many societies, persons with disabilities are unable to find steady employment due to discrimination (Bambra 2011). Social exclusion has been found to lead to premature death, increased illness, poor physical and mental health, and increased levels of societal violence. Conversely, social inclusion provides access to resources and social support networks, adequate housing, education, and transportation (Ruckert and Labonté 2014).

Being incarcerated is a literal form of social exclusion. The United States has the largest number of people in prison (2.2 million) and the world's highest incarceration rate at 716 per 100,000 population (Walmsley 2013), disproportionately affecting low-income and racial/ethnic minorities, many with mental health problems. Discriminatory policing and justice systems, such as heavy-handed police monitoring of minority and low-income areas, and mandatory minimum sentencing for small crimes (for instance not paying predatory fines), generate higher incarceration rates as well as perpetuating poverty, unemployment, disenfranchisement, and attendant higher illness and premature death rates among racialized groups (Travis, Western, and Redburn 2014). Moreover, all but two US states rescind voting rights from those incarcerated for a felony offense, often continuing during parole, probation, and even post-sentence (Chung 2015). The process of restoring these rights can be so complex that many ex-felons effectively lose voting rights permanently, with Black men especially subject to felony disenfranchisement (Alexander 2012).

It is not only those legally excluded from participating in the democratic process who lack political inclusion. The percentage of registered voters who cast votes in national elections ranges from a low of 40% in Switzerland and 43% in Chile to a high of 80% or more in Belgium, Turkey, and Sweden (Desilver 2015). In countries with high levels of participation, voting may be compulsory rather than reflecting trust in the political process or belief that one's interests are adequately represented. Across the board, those with the least education are least likely to vote (Hadjar and Beck 2010).

Welfare/Redistributive States as SDOH

To explain how social policies shape population health it is helpful to analyze a society's political/welfare state regime, government social spending, population coverage, benefit levels, and particular policies, including family allowances or old-age pensions (Bergqvist, Åberg Yngwe, and Lundberg 2013; Heins and Deeming 2015). Most social welfare policies are correlated with better population health and overall well-being. While these are important findings, they reveal little about the politics of redistribution at the national level or whether redistribution is largely economic or also addresses other dimensions of oppression including power differences by social group.

Welfare regime studies incorporate the political context of collective social policies in order to better understand how and why they affect health and health inequities. The welfare state refers to a set of "social rights of citizenship" (Marshall 1950), such as ". . .family benefits, health insurance, pension provisions, unemployment insurance, housing allowances, and welfare payments; engagement with other formal political institutions; and social movements" (Beckfield and Krieger 2009, p. 154). A product of working class and other struggles against brutal working and living conditions in industrializing countries in the late 19th and early 20th centuries, the welfare state has been recognized as a key determinant of population health and health equity due to its central functions of: ensuring income redistribution; protecting against immiseration, unemployment, and ill health; providing universal public health care and education; and improving occupational health and safety standards.

In order to better understand the arrangement of policies, programs, and entitlements purveyed by the state—and the tax and transfer mechanisms used to finance and deliver them—scholars have developed typologies of welfare states, typically referring to HICs (although germane to certain LMICs). Influential among these, Esping-Andersen's (1990) typology (with additions) of the relations among state, market, and family or household in capitalist countries includes:

- *Liberal welfare states*, which provide a minimum safety net (e.g., the United States, where benefits are concentrated among the elderly and certain indigent groups)
- *Wage earner welfare states*, which are more generous than liberal states and provide mostly employment-based (rather than citizenship-based) benefits (e.g., Australia)
- *Conservative-corporatist welfare states*, which are more generous than wage earner states and provide health and social services based on family status, religious affiliation, union membership, and residence (e.g., Austria)
- *Social democratic welfare states*, which are the most redistributive, providing universal benefits to all residents (e.g., Nordic states)

As one goes down the list there are increasing levels of redistribution (even as spending and benefit levels are nested in different ways). As one goes up the list, the family and market play a larger role. Though widely used, Esping-Andersen's classification has been critiqued for using too few regime types (i.e., there are wide variations within each) and paying insufficient attention to the content of policies implemented, whether they are provided as cash or services (decommodification), the role of women/gender roles in welfare provision (Bambra et al. 2009), and for being (Northern) Eurocentric. For example "Southern" European (e.g., Greece, Portugal) and certain Latin American (e.g., Argentina, Brazil) regimes are characterized by fragmented or stratified welfare systems and a more prominent role of the family and/or charitable/religious sectors. Similarly, "Confucian welfare states" (e.g., South Korea, Taiwan) (Walker and Wong 2005) place greater emphasis on filial obligations and kinship. Moreover, welfare states are not static, and post-Fordist restructuring (characterized by departure from a powerful working class, livable and rising wages, and near full employment) in the context of financial crises have led to neoliberal and neo-corporatist welfare states as well as welfare state expansions in some settings (Bambra 2009).

Generally, the more egalitarian a country is on political, economic, and social grounds, the fewer health inequities, pointing to the centrality of reducing unjust differences in social and economic conditions by social class, race/ethnicity, and other factors and redistributing societal resources via fair and representative political processes. There is also a high correlation between the strength of the welfare state and overall population health outcomes, including life expectancy and infant mortality (Muntaner et al. 2011).

While social democratic societies with universal, public, and comprehensive social security systems and strong unions, such as Sweden, experience less poverty and better health, on average, than less redistributive societies, class-based and other relative inequalities remain and redressing them is a prime societal concern (Mackenbach 2015). Still, even those who are in the lowest economic stratum in social democratic countries fare better (in health and poverty terms) than those in higher economic stratums in less redistributive societies (i.e., health-wise and poverty-wise it may be preferable to be among Sweden's lowest income group compared to middle-income or even higher stratums in Portugal).

Though there is limited systematic research on these questions outside HICs, the experiences of Cuba, Costa Rica, Kerala, and a few other settings also demonstrate the links between welfare-state redistribution and equitable and favorable health outcomes (see chapter 13).

The most successful welfare states—in terms of positive aggregate health outcomes (e.g., life expectancy)—are characterized by strong labor movements and socialist or social democratic political parties; high corporate taxes; progressive income taxes (people at lower income levels are taxed at lower rates than those with higher incomes); high expenditures on social security; high levels of employment, particularly in the public sector, and decent unemployment compensation; (near) universal and publicly-provided health and social services coverage; low rates of poverty and wage disparities; and—particularly important for reducing gender inequities—policies that support women's labor market participation and enforce shared responsibility of unpaid caregiving (dual-earner models), and adequate subsidies to single mothers and divorced women (Bergqvist, Åberg Yngwe, and Lundberg 2013; Borrell et al. 2013).

The pivotal welfare state mechanism enhancing population health and health equity is redistribution. This entails fair, progressive, and adequate income, property, and corporate taxation and the reallocation (transfer) of income and/or services back to the population through either universal or targeted measures. State revenues may be directly channeled to individual or family income (e.g., family allowances, child/maternity benefits, paid parental leave, disability or retirement pensions) or involve services (e.g., daycare, health care spending) (Beckfield et al. 2015), both of which significantly curb inequality and poverty. For instance, before taxes and transfers, the 2012 poverty rate was 29.2% in the United States and 35.6% in France. After redistribution, US poverty dropped by over 11 points to 17.9%, but in France poverty plunged by a far more dramatic 27.5 points to 8.1% (OECD 2015). Indeed, the limits to universality, redistribution, and the range of benefits in the United States (notwithstanding sizeable government spending) lead it to underperform in social welfare (and health outcomes), relative to its level of economic development. Other mechanisms used by (strong) welfare states include lower and upper limits of certain SDOH protections (e.g., minimum/living wage levels, ceilings on post-incarceration penalties) and buffers against adverse shocks to health (e.g., generous unemployment compensation) (Beckfield et al. 2015).

Many LMICs (and a growing number of HICs) face challenges in sustaining welfare states due to a combination of relatively few formal sector jobs (and large informal sectors only minimally contributing to the tax base) and tax evasion by domestic and foreign business interests and wealthy individuals. Economies unable to diversify beyond primary resources—and tied to the constraints of the global economic order—reinforce these patterns, underscoring the difficulties of sustaining universal and generous welfare provisions (Martínez Franzoni and Sánchez-Ancochea 2013).

Migration

Migration affects health in a variety of ways and is linked to many other SDOH, including discrimination, poor working and living conditions, political repression, stress, and poverty. Moving within and across borders permanently or temporarily—whether voluntarily or forced by war, economic, political, cultural, or environmental conditions—can have immediate and lifelong health repercussions.

In 2015, 244 million people—3% of the global population—were international migrants (UN-DESA 2016). These figures cover refugees but not undocumented migrants or the over 750 million people who are internal migrants (within their own countries) (Bell and Charles-Edwards 2013). In 2015 an ignominious milestone was met: 65.3 million people were refugees, asylum-seekers, or IDPs, the highest level since World War II (UNHCR 2016). Uprooted by global, regional, and local factors including armed conflict, political persecution, livelihood loss, famine, and ecological disasters, refugees and IDPs face a range of adverse health outcomes, from physical and psychological trauma to neonatal problems, nutrition, and waterborne diseases (Lori and Boyle 2015) (see chapter 8).

By contrast, certain groups of voluntary immigrants—particularly professionals who leave their homes seeking economic betterment, advanced education, family reunification, or cultural acceptance—may experience considerable positive health repercussions thanks to better employment conditions, options, and income, and greater social satisfaction.

But many more immigrants lack these advantages. From Mexico to the Mediterranean, thousands die along migrant routes every year (Brian and Laczko 2014). In new settings, migrants may experience racial and cultural discrimination, psychological stress, poor working conditions, loss of family and social support, incarceration under inhumane conditions, and lack of political representation or social benefits, all translating into adverse health effects. Migrant workers—such as seasonal agricultural workers and temporary laborers in the service and informal sectors—often face the synergistic effects of workplace exploitation, dangerous occupations, precarity, violence, and few social protections. Undocumented migrants—who may have crossed borders unofficially and lack legal status—are particularly subject to employer and police abuse as well as continuous threat of deportation, extremely limited legal protections, and family separation (Castañeda et al. 2015).

Those left behind are also affected. China's *hukou* system, which ties public services access to geographic origin, has led urban migrant workers to leave their children (approximately 60 million) in rural settings so they can attend school. Such family separation generates significant depression and unhealthy behaviors among these children compared with those in non-migrant households (Gao et al. 2010), even as migrant parents hope to improve their children's lives. Indeed, throughout the world, hundreds of billions of dollars in annual remittances (overwhelmingly from HICs to LMICs) sent by migrant family members abroad contribute to reduced child malnutrition and better health (Terrelonge 2014).

Poverty

According to UNICEF, 22,000 children under 5 years of age die from poverty every day. Extreme poverty is characterized by very low income and lack of access to the basic necessities of life—food, shelter, and water/sanitation. As discussed in chapter 3, living on less than PPP$1.25/day (or even PPP$3/day), the indicator of extreme poverty used by international agencies such as the World Bank, is a level so low as to prevent satisfaction of the most basic needs of survival. A higher cutoff of PPP$10/day or more depending on the cost of living would better measure destitution levels (Pritchett 2013) and support the efforts of minimum wage and living wage movements across many settings.

Poverty affects health through multiple channels, including: material deprivation and lack of access to life necessities and opportunities; discrimination, social exclusion, and stress; and unhealthful coping behaviors (e.g., narcotic use). Poverty at young ages also has important lifecourse effects, from stunting to arrested educational achievements (Raphael 2011). Poverty, often gauged by income below a certain level, is widely viewed as a quintessential determinant of health. In the United States it is estimated that where a modest one dollar increase above the federal minimum wage has been implemented, low birthweight births have fallen by 1%-2% and post-neonatal deaths by 4% (Komro et al. 2016). Yet income is intertwined with so many other determinants that we should be mindful of overstating its importance. Undoubtedly income is a crucial enabler of access to life necessities and material goods, but in some societies these may be furnished through transfers or community support that are not part of wage income. Moreover, poverty entails far more than lack of income, jeopardizing security, dignity, and social acceptance (Pogge and Sengupta 2015).

Recognizing the role of poverty in reproducing ill health, physicians adhering to a social medicine tradition have long incorporated food or social benefits as part of their treatment (Geiger 2013). Doctors with the Canadian advocacy group Health Providers against Poverty, for example, developed a clinical tool that instructs physicians to screen all patients for poverty by asking about their income security. Doctors who "diagnose" poverty then "prescribe" government benefits, connecting patients to social assistance, child subsidies, or other entitlements (Ontario College of Family Physicians 2013). Not only does this process generate needed resources, it also helps mobilize disenfranchised groups to exercise/claim their social rights. Another effort, BIEN (the Basic Income Earth Network), has advocated for over three decades for the right to a guaranteed income, unconditionally, regardless of employment status, with experiments in Finland and Québec and active chapters in Europe, the Americas, Southern Africa, the Pacific, and Southeast Asia.

Critically, improving income does not directly address the power inequities laid out in the previous chapter section, in terms of wealth distribution, global financial governance, discriminatory social structures, and so on. For example, many governments implement cash transfer programs to directly raise the incomes of the poorest groups (see chapter 13). Although such measures help lift people out of absolute poverty and reduce health inequity, the structures of concentrated political influence and power may remain largely intact. As such, a range of universal social policies—that are themselves both the result and the makings of greater equality in political power and wealth—are likely to have a far greater impact on health than income redistribution per se (Starfield and Birn 2007).

Education

Education is associated with better health through multiple channels that include but go beyond its effect on income: (1) greater range of employment possibilities at better pay (with higher likelihood of benefits, protection from workplace hazards, job security, and room for advancement); (2) specific health and hygiene

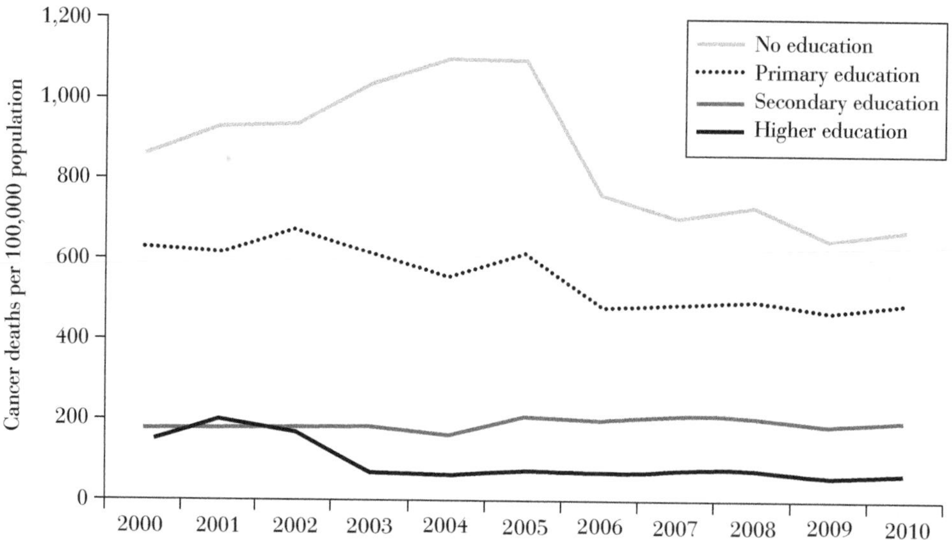

Figure 7-3: Age-adjusted cancer mortality rate among men over age 20 in Chile, by education level.
Source: Herrera Riquelme et al. (2015).

education, particularly salient in low-income settings with more limited sources of information; (3) development of cognitive, coping, and emotional skills to enable sound overall decisionmaking likely to enhance health, and the ability to take, or advocate for, protective health measures; (4) more time spent in school (especially for youth), which translates into fewer health-damaging activities such as harmful work or substance abuse; and (5) development of social connections that confer health advantages via professional networks, neighborhood ties, political engagement, and other factors (Glymour, Avendano, and Kawachi 2014).

Education has further lifecourse and intergenerational effects on health. Early childhood education can help ameliorate some of the negative effects of social disadvantage, with an impact throughout the life span (Hertzman et al. 2012). The positive effect of maternal education on child nutrition survival is also well-established (Makoka 2013; Monden and Smits 2013). In addition, higher educational attainment of parents is correlated with lower child poverty (Gornick and Jäntti 2012).

In general, more years of education (or greater literacy) are associated with lower levels of mortality and in some settings with cardiovascular and respiratory disease, unintentional injuries, and healthier behaviors (e.g., lower rates of smoking, heavy drinking, obesity, and drug use; higher rates of exercise and screening procedures; better management of stress and chronic health conditions) (Glymour, Avendano, and Kawachi 2014). For instance, in Chile, mortality rates from the three most prevalent cancers in women (breast, stomach, and gallbladder) and men (stomach, prostate, and lung) are inversely correlated with education level, also reflecting SES more generally (Figure 7-3 and Figure 7-4). Although Chile's system of Explicit Health Guarantees (Plan AUGE) enables universal access to treatment of many cancers, geographical differences in access and quality of care persist—contributing to late diagnosis in less educated and more socioeconomically disadvantaged groups (Herrera Riquelma et al. 2015).

In many LMICs and some HICs, loan conditionalities and austerity policies of the past three decades have plagued education with budget cuts. Widely employed enrollment and school supply fees exclude millions of children and youth from accessing education, especially girls and young women. Furthermore, educational systems have deteriorated due to emigration, civil conflict, and AIDS, together decimating the ranks of educators in some settings. For those who do complete school, translation of education into improved social (including health) conditions may be hampered by insufficient jobs commensurate with, or relevant to, training and skills demanded in the labor market (OECD 2014).

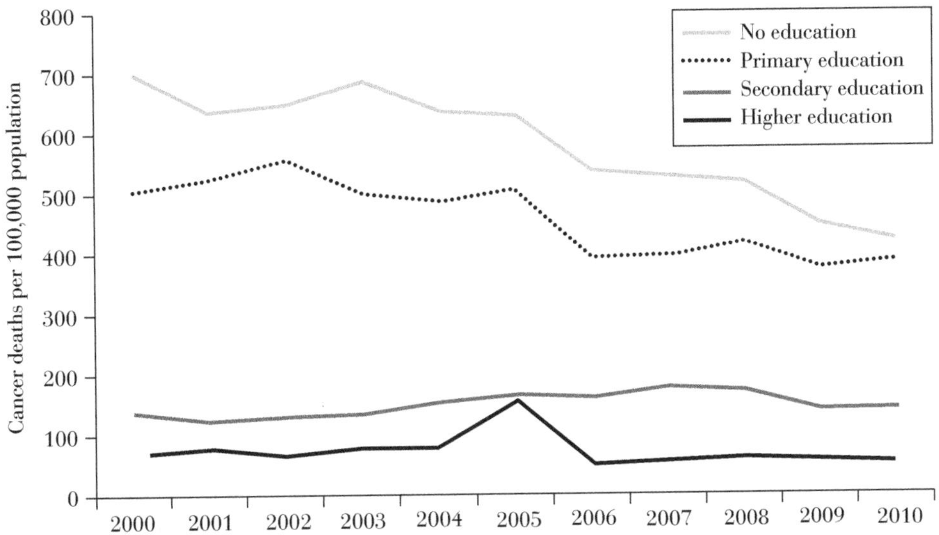

Figure 7-4: Age-adjusted cancer mortality rate among women over age 20 in Chile, by education level.
Source: Herrera Riquelme et al. (2015).

Employment and Work Conditions

The nature of work, its physical and psychosocial dimensions, structures of authority and control, and level of compensation and stability make work a key SDOH, with varied pathways and long-lasting effects. In addition to income, employment may confer social protections such as health benefits, sickness and unemployment coverage, pensions, education and training for advancement, as well as social networks, labor organizing, and solidarity.

Despite labor and social movement-driven improvements in work conditions in some settings, across numerous LMICs and HICs, work conditions have deteriorated in recent decades and are marked by miserable pay, long hours, child labor, hazardous exposures, few safety protections, and oppressive conditions. Moreover, neoliberal globalization (facilitating entry of TNCs) and the post-2008 global economic crisis have led to increasingly exploitative and precarious working environments, with consequent negative health effects (Benach et al. 2014) (see chapter 9).

Most workplaces are characterized by hierarchies of power and control, generating psychosocial stress. Stress is highest where there is low or no worker control, inadequate reward for amount of effort (in terms of fair pay, recognition, job security, advancement), lack of consideration for employee input (i.e., organizational injustice) (Bambra 2011), where unions are constrained or prohibited, and where there are gender-based, racial, ageist, ableist, and other forms of discrimination and harassment.

Stress, job strain, and exposure to (and lack of protections against) dangerous chemical, physical, and biological agents (including repetitive motion strain, unsafe equipment and activities, and toxins) lead to cancer, diabetes, heart disease, neurological, endocrinological, and mental disorders, as well as job-related disabilities (Berkman, Kawachi, and Theorell 2014). The most hazardous jobs are in the areas of farming, coal mining, sex work, construction, minibus driving in large cities, and work involving toxic chemicals (ILO 2015).

Globally, there are 315 million occupational injuries and over 2.3 million occupational deaths per year from work-related injuries (321,000) and diseases (2.02 million). An additional 160 million cases of non-fatal, job-related diseases add to the massive yearly occupational-related disease burden (ILO 2013). Those employed in the most dangerous sectors have the least workers' compensation benefits and protection by occupational health and safety laws (especially in LMICs, where very few workers are covered [Lucchini and London 2014]). All of these problems are exacerbated under conditions of precarious employment, characterized by short-term contracts, part-time work, little or no job security, and limited social and health benefits. Precarious and informal work is soaring in HICs and predominates in LMICs (Benach et al. 2014).

Unhealthy as precarious and hazardous employment is, unemployment can be worse, especially where there are few social welfare benefits. Since the 2008 crisis, documented unemployment has climbed to 204 million people (UNDP 2015). In HICs, the health effects of large-scale unemployment are most evidenced by short-term increases in suicides and homicides (Stuckler et al. 2009), with certain potentially favorable consequences due to lower production and disposable income (e.g., less pollution [CO_2 emissions have fallen in Europe and North America]; fewer occupational exposures; decreases in traffic fatalities, cardiovascular disease [CVD], and respiratory mortality) (Tapia Granados 2014). But in LMICs, where unemployment rates are approximately 30% compared with typical HIC rates of 4% to 12% (Benach et al. 2013), unemployment can spell loss of basic income, housing, and other key SDOH; worldwide it is associated with increased illness and suffering.

Food Production and Food Sovereignty

Food, together with water and shelter, is a primordial human need shaped by factors at all levels. Addressing issues of *food security*—the availability of and access to sufficient quantities of (nutritious) food—has driven the work of UN agencies such as FAO and, increasingly, global agribusiness. Posed in terms of access to global food markets, however, the concept and practices of food security may harm more than help (Gill and Bakker 2011).

Under the current political economy order, the most marginalized people, especially in LMICs, suffer the brunt of food-related health consequences of global power asymmetries. For example, the WTO's trade rules propelled under the Doha Development Round (see chapter 9) forces open LMIC markets to foreign imports by encouraging land investment and eliminating tariffs—pushing millions of farmers off the land—at the same time prolonging unfair HIC subsidies to domestic agricultural production (Dentico 2014). Loss of land tenure, driven by these global and national economic processes, adversely affects livelihoods as well as *food sovereignty*, that is: self-determination in the production and consumption of foods in ways socially, economically, and culturally consistent with local practices and conditions; protection from agricultural dumping; and the right to participate in agricultural policy decisions (Grey and Patel 2015).

Food production and consumption affect health in many other ways, influenced by national policies around land-use and environmental and safety regulations. Pesticide residues and industrial chemical run-off in soil and waterways (e.g., petroleum in the soil of the Niger Delta, mercury in North America's Great Lakes, and heavy metals in mining regions worldwide) lead to various cancers, organ diseases, and developmental problems. In addition, foodborne illnesses due to contamination in the production and distribution process kill 420,000 people and cause 600 million cases of illness each year (WHO 2015b).

Environmental Regulations and Conditions

Environmental problems and their health consequences derive from two key processes: depletion and contamination (see chapter 10). Depletion of water, forests, soil, and flora and fauna affect human health by reducing availability of and access to basic necessities such as drinking water and arable land, and impeding livelihoods. Contamination of air, water, and soil, which occurs through industrial extraction, production, transport, and consumption, leads to human exposure to a variety of chemical, biological, and physical agents, with endocrinological, physiological, genetic, and other effects (i.e., embodiment of environmental conditions). As well, high levels of greenhouse gas emissions due to human activity have accelerated climate change, affecting human health through extreme weather (i.e., heat waves) and population displacement due to disasters, food insecurity, and job loss (McMichael 2013).

Public Health and Medical Care

Numerous studies have sought to quantify the relative contribution of medicine (and public health)—as well as genetics, environmental factors, behavior, and social circumstances—to health and life expectancy, but such exercises are misleading (McGovern, Miller, and Hughes-Cromwick

2014). Because the determinants of health are interdependent and simultaneously shaped by a range of societal factors, teasing out the percentage share of different kinds of determinants in influencing health as though each operated independently and universally makes little sense. That said, it is essential to gauge whether health interventions are effective in identifying, preventing, treating, or alleviating ill health.

Perhaps nowhere have these questions been as hotly debated as in medical care and public health domains. While curative medical care can be a crucial determinant of health outcomes for certain conditions—such as high-risk pregnancy, rabies, poisonings, and traumatic injuries—in terms of overall population health, medical care works in concert with multiple other SDOH, not uniquely or in isolation (Braveman and Gottlieb 2014).

In particular, primary health care and public health, also integrated with and influenced by other determinants, have played a key role in up to half of infant mortality reductions over time (Macinko, Starfield, and Erinosho 2009). Because public health's role in preventing adverse effects is most noticeable when it falters, its visibility as a health determinant may be muted, even though past and present it has contributed significantly to reductions in mortality. Public health activities span food safety, disease surveillance, road safety; sanitation, clean water provision, and safe disposal of refuse; environmental and occupational protections; school health and meals; maternal and child health programs; and housing regulations and inspection, among others.

The health care system itself can also promote or jeopardize health, depending on how equitably it is financed and delivered (i.e., the presence or absence of user fees and national health insurance), whether it inflicts harm or discrimination, how it interacts with local healers and healing beliefs, its accessibility and quality (especially to rural populations and slum dwellers), and the extent to which it prioritizes preventive services and public health over curative services (Loewenson and Gilson 2012) (see chapters 11 and 12). To be sure, public health and medical care organization and access are strongly affected by national regulations and social protection policies (and how much these are governed by global trade and investment rules, as with pharmaceuticals). They also play out at the neighborhood level in terms of their availability and full implementation. As per other determinants, medicine and public health are also embodied, metaphorically and physically, through interventions and activities (or their absence), inscribed, for example, as a scar from a vaccine or a cognitive impairment due to inadequate monitoring of lead contamination in the water supply (Sellers 2016).

T-shirt Travels

Returning to our T-shirt example, what role do social policies play in the narrative of Disha and Dolores? The limited redistributive mechanisms in the United States mean that poverty remains high even after taxes and transfers. Moreover, real wages have not kept up with the cost of living (Desilver 2014), making families like Dolores's increasingly impoverished. In Bangladesh, despite targeted social safety net programs, poverty remains a chronic condition for millions (Masud-All-Kamal and Sahal 2014). The Bangladeshi garment industry pays among the lowest wages in the world, with almost no collective bargaining rights, and rampant unsafe and repressive working conditions (Khanna 2011). Not only is Disha constantly trying to stretch her earnings to cover her family's needs, she remains permanently concerned about her own safety in the overcrowded factory.

FROM LIVING CONDITIONS TO EMBODIED INFLUENCES

Key Questions:

- How are living conditions and social policies (at all government levels) linked?
- How do neighborhood factors become embodied in individual health and disease patterns?
- What are the health implications of community and household conditions?

Living conditions relate to multiple household and neighborhood characteristics: housing; availability of potable water and adequate sanitation; food quality and options; household roles; quality of and access to social services, such as public health and transportation; and social stress (and its mitigators, including leisure). Various cultural and religious aspects of health, which also manifest at national and regional levels, intertwine with and affect health at household and community levels.

While income can serve as a gateway to improving living conditions and increasing consumption levels of health-enhancing goods and activities, living conditions operate independently of income (whose level may be fleeting given the precarious nature of employment in most parts of the world). As noted, the intersection of class, race, and gender—and discrimination around these factors—all shape living conditions and health outcomes as do policies and possibilities at national and global levels.

Neighborhood Conditions

The features of the immediate surroundings (the "microcontext") are among the most evident determinants of health: without adequate housing, and access to clean water and plumbing, maintaining personal hygiene is extremely difficult. In addition, school attendance is affected by presence of schools, safety, and available/affordable transport at the neighborhood level. Unhealthy activities, namely smoking, drug use, excessive alcohol consumption, and poor diet, are shaped by a range of factors including access to these substances, peer pressure, family and community behavior, media influences, and local resources to relieve stress and boredom.

Physical characteristics and infrastructural and institutional resources for well-being are also key: schools, health and social services, parks/green spaces, stores, transport, and recreation and community spaces. Other less tangible neighborhood features such as unemployment rates, crime, community solidarity and organization, social, racial, and cultural tolerance, political empowerment, and civic engagement also affect health. Local access to physical activity resources and affordable healthy foods shapes exercise and healthy diets or lack thereof. Neighborhoods that are unsafe or possess little social cohesion have an adverse effect on mental health, particularly depression (Roux and Mair 2010).

In Africa, Asia, Latin America, and the Pacific, over 860 million people live in informal settlements or "slums" on the outskirts of cities (25% of the world's urban population, 33% of LMICs' urban population, and 60% of Africa's urban population). Over 600 million people living in these settlements have little or no access to clean water, sanitation, and other public services (UN-HABITAT 2014). Informal settlements may be marked by substandard housing, open sewers, stagnant water, rotting garbage, shoddy construction, toxic dumpsites, an unstable land base, abandoned lots and buildings, unpaved roads, intermittent electricity, overcrowding, gang and police violence, high eviction rates, and few legal protections. Because factories and waste facilities located near slums perennially evade regulations, air and soil in slums is often heavily polluted.

Though not all slum dwellers are poor, they include large numbers of destitute migrants from rural areas, and chronically precariously employed and exploited urban residents. These circumstances generate poor health from infectious diseases such as TB, HIV, and diarrhea, as well as cancer, trauma, and stress-related CVD. Salmonellosis, lung and skin infections, and plague and other diseases with rodent vectors particularly affect slum dwellers. The negative health impact of slums even seem to have reversed the urban health advantage, with child mortality in Kenyan slums (where most city residents live) now little better than in rural areas (Kimani-Murage et al. 2014).

"What good does it do to treat people's illnesses . . . then send them back to the conditions that made them sick?"—Michael Marmot, at "Tackling Health Inequalities" conference, London, October 2005.

In a contrary direction, those living in neighborhoods characterized by strong community mobilization experience health improvements, not only from realization of better neighborhood conditions but also due to the effects of collective action and political engagement. The very act of participating in community-led women's groups in India and Nepal, for instance, has been associated with lower neonatal mortality (without targeting behavior change or health services utilization). Instead, Paulo Freire's "critical consciousness" (see chapter 14) seems to be at play, whereby women's collective mobilization enables greater decisionmaking and resource control, in turn leading to better child health outcomes (albeit the exact mechanisms explaining how this transpires require further research) (Victora 2013).

Housing

Along with food and water, shelter is a basic human necessity, (ideally) enabling safety, stability, rest and leisure, food preparation, and hygiene that together foster physical and mental health. Poor housing not only inhibits these factors, for example due to unsafe plumbing, cooking, or sleeping facilities, but can also cause or exacerbate a range of health problems. Open or unventilated stoves used for heating or cooking with unclean fuels (e.g., biomass or kerosene) are associated with indoor air pollutants and high rates of respiratory illness. Additionally, housing that is cold, damp, and/or moldy can lead to upper- and lower-respiratory tract diseases, TB, asthma, and headaches (Firdaus and Ahmad 2013).

Overcrowding and inadequate ventilation, food storage, and sanitation facilitate the spread of airborne, food- and waterborne, and skin ailments, including TB, diarrhea, lice, and scabies, as witnessed with persistent housing deficiencies in Canada's Inuit and First Nations communities (Webster 2015). Flimsy structures provide little or no protection from storms, fires, and earthquakes, and recycled industrial materials and lead paint can cause fatal poisonings and severe neurological and cognitive problems. All of these aspects of housing also affect sleep, psychological well-being, health behavior, as well as school and work capacity.

A prime role of housing is to provide protection against the elements, animals, and violence. In areas with endemic malaria, dengue, and other vector-borne diseases, door and window screens (often prohibitively expensive) or bednets are the best impediment to mosquito bites. If there is no indoor plumbing or regular refuse collection, water storage containers serve as mosquito breeding sites (Olukolajo, Adewusi, and Ogungbenro 2013). In areas where Chagas disease is endemic, low-cost thatched roofs can pose a problem because triatomine bugs spend daylight hours hidden in them, descending and biting at night. Poor housing conditions, lack of privacy, and lack of control over where one lives are also associated with low self-reported general and mental health (Arku et al. 2011).

The most extreme housing problem is homelessness. Global estimates range from over 100 million homeless up to 1.6 billion people with inadequate or unstable housing (Habitat for Humanity 2015). In Germany, about 2% of the population has been homeless at some point in their lives, compared with 6% (16 million people) in the United States (Toro et al. 2007). On any given night nearly 600,000 Americans (0.2% of the population) lack shelter (National Alliance to End Homelessness 2015), double the rate in Spain (Busch-Geertsema et al. 2014). Homelessness "guesstimates" in LMICs go from less than 1% of the population in Paraguay to nearly 20% in Laos (UNDP 2014).

The death rate among homeless people is 3 to 13 times higher than among the non-homeless (Vuillermoz et al. 2014). Even societies with extensive social services for the homeless—including free health care, accessible shelters, food banks, and employment training programs—cannot compensate for the health effects of not having a permanent home (Hwang et al. 2011). In many locales, homeless people may be jailed or abused by the police. Children who live on the streets are subject to violence by shopkeepers, gangs, or political authorities. The desperate conditions of homelessness can also lead to drug use, sex work, and deterioration of mental health.

Beyond these material aspects of shelter (or homelessness) which are extremely important to population health outcomes, housing is also tied to identity, self-expression, and other socially and psychologically meaningful dimensions (this is why people decorate and adorn their homes). In fact, whether one takes pride in and enjoys being in one's home appears to be significantly tied to measures of self-reported physical and mental health (Dunn 2002).

Water and Sanitation

Water is fundamental to life, yet over one sixth of the world's population lives without an adequate supply of safe water. Even more appalling, one third of the world's population (2.4 billion people, mostly in rural areas) lacks access (unpaid or paid) to even the most basic sanitation and must resort to using pit latrines, fields, and ditches (UNICEF and WHO 2015). This leads to water and soil contamination and increased rates of communicable diseases, especially diarrhea (WWAP 2015). Water and sanitation-related illnesses kill at least 1.4 million people each year and are among the leading causes of preventable mortality and morbidity (Forouzanfar et al. 2015), including 842,000 annual deaths from diarrhea (Prüss-Ustün et al. 2014).

As shown in Figure 7-5, access to an in-house water connection is inversely related to infant mortality—in general, where piped water access is high, infant mortality is low, and vice versa. The countries above the line have higher than average infant mortality given the proportion of households with water connections, whereas those below the line have lower than average infant mortality for the water connection rate. This general trend is countered under some circumstances, as indicated by Figure 7-5's outliers. Although 74% of Botswana's population has piped water on premises, it has an infant mortality rate of 35 deaths/1,000 live births. Piped water and sanitation access are much higher in urban (96%) compared with rural areas (45%), but household water may not be potable, including for the country's majority urban population, or may require steep fees. Additionally, Botswana's poverty rates are extremely high (Lekobane and Seleka 2014). Sri Lanka, by contrast, where only 34% to 44% have an in-house water connection, infant mortality is 8.4 deaths/1,000 live births. Many among Sri Lanka's overwhelmingly rural population use protected dug wells or rainwater harvesting, and piped water is generally potable, so that 85% of the population is within 200 m of safe water sources (Fan 2015). Sri Lanka's many other social protections are also key determinants of low infant mortality (see chapter 13).

The UN estimates that since 1990 over 2.5 billion people have gained access to "improved water sources." However, it is important to read between the lines. By UN standards, "improved" means the separation of human use from animal use via access to a household connection, public standpipe, borehole, protected well, protected spring, or rainwater collection tank. This does not necessarily comply with the UN resolution on the human right to "safe, clean, accessible and affordable drinking water and sanitation" (UN General Assembly 2010). Meanwhile, charges for community latrines in numerous settings can reach up to 10% of daily earnings, forcing many to use forests, fields, and alleys, despite problems of disease and violence. Furthermore, some 1.9 billion people remain exposed to fecal contamination, including at least 10% of those using "improved water sources" (Bain et al. 2014). Consequently, the actual number of people without access to safe water may be as high as those without basic sanitation: 2.4 billion (WWAP 2015) (Figure 7-6).

The connection between water/sanitation and health is thus complex. For instance, hand washing can reduce diarrheal disease by 40%

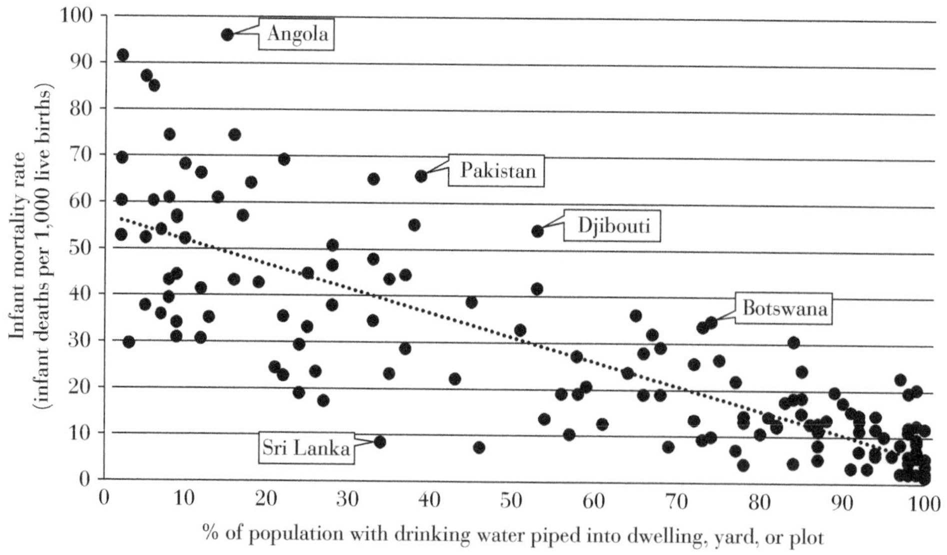

Figure 7-5: Piped water on premises and infant mortality rates, 2015.
Data Sources: UNICEF and WHO (2015); WHO (2016a).

(Freeman et al. 2014). This is not simply a matter of personal habits, but rather rests on sufficient access to clean water (and soap). Notably, almost half of the mortality decline in the United States during the first three decades of the 20th century can be attributed to water purification. Paradoxically, poorer populations tend to pay more for water use than richer ones, who typically live closer to utility systems (UNDP 2006). LMIC women, girls, and refugees are particularly affected by poor water supply (UNHCR 2011). They typically bear responsibility for collecting water, often over great distances, subjecting them to injury from heavy loads and assault, and jeopardizing school attendance and other activities. Moreover, women and girls are the primary caregivers for those who become sick from poor water sources, creating further burdens.

Nutrition and Access to Food

A healthy diet is essential to child development and growth and to overall human flourishing. Feeding is foremost a family/household responsibility, yet it is profoundly shaped by national measures influencing food sovereignty as well as global factors affecting land tenure and food production processes.

Nobel prize-winning economist Amartya Sen demonstrated that hunger and famines are caused more by the economics of maldistribution (political and economic) than by food shortages. For example, under British colonial rule, at least 3 million people died during Bengal's 1943 famine. Poor people starved because they lacked purchasing power (due to unemployment and wage declines), while excess food rotted in the storehouses of wealthy landowners and food retailers or was stockpiled for British soldiers (Keneally 2010). Over 60 years later, India under democracy has not experienced famine although rural undernutrition remains a grave concern.

In the past, both hunger and malnutrition were a matter of insufficient calories, protein, fresh fruits, and vegetables. Today, nearly 50% of child deaths still result from inadequate nutrition (UNICEF 2014a) and globally nearly 1 in 8 people (800 million, with over double that number hungry) are undernourished (FAO 2015; Hickel 2016). Yet malnutrition is increasingly associated with so-called "empty calories"—chemically processed foods with high sugar and fat content. These foods, due to HIC agricultural subsidies and mass production, are widely available, cheaper than fresh produce and nutritional foods, and heavily marketed in many societies (Rao et al. 2013).

In many poor urban neighborhoods, and even in places where fresh produce is abundant, healthy food selection in grocery stores or *bodegas* may be limited and expensive. At the same time, "junk food"

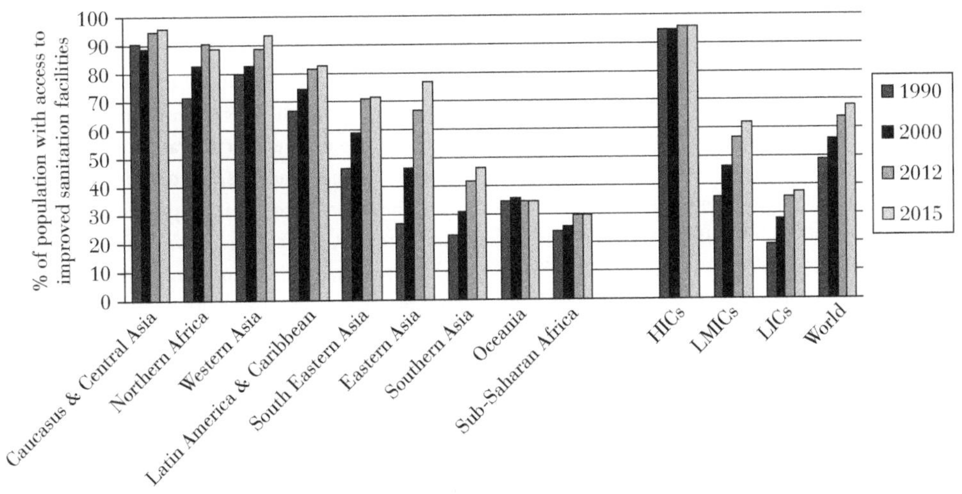

Figure 7-6: Percentage of population with access to "improved sanitation," 1990–2015.
Data Source: UNICEF and WHO (2015).

is targeted at low-income communities. For households with restricted food storage and cooking facilities, and/or in which household members work long hours or in non-coinciding shifts, junk food and "fast food" are indeed convenient (Fleischhacker et al. 2011). Not only does this food have little nutritional value, its consumption can lead to obesity, CVD, certain cancers, dental caries, low birthweight babies, diabetes, and vitamin deficiencies (WHO 2015a). In the United States, increasing consumption of fruits and vegetables through a combination of reforms to improve access to nutritious foods, such as investments in grocery stores and farmers markets, would prevent over 120,000 deaths per year from CVD alone and save US$17 billion annually in medical costs (O'Hara 2013).

Household Roles and Structure

Household size and structure—the number of persons living in a household and their respective roles and relations—may significantly influence health and well-being. In addition to societal-level effects of gender discrimination, household relations and expectations for girls and women may be deleterious to health. Despite increasing labor force participation, women are still responsible for the majority of unpaid caregiving for small children, the elderly, and extended family: women perform three quarters of all work that goes unpaid (UNDP 2015). (Also see Gender Inequality, Patriarchy, and Sexuality section.)

Transport

Transport influences health through multiple mechanisms: road injuries and fatalities, air quality and related respiratory illness (see chapter 10), green spaces for exercise and human interaction, interpersonal security, noise, cost, commuting time, and overall quality of life (Nieuwenhuijsen et al. 2016; Oliveira et al. 2015). As well, inadequate or unaffordable transport can affect other determinants, such as school attendance, employment, and preventive health care (e.g., prenatal care or control of chronic ailments). Most directly, road traffic collisions are the leading cause of death for 15- to 29-year-olds (and the second cause for children 5–14 years old) (WHO 2013b).

Traffic fatality and injury rates vary by SES and geography, with poor and working classes disproportionately affected. There has been a steady decline in traffic fatalities in high-income regions since the 1970s (due to a combination of improved road and automobile safety, legal restrictions and sanctions, and trauma care), but significant increases elsewhere. Much of the difference relates to safety measures: in HICs, most casualties are among drivers and passengers, whereas in LMICs, pedestrians, cyclists, and public transport passengers account for 90% of casualties, reflecting poor vehicle and road regulation. From Haiti to Nigeria, local transport vehicles are sardonically nicknamed "moving morgues" and "flying coffins."

Culture, Religion, and Health Practices

Culture is an oft-invoked determinant of health that is enormously complex and thus necessarily oversimplified in this discussion. Referring to socially transmitted frameworks of meaning, culture is the basis for how people interpret and engage with the world through personal and collective experience, including ways in which health and illness are defined, understood, and addressed. The cultural traditions, beliefs, and practices (involving values, politics, language, food, literature, music, and arts) of particular groups of people influence health both directly (e.g., through day-to-day customs of living and dietary and sanitary rituals) and indirectly.

Most people view health through perspectives other than the biomedical lens (see chapter 3) (which is itself an assemblage of cultural values, symbols, preferences, rituals, practices, and traditions). But biomedical ideas may also be appropriated from below and become part of local understandings (Menéndez 2009). Moreover, medical pluralism—the coexistence of multiple healing cultures, with people intermixing their use—is characteristic of virtually all settings.

Seeking to understand distinct cultural filters can help address SDOH, whether in culturally diverse populations or cross-nationally. In some cultures, pregnancy is medicalized and treated as though it were a disease; in others, it is understood in spiritual or kinship terms. Among the Maya, a fever may be considered an ailment rather than a symptom; in wine-loving France, general malaise is frequently referred to as a "liver crisis"; and in the United States, chronic fatigue syndrome is characterized as afflicting young urban professionals working long hours. Identifying cultural influences on health is fraught with issues of cultural relativism and misunderstanding. Even within a single cultural context, ways of viewing and addressing sickness and health may differ and also reflect larger policies (Das 2015).

Religion, which intersects with culture, also shapes health behavior, utilization of medical care, and understandings of well-being. Many religions call on prayer as a treatment (with Christian Scientists eschewing medical care); Muslims and Jews practice circumcision; and Jehovah's Witnesses refuse blood transfusions. The dietary practices of some religions, for instance the Jewish prohibition on eating pork, arose from ancient health concerns. Practices of hygiene, diet, and end-of-life care also vary among Hindus, Buddhists, Christians, and adherents to other religions, affecting health at the household and community level.

However, cultural and religious influences on health are often overemphasized, particularly when the illness and/or treatments are considered "exotic" or sensationalized by dominant actors. For example, most HIV prevention work in sub-Saharan Africa focuses on sexual practices, to the neglect of structural issues such as migration, immunological susceptibility due to poor nutrition and housing, unsafe employment, and inadequate social services, with attendant effects on relationships (see chapter 6).

T-shirt Travels

The T-shirt example also unfolds at the level of living conditions. While Disha works long hours in the factory, her children spend the day in their dilapidated home. With electricity costs high, they rely on a simple cookstove that burns biomass fuels, filling the poorly-ventilated home with smoke throughout the day. The smoke is inhaled by the children and has caused two of them to become asthmatic. The children also suffer recurrent bouts of diarrhea due to unclean drinking water in their informal settlement. Disha's long work hours and low wages rarely permit her to take them to the health clinic for treatment.

Dolores is also dealing with poor housing conditions but she fears complaining about her broken stove and pipes issuing brown water because her landlord—knowing she is an undocumented Latina migrant—may evict her, and the strapped Los Angeles social services agency can do little to help. She commutes over an hour to and from work each day and instructs her children to stay at home after school because the neighborhood is unsafe. This leads to further worries about their health: they get insufficient exercise and consume junk food and drink soda. Between the kitchen deficiencies and her work hours, her family must often rely on microwave dinners; moreover, she only visits a distant and expensive grocery store with fresh produce and other healthy options once per month, instead relying on neighborhood *bodegas*. With their partners frequently away working, both Disha and Dolores have primary caregiving roles, even as they lack time and resources to make better choices for their family.

Embodiment in Individuals of Contexts, Characteristics, and Experiences

To recapitulate how these SDOH are intertwined, we next explore how diabetes became Mexico's leading cause of death, examining the influence of factors at multiple levels—from global trade to government policies, food sovereignty, and living and household conditions—on the two faces of malnutrition in Mexico and the embodiment of diabetes.

Case Study: Two Faces of Malnutrition Driving Mexican Mortality

In a tragic twist, just a generation ago, Mexico's leading cause of death was malnutrition-related infant mortality. Since 2000 diabetes has been the primary cause of death (with a doubling in prevalence from 2000 to 2006, and 14 million cases of diabetic retinopathy—impaired vision) (Barquera et al. 2013), driven by widespread consumption of junk food, including ubiquitous soft drinks, fast food, and prepackaged energy-dense, low nutrition foods.

Mexico's 1994 entry with the United States and Canada into the North American Free Trade Agreement (NAFTA)—liberalizing trade and investment—shepherded this transformation with the "opening" of Mexico's agriculture and food market. Corn subsidies in the United States artificially lowered prices (and expanded the US share of the global market), while in Mexico, export-oriented agribusiness massively displaced small farms unable to compete with cheap imports. This created new dependency on imported maize, wheat, and other essential foodstuffs (Otero 2011). As a result, the traditional (and nutritionally ideal) Aztec/Nahuatl diet of corn tortillas, beans, chilies, and other fresh vegetables and fruits became less accessible, violating principles of food sovereignty even as food insecurity was addressed among Indigenous and low-income populations (insofar as processed foods became more affordable).

NAFTA's removal of domestic agriculture protections caused the agricultural labor force to fall by 1.8 million people between 1998 and 2007. Failure to absorb this labor force into other sectors accelerated rural-urban migration (initially to deregulated factory work in border areas) and undocumented migration to the United States, causing Mexico to lose its "labor sovereignty" (Otero 2011, p. 391).

As small farmers went out of business and traditional foods became more expensive, Big Food FDI poured into Mexico by the billions. By the early 2000s, processed foods accounted for about three quarters of total FDI. Massive food retailing and marketing expanded distribution of (and demand for) these unhealthy foods through chain supermarkets and small convenience stores (or *tiendas*), lubricating Big Food's penetration of Mexico's small towns and outskirt communities. Consequently, consumption of processed foods and beverages soared (Hawkes 2006). Migration also played a role, as remittances enable purchase of TNC-marketed foods, leading to higher obesity rates (Riosmena et al. 2012).

To add insult to injury (or disease, in terms of diabetes), the continued poor quality of the water supply, despite official figures to the contrary (Stigler-Granados et al. 2014), have made sugar-laden soft drinks a cheaper, more accessible, and safer (in the short run, at least relating to bacterial content) option than piped water in much of Mexico. A main ingredient in soft drinks, fructose, makes them addictive (Nestle 2015), similar to when cocaine was featured in Coca-Cola in the late 19th century. Not only do the sweeteners (ironically largely corn-based) in soft drinks represent the displacement of local crops and diet, they are a key factor leading to diabetes, as are sugars, independent of overweight and obesity (Basu et al. 2013) (Box 9-1).

Certainly the diabetes crisis in Mexico is not solely a function of biomedical factors and it is not only attributable to (and cannot be reversed simply by modifying) unhealthy food and beverage choices (as posited by the behavioral/lifestyle model). Nor can it be exclusively explained as a stress reaction to the social environment. As per the psychosocial model, unhealthy behaviors are triggered by the environment of many low-income Mexicans: increasing violence, job and economic insecurity, and deteriorating living conditions. Accordingly, cheap and widely available, junk food (not requiring time and resources of fuel, a kitchen, etc. for food preparation) and soft drinks are psychologically attractive and convenient.

Even a political economy model—which shows how the needs of the majority of Mexicans have been politically trumped by domestic elites and foreign interests, how NAFTA opened the floodgates to FDI penetration by food and beverage TNCs into Mexican markets, and how provision of clean water to low-income urban and rural populations has been politically deprioritized while big business interests are subsidized and undertaxed—may not fully explain the embodiment of ill health.

What ecosocial theory adds to this analysis is an understanding of how diabetes has become metabolically and physiologically inscribed on the bodies of tens of millions of Mexicans, not abstractly, but quite concretely and intergenerationally (given the importance, biologically and contextually, of pre-pregnancy maternal health

T-shirt Travels

Throughout the chapter we have highlighted societal determinants underlying the health problems that affect Disha, a garment worker in Bangladesh, and Dolores, a kitchen prep worker in the United States. We have identified macro, meso, and micro determinants—the constellation of factors that frame their lives and experiences of health and illness. Their stories are not unlike those of hundreds of millions of other people, showing how SDOH playing out at a personal level translate into health inequities on a population level. They also illustrate the intersection of various determinants—including class, gender, race/ethnicity, and migrant status—in shaping and constraining their agency.

Combined, Dolores's shift work, primary breadwinner and caregiving roles, inescapable poverty, and inadequate housing conditions, rather than her lack of nutritional knowledge, help explain why her children are overweight. Likewise, even with extended family caring for her children, Disha cannot eliminate the daily exposure to indoor smoke and unclean water, or the ensuing infections. What began as a story of a T-shirt tying one working mother to another depicts how global deregulation of work and trade, precarious employment and migration, and piecemeal social policies that do little to improve living conditions, commingle to affect health intergenerationally, over the lifecourse, and across borders. Disha and Dolores produce and consume products that reveal power asymmetries at local, national, and global levels. They and their children embody these inequities in the form of unsafe work and housing, day-to-day stress, exposure and susceptibility to adverse conditions, and their attendant health effects.

[Kim et al. 2012]), resulting in an embodied fructose nexus.

Having identified SDOH, understood how they are manifest in unequal and remediable health patterns (health inequities), sought explanation for what brings them about, and explored how and why health inequities add up to more than the sum of individual determinants; we turn to how health inequities might be addressed through public policies.

ADDRESSING HEALTH INEQUITIES AND THE SOCIETAL DETERMINANTS OF HEALTH

Key Questions:

- What do SDOH analyses tell us about how to improve both population health and health equity?
- How has WHO called for SDOH to be addressed and what kinds of approaches have been adopted by particular societies?

Policy Implications of Different Understandings of Health Inequities

The theoretical frameworks presented earlier in the chapter not only provide analytical value, they each have powerful, and contrasting, consequences on policymaking. A biomedical model points to health interventions to "treat" the effects of inequality. A lifestyle understanding focuses on changing habits and practices to promote health, whereas a psychosocial approach may involve workplace and community measures to increase social cohesion, as well as individual level interventions to enhance psychological well-being. Political economy and ecosocial approaches integrate the aforementioned measures with political struggles for structural changes in arrangements of power and distribution of resources that address inequity and social injustice in the community and at societal and global levels.

Why are prevailing approaches insufficient? In environments where there are few outlets for stress relief, more people abuse alcohol, food, and drugs, because these offer a means of coping with difficult circumstances (Okechukwu, Davison, and Emmons 2014). Where nutritious meal preparation is impeded by inadequate cooking facilities, neighborhood stores selling cheap convenience foods (in milieus where they are aggressively promoted), healthy foods are unavailable or expensive, and long, unpredictable, and non-coinciding work (and school) shifts, people tend to have worse diets, regardless of knowledge and volition to alter diet. Moreover, addressing one, but not all, of these circumstances may be futile. Similarly, long work hours, expensive childcare, dangerous and inconvenient transport, and parks that are in poor shape or unsafe all inhibit regular exercise (Raphael 2015). Despite this reality, health promotion policies mostly emphasize behavior change at the individual level, presuming that better knowledge influences attitudes and motivates behavior improvements, even as our all-too-real accounts of Disha and Dolores demonstrate otherwise. Indeed, carried out in a vacuum, without understanding and addressing the interlinked "causes of the causes of the causes," a behavioral policy approach can yield little (Mackenzie et al. 2016).

In bringing ecosocial and political economy policy approaches to fruition, various generic and global strategies merit attention (Bryant 2013). At the micro level, health care providers could be educated to see beyond a person's presenting problem to consider the conditions in which a patient lives, loves, works, and plays to advocate for social spending *as* health spending. Public health efforts could emphasize a range of collective protections, with favorable SDOH serving as a gauge of healthy societies. Government policy, at the fulcrum of SDOH, could be held to account to alleviate poverty and address discrimination in the context of broad tax redistribution and collective social welfare policies (Krieger 2007). At the global level, struggles around equitable systems of trade, investment, environmental protection, taxation, and other forms of socially just governance are warranted, focusing on fair distribution of political and economic power.

The WHO Commission on Social Determinants of Health

The confluence of longstanding and more recent burgeoning scholarship, political advocacy, public understanding, and mobilization of public health researchers and practitioners pushed WHO to address SDOH systematically through a special global Commission established in 2005. Its 2008 report, *Closing the Gap in a Generation: Health Equity through Action on the Social Determinants of Health*, opens with a compelling statement—"Social justice is a matter of life and death"—and follows with a comprehensive set of well-documented findings and bold calls to action.

All but unprecedented for WHO, which typically focuses on technical dimensions of disease control, *Closing the Gap* documents the living conditions—urban infrastructure and governance, early childhood development and education, employment conditions, social protection measures, and health care—as well as the larger political economy reforms relating to taxation and debt, market conditions, gender equity, global governance, and political empowerment—that are necessary to counter the killing fields of social injustice. It calls on governments, civil society, and multilateral institutions, including WHO itself, to proactively strive for equity in health via three over-arching recommendations (CSDH 2008, p. 2):

1. Improve daily living conditions;
2. Tackle the inequitable distribution of power, money, and resources;
3. Measure and understand the problem and assess the impact of action.

While offering a wholesale indictment of neoliberal economic policy, which has exacerbated social and health inequity over the past 30 years, *Closing the Gap* glosses over *how* market forces affect health equity (Birn 2009), misses the opportunity to link SDOH to health and human rights frameworks (Chapman 2011), does not take on the most powerful political and economic structure—market capitalism—that drives SDOH, and fails to translate its recommendations "into concrete, politically grounded processes and actions" (Satzinger and Birn 2014, p. 2643).

On a more promising front, *Closing the Gap's* emphasis on socioeconomic redistribution, fair taxation, expansion of welfare states, and universal services could go a considerable way in reducing health inequities. Alas, the report was released almost concomitantly with the financial crisis of 2008, which became an excuse for many governments not to adopt its recommendations; yet those that did, namely Iceland, saw significant benefits. Still, civil society movements have continued to push at both local and global levels for governments to take up *Closing the Gap*'s policies (PHM et al. 2014).

Government Frameworks to Address SDOH and Health Inequities: From National to Municipal Level Action

Closing the implementation gap around addressing SDOH—integrating socio-political reforms from social welfare, labor, health, and education policies to investment, emissions, and trade regulations—has thus far been disappointing: most countries have done little more than rhetorically invoke the need to incorporate SDOH into national health (but not other policy) agendas. Even the Rio Political Declaration on Social Determinants of Health (Otterson et al. 2014; WHO 2011) tiptoed around some of the most pressing political issues linked to global health: the need for public, comprehensive health care and social security systems and for financial, corporate, and government transparency and accountability regarding environmental degradation, poor work conditions, tax evasion, flouting of social protection laws, and so on, that perpetuate health inequities within and between countries. But the Declaration has been unable to redirect WHO (or most government) priorities.

A few countries spanning various economic levels serve as exceptions, harnessing intersectoral collaboration around health goals—also referred to as Health in All Policies (HiAP) (see chapter 13)—to engage multiple governmental departments and social and economic sectors to address the SDOH.

Finland is a prime example of how a decades-long commitment to intersectoralism enables collaboration across ministries and economic sectors and broad integration of health objectives. With WHO support, Finland transformed its 1970s health behavior focus (e.g., on smoking and nutrition) into a model promoting the EU Constitution's requirement to "protect health in all policies" (Melkas 2013, p. 3). Remarkably, Finland's HiAP approach was adopted during its 1990s recession (countering prevailing austerity approaches). By 2010, the Finnish Public Health Act institutionalized accountability mechanisms and mandated municipalities to promote health intersectorally. Finland's HiAP approach, guided by policies crafted inter-ministerially, has helped it become one of the world's healthiest societies, even as it continues to struggle against health and welfare inequities (Tello and Baez-Camargo 2015).

Turning to Bhutan, in 1970 the government developed a "gross national happiness" (GNH) indicator, distinguishing it from the dominant global emphasis on economic growth and GDP. This unique approach involves nine main policymaking domains: psychological well-being, time use, community vitality, culture, health (including SDOH), education, environmental diversity, living standard, and governance. In 2008, a GNH index was streamlined across government sectors, with every policy and project proposal screened for impact on equity, among other indicators, and directing reallocation of resources to address the unhappiest groups (WHO 2013c). Although Bhutan's per capita income is among the world's lowest, life expectancy has increased by 18 years, with infant mortality falling by 52% since the 1970s (Tobgay et al. 2011).

Scotland's more recent experience stems from government recognition of significant health and socioeconomic inequalities (see chapter 5) and its 2008 vow to confront them. Long-term measures include early childhood education, violence prevention, promoting equality and tackling discrimination, and investing in quality and affordable housing and neighborhood regeneration. Scotland's radical critique of health inequalities and commitment to solidarity measures involves ongoing monitoring, as well as acknowledgment of the direct impact on health inequity of inequalities in power and social status, such as growing income and wealth inequalities resulting from neoliberal macroeconomic policy. Its naming of the role of unfair distribution of power and resources—and the global economic forces driving inequality—makes Scotland stand out (NHS Health Scotland 2015).

Political and social empowerment has been at the heart of a 3-year action research project aimed at reducing child malnutrition and inequity in Mombasa, Kenya. With active participation from health care, women's, child and social development, education, agriculture, and water constituencies, as well as community members more generally, a working group has targeted extreme poverty, improved sanitation, and waste disposal in Chaani, one of Mombasa's informal settlements. Though the initiative is realized at the municipal level, Kenya's Ministry of Health is involved and has been inspired to form intersectoral committees at the national level (WHO 2013c).

While it is too soon to know whether these efforts are the harbinger of future, more widespread efforts, they offer illustrations of how leadership, social conscience, accountability, and solidarity can come together not only to address inequitable material conditions but to generate political expectations and involvement, thereby reducing power asymmetries at multiple levels.

CONCLUSION

Learning Points:

- The societal determinants/determination of health refers to the broad array of structural influences, processes, and relationships that take place simultaneously, synergistically, and dynamically at the level of global and national political and economic forces, government policies and actions, living conditions, and individual experience.
- There is considerable knowledge about SDOH but insufficient action.
- Though most global health analyses emphasize health inequalities between HICs and LMICs, there are persistent health inequities both *within* and *across* countries.
- Systemic and persistent differences in health by social class, gender, racial and ethnic group, occupation, and so on, are linked to inequities in power and resources.
- The explanatory model adopted (e.g., biological, lifestyle, psychosocial, political economy, or ecosocial) has significant policy implications in terms of how health inequities are explained and, as a consequence, addressed.
- An ecosocial framework examines both how underlying causal factors generate health inequities *and* how these conditions lead to different experiences of and reactions to physical, biological, social, and chemical exposures, focusing on the mechanisms through which societal conditions and biological processes interact to produce health or ill health.

In this chapter, we explored the concept of SDOH, drawing from various explanatory frameworks that grapple with how a range and confluence of determinants affect health and health equity.

Notwithstanding ample and growing evidence about health inequities, too few societies use this knowledge to shape social and economic policies. Is this because the evidence is not credible to policymakers? Or is it because the evidence challenges deeply entrenched ideological positions—with those wielding power unwilling to seriously consider changing societal patterns of distribution in order to begin to address health inequities? These are fundamentally *political* issues: whether societies adopt solidarity or retain skewed power arrangements as an organizing principle has repercussions for virtually every aspect of life. Social movements that battle for healthy and just social policies and against power inequities at local, national, and global levels can play a meaningful role in pushing governments and other societal institutions to reduce health inequity, but responsibility and accountability also rest at the level of elected officials and international agencies. We shall explore these matters further in chapter 13.

NOTES

1. To the extent that health outcomes involve biology, which they always do, gene expression is at play. But saying this in no way implies genetic determinism or biological determinism of any type—what matters is how societal and ecological conditions shape the expression of our biology (including via pathways involving gene expression) and create the social patterning of rates of disease and mortality at a given point in time and also changing rates over time.
2. From 1911 to 2001, the United Kingdom's Registrar-General collected routine mortality data by social class as measured by occupational category. It was then replaced with a larger socioeconomic classification based on employment relations and occupational conditions (Glymour, Avendano, and Kawachi 2014).
3. Documentation of these patterns began as far back as 1907 when Canada's medical officer responsible for inspecting residential schools, Peter Bryce, decried the almost one fourth of students who were dying. He was ignored and then removed from his position (Bryce 1922; Sproule-Jones 1996).

REFERENCES

Alexander M. 2012. *The New Jim Crow: Mass Incarceration in the Age of Colorblindness*. New York: The New Press.

Amnesty International. 2014. Twelve facts about the abortion ban in El Salvador. https://www.amnesty.org/en/latest/news/2014/09/twelve-facts-about-abortion-ban-el-salvador/. Accessed January 29, 2016.

Arku G, Luginaah I, Mkandawire P, et al. 2011. Housing and health in three contrasting neighbourhoods in Accra, Ghana. *Social Science and Medicine* 72(11):1864–1872.

Australian Institute of Health and Welfare. 2014. *Mortality and Life Expectancy of Indigenous Australians: 2008 to 2012*. Cat. no. IHW 140. Canberra: AIHW.

Bain R, Cronk R, Hossain R, et al. 2014. Global assessment of exposure to faecal contamination through drinking water based on a systematic review. *Tropical Medicine and International Health* 19(8):917–927.

Bambra C. 2009. Welfare state regimes and the political economy of health. *Humanity and Society* 33:99–117.

———. 2011. *Work, Worklessness, and the Political Economy of Health*. New York: Oxford University Press.

Bambra C, Pope D, Swami V, et al. 2009. Gender, health inequalities and welfare state regimes: A cross-national study of 13 European countries. *Journal of Epidemiology and Community Health* 63(1):38–44.

Barquera S, Campos-Nonato I, Aguilar-Salinas C, et al. 2013. Diabetes in Mexico: Cost and management of diabetes and its complications and challenges for health policy. *Globalization and Health* 9(1):3.

Basu S, Yoffe P, Hills N, and Lustig RH. 2013. The relationship of sugar to population-level diabetes prevalence: An econometric analysis of repeated cross-sectional data. *PLoS One* 8(2):e57873.

Beckfield J, Bambra C, Eikemo TA, et al. 2015. An institutional theory of welfare state effects on the distribution of population health. *Social Theory and Health* 13(3):227–244.

Beckfield J and Krieger N. 2009. Epi+ demos+ cracy: Linking political systems and priorities to the magnitude of health inequities—evidence, gaps, and a research agenda. *Epidemiologic Reviews* 31:152–177.

Beckfield J, Olafsdottir S, and Bakhtiari E. 2013. Health inequalities in global context. *American Behavioral Scientist* 57(8):1014–1039.

Bell M and Charles-Edwards E. 2013. *Cross-National Comparisons of Internal Migration: An Update on Global Patterns and Trends*. Population Division Technical Paper No. 2013/1. New York: UN Department of Economic and Social Affairs.

Bell R, Britton A, Brunner E, et al. 2004. *Work Stress and Health: The Whitehall II Study*. London: Public and Commercial Services Union.

Benach J, Muntaner C, Solar C, et al. 2013. *Employment, Work, and Health Inequalities: A Global Perspective*. Barcelona: Icaria Editorial SA.

Benach J, Vives A, Amable M, et al. 2014. Precarious employment: Understanding an emerging social determinant of health. *Annual Review of Public Health* 35:229–253.

Berer M. 2015. The history and role of the criminal law in anti-FGM campaigns: Is the criminal law what is needed, at least in countries like Great Britain? *Reproductive Health Matters* 23(46):145–157.

Bergad L. 2007. *The Comparative Histories of Slavery in Brazil, Cuba, and the United States*. London: Cambridge University Press.

Bergqvist K, ÅbergYngwe M, and Lundberg O. 2013. Understanding the role of welfare state characteristics for health and inequalities – an analytical review. *BMC Public Health* 13:1234.

Berkman LF and Kawachi I. 2014. A historical framework for social epidemiology: Social determinants of population health. In Berkman LF, Kawachi I, and Glymour MM, Editors. *Social Epidemiology*, Second Edition. New York: Oxford University Press.

Berkman LF, Kawachi I, and Theorell T. 2014. Working conditions and health. In Berkman LF, Kawachi I, and Glymour MM, Editors. *Social Epidemiology*, Second Edition. New York: Oxford University Press.

Birn A-E. 2009. Making it politic(al): Closing the Gap in a Generation: Health Equity Through Action on the Social Determinants of Health. *Social Medicine* 4(3):166–182.

Black SD and Research Working Group (Morris JN, Smith C, Townsend P). 1980. *Inequalities in Health: Report of a Research Working Group*. London: Department of Health and Social Security.

Boddy J. 2002. The female circumcision controversy: An anthropological perspective. *Journal of the Royal Anthropological Society* 8(1):181.

Borrell C, Palència L, Muntaner C, et al. 2013. Influence of macrosocial policies on women's health and gender inequalities in health. *Epidemiologic Reviews* 36:31–48.

Bowleg L. 2012. The problem with the phrase women and minorities: Intersectionality – an important theoretical framework for public health. *American Journal of Public Health* 102(7):1267–1273.

Bradshaw S, Nicol E, Pilay van Wyk V, et al. 2015. *2nd National Burden of Disease Study for South Africa: Maternal and Childhood Mortality Report 1997-2002*. Tygerberg: SAMRC Burden of Disease Research Unit.

Braveman PA, Cubbin C, Egerter S, et al. 2005. Socioeconomic status in health research: One size does not fit all. *JAMA* 294(22):2879–2888.

Braveman P and Gottlieb L. 2014. The social determinants of health: It's time to consider the causes of the causes. *Public Health Reports* 129(Suppl 2):19–31.

Breilh J. 2003. *Epidemiología Crítica: Ciencia Emancipadora e Interculturalidad*. Buenos Aires: Lugar Editorial.

Brian T and Laczko F 2014. *Fatal Journeys Tracking Lives Lost during Migration*. Geneva: IOM.

Bryant T. 2013. Policy change and the social determinants of health. In Clavier C and De Leeuw E, Editors. *Health Promotion and the Policy Process: Practical and Critical Theories*. Oxford: Oxford University Press.

Bryce P. 1922. *The Story of a National Crime, Being an Appeal for Justice to the Indians of Canada; The Wards of the Nation, Our Allies in the Revolutionary War, Our Brothers-in-Arms in the Great War.* Ottawa: J. Hope.

Busch-Geertsema V, Benjaminsen L, Hrast MF, and Pleace N. 2014. *Extent and Profile of Homelessness in European Member States EOH Comparative Studies on Homelessness Brussels – December 2014 A Statistical Update*. Brussels: EOH Comparative Studies on Homelessness.

Carvalho N, Hussein J, Goldie S, and Britten S. 2015. *Maternal Mortality Reported Trends in Afghanistan: Too Good To Be True?* London: British and Irish Agencies Afghanistan Group.

Castañeda H, Holmes SM, Madrigal DS, et al. 2015. Immigration as a social determinant of health. *Annual Review of Public Health* 36:375–392.

Center for Reproductive Rights. 2014. *Marginalized, Persecuted, and Imprisoned: The Effects of El Salvador's Total Criminalization of Abortion*. New York: Center for Reproductive Rights.

Chapman AR. 2011. Missed opportunities: The human rights gap in the report of the commission on social determinants of health. *Journal of Human Rights* 10(2):132–150.

Chung J. 2015. *Policy Brief: Felony Disenfranchisement*. Washington, DC: The Sentencing Project.

Coburn D. 2011. Global health: A political economy of historical trends and contemporary inequalities. In Teeple G and McBride S, Editors. *Relations of Global Power: Neoliberal Order and Disorder.* Toronto: University of Toronto Press.

———. 2015. Income inequality, welfare, class and health: A comment on Pickett and Wilkinson, 2015. *Social Science and Medicine* 146:228–232.

Connell R. 2012. Gender, health and theory: Conceptualizing the issue, in local and world perspective. *Social Science and Medicine* 74(11):1675–1683.

Corburn J. 2015. Urban inequities, population health and spatial planning. In Barton H, Thompson S, Burgess S, Editors. *The Routledge Handbook of Planning for Health and Well-Being: Shaping a sustainable and healthy future*. New York: Routledge.

Crammond BR and Carey G. 2016. Policy change for the social determinants of health: The strange irrelevance of social epidemiology. *Evidence & Policy: A Journal of Research, Debate and Practice* [Epub ahead of publication].

Crenshaw K. 1989. Demarginalizing the intersection of race and sex: A Black feminist critique of antidiscrimination doctrine, feminist theory and antiracist politics. *University of Chicago Legal Forum* 1989(1):139–167.

CSDH. 2008. *Closing the Gap in a Generation: Health Equity through Action on the Social Determinants of Health. Final Report of the Commission on Social Determinants of Health*. Geneva: WHO.

Czyzewski K. 2011. Colonialism as a broader social determinant of health. *The International Indigenous Policy Journal* 2(1).

Daniel A and Graf P. 2015. Gender and politics in Brazil between continuity and change. In de la Fontaine D and Stehnken T, Editors. *The Political System of Brazil*. Berlin: Springer-Verlag.

Das V. 2015. *Affliction: Health, Disease, Poverty*. The Bronx: Fordham University Press.

de Andrade LOM, Pellegrini A, Solar O, et al. 2015. Social determinants of health, universal health coverage, and sustainable development: Case studies from Latin American countries. *Lancet* 385(9975):1343–1351.

Deere DC, Alvarado GE, and Twyman J. 2012. Gender inequality in asset ownership in Latin America: Female owners vs. household heads. *Development and Change* 43(2):505–530.

Dentico N. 2014. Nutrition, pathologies of power and the need for health democracy. *Development* 57(2):184–191.

Desilver D. 2014. For most workers, real wages have barely budged for decades. *Pew Research Center*, October 9.

———. 2015. U.S. voter turnout trails most developed countries. *Pew Research Center*, May 6.

Domingues RMSM, Viellas EF, Dias MAB, et al. 2015. Adequacy of prenatal care according to maternal characteristics in Brazil. *Revista Panamericana de Salud Pública* 37(3):140–147.

Dorling D. 2015. *All that is Solid. How the Great Housing Disaster Defines Our Times, and What We Can Do About It*. London: Penguin UK.

Doshi S. 2013. The politics of the evicted: Redevelopment, subjectivity, and difference in Mumbai's slum frontier. *Antipode* 45(4):844–865.

Doyal L and Payne S. 2011. Gender and global health: Inequality and differences. In Benatar S and Brock G, Editors. *Global Health and Global Health Ethics*. Cambridge: Cambridge University Press.

Dunn JR. 2002. Housing and inequalities in health: A study of socioeconomic dimensions of housing and self reported health from a survey of Vancouver residents. *Journal of Epidemiology and Community Health* 56(9):671–681.

ECLAC. 2014. *Guaranteeing Indigenous People's Rights in Latin America: Progress in the Past Decade and Remaining Challenges (English Summary)*. Santiago: ECLAC.

Eslava-Schmalbach JH, Rincón CJ, and Guarnizo-Herreño CC. 2013. 'Inequidad' de la expectativa de vida al nacer por sexo y 'departamentos' de Colombia. *Biomédica* 33(3):383–392.

Esping-Andersen G. 1990. *The Three Worlds of Welfare Capitalism*. Princeton, NJ: Princeton University Press.

European Commission. 2014. *Roma Health Report Health status of the Roma population. Data collection in the Member States of the European Union*. Brussels: EC.

Fan M. 2015. *ADB South Asia Working Paper Series. Sri Lanka's Water Supply and Sanitation Sector: Achievements and a Way Forward*. Mandaluyong City: Asian Development Bank.

FAO. 2015. *The State of Food Insecurity in the World 2015: Meeting the 2015 International Hunger Targets: Taking Stock of Uneven Progress*. Rome: FAO.

Firdaus G and Ahmad A. 2013. Relationship between housing and health: A cross-sectional study of an urban centre of India. *Indoor and Built Environment* 22(3):498–507.

Fleischhacker SE, Evenson KR, Rodrigue DA, and Ammerman AS. 2011. A systematic review of fast food access studies. *Obesity Reviews* 12:e460–e471.

Forouzanfar MH, Alexander L, Anderson HR, et al. 2015. Global, regional, and national comparative risk assessment of 79 behavioural, environmental and occupational, and metabolic risks or clusters of risks in 188 countries, 1990–2013: A systematic analysis for the Global Burden of Disease Study 2013. *Lancet* 386(10010):2287–2323.

Freeman MC, Stocks ME, Cumming O, et al. 2014. Systematic review: Hygiene and health: Systematic review of handwashing practices worldwide and update of health effects. *Tropical Medicine and International Health* 19(8):906–916.

Friel S, Hattersley L, and Townsend R. 2015. Trade policy and public health. *Annual Review of Public Health* 36:325–344.

Friel S, Loring B, Aungkasuvapala N, et al. 2012. Policy approaches to address the social and environmental determinants of health inequity in Asia-Pacific. *Asia-Pacific Journal of Public Health* 24(6):896–914.

Gao Y, Li LP, Kim JH, et al. 2010. The impact of parental migration on health status and health behaviours among left behind adolescent school children in China. *BMC Public Health* 10:56.

Gates S, Hegre H, Nygård HM, and Strand H. 2012. Development consequences of armed conflict. *World Development* 40(9):1713–1722.

Geiger HJ. 2013. Contesting racism and innovating community health centers: Approaches on two continents. In Birn A-E and Brown T, Editors. *Comrades in Health: US Health Internationalists, Abroad and at Home*. New Brunswick, NJ: Rutgers University Press.

Gil-González D, Vives-Cases C, Borrell C, et al. 2014. Racism, other discriminations and effects on health. *Journal of Immigrant and Minority Health* 16(2):301–309.

Gill S and Bakker I. 2011. The global crisis and global health. In Benatar S and Brock G, Editors. *Global Health and Global Health Ethics*. Cambridge: Cambridge University Press.

Glymour MM, Avendano M, and Kawachi I. 2014. Socioeconomic status and health. In Berkman LF, Kawachi I, and Glymour MM, Editors. *Social Epidemiology*, Second Edition. New York: Oxford University Press.

Gornick JC and Jäntti M. 2012. Child poverty in cross-national perspective: Lessons from the Luxembourg Income Study. *Children and Youth Services Review* 34(3):558–568.

Gracey M. 2014. Why closing the Aboriginal health gap is so elusive. *Internal Medicine Journal* 44(11): 1141–1143.

Gras C. 2009. Changing patterns in family farming: The case of the Pampa Region, Argentina. *Journal of Agrarian Change* 9(3):345–364.

Grassi D and Luppi F. 2014. *Do We Live Longer and Healthier Lives under Democracy? A Configurational Comparative Analysis of Latin America (Working Paper 2014-78)*. Houston: COMPASSS Working Papers Series.

Grey S and Patel R. 2015. Food sovereignty as decolonization: Some contributions from Indigenous movements to food system and development politics. *Agriculture and Human Values* 32(3):431–444.

Gupta N, Goel K, Shah P, and Misra A. 2012. Childhood obesity in developing countries: Epidemiology, determinants, and prevention. *Endocrine Reviews* 33(1):48–70.

Habitat for Humanity 2015. World Habitat Day 2015 key housing facts. http://www.habitat.org/getinv/events/world-habitat-day/housing-facts. Accessed February 19, 2016.

Hadjar A and Beck M. 2010. Who does not participate in elections in Europe and why is this? A multilevel analysis of social mechanisms behind non-voting. *European Societies* 12(4):521–542.

Hardoon D, Ayele S, and Fuentes-Nieva R. 2016. *An Economy For the 1%: How Privilege and Power in the Economy Drive Extreme Inequality and How This Can Be Stopped*. Oxford: Oxfam International.

Harris R, Cormack D, Tobias M, et al. 2012. The pervasive effects of racism: Experiences of racial discrimination in New Zealand over time and associations with multiple health domains. *Social Science and Medicine* 74(3):408–415.

Harvey D. 2006. *Spaces of Global Capitalism: Towards a Theory of Uneven Geographical Development*. London & New York: Verso.

Hawkes C. 2006. Uneven dietary development: Linking the policies and processes of globalization with the nutrition transition, obesity and diet-related chronic diseases. *Globalization and Health* 2(1):4.

Heins E and Deeming C. 2015. Welfare and well-being–inextricably linked. *In Defence of Welfare* 2:13–15.

Heise L and Kotsadam A. 2015. Cross-national and multilevel correlates of partner violence: An analysis of data from population-based surveys. *Lancet Global Health* 3:e332–e340.

Herrera Riquelme CA, Kuhn-Barrientos L, et al. 2015. Tendencia de la mortalidad por cáncer en Chile según diferencias por nivel educacional, 2000-2010. *Revista Panamericana de Salud Pública* 37(1):44–51.

Hertzman C, Irwin L, Siddiqi A, et al. 2012. Early childhood strategies for closing the socioeconomic gap in school outcomes. In Heymann J and Cassola A, Editors. *Lessons in Educational Equality: Successful Approaches to Intractable Problems around the World*. New York: Oxford University Press.

Hickel J. 2016. The true extent of global poverty and hunger: Questioning the good news narrative of the Millennium Development Goals. *Third World Quarterly* 37(5):749–767.

Hoffman B. 2013. *Behind the Brands: Food Justice and the "Big 10" Food and Beverage Companies*. Oxford: Oxfam International.

Human Rights Watch. 2012. *"Waiting Here for Death": Forced Displacement and "Villagization" in Ethiopia's Gambella Region*. New York: Human Rights Watch.

Hwang SW, Gogosis E, Chambers C, et al. 2011. Health status, quality of life, residential stability, substance use, and health care utilization among adults applying to a supportive housing program. *Journal of Urban Health* 88(6): 1076–1090.

ILO. 2013. *The Prevention of Occupational Diseases*. Geneva: ILO.

———. 2015. Hazardous work. http://www.ilo.org/safework/areasofwork/hazardous-work/lang--en/index.htm. Accessed December 22, 2015.

Jaumotte F and Buitron CO. 2015. *Inequality and Labor Market Institutions*. Washington, DC: IMF.

Joshi DK. 2015. The inclusion of excluded majorities in South Asian parliaments: Women, youth, and the working class. *Journal of Asian and African Studies* 50(2):223–238.

Kapilashrami A, Hill S, and Meer N. 2015. What can health inequalities researchers learn from an intersectionality perspective? Understanding social dynamics with an inter-categorical approach?. *Social Theory and Health* 13:288–307.

Kawachi I and Subramanian SV. 2014. Income inequality. In Berkman LF, Kawachi I, and Glymour MM, Editors. *Social Epidemiology*, Second Edition. New York: Oxford University Press.

Keneally T. 2010. *Three Famines: Starvation and Politics*. New York: PublicAffairs.

Khanna P. 2011. Making labour voices heard during an industrial crisis: Workers' struggles in the Bangladesh garment industry. *Labour, Capital and Society* 44(2):106–129.

Kim SY, Sharma AJ, and Callaghan WM. 2012. Gestational diabetes and childhood obesity: What is the link? *Current Opinion in Obstetrics and Gynecology* 24(6):376–381.

Kimani-Murage EW, Fotso JC, Egondi T, et al. 2014. Trends in childhood mortality in Kenya: The urban advantage has seemingly been wiped out. *Health and Place* 29:95–103.

Kindig DA. 2007. Understanding population health terminology. *Milbank Quarterly* 85(1):139–161.

Koivusalo M. 2011. Trade and health: The ethics of global rights, regulation and redistribution. In Benatar S and Brock G, Editors. *Global Health and Global Health Ethics*. Cambridge: Cambridge University Press.

Komro KA, Livingston MD, Markowitz S, and Wagenaar AC. 2016. The effect of an increased minimum wage on infant mortality and birth weight. *American Journal of Public Health* 106(8):1514–1516.

Krieger N. 2007. Why epidemiologists cannot afford to ignore poverty. *Epidemiology* 18(6):658–663.

———. 2008. Proximal, distal, and the politics of causation: What's level got to do with it? *American Journal of Public Health* 98(2):221–230.

———. 2011. *Epidemiology and the People's Health: Theory and Context*. New York: Oxford University Press.

———. 2014a. Discrimination and health inequities. *International Journal of Health Services* 44(4):643–710.

———. 2014b. Got Theory? On the 21st c. CE rise of explicit use of epidemiologic theories of disease distribution: A review and ecosocial analysis. *Current Epidemiology Reports* 1(1):45–56.

Krieger N, Chen JT, Coull B, et al. 2013. The unique impact of abolition of Jim Crow laws on reducing inequities in infant death rates and implications for choice of comparison groups in analyzing societal determinants of health. *American Journal of Public Health* 103(12):2234–2244.

Krieger N, Williams D, and Moss N. 1997. Measuring social class in US public health research: Concepts, methodologies and guidelines. *Annual Review of Public Health* 18:341–378.

Kubzansky LD, Winning A, and Kawachi I. 2014. Affective states and health. In Berkman LF, Kawachi I, and Glymour MM, Editors. *Social Epidemiology*, Second Edition. New York: Oxford University Press.

Lekobane KR and Seleka TB. 2014. *BIDPA Working Paper 38: Determinants of Household Welfare and Poverty in Botswana, 2002/03 and 2009/10*. Botswana: Botswana Institute for Development Policy Analysis.

Levy BS and Sidel VW. 2013. War and other forms of armed conflict (Box 17–1). In Levy BS and Sidel VW, Editors. *Social Injustice and Public Health*. London: Oxford University Press.

Lewis K and Burd-Sharps S. 2013. *American Human Development Report: The Measure of America 2013-2014*. Brooklyn: Measure of America.

Loewenson R and Gilson L. 2012. The health system and wider social determinants of health. In Smith RD and Hanson K, Editors. *Health Systems in Low- and Middle-Income Countries: An economic and policy perspective*. New York: Oxford University Press.

Logie C. 2012. The case for the World Health Organization's Commission on Social Determinants of Health to address sexual orientation. *American Journal of Public Health* 102(7):1243–1246.

Lori JR and Boyle JS. 2015. Forced migration: Health and human rights issues among refugee populations. *Nursing Outlook* 63(1):68–76.

Lucchini RG and London L. 2014. Global occupational health: Current challenges and the need for urgent action. *Annals of Global Health* 80(4):251–256.

Lynch J and Smith GD. 2005. A lifecourse approach to chronic disease epidemiology. *Annual Review of Public Health* 26:1–35.

Macinko J, Starfield B, and Erinosho T. 2009. The impact of primary healthcare on population health in low-and middle-income countries. *Journal of Ambulatory Care Management* 32(2):150–171.

Mackenbach JP. 2015. Socioeconomic inequalities in health in high-income countries: The facts and the options. In Detels R, Gulliford M, Karim QA, and Tan CC, Editors. 2015. *Oxford Textbook of Global Public Health*. New York: Oxford University Press.

Mackenzie M, Collins C, Connolly J, et al. 2016. Working-class discourses of politics, policy and health: 'I don't smoke; I don't drink. The only thing wrong with me is my health'. *Policy and Politics* [Epub ahead of publication].

Makoka D. 2013. *The Impact of Maternal Education on Child Nutrition: Evidence from Malawi, Tanzania, and Zimbabwe*. DHS Working Papers: USAID.

Marmot MG. 2004. *The Status Syndrome: How Social Standing Affects Our Health and Longevity*. London: Macmillan.

———. 2005. The social determinants of health inequalities. *Lancet* 365(9464):1099–1104.

Marmot M and Brunner E. 2005. Cohort profile: The Whitehall II study. *International Journal of Epidemiology* 34(2):251–256.

Marshall TH. 1950. *Citizenship and Social Class and Other Essays*. Cambridge: Cambridge University Press.

Martínez Franzoni J and Sánchez-Ancochea D. 2013. Can Latin American production regimes complement universalistic welfare regimes? Implications from the Costa Rican case. *Latin American Research Review* 48(2):148–173.

Masud-All-Kamal M and Saha CK. 2014. Targeting social policy and poverty reduction: The case of social safety nets in Bangladesh. *Poverty and Public Policy* 6(2):195–211.

Math SB and Seshadri SP. 2013. The invisible ones: Sexual minorities. *The Indian Journal of Medical Research* 137(1):4–6.

Mathews TJ, MacDorman MF, and Thoma ME. 2015. Infant mortality statistics from the 2013 period linked birth/infant death data set. *National Vital Statistics Reports* 64(9):1–30.

Matthews KA and Gallo LC. 2011. Psychological perspectives on pathways linking socioeconomic status and physical health. *Annual Review of Psychology* 62:501–530.

McGovern L, Miller G, and Hughes-Cromwick P. 2014. Health Policy Brief: The relative contribution of multiple determinants to health outcomes. *Health Affairs*, August 21.

McGuire JW. 2010. *Wealth, Health, and Democracy in East Asia and Latin America*. Cambridge: Cambridge University Press.

McMichael AJ. 2013. Globalization, climate change, and human health. *NEJM* 368(14):1335–1343.

Melkas T. 2013. Health in all policies as a priority in Finnish health policy: A case study on national health policy development. *Scandinavian Journal of Public Health* 41(Suppl 11):3–28.

Menéndez EL. 2009. *De sujetos, saberes y estructuras. Introducción al enfoque relacionalen el estudio de la salud colectiva*. Buenos Aires: Lugar Editorial.

Monden CW and Smits J. 2013. Maternal education is associated with reduced female disadvantages in under-five mortality in sub-Saharan Africa and southern Asia. *International Journal of Epidemiology* 42(1):211–218.

Morales-Borrero C, Borde E, Eslava-Castañeda JC, and Concha-Sánchez SC. 2013. ¿Determinación social o determinantes sociales? Diferencias conceptuales e implicaciones praxiológicas. *Revista de Salud Pública* 15(6):797–808.

Muntaner C, Borrell C, Ng E, et al. 2011. Review article: Politics, welfare regimes, and population health: Controversies and evidence. *Sociology of Health and Illness* 33(6):946–964.

Muntaner C, Borrell C, Vanroelen C, et al. 2010. Employment relations, social class and health: A review and analysis of conceptual and measurement alternatives. *Social Science and Medicine* 71(12):2130–2140.

Muntaner C, Ng E, Chung H, and Prins SJ. 2015. Two decades of Neo-Marxist class analysis and health inequalities: A critical reconstruction. *Social Theory and Health* 13(3-4):267–287.

National Alliance to End Homelessness. 2015. *The State of Homelessness in America 2015*. Washington, DC: National Alliance to End Homelessness.

Nestle M. 2015. *Soda Politics: Taking on Big Soda (and Winning)*. New York: Oxford University Press.

Ng E and Muntaner C. 2014. A critical approach to macrosocial determinants of population health: Engaging scientific realism and incorporating social conflict. *Current Epidemiology Reports* 1(1):27–37.

NHS Health Scotland. 2015. *Health Inequalities: What Are They? How Do We Reduce Them?*. Edinburgh: NHS Health Scotland.

Nieuwenhuijsen MJ, Khreis H, Verlinghieri E, and Rojas-Rueda D. 2016. Transport and health: A marriage of convenience or an absolute necessity. *Environment International* 88:150–152.

OECD. 2014. *Promoting Better Labour Market Outcomes For Youth: Report on Youth Employment and Apprenticeships Prepared for the G20 Labour and Employment Ministerial Meeting*. Melbourne: OECD.

———. 2015. OECD Income Distribution Database (IDD): Gini, poverty, income, Methods and Concepts. http://www.oecd.org/social/income-distribution-database.htm. Accessed July 16, 2015.

Office for National Statistics. 2015. *ONS Longitudinal Study (LS) based estimates of Life Expectancy (LE) by the National Statistics Socioeconomic Classification (NS to SEC): England and Wales, between 1982 to 1986 and 2007 to 2011*. Datasets and reference tables. http://www.ons.gov.uk/ons/datasets-and-tables/index.html. Accessed November 23, 2015.

Office of Disease Prevention and Health Promotion. 2016. Social determinants of health. http://www.healthypeople.gov/2020/topics-objectives/topic/social-determinants-health. Accessed January 9, 2016.

O'Hara J. 2013. *The $11 Trillion Reward: How Simple Dietary Changes Can Save Lives and Money, and How We Get There*. Cambridge: Union of Concerned Scientists.

Okechukwu C, Davison K, and Emmons K. 2014. Changing health behaviors in a social context. In Berkman LF, Kawachi I, and Glymour MM, Editors. *Social Epidemiology*, Second Edition. New York: Oxford University Press.

Oliveira R, Moura K, Viana J, et al. 2015. Commute duration and health: Empirical evidence from Brazil. *Transportation Research Part A: Policy and Practice* 80:62–75.

Olukolajo MA, Adewusi AO, and Ogungbenro MT. 2013. Influence of housing condition on the health status of residents of urban core of Akure, Nigeria. *International Journal of Development and Sustainability* 2(2):1567–1579.

Ontario College of Family Physicians. 2013. Poverty: A clinical tool for primary care in Ontario. http://ocfp.on.ca/docs/default-source/poverty-tool/poverty-a-clinical-tool-2013-(with-references).pdf?sfvrsn=2. Accessed May 20, 2015.

Otero G. 2011. Neoliberal globalization, NAFTA, and migration: Mexico's loss of food and labor sovereignty. *Journal of Poverty* 15(4):384–402.

Otterson OP, Dasgupta J, Blouin C, et al. 2014. The political origins of health inequity: Prospects for change. *Lancet* 383(9917):630–667.

Panitch L and Gindin S. 2012. *The Making of Global Capitalism: The Political Economy of American Empire*. New York: Verso Books.

Paradies Y, Ben J, Denson N, et al. 2015. Racism as a determinant of health: A systematic review and meta-analysis. *PLoS One* 10(9):e0138511.

Pinzon-Rondon AM, Attaran A, Botero JC, and Ruiz-Sternberg AM. 2015. Association of rule of law and health outcomes: An ecological study. *BMJ Open* 5(10):e007004.

Pogge T and Sengupta M. 2015. The Sustainable Development Goals: A plan for building a better world?.*Journal of Global Ethics* 11(1):56–64.

Pritchett L. 2013. Monitoring progress on poverty: The case for a high global poverty line. *Development Progress*, May 16.

Prüss-Ustün A, Bartram J, Clasen T, et al. 2014. Burden of disease from inadequate water, sanitation and hygiene in low-and middle-income settings: A retrospective analysis of data from 145 countries. *Tropical Medicine and International Health* 19(8):894–905.

Radhakrishnan R and Andrade C. 2012. Suicide: an Indian perspective. *Indian Journal of Psychiatry* 54(4):304–319.

Rambotti S. 2015. Recalibrating the spirit level: An analysis of the interaction of income inequality and poverty and its effect on health. *Social Science and Medicine* 139:123–131.

Rao M, Afshin A, Singh G, and Mozaffarian D. 2013. Do healthier foods and diet patterns cost more than less healthy options? A systematic review and meta-analysis. *BMJ Open* 3(12):e004277.

Raphael D. 2011. *Poverty in Canada: Implications for Health and Quality of Life*. Toronto: Canadian Scholars' Press.

———. 2015. The parameters of children's health: Key concepts from the political economy of health literature. *International Journal of Child, Youth and Family Studies* 6(2):186–203.

Reddy DN and Mishra S, Editors. 2010. *Agrarian Crisis in India*. New Delhi: Oxford University Press.

Riosmena F, Frank R, Akresh IR, and Kroeger RA. 2012. US migration, translocality, and the acceleration of the nutrition transition in Mexico. *Annals of the Association of American Geographers* 102(5):1209–1218.

Robinson WI. 2014. *Global Capitalism and the Crisis of Humanity*. Cambridge: Cambridge University Press.

Rose G and Marmot MG. 1981. Social class and coronary heart disease. *British Heart Journal* 45(1):13–19.

Roux AV and Mair C. 2010. Neighborhoods and health. *Annals of the New York Academy of Sciences* 1186(1):125–145.

Ruckert A and Labonté R. 2014. The social determinants of health. In Brown GW, Yamey G, and Wamala S, Editors. *The Handbook of Global Health Policy, First Edition*. Hoboken: John Wiley & Sons, Ltd.

Rudin J and Sanders D. 2011. Debt, structural adjustment and health. In Benatar S and Brock G, Editors. *Global Health and Global Health Ethics*. Cambridge: Cambridge University Press.

Satzinger F and Birn A-E. 2014. Social and societal determinants of health. In Jennings B, Editor. *Encyclopedia of Bioethics*, 4th Edition. Farmington Hills, MI: Macmillan.

Say L and Raine R. 2007. A systematic review of inequalities in the use of maternal health care in developing countries: Examining the scale of the problem and the importance of context. *Bulletin of the World Health Organization* 85(10):812–819.

Sehgal M and Krishnan A. 2013. *Indoor Air Pollution and Child Health in India. Child Poverty Insights*. New York: UNICEF.

Sellers C. 2016. Piping as poison: The Flint water crisis and America's toxic infrastructure. *The Conversation*, January 25.

Shaw M, Galobardes B, Lawlor DA, et al. 2007. *The Handbook of Inequality and Socioeconomic Position: Concepts and Measures*. Bristol: The Policy Press.

Spiegel JM, Breilh J, and Yassi A. 2015. Why language matters: Insights and challenges in applying a social determination of health approach in a north-south collaborative research program. *Globalization and Health* 11:9.

Sproule-Jones M. 1996. Crusading for the forgotten: Dr. Peter Bryce, public health, and prairie Native residential schools. *Canadian Bulletin of Medical History* 13(1996):199–224.

Starfield B and Birn A-E. 2007. Income redistribution is not enough: Income inequality, social welfare programs, and achieving equity in health. *Journal of Epidemiology and Community Health* 61(12):1038–1041.

Stigler-Granados P, Quintana PJ, Gersberg R, et al. 2014. Comparing health outcomes and point-of-use water quality in two rural Indigenous communities of Baja California, Mexico before and after receiving new potable water infrastructure. *Journal of Water Sanitation and Hygiene for Development* 4(4):672–680.

Stuckler D, Basu S, Suhrcke M, et al. 2009. The public health effect of economic crises and alternative policy responses in Europe: An empirical analysis. *Lancet* 374(9686):315–323.

Susuman AS, Lougue S, and Battala M. 2014. Female literacy, fertility decline and life expectancy in Kerala, India: An analysis from census of India 2011. *Journal of Asian and African Studies* 51(1):32–42.

Tapia Granados J. 2014. In conversation: Health and economic crisis. *The Brooklyn Rail*, October 3.

Tarantola D and Gruskin S. Human rights approach to public health policy. 2013. In Grodin MA, Tarantola D, Annas GJ, and Gruskin S, Editors. *Health and Human Rights in a Changing World*. New York: Routledge.

Teerawichitchainan B. 2014. Gender and health status among older adults in Vietnam. In Devasahayam TW, Editor. *Gender and Ageing: Southeast Asian Perspectives*. Singapore: Institute of Southeast Asian Studies.

Tello J and Baez-Camargo C. 2015. *Strengthening Health System Accountability: A WHO European Region Multi-Country Study*. Copenhagen: WHO Europe.

Terrelonge SC. 2014. For health, strength, and daily food: The dual impact of remittances and public health expenditure on household health spending and child health outcomes. *Journal of Development Studies* 50(10):1397–1410.

Thrasher SW. 2015. Income inequality happens by design. We can't fix it by tweaking capitalism. *The Guardian*, December 5.

Tobgay T, Dorji T, Pelzom D, and Gibbons RV. 2011. Progress and delivery of health care in Bhutan, the land of the thunder dragon and gross national happiness. *Tropical Medicine and International Health* 16(6):731–736.

Toch M, Bambra C, Lunau T, et al. 2014. All part of the job? The contribution of the psychosocial and physical work environment to health inequalities in Europe and the European health divide. *International Journal of Health Services* 44(2):285–305.

Toro PA, Tompsett CJ, Lombardo S, et al. 2007. Homelessness in Europe and the United States: A comparison of prevalence and public opinion. *Journal of Social Issues* 63(3):505–524.

Travis J, Western B, and Redburn S. 2014. *The Growth of Incarceration in the United States: Exploring Causes and Consequences*. Washington, DC: National Research Council.

Truth and Reconciliation Commission of Canada. 2015. *Honouring the Truth, Reconciling for the Future: Summary of the Final Report of the Truth and Reconciliation Commission of Canada*. Winnipeg: TRC.

UN. 2015. *The Millennium Development Goals Report 2015*. New York: UN.

UN-DESA [Department of Economic and Social Affairs of the United Nations]. 2014. World's population increasingly urban with more than half living in urban areas. https://www.un.org/development/desa/en/news/population/world-urbanization-prospects.html. Accessed December 18, 2015.

———. 2015. *State of the World's Indigenous Peoples, 2015, 2nd Volume, Indigenous Peoples' Access to Health Services*. New York: UN-DESA.

———. 2016. *International Migration Report 2015*. New York: UN.

UNDP. 2006. *Human Development Report 2006. Beyond Scarcity: Power, Poverty and the Global Water Crisis*. New York: UNDP.

———. 2014. *Human Development Report 2014. Sustaining Human Progress: Reducing Vulnerabilities and Building Resilience*. New York: UNDP.

———. 2015. *Human Development Report 2015: Work for Human Development*. New York: UNDP.

UN General Assembly. 2010. Resolution adopted by the General Assembly on 28 July 2010. A/RES/64/292.

UN-HABITAT. 2014. *Background Paper on World Habitat Day 2014*. Nairobi: UN-HABITAT.

UNHCR. 2011. Refugee women – "survivors, protectors, providers." http://www.unhcr.org.uk/resources/monthly-updates/november-2011-update/refugee-women-survivors-protectors-providers.html. Accessed November 11, 2014.

———. 2016. *Global Trends: Forced Displacement in 2015*. Geneva: UNHCR.

UNICEF. 2014a. *Committing to Child Survival: A Promise Renewed. Progress Report 2014*. New York: UNICEF.

———. 2014b. *Ending Child Marriage: Progress and Prospects*. New York: UNICEF.

———. 2014c. *Hidden in Plain Sight: A statistical analysis of violence against children*. New York: UNICEF.

———. 2016. *Female Genital Mutilation/Cutting: A Global Concern*. New York: UNICEF.

UNICEF and WHO. 2015. *Progress on Sanitation and Drinking Water – 2015 Update and MDG Assessment*. Geneva: WHO.

Van de Poel E, O'Donnell O, and Van Doorslaer E. 2007. Are urban children really healthier? Evidence from 47 developing countries. *Social Science and Medicine* 65(10):1986–2003.

Victora CG. 2013. Commentary: Participatory interventions reduce maternal and child mortality among the poorest, but how do they work?. *International journal of epidemiology* 42(2):503–505.

Vuillermoz C, Aouba A, Grout L, et al. 2014. Estimating the number of homeless deaths in France, 2008-2010. *BMC Public Health* 14(1):690.

Walker A and Wong C. 2005. Conclusion: from Confucianism to globalisation. In Walker A and Wong C, Editors. *East Asian Welfare Regimes in Transition: From Confucianism to Globalisation*. Bristol: The Polity Press.

Walker SP, Wachs TD, Grantham-McGregor S, et al. 2011. Inequality in early childhood: Risk and protective factors for early child development. *Lancet* 378(9799):1325–1338.

Walmsley R. 2013. *World Prison Population List (Tenth Edition)*. London: International Centre for Prison Studies.

Walters KL, Mohammed SA, Evans-Campbell T, et al. 2011. Bodies don't just tell stories, they tell histories. *Du Bois Review: Social Science Research on Race* 8(01):179–189.

Webster PC. 2015. Housing triggers health problems for Canada's First Nations. *Lancet* 385(9967):495–496.

Whitehead M. 1992. *The Concepts and Principles of Equity and Health*. Copenhagen: WHO EURO.

Whitmee S, Haines A, Beyrer C, et al. 2015. Safeguarding human health in the Anthropocene epoch: Report of The Rockefeller Foundation-Lancet Commission on planetary health. *Lancet* 386:1973–2028.

WHO. 2011. Rio Political Declaration on Social Determinants of Health. World Conference on Social Determinants of Health. October 21. Rio de Janeiro: WHO.

———. 2013a. *Global and Regional Estimates of Violence against Women: Prevalence and Health Effects of Intimate Partner Violence and Non-Partner Sexual Violence*. Geneva: WHO.

———. 2013b. *Global Status Report on Road Safety 2013: Supporting a Decade of Action*. Geneva: WHO.

———. 2013c. *Moving towards Health in All Policies: a Compilation of Experiences from Africa, South-East Asia and the Western Pacific*. Geneva: WHO.

———. 2014. *Global Status Report on Violence Prevention 2014*. Geneva: WHO.

———. 2015a. Healthy diet: Fact sheet. http://www.who.int/mediacentre/factsheets/fs394/en/. Accessed February 9, 2016.

———. 2015b. *WHO Estimates of the Global Burden of Foodborne Diseases*. Geneva: WHO.

———. 2016a. Global Health Observatory (GHO) data: Health Equity Monitor. http://www.who.int/gho/health_equity/en/. Accessed January 28, 2016.

———. 2016b. Preventing unsafe abortion: Factsheet. http://www.who.int/mediacentre/factsheets/fs388/en/. Accessed July 21, 2016.

———. 2016c. *WHO Guidelines on the Management of Health Complications from Female Genital Mutilation*. Geneva: WHO.

Wilkinson R and Pickett K. 2009. *The Spirit Level: Why More Equal Societies Almost Always Do Better*. New York: Bloomsbury Press.

———. 2015. Income inequality and health: A causal review. *Social Science and Medicine* 128:316–326.

Williams DR and Mohammed SA. 2013. Racism and health I: Pathways and scientific evidence. *American Behavioral Scientist* 57(8): 1152–1173.

World Bank. 2015. World Development Indicators. http://data.worldbank.org/data-catalog/world-development-indicators. Accessed July 10, 2015.

Wright EO. 1998. *Debate on Classes*. London: Verso.

WWAP [United Nations World Water Assessment Programme]. 2015. *The United Nations World Water Development Report 2015: Water for a Sustainable World*. Paris: UNESCO.

Zhou M, Wang H, Zhu J, et al. 2015. Cause-specific mortality for 240 causes in China during 1990–2013: A systematic subnational analysis for the Global Burden of Disease Study 2013. *Lancet* 387(10015):251–272.

8

HEALTH UNDER CRISES AND THE LIMITS TO HUMANITARIANISM

Key Questions:

- What are the different types of humanitarian crises and in what ways are they affected by human action?
- How does responding to health under crisis situations differ from addressing ongoing health needs?
- What should be the responsibility of global health humanitarians in the face of war and militarism?

In January 2010 a 7.0 magnitude earthquake (and 52 aftershocks) struck Léogâne, Haiti, just west of the capital, killing an estimated 220,000 people, injuring more than 300,000, and displacing 2.3 million in the deadliest disaster in recent years (UNOCHA 2011). One year later, in New Zealand's costliest ever disaster, a 6.3 earthquake, also as measured on the Richter scale, struck the city of Christchurch, causing 185 deaths and 6,800 injuries. Why was there such a marked disparity in casualties between these two earthquakes? No doubt differences in intensity, geology, population density, and timing were all important, but even these factors are insufficient to explain the extent of the differential impact.

As this chapter will explore, a crucial set of factors has to do with social conditions and physical infrastructure, in turn shaped by historical and political contexts. In addition, inequalities in preparedness between and within countries are reflected in differential disaster responses. Most, but not all, high-income countries (HICs) invest in public health and emergency preparedness, whereas many low- and middle-income countries (LMICs), especially the lowest-income, lack resources to mitigate and address disasters (Spiegel 2005). In the case of Haiti, as examined ahead, the earthquake came atop a legacy of centuries of slavery, political and economic oppression by foreign and domestic elites, sanctions, and structural adjustment programs. New Zealand, by contrast, has among the world's strongest building codes (upgraded again since the Christchurch earthquake), undergirded by among the oldest (albeit eroding in recent decades) comprehensive welfare states.

The role of political economy factors in provoking or worsening these crises rarely receives attention. While many disasters are termed "natural," the context and consequences of these events are anything but (Page 2003). Simply put, ecological disasters may be inevitable, but calamitous outcomes are preventable.

Even more important (if commonly attracting less media attention) than ecological disasters in terms of their scale and impact are the human-made crises shaped by militarism, contests for power, and contemporary and longstanding conflicts over access to land, minerals, and other resources. The humanitarian emergencies set off by war and violence feature death, disease, and displacement for tens of millions each year, and accompanying untold human suffering. For example, the 2003–2011 US war on Iraq, linked to access and control of oil reserves, terrorism, and geopolitical alliances, led to almost half a million deaths; it has now expanded through the Levant region, killing hundreds of thousands more, and forcing half of Syria's 22 million inhabitants from their homes in just 4 years.

Tending to the enormous needs generated under such conditions brings many people into the global health field, but understanding the political economy context of crises and the political factors aggravating (many well-intentioned) responses may not be part of people's training.

Much of this textbook has focused on the ongoing health consequences of poor living and working conditions, racial, class, and gender oppression, and a host of other policies, processes, and forces operating at the household, societal, and global levels. Here we examine what happens to health when already dire circumstances are greatly intensified by additional crises (for guiding definitions see Box 8-1). We begin with an examination of a series of recent ecological disasters, their health implications, and the international responses to these events. The chapter continues with an analysis of hunger and famine and the politics surrounding them. Next, we turn to: militarism, war, terrorism, and public health; the effects of nuclear, chemical, and biological weapons; and the escalating crises of refugees and displaced populations. We then explore complex humanitarian emergencies (CHEs), their scope and impact on nutrition, mental health, vulnerable groups, and population displacement, homing in on several illustrative case studies. The chapter concludes with reflections on the reach, dilemmas, and limits of humanitarianism and contemplates the potential role of a political

Box 8-1 Definitions and Classifications

Crisis—a critical incident that involves death, serious injury, or threat to a significant number of people or animals, or damage to the environment.

Humanitarian emergency—a crisis characterized by large population displacement, food shortages, and social disruption, necessitating a humanitarian response.

Complex humanitarian emergency (CHE)—a situation of civil strife, armed conflict or war, or political instability resulting in social upheaval and excess mortality (Brennan and Nandy 2001). Although called emergencies, CHEs may be protracted in duration.

Refugee—as defined by the 1951 UN Convention Relating to the Status of Refugees, a person who has fled their own country because of well-founded fears of persecution based on race, religion, nationality, membership of a particular social group, or political affiliation (UNHCR 2000).

Asylum-seeker—a person who enters a country and appeals to State authorities for refugee status (UNHCR 2000).

Internally displaced person (IDP)—a person who has been forced from his/her home for similar reasons as a refugee, but who remains within the internationally recognized borders of his/her country. IDPs are not protected by the UN refugee convention but are protected by international human rights law, domestic law, and by international humanitarian law if they are located in armed conflict situations (without participating directly) (ICRC 2004).

Disaster—"A disaster is a sudden, calamitous event that seriously disrupts the functioning of a community or society and causes human, material, and economic or environmental losses that exceed the community's or society's ability to cope using its own resources. Though often caused by nature, disasters can have human origins" (IFRC 2014).

Ecological disaster—disastrous consequences to organisms (including humans) and the environment caused by concomitant "natural" events (hydro-meteorological, biological, and geophysical) and human-induced events (e.g., climate change or social policies that lead to poorly-constructed housing in geologically vulnerable areas).

economy approach in preventing crises and transforming humanitarian responses.

ECOLOGICAL DISASTERS AND THEIR IMPLICATIONS

Key Questions:

- What are the public health implications of hurricanes, tsunamis, cyclones, typhoons, floods, earthquakes, droughts, and related disasters?
- What is the role of international actors and agencies in disaster assessment, response, preparedness, and mitigation?

Ecological disasters,[1] provoked by so-called "natural events" such as major storms and earthquakes, can cause a great deal of suffering—mortality, disability, and displacement—and typically elicit (at least in the short-term) a highly visible global response from the public, governments, multilateral agencies, and a range of humanitarian and nongovernmental organizations (NGOs) and donors. Ecological disasters lay bare miserable social conditions that are otherwise not top public health priorities locally or globally.

LMICs undergo approximately the same number and intensity of ecological shocks as richer nations, but experience many more deaths. Moreover, within countries, poorer regions suffer disproportionate deaths and disability from disasters as well as far greater suffering and loss of possessions and livelihoods (Strömberg 2007). Disasters exacerbate the pre-existing deprivation experienced by disadvantaged communities, as witnessed in Nepal's severe April 2015 earthquake and aftershocks, which killed more than 7,600 people, injured 16,000, destroyed 300,000 homes, and displaced over 3 million people (Shrestha 2015). The extensive and long-term damages that accompany many crises (and often go unaddressed) contribute to cycles of poverty, disaster, disease, and death.

Nonetheless, the scale of disasters can be deceptive. Despite Western media sensationalizing, with few exceptions, disasters have a large impact locally and may provoke significant morbidity and social disruption while contributing only a small fraction of global or even local mortality. The nearly 6 million children under five who die annually from preventable causes (roughly 16,000 per day) are the daily equivalent of over twice the number who died in the 2015 Nepal earthquake. In Nepal alone, about 20,000 children under 5 died in 2015 (WHO 2016). Yet this news did not enter into mainstream media coverage. This is not to diminish the importance of crises but to put them in perspective, especially in the context of the limited attention garnered by ongoing needs as opposed to emergencies.

In this section we review two kinds of ecological disasters—water-related and earthquakes (heat waves are discussed in chapter 10)—and explore the health implications of and responses to these events.

Major Storms, Floods, and Tsunamis

Water disasters, whether provoked by major storms and waterway breaks or even minor rainfall alterations, can wipe out a community's entire infrastructure, including housing, schools, roads, workplaces, and health centers. In the 1930s almost 5 million people are estimated to have died in a series of floods in China; in 1999 over 20,000 people died in a single mudslide in Venezuela; Cyclone Nargis killed some 140,000 people in Myanmar in 2008; Typhoon Haiyan killed over 6,300 people in the Philippines in 2013, affecting 14 million people; and severe flooding and displacement are a perennial occurrence in Assam, other northern Indian states, and parts of Bangladesh and Pakistan. As the following cases show, the effects of major storms and flooding are most devastating to vulnerable populations, whose lodgings, neighborhood infrastructure, and surrounding conditions are already precarious, who receive the least attention from governments, and who have the fewest resources to escape and mitigate the effects of disasters and rebuild afterward.

Tsunami in South Asia

The Indian Ocean tsunami (massive wave/s triggered by an undersea earthquake) that struck a band of 14 countries on December 26, 2004, killing upwards of 227,000 people in a single day (and thousands more subsequently), is an extreme example of water devastation (Telford and Cosgrave 2006). Entire coastal communities were taken by surprise and leveled in seconds by the force of the wall of water. The impact of the wave was over in a matter of minutes, but in many areas coastal flooding continued for days.

Indonesia was hardest hit, with an estimated 200,000 people confirmed dead or missing. Sri Lanka saw 35,000 deaths, India 18,000, and at least half a million people were displaced and lost all of their possessions in each of the three countries, with grief and rebuilding struggles continuing for over a decade. The first to respond were the affected communities themselves, followed by government and civic groups.

In hardest hit Aceh province, the Indonesian army and marines already present (enforcing a repressive military occupation since a late 1980s independence movement) delivered supplies of food and water, cleared roads, and repaired bridges in the immediate aftermath of the disaster. That the most capable responders were the same military forces that had committed widespread human rights abuses causing thousands of civilian deaths substantially complicated these efforts (Fletcher, Stover, and Weinstein 2005).

News of the tsunami sparked a huge outpouring of international assistance. Governments of 13 countries deployed military contingents to Aceh, sparking concerns over humanitarian "neutrality." Survivor assistance agencies arrived in droves, with the few experienced and well-equipped NGOs vastly outnumbered by a plethora of amateur outfits. Many privately funded organizations failed to coordinate with UN agencies or other NGOs, leading to duplication and confusion. Disaster supply routes, as invariably, were clogged with inappropriate donations of clothing, perishables, and other unnecessary items.

The UN's Office of Coordination of Humanitarian Affairs (OCHA) was created in the 1990s to help organize such responses, yet as seen in the tsunami response, it often has little command—even of UN organizations—due to conflicting interests among multiple agencies and inter-organizational competition over donor and media attention, as well as the challenges of coordinating strategic versus long-term operational responses (Stumpenhorst, Stumpenhorst, and Razum 2011).

Compared with ongoing emergencies elsewhere, the tsunami response was extremely well funded. In total, US$14 billion was committed to the relief effort from across the globe (UNICEF 2009b). Médecins Sans Frontières (MSF) even took the rare step of no longer accepting earmarked donations for the tsunami response (Krause 2014).

Extensive media coverage of the tsunami propagated several myths associated with sudden impact disasters: that unburied human remains pose outbreak threats; that survivors face severe epidemics; and that the most urgent needs are international medical teams and equipment. However, the risk of infection from unburied corpses is overstated (Kirkis 2006), with specific precautions only required for deaths from cholera or hemorrhagic fevers. As well, though communicable disease transmission among the displaced is a legitimate concern, the risk may be overemphasized (Kouadio et al. 2012). Finally, the most urgent needs are not only for medical and trauma care, but also for potable water and food, the provision of which reduces outbreak occurrence (Watson, Gayer, and Connolly 2007).

Storms of the Caribbean and Central America

On August 29, 2005, Hurricane Katrina struck the US Gulf coastline. The hurricane caused a storm surge of over 20 feet, resulting in large-scale damage to the states of Louisiana and Mississippi. More than 75% of New Orleans's 500,000 residents became internally displaced within hours. The following day, Lake Pontchartrain's waters breached the levees and flooded most of the city. While tens of thousands of people fled before the storm hit, many more had no immediate means of transportation, particularly poor and elderly people living alone. As the water level rose, residents in flooded neighborhoods were forced into enclosed attics, hacking holes to escape onto rooftops to await rescue.

The hurricane killed over 1,200 people (including many who drowned in their own homes or trying to escape) and destroyed many local hospitals, clinics, and public health facilities, plus thousands of homes. Katrina was the deadliest US hurricane since 1928, and became the country's costliest disaster on record (over US$200 billion in losses) (CDC 2006), albeit enormously profitable for private contractors, many of whom were already enjoying a large role in the Iraq war (Klein 2007).

Full-scale disaster assistance was slow and ineffectual, prompting criticism of the US government's Federal Emergency Management Agency (FEMA). FEMA director Michael Brown retorted: "I don't make judgments about why people chose not to leave, but, you know, there was a mandatory evacuation of New Orleans" (CNN 2005), implying that those left stranded had only themselves to blame. Outrageously, Brown disregarded the fact that the local government and FEMA all but abandoned the city's vulnerable groups. Indeed, news reporters reached stranded residents more quickly and efficiently than official government rescue teams, which took several days to arrive.

Katrina was a disaster waiting to happen, but hardly a natural one (Smith 2006). Over the years, large tracts of marshland designed to protect against a storm surge were drained and paved for short-term profit. The levee system, built to protect New Orleans from flooding, was only designed to withstand a category 3 storm. One year before Katrina, the US Army Corps of Engineers' request for US$100 million to repair the levees was only funded at US$40 million, typical of the US's public infrastructure neglect at the time. City administrators had done no serious disaster planning despite repeated warnings from the scientific community and a 2001 US government report listing a hurricane striking New Orleans as the country's third most likely disaster (after an earthquake in San Francisco and a terrorist attack in New York City) (Krugman 2005).

One country with an exceptional record of coping with hurricanes is Cuba. Like other Caribbean islands, Cuba, with a per capita income around one third of the US's is hit by tropical storms of varying severity every year. In 2004's Hurricane Jeanne, over 3,000 Haitians died from flooding and mudslides. But in neighboring Cuba no one died. Cuba performs several storm preparation exercises every year, encouraging universal participation. As a result, hurricane casualties remain very low notwithstanding Cuba's material shortages resulting from a decades-long US embargo (see chapter 13). The UN has praised Cuba's Civil Defense System as a model for LMICs (Bermejo 2006). Cuba sought to extend its disaster response expertise to the Katrina-affected region, with President Castro proposing to send over 1,500 medical personnel, but the US government rejected the offer (MEDICC Review 2015) (though it did accept donations from other LMICs).

Hurricane Katrina exposed New Orleans's deep underlying inequalities. The disaster was provoked by a storm and exacerbated by infrastructure neglect, but social forces—a toxic mix of racism and classism—determined who lived and who died (Hartman and Squires 2006). The vast majority of those who could not escape the storm were low-income African-Americans, for whom the catastrophe is ongoing. Ten years later, residents were still struggling to rebuild their lives (Hobor 2015). In addition to lost jobs, homes, disrupted education, and family separation, longtime community institutions and organizations were wiped out. Returning residents found a city only half its previous size, and moneyed interests forced privatization on public housing and schools (Gotham 2012). As a Congressman from Baton Rouge put it, "We finally cleaned up public housing in New Orleans. We couldn't do it, but God could" (Arena 2012, p. 145).

Atlantic hurricanes and other "acts of God" frequently hit Central America too. A prime example is 1998's Hurricane Mitch. The interplay among historical, political, and ecological factors is key to understanding the scale of devastation. Starting in the 19th century, much of the region was turned into fruit plantations owned by US conglomerates, domestic elites, and complicit politicians. Over decades, wide swaths of land were stripped of indigenous flora and over-farmed to make way for export-based profiteering, and the US military invaded and occupied whenever US economic (and under the Cold War, political-ideological) interests were threatened. For example, in 1954, after Guatemala's president Jacobo Arbenz sought to redistribute United Fruit Company lands to peasants, the US Central Intelligence Agency (CIA) orchestrated a coup against him and reversed the reforms, opening the way for further Western corporate investment. In Nicaragua, longtime dictator Anastasio Somoza himself owned 20% of the country's farmland, while tens of thousands lived on riverbanks that routinely flooded during storms.

Compounding these problems, two decades of structural adjustment policies (see chapters 2 and 9) hollowed out government social programs and depleted funding for evacuations, emergency supplies, vaccines, and secure housing, leaving much of the region's population further exposed to annual storms. The simultaneous growth of export-oriented agribusiness forced hundreds of thousands of farmers in Honduras to migrate to precarious shantytowns and mountainsides, where their agricultural practices led to deforestation (Ensor and Ensor 2009; Smith 2013).

Political economy factors did not decide the timing or intensity of Hurricane Mitch (though climate change may have played a role), but they magnified its effects and were instrumental in determining the extent of human and physical destruction (Cockburn, St. Clair, and Silverstein 1999). When the hurricane hit, barren hillsides gave way to destructive landslides: approximately 10,000 people were killed, over 13,000 injured, and more than 9,000 went missing in Honduras, Nicaragua, and Guatemala, with 1.5 million people displaced (Ensor and Ensor 2009).

Earthquakes

Second to water disasters, earthquakes are the ecological disasters that cause the greatest damage to people and infrastructure. Earthquakes affect most regions from the Americas and Caribbean to Europe and Asia, where China's 2008 Sichuan earthquake killed up to 90,000 people. Infrastructural prevention and preparedness play key roles in mitigating the impact. For example, a December 2003 earthquake struck Bam, Iran killing an estimated 50,000 of the city's 200,000 residents, leaving over 100,000 homeless, and destroying approximately 60% of the city's buildings, many made of mud bricks (including the 2,000-year old Citadel). The high death toll was attributed to lax enforcement of municipal construction regulations (Kenny 2009).

Illustrating the complexities of response is the massive 2005 7.6 magnitude earthquake that struck Kashmir (a territory claimed by both India and Pakistan, and beset by ongoing struggles for self-determination against an increasingly militarized Indian presence). Due to the remote, widespread, and mountainous earthquake zone—and Pakistan's refusal of assistance from Indian defense force helicopters unless they were loaned and flown by Pakistani pilots—rescue assistance was delayed (McGirk 2005). Yet hostilities also gave way to mutual cooperation during the relief effort (Rajagopalan 2006). An estimated 75,000 people lost their lives, with 76,000 injured, 2.8 million left homeless, and 2.3 million lacking secure access to food and essential goods (Brennan and Waldman 2006) in an area marked by poverty and a dearth of health infrastructure. Emergency response crews undertook mass vaccination for measles and sought to establish water and sanitation services. With over half the region's health facilities destroyed, provision of health care—with special attention to women's access—became a primary focus of relief. Yet overcrowding, poor sanitation, and limited access to potable water remained ongoing impediments.

Because lack of coordination had been identified as a contributing cause of death in prior disasters, the UN's OCHA implemented a new "cluster" approach in Kashmir. A lead agency was identified within each sector to improve coordination, quality, consistency, and predictability of the relief effort. Clusters were established to address health, emergency shelter, water and sanitation, logistics, camp management, protection, food security, nutrition, telecommunications, education, and reconstruction. While the cluster approach has been cited as increasing effectiveness of humanitarian aid thanks to greater coordination, it has also been marred by turnover in on-the-ground leadership, limits on inclusiveness, and inadequate accountability to affected populations (Humphries 2013).

Concerns mounted in Kashmir as winter set in and millions faced food deprivation and exposure to the cold. The efforts were also hampered by "relief fatigue," as the Indian Ocean tsunami that struck 10 months earlier had occupied so much attention on the global stage. Though the earthquake caused an estimated US$5 billion in damages, the World Bank delivered just US$470 million in recovery aid.

Shifting from Response to Preparedness

The UN General Assembly declared the 1990s the International Decade for National Disaster Risk Reduction to highlight the need to increase preparedness and response capacity. Disaster risk reduction's prevention component involves actions that lessen the chances of a disaster occurring. For example, aiding farmers to diversify their crops and sources of income may prevent occurrence of famine. The companion preparedness component encompasses activities that reduce the impact of the disaster when it happens (CARE 2001), such as making a disaster plan, building seawalls, and requiring buildings to be earthquake-proof. The Pan American Health Organization (PAHO) has an extensive disaster preparedness unit that supports member states in training around emergency response, risk communication, health logistics, mass casualty management, emergency care and treatment, and other competencies (PAHO 2010). Preparedness also rests on ongoing societal attention to redressing racial/ethnic, class, gender, and geographic inequities in education, housing, nutrition, transport, and other domains, because the most marginalized populations are usually hit hardest by disaster. Especially when humanitarian organizations are involved, preparedness activities can be difficult to plan, fund, and implement because they blur the lines between relief and development, domains that are often organized into narrowly focused silos (Kopinak 2013).

Furthermore, local politics and economic interests can clash with preparedness priorities. Take, for example, Sanjoy Ghosh, an Indian aid worker with the Association of Voluntary Agencies for Rural Development for the North East, who was making great strides erecting permanent flood protections and lessening flood impact on local populations in Assam (Mahanta 2013). His 1997 abduction and assassination by the United Liberation Front of Assam was likely linked to the logging industry, which saw sizeable revenues from constructing annual flood barriers and considered Ghosh's efforts a business menace.

At the international level, early warning systems have expanded in recent years. Volcano monitoring systems have enabled timely evacuations and are credited with averting disasters in Iceland, Chile, and elsewhere. Following the 2004 Indian Ocean tsunami, the UN launched a multi-hazard International Early Warning Programme, building on existing tsunami warning systems. But these systems are not perfect. Despite Japan's sophisticated tsunami warning technology, scientists underestimated the potential impact of the March 2011 tsunami waves (which left 20,000 people dead or missing and caused hundreds of billions of dollars of damage), in part because the magnitude of the undersea Tohoku earthquake (9.0) was unprecedented.

In sum, preparedness efforts interact with ongoing prevention and existing societal conditions. As we shall see next, surveillance systems for hunger and famine that monitor rainfall, crop production, and market prices, and map priority zones, can contribute to preparedness for groups vulnerable to hunger. But these constitute only part of the story.

FAMINE AND FOOD AID

Key Question:

- Why and how are famine and food aid political issues?

Though typically instigated by flooding, drought, or soil depletion/desertification—generating crop failure—famines are not sudden ecological disasters but rooted in political and economic circumstances linked to lack of land tenure, lack of democracy, poverty and indebtedness, war, and forced displacement. Precursor to famine is food insecurity, experienced daily by hundreds of millions of people whose nutritional intake is limited by problems of availability, access, quality, utilization, or stability over time. Chronic food insecurity generates vulnerability to hunger and famine as well as illness or death. Transitory food insecurity can lead to acute malnutrition, wasting, and illness, and chronic food shortages can cause micronutrient deficiency diseases, stunting in children, and increased mortality.

As discussed in chapter 7, central to food security is food sovereignty, that is, autonomy of decisions around production and consumption of food, contextualized socio-culturally. Food sovereignty addresses the political and economic underpinnings of much food insecurity, from land grabbing and land degradation to maldistribution, and inappropriate, unsustainable, and inequitable food production—involving monoculture, overcropping, and the use of damaging pesticides, fertilizers, and seeds. These problems, in turn, derive from agribusiness and export-oriented pressures, corruption, inadequate infrastructure, and oppression of poor, rural populations. Importantly, ensuring food security requires that people be fed, regardless of the source or kind of food, whereas food sovereignty also addresses long-term prevention in the context of local farming and preferences. For this reason, international responses to famine and food insecurity often aggravate lack of food sovereignty, creating dependence on foreign food supplies and impeding return to local production.

Root Causes of Famines and Hunger

Approximately 800 million people are chronically malnourished (though actual numbers of people experiencing hunger may exceed 2 billion), with recent increases to almost 230 million people in sub-Saharan Africa alone (UN 2015b; FAO, IFAD, and WFP 2014). A range of places in Africa and Asia have faced extreme food crises or famines in recent years, including various countries across the Sahel (Devereux and Berge 2000; FAO 2015) and in Southern Africa, where 40 million people faced food insecurity in 2016 due to drought (UNOCHA 2016a). In North Korea, a combination of unsustainable agricultural practices, loss of food sources, rising global food prices, floods, internal displacement, conflict and delays around food aid, and poor government planning resulted in up to 3 million deaths in the late 1990s (Noland, Robinson, and Wang 2001). In Somalia, over 250,000 people died in a 2011–2012 famine amid rising costs of food imports, drought, internal conflict and terrorism, and large-scale internal displacement (Maxwell and Fitzpatrick 2012).

Sparsely settled Niger, with the world's lowest HDI ranking and subject to recurring famines, exemplifies how famine can unfold. A 2005 food crisis left 2.5 million people food insecure and over 15% of children suffering from moderate to severe acute malnutrition. Food scarcity was blamed on locusts and drought, yet the 2004 crop yield was only 9% lower than previous years. A deeper analysis points to the Niger government's adherence to free market economics: it eliminated key regulations of the import-oriented cereal market, leading to large price fluctuations amid currency devaluation, new taxes on foodstuffs, and little attention to food relief (Cornia and Deotti 2015). Incredibly, Niger exported food during this time of food deficits. By 2010 more than seven million people were affected by food shortages (IFRC 2011b), exacerbated by an influx of refugees fleeing terrorism in Mali and Nigeria. Although the Niger government called for help more swiftly in 2010 than in 2005, enabling a better coordinated and effective response, the underlying causes of famine persist.

In southeast Africa, landlocked and subsistence-farming-based Malawi has experienced years of cyclical food shortages, with a 2001–2002 famine causing up to 1,000 deaths and severe food shortages. After the 2005 harvest ranked as the worst on record, with almost 5 million of the country's 12 million people requiring emergency food aid, Malawi's President Bingu wa Mutharika vowed not to let it happen again. For years the World Bank pressured small countries to eliminate fertilizer subsidies (while many HICs continue to heavily subsidize their own farming industries; see chapter 9). Breaking with these recommendations, the president increased fertilizer subsidies in 2004–2005, enabling widespread soil enrichment among smallholders (Dugger 2007). The subsidies had a notable impact: small farmers increased their yields, and Malawi generated a food surplus, though it exported grain even as it continued imports (Chirwa and Dorward 2013). However, after a few years Malawi again faced crisis due to rising food and agricultural input prices, insufficient rain, currency devaluation and inflation, a general economic downturn, and the same president's corrupt and autocratic turn. In 2012 more than 11% of the population (1.6 million people) experienced severe food shortages (UN Africa Renewal 2015).

Politics of Food Aid

The World Food Programme (WFP) is the UN's food relief agency, the largest humanitarian organization of its kind. It is entirely reliant on annual food and cash pledges plus emergency appeals. Despite recognizing the causes of hunger to include such socio-political factors as poverty, war and human displacement, and unstable food prices (WFP 2015), WFP's ability to address these underlying issues is constrained by tied donations from governments, corporations, and individuals.

Informing the political act of declaring a famine and WFP's decision to act, the Famine Early Warning Systems Network monitors food security in 36 countries. According to the UN, only extreme instances of food insecurity should prompt declaration of a famine. The criteria are: 20% or more of households facing extreme food shortages with a limited ability to cope; acute malnutrition rates over 30%; and death rates exceeding two people per day per 10,000 people (UN News Centre 2011a). With governmental consent, the food aid system kicks into action. The UN can declare famines if governments fail to do so, as happened in Somalia in 2011 (UN News Centre 2011b).

Most large bilateral aid agencies are involved in food aid, which comprises the largest proportion (25%–30%) of humanitarian assistance (Harvey et al. 2010). The WFP and UN Food and Agricultural Organization (FAO) provide emergency food assistance, daily food programs, and technical assistance in food and agricultural production and distribution. These and other agencies deliver food aid to the *most vulnerable* groups, but this approach neglects groups *less vulnerable but still in need.*

While food aid may be needed at particular moments, recipient countries are often worse off after receiving food donations. In addition to displacing local production and jeopardizing the livelihoods of local farmers, food aid is linked to dumping, crowding out of other exporters, transnational companies using their donations to capture new markets, and profiteering (Kripke 2005). Most countries give food aid in grant form rather than tied to donor agri-industry, but the majority of US food aid is "monetized" (i.e., sold in recipient countries to generate cash)—almost 70% in 2009—though this proportion is now declining (Clapp 2012). The United States has been the only country to "sell" food aid to recipients through concessional financing or export credit guarantees (Kripke 2005).

Food aid can create dependence, especially when not accompanied by sustainable agricultural support: for example, in 2008, the United States donated US$460 million to Ethiopia for food aid, but just US$7 million for agricultural development (Perry 2008). Additionally, food aid may be requisitioned by particular political factions or coopted by military forces: in Somalia, al-Shabab militants extort a US$20,000 security fee from WFP every 6 months (Nunn and Qian 2014).

For the United States the provision of food aid is as much a political decision as a humanitarian one. US food production, though privately owned and operated, is heavily government-subsidized, in part through food aid. This system allows private interests to profit from the production, procurement, packaging, transport, and distribution of food aid, and via the sale of food surpluses. The US government requests bids from a limited list of prequalified companies, and arranges for transport on US-flagged ships. The bidding process results in expenses that are higher than market costs, with a handful of transnational companies benefiting—from 2004 to 2007, more than half of Food for Peace's food aid came from just four corporations: Archer Daniels Midland, Bunge, Cargill (which control the US wheat industry, together with Louis Dreyfus), and Cal Western Packaging (Clapp 2012).

There are growing efforts to reform the food aid system. In 2007 the NGO CARE took the bold step of refusing US government support (US$45 million per year) to deliver food aid, claiming that US programs risked harming the very people they purported to help. CARE held that not only was purchasing food at local markets more efficient, but it helped sustain local farmers, many of them women (CARE 2013). The shakeup in food aid has also led to increasing challenges to monetization, emergence of new donors beyond HICs, food aid being gradually untied from donor country industries, and greater local and regional food procurement, which can shorten arrival time by 70 to 100 days (Elliott and McKitterick 2013). These changes have repercussions not only in the context of ecological disasters but also under war conditions, for CHEs, and in refugee camps.

WAR, MILITARISM, AND PUBLIC HEALTH

Key Questions:

- What is the impact of militarism and war on public health?
- Why should nuclear, chemical, and biological weapons be banned?

As we have seen, the political economy context substantially shapes the susceptibility to, responses around, and health outcomes of disasters. Yet its

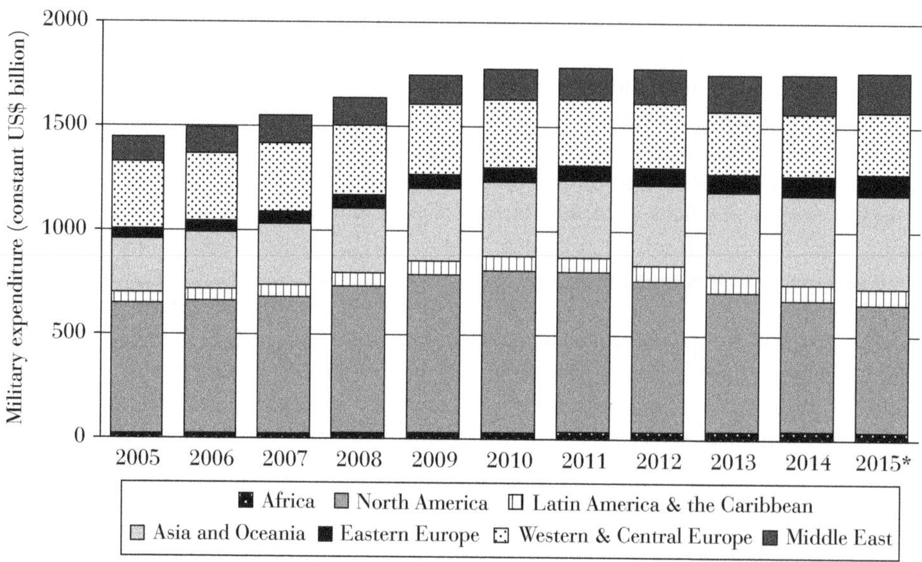

*Note: Data for the Middle East region were not available for 2015; instead the 2014 data were used again.

Figure 8-1: World military expenditures, 2005–2015 (constant 2014 US$ billion).
Data Source: SIPRI Military Expenditure Database 2015, https://www.sipri.org/databases/milex.

explanatory resonance in "human-manufactured" crises, most notably wars, is even more profound (the health toll of other kinds of "human-made" crises, such as environmental disasters and climate change, are discussed in chapter 10).

In the course of human history, more so now than ever, wars have been an integral part of the political economy of societies. The causes of war are complex, relating to local and far larger struggles linked to ethnic and class conflicts, longstanding animosities, corruption, repression, and colonial legacies of exploitation and oppression; war is often inflamed when abundant resources are controlled by a few.

Development, manufacturing, and sale of arms, maintenance of military forces and capabilities—together constituting the "military-industrial complex"—and mobilization of the population for military goals and policies take up a large portion of nations' resources, diverting attention and money from other societal needs around income security, education, and health equity. In the last century, wars became a preferred solution to a range of social, political, and economic issues (both local and global), and militarism—the subordination of the ideals or practices of a nation's government or of its civil society to military goals and policies—became a dominant ideology of modern societies.

Albeit with variations among major spenders (Figure 8-1), military expenditures have risen in both absolute and real terms since 1996, following a short-lived "peace dividend" after the Cold War. In 2015, world military expenditures amounted to an estimated US$1.8 trillion, 2.5% of global GDP. The United States is overwhelmingly the largest actor, contributing 34% of world military spending in 2015, with over US$15 trillion in military expenditures since the end of World War II (SIPRI 2015).

Weapons manufacture and sales are concentrated in the hands of a small group of powerful countries. Between 2004 and 2011 the five permanent members of the UN Security Council (China, France, the Russian Federation, the United Kingdom, and the United States) produced and sold 85% of the world's arms (Global Issues 2013).

World expenditures on weapons research exceeds the combined spending on developing new energy technology, increasing agricultural productivity, and controlling pollutants. Some military discoveries spill over into the civilian sector, including the development of the Internet, antimalarial insecticides, drones, and advances in surgery and field medicine. But not only does militarism lead to huge expenditures on the development, production, and testing of nuclear and conventional weapons, the enormous sums going to financial and human resources for military services diverts from social investments in improving the quality of life.

Moreover, promotion of violence as an acceptable way to resolve conflicts contributes to increased violence worldwide (Levy and Sidel 2008). Newer technologies such as unmanned drones heighten tensions and generate civilian casualties even without declaration of war (Kolsy 2015). Countries marked by militarism, for instance the United States, Honduras, Afghanistan, and South Africa, also tend to have the highest rates of gun violence (Geneva Declaration 2015). In such settings, the political forces advocating gun ownership may garner such power that they can paralyze efforts to limit access to guns or even study the consequences of gun use. For example, since 1996 the US Congress has refused to fund the Centers for Disease Control and Prevention to carry out research on gun violence as a public health issue (Kellermann and Rivara 2013). Militarized societies normalize police violence and fragment communities, especially in contexts of poverty and discrimination. In

Box 8-2 Drug Wars

Narco-trafficking generates enormous violence, mortality, and disability: drug wars involve not only military and police forces and battling drug cartels, but also entail targeted killings of civilians and terrorizing of local populations. The lucrative illegal drug trade (worth hundreds of billions of dollars per year) has long plagued the Americas (especially due to cocaine-trafficking) and Central Asia (with Afghanistan producing 80% of the world's heroin [UNODC 2014b]). Of the approximately 1,000 tons of cocaine produced annually (mostly in Colombia, Peru, and Bolivia), half goes to North America, and just under half to Europe (UNODC 2008), where domestic and transnational crime syndicates control distribution. Though international markets generate demand, the brunt of violence is suffered by those in producing and transporting countries caught amid competition between cartels (Mejia and Restrepo 2013).

Poverty and inequality undergird crime in much of Latin America, but drug trafficking has brought gang violence to a new level, involving soaring homicide rates and widespread corruption and money laundering, jeopardizing the economy and governance of various countries (UNODC 2008). Colombia experienced an estimated 90,000 drug-related homicides between 1994 and 2008 (Mejia and Restrepo 2013), and tiny El Salvador has more violence-related casualties today (due to drug violence) than during its deadly civil war in the 1980s. Likewise, from 2006 to 2012, there were approximately 60,000 deaths (with up to 20,000 more in 2013–15) and spiraling crime linked to Mexico's booming drug trade corridor (Espinosa and Rubin 2015). The violence has led hundreds of thousands of Central Americans, including tens of thousands of unaccompanied children, to flee northward via clandestine routes; large numbers face deportation from the United States and Mexico back to the very dangers they sought to escape.

Traffickers have become increasingly militarized, with rising gun violence alongside militarized state responses and complicit politicians, all acting with impunity. In 2014, 43 students in Ayotzinapa, Mexico were forcibly "disappeared," with the federal government's blaming of a local drug cartel discredited by human rights investigators, who found a flagrant cover-up of police and military involvement and torturing of witnesses and suspects (Valencia Villa et al. 2016).

Efforts on the part of the US government to stem the drug trade have been critiqued for overlooking the role of US actors in drug money laundering, and for supporting government and military repression (Mercille 2011). In sum, the illegal drug trade has created war-like conditions in some places, with a huge localized cost in human suffering, escalating militarism on all sides, and inadequate responsibility taken by outside actors (Laurell 2015).

Baltimore, USA, poor African-American neighborhoods have experienced decades of social disinvestment while being "hyper-targeted" by the police force's "war on drugs," together contributing to high stress rates and poor health (Gomez 2016). (For more on drug wars see Box 8-2.)

Although militarism is not identical to war, it is war's precursor and companion, readying societies logistically, technically, practically, politically, psychologically, socially, and economically. The effects of militarism are particularly detrimental in LMICs. Every yuan, real, and rand that goes to armed forces and weapons means neglect or underfunding of nutrition, housing, education, and health services. Arms spending can destabilize governments, as during the destructive civil wars in Liberia and Sierra Leone through the 1990s, in which the harvesting of raw diamonds subsidized the weapons used in the fighting, in turn fueling further conflict. Wars are also ecologically devastating and a windfall for weapons contractors and arms manufacturers.

Militarism's immense burden on civilians is even evidenced in approaches framed as alternatives to militarism. Sanctions and embargoes have been used by high-income powerful nations to impose penalties on countries whose foreign and domestic policies they oppose. Embargoes were once considered a "safe" way to punish a country's leadership, but research shows they have serious effects on the health and well-being of the most disadvantaged populations (Thoms and Ron 2007). Before the first Gulf War in 1991, embargo-related shortages of food and the deterioration of infrastructure significantly increased infant and child mortality in Iraq (Garfield and Daponte 2000). Ultimately, the impact of sanctions was greatest not on leaders, but on those least able to bear the burden.

Perhaps most importantly, the deep integration and normalization of war into the world's political and economic order has blurred the traditional line between military personnel and civilians, making

Box 8-3 The Movement Against Landmines

Landmines and unexploded ordnance (bombs, shells, grenades) kill or wound thousands of people annually, even decades after conflicts resolve. There are undetonated landmines in over 59 countries, concentrated in Afghanistan, Cambodia, Colombia, Myanmar, Pakistan, and South Sudan (Duttine and Hottentot 2013). In 2014, there were over 3,600 landmine casualties, comprising at least 1,243 deaths and 2,386 injuries (International Campaign to Ban Landmines 2015). Cheap, durable, effective, and easy to make, landmines are designed to kill or injure. The blast and shrapnel cause traumatic wounds to the extremities, chest, genitals, and face; need for amputation is common.

Because landmines remain buried after hostilities cease, farmers, civilians looking for firewood, and children playing can all inadvertently activate the mechanism. Women and girls are particularly subject to landmine injuries given their responsibilities for collecting water or firewood. Over 400,000 landmine survivors require care, rehabilitation services, and significant hospital resources in affected countries. Civilians who lose limbs may have limited access to proper prostheses. Amputees may suffer discrimination and are often considered unemployable.

The only certain way to prevent casualties from landmines is to ban them. In the late 1980s, NGOs drew attention to the deadly ongoing effects of landmines in Afghanistan and Cambodia (Stover, Cobey, and Fine 1997), and in 1991 an international movement started by Physicians for Human Rights and Human Rights Watch, among other groups, called for an unconditional ban on all landmines that detonate on contact. In 1992, the United States and EU member states agreed to a 5-year moratorium on the sale, transfer, production, or export of antipersonnel mines (Cobey and Raymond 2001), preceding development of the the 1997 Mine Ban Treaty. As of 2015, 162 countries had ratified the treaty, but the United States (in spite of its 1992 promise), China, and Russia have not signed. The number of countries producing mines has dropped from 54 to 11, although six of them, including India, Pakistan, China, and Russia, have formal moratoriums on their export (International Campaign to Ban Landmines 2015).

the latter a "legitimate" target for military actions. The 20th century was the deadliest on record, with an estimated 45 million combat casualties. Yet civilian losses were three times higher, reaching a staggering 146 million people. The civilian toll now comprises 80% to 90% of war-related deaths (Roberts 2010).

Since the end of World War II, at least 30 million people have died in 250 armed conflicts, often driven by the interests of international arms producers and traders (Mahmudi-Azer 2011). War's indirect effects on civilians include population displacement, loss of social services, unstable food sources, destruction of infrastructure, and the long-term impact of leftover landmines (Wiist et al. 2014) (Box 8-3).

Nuclear, Chemical, and Biological Weapons

The industrialization of war during the 20th century led to the development of new kinds of armaments—chemical, biological, and nuclear weapons of mass destruction (WMD). During World War I, military, political, and corporate leaders in the major warring nations, particularly Germany, developed chemical weapons (CW) (e.g., mustard gas and chlorine) that were responsible for the deaths of thousands of soldiers (Box 8-4). Various countries also sponsored research on biological weapons (BW). Revulsion against the use of CW provided impetus for the Geneva Protocols of 1925 banning the use of chemical and biological weapons (CBW) in warfare. However, the Geneva Protocols did not prohibit the development, production, stockpiling, and transport of such armaments, and between the two world wars, major military powers utilized this loophole to develop CBW programs.

BW programs expanded during World War II, with the United States, Japan, and Great Britain weaponizing anthrax and other pathologic organisms, and culturing microorganisms and insect vectors. Japan performed grisly experiments with biological agents on captured prisoners of war and civilians, and used chemical agents freely in the Manchurian war from 1937 to 1945. In addition, Japanese airplanes dropped various infectious agents, including plague bacteria, on numerous Chinese cities, with reported outbreaks of disease among the civilian population.

By far the world's most deadly and egregious use of CW was by the Nazis during World War II: upwards of 1 million Jews plus at least 100,000 others were gassed using Zyklon B in concentration camps; and more than 1.7 million Jews, 90,000 people with disabilities, over 4,000 Roma, and untold numbers (probably in the millions) of Soviet prisoners of war and Soviet civilians were killed in stationary chambers and vans with carbon monoxide.[2]

Since then, intentional military use of CBW has involved: napalm deployed in wars in Korea (1950–1953) and, especially, Vietnam (1955/61–1975), where it caused widespread destruction of foliage and infrastructure and innumerable deaths from horrible burns (Neer 2013); mustard and nerve gas, used in the 1980s Iran–Iraq war (Ali 2001); and, according to the Organisation for the Prohibition of Chemical Weapons, use of chlorine and other poisonous gases in the ongoing war in Syria (2011–present), killing up to 1,500 people. There has also been isolated CBW use for terrorizing purposes, such as in the 1995 Tokyo subway sarin attacks. Although not included in the international conventions, tear gas and pepper spray, causing severe eye, lung, and mucous membrane irritation (and unknown long-term effects) are routinely deployed by police forces around the world against public protesters.

During World War II, the United States developed the world's first nuclear weapon—the atomic bomb. Its use against Japan in August 1945 is the only instance of nuclear weapons directed at civilian or military populations. The bombs, dropped on Hiroshima and Nagasaki, killed 118,000 people and injured 30,000 in the first year alone, with 95% of casualties occurring within a 1.3 mile radius of the explosions, and up to 300,000 deaths overall (Yokoro and Kamada 1997). The bombs caused the near complete destruction of the physical infrastructure and populations of the two cities and generated long-term health effects of radiation and deep psychological trauma among survivors. Delayed effects included fetal deaths in 1946, elevated rates of leukemia in the 1950s, thyroid cancer in the 1960s, and breast and lung cancer in the 1970s.

Within a few years, the Soviets also developed nuclear weapons, leading the Cold War rivals to produce tens of thousands of nuclear warheads. Over time the horizontal proliferation of nuclear weapons

Box 8-4 Chemical Weapons and Environmental Health

The first recorded use of a weapon of mass destruction was in 1915 in Ypres, Belgium amid World War I. Experiencing a shortage of explosives, Germany released 180 tons of liquid chlorine into the air. The resulting asphyxiation affected 15,000 Allied solders—one third of whom died.

During World War II it was discovered that certain chemicals were as toxic to plants as the new nerve gases were to people. These new defoliant herbicides were used as weapons in several conflicts in Africa and Southeast Asia during the 1950–1975 period, targeted against food crops and forest vegetation that provided concealment (WHO 2004).

A notable example is the extensive spraying of the herbicide Agent Orange by US forces during the Vietnam War. Agent Orange contains dioxin—one of the most toxic chemicals known—which causes: immune, reproductive, developmental, and nervous system damage; endocrine disruption; cancer; altered lipid metabolism; liver damage; birth defects; and skin lesions. Approximately 12 million gallons of Agent Orange were sprayed during the war in southern Vietnam, damaging two million hectares (Martin 2012) and multitudes of people, the largest dioxin contamination known to date. The environmental impact is still apparent, with elevated dioxin levels found in Vietnamese populations whose diet is fish based and among the children of those exposed (Allukian and Atwood 2008). In 2012, the United States made a belated commitment of US$43 million to reduce contamination around Danang airport, the primary dioxin storage site during the Vietnam War (Fuller 2012). This marks the first cleanup effort by the United States after decades of denial of responsibility. A US District Court dismissed a 2005 class action lawsuit on behalf of millions of Vietnamese against the companies that supplied the chemicals, citing that dioxin spraying was not chemical warfare and that more substantial evidence for a causal connection to health problems was necessary. Even the US government's paltry US$11.4 million program to help Vietnamese people with disabilities was not formally linked to Agent Orange. The number of Vietnamese affected continues to be debated, but the 2005 lawsuit claimed that 3 million Vietnamese were exposed, and 800,000 suffered from serious health problems, including 150,000 children born with severe birth defects (Allukian and Atwood 2008).

More recently, US and Colombian "war on drugs" programs have sprayed rural areas in Colombia with the herbicide glyphosate in attempts to eradicate coca production. Hundreds of thousands of kilometers^2 have been sprayed, with 172,000 hectares sprayed in 2006 alone (Mejía 2012). While proponents claim that glyphosate is safe, numerous environmental organizations argue that these sprayings are linked to human and livestock health problems (AIDA 2007). In May 2015 Colombia banned glyphosate following the WHO International Agency for Research on Cancer's labeling of glyphosate as "probably carcinogenic to humans" (Fritschi et al. 2015).

programs has expanded beyond a core group of states (United States, Russia, the United Kingdom, France, and China) to include India, Pakistan, North Korea, and Israel (undeclared). South Africa, Ukraine, Belarus, and Kazakhstan have acceded to the Nuclear Non-Proliferation Treaty and no longer have weapons, and Iran agreed in 2015 to make its nuclear program exclusively peaceful.

Collective agreements to control WMD are one way of preventing their health hazards. A 1975 Biological Weapons Convention (BWC), calling for the elimination of all biological weapons programs, currently has 173 parties, with 14 UN member states having neither signed nor ratified the convention (UNOG 2015). Originally proposed by the United States to keep states without nuclear weapons from developing BW programs, the United States ensured the BWC would allow stockpiled biological agents for "defensive" purposes, such as vaccines and countermeasures. In 2001 the US government spurned a tentative global accord on a more vigorous BWC, due to pressure from the US pharmaceutical industry regarding loss of proprietary information, and US desire to expand its own "biodefense" programs in potential violation of the BWC. But in 2011, the US administration agreed to the terms of the seventh BWC review conference (The White House Office of the Press Secretary 2011).

Similar concerns about CW, underscored by their use during the Iran–Iraq war, led to the ratification and entry-into-force of the Chemical Weapons Convention (CWC) in 1997, with 190 parties. Enforcement of the CWC has been constrained by inadequate funding for inspections. Of note, while Syria acceded to the CWC in 2013 following international pressure, it was since found to have used CW, highlighting the difficulty of enforcing such treaties. Moreover, technical challenges surrounding the safe destruction of stockpiles have delayed elimination of the vast and dangerously deteriorating CW arsenals of the United States and Russia. Neither country met the CWC's 2012 deadline for stockpile destruction, and both received extensions. The United States now projects a 2023 completion date, and Russia a 2020 date (Arms Control Association 2014). Iraq has also missed its 2012 deadline for destruction of its small stockpile.

Most daunting are global efforts to control and end the dangerous and ever-costly nuclear arms race, on which US spending alone amounted to US$7.5 trillion (in 2005 dollars) from 1940 to 2005 (Cirincione 2005). Huge volumes of toxic and radioactive waste generated by global nuclear weapons manufacture has poisoned countless workers and communities, threatening public and environmental health for future generations (see chapter 10).

The Nuclear Non-Proliferation Treaty of 1968, to which all but five nations are signatories, commits nuclear weapons states to move speedily through disarmament and the eventual elimination of their nuclear weapons stockpiles. Toward this end, the 1996 Comprehensive Test Ban Treaty (CTBT), still not ratified by 32 countries including the United States, would end all nuclear weapons testing. The Nobel prize-winning activist medical group International Physicians for the Prevention of Nuclear War was instrumental in finalizing the CTBT. There is renewed attention to creating a Nuclear Weapons Convention, supported by the United Nations and the International Committee of the Red Cross (ICRC), to extend the principles of the CWC and BWC to the nuclear realm, given the "catastrophic humanitarian consequences of any use of nuclear weapons" (Maurer 2015).

Terrorism and Public Health

On September 11, 2001, two hijacked planes crashed into the twin World Trade Center (WTC) towers in New York City. The buildings quickly collapsed due to enormous fires, trapping several thousand office workers unable to escape. The hijackers crashed a third airliner into US Department of Defense headquarters, and a fourth plane, also heading to Washington, D.C., plunged into a field after passengers battled the hijackers. In addition to the 19 hijackers, 2,997 people died, comprising office workers, airline passengers, and rescue workers.

The 9/11 attacks caused the single largest loss of civilian life from a coordinated act of terrorism. New York City's Department of Health mobilized a month-long emergency response, then shifted to worker-injury prevention and surveillance, bioterrorism surveillance, environmental health monitoring and cleanup, and ensuring food and water safety, rodent and vector control, and related public education (Holtz et al. 2003).

Immediately following the attacks, nearly 10% of Manhattan residents showed signs of acute traumatic stress and other mental health problems (Galea et al. 2002). Thousands of tons of WTC debris containing high levels of toxins, including known carcinogens (dioxins, cadmium), have led to a range of illnesses. Several thousand emergency responders have either retired on disability or experienced chronic health problems as a result of their exposure at the scene (Yip et al. 2016). The longer term effects are being monitored through a 20-year registry of over 70,000 people (Brackbill et al. 2006).

Although the long-term psychological and carcinogenic consequences of 9/11 remain significant, the US-led "war on terrorism" has generated far larger consequences globally, with terror begetting more terror in an escalating cycle. The war waged on al-Qaeda (the Jihadist group responsible for 9/11) and on Iraq and Afghanistan has not only caused massive civilian mortality and destruction, it also helped spawn the more decentralized Wahhabi Sunni group Daesh (which calls itself ISIS, also referred to as Islamic State group). Daesh operates on an ever more diffuse and deadly scale involving extremist factions in multiple countries throughout the region and beyond, affecting, directly and indirectly, much of the world. This situation of seemingly intractable complexity has been facilitated and worsened by the West's militarized approach, which ignores extremism's social, political, and historical roots, from imperial exploitation to nefarious Cold War and commodity-driven calculations and alliances.

In addition to terrorism linked to the wars the United States launched in Afghanistan (2001–present, with up to 100,000 casualties) (Crawford 2015) and Iraq, spilling into Syria (see ahead for both), in recent years there have been repeated Daesh-inspired group bombings and automatic weapon and vehicle assaults in Belgium, France, Germany, and elsewhere across Europe, in Turkey, Indonesia, Lebanon, Iraq, of a Russian airliner, among other incidents, each causing up to hundreds of casualties and generating military counter-attacks with huge death tolls among civilians and medical facilities, and in turn sparking Daesh retaliation. Other conflicts, such as between Pakistan and India (dating from imperial Britain's exit from India and its 1947 partition, which uprooted some 15 million people and led to the deaths of up to 1 million), Russia and Chechnya, Palestine and Israel, and civil wars in Lebanon, Libya, and Algeria, have also seen multiple deadly terrorist acts in recent decades.

Terrorism is not new, but it has accelerated since 9/11, with no country (outside direct war zones) more affected than Pakistan. From 2003 until mid-2016, over 21,000 Pakistani civilians died from terrorist attacks, involving hundreds of bombings, suicide attacks, and railway assaults (Institute for Conflict Management 2016). HICs are highly concerned about terrorism strikes within their borders, propagating a culture of fear and heightened militarism, but only 5% of the estimated 107,000 terrorist fatalities from 2000 through 2014 occurred in OECD countries. In 2013, 82% of the almost 18,000 deaths from terrorist attacks occurred in Iraq, Afghanistan, Pakistan, Nigeria, and Syria. Iraq, bearing the heaviest brunt of terrorism that year, had 2,492 incidents.

In sub-Saharan Africa, the Somalia-based militant Islamist group al-Shabab has carried out deadly attacks in Kenya and Uganda. In Mali, al-Qaeda terrorized the country's north and took over the storied city of Timbuktu in 2013, swiftly eliciting French bombing and ever more attacks and hostage-takings, even as Mali's pleas for debt relief and social development to address deep impoverishment were long spurned by Western donors and bankers (Prashad 2015). Meanwhile, Boko Haram, resurgent since 2009, has terrorized parts of Nigeria and Cameroon through frequent deadly attacks affecting thousands of people, the abduction and rape of hundreds of women and schoolgirls, and kidnappings of business leaders, police officers, and soldiers, in seeking to create a "pure" Islamic state in Nigeria's north (Institute for Economics and Peace 2014).

The impact of these events reverberates widely for those directly affected, for those living in circumstances of danger and anxiety, and for much of humanity living under conditions of heightened militarism, uncertainty, and increasing violations of human rights. Yet beyond the reported number of casualties, little is known about the long-term effects of terrorism on health in "non-Western" settings: the security concerns of Western powers privilege the suffering of their "innocent" populations over comparable horrific realities among much larger numbers of affected "innocents" in "counter-terrorism" target countries. All suffering merits public health attention, but the global health community has an important role to play in ensuring equity in care and research on the health effects of terrorism across the world.

The "war on terror" has harmed public health in other ways. In 2013, the CIA allegedly organized a fake vaccination campaign as part of its hunt for al-Qaeda leader Osama bin Laden in Abbottabad, Pakistan, recruiting (or duping) Pakistani physician Shakil Afridi (imprisoned by Pakistani authorities) to go door-to-door offering hepatitis B vaccinations. Purportedly the campaign's real goal was to collect DNA evidence from bin Laden's offspring to identify his presence (Mullaney and Hassan 2015). True or not, once uncovered this story destroyed trust in vaccination campaigns in the area, particularly jeopardizing polio vaccination efforts: in the years following the deception, 78 vaccination workers were killed by militants accusing the eradication program of espionage (Agence France-Presse 2015). In 2013, Deans of 12 prominent US schools of public health wrote an outraged letter to US President

Obama decrying the use of vaccination programs for intelligence purposes.

REFUGEES AND INTERNALLY DISPLACED PERSONS: NUMBERS, TYPES, AND PLACES

Key Questions:

- Where are the recent "hot spots" for refugees and internally displaced persons (IDPs)?
- Why are their numbers growing?

Together with the toll of death, illness, and injury, militarism and wars lead to massive displacement within and beyond borders. According to the United Nations High Commissioner for Refugees (UNHCR), the UN agency charged with the protection of "populations of concern," in 2015 there were 65.3 million people forcibly displaced around the world, a number that has been rising steadily since 2000 (Figure 8-2). The total number of displaced persons consists of refugees (21.3 million, including 5.2 million Palestine refugees), IDPs (40.8 million), and asylum-seekers (3.2 million) (UNHCR 2016a).

Although refugee numbers declined from the early 1990s until recently due to fewer armed conflicts and several large repatriations, such as the return home of displaced Guatemalans from Mexico, Liberians from Ghana, and Hutus to Rwanda, since 2010 the total number of refugees has soared again (UNHCR 2016a).

In 2015 alone, there were 12.4 million newly displaced individuals (including 8.6 million IDPs, the highest number on record [Figure 8-3], and 1.8 million refugees), quadrupling the number of newly displaced persons in just 4 years (UNHCR 2016a) (Table 8-1). This worst year for displacement since World War II has created a "post-apocalyptic" situation in camps, major receiving communities, and along routes of flight (Feffer 2015). The largest recent surge of refugees and IDPs stems from the war in Syria that risks engulfing the entire Levant. The Syrian war is itself linked to the protracted Iraq War (and "Coalition of the Willing" occupation). It has involved continuing use of drones and airstrikes—against Daesh among other targets—by the United States, France, United

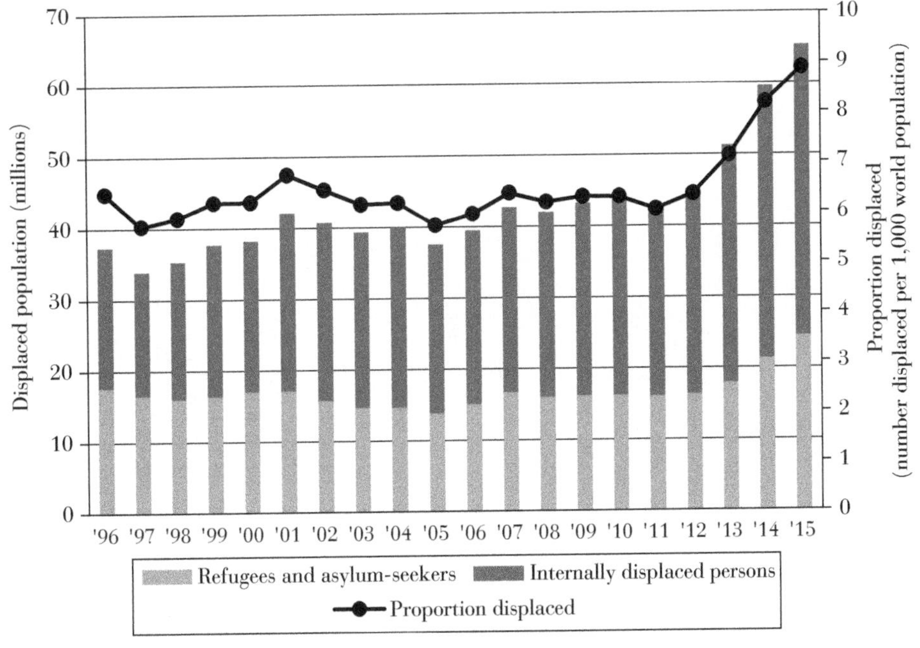

Figure 8-2: Trend of global displacement and proportion of world population displaced, 1996–2015.
Source: UNHCR (2016).

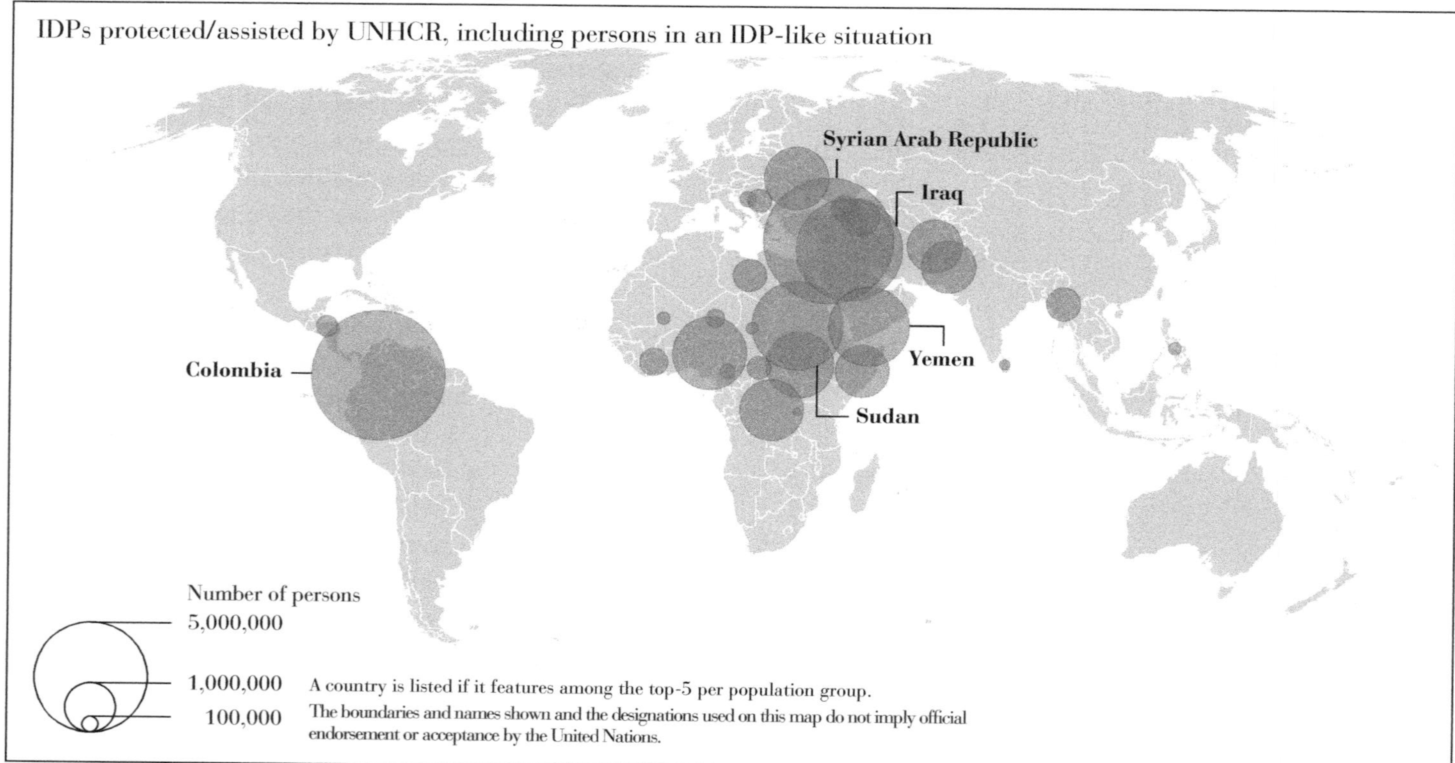

Figure 8-3: Map of complex humanitarian emergencies causing internal displacement, 2015.
Source: UNHCR (2016).

Table 8-1 Main Origins of the World's Refugees, 2015

Place of Origin	Estimated Persons
Palestinian Territories[a]	5,149,742
Syria	4,850,792
Afghanistan	2,662,954
Somalia	1,123,022
South Sudan[b]	778,629
Sudan	622,463
Democratic Republic of Congo	541,291
Central African Republic	471,104
Eritrea	379,766
Ukraine	321,014
Vietnam	313,155
Burundi	292,764
Rwanda	286,366
Pakistan	277,344
Iraq	261,107
China	212,911
Myanmar	198,685

[a]For Palestine, number of refugees reflects those under United Nations Relief and Works Agency for Palestine Refugees in the Near East (UNRWA) mandate; for the other countries, numbers reflect those under UNHCR mandate.

[b]Refugees from South Sudan may be included under Sudan due to lack of separate statistics.

Data Source: UNHCR (2016a); UNRWA (2015).

Kingdom, and other NATO countries, as well as Russia, the Syrian government, and certain Gulf States. Since 2011, almost 5 million Syrian refugees have fled to Turkey, Jordan, Lebanon, and other countries, with 6.6 million internally displaced (UNHCR 2016a), living in crowded settlements with water and electricity shortages, and limited health services (Bashour 2015). Turkey is now the biggest host of refugees (2.5 million), followed by Pakistan (1.6 million), Lebanon (1.1 million), and Iran (~1 million) (UNHCR 2016a). This is why Asia is currently the site of the world's largest "population of concern" (Table 8-2).

A large proportion of UNHCR's "populations of concern" are young people (over 50% are under 18 years old, with many under age 5). Dubbed the "year of fear," 2015 became the most dangerous year for children since 1945 (Tisdall 2015). Children and adolescents, especially unaccompanied children who have been separated from families during war or refugee flight, are extremely vulnerable to forced labor, abuse and violence, recruitment into armed groups, sexual exploitation, HIV, and trafficking (with children constituting one third of trafficked persons). Refugee and displaced children are often denied access to education, basic assistance, and asylum (UNODC 2014a).

Unfolding Refugee Situations and HIC Negligence

Refugee and IDP crises are proliferating in multiple parts of the world simultaneously. Since 2012 the Central African Republic (CAR) has been in turmoil, lacking a functional government, and facing ongoing civil conflict. Almost one million people (one fifth of the population) are refugees or IDPs (UNHCR 2016a), and virtually all of the country's children have witnessed violence and fear for their lives (Jones 2015). Both the African Union and the United Nations have deployed peacekeepers to CAR but humanitarian

Table 8-2 Total Population of Concern to UNHCR by Region of Asylum, 2015

Region	Refugees	Asylum-Seekers	Returned Refugees	IDPs of Concern	Others of Concern	*Total Population of Concern*
Africa	4,769,513	1,367,409	130,781	11,197,751	2,811,708	20,277,162
Asia	8,366,000	396,662	68,372	17,265,028	3,607,984	29,704,046
Europe	1,808,289	1,083,567	468	1,918,326	676,942	5,487,592
Latin America & the Caribbean	87,294	44,887	1,794	7,113,067	412,102	7,659,144
North America	409,090	305,810	–	–	–	714,900
Oceania	43,707	21,606	–	–	4,581	69,894
Total	**15,483,893**	**3,219,941**	**201,415**	**37,494,172**	**7,513,317**	**63,912,738**

Data Source: UNHCR (2016a).

organizations are being denied access to parts of the country by local militias (UN 2015a).

Meanwhile, though most attention to the military conflict in eastern Ukraine has focused on political dimensions, there has been a rapid swelling of over 1.3 million asylum-seekers to Russia, Belarus, Moldova, Poland, Hungary, and Romania (UNHCR 2016c) and 1.5 million IDPs within Ukraine (UNHCR 2015b).

Two other ongoing humanitarian crises, involving large numbers of refugees fleeing war, oppression, and dire economic conditions and making perilous journeys to seek asylum, demonstrate that many HIC governments have a tendency to raise alarms only when their own borders are breached. In recent years millions of political and economic refugees from Syria, Afghanistan, Iraq, Eritrea, Somalia, Nigeria, Gambia, and elsewhere in Africa and the Middle East have made their way to Libya (where civil war has both reduced employment opportunities and facilitated human smuggling) and crossed the Mediterranean Sea in flimsy boats to seek asylum in Europe. In 2015 alone, over 1 million people made the crossing and nearly 3,800 died or went missing. By September 2016, over 310,000 more people had made the trip, with more than 3,600 dead or missing (UNHCR 2016b). Those continuing to make this risky passage, many young and educated professionals, face crowded conditions, violence, and precarious prospects, while those left behind are disproportionately elderly and poor (Morabia and Benjamin 2015). Migrants and asylum-seekers also face tremendous mental health distress, a problem poorly addressed by recipient countries (MSF 2016).

Italy and, especially, Greece are the main frontline recipients of these migrants, many of whom hope to reach Northern Europe via increasingly reluctant Eastern European countries. Though Germany registered over 1 million asylum-seekers in 2015 and Sweden accepted hundreds of thousands (the highest per capita in Europe), the situation remains contentious (European Council on Foreign Relations 2016). Among controversial responses are plans to send migrants rejected by European countries back to Turkey. Failing to provide a collective humanitarian response, the EU is focusing on forestalling migrants at sea and fighting human traffickers, with pledges to provide financial support to sending countries (Casinge 2015). North America, by contrast, has welcomed few Syrian refugees, though in late 2015 Canada began resettling almost 30,000 refugees.

Another crisis concerns the Rohingya, a persecuted Muslim ethnic group totaling over 800,000 people and considered stateless, who are fleeing Myanmar and Bangladesh to Indonesia, Thailand, and Malaysia (Parnini 2013). Conflict in 2012 left hundreds dead and 140,000 homeless. An estimated 100,000 Rohingya have faced exploitation by ruthless smugglers (UNHCR 2015a). Thousands of refugees were stranded at sea, with surrounding governments slow to act. In 2015 Australian politicians rejected asylees outright, claiming a war on human smugglers (Iltis 2015).

In recent years the number of environmental/climate refugees (not documented by UNHCR) has also mounted, stemming from the complex interplay among economic forces, human settlement patterns, and ecological change (see chapter 10). For example, international demand for timber leads to excess logging and loss of forest cover, increasing flood magnitude along rivers and causing dislocation of entire communities from their homes. In 2011 almost 15 million people were internally displaced due to water disasters, largely in Asia. It is estimated that by 2050 there could be 200 million environmental migrants (Warner et al. 2009).

Refugees and IDPs experience high rates of human rights violations such as exploitative working conditions, sometimes lasting for decades, as in the case of Palestinians (Giacaman 2015) (see ahead). Their vulnerability, due to displacement from known surroundings, makes their rights to food, housing, and medical care all the more pressing. Threats to refugee rights range from abuse in the hands of foreign authorities to theft, assault, domestic violence, child abuse, rape, and human trafficking.

COMPLEX HUMANITARIAN EMERGENCIES

Key Questions:

- How does a CHE differ from other types of crises and disasters?
- What are the political economy of health dimensions of CHEs?
- What specific threats are faced by women and children during CHEs?

Protracted military conflicts frequently deteriorate into CHEs, which involve "total or considerable breakdown of authority resulting from internal or external conflict," leading to severe health and social consequences and requiring "an international response that goes beyond the mandate or capacity of any single agency" (IFRC 2011a). CHEs can last for years or even decades, as happened in Sudan, Somalia, and the Democratic Republic of Congo (DRC), contributing to huge numbers of IDPs (Centre for Research on the Epidemiology of Disasters 2013).

It is important to note that while the standard CHE definition describes visible circumstances, it omits key dimensions related to the history of colonialism and ongoing imperialism, asymmetric political and economic power, and social relations that determine who is affected and in what ways. Most recent CHEs arise from civil wars connected to failure in the political and diplomatic arena, yet many of these "internal" conflicts are spurred by competition among and between local and external forces for land or valuable natural resources such as gold, diamonds, or coltan. Such economic interests often become conflated with and heighten ethnic, regional, and class divisions, with civilians recruited and manipulated on behalf of foreign interests into killing, terrorizing, and pillaging entire communities in order to ensure access to resources (Mining Watch Canada 2003).

As with famines, declaring a CHE can be fraught with dilemmas, because it opens the door to UN presence and, increasingly, military intervention. An initial technical indicator of a humanitarian emergency is a doubling of the crude mortality rate (CMR; see chapter 5). Where prior data are not available, the baseline CMR is assumed to be one death per 10,000 people per day, so 2 or more deaths per 10,000 per day is deemed a humanitarian emergency (Sphere Project 2011b). Such quantitative indicators, even when based on incomplete data, allow for comparisons of different emergencies and for monitoring trends within an emergency. A CHE goes beyond a humanitarian emergency, typically involving political and/or sectarian violence, breakdown of social cohesion, disease outbreaks, severe food insecurity, and large-scale population displacement.

The contemporary concern with humanitarian emergencies arose in the context of the 1967–1970 conflict in Biafra, Nigeria. Following Nigerian independence from Britain, the Igbo people sought to secede from the colonially constructed state. Turmoil turned into civil war, resulting in the death of up to three million people (Uzokwe 2003), mostly due to hunger and disease generated by mass displacement and impeded food distribution (Noji and Toole 1997). Responses to this conflict, including the founding of MSF (see ahead), spurred the beginnings of a more outspoken and systematic (public health) approach to such crises. Other instances of prolonged civil strife, food shortages, and significant population dislocation shaping humanitarian responses include: Bangladesh's 1971 liberation war from Pakistan atop the devastation of Cyclone Bhola (with 300,000–500,000 deaths and over 4 million people displaced); the US bombings of hundreds of thousands of Cambodians followed by the 1975–1979 Khmer Rouge terror that led millions of refugees to flee to Thailand (Haas 1991); and the millions of Afghans who fled to Pakistan during the 1979–1989 Soviet-Afghan war.

Particularly horrific, the Rwandan genocide illustrates the sheer dimensions of a CHE and its inseparability from the political economy context. In April 1994, long-festering inter-ethnic tensions, largely deriving from colonial hierarchies, spiraled out of control, and the Interahamwe militia and Rwandan Armed Forces launched a 100-day massacre of approximately 1 million people—mostly Tutsis as well as moderate Hutu sympathizers—in their homes, places of worship, and hiding places in forests and marshes. Roughly 11% of the population, including 85% of all Tutsis in Rwanda, were exterminated, with half a million injured and hundreds of thousands of women and girls raped. The "unimaginable carnage" was essentially ignored by the United States, which did not consider it of immediate national interest. The UN meekly ceded to the Security Council's refusal to recognize the genocide and sabotaged its own peacekeeping force (Orbinski 2009). Belgium and France, former colonial powers with ongoing strategic and business interests in Rwanda, have been accused of complicity, with France secretly sending arms to the Rwandan government (Dallaire and Beardsley 2004).

After the genocide, with the Tutsis now in power, over 2 million people (mostly Hutus) fled to neighboring countries, especially the DRC (then called Zaire), Burundi, and Tanzania, with another one to two million persons displaced within Rwanda. Goma, in Eastern Congo, received masses of refugees, both perpetrators and victims. The CHE saw renewed killings on both sides and severe outbreaks of cholera and dysentery (Van Damme 1995). After just one month, 50,000 refugees died of these preventable diseases, with one of the highest CHE mortality rates (60 times the baseline) ever documented (Goma Epidemiology Group 1995). With the Interahamwe taking control of many camps, the slaughter continued: UNHCR called Zairian refugee camps a "virtual state of war" (Seybolt 1997). Some NGOs (e.g., MSF) withdrew from certain camps in protest of the misappropriation of humanitarian aid; camps were so unsafe that Zairian forces pulled out a few months after agreeing to provide security. UN agencies provided strategic and operational leadership and organized delivery of goods (albeit with numerous donations not matching needs) for the 200 NGOs on the ground to distribute. Many refugees were forcibly returned to Rwanda after outbreak of war in Congo in 1996; most refugees have left the camps in DRC and elsewhere, but given Rwanda's extreme poverty and post-genocide context, the challenges of repatriation persist.

Simultaneous to the Rwandan genocide, another set of humanitarian crises garnering inadequate international response was taking place in the Balkans. Following the post-Cold War breakup of Yugoslavia, in the early 1990s the region experienced a series of civil wars that escalated into CHEs. Involving shifting protagonists pandering to extremist nationalism and engaged in "ethnic cleansing"—often with problematic UN, NATO, and EU military and humanitarian participation—the region was engulfed in conflict for over a decade. In Bosnia-Herzegovina, for example, 2.6 million people became refugees in less than 3 months, with Sarajevo under siege for almost 4 years and requiring a protracted airlift. By the time a peace agreement was signed in 1995, between 97,000 and 200,000 were dead, including some 8,000 people in that year's Srebrenica genocide, and over half the population was displaced (Ahmetasevic 2007; Young 2001). In the Kosovo conflict in the late 1990s, ethnic/racial oppression and violence led to another 12,000 deaths. Throughout, refugees became a target—not only a consequence—of war, with denial of humanitarian assistance used as a weapon (Goodwin 2002). A UN peacekeeping force, UNPROFOR, was meant to enable a humanitarian response, but security problems plagued the 250 relief missions coordinated under UNHCR's lead (Cutts 1999).

Syria and Yemen serve as tragic contemporary examples of CHEs. After years of expanding armed conflict, upwards of 250,000 Syrian men, women, and children have been killed, with many more seriously wounded and traumatized, and over half of the population living in extreme poverty, thousands facing siege and starvation, and nearly 12 million uprooted (UNOCHA 2016b). The deliberate destruction of health facilities has left 13.5 million people in dire need and wholly dependent on humanitarian assistance for survival (UNOCHA 2016b). Strife-ridden Yemen is also facing catastrophe: 21.2 million people rely on humanitarian assistance; hundreds of medical facilities have been shuttered; and millions of children risk dying from pneumonia and diarrhea (UNOCHA Yemen 2016).

CHEs, Public Health, and Mental Health

The health impact of CHEs is greatest where the public health infrastructure is already tenuous, especially when IDPs and refugees arrive into unprepared settings. Countries wracked by war, chronic food insecurity, economic exploitation, political oppression, and net extraction of wealth have limited ability to cope with a massive influx of people. It is precisely these political contexts that have generated the world's most pressing refugee situations.

The acute, or emergency, phase of the displacement of large numbers of people is usually characterized by the highest morbidity and mortality, most commonly due to diarrheal diseases, acute respiratory infections, and malaria, exacerbated by concomitant acute malnutrition. Diarrheal diseases can account for over 50% of deaths during a CHE's acute phase, mainly from inadequate quality and quantity of water, substandard sanitation, overcrowding, poor hygiene, and a scarcity of soap. CHE responses typically emphasize clinical care and vaccination campaigns to prevent outbreaks of cholera, measles, and other outbreak-prone diseases, but these efforts cannot compensate for hazardous living conditions.

Increasingly, populations displaced by CHEs seek refuge in towns and cities rather than refugee camps (Crisp, Morris, and Refstie 2012). However, medical care quality and access inside long-established camps are frequently greater and better funded (and have lower mortality) than services for local populations.

Where there is inadequate health infrastructure, CHEs feature poor maternal outcomes and high neonatal death rates (Morof et al. 2014). As well, ongoing health concerns of tuberculosis, malaria, diabetes, HIV, and other diseases require attention just as they do in non-emergency settings (Sphere Project 2011a).

To help address child health under conflict conditions, in the mid-1980s PAHO pioneered the "Health as (a) Bridge for Peace" program in Central America. Amid El Salvador's civil war, PAHO worked with UNICEF, the Red Cross, and the Catholic Church, among others, to negotiate 1-day, and later 3-day, cease-fires between the government and rebel forces that enabled child immunization against polio, tetanus, diphtheria, and other diseases (de Quadros and Epstein 2002). This approach—involving large-scale social mobilization and the work of thousands of volunteers, health personnel, and guerilla forces as vaccinators during "days of tranquility"—was subsequently adopted by WHO and implemented in Peru, Angola, the DRC, Afghanistan, Croatia, Indonesia, Sri Lanka, and elsewhere.

Mental health is also a leading CHE concern. Most refugees and IDPs exhibit remarkable resiliency, yet the mental health consequences of CHEs can be significant. According to contemporary Western definitions, up to 21% of those who lived through the 1970s Cambodian conflict, for example, experience posttraumatic stress disorder (PTSD) (Mollica et al. 2014). However, applying Western psychiatric understandings and treatment via individualized psychiatric care (e.g., "debriefing") is problematic: such assessments may lack cultural validation (Ertl et al. 2010) and whether these framings are relevant in war contexts or are ever preferable to local understandings and forms of healing is contested (Bracken, Giller, and Summerfield 2016; Fernando 2014; Summerfield 2000). The social construction of PTSD, for instance, is subject to intense debate in multiple contexts (Akyeampong et al. 2015).

The Inter-Agency Standing Committee that coordinates humanitarian assistance across sectors has developed Guidelines on Mental Health and Psychosocial Support in Emergency Settings (IASC 2007) to address some of these concerns. In addition to "cultural competence," listening to communities, and integrating humanitarian mental health care with existing healing services, mental health "first aid" includes ensuring basic needs and mobilizing a gamut of social services.

Nevertheless, humanitarian responses alone cannot possibly address the near complete destruction of society and its institutions that occurs with a CHE. Even where a comprehensive mental health plan supports the normalization of everyday life through reestablishment of sociocultural and economic activities, family reunification, and protection from violence (Mollica et al. 2004), restoring tolerance and peaceful coexistence remains a tremendous political challenge. Healing is a profoundly complex matter and can take generations, if not centuries. For example, although two decades later, the unspeakable genocide in Rwanda seems to have given way to a more stable society with attempts at equity-oriented health and social policies, poverty is growing and under the surface there remain high levels of psychological distress that were likely exacerbated by village level truth and reconciliation tribunals (Brounéus 2010).

Gender-Based Violence and Gendered Economic Consequences of CHEs

At least one in five women have experienced gender-based violence (GBV) in CHEs since the 1990s—in Uganda, Liberia, Sierra Leone, Bosnia, Rwanda, the DRC, Darfur, Syria, and elsewhere (Vu et al. 2014). The problem of rape and abuse during war is hardly new. During World War II, Japanese troops abducted between 100,000 and 200,000 Korean, Chinese, Filipina, Indonesian, and Burmese women to serve as "comfort women" (sex slaves) to the Japanese army (Ashford and Huet-Vaughn 1997). Only 10% of these female prisoners survived the war, and few were alive to receive Japan's formal apologies starting in 1993.

During wartime, public rape is used to terrorize entire communities, forcing flight or submission to captors (Ward and Marsh 2006). During the 1994 Rwandan genocide, Hutu men were urged to rape Tutsi women as an expression of ethnic hatred. The trauma of this humiliation and its long-term psychological effects was magnified for the many women who became pregnant as a result of assault, and/or have suffered from sexually transmitted diseases including HIV (reportedly intentionally spread as further torment) and reproductive health problems.

The social upheaval of CHEs worsens the everyday injustices many women experience, from systematic bias and discrimination leading to smaller provisions of water, food, and soap, to withholding of food for sex and high rates of intimate partner violence. In refugee settings there are particularly high rates of GBV. Hastily erected camps often ignore the security concerns of women and girls, who may be forced to travel unprotected and walk at night to latrines or in search of food, water, and firewood (Leatherman and Griffin 2014). Without the protection of family and friends, they can become sexual prey for refugees, camp guards, and humanitarian relief workers. Gender-based crimes are heavily stigmatized in most countries and thus underreported (see chapter 7), with many women and girls remaining silent due to shame and fear of being shunned by their communities.

While GBV can be reduced in camps through better planning, training, and allocation of supplies, the longer-term economic consequences of CHEs for women and girls is rarely addressed by humanitarian efforts. CHEs leave large numbers of women solely responsible for their families, debt ridden, and with no access to employment. Although humanitarian agencies are rarely equipped to deal with the lasting effects of CHEs, failure to address the material side of survival (and lack of sensitivity to economic realities) means that the lot of women and communities can be forgotten once the acute phase of a CHE is over.

Effects of Violence and War on Children

Presently, 250 million children live in countries affected by conflicts (UNICEF 2016), with an estimated 15 million children directly caught up in the violence of CAR, Iraq, South Sudan, Palestine, Syria, and Ukraine (UNICEF 2014).

The proliferation of deadly warfare technologies such as landmines and small arms has had dramatic consequences for morbidity and mortality: in conflict zones, for every child who dies from armed attacks, three times as many are left severely wounded. Over the last decade, conflict-related wounds have left approximately 4 million children with disabilities; millions more have experienced war-related psychological distress (Schauer and Elbert 2010).

For children, war represents not only acute risk of personal physical and psychological endangerment, but also extreme disruption to normal childhood development, with long-term mental health consequences (Betancourt et al. 2011). In addition to the loss of security, predictability, and the structure of daily life, many children experience infrastructure devastation and family separation; witness atrocities such as rape or killing of friends and family; and directly experience acts of violence, from torture and rape to abduction or forced recruitment as soldiers (UNICEF and United Nations 2009).

An estimated 250,000 "child soldiers" are active in conflicts around the globe. Child soldiers have been used in almost 20 countries, including Afghanistan, Myanmar, CAR, Chad, Colombia, DRC, India, Iraq, Palestine, Philippines, Sierra Leone, Somalia, Sri Lanka, Sudan, Syria, Thailand, and Uganda (Schauer and Elbert 2010). Children conscripted with fighting forces may be forced into combat roles, involved in pillaging villages and mass rapes, or work as porters, cooks, servants, human shields, and sexual slaves (Walk Free Foundation 2014). Child soldiers frequently face torture, forced alcohol and substance use, and persistent psychological threats from their captors (Schauer and Elbert 2010). Abducted girls comprise a significant proportion of child soldiers and can face years of sexual violence, abuse, and unwanted pregnancy (Coulter 2015).

Current and former child soldiers show extremely elevated rates of mental distress, with between one third and almost all affected (Schauer and Elbert 2010). The stigma and discrimination experienced upon returning to their communities further compounds these problems and inhibits reintegration into home communities (Newman 2014).

Ongoing Challenges in Responding to CHEs

While humanitarian aid, often a last resort, may be morally justified, it is not a panacea (Orbinski 2009). Even where need is great, assistance may be limited to a few areas, typically around major hubs, potentially leaving those most vulnerable without assistance. There are further practical questions, particularly in acute conflict settings, regarding treatment of chronic communicable diseases (such as tuberculosis and HIV) whose interruption could exacerbate these conditions (Waldman 2008).

Humanitarian responses have been complicated over the past decade by the UN's endorsement of the "Responsibility to Protect (R2P)" norm authorizing international military intervention to prevent genocide in contexts where sovereign states are unable or unwilling to protect their populations. Invoked in CHEs marked by pervasive violence, for instance Mali, Northern Nigeria, Somalia, and Syria, R2P is "often misconstrued as a mandate for military action" (Moore 2014). The 2011 NATO military action in Libya, for example, is widely considered in the Majority World to have been an abuse of R2P (Adebajo 2016). Humanitarian organizations remain divided on R2P: while protection of civilians and relief workers is a laudable aim, MSF has argued that militarizing aid constitutes an act of war (and war's rationalization) in itself and transforms relief efforts into military targets (Weissman 2010).

Even non-militarized CHE responses can cause harm alongside any good. Food drops were used extensively during the 1990s, but their benefits have come into question because centralized distribution of food attracted people to places with poor sanitation where communicable diseases flourished. Food-based interventions that neglect preventive health services, as during the Sudan emergency during the 1990s, can contribute to outbreaks of vaccine-preventable disease such as measles (Deng 2002).

In 2000, a coalition of humanitarian agencies and disaster experts cooperated to produce the *Sphere Project Handbook*. Proposing a core humanitarian standard, its Charter states that all people in all circumstances have the right to live with dignity and to protection and assistance as described in international humanitarian law, refugee law, and human rights instruments (Sphere Project 2011a). Some NGOs argue that the handbook is too technical and does not place enough emphasis on political solutions and the international community's obligation to provide protection.

Indeed, despite improvements in guidelines and resources for addressing CHEs and protecting affected populations, CHE responses rarely tackle the underlying structural factors and conditions that make these crises so devastating. On one level this may be understandable. Humanitarian organizations and their staffs are trained, organized, and committed to addressing existing suffering and need, not to engage in conflict resolution or advance social and economic policies. But they should at least be aware of the politics of humanitarianism.

Taking a political stance decrying the perpetrators based on evidence at hand is one approach to addressing the underlying causes of CHEs or at least mitigating them once they have started. But this is controversial for groups that wish to maintain "neutrality," may be dangerous for humanitarian workers and UN peacekeepers, and does not guarantee that the world will listen or respond (Magone, Neuman, and Weissman 2012). For example, Roméo Dallaire, Force Commander for the UN Assistance Mission for Rwanda during the genocide repeatedly requested UN reinforcements before the violence escalated out of control, but was met with a pullback of forces instead (Orbinski 2009).

Case Studies of Conflict, CHEs, and Public Health

Wars in the Democratic Republic of Congo (First and Second Congo Wars, or African World War): Colonial and Transnational Origins

From 1884 to 1908, King Léopold II of Belgium considered Congo his personal property. He ran a ruthless economic system based on forced labor—leading the population to plunge from approximately 20 million to 10 million people—until he was forced to formally relinquish control of the Congo Free State to the government of Belgium. Under ensuing colonial rule, brutal economic exploitation and political repression continued, with various European and US interests acquiring a stake in the Congo's enormous natural wealth in diamonds, uranium, and other minerals (Hochschild 1998).

After a violent struggle, Congo won its independence from Belgium in June 1960, under the leadership of Patrice Lumumba, an impassioned critic of colonial oppression and advocate of Congolese unity and pan-Africanism. Shortly after Lumumba was democratically elected the country's first prime minister, the United States and Belgium plotted to eliminate him, allegedly fearing that Congo's valuable mineral resources would get into Soviet hands. The CIA-sponsored assassination was carried out by Belgian and local accomplices with UN and British complicity (de Witte 2002).

In 1965, army leader Joseph Mobutu (later called Mobutu Sese Seko) staged a coup d'état and installed himself as president of the country (subsequently known as Zaire). One of the world's most infamous dictators, Mobutu ruled the country for three decades with Washington's firm backing, pocketing billions of foreign aid dollars along the way. He was overthrown in May 1997 by strongman Laurent-Désiré Kabila, succeeded by his son Joseph in 2001. From 1996 and for over a decade, war raged in eastern and southern Congo among dozens of factions involving nine countries, and including both Hutu and Tutsi militias continuing their conflict in and around the post-Rwandan genocide refugee camps in eastern Congo, all with utter disregard for the local population.

Fighting was also driven by competition over control of lucrative gold, tin, diamond, uranium, copper, zinc, and coltan (used for consumer electronics) deposits, involving both national and transnational corporate interests (Van Reybrouck 2014). A UN Security Council Panel of Experts found that the commercial activities of over 100 transnational mining companies contributed to and benefited from the DRC wars, but Canada and other OECD governments where mining companies are based have failed to investigate the role of these corporations in the conflict (Kneen 2009).

The magnitude of death during the Congo Wars is unfathomable. Four surveys (including one with 19,500 households in 750 clusters) conducted in the DRC determined that 5.4 million people died due to the conflict between 1998 and 2007, a loss of roughly 9% of the 2007 population of 57 million. The overwhelming majority of deaths were due to infectious and malnutrition-related diseases: respiratory infections, diarrhea, and malaria, plus neonatal and pregnancy-related conditions, the latter reflecting health services breakdown. In eastern regions, a shocking 9.9% of deaths in children under 5 were reportedly caused by measles, with rates as high as 15% where conflict was concentrated, reflecting patterns of inordinately high child and overall deaths in war zones (Coghlan et al 2009) (Table 8-3). Extreme sexual violence against women and girls was rampant, leaving up to 2 million mutilated, shunned,

Table 8-3 Comparison of Mortality Before and During War: Violence in the DRC and Iraq

	Crude Mortality Rate	Under-5 Crude Mortality Rate
Pre-war period (2001-2003) in Iraq[b]	2.89	NA
War time (2003-2011) in Iraq[b]	4.55	NA
Pre-war period (1984) DRC[a]	1.3	NA
War time (2004) DRC[a]	2.1	4.5
Health zones in DRC not reporting violence (2003–2004)[a]	1.7	3.1
Health zones in DRC reporting violence (2003–2004)[a]	3.0	6.4
Ongoing post-war conflict in DRC (2007)[a]	2.2	5.0

[a]Deaths per 1,000 people per month for crude mortality rate. For under-5 crude mortality, the denominator of total children under-5 is much larger than the standard denominator of 1,000 live births per year, necessitated by deficient birth registration data. The figures nonetheless show that child mortality in violent zones was over twice the rate in non-violent zones (the latter roughly equivalent to overall under-5 mortality in West and Central Africa at the time).

[b]Deaths per 1,000 people per year

Sources: Coghlan et al. (2006); Coghlan et al. (2009); Hagopian et al. (2013).

and with long-term disabilities (Peterman, Palermo, and Bredenkamp 2011).

With a death toll far exceeding those of other recent CHEs, for instance the crisis in Darfur, Sudan (up to 400,000 dead; Sudan's leader stands accused of genocide in the International Criminal Court), as well as ongoing war in Syria—the Congo Wars constitute the deadliest conflict since World War II. As in the Bosnian and Rwandan genocides, the international response to Congo's CHE was abysmal. Most deaths were due to starvation and disease: humanitarian agencies were unable to provide simple yet lifesaving interventions such as food, safe water, sanitation, vaccination, and effective medical care. Not only was the area at war extremely difficult to reach, the level of violence made aid provision highly dangerous for humanitarian aid workers, many of whom were kidnapped and killed (MSF 2013b).

Countering a Rationalization for War in Iraq: The Politics of Epidemiology

One claim by warring parties is that "collateral damage" (the civilian death toll) cannot be clocked as conflict is unfolding. Just as there is a breakdown in health care systems in most conflict settings, vital statistics capacity is also disrupted. But as shown in Iraq, there are other means of counting civilian deaths that can play an important role in countering official pronouncements on the civilian protection rationale for armed invasion.

Shortly after the "Coalition Forces" (led by the United States and the United Kingdom) launched the Iraq War (justified by the purported existence of never proven WMD) in March 2003, a team of US epidemiologists undertook a classic household cluster sample survey. This involved interviews about births, deaths, and circumstances of violent death in 33 clusters of 30 households to enable "before–after" assessments of the war's impact on civilian mortality (Roberts et al. 2004). The study team found the risk of mortality to be 2.5 times higher after the invasion compared with before; most of the violent deaths occurred among women and children. Two years later the team attributed 650,000 excess deaths to the war, producing epidemiologic evidence that Iraqi civilians were dying at more than twice the rate as before the war (Burnham et al. 2006).

Although these studies were challenged on methodological grounds, it was clear that far more civilians were dying than the Coalition Forces occupying the country acknowledged, and that, despite their claims that the invasion was partially motivated on humanitarian grounds, they were failing to protect civilians (Thoms and Ron 2007). This was in violation of Convention IV, Part III, Section

I, Article 27 of the Geneva Conventions, which states that "protected persons shall at all times be humanely treated, and shall be protected especially against all acts of violence or threats thereof and against insults and public curiosity."

Notwithstanding controversy around the studies, they showed that even during wartime and difficult circumstances, the collection of valid public health data was possible (albeit with limited precision, as the authors noted). A more definitive study using random two-stage cluster sampling was carried out at war's end in 2011, finding the death rate over 50% higher during the war than for the 2 years preceding invasion (Table 8-3). This amounted to approximately 405,000 "excess deaths attributable to the conflict," with 60% due to direct violence and the remaining linked to infrastructure (e.g., sanitation system) collapse and related causes (Hagopian et al. 2013). Conflict epidemiology is now considered an important arena bringing together public health, human rights, and international law.

Ongoing Conflict in the Palestinian Occupied Territories

The Palestinian Occupied Territories includes the West Bank, comprised of almost 2.8 million people dispersed over 6,000 km², and the Gaza Strip, with over 1.7 million people concentrated in just 365 km². The Israeli occupation of Palestine since 1967 has resulted in the destruction of Palestinian institutions and infrastructure, violation of mobility and other human rights, deprivation of medical care, inadequate water and sewage maintenance, chronic poverty, long-term unemployment, food insecurity, and electricity and fuel disruptions—all atop a decades-long refugee crisis (Giacaman 2015).

These factors, together with the effects of militarism and the stifling Gaza blockade, have resulted in elevated rates of physical and mental illness. Amid the occupation, there have been multiple periods of extreme violence during the first intifada from 1987 to 1993, which ended with the Oslo Declaration (though violence continued), the second intifada in 2000, the 2008–2009 Gaza war, and the Israel-Gaza conflict in 2014. While violence is experienced on both sides of the border, it is asymmetric, with far greater Israeli military capacity and use of collective punishment against all Palestinians when it is only some who engage in violence (Gallo and Marzano 2009).

The 2010 Palestinian Family Survey reported that 18% of the population over age 18 had at least one chronic disease compared with 12% in 2006 (Palestinian Central Bureau of Statistics 2013), and Palestinian life expectancy gains are slower than in other countries in the region (Qlalweh, Duraidi, and Brønnum-Hansen 2012). Because of their lifelong and intergenerational exposure to the violence and effects of occupation, children—who make up more than half of Gaza's population—bear the brunt of the effects, also comprising one third of deaths and injuries in the 2008 conflict (UNICEF 2009a). One third of preschoolers in the Gaza strip suffer from anemia (Sirdah, Yaghi, and Yaghi 2014), with significant levels of stunting. Palestinians of all ages experience high rates of mental health problems associated with the loss of family members, exposure to military violence, and injury (Giacaman et al. 2011). (Mental health effects are also evident in Israel, where there is greater monitoring capacity: PTSD has been found in 38% of Israeli children living close to the Gaza strip [Feldman and Vengrober 2011].)

Restrictions on the freedom of movement of Palestinians due to Israeli military checkpoints, closures, and blockades pose severe barriers to medical care, exacerbating the shortages of medicine, equipment, and health workers within Palestine. Many villages are cut off from urban centers and ambulances are regularly detained at checkpoints, resulting in numerous preventable deaths—extending to six patients from Gaza who died in 2011 awaiting permits to access health care (Vitullo et al. 2012). Health workers, particularly ambulance drivers, have also been subject to violence and harassment while on duty (Sousa and Hagopian 2011).

Political sanctions prevent the government from consistently paying Gaza's 42,000 public sector workers, including health personnel, and the Palestinian Ministry of Health has had to increase its referrals for unavailable specialized care (e.g., cancer treatment) to private and foreign facilities more than seven-fold since 2000 (WHO 2014b).

The conflict in the Palestinian Occupied Territories shows no sign of abating. Periodic flares in violence, such as in 2014, resulted in over 2,200 dead, 11,000 injured, and 500,000 displaced persons (de Ville de Goyet et al. 2015). Twenty-three health care workers were killed and 83 were injured (WHO EMRO 2014). One hospital and five PHC clinics were destroyed, with almost half of health facilities damaged or closed during the conflict (WHO 2014a).

A movement to isolate Israel over its treatment of the Palestinian people, which began in 2005, advocates for a boycott, divestment, and sanctions (BDS) against the state of Israel until it complies with international law and human rights principles. Similar to the campaign against apartheid South Africa in the 1980s, BDS has garnered both international solidarity (Bakan and Abu-Laban 2009) and strong detractors. An intense controversy surrounding "An open letter to the people of Gaza" published in *The Lancet* (2014) regarding the civilian medical impact of the Israeli attack shows that the occupation (and conflict) remains one of the most contentious issues in health and humanitarian work of our era.

Campaigns to enable access to health care and the right to health for Palestinians have been taken up by regional and transnational activist groups, such as Physicians for Human Rights-Israel, which involves both Israeli and Palestinian physicians (Right Livelihood Award Foundation 2010). Palestinian physician Izzeldin Abuelaish, who in 2009 suffered the unspeakable loss of three of his daughters in an Israeli missile strike on his home, has taken the courageous stance of seeking to heal through peace and reconciliation, rather than fomenting hate (Abuelaish 2010).

POLITICAL ECONOMY OF DISASTERS AND CHEs: WHERE DOES HUMANITARIANISM FIT IN?

Key Questions:

- What dangers do humanitarian aid workers face when working in conflict zones and how should these be addressed?
- Why is humanitarianism an insufficient means of addressing emergencies?

Dangers and Dilemmas of Humanitarian Aid

Humanitarian workers face significant dangers when they enter conflict-ridden environments, even if incomparable to the suffering of those they are aiding. Sometimes humanitarian workers are targeted because they work with international peacekeeping or foreign intervention forces. Usually unarmed, they are easy targets, though their presence can also discourage attacks on the displaced. In 2015, there were 148 attacks on 287 humanitarian aid workers (mostly local), resulting in death (109 people), injury (110), and kidnapping (68). Most of these attacks took place in Syria, South Sudan, Afghanistan, Somalia, and Yemen (Humanitarian Outcomes 2016).

Health care facilities are often deliberately attacked to deprive enemy combatants of medical support, to acquire drugs and equipment, and for military advantage, affecting both local and foreign health care workers (ICRC 2011). For instance, between October 2015 and September 2016 there were numerous airstrikes on hospitals in Aleppo, Syria, Kunduz, Afghanistan, and northern Yemen, killing dozens of health workers, patients, and others. As of mid-2016, increasingly frequent assaults had resulted in at least 370 medical facilities being attacked and 750 health care workers killed in Syria alone (Physicians for Human Rights 2016).

Humanitarian aid workers may also experience mental health effects from working in situations of mass violence. Up to 14% of aid workers in the Kosovo conflict exhibited symptoms of depression and anxiety (Lopes Cardozo et al. 2005). As well, those who document human rights abuses in the field and collect stories of trauma and abuse may experience vicarious or "second-hand" traumatization (Holtz et al. 2002).

In the past, relief organizations maintained control and leadership over CHE responses, adhering to the principle of neutrality. Since the Balkan wars, however, military forces have become increasingly involved in community health and food programs during CHEs. Instead of improving security, increased military engagement potentially worsens it by blurring the line between civilian and military populations, eroding trust, and associating relief organizations with armed forces (Pringle 2008).

This has been accompanied by a rising corporate penetration of war and disaster relief (Klein 2007). In 2003, NGOs voiced concern regarding the US military's decision to coordinate relief efforts in Iraq, given the potential to undermine their impartiality; still, many of the largest US and European NGOs were forced to comply with this directive (Burkle and Noji 2004).

The US Pentagon's ill-conceived foray into the aid business offers a telling illustration. In 2001, amid a bombing campaign in Afghanistan, US warplanes dropped food packages as humanitarian relief. But cluster bombs that were also being dropped had an almost identical appearance to the food canisters. As a result, an unknown number of persons were maimed or killed, with uproar forcing the Pentagon to suspend this practice (Human Rights Watch 2001).

The threats faced by humanitarian workers raise important questions about the role of the military and intelligence/security forces in purveying relief. Humanitarian organizations have traditionally distanced themselves from military forces, except for cooperation around ecological disasters. Yet rapidly deployable military and security forces may be the sole entity able to meet the reconnaissance, evacuation, and supply needs of certain emergency responses (see chapter 4).

In sum, working with military and intelligence forces, even when they provide essential logistical and security support, presents moral dilemmas for relief organizations and imposes substantial risks for both beneficiaries and aid workers, many of whom argue for humanitarian independence or consider the military to be part of the problem.

Whither Humanitarianism?

The human impulse to do good and serve those in need drives much humanitarian work and has attracted many to the global health field in the first place. Both the nobility and the limits of this aim are evident in the story of MSF, one of the most effective and ubiquitous organizations involved in CHE and disaster responses. Founded in 1971 in Paris by 13 doctors and journalists outraged at the inadequate government and ICRC response to the conflict and famine in Biafra, MSF quickly grew to 300—now 30,000—volunteer doctors, nurses, and staff in 28 countries (see chapter 4). MSF's first mission was to Nicaragua in the aftermath of a 1972 earthquake, and by 1975 it developed a large-scale medical program for Cambodian refugees in Thailand (MSF 2013a). In 1979 the organization fractured: those preferring more formal structure and organization, while retaining a tempered if still powerful principle of "speaking out" against atrocities, remained in MSF; those seeking to serve as practitioners of social justice-oriented "guerrilla medicine" and more outspoken activist witnessing formed Médecins du Monde (Fox 2014). MSF grew far more rapidly and was awarded the Nobel peace prize in 1999.

Questions of neutrality versus bearing witness have troubled the humanitarian field since its beginnings. Legendary founder of modern nursing Florence Nightingale famously warned in the 1860s that the newly founded ICRC's volunteer medical caregivers for the war wounded and sick would relieve governments of their responsibilities and thus "render war more easy." In the 20th century, and despite the horrific human impact of conflict in Europe, Asia, and beyond, the ICRC continued its refusal to take a stance against war, in part arguing that this would limit its access to the wounded and suffering on all sides of conflagrations (and thus constrain its institutional utility). In remaining silent while aligning itself with nationalism and militarism—witnessing barbarism without denouncing it—the ICRC sidestepped founder Henri Dunant's espousal of pacifism (Hutchinson 1996).

In its founding and early forays, MSF sought to resolve such dilemmas (Redfield 2013). Navigating moral legitimacy, neutrality, and speaking out to justify its cause, MSF was expelled from Ethiopia in the 1980s after its French section accused the regime of using famine and food aid to force resettlement (DeChaine 2002). And in Rwanda, MSF's call for collective action was articulated in its bitter refrain "you can't stop genocide with doctors" (Bortolotti 2010, p. 282).

Of course, humanitarian aid organizations are circumscribed by their missions and ambits. MSF, for example, notes that notwithstanding their provision of health services in Gaza, they are unable to ". . . open borders or end violence" in the Palestine-Israel impasse (Whittall 2014). Humanitarian organizations do not serve the same role as diplomats or politicians, though they can report and decry violence to authorities.

Can humanitarian aid workers ever play a role in upending or preventing humanitarian emergencies altogether? In other words, can an emergency response be mounted that also deals with underlying causes? One illustration of a missed opportunity can be found in MSF's response to a severe childhood lead poisoning outbreak in impoverished communities in northern Nigeria in 2010. The outbreak, which resulted in hundreds of child deaths and many more exposed, was linked to the rise of artisanal gold mining (which through the grinding process released large quantities of lead dust), fueled by soaring gold prices, the collapse of subsistence farming, and the economic crisis that began in 2008. In the absence of Nigerian government action, MSF provided chelation therapy in what would be the "world's first population-level treatment of severe lead poisoning," and by helping to coordinate environmental remediation and safer mining practices (Pringle 2014b, p. 301). MSF's efforts were deemed successful because of the drastic reduction in mortality (Thurtle et al. 2014).

But as John Pringle, an MSF responder in the outbreak, argues, in leaving "unjust political structures" untouched, the "humanitarian response may have created apathy by allowing political structures to gloss over a sense of urgency. Years later, MSF, which has failed to speak out on the political determinants of the lead poisoning outbreak, is still spearheading the medical response, and prospects for a generation of severely lead-affected children seem grim" (Pringle 2014b, p. 304).

Little discussed, but with ongoing salience, is how (medical) humanitarianism was historically enmeshed with the colonial enterprise (Paulmann 2016). Humanitarianism continues to be viewed in some contexts as an accomplice to imperialism through its appropriation by warring parties and its own role in perpetuating dependency and charity over solidarity and human rights (Drayton 2013; Klein 2007; Murdoch 2015).

Like all institutions, humanitarian organizations must also focus on their own survival. Unlike the military, which expects casualties as part of its role, humanitarian organizations may (plan to) evacuate aid workers when they face danger (Karunakara and Dollé 2013). On a different note, use of media and storytelling by UN and humanitarian organizations is a key fundraising strategy that may skew public perceptions of conflicts, disasters, and how they can be addressed (DeChaine 2002). Humanitarian assistance in 2015 grew to US$28 billion (3/4 in government contributions, 1/4 private), about half channelled through multilateral organizations, 40% through NGOs and the ICRC, and just 6% via the public sector (Development Initiatives 2016).

In the end, Nightingale's concern, amplified, may still stand, more than 150 years later. Some even argue that humanitarian aid that does not address the political economy context on some level may serve to legitimize the status quo, alleviating the responsibilities of governments (including current and former imperial powers) to preempt crisis and excusing their mismanagement, nefarious ties with elite interests, and failure to avert harm and conflict from the other powerful entities in the chain of political and societal determination of health: corporate perpetrators of exploitation of people and resources and international financial actors and their national counterparts, who tolerate or encourage tax evasion, capital flight, deregulation, indebtedness, poverty and inequality, disinvestment in infrastructure, unfair trade rules, and so on (Polman 2010).

While humanitarian organizations alone cannot possibly take on such forces, perhaps there remains a special onus on those who engage in action on the ground and respond firsthand to the needs of the poor and downtrodden—a quid pro quo of providing a lens on atrocities and disasters—conferring responsibilities of speaking out and advocating for political and economic accountability. Here we join the small chorus of voices who call for a social justice response for transformative change that complements, and in the long term transcends the need for, emergency humanitarian responses.

CONCLUSION

Learning Points:

- The human cost in death, disability, and displacement from ecological disasters such as hurricanes, tsunamis, and earthquakes, as well as from droughts and famines, depends on the political economy of prevention and response efforts well beyond the actual events.

- Wars and civil conflict are a central part of the world political economy and require both immediate responses as well as critical preventive measures, including ending militarism and eliminating CBW and nuclear weapons.
- The civilian toll of conflict is higher now than ever before. Soaring numbers of refugees and IDPs constitute a grave public health concern and warrant far more sustained and integrated attention and responsibility across societies.
- CHEs require a broad range of measures in the short term, including housing and sanitation, communicable disease prevention, mental health care, nutrition, and ensuring security, particularly for women and children. At the same time, long-term, political commitment to preventing future CHEs is crucial and ought not be ignored by humanitarian efforts.
- Humanitarianism, while an essential and noble response to human suffering, is constrained by the political and economic context of conflicts.

This chapter opened with the Haitian earthquake of 2010 and so we close with a political economy analysis of this catastrophe. The humanitarian disaster following the earthquake was in many ways the product of the country's history, with chronic debt, worker exploitation, and foreign military, political, and economic intervention all contributing to the inadequate infrastructure that caused high levels of misery and exacerbated the death toll (Danner 2010).

A remarkable 1790s slave revolt and liberation movement led by Toussaint L'Ouverture, a former slave, resulted in the abolition of slavery and then Haiti's independence from France (having been its richest colony thanks to lucrative sugar plantations) in 1804. Haiti was the first independent Black republic and second independent nation in the Western Hemisphere. But a combination of military reprisals, steep French reparations, US and European trade embargoes, perennial threats of invasion, continued labor exploitation, a 20-year US occupation (1915–1934) and land grabs to enrich and protect corporate interests, crippling debt repayment, and corrupt leaders allied with foreign interests and domestic elites generating extreme concentration of wealth, all stymied Haitian development well into the 20th century (Dubois 2012). In the 1950s François "Papa Doc" Duvalier came to power and, succeeded by his son, ran a 30-year dictatorship generously armed and backed by the United States amid Cold War fears of Cuba's socialist influence in the region.

Under their harsh rule, enforced by the Tonton Macoutes paramilitary who killed 30,000 people and drove hundreds of thousands into exile, the Duvalier family enriched themselves and a few cronies and further impoverished the country, letting its scant infrastructure crumble. "Baby Doc" Duvalier was finally forced out by popular uprisings in 1986, leaving the country impoverished and in turmoil.

In 1990, Haiti held its first fair elections, and Jean-Bertrand Aristide, a former Catholic priest who championed the rights of the poor, was voted President. Aristide's attempts to democratize economic institutions, demobilize the army, and improve social services were met with several US-backed coups. Re-elected and forced into exile multiple times, he was temporarily reinstated under the condition that he implement structural adjustment policies and allow US food imports, which together devastated local rice production (Drobac et al. 2013). The country remained beleaguered by political instability, debt, and harmful trade sanctions, causing a decline in income, rising unemployment and violence, worsened nutrition, increases in child mortality, and a breakdown in the education system and family cohesion (Gibbons and Garfield 1999). Haitians coped by decreasing their caloric intake, moving in with relatives, selling domestic goods, taking children out of school to work, beg on the streets, or be lent out as indentured servants. With Haiti the poorest country in the Americas, the majority of the population survived on remittances and worked on increasingly degraded land, in abusive Dominican sugar plants, or in low-wage garment production. Since 2004, the country has effectively been run by UN peacekeepers and US "oversight" that, together with the heavy presence of NGOs, have impeded development of the public sector.

That hundreds of thousands of Haitians were living in substandard housing with inadequate infrastructure when the 2010 earthquake struck is thus not surprising, even as the extent of devastation was shocking. Accompanying massive death and displacement, an already weak and ineffective government literally collapsed, with most of its buildings destroyed and 20% of its workforce perishing in the quake (Petchesky 2012). To add hardship to misery, a cholera epidemic broke out in October 2010—the first in Haiti in over 50 years—which had killed almost 10,000 people as of mid-2016 (PAHO 2016). Brought to the island via UN peacekeepers, the outbreak has compounded a second disaster on top of the first (and a third with October 2016's Hurricane Matthew), stretching international aid efforts beyond capacity and raising fury among the Haitian population.

The international response to the earthquake has all but overlooked this historical and political context and why it continues to impede recovery (Pinto 2010). In 2012, 500,000 people were still living in dangerous shanties without proper sanitation, water, or hygiene, and only 43% of promised aid had been distributed (Petchesky 2012). With the exception of over 1,000 Cuban medics, whose solidarity-oriented training and health system-building activities predated the earthquake by more than a decade, foreign assistance has been hampered by mismanagement, delays, exorbitant NGO overhead costs, and aid workers who do not speak French or Creole (Edmonds 2013). The American Red Cross raised US$500 million, passing much of it to other groups (while retaining an outrageous 25% for "overhead"), but failed to document how much of it was spent (Grassley 2016). For example, it pledged to provide homes to 130,000 people in Port-au-Prince; however, land disputes have blocked all except six houses from being built (Elliott and Sullivan 2015). With humanitarian organizations raising colossal sums, many have reached beyond their expertise and management capacity, leaving Haitians to continue suffering while the international community erroneously assumes that resources are reaching them. Shamefully, just 1% of US$1.5 billion in USAID monies have gone directly to Haitian organizations, even as Haiti's Health Ministry, for example, has been highly effective at implementing post-earthquake programs, using donor funding to increase vaccination rates and access to HIV treatment (Knox 2015).

In sum, though many people are drawn into global health through humanitarian work in the context of CHEs and ecological disasters, they are often naïve about what underlies and exacerbates these situations. Without a larger understanding of the political, economic, racial/ethnic, environmental, and other drivers of CHEs and the inadequate ability to mitigate the consequences of disasters, humanitarianism becomes justified as a logical component of addressing global health and equity, a temporary yet perpetual stopgap when needed. While some humanitarian organizations hope that they will one day be put out of work, many have been swept into the neoliberal establishment (and are now unwilling to challenge the status quo), which depends on these organizations to attenuate the human suffering caused by the persistence of gross exploitation and imbalances of power that have in turn been built on long colonial and post-colonial legacies, militarism, and (neoliberal) capitalism (Pringle 2014a).

Ecological disasters are important causes of morbidity, displacement, and disability worldwide. While relatively few disasters result in significant mortality, they often have a large and enduring economic impact. Meanwhile, global responses to ecological disasters have improved in recent decades, limiting casualties in some places. Local and international public health agencies, such as PAHO, regularly conduct preparedness exercises and train public health professionals in both HICs and LMICs about how to handle injuries and deaths due to earthquakes and major storms. Unfortunately given the effects of climate change, there will likely be greater frequency of disasters in the coming years. Where there is little preparedness, for instance lack of flood abatement or resettlement in areas with perennial threats—as in Pakistan in 2010, when monsoon-provoked floods covering one fifth of the land mass killed nearly 2,000 people, with almost 20 million affected by disease, displacement, and livelihood loss (Shabir 2013), plus repeat flooding in 2011—problems are bound to recur.

Although ecological disasters are among the most visible rationales for global health aid, CHE consequences on health can be far more catastrophic, with high rates of infectious disease and malnutrition claiming more lives than the immediate situation causing people to flee. The challenge is how to prevent crises from turning into CHEs and, when this is not possible, how to reduce the lasting impact. Organized and prioritized interventions, such as those laid out by the Sphere Project (2011a) may help alleviate suffering.

Yet in many ways, such organized responses indicate a grand failure rather than a success. Humanitarian aid, while arguably necessary, is neither comprehensive nor can it provide cost-effective or long-term solutions (Redfield 2013). The chronic underfunding of public infrastructure and near collapse of public health systems in many countries lead to unnecessary loss of life when disasters and CHEs strike. How many lives are lost, as we have seen, is determined as much by how well government social and health programs have stood up to neoliberal capitalism as by the magnitude of the actual events. Under austerity conditions, disaster preparation and prevention are commonly left by the wayside.

Even more appalling, CHEs wrought by war plague the human race at an unending pace. Over 60 million refugees and IDPs are in continual need of assistance. Militarism must be challenged with as much vigor as deadly epidemics. This entails nuclear disarmament and the destruction of biological and chemical weapons. Military conflicts are often related to commodities or land that have enormous value on the international market and build upon colonial-era acrimony. Moreover, "disaster capitalism," as journalist Naomi Klein has dubbed it, has itself become a powerful force that impedes peace and preparedness and, like the military-industrial complex during the Cold War, feeds into a global political, economic, and security order.

In the end, the best way of ending conflicts and preventing future ones is to contest the underpinnings of the world order by promoting peace building and conflict avoidance, including via the peace through health movement that works toward creating equitable societies (Abuelaish et al. 2013; Arya and Santa Barbara 2008). Even as humanitarian responses to crises and emergencies constitute a moral imperative to relieve human suffering, they should not distract from nor impede the much broader moral and political global health imperative of struggling for social justice over the long term.

NOTES

1. By contrast, environmental disasters are set off by human-induced harms to the natural environment (contamination, depletion, misuse) resulting in actual or impending disease and death of flora and fauna, including humans. Environmental disasters (including oil spills and nuclear disasters [see chapter 10]) differ from ecological disasters in that the latter are triggered by a "natural" event (e.g., an earthquake).
2. Numbers derived from a compilation of sources by Peter Black, Senior Historian, US Holocaust Memorial Museum, E-mail correspondence June 28–30, 2015.

REFERENCES

Abuelaish I. 2010. *I Shall Not Hate: A Gaza Doctor's Journey on the Road to Peace and Human Dignity.* Toronto: Random House Canada.

Abuelaish I, Fazal N, Doubleday N, et al. 2013. The mutual determinants of individual, community, and societal peace and health. *International Journal of Peace and Development Studies* 4(1):1–7.

Adebajo A. 2016. The revolt against the West: Intervention and sovereignty. *Third World Quarterly* 37(7):1187–1202.

Agence France-Presse. 2015. Pakistan sees huge drop in polio cases. *The Guardian*, June 4.

Ahmetasevic N. 2007. Justice Report: Bosnia's Book of the Dead. http://www.balkaninsight.com/en/article/justice-report-bosnia-s-book-of-the-dead. Accessed July 28, 2016.

AIDA. 2007. Environmental and health impacts. http://www.aida-americas.org/aida.php?page=plancolombia_enviroandhhdamages. Accessed August 8, 2007.

Akyeampong E, Hill AG, and Kleinman A, Editors. 2015. *The Culture of Mental Illness and Psychiatric Practice in Africa.* Bloomington: Indiana University Press.

Ali J. 2001. Chemical weapons and the Iran-Iraq war: A case study in noncompliance. *Nonproliferation Review* 8(1):43–58.

Allukian M and Atwood PL. 2008. The Vietnam War. In Levy BS and Sidel VW, Editors. *War and Public Health*, Second Edition. New York: Oxford University Press.

Arena J. 2012. *Driven from New Orleans: How Nonprofits Betray Public Housing and Promote Privatization.* Minneapolis: University of Minnesota Press.

Arms Control Association. 2014. Chemical and Biological Weapons Status at a Glance. http://www.armscontrol.org/factsheets/cbwprolif. Accessed June 2, 2015.

Arya N and Santa Barbara J, Editors. 2008. *Peace through Health: How Health Professionals Can Work for a Less Violent World.* New York: Kumarian Press.

Ashford M and Huet-Vaughn Y. 1997. The impact of war on women. In Levy BS and Sidel VW, Eds. *War and Public Health*. New York: Oxford University Press.

Bakan AB and Abu-Laban Y. 2009. Palestinian resistance and international solidarity: The BDS campaign. *Race & Class* 51(1):29–54.

Bashour H. 2015. Let's not forget the health of the Syrians within their own country. *American Journal of Public Health* 105(12):2407–2408.

Bermejo PM. 2006. Preparation and response in case of natural disasters: Cuban programs and experience. *Journal of Public Health Policy* 27(1):13–21.

Betancourt TS, Borisova II, de la Soudiere M, and Williamson, J. 2011. Sierra Leone's child soldiers: War exposures and mental health problems by gender. *Journal of Adolescent Health* 49(1):21–28.

Bortolotti D. 2010. *Hope in Hell: Inside the World of Doctors Without Borders* (3rd ed.). Buffalo: Firefly Books.

Brackbill RM, Thorpe LE, DiGrande L, et al. 2006. Surveillance for World Trade Center disaster health effects among survivors of collapsed and damaged buildings. *Morbidity and Mortality Weekly Report Surveillance Summary* 55(2):1–18.

Bracken P, Giller J, and Summerfield D. 2016. Primum non nocere: The case for a critical approach to global mental health. *Epidemiology and Psychiatric Sciences* [Epub ahead of publication].

Brennan RJ and Nandy R. 2001. Complex humanitarian emergencies: A major global health challenge. *Emergency Medicine* 13(2):147–156.

Brennan RJ and Waldman RJ. 2006. The South Asian earthquake six months later—an ongoing crisis. *NEJM* 354(17):1769–1771.

Brounéus K. 2010. The trauma of truth telling: Effects of witnessing in the Rwandan Gacaca courts on psychological health. *Journal of Conflict Resolution* 54(3):408–437.

Burkle FM and Noji EK. 2004. Health and politics in the 2003 war with Iraq: Lessons learned. *Lancet* 364(9442):1371–1375.

Burnham G, Lafta R, Doocy S, and Roberts L. 2006. Mortality after the 2003 invasion of Iraq: A cross-sectional cluster sample survey. *Lancet* 368(9545):1421–1428.

CARE. 2001. *Emergency Preparedness Planning Guidelines*. Atlanta: CARE.

———. 2013. Support food aid reform. http://www.care.org/work/advocacy/food-aid. Accessed June 26, 2015.

Casinge E. 2015. Wrap-up: Special EU summit on the Mediterranean crisis. EurActiv. http://www.euractiv.com/sections/justice-home-affairs/live-special-eu-summit-mediterranean-crisis-314025. Accessed May 31, 2015.

CDC [Centers for Disease Control and Prevention]. 2006. Public health response to hurricanes Katrina and Rita—United States, 2005. *Morbidity and Mortality Weekly Report* 55(9):229–231.

Centre for Research on the Epidemiology of Disasters. 2013. *People Affected by Conflict 2013: Humanitarian Needs in Numbers*. Brussels: Centre for Research on the Epidemiology of Disasters.

Chirwa E and Dorward A. 2013. *Agricultural Input Subsidies: The Recent Malawi Experience*. Oxford: Oxford University Press.

Clapp J. 2012. *Hunger in the Balance: The New Politics of International Food Aid*. Ithaca: Cornell University Press.

CNN. 2005. FEMA chief: Victims bear some responsibility. http://www.cnn.com/2005/WEATHER/09/01/katrina.fema.brown/index.html. Updated September 1, 2005. Accessed October 25, 2007.

Cobey JC and Raymond NA. 2001. Antipersonnel land mines: A vector for human suffering. *Annals of Internal Medicine* 134(5):421–422.

Cockburn A, St. Clair J, and Silverstein K. 1999. The politics of 'natural' disaster: Who made Mitch so bad? *International Journal of Health Services* 29(2):459–462.

Coghlan B, Brennan RJ, Ngoy P, et al. 2006. Mortality in the Democratic Republic of Congo: A nationwide survey. *Lancet* 367(9504):44–51.

Coghlan B, Ngoy P, Mulumba F, et al. 2009. Update on mortality in the Democratic Republic of Congo: Results from a third nationwide survey. *Disaster Medicine and Public Health Preparedness* 3(02):88–96.

Cornia GA and Deotti L. 2015. Niger's 2005 Food Crisis and Child Malnutrition: the Role of Exogenous and Policy Factors. Italian Development Economists Association Working Paper No. 01.

Coulter C. 2015. *Bush Wives and Girl Soldiers: Women's Lives Through War and Peace in Sierra Leone*. Ithaca: Cornell University Press.

Crawford N. 2015. *War-related Death, Injury, and Displacement in Afghanistan and Pakistan 2001-2014*. Providence: Brown University Watson Institute, Costs of War project.

Crisp J, Morris T, and Refstie H. 2012. Displacement in urban areas: New challenges, new partnerships. *Disasters* 36(s1):S23–S42.

Cutts M. *Working Paper No. 8: The Humanitarian Operation in Bosnia, 1992-95: Dilemmas of*

Negotiating Humanitarian Access. Geneva: Policy Research Unit, UNHCR.

Dallaire R. and Beardsley B. 2004. *Shake Hands with the Devil: The Failure of Humanity in Rwanda*. Toronto: Vintage Canada.

de Quadros CA and Epstein D. 2002. Health as a bridge for peace: PAHO's experience. *Lancet* 360:s25–s26.

De Ville de Goyet C, Manenti A, Carswell K, and van Ommeren M. 2015. *Report of a Field Assessment of Health Conditions in the Occupied Palestinian Territory (oPt)*. Geneva: WHO.

De Witte L. 2002. *The assassination of Lumumba*. Brooklyn: Verso.

DeChaine DR. 2002. Humanitarian space and the social imaginary: Médecins Sans Frontières/ Doctors Without Borders and the rhetoric of global community. *Journal of Communication Inquiry* 26(4):354–369.

Deng L. 2002. The Sudan famine of 1998: Unfolding the global dimensions. *Institute of Development Studies Bulletin* 33(4):28–38.

Development Initiatives. 2016. *Global Humanitarian Assistance Report 2016*. Bristol: Development Initiatives.

Devereux S and Berge K. 2000. *Famine in the Twentieth Century* (Vol. 105). Brighton: Institute of Development Studies.

Drayton R. 2013. Beyond humanitarian imperialism: The dubious origins of 'humanitarian intervention' and some rules for its future. In Everill B and Kaplan J, Editors. *The History and Practice of Humanitarian Intervention and Aid in Africa*. London: Palgrave Macmillan.

Drobac P, Basilico M, Messac L, et al. 2013. Building an effective rural health delivery model in Haiti and Rwanda. In Farmer P, Kim JY, Kleinman A, and Basilico MT, Editors. *Reimagining Global Health: An Introduction*. Berkeley: University of California Press.

Dubois L. 2012. *Haiti: The Aftershocks of History*. London: Macmillan Publishers.

Dugger C. 2007. Ending famine, simply by ignoring the experts. *New York Times*, December 2.

Duttine A and Hottentot E. 2013. Landmines and explosive remnants of war: A health threat not to be ignored. *Bulletin of the World Health Organization* 91(3):160–160A.

Edmonds K. 2013. Beyond good intentions: The structural limitations of NGOs in Haiti. *Critical Sociology* 39(3):439–452.

Elliott J and Sullivan L. 2015. Confidential documents: Red Cross itself may not know how millions donated for Haiti were spent. https://www.propublica.org/article/confidential-documents-red-cross-millions-donated-haiti. Accessed August 29, 2015.

Elliott KA and McKitterick W. 2013. Food aid for the 21st century: Saving more money, time, and lives. http://www.cgdev.org/sites/default/files/archive/doc/full_text/CGDBriefs/3120442/food-aid-for-the-21st-century.html. Accessed May 30, 2015.

Ensor BE and Ensor MO. 2009. Hurricane Mitch: Root causes and responses to the disaster. In Ensor M, Editor. *The Legacy of Hurricane Mitch*. Phoenix: University of Arizona Press.

Ertl V, Pfeiffer A, Saile R, et al. 2010. Validation of a mental health assessment in an African conflict population. *Psychological Assessement* 22(2):318–324.

Espinosa V and Rubin DB. 2015. Did the military interventions in the Mexican drug war increase violence? *The American Statistician* 69(1):17–27.

European Council on Foreign Relations. 2016. European responses to the refugee crisis. http://www.ecfr.eu/refugee_crisis. Accessed May 31, 2016.

FAO. 2015. Countries requiring external assistance for food. http://www.fao.org/Giews/english/hotspots/index.htm. Accessed May 30 2015.

FAO, IFAD, and WFP. 2014. *The State of Food Insecurity in the World 2014: Strengthening the Enabling Environment for Food Security and Nutrition*. Rome: FAO.

Feffer J. 2015. Our refugee world. *Foreign Policy in Focus*, June 24.

Feldman R and Vengrober A. 2011. Posttraumatic stress disorder in infants and young children exposed to war-related trauma. *Journal of the American Academy of Child & Adolescent Psychiatry* 50(7):645–658.

Fernando S. 2014. *Mental Health Worldwide: Culture, Globalization and Development*. London: Palgrave Macmillan.

Fletcher L, Stover E, and Weinstein H. 2005. *After the Tsunami: Human Rights of Vulnerable Populations*. Berkeley: Human Rights Center, University of California.

Fox RC. 2014. *Doctors Without Borders: Humanitarian Quests, Impossible Dreams of Médecins Sans Frontières*. Baltimore: Johns Hopkins University Press.

Fritschi L, McLaughlin J, Sergi CM, et al. 2015. Carcinogenicity of tetrachlorvinphos, parathion, malathion, diazinon, and glyphosate. *Red* 114.

Fuller T. 2012. 4 Decades on, U.S. Starts Cleanup of Agent Orange in Vietnam. *New York Times*, August 9.

Galea S, Ahern J, Resnick H, et al. 2002. Psychological sequelae of the September 11 terrorist attacks in NYC. *NEJM* 346(13):982–987.

Gallo G and Marzano A. 2009. The dynamics of asymmetric conflicts: The Israeli-Palestinian case. *Journal of Conflict Studies* 29:33–49.

Garfield R and Daponte BO. 2000. The effect of economic sanctions on the mortality of Iraqi children prior to the 1991 Persian Gulf War. *American Journal of Public Health* 90(4):546–552.

Geneva Declaration. Global burden of armed violence 2015: Interactive map and charts. http://www.genevadeclaration.org/measurability/global-burden-of-armed-violence/gbav-2015/interactive-map-charts.html. Accessed June 26, 2015.

Giacaman R. 2015. Syrian and Iraqi refugees: A Palestinian perspective. *American Journal of Public Health* 105(12):2406–2407.

Giacaman R, Rabaia Y, Nguyen-Gillham V, et al. 2011. Mental health, social distress and political oppression: The case of the occupied Palestinian territory. *Global Public Health* 6(5):547–559.

Gibbons E and Garfield R. 1999. The impact of economic sanctions on health and human rights in Haiti, 1991–1994. *American Journal of Public Health* 89(10):1499–1504.

Global Issues. 2013. The arms trade is big business 2013. http://www.globalissues.org/article/74/the-arms-trade-is-big-business. Accessed July 1, 2015.

Goma Epidemiology Group. 1995. Public health impact of Rwandan refugee crisis: What happened in Goma, Zaire, in July 1994? *Lancet* 345(8946):339–344.

Gomez MB. 2016. Policing, community fragmentation, and public health: Observations from Baltimore. *Journal of Urban Health* 93(Suppl 1):154–167.

Goodwin D. 2002. *Negotiation in International Conflict: Understanding Persuasion*. Boca Raton: Taylor & Francis.

Gotham KF. 2012. Disaster, Inc.: Privatization and post-Katrina rebuilding in New Orleans. *Perspectives on Politics* 10(03):633–646.

Grassley C. 2016. Grassley releases memo on Red Cross' Haiti earthquake relief response. http://www.grassley.senate.gov/news/news-releases/grassley-releases-memo-red-cross%E2%80%99-haiti-earthquake-relief-response-finds-red. Accessed July 28, 2016.

Haas M. 1991. *Genocide by Proxy: Cambodian Pawn on a Superpower Chessboard*. New York: Praeger Publishers.

Hagopian A, Flaxman AD, Takaro TK, et al. 2013. Mortality in Iraq associated with the 2003–2011 war and occupation: Findings from a national cluster sample survey by the university collaborative Iraq mortality study. *PLoS Medicine* 10(10):e1001533.

Hartman C and Squires G. 2006. *There is No Such Thing as a Natural Disaster: Race, Class, and Hurricane Katrina*. New York: Routledge Press.

Harvey P, Proudlock K, Clay E, et al. 2010. *Food Aid and Food Assistance in Emergency and Transitional Contexts: A Review of Current Thinking.* London: Overseas Development Institute.

Hobor G. 2015. New Orleans' remarkably (un)predictable recovery: Developing a theory of urban resilience. *American Behavioral Scientist* 59(10):1214–1230.

Hochschild A. 1998. *King Leopold's Ghost: A Story of Greed, Terror, and Heroism in Colonial Africa*. New York: Houghton Mifflin Books.

Holtz TH, Leighton J, Balter S, et al. 2003. The public health response to the World Trade Center disaster. In Levy BS and Sidel VW, Editors. *Terrorism and Public Health*. New York: Oxford University Press.

Holtz TH, Salama P, Lopes Cardozo B, and Gotway CA. 2002. Mental health status of human rights workers, Kosovo 2000. *Journal of Traumatic Stress* 15(5):389–395.

Human Rights Watch. 2001. *Cluster Bombs in Afghanistan: A Human Rights Watch Backgrounder.* New York: Human Rights Watch.

Humanitarian Outcomes. 2016. *Aid Worker Security Report 2016: Figures at a Glance*. London: Humanitarian Outcomes.

Humphries V. 2013. Improving humanitarian coordination: Common challenges and lessons learned from the cluster approach. *Journal of Humanitarian Assistance*, April 30.

Hutchinson J. 1996. *Champions of Charity: War and the Rise of the Red Cross.* Oxford: Westview Press.

IASC 2007. *Guidelines on Mental Health and Psychosocial Support in Emergency Settings.* Geneva: IASC.

ICRC. 2004. How does humanitarian law protect refugees and internally displaced persons? https://www.icrc.org/eng/resources/documents/misc/5kzlzb.htm. Accessed June 26, 2015.

———. 2011. *Health Care in Danger: Making the Case.* Geneva: ICRC.

IFRC. 2011a. Complex/manmade hazards: complex emergencies. https://www.ifrc.org/en/what-we-do/disaster-management/about-disasters/definition-of-hazard/complex-emergencies/. Accessed June 26, 2015.

———. 2011b. Niger - Background to a food crisis. http://www.ifrc.org/en/news-and-media/features/niger—background-to-a-food-crisis/. Accessed 30 May 2015.

———. 2014. What is a disaster? https://www.ifrc.org/en/what-we-do/disaster-management/

about-disasters/what-is-a-disaster/. Accessed May 27, 2015.

Iltis T. 2015. Australia's War on People Smugglers Is Really a War on Refugees. http://www.truth-out.org/news/item/31466-australia-s-war-on-people-smugglers-is-really-a-war-on-refugees. Accessed June 27, 2015.

Institute for Conflict Management. 2016. Fatalities in Terrorist Violence in Pakistan 2003-2016. http://www.satp.org/satporgtp/countries/pakistan/database/casualties.htm. Accessed July 28, 2016.

Institute for Economics and Peace. 2014. *Global Terrorism Index 2014*. Sydney, New York, Mexico City: Institute for Economics and Peace.

International Campaign to Ban Landmines. 2015. *Landmine Monitor 2015*. Geneva: Landmine and Cluster Munition Monitor.

Jones S. 2015. Extreme violence 'blighting a generation' in Central African Republic. *The Guardian*, May 26.

Karunakara U and Dollé J-C. 2013. The limits of humanitarian aid: MSF and TB in Somalia. http://blogs.plos.org/speakingofmedicine/2013/10/23/the-limits-of-humanitarian-aid-msf-and-tb-in-somalia/. Accessed June 26, 2015.

Kellermann AL and Rivara FP. 2013. Silencing the science on gun research. *JAMA* 309(6):549–550.

Kenny C. 2009. *Why Do People Die in Earthquakes? The Costs, Benefits and Institutions of Disaster Risk Reduction in Developing Countries*. Washington, DC: World Bank.

Kirkis EJ. 2006. A myth too tough to die: The dead of disasters cause epidemics of disease. *American Journal of Infection Control* 34(6):331–334.

Klein N. 2007. *The Shock Doctrine: The Rise of Disaster Capitalism*. London: Macmillan.

Kneen J. 2009. Mining in the Democratic Republic of Congo. *MiningWatch Canada Blog*, May 6.

Knox R. 2015. 5 Years After Haiti's Earthquake, Where Did The $13.5 Billion Go? *NPR*, January 12.

Kolsy N. 2015. Five signs the drone war is undermining the 'war on terror'. *Foreign Policy in Focus*, November 24.

Kopinak JK. 2013. Humanitarian aid: Are effectiveness and sustainability impossible dreams? *Journal of Humanitarian Assistance*, March 10.

Kouadio IK, Aljunid S, Kamigaki T, et al. 2012. Infectious diseases following natural disasters: prevention and control measures. *Expert Review of Anti-Infective Therapy* 10(1):95–104.

Krause M. 2014. *The Good Project: Humanitarian Relief NGOs and the Fragmentation of Reason*. Chicago: University of Chicago Press.

Kripke G. 2005. Food aid or hidden dumping? Separating the wheat from chaff. In *Oxfam Briefing Paper*. Oxford: Oxfam International.

Krugman P. 2005. A Can't Do Government. *New York Times*, September 2.

Lancet. 2014. Published responses to the Gaza open letter. http://www.thelancet.com/gaza-letter-2014-responses. Accessed June 28, 2015.

Laurell AC. 2015. Three decades of neoliberalism in Mexico: the destruction of society. *International Journal of Health Services* 45(2):246–264.

Leatherman J and Griffin N. 2014. Unsafe spaces: Trends and challenges in gender-based violence. *World Politics Review*, March 25.

Levy BS and Sidel VW. 2008. The impact of military activities on civilian populations. In Levy BS and Sidel VW, Editors. *War and Public Health*, Second Edition. New York: Oxford University Press.

Lopes Cardozo B, Holtz TH, Kaiser R, et al. 2005. The mental health of expatriate and Kosovar Albanian humanitarian aid workers. *Disasters* 29 (2):152–170.

Magone C, Neuman M, and Weissman F, Editors. 2012. *Humanitarian Negotiations Revealed: The MSF Experience*. New York: Columbia University Press.

Mahanta NG. 2013. *Confronting the State: ULFA's Quest for Sovereignty*. New Delhi: SAGE Publications India.

Mahmudi-Azer S. 2011. The international arms trade and global health. In Benatar S and Brock G, Editors. *Global Health and Global Health Ethics*. Cambridge: Cambridge University Press.

Martin MF. 2012. *Vietnamese Victims of Agent Orange and U.S.-Vietnam Relations*. Washington, DC: Congressional Research Service Report for Congress.

Maurer P. 2015. Nuclear weapons: Ending a threat to humanity. https://www.icrc.org/en/document/nuclear-weapons-ending-threat-humanity. Accessed August 3, 2015.

Maxwell D and Fitzpatrick M. 2012. The 2011 Somalia famine: Context, causes, and complications. *Global Food Security* 1(1):5–12.

McGirk J. 2005. Kashmir: the politics of an earthquake. https://www.opendemocracy.net/conflict-india_pakistan/jihadi_2941.jsp 9. Accessed November 28, 2015.

MEDICC Review. 2015. Facts and figures: Cuba's global health cooperation. *MEDICC Review* 17(3):1–4.

Mejía D. 2012. The war on drugs under Plan Colombia. In Sedillo E and Wheeler H, Editors. *Rethinking the "War on Drugs" Through the US-Mexico Prism*. New Haven: Yale Center for the Study of Globalization.

Mejia D and Restrepo P. 2013. *Bushes and Bullets: Illegal Cocaine Markets and Violence in Colombia.* Bogotá: Universidad de los Andes–Facultad de Economía–CEDE.

Mercille J. 2011. Violent narco-cartels or US hegemony? The political economy of the 'war on drugs' in Mexico. *Third World Quarterly* 32(9):1637–1653.

MiningWatch Canada. 2003. Canadian companies accused of pillaging Congo — United Nations report. http://www.miningwatch.ca/canadian-companies-accused-pillaging-congo-united-nations-report. Accessed June 27, 2015.

Mollica RF, Lopes Cardozo B, Osofsky HJ, et al. 2004. Mental health in complex emergencies. *Lancet* 364(9450):2058–2067.

Mollica RF, Brooks R, Tor S, et al. 2014. The enduring mental health impact of mass violence: A community comparison study of Cambodian civilians living in Cambodia and Thailand. *International Journal of Social Psychiatry* 60(1):6–20.

Moore J. 2014. The responsibility to protect in the Ebola outbreak. *Oxford University Press Blog,* September 22.

Morabia A and Benjamin GC. 2015. The refugee crisis in the Middle East and public health. *American Journal of Public Health* 105(12):2405–2406.

Morof DF, Kerber K, Tomczyk B, et al. 2014. Neonatal survival in complex humanitarian emergencies: Setting an evidence-based research agenda. *Conflict and Health* 8(1):8.

MSF. 2013a. Founding of MSF. http://www.doctorswithoutborders.org/founding-msf. Accessed June 26, 2015.

———. 2013b. International Activity Report 2013 - Democratic Republic of Congo. http://www.msf.org/international-activity-report-2013-democratic-republic-congo. Accessed March 15, 2015.

———. 2016. *Asylum Seekers in Italy: An Analysis of Mental Health Distress and Access to Healthcare.* Rome: MSF Italia.

Mullaney A and Hassan SA. 2015. He led the CIA to bin Laden-and unwittingly fueled a vaccine backlash. *National Geographic,* February 27.

Murdoch N. 2015. *Christian Warfare in Rhodesia-Zimbabwe: The Salvation Army and African Liberation, 1891-1991.* Eugene: Pickwick Publications.

Neer RM. 2013. *Napalm.* Cambridge: Harvard University Press.

Newman C. 2014. No one to stand by us: Reintegrating formerly abducted child-mothers in Uganda. *Journal of Intervention and Statebuilding* 8(4):357–380.

Noji EK and Toole MJ. 1997. The historical development of public health responses to disaster. *Disasters* 21(4):366–376.

Noland M, Robinson S, and Wang T. 2001. Famine in North Korea: Causes and cures, *Economic Development and Cultural Change* 49(4):741–767.

Nunn N and Qian N. 2014. US food aid and civil conflict. *American Economic Review* 104(6):1630–1666.

Orbinski J. 2009. *An Imperfect Offering: Humanitarian Action in the Twenty-first Century.* London: Walker Books.

Page M. 2003. The unnatural history of natural disaster (review essay). *Journal of Planning History* 2(4):356–361.

PAHO. 2010. Emergency preparedness and disaster relief: Health logistics course. http://www.paho.org/disasters/index.php?option=com_content&view=category&layout=blog&id=864&Itemid=815&lang=en. Accessed June 26, 2015.

———. 2016. *Epidemiological Update, Cholera: 27 May 2016. Cholera in the Americas—Situation Summary. Epidemiological Alerts.* Washington, DC: PAHO.

Palestinian Central Bureau of Statistics. 2013. *Final Report of the Palestinian Family Survey 2010.* Ramallah: Palestinian Central Bureau of Statistics.

Parnini SN. 2013. The crisis of the Rohingya as a Muslim minority in Myanmar and bilateral relations with Bangladesh. *Journal of Muslim Minority Affairs* 33(2):281–297.

Paulmann J, Editor. 2016. *Dilemmas of Humanitarian Aid in the Twentieth Century.* Oxford: Oxford University Press.

Perry A. 2008. Why Africa is still starving. *Time,* August 18.

Petchesky R. 2012. Biopolitics at the crossroads of sexuality and disaster: The case of Haiti. In Schrecker T, Editor. *The Ashgate Research Companion to the Globalization of Health.* Farnham: Ashgate Publishing.

Peterman A, Palermo T, and Bredenkamp C. 2011. Estimates and determinants of sexual violence against women in the Democratic Republic of Congo. *American Journal of Public Health* 101(6):1060–1067.

Physicians for Human Rights. 2016. *Anatomy of a Crisis: A Map of Attacks on Health Care in Syria.* New York: Physicians for Human Rights.

Pinto AD. 2010. Denaturalizing "natural" disasters: Haiti's earthquake and the humanitarian impulse. *Open Medicine* 4(4):e193.

Polman L. 2010. *The Crisis Caravan: What's Wrong with Humanitarian Aid?* New York: Henry Holt and Company.

Prashad V. 2015. We are in pitiless times. https://opendemocracy.net/vijay-prashad/we-are-in-pitiless-times. Accessed December 3, 2015.

Pringle JD. 2008. The military invasion of humanitarian space. http://med.stanford.edu/oih/militaryinvasion.html. Accessed June 26, 2015.

———. 2014a. *Charity Medicine for the Global Poor: Humanitarian Ethics and the Nigerian Lead-Poisoning Outbreak*. PhD [dissertation]. Toronto: Dalla Lana School of Public Health, University of Toronto.

———. 2014b. The unprecedented lead-poisoning outbreak: Ethical issues in a troubling broader context. *Public Health Ethics* 7(3):301–305.

Qlalweh K, Duraidi M, and Brønnum-Hansen H. 2012. Health expectancy in the occupied Palestinian territory: Estimates from the Gaza Strip and the West Bank: Based on surveys from 2006 to 2010. *BMJ Open* 2:e001572.

Rajagopalan S. 2006. Silver linings: Natural disasters, international relations and political change in South Asia, 2004–5. *Defense & Security Analysis* 22(4):451–468.

Redfield P. 2013. *Life in Crisis: The Ethical Journey of Doctors Without Borders*. Berkeley: University of California Press.

Right Livelihood Award Foundation. 2010. Physicians for Human Rights-Israel (2010, Israel). http://www.rightlivelihood.org/phri.html. Accessed June 20, 2015.

Roberts A. 2010. Lives and statistics: Are 90% of war victims civilians? *Survival* 52(3):115–136.

Roberts L, Lafta R, Garfield R, et al. 2004. Mortality before and after the 2003 invasion of Iraq: Cluster sample survey. *Lancet* 364(9448):1857–1864.

Schauer E and Elbert T. 2010. The psychological impact of child soldiering. In Martz E, Editor. *Trauma Rehabilitation after War and Conflict*. New York: Springer.

Seybolt TB. 1997. *Coordination in Rwanda: Humanitarian Response to Genocide and Civil War*. Cambridge: Conflict Management Group.

Shabir O. 2013. A summary case report on the health impacts and response to the Pakistan floods of 2010. *PLoS Currents* 5.

Shrestha D. 2015. UNHCR flies in shelter materials for quake-displaced in Nepal. *UNHCR News Stories*, May 7.

Sirdah MM, Yaghi A, and Yaghi AR. 2014. Iron deficiency anemia among kindergarten children living in the marginalized areas of Gaza Strip, Palestine. *Revista Brasileira de Hematologia e Hemoterapia* 36(2):132–138.

Smith N. 2006. There's no such thing as a natural disaster. http://understandingkatrina.ssrc.org/Smith/. Accessed July 20, 2016.

Smith WC. 2013. Hurricane Mitch and Honduras: An illustration of population vulnerability. *International Journal of Health System and Disaster Management* 1(1):54.

Sousa C and Hagopian A. 2011. Conflict, health and professional perseverance: Effects of military occupation on healthcare delivery in the West Bank. *Global Public Health* 6(5):520–533.

Sphere Project. 2011a. Humanitarian Charter and Minimum Standards in Humanitarian Response. http://www.sphereproject.org. Accessed June 27, 2015.

———. 2011b. *Sphere Handbook: Humanitarian Charter and Minimum Standards in Disaster Response, 2011*. Southampton: Practical Action Publishing.

Spiegel PB. 2005. Differences in world responses to natural disasters and complex emergencies. *JAMA* 293(15):1915–1918.

SIPRI [Stockholm International Peace Research Institute]. 2015. SIPRI Military Expenditure Database. https://www.sipri.org/databases/milex. Accessed July 20, 2016.

Stover E, Cobey JC, and Fine J. 1997. The public health effects of land mines: Long-term consequences for civilians. In Levy BS and Sidel VW, Editors. *War and Public Health*. New York: Oxford University Press.

Strömberg D. 2007. Natural disasters, economic development, and humanitarian aid. *Journal of Economic Perspectives* 21(3):199–222.

Stumpenhorst M, Stumpenhorst R, and Razum O. 2011. The UN OCHA cluster approach: Gaps between theory and practice. *Journal of Public Health* 19(6):587–592.

Summerfield D. 2000. War and mental health: A brief overview. *BMJ* 321:232–235.

Telford J and Cosgrave J. 2006. *Joint Evaluation of the International Response to the Indian Ocean Tsunami: Synthesis Report*. London: Tsunami Evaluation Coalition.

Thoms O and Ron J. 2007. Public health, conflict and human rights: Toward a collaborative research agenda. *Conflict and Health* 1(11).

Thurtle N, Cooney L, Amitai Y, et al. 2014. Description of 3,180 courses of chelation with dimercaptosuccinic acid in children ≤5 y with severe lead poisoning in Zamfara, northern Nigeria: A retrospective analysis of programme data. *PLoS Medicine* 11(10):e1001739.

Tisdall S. 2015. 2015 is 'year of fear' for children worldwide, warns Gordon Brown. *Guardian,* May 26.

UN. 2015a. Office of the Special Representative of the Secretary General for Children and Armed Conflict: Central African Republic. https://childrenandarmedconflict.un.org/countries/central-african-republic/. Accessed June 27, 3015.

———. 2015b. *The Millennium Development Goals Report 2015*. New York: UN.

UN Africa Renewal. 2015. What went wrong? Lessons from Malawi's food crisis. http://www.un.org/africarenewal/magazine/january-2013/what-went-wrong-lessons-malawi%E2%80%99s-food-crisis. Accessed May 30, 2015.

UN News Centre. 2011a. When a food security crisis becomes a famine. http://www.un.org/apps/news/story.asp?NewsID=39113#.VWmTIcguk. Accessed 30 May, 2015.

———. 2011b. UN declares famine in two regions of southern Somalia. http://www.un.org/apps/news/story.asp?NewsID=39086#.VXhbielViko. Accessed June 26, 2015.

UNHCR. 2000. *Protecting Refugees: A Field Guide for NGOs*. Geneva: UNHCR.

———. 2015a. Myanmar: 2015 UNHCR country operations profile. http://www.unhcr.org/pages/49e4877d6.html. Accessed June 3, 2015.

———. 2015b. *Ukraine Situation: UNHCR Operational Update, 7-22 October 2015*. Geneva: UNHCR.

———. 2016a. *Global Trends: Forced Displacement in 2015*. Geneva: UNHCR.

———. 2016b. Refugees/Migrants Emergency Response – Mediterranean. http://data.unhcr.org/mediterranean/regional.php. Accessed October 6, 2016.

———. 2016c. *Ukraine: UNHCR Operational Update 2–22 April 2016*. UNHCR: Geneva.

UNICEF. 2009a. Beyond School Books - a podcast series on education in emergencies. http://www.unicef.org/infobycountry/oPt_48758.html. Accessed June 28, 2015.

———. 2009b. *Tsunami Five-Year Report Q&A*. New York: UNICEF.

———. 2014. *Children and Emergencies in 2014: Facts & Figures*. New York: UNICEF.

———. 2016. Humanitarian action for children 2016. http://www.unicef.org/hac2016/. July 20, 2016.

UNICEF and United Nations (Office of the Special Representative of the Secretary-General for Children and Armed Conflict). 2009. *Machel Study 10-Year Strategic Review: Children and Conflict in a Changing World*. New York: UNICEF.

UNOCHA. 2011 Haiti: one year later – the crisis at a glance. http://www.unocha.org/issues-in-depth/haiti-one-year-later. Accessed August 3, 2015.

———. 2016a. El Niño: Southern Africa faces its worst drought in 35 years. http://www.unocha.org/top-stories/all-stories/el-ni%C3%B10-southern-africa-faces-its-worst-drought-35-years. Accessed July 20, 2016.

———. 2016b. Syrian Arab Republic. http://www.unocha.org/syria. Accessed July 20, 2016.

UNOCHA Yemen. 2016. *Humanitarian Response Plan: January-December 2016*. Sana'a: UNOCHA Yemen.

UNODC. 2008. *The Threat of Narco-Trafficking in the Americas*. Vienna: UNODC.

———. 2014a. *Global Report on Trafficking in Persons 2014*. Vienna: UNODC.

———. 2014b. *World Drug Report 2014*. Vienna: UNODC.

UNOG. 2015. Membership of the Biological Weapons Convention. http://www.unog.ch/—80256ee600585943.nsf/(httpPages)/7be6cbbea0477b52c12571860035fd5c?OpenDocument&ExpandSection=3%2C2%2C1#_Section3. Accessed June 26, 2015.

UNRWA. 2015. *In Figures 2015*. Jerusalem: UNRWA.

Uzokwe AO. 2003. *Surviving in Biafra: The Story of the Nigerian Civil War: Over Two Million Died*. Bloomington: iUniverse.

Valencia Villa A, Buitrago AM, Beristain CM, et al. 2016. *Final report: Ayotzinapa Report 2: Advances and New Conclusions*. Washington, DC: Inter-American Commission of Human Rights, Grupo Interdisciplinario de Expertos Independientes.

Van Damme W. 1995. Do refugees belong in camps? Experiences from Goma and Guinea. *Lancet* 346:360–362.

Van Reybrouck D. 2014. *Congo: The Epic History of a People*. New York: Harper Collins.

Vitullo A, Soboh A, Oskarsson J, et al. 2012. Barriers to the access to health services in the occupied Palestinian territory: A cohort study. *Lancet* 380:S18–S19.

Vu A, Adam A, Wirtz A, et al. 2014. The Prevalence of Sexual violence among female refugees in complex humanitarian emergencies: A systematic review and meta-analysis. *PLoS Currents* 6.

Waldman RJ. 2008. The roles of humanitarian assistance organizations. In Levy BS and Sidel VW, Editors. *War and Public Health*, Second Edition. New York: Oxford University Press.

Walk Free Foundation. 2014. *The Global Slavery Index 2014*. Nedlands: Walk Free Foundation.

Ward J and Marsh M. 2006. Sexual violence against women and girls in war and its aftermath: Realities, responses and required resources: Symposium on Sexual Violence in Conflict and Beyond, June 21-23. Brussels: UNFPA, the European Commission and the Government of Belgium.

Warner K, Ehrhart C, de Sherbinin A, et al. 2009. *In Search of Shelter: Mapping the Effects of Climate Change on Human Migration and Displacement.* Atlanta: CARE.

Watson JT, Gayer M, and Connolly MA. 2007. Epidemics after natural disasters. *Emerging Infectious Diseases* 13(1):1–5.

Weissman F. 2010. Not in our name: Why MSF does not support the Responsibility to Protect. http://www.doctorswithoutborders.org/news-stories/ideaopinion/not-our-name-why-msf-does-not-support-responsibility-protect. Accessed May 31, 2016.

White House Office of the Press Secretary. 2011. *Fact Sheet on the Successful Conclusion of the Seventh Review Conference of the Biological and Toxin Weapons Convention.* Washington, DC.

Whittall J. 2014. Opinion and debate: The limits of humanitarianism in Gaza. http://www.msf.org.uk/article/opinion-and-debate-limits-humanitarianism-gaza. Accessed May 31, 2015.

WHO. 2004. *Public Health Response to Biological and Chemical Weapons,* Second Edition. Geneva: WHO.

———. 2014a. *Gaza Strip Joint Health Sector Assessment Report: Prepared by the Health Cluster in the occupied Palestinian territory.* Geneva: WHO.

———. 2014b. *Right to health: Crossing barriers to access health in the occupied Palestinian territory.* Geneva: WHO.

———. 2016. Global Health Observatory data repository. http://apps.who.int/gho/data/. Accessed July 20, 2016.

WHO EMRO. 2014. WHO appeals for US$8.7 million to rejuvenate, improve Gaza's health system. http://www.emro.who.int/pse/palestine-news/health-system-appeal.html. Accessed June 20, 2015.

WFP. 2015. What causes hunger? https://www.wfp.org/hunger/causes. Accessed May 30, 2015.

Wiist WH, Barker K, Arya N, et al. 2014. The role of public health in the prevention of war: Rationale and competencies. *American Journal of Public Health* 104(6):e34–e47.

Yip J, Zeig-Owens R, Webber MP, et al. 2016. World Trade Center-related physical and mental health burden among New York City Fire Department emergency medical service workers. *Occupational and Environmental Medicine* 73:13–20.

Yokoro K and Kamada N. 1997. The public health effects of the use of nuclear weapons. In Levy BS and Sidel VW, Editors. *War and Public Health.* New York: Oxford University Press.

Young K. 2001. UNHCR and ICRC in the former Yugoslavia: Bosnia-Herzegovina. *Revue Internationale de la Croix-Rouge/International Review of the Red Cross* 83(843):781–806.

9

GLOBALIZATION, TRADE, WORK, AND HEALTH

Idris is a 10-year-old boy growing up in Dhaka, Bangladesh. As portrayed in the documentary "A Kind of Childhood," Idris works at a garment factory in order to support his family because his blind father is unemployed. When a nongovernmental organization (NGO) campaigns against child labor, however, Idris loses his job and the family its income. Local NGOs, with international support, help Idris and other former child laborers attend school by covering their fees. Idris is a dedicated student, but because his family relies on his wages, he begins to work as a fare collector on a three-wheeled minibus, facing the triple perils of treacherous traffic, stress, and extremely contaminated air.

When the school schedule changes, Idris is forced to drop out and transforms his dream of education into one of minibus driver. Then his minibus crashes: injury and financial stress ensue; he also begins experiencing respiratory problems. As the film progresses, we see Idris age before our eyes. He becomes severely ill at the age of 14, already seeming like an old man (Masud and Masud 2003). As this chapter illustrates, the factors involved in Idris's plight, including poverty, child labor, unsafe working conditions, global markets for cheap consumer goods, international advocacy and aid—as well as inadequate health and social protections—are all linked to globalization processes.

The term *globalization* is omnipresent—used to describe developments in arenas as diverse as communications, culture, technology, business, travel, finance, and social movements. But what *is* globalization and how does it affect health? This chapter explores the concept of globalization and outlines its implications for trade, work, and human health and well-being. We begin by discussing different types of globalization, emphasizing its dominant form within the current stage of capitalism, known as *neoliberal globalization*. Then we focus on the causal pathways that link neoliberal globalization to patterns of illness, death, and injury: debt and financial crises; financial liberalization; "free" trade, investment, and the penetration of transnational corporations (TNCs); and reorganization of production, and deregulation of worker and environmental protections. The next part of the chapter concentrates on the crucial global health issue of work under neoliberal globalization. We examine the effects of changing labor and production patterns—and the role of occupational safety and health measures—on the health of workers, including women and children. We conclude with a discussion of governmental, transnational, and local social movement challenges to neoliberal globalization in the realm of health.

GLOBALIZATION AND ITS (DIS)CONTENTS

Key Questions:

- Which dimensions of contemporary globalization are old and which are new?

- What is neoliberal globalization and what are its key features? Where does capitalism fit in?

Generally speaking, globalization is "... a *process* of greater integration within the world economy through movements of goods and services, capital, technology and (to a lesser extent) labor, which lead increasingly to economic decisions being influenced by global conditions" (Jenkins 2004, p. 1). Although people and societies have traded goods and ideas throughout human history—as well as slaves and other forced laborers—the pace of contemporary globalization marks it as a distinct historical phenomenon. Globalization is not inherently "good" or "bad" and goes beyond economic issues: it might engender enhanced cultural understanding or political solidarity among oppressed groups. Still, globalization's contemporary manifestation under capitalism's neoliberal period involves the internationalization of finance at record-breaking speed, with accompanying extreme, sometimes overnight, effects on social inequality. It has affected virtually all people: there are clear "winners" and "losers" based on *how* globalization has unfolded and on *whose* terms.

Briefly, neoliberal globalization is a particular configuration of the 250-year-old economic system of capitalism, in which investment in and ownership of the means of production (property), distribution, and exchange of wealth is made and maintained chiefly by private individuals or corporations, as opposed to cooperative or state-owned arrangements. This system of private property and exchange forces virtually all economic actors to depend on the market (Brenner 2006). Capitalism is characterized by the existence of and relations between a ruling class of owners and managers and a subordinate class of wage and salary earners (workers) plus dependents and retirees. While unemployed and self-employed persons are not technically subject to capitalist relations, they still operate within the capitalist system: the unemployed serve as a "reserve army" of potential workers, and self-employed persons must nonetheless buy and sell goods and services within a capitalist market. By contrast, certain Indigenous groups and other people living in communal or shared economy situations may remain outside the capitalist system.[1]

The subordinate class does the work (making goods or producing services) for the reproduction of the ruling class. Not only are workers exploited (meaning that the products of their labor, and associated profits, go not to themselves but to the owners), they end up working to reproduce the very conditions of their own subordination. The more exploited the workers are (the more surplus is extracted from them), the wealthier the owners and the lower the standard of living of the subordinate class (Shaikh 1990).

With profitability the ultimate goal of capitalists (and essential to succeeding in the market), the drive for profits depends on ever-expanding economic growth and consumption, in turn derived from extraction, exploitation, depletion, and contamination of natural and human resources, as well as other forms of accumulation such as land dispossession. War (and under colonialism, territorial expansion and domination) is partner to capitalism in assuring control over resources and capital accumulation (Panitch and Gindin 2012) (see chapters 1 and 8).

Ensuring profits requires continuous technological innovation, productivity gains, financialization, and speculation carried out in new ways and in new places (Harvey 2014). Capitalism also faces periodic crises of capital accumulation (often benignly called business cycles), including the Great Depression of the 1930s, a crisis so large that it upended the relationship among the state, society, and market, but preserved capitalism itself.

Modern globalization under capitalism has taken place in several waves. Comparing the period from the 1870s to the 1930s with the last 4 decades, the earlier period experienced a highly internationalized economy as measured by the sum of exports plus imports as a percentage of gross national product (GNP) (Hirst, Thompson, and Bromley 2009). This "globalization index" declined sharply in the 1930s and only recovered after the 1960s, then grew rapidly as of 1990, leading to the phenomenon we see today.

Likewise, the mobility of capital (the international flow of money) for major trading countries was even higher in the 1890s than in recent years. Just as today, technology, means of communications (telegraph, telephone, media), and transportation (railroads, steamships) were evolving rapidly during the late 19th century (together with accelerated business and cultural transnationalism), as finance overtook labor in its ability to move across borders easily. In fact, many features of 19th century globalization persist, underwritten by capitalist ideology and

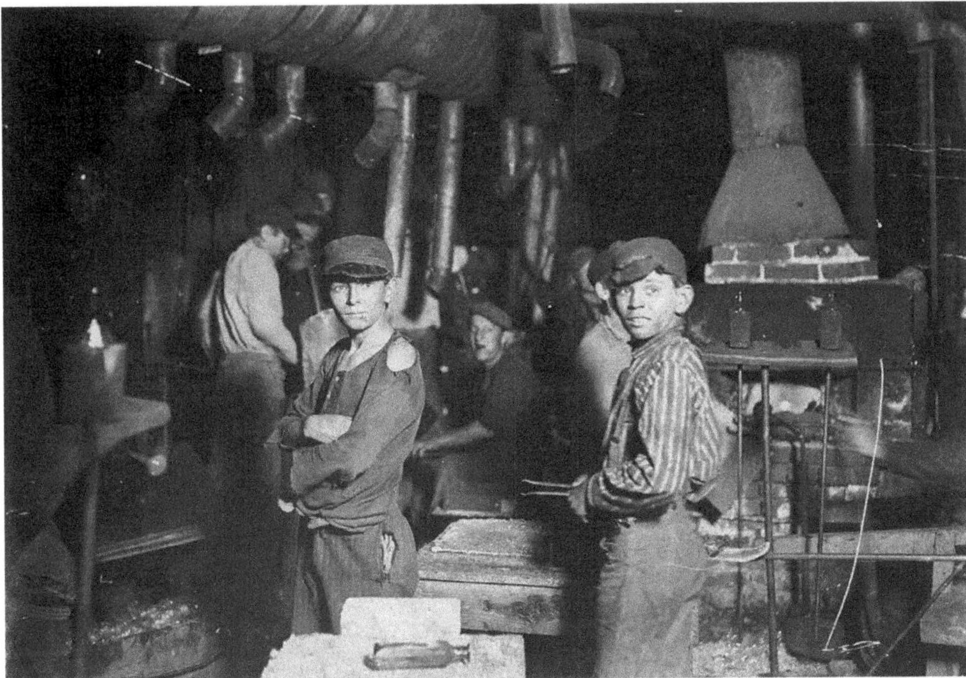

Figure 9-1: Child laborers at Indiana Glass Works, at midnight, 1908.
Photograph by Lewis Hine. Source: Library of Congress, Prints & Photographs Division, National Child Labor Committee Collection, [LC-DIG-nclc-01151].

practices. The image of child laborers in a US factory circa 1900 (Figure 9-1) is eerily echoed in appalling working conditions for children in India and many other places today (Figure 9-2).

The earlier period saw Europe's colonial powers—joined by the United States in the late 19th century—promote global economic expansion as the key to progress, shepherded by big business and corporate trusts and enabled by territorial expansion. Such imperial domination (which in the case of the United States was only partially based on direct colonial control) propelled the extraction of precious raw materials, exemplified by the asymmetrical power relationship between US rubber giant Firestone and the small country of Liberia. A 1926 rubber concession gave the company an option of leasing up to 1 million acres, also requiring the Liberian government to take out a large loan (from, it turned out, a Firestone subsidiary) to cover outstanding debts to other creditors (in order to protect Firestone's capital investment). Even more burdensome were the terms of the loan agreement, which gave a US auditor extensive oversight over Liberian government spending, and prohibited it from issuing its own debt, making certain that US appointees would oversee customs and revenue collections, with disputes resolved in US-stacked panels! In sum, "Firestone was determined to ensure that no nation or business other than his own could exercise control over many of the essential functions of the Liberian government" (Mitman and Erickson 2010, p. 65). As we shall see, this multinational-finance-government nexus present a century ago has remarkable contemporary parallels under neoliberal globalization, with considerable health implications.

But between these two periods, the world was governed by a contrasting political economy arrangement. Governments forged policies to address capitalism's largest ever crisis—the Great Depression—modifying market rule with an unprecedented level of state intervention (known as regulated capitalism) in the economy, an approach lasting for over three decades following World War II. This shift heeded principles of government fiscal

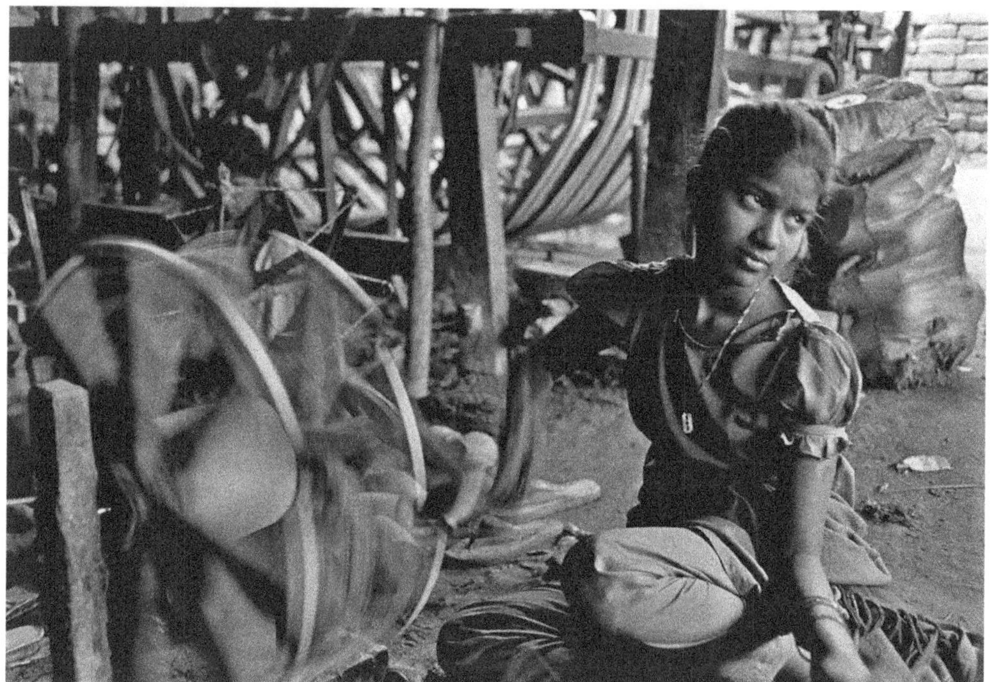

Figure 9-2: Child spinning wool, India.
Photo courtesy of David Parker.

management, progressive taxation, redistributive social spending, and a large public sector within a mixed economy, simultaneously responding to pressure from ever greater working class power.

During these years—amid decolonization and Cold War tensions between capitalist and communist ideologies—Western powers, the Soviet bloc, and some Third World settings experienced an expansion of welfare states (see chapter 7), building on prior struggles to improve living, working, and political conditions. Social security systems and other government protections spurred reductions in poverty and inequity, although social struggles for gender, class, and racial justice were uneven and incomplete. Despite fears around nuclear escalation—as well as brutal proxy wars in the remains of the Belgian, British, Dutch, French, and Portuguese colonial empires—there were certain benefits stemming from the US-Soviet rivalry for many non-aligned countries. As the two superpowers sought to garner allies, foreign aid investments in infrastructure, education, health, and other social arenas flowed in (though much aid was harmful, irrelevant, or patronizing—see chapter 2).

By the 1980s, however, these developments reversed course as neoliberal globalization took hold. As presented in chapter 2, neoliberal ideology is linked to reorganization of state institutions, production processes, and state power (including military and police), with the state undergirding the market through privatization and reorientation to favor foreign and domestic elites. This has transpired through legislation protecting (transnational) corporate interests and trade at the expense of workers, lowering of corporate/wealth taxes, redistribution upwards instead of downwards, and an overall retrenchment of the welfare state (Schrecker and Bambra 2015; Ward and England 2007). With the US-backed Chilean military dictatorship led by Augusto Pinochet serving as a policy incubator starting in the 1970s, neoliberal ideology flourished under the 1980s regimes of UK Prime Minister Margaret Thatcher and US President Ronald Reagan and, spread through the resurgence of a globalized economy as the Cold War was waning. These policies were crystallized and applied to low- and middle-income countries (LMICs) via the Washington Consensus development orthodoxy (see chapter 2) marshaled by international financial institutions (IFIs) (Stiglitz 2002).

Meanwhile, the dissolution of the USSR and collapse of the Soviet bloc in the early 1990s facilitated neoliberal capitalism's aim of integrating all countries into a global market. This also reinforced the tendencies toward privatization and deregulation (of health, safety, etc.) and purportedly "proved" that state regulation did not "work" (even as the countries of the former USSR, now capitalist and with social protections stripped down, faced a major crisis of increasing mortality—see chapter 3).

Notwithstanding similarities between 19th century and contemporary global capitalism around intensification of trade and labor exploitation, technological and communications revolutions, and market and cultural transnationalism, the present period marks a departure in terms of the extent of internationalization of finance and speculation (resulting in potentially sudden huge economic and social effects), as well as a "profound reorganization of the production process . . .—the fragmentation and decentralization across the globe of vast production chains" (Robinson 2014, p. 160).

The current neoliberal stage of capitalism (Wood 1999) has already undergone several phases. First has been the rise of the neoliberal model rearranging the relations among the state, labor, and market, as described earlier. Second is financialization—the growing role of financial motives, markets, actors, and "institutions in the operation of the domestic and international economies" (Epstein 2005, p. 3)—with profit and accumulation increasingly derived from the speculative (non-productive) sectors of banking, insurance, and real estate rather than through trade and production of commodities. Third is the globalization of austerity following the 2008 global financial crisis, as manifested in a hollowing out of the public sector and accelerating economic and social inequality in high-income countries (HICs) and LMICs alike. That is, instead of delegitimizing neoliberalism, the 2008 crisis has reinforced it, so that all three phases are presently pervasive, albeit with some signs of resistance (Harvey 2014; PHM et al. 2014).

Accordingly, trade and finance under neoliberal globalization have multiple implications. To a currency trader in Singapore or London, it might mean the lightning speed at which multimillion dollar transactions are completed anywhere in the world, at any time of day. To a small farmer in rural Ethiopia, neoliberal globalization might result in a new toll road linking him to the market to sell his crops, but also the arrival of low-priced competitor crops. It also signifies more expensive seeds and credit, indebtedness, and the increasing likelihood that his plot will be bought by a wealthier farmer or a foreign-owned agribusiness producing for export. To a second-generation nurse in Madrid or Montreal, it might mean a precarious job (or several) with no benefits or security, lower earning prospects than his mother had, and mounting debt. To a low-wage auto parts worker in Honduras, neoliberal globalization might mean (barely) being able to pay rent and support family members thanks to a job that lacks adequate safety precautions and the right to unionize. This work, likely outsourced from a higher paid setting in North America, may soon be shifted to Southeast Asia, where wages and factory conditions are even worse. In either setting, drinking a globally-marketed bottle of Pepsi may be cheaper and safer than a glass of municipal water.

How has this transpired? According to economic historian Ha-Joon Chang (2002), the free trade cornerstone of Washington Consensus policy has been uniquely detrimental to LMICs. Chang argues that from the 18th to the mid-20th centuries, currently affluent nations made extensive use of tariffs, supports, and other interventionist policies promoting domestic industries to enable growth.

Yet these now wealthy nations and the institutions they established and influence, including the World Trade Organization (WTO) and the International Monetary Fund (IMF), today insist that poorer nations abandon such measures and implement comprehensive free trade policies, inviting foreign capital to partake in local riches while leaving little behind. This is particularly true and hypocritical of countries that are strong advocates of removing trade barriers, like the United States and United Kingdom. Both of these nations used tariffs and subsidies well into their peak industrialization eras to foster the growth of nascent sectors. Such a blatantly contradictory changing of the rules of the game (stated more politely by Chang [2002] as "policy inconsistency") amounts to wealthy nations "kicking away the ladder" they climbed up. In following neoliberal globalization's canons, LMICs are compelled to jeopardize both economic conditions and, as we shall see, health.

In fact, those LMICs held up as globalization success stories, for instance South Korea, Taiwan, and Singapore, experienced much of their poverty-reducing growth (and health improvements) before they began to open up their economies, reduce their import tariffs, and invite foreign investment (Rapley 2007). Their more recent but larger counterparts, India and China, shepherded limited economic growth under import protection measures and strict controls over banking and investment, not full-fledged integration. Likewise, their largest health gains (due to infant mortality declines) preceded rapid economic growth under neoliberal globalization in the 1980s (China) and 1990s (India) (Cutler, Deaton, and Lleras-Muney 2006).

Ultimately, how globalization affects the health of people around the world depends on who controls the flow of capital, labor, and knowledge, and who benefits and suffers. Power and politics—and their complex relationships with the economy—are thus central to understanding the effects of globalization (see key definitions in Table 9-1). Still, Chang's call for LMIC sovereignty and domestic protections does not challenge the asymmetries in power and resources inherent in capitalism, which would require a large-scale realignment of power both within and across settings (Tapia Granados 2013).

Table 9-1 Key Definitions Relating to Globalization, Trade, and Work

Term	Definition
Capital	Wealth (financial and physical resources); may also refer to owners/investors
Currency devaluation; inflation	A reduction in the value of a currency with respect to other monetary units (often to stimulate exports); contrasted with inflation, which is a sustained rise in the price of goods and services. Both may affect purchasing power, especially of low-income groups
Deregulation/reorientation of the state	Reduction of the role of the state in the labor market and in protecting health, safety, and the environment; and simultaneous reorientation and strengthening of state regulations to facilitate private capital accumulation (and manage crises in favor of financial interests)
Foreign direct investment (FDI)	Controlling ownership in a business enterprise in one country by an entity based in another country
Foreign reserves	The foreign currency deposits held by central banks and monetary authorities
Free trade	A market model in which trade in goods and services between countries flows unhindered by tariffs, subsidies, or other government measures. In reality, most "free" trade is not truly unfettered, as governments often create regulations and loopholes that favor some industries over others, or TNCs at the expense of workers and the environment.
Free trade zones/export processing zones (EPZs)	Areas of a country where tariffs and domestic content quotas are eliminated and regulations and labor protections are lowered in hopes of attracting new business and FDI. Most free trade zones are labor-intensive manufacturing centers that involve the import of raw materials and the export of factory products.

Table 9-1 Continued

Gross Domestic Product (GDP) and Gross National Product (GNP)	Measures of national income and output that estimate the value of all goods and services produced in an economy. GDP consists of personal and governmental expenditures, private domestic investment, and exports minus imports. GNP comprises GDP plus income earned by residents from investments abroad (which for some countries can be substantial), minus income earned in the domestic economy by foreign residents. Neither takes remittances into account.
Informal sector	Work carried out outside official legal and social institutions (not taxed, monitored, or accounted for)
Labor	Work; or workers
Liberalization (economic/financial and trade)	Policies allowing market forces to determine key elements of the economy, including: exchange rates, interest rates, minimum wages; lifting barriers to trade and investment such as tariffs and FDI controls; "opening" banking and financial sectors; reducing subsidies that keep prices of some essential goods low to protect consumers or industries
Multinational/transnational corporations (TNCs)	Legally incorporated enterprises (obliged to maximize profits of shareholders) that own, manage, or subcontract production and deliver goods and services in at least two countries
Precariat	Class of workers (increasingly semi-skilled or skilled) with minimal job security or work predictability (experiencing frequent periods of unemployment or uneven employment); increasingly replaces proletariat—the industrial working class
Privatization	Selling of government assets and state-owned enterprises to private sector entities
Progressive taxation	A taxation policy in which the effective tax rate increases as income/earnings rise (i.e., people with a higher income pay a higher percentage of their income in taxes)
Protectionism	An economic policy to protect national industries through tariffs on imported goods, quotas, and other governmental regulations that discourage (competition from) imports
Subsidiary/foreign affiliate	A business entity that is controlled by another—often foreign—entity
Subsidies	Governmental financial assistance, usually in the form of grants, tax breaks, or trade barriers, to encourage production or facilitate purchase (lower consumer costs) of particular goods
Tariffs and duties	Tariffs are taxes on foreign goods upon importation. Duties also refer to taxes on exports or goods in transit. Tariffs and duties can be a set amount, a percent of the total value of the goods, or vary according to weight or quantity of goods.

HEALTH EFFECTS OF NEOLIBERAL GLOBALIZATION

Key Questions:

- What are the major pathways through which neoliberal globalization affects health?
- How have LMICs been affected by debt, foreign direct investment (FDI), capital flight, tax evasion, and structural adjustment "remedies" since the 1980s?
- How does the leadup to the 2008 financial crisis and the Great Recession's austerity measures in HICs compare to prior LMIC experiences?
- What are the effects of WTO agreements and regional trade and investment treaties on public health?

Proponents of (neoliberal) globalization argue that, at the aggregate level, global integration improves health thanks to economic growth, alongside social and political benefits (Dollar 2001). Some contend that the various economic (e.g., increased trade and capital flows; reduction in trade barriers), social (e.g., levels of media and information flows), and political (e.g., participation in international treaties and organizations) aspects of globalization are associated with lower infant and child mortality and higher life expectancy, independent of gross domestic product (GDP) per capita (with little clarity on the specific mechanisms) (Mukherjee and Krieckhaus 2012).

Remarkably, Richard Feachem (2001), the first director of the Global Fund to Fight AIDS, Tuberculosis and Malaria—charged with expanding access to therapeutics in LMICs—concluded that globalization's contribution to increasing the incomes of the poor overshadowed any of its ill effects (even though at the time literally millions of people were dying from AIDS due to rapacious antiretroviral [ARV] medication prices on the free market).

To be sure, such assertions and aggregate correlations between globalization and improved health do not demonstrate causality: the postulated mechanisms are unsubstantiated and the statistical results flawed by failing to disaggregate data over time, space, and in terms of equity effects within populations. Contesting Feachem's line of thinking, a range of powerful assessments show a decidedly deleterious impact of globalization upon health (Labonté et al. 2009; Schrecker 2012).

Countering its proponents' claims, unbridled economic integration has been shown to negatively affect the economies and health of many poorer countries. From 1980 to 2000—a period of rapid neoliberal globalization—economic growth was considerably slower than between 1960 and 1980 for countries at almost every income level. Among the world's 17 poorest countries, the rate of growth from 1960 to 1980 was a healthy 1.9%. During neoliberal globalization's surge between 1980 and 2000, these same countries experienced net negative growth and a decline of real per capita GDP (Weisbrot et al. 2002). Across sub-Saharan Africa, poverty nearly doubled during this period and life expectancy at birth fell by almost 9 years—amid liberalized markets, detrimental loan conditionalities, and the HIV epidemic (Schrecker, Labonté, and de Vogli 2008).

In subsequent years, trade in commodities helped improve economic performance in some countries, but this was not necessarily accompanied by health gains. For example, Africa grew on average 5% per year between 1996 and 2014 (including oil exporting nations Chad, Angola, Sudan, Nigeria, and Gabon) (UN Economic Commission for Africa 2014). Yet poverty and mortality rates in these countries remain among the highest in the world.

This leads to the second and even more problematic assumption by neoliberal globalization's advocates—that the benefits of increased trade and foreign investment are shared across and within societies via wealth distribution and sustained social services spending. If anything, with neoliberal globalization's onset in the 1980s, most countries have experienced a marked deterioration in public social services and an increase in wealth and income inequality. Despite some improvements in between-country GDP per capita inequality in the early 2000s, global wealth inequality has remained consistently extremely high (Milanovic 2012), and within many countries, such as the United States, there has been a significant increase in wealth and income inequality since the late 1970s, particularly driven by the wealthiest 0.1% (Saez and Zucman 2014) (see chapter 7).

In sum, the premise that neoliberal globalization levels the playing field simply does not stand up to scrutiny. As discussed in chapter 3, contrary to UN assessments, LMIC poverty rates have barely budged in 25 years, once China is excluded or the magnitude of poverty is appropriately gauged. Moreover, inequality grows faster with higher economic growth (Piketty 2013): promoting faster growth thus implies faster growth in inequality.

Flawed logic regarding neoliberal globalization's putative benefits aside, there is growing agreement that "global inequalities in income and living standards have reached grotesque proportions" (UNDP 1999, p. 104). Even Christine Lagarde (2014), the IMF's Managing Director (noting that IMF policies have played no small part in worsening inequality over the past 4 decades) admits, "There has been a staggering rise in inequality—7 out of 10 people in the world today live in countries where inequality has increased over the last three decades".

But recognizing the existence of inequality and understanding its roots and effects—as well as its remedies—are very different things. Accordingly, this chapter examines how the configuration of the global economic system, including labor market patterns, influences health. It also offers some prospects for resistance that will be explored further in chapters 13 and 14.

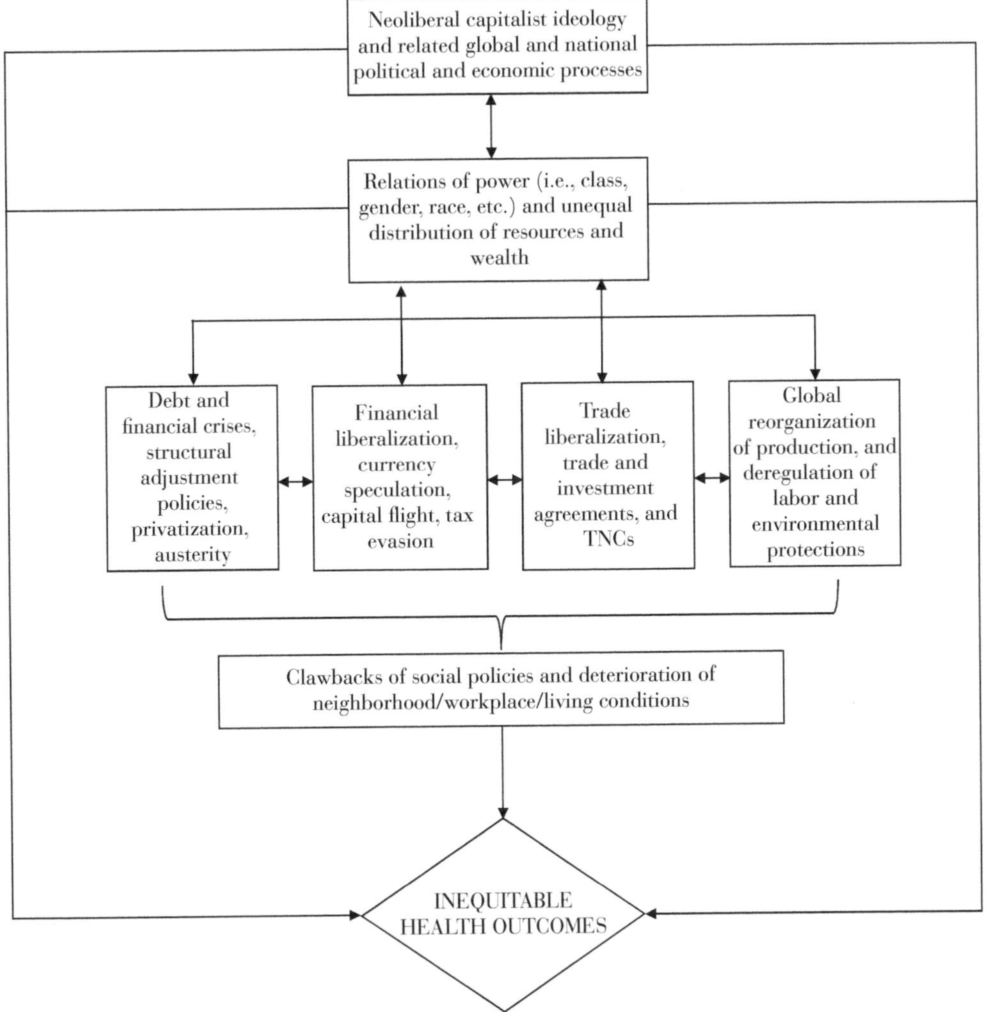

Figure 9-3: Pathways of neoliberal globalization and effects on health.
Source: Adapted from Labonté and Schrecker (2007, p. 5).

We continue with analysis of how neoliberal globalization affects health and health inequities via four major pathways (Figure 9-3):

1. Debt and financial crises, international financial instruments, including loan conditionalities, policy implications and consequences, such as privatization and austerity
2. Financial liberalization, currency speculation, capital flight and tax evasion
3. Trade liberalization, trade and investment agreements, and TNCs
4. Global reorganization of production/ deregulation of worker and environmental protections

Debt, Financial Crises, International Financial Instruments, Policy Responses, and their Consequences

Debt and Structural Adjustment

In the early 1980s a debt crisis that swept LMICs served to jump-start the contemporary wave of globalization. Understanding how this came about requires revisiting the decolonization process. In the aftermath of World War II, European colonial powers were faced with depleted coffers and renewed liberation struggles across Africa and Asia (later the Caribbean). Whereas France fought brutally to stave off Algerian independence, for example, other colonial powers left more willingly. Either way, dismantling colonialism's costly administrative apparatus did not remove one of its key rationales—access to profitable resources.

The former imperial powers inaugurated a new form of dependence through a quid pro quo arrangement that extended credit and loans to the newly liberated countries in exchange for continued business investment and access to primary resources. A cascade of loans was granted for infrastructure and institutional development, while foreign-controlled resources and profits flowed out, frequently skirting the law. In numerous locales, loan monies went into the hands of corrupt leaders, whose often brutal regimes were backed by the Cold War rivals in exchange for economic and political loyalty. Within a few decades, most former colonies, including those that genuinely invested in human need, found themselves shackled by debt and dependency (Toussaint and Millet 2010). By the 1970s, soaring oil prices, the breakdown of the Bretton Woods currency stabilization measures, and a huge US interest rate hike, put a swath of countries in dire indebtedness straits, straits that were very much manufactured (Prashad 2014) (see chapter 2).

Latin America, which (though decolonized from Spain and Portugal in the 19th century and despite import substitution and economic sovereignty attempts in the 20th) was dominated by US interests, had larger loans and was hit first by the debt crisis and its "remedies." The prescriptions were structural adjustment loans (SALs), aimed at restoring financial stability and ensuring the necessary economic growth and revenues to repay loans owed to private banks in HICs. Unleashed on more than 75 LMICs, SALs and subsequent loan programs from the World Bank and IMF compelled major economic reforms (known as structural adjustment programs or policies—SAPS) designed to reduce the size of government, open domestic markets to foreign penetration, expand the private sector, and stimulate low-cost exports.

Conditionalities accompanying these loans (rules governing their acceptance) included: deep cuts in government spending (in benefits and in health, sanitation, water, housing, and other social sectors), removal of trade tariffs and of agricultural and other basic goods subsidies, labor market reforms, lifting of restrictions on foreign investment in domestic industries (especially mining and agriculture), financial-sector liberalization, currency devaluation, and privatization of state enterprises (SAPRIN 2002). The top 20 SAL recipient countries received an average of 19 loans each between 1980 and 1999, without evidence that they were achieving either macroeconomic stability or sustained economic growth (Easterly 2005).

FDI flowed into countries under favorable (for the investor) conditions, but far more money left through tax evasion and capital flight, again with Latin America initially hit hardest. Simultaneously, currency devaluation—forced by conditionalities to encourage exports and obtain foreign currency to service debt—had enormous social consequences. Escalating inflation—over 500% annually in Brazil between 1985 and 1990 (Roberts 2014)—caused the cost of goods, including food basics, to double or triple overnight. Those with bank accounts lined up to retrieve cash each morning, quickly spending it even as inflation continued through the day. Those without accounts had little means of shielding themselves against rising prices. Poverty rates skyrocketed to over 50% (not returning to prior levels until after 2000) (Ocampo 2013), with the most vulnerable populations (children, women, Indigenous groups, and small farmers) disproportionately affected.

The effects of SAPs on health and its determinants have been debated (Breman and Shelton 2007), but even a World Bank-sanctioned review found that during the 1980s and 1990s SAP-induced declines in government spending decreased availability and quality of public-sector health care, with access further jeopardized by user fees and privatization (SAPRIN 2002). In 1980s Ecuador, for instance, per capita Ministry of Health spending fell by more than half, the number of private clinics grew by 75%, and the number of physicians working in the private sector increased 2.5 times, leaving the growing poor population to face prohibitive payments in private clinics or seek care in the overcrowded public sector (where fees were also often charged) (Peabody 1996).

The IMF claimed that health spending would rise with adherence to SAPs; however, the evidence suggests otherwise. Between 1985 and 2009, government expenditure on health in countries participating in SAPs decreased or stagnated everywhere except sub-Saharan Africa—where spending before this period was abysmally low (Kentikelenis, Stubbs, and King 2015). The IMF's argument that SAPs would attract donors to the health sector proved erroneous. From 1996 to 2006, countries that had *not* borrowed from the IMF channeled an additional US$0.45 to their health care system for every US$1 received in development assistance for health (DAH). Meanwhile, IMF borrowers channeled less than US$0.01 to their health care system for every US$1 received in DAH, due to IMF advice that rather than going to health, DAH be used to build up reserves, policies also conducive to keeping public sector spending low and inflation controlled (Stuckler, Basu, and McKee 2011). Moreover, until 2009, IMF-imposed ceilings on public sector wages pushed many health workers into the private sector or to emigrate, leading to huge health worker shortages, especially in sub-Saharan Africa (see chapter 11).

In sum, SAPs have generated adverse health effects in most settings where they were applied. In countries that signed an IMF loan between 1985 and 1989, overall death and disability rates increased through the 1990s (Hoddie and Hartzell 2014). Sub-Saharan African countries under World Bank-administered SAPs between 1990 and 2005 experienced worse child mortality; higher debt servicing was also associated with higher child mortality (Shandra, Shandra, and London 2011). IFI policies also had a devastating role in the inadequate initial response to the HIV pandemic in sub-Saharan Africa (Baker 2010). Similarly, former centrally-planned economies that underwent IMF reforms experienced health care system cuts and significantly higher TB incidence and mortality than non-IMF-affected counterparts (Stuckler and Basu 2009).

As discussed in chapter 3, SAPs' multiple failings led the IFIs to replace them with new debt relief programs and instruments, such as Poverty Reduction Strategy Papers (PRSPs). Despite tinkering on the margins to address the social impact of conditionalities, PRSPs, according to the World Health Organization (WHO), "do not systematically identify those health issues which are the biggest contributors to poverty . . . Nor do they look systematically at the health situation of the poor . . . Finally, it is clear . . . that PRSPs will not result in large increases in resources available for health" (WHO 2004, p. 18). In the end, PRSPs remain donor-driven, limiting domestic control over social and economic policymaking (Dijkstra 2011): they "put new wrappings on . . . old policies" (Baker 2010, p. 353). Yet similar loans and agreements have continued to proliferate in recent years (Bretton Woods Project 2015), entrenching privatization, liberalization, and deregulation policies long promoted by SALs (Ruckert, Labonté, and Parker 2015).

Global Financial Crisis, Austerity, and Health

> "We are meeting at a time of crisis. We face a fuel crisis, a food crisis, a severe financial crisis, and a climate that has begun to change in ominous ways. All of these crises have global causes and global consequences. All have profound, and profoundly unfair, consequences for health. Let me be very clear at the start. The health sector had no say when the policies responsible for these crises were made. But health bears the brunt." – Margaret Chan, WHO Director-General (Chan 2008)

Though North America and Europe also underwent neoliberal reforms, it would take yet another crisis of capital accumulation for financialization to play out on a global scale (Kotz 2015) and for the neoliberal policies rampant in many LMICs to fully reach HICs (Navarro and Muntaner 2014). The 2008 financial crisis may be seen as a direct result of the state "disentwining itself from the financial market" in the prior decade as one means of restoring profitability to the capitalist system (Weiss 2012, p. 36). This financial sector "self-regulation" opened the door to ever riskier and shadier lending and borrowing practices, such as credit default swaps (trading on bankruptcies) and derivatives ("securities" with no intrinsic value that are entirely based on an underlying asset or index), essentially creating a shadow banking sector with almost no oversight.

By 2006–2007, deflation in US housing prices following predatory bank lending led to large-scale defaults on mortgages and a massive devaluation of housing-related securities (stocks, bonds, and other assets), straining what was then the world's largest economy. The threat of collapse of financial institutions across HICs led to stock market declines, triggering the 2008–2012 global recession (Great Recession) and the European sovereign-debt crisis. Across multiple regions, economies slowed, unemployment soared, credit tightened, and international trade declined, sparking the worst economic downturn since the Great Depression. In the United States alone, over 5 million homes (and associated life savings) were lost to foreclosure, disproportionately affecting working class, low-income, and minority populations. Across much of the world, both the urban and rural poor, already suffering from a 2007–2008 food and fuel crisis, became even more susceptible to malnutrition and further impoverishment due to price spikes and financial shocks (Ruel et al. 2010).

Several European countries entered depression (sustained economic slowdown), hitting those with large trade deficits and heavily financialized economies (reliant on debt as a prime driver of the economy)—Spain, Portugal, Ireland, and Greece—particularly hard. Facing balance of payment crises, governments were pressed to apply harsh austerity measures, cutting services and benefits, thereby evaporating pensions and household budgets. Meanwhile these governments applied an "internal devaluation" by forcing wage cuts, purportedly to spur competitiveness but mostly resulting in increased corporate profits (Toussaint 2013). The reforms that the European Commission (EC), the European Central Bank (ECB), and the IMF obliged Greece to implement in return for loan packages averting default and exit from the Eurozone have created a circle of ongoing recession, repayment, and loan conditionalities leading to unemployment levels of over 25% in 2014 (an astounding 50% among youth) (OECD 2016), mounting poverty, and strangling the lower middle class and small- and medium-sized enterprises.

Though less time has elapsed than since the 1980s LMIC debt crisis, the health and social effects of austerity policies have begun to emerge. Between 2008 and 2010 there were an estimated 10,000 excess suicides in Europe and North America (Reeves, McKee, and Stuckler 2014). Austerity-driven social suffering in Greece and other countries—involving, for instance, drastic cuts to housing, disability, child, and unemployment benefits in the United Kingdom (O'Hara 2015)—has been magnified among the most disadvantaged groups. Economic hardship has been linked to increases in the prevalence of major depression in Greece and Spain, with household income insecurity leading to higher child malnutrition (Karanikolos et al. 2013).

The fiscal situation caused a partial collapse of Greece's health care system, with a 25% reduction in health care spending, more than 2.3 million people uninsured compared with 500,000 in 2008, shortages of pharmaceuticals and medical equipment (especially in rural areas), and shifting of health care costs to patients (Kentikelenis et al. 2014). Health care access for the poorest groups has been undermined, even as the wealthiest quintile have enjoyed a decline in unmet health care needs (Karanikolos and Kentikelenis 2016). There was also a large-scale exodus of doctors, particularly to Germany, the United Kingdom, and Sweden (Ifanti et al. 2014). Reduced access to care—including prenatal services—combined with the deterioration in social and economic circumstances may also be responsible for a 2008–2010 rise in low birthweight babies, stillbirths, and infant mortality (Kentikelenis et al. 2014). Large cuts in health care spending have also occurred in Ireland, Spain, and Portugal, where governments adopted strict austerity policies (Karanikolos et al. 2013).

Yet Greece, at least in the short term, did not experience overall worse mortality than Iceland or Finland, which did not pursue austerity cuts (Tapia Granados and Rodriguez 2015). While mortality (or life expectancy) is not the only indicator of population health—and an austerity-induced mortality crisis could still materialize—the buffer provided by longtime welfare states (even those facing severe cuts) may well differentiate the effects of crisis in Europe compared with LMICs in the 1980s and 1990s.

The EC-ECB-IMF troika-imposed Greek response to the recession turned a bad economic situation drastically worse (Toussaint 2013). But other alternatives existed: Iceland rejected austerity through a referendum. Although the devaluation of the krona dramatically increased the price of imports and reduced household income, suicides did not rise and the impact on well-being has been minimal. Instead of following IFI advice on cutbacks and deregulation, Iceland invested in social protection and is the only country to have prosecuted and imprisoned bankers responsible for the crisis. On another front, the high price of imports prompted the exit of McDonald's from the country, benefiting the domestic fishing economy and favoring healthier home-cooked meals (Karanikolos et al. 2013).

Iceland's example shows that economic crises can sometimes have positive health and social effects. As with the 1990s experiences under Japan's decade-long recession and Cuba after the collapse of Soviet support (see chapter 13), countries that pursue more egalitarian policies, notwithstanding overall economic conditions, can protect against mortality under conditions of "healthy de-growth" (De Vogli and Owusu 2015).

For the most part, however, the crisis has entailed a colossal realignment of power and capital in the hands of private financial interests across HICs. In the United States, taxpayers are underwriting ongoing government subsidies of up to US$17 trillion in secretive, conditionality-free taxpayer bailouts of banks "too big to fail," whereas social programs face massive cuts now and into the future (Collins 2015). Thus, governments purportedly too cash-strapped to ensure basic well-being to those "too small to save" (the majority of the population) have untold resources funded by those "too small" in order to resolve the capital side of the 2008 financial crisis, itself an outgrowth of a deliberately under-regulated financial system (Gindin 2013). The rescue packages also helped to replenish IMF coffers with US$750 billion to rescue big investors (De Vogli 2011).

The ripple effects globally are still playing out. Initially Brazil and China, for example, recovered quickly, though both countries are currently facing serious economic downturns amid dropping commodity prices and declining demand for goods. The International Labour Organization (ILO) has estimated that the Great Recession caused over 60 million people to lose their jobs (ILO 2015a), with hundreds of millions of people in LMICs forced into poverty. Meanwhile the neoliberal agenda has been strengthened and justified, with banks and their unpunished executives ever wealthier (De Vogli 2011).

Financial Liberalization, Currency Speculation, Capital Flight, and Tax Evasion

Financial Liberalization and Currency Speculation

Financial liberalization—reorienting the role of the state to favor private capital and opening up banking and financial systems to world markets—is a key aspect of neoliberal globalization, justified as a stimulus to economic growth. Yet even mainstream economists cannot provide empirical evidence about whether financial liberalization and growth are positively correlated (Bumann et al. 2013).

By definition, financial liberalization exposes national economies to the uncertainties created by large and volatile capital. The over US$5 trillion in daily currency transactions (communication technology enables round-the-clock currency trading and finance capital exchanges) have caused enormous instability, with transactions dwarfing the foreign currency reserves of many governments.

Much of this capital flow is speculative rather than investment in productive capacity. Speculative finance has made some investors, such as George Soros, spectacularly rich from betting on currency devaluations, in turn contributing to commodity price volatility and the attendant social and economic effects (UNCTAD 2012). On the whole, many of the countries (and entire regions) most exposed to financial liberalization have experienced socially disruptive crises in the past quarter century, including Mexico (1994–1995), South Asia (1997–1998), Russia (1998), Argentina (2001–2002), Ireland (2008), and Greece (2010–present). Sudden financial crises and currency devaluations can evaporate purchasing power overnight and undermine the livelihoods and health of hundreds of millions of people for years following these events.

Capital Flight and Tax Evasion (Illicit Financial Flows)

Capital flight and tax evasion have long been partners to global capitalism, as per the story of Firestone in Liberia—involving manipulation of accounting, trade, tax, and investment rules, corporate-related activity constitutes the bulk of global corruption (Sachs 2011). Capital flight refers to financial outflows that are not officially recorded in a country's balance of payments. This money may be: illegally acquired (e.g., from criminal activity); moved out of a country to escape economic instability, currency risk, or to pursue higher returns; intentionally hidden abroad to avoid paying taxes; or part of elaborate TNC accounting gymnastics that shift profits to countries with low tax rates and report expenditures in high-tax settings in order to offset taxes (Ajayi and Ndikumana 2015; Tax Justice Network 2016). Although capital flight predates neoliberal globalization, "it has been facilitated by financial liberalization and deregulation and the provision of shelters for flight capital in the financial institutions (and real estate markets) of high-income countries and offshore financial centers" (Schrecker 2014, p. 398).

The more recent concept of illicit financial flows, extensively overlapping with capital flight, encompasses illegal trans-border movement of capital, including all forms of money laundering, the transfer of money illegally obtained (e.g. from smuggling, trafficking, tax evasion, bribes), unlawful bulk transfer of cash, trade misinvoicing (i.e. "deliberately misreporting" the value of commercial transactions), and balance-of-payment "leakages" (i.e. improperly maintained international transaction records). Conservatively estimated, illicit financial outflows from LMICs amounted to US$1.1 trillion in 2013 (Kar and Spanjers 2015).

Tax evasion is a major part of capital flight/illicit financial flows, involving money that is illegally transferred internationally to escape taxation/detection and thus permanently lost to tax collection. An estimated US$156 billion is lost in potential tax revenues to LMICs every year, and globally between US$21 and US$32 trillion in capital is stashed in tax havens (Kedir 2015).

A fellow traveler to tax evasion is tax avoidance, referring to technically legal cross-border transfers of wealth in order to benefit from lower tax rates. This phenomenon has been stimulated by tax competition, whereby countries (some in the EU, such as Ireland, and a growing number of LMICs) engage in a "race to the bottom" by lowering tax rates to attract or retain large corporate and individual investors. Yet tax avoidance derives from preferential laws and obfuscatory loopholes devised specifically for corporate and other monied interests to flout fair and democratic tax policies—ultimately to dodge taxes. Thus, tax evasion and avoidance may be more appropriately considered together under the rubric *tax abuse* (Tax Justice Network 2016). The 2016 Panama Papers leak revealed the mammoth scale of tax abuse, with tax havens harboring up to 14% of global wealth. Panama's Mossack Fonseca firm, only the fourth largest in the world, holds accounts for several hundred thousand shell companies, trusts, and foundations, hiding the owners' identities and thus shielding them from taxation. Indeed, Fortune 500 corporate tax cheats park over US$2 trillion offshore, amounting to approximately US$620 billion in lost US taxes (FACT Coalition 2015). All forms of tax abuse have damaging effects on health by reducing revenues available for domestic spending on health care and on other societal determinants of health.

Damning as US figures are, the situation of illicit flows is even worse for LMICs, where missing resources have the most palpable impact. Whereas Latin America experienced the highest rates of capital flight in the 1970s and 1980s, then amounting to hundreds of billions of dollars, today Africa is in the lead, thanks to both foreign and domestic elites. The capital flight numbers out of Africa—reaching almost US$300 billion from 39 countries for 2005 to 2010 (or over US$1 trillion spanning the 1970 to 2008 period) (Ndikumana, Boyce, and Ndiaye 2015)—offer a stark illustration of why there are so few resources available for domestic investment in physical and social infrastructure (including health and education) despite economic growth. By comparison, development assistance pledges to Africa in recent years have amounted to roughly half of capital flight outflows (besides, 60% of aid ends up as capital flight) (Ndikumana and Boyce 2011). To focus attention on the magnitude of the problem and the shared governance responsibilities of both origin and destination countries, a High-level Panel on Illicit Financial Flows was established in 2012 by the Economic Commission for Africa and the African Union Commission. Whether the outflows can be tracked, halted, and monies recouped is uncertain.

Capital flight has an enormous direct and indirect bearing on health and its determinants. It shrinks the size of public treasuries through lost tax revenues, which in turn leads to more debt (not adequately compensated by debt forgiveness programs) and external borrowing, less investment available for domestic spending, greater inequality, and governance problems (Nkurunziza 2015). For instance, had the hundreds of billions funneled out of sub-Saharan Africa been invested in public health, some 77,000 excess infant deaths per year could have been prevented (Ndikumana and Boyce 2011). Countries with governments elected on platforms calling for combating tax abuse, higher tax rates on the wealthy, and redistributive social investment may experience preemptive capital flight, whereby wealthy elites pull out their capital before it can be taxed.

Furthermore, "the distributional effects of capital flight are inherently regressive: it is by definition available only to a [minority of the] minority of the population. . . with investable assets" of over US$30 million, that is less than .0015% of the world's population of 7 billion people (Schrecker 2014, p. 399). In sum, whereas "capital flight enables elites to socialize the cost of accumulating private fortunes," entire populations are strangled by debt burdens "directly or in the form of lost services and transfers, as governments give priority to repaying creditors" (ibid).

Trade Liberalization, Trade and Investment Agreements, and TNCs

Global Trade and the WTO

Trade in goods and services, together with unfettered movement of capital, are the central components of globalization. Trade liberalization entails opening up economies to foreign investment, as well as reducing trade barriers, such as tariffs, and subsidies for domestic industries. With the end of the Cold War, the neoliberal order became institutionalized at the global level through the WTO, formed in 1995 as the standard bearer of free market principles and the main overseer of global trade (see chapter 4 for details). Distinct from other international organizations, it has a supranational dispute resolution body that sanctions binding fines or monetized trade concessions. The WTO governs all forms of trade among its 164 signatory countries (as of July 2016), including intellectual property (IP), services, and goods, and also has bearing on environmental and other regulations construed as trade barriers.

According to the WTO, the trading system should be: *"without discrimination"*—a country should not differentiate among its trading partners or between foreign and domestic products and services, treating all equally; *"freer"*—working toward reducing trade barriers; *"predictable"*—trade barriers should not be arbitrarily raised; *"more competitive"*—export subsidies, product dumping, and other "unfair" practices should be discouraged; and *"more beneficial for less developed countries*—giving them more time to adjust, greater flexibility, and special privileges" (WTO 2016).

WTO trade agreements contain rules for dispute resolution between governments on matters of trade. Trade charges must be brought by national governments and undergo an internal panel ruling, endorsement or rejection by the WTO membership, and may be appealed. However, WTO decisions are binding in that they authorize winners to levy duties on imports from losing parties, inflicting particular hardship on small, export-oriented LICs.

Proponents claim that the WTO treats all members equally and operates on a consensus basis among members. By contrast, critics argue that the WTO is fundamentally undemocratic because poor countries cannot afford to defend themselves against trade disputes brought to the WTO. Not only do WTO rules undermine sovereign decision-making, but corporate interests enjoy insider access to negotiations—which are kept secret—while the public interest is routinely ignored. Moreover, "WTO rules put the 'rights' of corporations to profit over human and labor rights. . . . it is illegal for a government to ban a product based on the way it is produced, such as with child labor" (Global Exchange 2015). In essence, according to Nobel Prize-winning economist Joseph Stiglitz (2002) (who was forced from the World Bank), free trade agreements supporting globalization are really a corporate bill of rights harming working and poor people across the globe.

The WTO's Doha Development Round of negotiations, which began in Qatar in 2001, has sought to further lower trade barriers, open markets, and expand IP protections. But subsequent meetings in Cancun (2003) and Hong Kong (2005) stalled due to disagreements between a set of HICs (the United States, the European Union, and Japan) and LMICs (led by India, Brazil, South Africa, and China). At the Bali meeting (2013), an agreement on measures to reduce bureaucratic impediments to trade (Wilkinson, Hannah, and Scott 2014) was formally countered by Bolivia, Cuba, Ecuador, Nicaragua, and Venezuela, arguing that these provisions favored HICs by preserving unfair terms of trade, particularly in agriculture (WTO 2013). Agricultural subsidies in Europe and the United States total US$148 billion per year (OECD 2016), even as HICs hypocritically demand that LMICs end agricultural subsidies that aim to help poor farmers and reduce rural hunger. HICs were supposed to eliminate all agricultural subsidies by 2013 (agreed in Hong Kong), but the Nairobi meeting (2015) continued to favor HIC interests by extending the elimination deadline to 2020 (with major loopholes for processed products and the dairy industry, and few concessions made for fairness to LMICs) (Jafri 2015).

A related problem is agricultural dumping—the flooding of markets with cheap foreign products to drive down local prices and prevent local producers from competing. For example, between 1997 and 2005, US soybeans, corn, wheat, rice, and cotton were exported at 12% to 47% below production cost (in part thanks to US government subsidies). Mexican producers alone lost nearly US$13 billion due to lower crop prices (Wise 2013). This practice also hinders progress toward food sovereignty (see chapter 7). Incredibly, the WTO does not consider this unfair competition and only "disciplines anti-dumping actions" (WTO 2015a), invariably favoring HIC dumpers against LMIC challengers.

Health Implications of WTO Agreements

Neoliberalized trade (as opposed to trade that is both fair and protective of health and well-being) affects health and its determinants in a variety of ways. It exacerbates chronic diseases through the marketing, tax advantages, and dumping of unhealthy products such as tobacco, alcohol, or processed, energy-dense foods and beverages (Labonté, Mohindra, and Lencucha 2011). Trade can also damage health by reducing the provision and distribution of health-related goods, services, and personnel. For instance, extended patent protection may lead to decreased access to medicines and technologies, and trade treaties may restrict national governments from investing in or regulating health care. Relaxed trade rules can also result in the importation of insufficiently regulated—or biologically or chemically contaminated—goods.

Various WTO agreements directly influence the health of the poor (Table 9-2) and the "domestic policy space for health," that is "the freedom, scope, and mechanisms that governments have to choose, design, and implement public policies to fulfill their aims" (Koivusalo, Schrecker, and Labonté 2009, p. 105). Most prominent is the Agreement on Trade-Related Aspects of Intellectual Property Rights (TRIPS), which protects many forms of IP, including patented pharmaceuticals, processes, and medical technologies (as well as copyright, trademarks, and new botanical patents). Enacted in January 1995 (with a compliance deadline of 2000 for most LMICs), TRIPS stipulates that all WTO member states must abide by IP patents wherever they are issued for a minimum period of 20 years. This means that within the period of patent protection, a manufacturer can only produce patented drugs and technologies if they obtain a costly license from the patent holder. Essentially this gives monopoly rights to pharmaceutical corporations, mostly based in wealthy countries (also see chapter 11).

Although Big Pharma and its allies contend that IP rights provide crucial incentives to research and development (R&D), this position is contradicted by countless innovations from the past. To name just one example, Jonas Salk, who developed a polio vaccine, was not motivated by profit per se. The claim that IP rights drive R&D has also been demonstrated erroneous for low-income countries

Table 9-2 Selected WTO Trade Agreements and their Influence on Health

Agreement	Health Effects from Loss of Domestic Regulatory Space
Agreement on Trade-Related Aspects of Intellectual Property Rights (TRIPS)	Expanded patent protection drives up drug prices, limiting access to essential medicines and draining money from primary health care (PHC) and other health spending.
Agreement on Sanitary and Phytosanitary Measures (SPS)	Circumscribes domestic public health standards around food and drug safety when assessments treat foreign goods differently from domestic goods.
Technical Barriers to Trade Agreement (TBT)	Requires that any regulatory barriers impeding free flow of goods for security, health, or environmental protection not create "unnecessary obstacles" for trade. Many trade disputes over domestic health and safety regulations have invoked TBT.
General Agreement on Trade in Services (GATS)	Opens health-related services (e.g., health care, education, water and sanitation services) to commercialization, with profiteering detrimental to equity, access, quality, and comprehensiveness of care.

Source: Adapted from Labonté, Blouin, and Forman (2009).

(LICs) that joined TRIPS over its initial 15 years (Kyle and McGahan 2012).

Most importantly, TRIPS threatens health and human rights: 2 billion people lack access to essential medicines largely due to prohibitive costs, with patents the principal determinant of high drug prices. TRIPS places restrictions both on producers of generic medications, vital for LMICs, and on purchasers—especially jeopardizing governments that cannot afford patented drugs (Forman and MacNaughton 2015). For example, the high prices charged by Big Pharma drastically limited the availability of lifesaving ARVs for millions of people living with HIV until they began to be produced generically in countries like Brazil, China, and India.

How did this come about? First, some countries bravely challenged patent protection solo. Then, in 2001, advocates argued that TRIPS and proposed new Doha Development Round rules interfered with domestic policies, including access to generic drugs. Faced with intense public-interest pressure, the Doha Declaration conceded that TRIPS should be implemented in a manner that supports the right of countries "to protect public health and, in particular, to promote access to medicines for all" (WTO 2001, p. 1) in times of emergency. In the interest of public health, countries can overcome patent barriers using TRIPS "flexibilities" by granting compulsory licenses for production or import of generic medicines without the patent holder's consent, or through parallel imports of cheaper patented medicines in the absence of sufficient domestic manufacturing capacity. The Doha Declaration also delayed the deadline for TRIPS compliance for the 30 lowest income countries until 2016, subsequently extended to 2033 (Third World Network 2015).

Various countries have used TRIPS "flexibilities" to challenge the high cost of patent-protected drugs. Zimbabwe's government declared a public health emergency in 2002 (initially for 6 months and then extended to 2008), enabling immediate compulsory licensing for local manufacture and importation of generic ARVs. With greater reliance on generics, the price of ARVs was halved, but Zimbabwe's government, unlike India's, has not been consistently supportive of domestic production (Russo and Banda 2015). Mozambique, Brazil, India, Kenya, South Africa, and Thailand have also employed these provisions. As a result of pressure from activists as well as demands from governments, some 30 compulsory licenses have been issued for ARVs (Beall, Kuhn, and Attaran 2015). In some instances where countries have threatened to invoke compulsory licenses, pharmaceutical companies have relented and reduced prices. However, an ongoing challenge is to ensure that compulsory licenses be used for other new and expensive drugs, including new TB drugs. India and Thailand have employed these approaches for cancer drugs, albeit in a limited fashion (Mezher 2015).

Despite some gains, implementing TRIPS flexibilities is undermined by corporate litigation and governmental trade sanctions pursued by Big Pharma and their home bases—particularly the US and EU governments—seeking to dissuade their use. Pharmaceutical companies also try to block market access for generic companies through "evergreening" (i.e., making minor chemical changes to existing drugs) to extend patent protection and by suing countries to prevent parallel importing of cheaper drugs—especially harming residents of countries that lack manufacturing capacity. In sum, TRIPS still limits domestic policy options for ensuring and protecting access to affordable medicines, and the use of TRIPS flexibilities remains challenging and extremely rare (Forman and MacNaughton 2015).

Another WTO instrument, the Agreement on Sanitary and Phytosanitary Measures (SPS), allows each country to set its own standards for food and drug safety but requires regulations to be based on scientific risk assessment without discriminating between domestic and imported food products. For example, in 2015, Japan launched a WTO dispute to compel South Korea to lift a ban on the importation of certain food products put in place following the 2011 Fukushima nuclear disaster due to concerns around radioactive contamination. Japan is citing various SPS articles to build its case in the ongoing dispute (WTO 2015b).

The Technical Barriers to Trade Agreement (TBT) stipulates that all "like products" be treated alike, and that all domestic regulations be "least trade restrictive." Canada used the TBT to challenge France's ban on asbestos products as discriminatory, arguing that asbestos was "like" glass fibers permitted in France. Canada lost both the initial case and its 2001 appeal, in a rare example of a WTO decision favoring health over trade (Labonté, Blouin, and Forman 2009).

The General Agreement on Trade in Services (GATS) is potentially the most insidious of all WTO agreements, encouraging liberalization—private investment in and deregulation of worker and environmental protections—of a wide spectrum of services. GATS locks in existing levels of private provision of services and prevents them from being nationalized, thus incentivizing foreign investors to lobby for privatization of a wide range of services. Government-purveyed services are excluded from the treaty, but this does not extend to publicly funded services that are privately delivered. This inordinately complex agreement enables countries to decide which sectors to liberalize; however many LMICs made early commitments that may prove difficult to revert without compensating investors (Labonté, Blouin, and Forman 2009). By contrast, more powerful countries (such as EU member states) have been able to exclude certain services (e.g., utilities and social security) from GATS (Koivusalo 2014).

Bilateral and Regional Trade Agreements and Investor Privileges

Although the WTO was envisioned as *the* handmaiden to neoliberal globalization, its proponents have been dissatisfied with its pace and reach. With the Doha Development Round deadlocked, a proliferating number of bilateral and regional trade agreements are going beyond the baseline established by WTO agreements. Referred to as *WTO-plus*, over 400 regional agreements in goods or services (WTO 2015c) and approximately 3,000 bilateral investment treaties or trade agreements with investment provisions (UNCTAD 2015) are now active. Public health concerns around trade agreements center on the inclusion of enhanced IP features and investment protection provisions, as well as limitations on domestic policy space in relation to health services, pharmaceuticals, and medical devices vis-à-vis foreign investor interests. These issues matter a great deal because governments must comply with legally binding global trade and investment treaties (Koivusalo and Tritter 2014).

Indeed, a distinguishing characteristic of many trade agreements (usually more important than lowering already low trade barriers) is the investor-state dispute settlement (ISDS) mechanism. ISDS is similar to WTO dispute settlement except that instead of fielding country-to-country complaints, it allows foreign entities to file complaints against governments—whenever public policies imperil profits—via the International Centre for Settlement of Investment Disputes (ICSID, part of the World Bank group) and other privatized, pro-corporate tribunals. Sovereign laws and national judicial systems can be subordinated to these tribunals, which have no appeals process. Only foreign investors can sue countries and win cases via ISDS, not vice-versa. Thus, the best outcome countries can seek is to have cases dismissed (Olivet and Villareal 2016), but only after considerable time and money have been spent. In 2014, 60% of 42 total cases were brought against LMICs, with three inter-related cases that year resulting in the highest compensation ever granted to investors: US$50 billion (UNCTAD 2015).

The 1994 North American Free Trade Agreement (NAFTA) among the United States, Canada, and Mexico is one of the earliest and most frequently invoked agreements sanctioning corporate enforcement claims against governments, involving ISDS claims that endanger food safety, health, environmental, and other regulations (Weisbrot 2015). For example, two thirds of claims brought by American corporations against Canada (the country most sued under NAFTA) have challenged its environmental protection and natural resource management policies (Barlow 2015).

As with WTO dispute settlement processes, ISDS claims pose a particular menace to public health. A prime example was a 2010 case launched against Uruguay by Philip Morris, one of the largest tobacco companies in the world, with annual revenues nearly US$30 billion more than Uruguay's GDP. Since 2005, Uruguay has made laudable policy advances in line with the WHO's Framework Convention on Tobacco Control (FCTC) (see chapter 13) to curtail cigarette smoking. Among other measures, Uruguay's Ministry of Health mandated health warnings to cover 80% of cigarette packages, beyond the FCTC-specified 50% minimum. Headquartered in Switzerland, Philip Morris used the ISDS process under the Switzerland–Uruguay bilateral investment treaty to argue in a US$25 million suit that Uruguay's tobacco control measures violate this treaty (Armitage 2014). In another instance, after El Salvador denied digging rights to Australian/Canadian mining conglomerate OceanaGold (formerly Pacific Rim) for regulatory and environmental assessment violations (amid widespread public opposition to mining contamination of the country's main drinking water source), the company filed an ISDS suit demanding up to US$301 million in compensation (Blue Planet Project et al. 2014). In 2016, after seven years, the ICSID dismissed the case and ordered OceanaGold to pay El Salvador US$8 million to cover (two thirds of) its legal fees. Although Uruguay, too, eventually prevailed and Philip Morris was ordered to repay US$7 million (of 10 million the country spent) in legal costs, the effects of these suits are chilling. ISDS cases (numbering almost 700) are proliferating, enriching corporate lawyers and frightening governments away from healthy public policies that might raise the ire of TNCs and embroil them in lengthy and expensive suits (Olivet and Villareal 2016).

Other health harms stem from regional and bilateral trade agreements that exert even greater IP protection than TRIPS (so-called *TRIPS-plus* provisions), such as longer patent periods, restrictions on generic competition, and provisions undermining use of TRIPS flexibilities (PHM et al. 2014). The United States has employed TRIPS-plus in the Central America Free Trade Agreement (CAFTA) (Shaffer and Brenner 2009) and in its bilateral agreements with Australia, Chile, Bahrain, Egypt, Jordan, Morocco, Tunisia, Vietnam, Singapore, Laos, and others (Lindstrom 2010).

Such pro-corporate features are embedded in the very conceptualization of trade and investment treaties. Major regional agreements recently under consideration, for instance the Transatlantic Trade and Investment Partnership (TTIP, between the EU and the United States) and the Trans-Pacific Partnership (TPP, among 12 countries around the Pacific Rim), have welcomed industries such as pharmaceuticals, tobacco, energy, processed foods, and health insurance to the negotiation table, whereas public health representatives are largely shut out (Shaffer and Brenner 2014). Consequently, these agreements incorporate TRIPS-plus provisions and increased burdens of scientific justification for food protection standards, among other measures (Labonté, Schram, and Ruckert 2016).

Because TNCs operate globally, they have a great interest in how trade agreements are negotiated, particularly around harmonization of trade-related standards and requirements. At the same time, the power that TNCs exert over national policymakers and priorities fundamentally challenges public accountability, including for health. Incorporation of ISDS provisions into new agreements would extend TNCs' ability to dilute standards on worker health and safety, employment security, and the environment if these affect the corporate bottom line. As well TNCs would be able to penetrate public national health care systems by commercializing health services (Koivusalo and Tritter 2014), threatening quality, safety, efficiency, effectiveness, and equity (see chapter 11). The upcoming generation of trade and investment agreements provide considerable scope for clawed-back government regulatory measures under heightened investor "protection."

Yet another regional agreement under secretive negotiation, the Trade in Services Agreement (TiSA), encompasses 22 countries plus the EU. It builds on and is likely to be integrated with WTO's GATS framework, seeking to expand deregulation and privatization of service suppliers, allowing TNC takeovers in sectors such as electricity and water management, services for agriculture and forestry, and transportation management (James 2015). A clear implication for health care systems is the commodification of health care services in a global marketplace, facilitating purchase of services abroad, at least partially funded by the home country. Such "offshoring" would lead to disinvestment in home country and foreign health care systems alike. Akin to medical tourism (see Box 12-2), overseas health care markets increasingly orient (mostly LMIC) health care systems to foreign payers, eroding quality of public services and aggravating health inequities (Kelsey 2015).

Activist groups concerned about the repercussions for labor (unions), agriculture (e.g., the Institute for Agriculture and Trade Policy), the environment (e.g., Friends of the Earth), access to medicines (e.g., Médecins Sans Frontières), of increasing corporate globalization (e.g., Our World Is Not for Sale network), and others have been struggling hard against proposed regional agreements, with some gains, but so far things do not look favorable for health and well-being (Citizens Trade Campaign 2015).

TNCs and Health

Corporations, transnational or national, differ from other businesses in that they are established as legal entities separate from the owners (called shareholders), who are not personally liable for the corporations' actions or debts. Corporations are controlled by executives and corporate boards, and ultimately, shareholders, to whom corporations are obliged to deliver the largest profits possible. TNCs (also called multinational corporations) operate in two or more countries and may be organized as a single company or as a tightly or loosely knit set of companies bound by legal and financial ties. They are active in areas such as manufacturing, raw material extraction, agriculture, power generation, and services (e.g., health care and insurance). There are an estimated 100,000 TNCs operating globally, with over 890,000 foreign affiliates. The 500 largest TNCs amassed over US$31 trillion in revenues in 2013 alone (Jaworek and Kuzel 2015).

Like global trade overall, TNCs affect health both directly—through the marketing of harmful products (e.g., tobacco and unhealthy food and beverages) (Box 9-1); hazardous production processes (e.g., chemical or bacterial contamination, toxic mining tailings, labor and other human rights violations), prohibitive pricing of/access to health-enhancing products (e.g., pharmaceuticals)—and indirectly, through their impact on (lower/evaded) tax revenues, government regulations on worker, environmental, and consumer safety, living conditions, overall equity, and by misinterpreting and suppressing scientific evidence to make products appear safer and more efficacious than they are (e.g., pharmaceuticals, devices) (Baum et al. 2016; Freudenberg 2014).

TNC champions hail their impact on economic development, job creation, quality of life, and indirect promotion of civil and political rights (Sikka 2011), also citing that TNC tax revenues are used to fund social programs. Each of these assertions may be contested for their inequitable impact, but the tax contribution claim is especially duplicitous. As discussed, TNCs are a major tax evasion culprit, particularly stemming from transfer pricing manipulation,

Box 9-1 Is Sugar the New Tobacco?

This is the question asked by many, given the relationship between sugar and soaring global rates of obesity and noncommunicable diseases (NCDs). In 2014 nearly 2 billion adults were estimated overweight (including 41 million children under 5), with more than 600 million obese (WHO 2015). While HICs have higher child obesity rates (one third of US children are overweight or obese; children weigh over 5 kg more today than three decades ago) (Lobstein et al. 2015), LMICs have experienced faster increases (for instance Mexico's child obesity rate is even higher than the United States's) (WHO 2015).

A major contributing factor is consumption of sugar, due to its addictive properties and endocrinological effects on blood pressure and blood glucose (Imamura et al. 2015; Lustig 2012). Between 1977 and 2010, sugar intake among US adults rose by almost one third, and among children by 20% (Powell 2014), increases mirrored around the world. Though candy and other sweets consumption is widespread, sugar intake is largely passive, with fructose (corn syrup and other sweeteners) added to most processed foods, ranging from breakfast cereals to canned fruits and vegetables, bread, snacks, cold cuts, condiments, microwave and ready meals, juices, and, especially, soft drinks (NHS 2014). Annually, over 180,000 obesity-related deaths are attributed to sugary soft drinks, almost 80% in LMICs, three quarters due to diabetes, with heart disease and cancer as other principal causes (Singh et al. 2015).

The increase in global obesity and sugar consumption is intimately related to neoliberal globalization and transnational food corporations (TFCs), which may be considered "vectors for the global spread of NCD risks" (Stuckler et al. 2012). Just a handful of conglomerates, such as PepsiCo, Coca-Cola, Nestlé, and Kellogg, now dominate world markets, including in the Global South (Monteiro and Cannon 2012).

For example, trade liberalization under CAFTA and NAFTA has enabled large-scale TFC penetration, in turn influencing the rapid shift from traditional diets to processed food consumption in Mesoamerica (Thow and Hawkes 2009). These and other trade agreements facilitate FDI in both food processing and food retailers (i.e., fast food restaurants and supermarket chains), as well as widespread distribution of soft drinks and "junk food" to small town convenience stores (Labonté, Mohindra, and Lencucha 2011).

In South Africa, per capita consumption of Coca-Cola products (which constitute half the soft drink market) doubled from 1992 to 2010 amid growing TFC penetration (Igumbor et al. 2012). By contrast, Venezuela, which does not have a free trade agreement with the United States, maintained a steady level of soft drink consumption through the 1990s and 2000s (Stuckler et al. 2012).

In the context of trade pacts, government regulations on marketing, distribution, and pricing of TFC products may be considered interference or potential violations of free trade. Mexico—which has the world's highest sugar-sweetened beverage consumption rate (over 120 liters per person annually), as well as the highest absolute and proportional death rate attributable to soda consumption (Singh et al. 2015)—was compelled to address the problem due to its cost to society (Nestle 2015). In 2014 it became the first country in the world to enact a national soda tax, a blow to the soft drink industry, whose cozy relations with politicians (former Mexican President Vicente Fox was previously a Coca-Cola executive responsible for making Coca-Cola the market leader) has long impeded any restrictions on its business. So far, the tax has led to a 6% decline in soda purchases, with higher declines among the poor and an expected lowering of obesity (Escobar et al. 2013), but there is already pushback from industry (Kilpatrick 2015).

A 2011 UN high-level meeting and declaration to address the rise in NCDs tiptoed around trade liberalization and TFC interests, focusing instead on individual-level preventive behaviors (i.e., tobacco and alcohol use, unhealthy diets, and exercise) (Glasgow and Schrecker 2015). While health professionals and advocates call for restrictions on TFCs in national/local food systems and stricter regulations on unethical marketing of unhealthy foods to children (Swinburn et al. 2015), WHO remains bullied by the US$8 billion US sugar industry (see chapter 4). Moreover, TFCs deflect attention from their unhealthy products by operating high-visibility wellness programs and funding NGOs to address "other causes" of NCDs, such as inadequate exercise: soda companies, like tobacco TNCs previously, remain ubiquitous sponsors of sports events.

the deliberate over-pricing of imported goods or under-pricing of exports between subsidiaries of the same TNC (which comprises almost two thirds of all trade) in order to lower their tax bill. In 2010 alone, TNCs avoided paying US$11 billion in taxes and duties across Africa (Oxfam International 2015). Other shady TNC tax evasion techniques, in addition to using tax havens, involve profit-stripping—shifting profits from high-tax to low-tax jurisdictions via loans to subsidiaries with deductions for interest paid.

TNC claims around job creation also need to be balanced against harmful effects on human health and rights (Ottersen et al. 2014). For decades, TNCs have deliberately relocated operations to host countries with tariff exemptions, near absence of unions, weak tax collection, poverty wages, internal conflict, corruption, poor environmental regulation, inadequate enforcement of labor standards, and lack of compensation for workplace-related illness and disability. Moving hazardous and low-wage industries to such contexts of course makes good business sense, atop TNC strategies of tax evasion and flouting workplace and environmental laws. Moreover, as discussed ahead, TNCs have displaced countless local industries in host countries, devastating small and medium enterprises and lowering employment in agriculture and other sectors.

Worldwide awareness of the harms wrought by TNCs and their government accomplices grew markedly after the Bhopal disaster (Box 9-2), thanks to the committed work of activist groups urging greater TNC accountability. More

Box 9-2 The Union Carbide Disaster in Bhopal: A Case Study of TNC Impunity

One of the worst industrial disasters in history was a 1984 chemical leak at a Union Carbide plant in Bhopal, India. Within a 2-hour period, more than 27 tons of deadly methyl isocyanate gas escaped out of a pesticide plant owned by the US-based TNC. An estimated 3,800 people died immediately, mostly residents of neighboring slums. Tens of thousands more persons experienced serious health effects and premature death (Broughton 2005). Thirty years later, the Bhopal leak has been linked to over 22,000 deaths, with 500,000 people suffering long-term effects, from chronic inflammation of the eyes and lungs to reproductive (spontaneous abortions), genetic (chromosomal abnormalities), and neurobehavioral and cognitive problems.

Union Carbide (now owned by Dow Chemical) immediately sought to dissociate itself from the incident, denying legal responsibility and instead blaming local plant operators and Indian government regulators. Although India's Supreme Court eventually mediated a legal settlement with Union Carbide accepting "moral"—but not criminal—liability for the incident, there remains heated debate about the company's role and the government's weak response. The plant's operations were discontinued and the company paid US$470 million in compensation to victims and relatives, but the site continues to leak toxic chemicals and metals into soil and groundwater. Meanwhile, India's government has failed to evaluate the extent of contamination and has underestimated the death and disability toll (Amnesty International 2014).

than 600 civil society organizations pressed the UN's Human Rights Council to a 2014 commitment to elaborate a legally binding instrument on TNCs and human rights. Many TNCs now claim to prohibit "double standards" (different policies for home and host countries) in health, safety, and environmental protections. Yet improvements are perforce dependent on strong regulatory environments that conflict with trade liberalization. Abundant recent examples show that TNCs continue to violate human rights through use of child labor, sweatshop conditions, inhumane wages, repression of citizen protest, and environmental pollution, with demonstrated adverse effects on health (Table 9-3).

Table 9-3 Recent Examples of Human Rights Violations Linked to Transnational Corporate Activity

Issue and Year(s)	Description
Killings at mining sites and targeting of activists	Canadian-owned Barrick Gold's subsidiary Acacia Mining (formerly African Barrick Gold) was cited for human rights abuses of villagers in its North Mara Gold Mine in Tanzania. Company security forces and police violently attacked artisanal miners (who had paid to access waste rock dumps), resulting in numerous injuries and at least ten deaths by gunshot in 2014. Only a few individuals and families have been compensated, which requires them to forfeit further legal action against the company (MiningWatch Canada and RAID 2014). Other mining TNCs, often protected by the Canadian government, have been associated with repression and killing of anti-mining activists across the Americas (MiningWatch Canada 2015).
Child labor abuses	The Democratic Republic of Congo supplies more than half the world's cobalt, used to manufacture rechargeable batteries for cellphones, laptops, and other devices. An estimated 40,000 child artisanal miners scavenge for cobalt in discarded rocks from industrial mines, enduring physically demanding work and toxic exposures, seldom with protective equipment. Many report health problems, including respiratory illness and back and hip pain, and are deprived of an education. One of the largest companies involved is a subsidiary of China-based Huayou Cobalt, which sells processed cobalt to suppliers of some of the most well-known electronics TNCs such as Apple, Dell, HP, LG, Microsoft, Samsung, and Sony (Amnesty International 2016).
Workers' rights violations and hazardous working conditions	On April 24, 2013, the eight-story Rana Plaza factory building in Savar, Bangladesh collapsed, killing 1,137 workers. Rana Plaza's factories supplied garments to 32 North American and European retailers including Primark, Walmart, the Children's Place, and Joe Fresh. The morning of the tragedy, workers had resisted entering the building due to clearly visible cracks on exterior walls but were physically assaulted and threatened with withholding of pay. The paltry ex-post facto donations to workers' families made by many of these companies are little recompense for these extreme violations (Institute for Global Labour and Human Rights 2014).

Extractive industries (petroleum, gas, mining) operating in LMICs are often the worst perpetrators of civil and health rights abuses, routinely abetted or overlooked by host governments. Responsibility for these abuses also resides with the home countries of TNCs. In 2015, the 40 largest mining transnationals (representing 80% of the market) had US$539 billion in revenues (PricewaterhouseCoopers 2016). Two thirds of mining companies are based in Canada, an industry haven because of lax liability laws for overseas subsidiaries, plus favorable tax shelters, government subsidies, and other corporate protections (Déneault and Sacher 2012). Seeking to counter such flagrancy and enhance the likelihood that oil, gas, and mining benefits accrue to local populations, a group of civil society organizations, including the anti-corruption NGO Global Witness, pushed governments and TNCs to found the Extractive Industries Transparency Initiative in 2003 (EITI 2015). Although 51 countries participate in EITI, extraction giants such as Canada, Russia, Argentina, Chile, and South Africa are not members. Moreover, properly reporting revenues is only part of the story.

Faced with rising resistance, TNCs increasingly tout their corporate social responsibility (CSR) pledges. This, too, is deceptive: TNCs exist for one purpose—to maximize profits for their shareholders. Because this condition is a fiduciary responsibility, any impediments to profit-making are subject to shareholder scrutiny, objection, or legal action. As such, "goodwill" or voluntary measures provide patently insufficient protection for human or environmental health.

Time and again, CSR and self-governance—not to mention trade and investment agreements—have proved inadequate to protect social well-being. Yet TNCs disingenuously leverage CSR rhetoric to legitimize their presence in global governance bodies such as the UN's Global Compact (see chapter 3) and in global health forums (e.g., FCTC discussions) (Gilmore et al. 2015). As Nobel Prize-winning economist Milton Friedman (2006) portrayed this absurdity, "asking a corporation to be socially responsible makes no more sense than asking a building to be."

In a nutshell:

> TNCs use public relations to present a positive impression, even if practices damage human health or the environment. They engage in philanthropy and corporate social responsibility programs and use a range of sometimes misleading marketing strategies, including new technologies and targeting of specific sectors that include vulnerable populations [Box 9-3]. To protect profits, corporations have developed legal, scientific, and public relations tactics. They form strategic alliances with nonprofit organizations and masquerade as 'grassroots' operations. They effectively suppress public health messages through global advertising, discredit critics, influence research, and access the policymaking process (Baum and Anaf 2015, pp. 354–355).

Global Reorganization of Production/ Deregulation of Worker and Environmental Protections

Reorganization and Deregulation of Work

Trade liberalization has (had) a profound effect on employment patterns across the world, with TNCs upping their global competitiveness—read profits—by reorganizing ("outsourcing") production to where labor costs are lowest (Schrecker and Labonté 2011). Since the 1980s, tens of millions of manufacturing and service support jobs and entire industries (such as garment-making) have relocated from HICs to LMICs to take advantage of lax regulation, poor working conditions, an anti-union climate, and absent social safety nets. With some industries relocating multiple times, this has led to downward wage pressures in all settings (Khanna 2011). Half of all working families in LMICs get by on less than US$4 a day (UNDP 2015), which leaves them experiencing hunger, inadequate shelter, and other dimensions of extreme poverty.

Neoliberal globalization has accelerated the growth of export processing zones (EPZs)—special tariff-free production areas where TNCs are exempt from many hard-earned regulations safeguarding workers and the environment (McCallum 2011). Labor protection roll-backs and union suppression have resulted in high rates of on-the-job and union-organizer deaths and injuries. EPZs thus offer an added (legal) pretense for workplace abuse and minimal protections

Box 9-3 Transnationals, the WTO, and Infant Formula: A Case Study of Unethical Practices

WHO estimates that 800,000 children die each year because they are not optimally breastfed (i.e., exclusively breastfed from birth to 6 months, then breastfed until at least 2 years of age, complemented by introduction of safe and nutritional solid foods) (WHO 2016). A major cause of death in non-breastfed infants is diarrhea resulting from powdered infant formula (PIF) mixed with contaminated water (there is often no other option) or because of "intrinsic contamination" associated with its manufacturing (WHO and FAO 2007). Presently, only 37% of infants in LMICs (as low as 20% in HICs) are exclusively breastfed (Victora et al. 2016), despite the high costs of PIF and fuel to boil unclean water. Worldwide, new mothers face a constant barrage of misleading ads and tactics promoting the benefits of infant formula, even as they lack skilled breastfeeding support. Moreover, in many settings women do not have adequate maternity protections, such as paid maternity leave and breastfeeding breaks in the workplace.

During the 1960s, declining birthrates in the West led PIF manufacturers to seek new markets in LMICs. Marketers dressed as nurses handed out free samples of formula to new mothers, encouraging them—during this most vulnerable time—to use formula instead of breastfeeding. Corporations were found responsible for promoting skyrocketing formula use, with Nestlé the most aggressive marketer. A worldwide campaign—with strong advocacy from the International Baby Food Action Network (IBFAN, founded 1979)—against these unethical practices led to the 1981 World Health Assembly's adoption by vote of the WHO-UNICEF International Code of Marketing of Breast-Milk Substitutes (only the United States opposed it, until 1994). The code is not legally binding, however, and, unlike WTO rulings, it is widely ignored, with just 70 countries having legal measures in place that partially or comprehensively implement the Code (WHO, UNICEF, and IBFAN 2016). IBFAN has documented innumerable examples from around the world demonstrating that Nestlé and other TNCs continue to market infant formula and other breastmilk substitutes with impunity in spite of the WHO-UNICEF code (Freudenberg 2014). International boycotts have intermittently put pressure on breastmilk substitutes manufacturers, but it remains a powerful US$45 billion annual business (WHO, UNICEF, and IBFAN 2016).

The fight to safely promote breastfeeding in Guatemala is a case in point. A 1983 law aimed at reducing infant mortality implemented key elements of the WHO/UNICEF marketing code, which prohibited use of the words "equivalent to breast milk," banned visual depictions of fat, healthy infants encouraging the use of bottle-feeding, and forbade direct marketing and free distribution of samples (Government of Guatemala 1983). Although other companies abided by the law (leading to infant mortality declines), US-incorporated Gerber Products Company continued marketing its formula to new mothers, providing free samples to daycare centers and failing to remove the pudgy "Gerber Baby" from its label. In 1992 the Guatemalan Food and Drug Registration Agency requested that Gerber change its proposed packaging to include the words "breast milk is the best for baby" in accordance with national law. Gerber refused to comply, also arguing that the "Gerber Baby" is integral to their trademark. Gerber subsequently took the case to the WTO and won. Guatemala was forced to exempt imported baby food products from its stringent infant food labeling policy, reversing prior gains (Wallach and Woodall 2004). Today, Nestlé (Gerber is now its subsidiary) still promotes its products in violation of Guatemala's code and continues such practices elsewhere (e.g., China, Costa Rica, Greece, and the United States) (IBFAN 2014).

(Khanna 2011). The excess labor force available for such employment is linked to decline in rural livelihoods in countries where agribusiness has squeezed out small farmers (Tandon 2010). Those most negatively affected—having lost work in domestic jobs or farming—end up in the unregulated informal economy or as part of the *precariat,* those on the margins of work (Standing 2011). Even the World Bank concedes that unskilled workers are being left further and further behind (World Bank 2015b), with consequent mounting inequality and health deterioration. The impact of these global changes on workplace health is further explored ahead.

Environmental Degradation

As discussed in chapter 10, environmental contamination and depletion have accelerated since the

Box 9-4 Trade Liberalization and the Export of Hazard

The global reorganization of production has been accompanied by the export of hazard—waste dumping in low-income settings or in the open ocean. In an infamous leaked 1991 internal memorandum, then World Bank economist Lawrence Summers provided striking insight into the neoliberal logic behind this practice. Advocating the transfer of waste and dirty industries from HICs to LMICs, Summers argued:

> Just between you and me, shouldn't the World Bank be encouraging more migration of the dirty industries to the LDCs [least developed countries]? I can think of [various] reasons: 1) The measurements of the costs of health-impairing pollution depends on the foregone earnings from increased morbidity and mortality . . . I think the economic logic behind dumping a load of toxic waste in the lowest wage country is impeccable and we should face up to that. 2) . . . I've always thought that under-populated countries in Africa are vastly under-polluted, their air quality is probably vastly inefficiently low compared to Los Angeles or Mexico City (Summers cited in Economist 1992, p. 82).

Summers also recognized that "[T]he arguments against all of these proposals for more pollution in LDCs . . . could be turned around and used more or less effectively against every Bank proposal for liberalization" (ibid). He later claimed that the memo was meant to be ironic, but its realpolitik is all too tragic.

Among the most notorious examples of global hazardous waste dumping involved the *Khian Sea,* which set sail from the United States in 1986 loaded with nearly 14,000 tons of toxic fly-ash from Philadelphia's municipal waste incinerator (Parayre 2006). After unsuccessfully attempting to dump the ash in the Bahamas, the ship sailed around the Caribbean for over 16 months in search of a port that would accept the waste. The crew was finally authorized to unload the cargo in Haiti as "topsoil fertilizer," but when its true content was revealed, the Haitian government ordered it removed and banned all waste imports. Nonetheless, an estimated 4,000 tons of ash was left on the beach adjacent to a wharf in Gonaives, Haiti, where it leaked toxins for 10 years. Eventually a deal was brokered with the United States for its safe removal. The crew vainly sought to dispose of the remaining ash back in Philadelphia, and in West Africa, the Philippines, and Yugoslavia. Then the ash mysteriously disappeared from the ship. In 1994 the ship's captain admitted to having dumped more than 10,000 tons of ash into the Atlantic and Indian Oceans. Although the owners of the *Khian Sea* were convicted of perjury, they were never tried for the dumping in Haiti, and the city of Philadelphia was never fined or punished. This incident led to the creation of the 1989 UN Basel Convention governing the transboundary movement and disposal of hazardous waste. However, such illegal disposal continues, with waste producers and smugglers enabled by fractured and inadequate enforcement of the convention (UNEP 2015).

Industrial Revolution and especially since World War II. While there were improvements in environmental regulations in some settings in the 1960s and 1970s, the subsequent rise of neoliberal globalization has been marked by worsened environmental conditions due to: (1) deregulation and failure to monitor/strengthen environmental standards; (2) export of hazard (Box 9-4); (3) a commodities boom that has fueled extractive industries; and (4) trade agreements that privilege TNCs and other investors over health and the environment.

A crucial issue is whether environmental protection and trade under neoliberal globalization are ever compatible. Several dozen multilateral environmental agreements (MEAs) contain trade provisions or are designed to regulate trade in environmentally harmful substances (see chapter 10). MEAs arguably conflict with WTO rules on equal treatment, particularly when a WTO member party to an MEA applies trade restrictions against a WTO country that has not signed the MEA. The WTO's power and reach serve as a deterrent to compliance or even participation in MEAs, and its dispute resolution process is significantly more robust than MEA enforcement mechanisms (Clapp and Dauvergne 2011).

A great deal of environmental damage is propagated by TNCs, with environmental abuses constituting one third of the hundreds of TNC transgressions reported to the UN Special Representative on human rights and business in 2011 (Knox 2014). Extractive industries are particularly culpable, accelerated by the primary commodities boom since the 1990s, in turn driven by growing demand for natural resources from rapidly industrializing countries, most of all China and India, and continuing demand from HICs. Between 1990 and 2008, the average real price of crude oil more than tripled, declining after the contraction of the global economy—though still well above 1990s levels—and increasing again then declining precipitously after 2014 (World Bank 2015c). The boom cycles intensified the TNC grab for land and resources across LMICs (Petras and Veltmeyer 2014), with attendant livelihood and health consequences, in addition to the pollution generated by energy extraction and combustion.

Mining in Latin America and elsewhere has similarly caused high levels of air, water, and ground contamination, as well as the forced environmental displacement of Indigenous peoples (Working Group on Mining and Human Rights in Latin America 2014). For example, Canadian TNC Goldcorp's subsidiary Marlin Mine, located in an Indigenous Guatemalan community, has been linked to local river contamination with toxic heavy metals (Basu and Hu 2010) as well as livelihood loss, violence, and mental health problems (Cajax et al. 2014).

WORK AND OCCUPATIONAL HEALTH AND SAFETY ACROSS THE WORLD

Key Questions:

- What makes the workplace a hazardous environment?
- How have processes of globalization affected workplace health conditions?
- What social and political forces are necessary to improve worker safety and health in LMICs?

Approximately 63% of the world's population over 15 years of age participates in the labor force (World Bank 2016b), and work is a key determinant of health (see chapter 7). Healthy work conditions (as laid out in Article 23 of the Universal Declaration of Human Rights) are also among the most important rights that employers, communities, and governments can cultivate. Conducive work environments contribute to improved living conditions, fulfillment, and overall well-being of individuals and families. By contrast, deleterious work environments can lead to job and household stress, ill health, low living standards, toxic exposures, and an overall poor quality of life.

Precarious Work and Hazardous Working Conditions across the World

Precarious employment—job insecurity and unpredictability—derives from "flexible forms of employment (e.g., short-term contracts, temporary work, part-time work, and daily work) . . . [featuring problems of] continuity (i.e., temporality), vulnerability (i.e., powerlessness), protection (i.e., lack of benefits), and income (i.e., low levels of earnings)"

(Kim et al. 2012, p. 100). Since the mid-1970s, the trend toward euphemistically-termed "flexible employment" in both LMICs and HICs underscores the role of neoliberal globalization in the rise of precarious work: just as barriers to trade are deemed a hindrance to economic growth and prosperity, so too are the "alleged rigidities" of employment protection. Under debt and financial crises, secure employment has further deteriorated with workforce downsizing, dramatic increases in unemployment, and the replacement of quality jobs with low wage, low control work, for instance through outsourcing. The health effects of precarious work include chronic stress related to fear of job loss and diminished workplace rights and control—contributing to chronic diseases ranging from cardiovascular disease to musculoskeletal pain (Benach et al. 2014) (also see chapter 7). A decline in secure, well-paid jobs in the United States, for example, is coterminous with health deterioration: maternal mortality rose by 65% from 2005 to 2013 (WHO et al. 2014).

The informal sector, involving perhaps 2 billion unofficial workers, independent contractors, and small family-run businesses, accounts for more than half of non-agricultural work in LMICs and over 12% in HICs (Siqueira 2016). In virtually every city in the Majority World, thousands of people hawk goods on the street—selling candy, drinks, small meals, or household goods to passing motorists or pedestrians. In South Asia 82% of the adult workforce is in the informal sector, in sub-Saharan Africa 66%, East and Southeast Asia 65%, and Latin America 51% (UNDP 2015).

Although an integral part of many economies, the informal sector generates few taxes, leading governments to care little about the welfare of these workers, who, like precarious workers typically lack social security, decent working conditions, and union representation. Employers may deliberately turn to informal work to avoid paying taxes, while workers may also favor informal work where social security protections are paltry (Chen 2016). Conversely, countries that have increased work formalization in the context of ample social benefits, such as Argentina, have realized decreases in income inequality (Damodaran 2015).

For those employed in EPZs, either formally or informally, work is frequently performed in cramped and unventilated conditions with outdated machinery, and limited personal protective equipment. Acute health hazards in EPZs consist of harmful ergonomic conditions (e.g., repetitive work, prolonged standing); noise pollution; excessive heat or cold; and exposure to toxic chemicals, dust, and fumes. These contribute to gastrointestinal, musculoskeletal, reproductive, and skin disorders, as well as psychosocial problems (Lu 2008). The expansion of export-led chemical, electronic, and biotechnology sectors has added new hazards to those already prevalent in many LMICs. For example, workers in computer chip manufacturing plants are exposed to solvents, glues, and heavy metals without adequate safety measures or supervision.

All told, some 30% to 50% of workers worldwide, including in HICs, are exposed to hazardous agents or to unreasonably heavy loads that are harmful to health. Up to one third of workers experience a work-related injury every year, leading to disability and, potentially, premature death. Workers in extractive industries, forestry, construction, and agriculture are most likely to be injured or die on the job (Box 9-5).

As many as 315 million occupational injuries and over 2 million deaths from occupation-related diseases and injuries occur every year (ILO 2013b), generating direct and indirect costs of up to 4% of global GDP or US$2.8 trillion (Takala et al. 2014). Moreover, approximately 70% of workers lack access to compensation for occupational disease or injury (WHO 2014). High rates of occupational illness, injury, and death mirror immense inequalities in political power.

Amid the growing worldwide convergence of precarious and dangerous working conditions, LMICs continue to experience particularly high rates of workplace illness and death. There are five main reasons for this. First, where primary commodities and warmer climates are present, hazardous extractive industries and agriculture figure prominently in the overall economic picture (Lucchini and London 2014). Second, work begins at an earlier age and extends later in life than in HICs due to educational barriers, household income needs, and more limited social security. In LMICs, 42% of men over age 65 and 22% of women over 65 are in the workforce compared with 11% of men and 6% of women in HICs (UN-DESA 2013). Third, in most LMICs there are fewer human and material resources—including inspectors, and safety and monitoring equipment—to prevent and treat job injuries. Fourth, hazardous jobs are increasingly outsourced to

Box 9-5 Farming and Mining as Hazardous Occupations

Nearly 1 billion people work in agriculture (UNDP 2015), and farming is one of the world's most dangerous occupations, accounting for half of all workplace fatalities every year. In addition to rampant machine and tool injuries, farming practices and conditions—from use of dangerous pesticides to lack of protective equipment—lead to approximately one million deaths and tens of millions of illnesses due to respiratory ailments, zoonotic diseases, cancers, hearing deficits, musculoskeletal problems, and skin conditions, as well as poor water quality and other features of harmful living and working circumstances (Padilla 2013).

Pesticide imports in LMICs have accelerated under neoliberalized trade conditions, even as there have been important struggles to counter toxic trade (Bohme 2015) (see chapter 10). In Tanzania, most of these chemicals are used by small-scale farmers who apply pesticides, insecticides, herbicides, and fungicides using hand-held tank sprayers or knapsack sprayers. Few farmers are adequately trained in their use and application, and most do not have proper protective equipment (Ngowi, Mrema, and Kishinhi 2016). To this day, children can be seen selling pesticides on the streets or in open markets, in violation of the country's Pesticides Law.

Extractive industries, particularly mining, are also associated with high rates of workplace injury and illness. With poor ventilation in underground shafts, miners are exposed to harmful gases, dust, toxins, and heat, leading to pneumoconiosis or "black lung disease" in coal miners (lung damage from exposure to coal dust), chronic obstructive lung disease, heat stroke, and cancer. In China alone, almost 6 million people have pneumoconiosis. In Russia, uranium miners face elevated levels of lung cancer, silicosis and, together with populations surrounding mines, are exposed to radiation, causing birth defects, immune system impairment, and cancer (Zhukovsky, Varaksin, and Pakholkina 2014).

The dangers of extractive industries are compounded by inadequate engineering controls, lack of protective equipment and respirators, poor medical surveillance, and a high prevalence of concurrent diseases, as with TB in southern Africa (Basu et al. 2009). Pointing to just a few incidents: in May 2014 fire killed 301 miners from carbon monoxide poisoning at the Soma Holding Eynez coal mine in western Turkey (Human Rights Watch 2015), and underground explosions of methane and other gases trap and kill thousands of coal miners in China every year. The Chinese government reported 589 mining accidents and 1,049 people dead or missing in 2013 alone, though labor rights advocates believe there is substantial underreporting of deaths (Al Jazeera 2014).

LMICs through subcontracting or subsidiaries. Fifth, in many LMICs there is weaker government enforcement of labor and occupational health and safety laws (Quinlan and Sheldon 2011), in both domestic and foreign-controlled industries.

Social Effects of Labor Market Shifts

Women in the Global Labor Market

Work inequities are a major contributor to the feminization of poverty. In low-income industrializing areas, women have higher rates of employment than men, but are paid lower wages and work under worse conditions. Beyond wage labor, women carry out most unpaid work in the home (e.g., child care, housekeeping, and food preparation), and girls are more likely than boys to be withdrawn from school to work at home or elsewhere (UNFPA and UNICEF 2010). Certain industries are decidedly gendered, such as floriculture, exposing mostly young women to neurotoxic and endocrine-disrupting pesticides and chemicals (see Box 10-4) and high levels of violence and abuse (Benach et al. 2013).

Women comprise the primary labor force in EPZs—dominated by textiles and electronics—because: their fingers are considered more "nimble" for garment and assembly work; they may be less likely to organize; and employers get away with paying them 60% to 80% of men's wages. EPZ jobs, sometimes called "wage labor slavery," rarely improve the lot of women or men. Yet miserable as EPZ jobs are, they may be preferable to other local economic options, especially for women (Kabeer and Mahmud 2004).

Child Labor

Child labor is not new, but the changing patterns of work performed by children (as with adults) is shaped by global economic forces. Child labor (contrasted with work done by children in and around their home/land assisting the family) reflects (lack of) societal adherence to social rights: no child under the age of 16 should have to work for a living. According to ILO Convention 138, the term "child labor" refers to children below 12 years of age working in any economic activities, those aged 12 to 14 years engaged in harmful work, those aged 15 to 17 in hazardous work, and all children who are enslaved, forcibly recruited, prostituted, trafficked, and made to work in illegal activities.

Most child labor occurs in LMICs, where poverty and weak legal enforcement prevent local and international efforts from stopping it. The story of Idris opening this chapter is just one of innumerable accounts of children compelled to work, jeopardizing their health, schooling, and lives, and with few facile remedies. Although numbers have declined by up to one third in recent years, the ILO estimates that globally there are 168 million child laborers aged 5 to 17; 144 million are under 15, with 85 million involved in hazardous work (ILO 2015b). Altogether, an estimated 10.6% of the world's children are child laborers, ranging from 21.4% in sub-Saharan Africa to 8.8% in Latin America and the Caribbean. Almost half of child laborers are in Asia. Child labor is concentrated in agriculture (59%), followed by services (32%), and industry (7%) (Diallo, Etienne, and Mehran 2013).

Exploitative child labor is not exclusive to LMICs. Across the United States, for example, farms employ some 260,000 laborers under age 16, even children as young as 5 years old, with similarly high numbers in the parts of Europe most affected by austerity and in former Soviet bloc countries (Muižnieks 2013). On tobacco farms, young farmworkers are exposed to pesticides and nicotine, endure long hours of work in extreme heat, and may work without adequate drinking water and sanitation facilities. Documented health effects include cuts, burns, musculoskeletal injuries, nausea and headaches (associated with nicotine poisoning), and death. In 2012, an estimated 38 US farmworker children suffered an injury every day with one child dying every three days (Grossman 2015).

Children are the most oppressed of all workers, less able to defend themselves physically, psychologically, and legally. Children's health is particularly affected by harmful exposure to toxins, machinery, long work hours, and stress. Denied their human rights, child laborers are forced to sacrifice play, family life, and the vital role of education in equipping them with knowledge, life skills, and experience in community engagement. As older youth, they often become vulnerable to hazardous work or unemployment (ILO 2015b).

Marking the importance of protecting children's rights, the 2014 Nobel Peace Prize was awarded jointly to Kailash Satyarthi and Malala Yousafzai "for their struggle against the suppression of children and young people and for the right of all children to education" (Nobel Media 2014). In 1980 Satyarthi founded Bachpan Bachao Andolan (BBA—Save the Childhood Movement) in India. Aimed at ending child labor, trafficking, and slavery, and promoting education, BBA has rescued over 80,000 children. As a teenage schoolgirl in Pakistan, Malala Yousafzai was shot in the face by Taliban gunmen for advocating for girls' rights to education; at 17 she became the youngest recipient of a Nobel, and her continued efforts are enormously inspiring.

Youth Unemployment

While almost 170 million school-aged children are forced to work, young adults face inordinately high levels of unemployment, reaching 13% in 2014 worldwide, totaling 74 million people aged 15 to 24. This constitutes three times the unemployment rate for adults over 25 (ILO 2015a). In both HICs and LMICs, spiraling numbers of young people lack work prospects. The Middle East and North Africa have the highest youth unemployment with a significant gender gap: 24.5% for young men versus 42.6% for young women (ILO 2013a). When youth are working, they are more likely to be in insecure, low-quality jobs. Over three quarters of youth employment in Cambodia, Liberia, Malawi, and Peru is in the informal sector, lacking health and social protections, and adequate working conditions (ILO 2013a).

Migrant Workers

Although millions of people are uprooted each year due to war and ecologic disasters (see chapter 8), the vast majority of the currently over 240 million international migrants (numbers underestimated due to difficulties capturing seasonal and undocumented migration) and 750 million internal migrants have left their homes seeking work. About three quarters of international migration originates from LMICs, almost equally split between migration to HICs and to other LMICs (ILO 2014; World Bank 2016a). Labor migration often takes place through undocumented channels, with thousands dying each year on illegal transport routes, and hundreds of thousands subject to ruthless smugglers, labor exploitation, and human trafficking (ILO 2010).

Most are escaping repression or misery (with a growing number joining the brain drain). Labor migrants' economic significance has soared, with HIC-to-LMIC migrant remittances increasing 10-fold in the last 20 years. Now surpassing US$430 billion annually, remittances exceed 10% of GDP in some countries (e.g., El Salvador, Lebanon, the Philippines), reaching 20% of GDP in others (e.g., Haiti, Liberia, Moldova, Tajikistan) (World Bank 2016a). Furthermore, many undocumented workers must pay into—thus shoring up—social security systems while receiving no benefits, as in the United States, where undocumented workers contribute US$12 billion more than they receive (Goss et al. 2013).

In Qatar, migrant workers make up half of the 2.1 million population and over 90% of the workforce. Many are exposed to hazardous working conditions, are prohibited from unionizing, have no rest days, and are paid late (Human Rights Watch 2014). Construction for the 2022 FIFA World Cup in Qatar is heavily dependent on migrant laborers from Nepal and India, approximately 400 of whom die each year from workplace injuries, heart attacks, and illness associated with squalid living conditions. By the time of the World Cup, over 4,000 construction workers will have died (International Trade Union Confederation 2014).

Human Trafficking

Receiving insufficient attention are the estimated 21 million people subject to human trafficking (and millions more facing various other forms of enslavement [Walk Free Foundation 2016]) at any given time, particularly women and children forced to become slave laborers on plantations, in mines, factory sweatshops, domestic settings, and as sex workers. Human trafficking has long existed, but it has grown under neoliberal globalization, as grim economic conditions and greater mobility bring more poor people into this form of exploitation, and deregulation lessens government vigilance (although countries that have opened to trade may also have less forced labor and improved economic rights of women [Neumayer and De Soysa 2007]).

Most persons identified as trafficked are subject to sexual exploitation (almost 5 million people, overwhelmingly women, over one fifth children) (ILO 2012); an increasing number are trafficked for forced labor (UNODC 2014). The prostitution of children involves traffickers offering the sexual services of a child (under 18) or inducing a child to perform sexual acts for financial or nonfinancial compensation (UNODC 2014). Prostitution differs from sexual abuse in that it entails commercial gain. Those trafficked are often trapped by obligations to provide remittances to the families who sold them.

With most going undetected, there may be as many as 5 million prostituted children worldwide (ILO 2012) (Table 9-4). The main prostitutors of children are local men, with foreign pedophiles driving the "sex tour" market. Organized criminal elements are commonly involved, employing addictive drugs to control children. Highly profitable, human trafficking—spanning sexual and labor exploitation and illicit organ trade—generates over US$30 billion yearly (Smith, Martin, and Smith 2014).

Prostituted children have a high risk of acquiring sexually-transmitted diseases such as HIV, syphilis, and gonorrhea, of becoming pregnant and suffering complications from attempted abortion, as well as experiencing mental illness, substance abuse, and violence (Rafferty 2013). Programs to rescue and provide services to trafficked children operate in most major countries, but they are under-resourced. Criminalizing sex tourism and enforcing local laws that prohibit the prostitution of children are critical legal measures needed to end this horrendous practice.

Table 9-4 Estimated Number of Children Exploited through Prostitution

Country	Estimated Number of Children Exploited through Prostitution, (2011–2013)
Bangladesh	10,000–29, 000
Brazil[a]	500,000
Cambodia	12,000–35,000
India	1,200,000
Nepal	7,000–12,000
Philippines	60,000–75,000
Russia	16,000–32,500
Thailand	60,000
South Africa	28,000–30,000
United States	100,000

Data Sources: Serafini (2012)[a]. See country reports at ECPAT (2016).

International and National Labor Standards and Occupational Safety and Health

Working conditions for many of the world's poor and socially/economically excluded people are abysmal, with occupational safety and health standards woefully legislated or enforced, despite the range of worker rights stipulated in many international human rights treaties and international labor standards (London 2011). With limited access to occupational health services, a major problem is the failure to properly inform and train workers on hazards associated with their work and on safety protocols, particularly in the informal economy (including in HICs) (Lucchini and London 2014).

The sine qua non for successfully addressing global occupational health and safety concerns revolves around the right to bargain collectively and organize for social and workplace rights. The ILO, founded in 1919, sets minimum standards for international work conditions, covering ethical and human rights protections. ILO conventions, which have legal standing where they have been ratified, heavily stress occupational safety and health (OSH) issues:

No. 81—labor inspection

No. 98—freedom to organize and bargain collectively

No. 105—freedom from forced labor

No. 155—occupational safety and health

No. 161—occupational health services

No. 174—prevention of major industrial accidents

Other ILO conventions address health and safety in specific economic sectors (e.g., construction, mining, and agriculture). But, for example, only 32 countries have ratified the Convention on Occupational Health Services. Moreover, the ILO has no enforcement authority. Shamefully, working conditions for the majority of the world's workers do not meet the basic minimum standards and guidelines.

WHO is responsible for the technical aspects of OSH, such as the promotion of medical and hygienic standards and medical examinations, but a minuscule budget impedes it from providing needed support. Incomprehensibly, given the centrality of work conditions to health, WHO's Program for Occupational Health has just a handful of staff covering the entire world!

Protective legislation is generally weaker in LMICs than in HICs, albeit with certain exceptions, for instance Brazil's workplace health and safety laws and recent improvements in addressing OSH in India, Laos, Papua New Guinea, and South Africa. Occupational safety and health laws and their enforcement, as well as pay, are typically better where workers are unionized (Mishel

2012), with notable gains for union members in the Majority World (Groll 2013). Still, only 5% to 10% of workers in LMICs and 20% to 50% of workers in HICs have access to occupational health services, treatment, and rehabilitation (Lucchini and London 2014). There remains much to be done, ranging from OSH training for medical personnel to national inspection programs (especially in hazardous industries), all essential to monitoring, preventing, and treating occupational disease and injury (ILO 2013b).

Building on ILO standards, Table 9-5 outlines key policy approaches that would help protect health in the workplace and restrict hazardous and precarious work across the world.

Table 9-5 Key Labor Policies and OSH Measures to Improve Working Conditions and Protect Workers' Health

LABOR PROTECTIONS AND POLICIES (NATIONAL AND INTERNATIONAL)	
Strengthen governance and policy frameworks	• Increase public capacity for regulation and control of employment conditions. • Integrate OSH into PHC and public health systems, as well as intersectoral policies. • Include OSH in collective bargaining (e.g., "right to know" provisions about presence of hazards; safety protections). • Expand coverage of occupational health services to temporary workers, self-employed, and small businesses.
Promote equal access to labor market	• Develop full employment policies to provide more stability and reduce insecurity and health inequalities associated with unemployment, temporary and precarious employment, and informal work. • Develop active labor market policies to facilitate access to employment among women, youth, and older workers.
Ensure fair employment and social inclusion	• Expand social security to provide fair wages, unemployment insurance, and social protections to informal sector workers and home-makers. • Strengthen occupational protections in social security and insurance mechanisms. • Promote work schedule flexibility ("flextime," enabling family care). • Strengthen regulatory controls on downsizing, subcontracting, and outsourcing (including supply chain regulation) and enact laws placing limits on precarious employment.
Give more power to workers	• Support the creation of precarious and informal workers' organizations based on shared features such as: occupation (domestic workers, taxi drivers, etc.); workplace location (farmers' markets, streets); and migrant status. • Remove anti-union laws and practices and increase the rights of workers and unions, protecting the right to organize. • Support solidarity economies, worker co-management in manufacturing, and popular participation in labor/employment policies.

Table 9-5 Continued

Protect against exploitation and discrimination	• Reinforce laws against forced, bonded, and child labor. • Enhance and enforce national and international laws and controls to eliminate slavery and human trafficking. • Implement measures to counter discrimination against foreign-born, migrant, and other vulnerable workers. • Protect workers' right to refuse hazardous work.
Protect against negative impact of globalization	• Protect the rights to safe and healthy work environments from violations by third parties (e.g., TNCs) by developing, adopting, and enforcing health and safety regulations. • Cover OSH protections in regional trade agreements and oppose agreements that reduce access to safer technologies. • Prohibit free trade zones/trade treaties that flout labor and OSH protections. • Ensure that TNCs abide by all international and national environmental and OSH standards and regulations. • Include OSH in subcontracting and outsourcing regulations.
OSH MEASURES (NATIONAL, LOCAL, AND WORKPLACE LEVEL)	
On-site safety and oversight	• Ensure safety and protective measures against physical, biological, and chemical hazards. • Prohibit excessive work hours and ensure adequate breaks. • Improve ergonomic standards and temperature, hearing, ventilation, and respiratory controls and protections. • Rigorously enforce worker health and safety regulations and legislation (e.g., inspection, sanctions, and follow-up). • Establish occupational health offices to monitor and address occupational diseases, injuries, and worker complaints.
Awareness and knowledge on occupational health and safety, and workers' rights	• Provide workers and trainees with the tools to participate in the analysis, evaluation and modification of health damaging work exposures, hazards, and processes. • Raise parents' awareness about the social and health problems caused by child labor. • Promote awareness of human rights among workers.
Worker participation and control	• Promote worker participation and the action of safety representatives to prevent occupational hazards. • Incorporate social movements and grassroots community activities into efforts to reach fair employment (e.g., living wage campaigns). • Expand worker control over the labor process and over the setting, implementation, and enforcement of workplace organization/decisions/policies.

Source: Adapted, with permission, from Benach et al. (2013).

SIGNS OF HOPE FOR THE FUTURE: RESISTANCE TO NEOLIBERAL GLOBALIZATION

Key Questions:

- What kinds of efforts are able to challenge neoliberal globalization?
- What makes these policies and movements effective?

While neoliberal globalization has jeopardized health and exacerbated health and wealth inequities, digital technologies, the Internet, and social media have also enhanced information access and exchange, fostering local and transnational solidarity-oriented forms of globalization that are beneficial for health and social justice. In this section we highlight a few of the myriad ways the "global village" of social advocates and activists acting in the public interest have challenged prevailing neoliberal orthodoxy, managing to attenuate—or even reverse—some of its detrimental (health) effects.

LMIC Governments versus Big Pharma

Notwithstanding the pressures of neoliberal globalization, a number of LMIC governments, bolstered by social movements, have taken concrete measures to protect the health and well-being of their populations. Illustrative are actions taken to ensure the production of safe and affordable generic drugs by the governments of India, Thailand, and Brazil, which have stood up to Big Pharma, the WTO, and US government lobbying.

India has long been known as the "pharmacy of the developing world," furnishing large quantities of inexpensive generic medicines to a range of LMICs (Gabble and Kohler 2014). For example, India's generic ARVs—produced at four to eight times below brand prices—supply over 80% of donor-funded ARVs in LMICs and 90% of pediatric ARVs (Waning, Diedrichsen, and Moon 2010). This is enabled by the government's wide interpretation of the flexibilities of the TRIPS regime to suit domestic policy preferences. In order to obtain a patent in India, companies must reach a high threshold of "novelty"—each new drug must bring significant efficacious benefit to patients beyond existing drugs—one of the most restrictive standards in the world. After Swiss pharmaceutical giant Novartis brought a patent denial case to the Indian High Court charging violation of the TRIPS Agreement, the Court ruled in 2007 that it had no jurisdiction over this issue, leaving India's policies intact. This was repeated in 2013 with another challenge by Novartis, regarding a patent denial for a cancer drug. The court ruled against Novartis, deeming that the drug was not innovative but "evergreened" and thus did not require patent protection (Gabble and Kohler 2014). Argentina and the Philippines have also passed laws against "evergreening" patents, and Brazil and South Africa are developing similar provisions (PHM et al. 2014). Even so, India was compelled in 2005 to change its Patent Law to abide by TRIPS, preventing generic production of new patented drugs thereby making these medicines "beyond the reach of most Indian patients" (Sengupta 2013, p. 3).

On the other side of the world, Brazil has also fought to reduce drug prices and assure access to patented pharmaceuticals. Despite pressure from the US government in the early 2000s, the Brazilian government made full use of TRIPS Agreement flexibilities ('t Hoen et al. 2011). Brazil expertly employed TRIPS's compulsory licensing clause as an effective tool on two fronts: first, by including a provision under Brazil's IP law stipulating that—unless locally manufactured—pharmaceutical products are subject to compulsory licensing, it has compelled drug companies to substantially lower prices of ARVs; and second, thanks to its production capacity, by actually issuing a compulsory license (in 2007) to manufacture a patented ARV drug domestically (Chan 2015). In so doing, Brazil serves as an international role model of how to ensure that the rules and arrangements under globalization do not undercut domestic social policies.

NGOs Working on Trade and Health

Various public interest NGOs actively challenge the status quo around trade and health issues. Global Trade Watch (GTW) was founded in 1995 as part of Public Citizen (started in 1971 by longtime US political activist Ralph Nader). GTW disputes current mechanisms of globalization (as neither based on free trade, nor inevitable) and strives to ensure that communities enjoy "economic security, a clean environment, safe food, medicines and products, access to quality affordable services such as health" (Public Citizen 2015). Advocating both government and corporate accountability, it lobbies the US Congress on behalf of the public. GTW was a chief organizer of the first large-scale protest against the WTO at its 1999 meeting in Seattle. Also US-based, CPATH (Center for Policy Analysis on Trade and Health) conducts research and advocacy around health dimensions of trade agreements, including tobacco control, access to medicines, and corporate influence on trade negotiations.

In the Majority World, the Regional Network on Equity in Health in Southern Africa (Equinet) carries out analysis, training, and research on the health equity dimensions of economic and trade policies especially related to TRIPS. Focus on the Global South, based in Thailand, has been at the forefront of struggles against the WTO in Asia, advocating for alternatives to neoliberal globalization. Among its recent activities are reports on the impact of trade agreements on agriculture, health, and access to medicines.

Scientific Evidence, Industry Power, and Social Movement Activism: The Case of Canadian Asbestos Production

Asbestos is a naturally occurring mineral found in numerous countries and widely used in building materials for heat and acoustic insulation because it is light, strong, durable, and noncombustible. The dangers of all forms of asbestos were recognized in the 1920s, and in 1963 scientists demonstrated the link between asbestosis (scarring of the lung tissue caused by inhaling asbestos) and mesothelioma (a type of lung cancer) (Castleman and Tweedale 2012). Beginning in the 1970s, asbestos products were discontinued and asbestos abatement began in many HICs and some LMICs. However, an estimated 2 million tons of asbestos continue to be used, and WHO and ILO estimate that 125 million workers are exposed to asbestos and 100,000 die from asbestos-related causes annually (Ogunseitan 2015).

Though use of asbestos was restricted in Canada in 1973 under the *Hazardous Products Act,* virtually ending its domestic use, Canada remained one of the world's leading producers and exporters of chrysotile asbestos (the most common form of asbestos) until 2012, when the government of the province of Québec stopped supporting the industry, and Canada's last two asbestos mines closed. Until then 95% of Canadian asbestos was exported to LMICs that had not yet banned its use, including India, Thailand, Indonesia, and Vietnam. In a hypocritical double standard, asbestos was deemed harmful to Canadians but not to LMIC residents.

What changed? Starting in 2008 an intense social activism campaign was carried out through the human rights group RightOnCanada.ca, which mobilized thousands of health activists, civil society organizations, asbestos victims, and health professionals to press the Canadian and Québec governments to stop mining and exporting asbestos. They exposed and challenged government financing of the asbestos industry's influential lobby organization, forcing it to close. Over one hundred medical experts filed an ethics complaint against the Québec Minister of Health for spreading medical misinformation about the health effects of asbestos, bringing the irresponsible and harmful collusion of government and industry to public attention. This range of civil society activists succeeded in ending the government's financial support and eventually stopping the mining and export of asbestos (Ruff 2012).

While an important advance, more remains to be done. In spite of decades-long global consensus that all types of asbestos are carcinogenic and all levels of asbestos exposure extremely toxic, at the 2011 meeting of the Rotterdam Convention, Canada singlehandedly blocked the recommendation to place chrysotile asbestos on the Convention's list of hazardous substances, insisting that it is less harmful than other forms of asbestos and, when handled properly, can be used safely. At the 2013 and 2015 convention meetings, Canada stayed silent, but Russia—which mines and exports approximately two thirds of all asbestos, together with a handful of other countries—blocked the listing of asbestos. Canada has continued to send a terrible message to the rest of the world by opposing responsible trade, rejecting scientific evidence, and obstructing international cooperation to build a safer world (Frank and Joshi 2014).

Legal Challenges to Corporate Impunity

Increasingly, workers themselves courageously challenge corporate impunity. The residents of

Paulínia, (São Paulo state) Brazil have spent years struggling against the transnational chemical industry. In the late 1970s, Shell installed a chemical plant in Paulínia, which it sold to American Cyanamid in 1992. As required by local regulations, Shell paid for an environmental assessment, which revealed that water in the residential areas surrounding the plant was contaminated with pesticides and unfit for human consumption. Shell agreed to provide drinking water to residents but routinely sourced it from contaminated wells. American Cyanamid was eventually acquired by BASF, one of the largest chemical manufacturers in the world. BASF concealed ongoing worker exposure to organochlorine pesticides until 2002, when the Brazilian government closed the site based on its own findings of contamination. A 2005 Ministry of Health assessment concluded that the plant's employees faced increased cancer risks linked to years of hazardous exposure. A lawsuit filed by the District Attorney of São Paulo resulted in a 2013 settlement of US$316 million to compensate 1,000 exposed workers and for "collective moral damages" (Murphy 2013). While an important victory for workers, separate lawsuits filed by residents living in exposed areas are ongoing.

This movement, among others, has pushed the Brazilian government to respond more swiftly and effectively against corporate violations. After a massive 2015 mudslide caused by a burst dam at an iron ore mine in the state of Minas Gerais killed 19 people, contaminated an 800-km river, and destroyed hundreds of homes, within 2 weeks the government fined the company, Samarco, US$6 billion. When a judge determined that Samarco was unable to cover the fine, he froze the assets of its parent companies, mining giants Vale and BHP until they agreed to pay for environmental restoration and community rebuilding. Federal prosecutors have since filed a US$44 billion civil suit, arguing that the settlement was insufficient to cover the costs of Brazil's worst ever environmental disaster.

Struggles Around Water Privatization

A prime example of the impact of neoliberal globalization on social rights is water privatization. Cities and provinces in Benin, India, Kenya, Niger, the Philippines, and many other settings have undergone water privatization over recent decades under pressure from IFIs and corporate interests (Blue Planet Project 2012). The public provision of water in many LMICs has long suffered from inadequate funding, yet privatization has brought worse problems, threatening safety, quality, and the very human right to water access, all in the name of profits (Barlow 2011). Despite evidence of dire outcomes from commodifying water, since 1990 the World Bank has financed some 950 water and sewerage privatization projects in 64 countries (World Bank 2015a). It has encouraged prepaid water across sub-Saharan Africa, as well as in Palestine, to enable "cost recovery" (Moyo 2015).

When water was privatized in KwaZulu-Natal, South Africa in 2000, over 100,000 cases of cholera were reported during a 6-month period, causing hundreds of deaths. Although water had previously been provided free of charge and South Africa's post-apartheid constitution guaranteed the right to water, private mega-companies imposed a water connection fee of 51 rands (then US$7), an amount categorically unaffordable (Bond 2004). Just weeks later, local authorities began shutting off water to residents who were unable to pay their bills, and cholera broke out as thousands resorted to using polluted river water.

Various collective movements to resist privatization of water have had remarkable effects. In 2004, an overwhelming majority of Uruguay's population voted for a constitutional amendment to protect water as a natural—and public—resource necessary for life, declaring that access to potable water and sanitation was a fundamental human right. Despite corporate retribution, between 2000 and 2014, 136 cities in HICs and 44 cities in LMICs remunicipalized water provision, from Dar es Salaam, Tanzania to Kuala Lumpur, Malaysia and all of Ghana (Lobina, Kishimoto, and Petitjean 2014).

In Jakarta, Indonesia, notwithstanding constitutional recognition of the right to water and sanitation, water provision was privatized in 1997 via a public–private partnership with French multinational Suez and Indonesian company Aetra, causing rate hikes and suspension of the water supply even when bills were paid. Civil society activists challenged the constitutionality of the water privatization, and in 2015, after a prolonged struggle, the Central Jakarta District Court found Suez and Aetra negligent and annulled their contracts (Transnational Institute 2015).

Most famously, in the late 1990s, the Bolivian government, pressured by the World Bank, agreed to privatize water management under foreign investors. A 1999 law ended guaranteed public water provision, prohibiting autonomous water systems, wells, and even rainwater collection, while a 40-year concession for Cochabamba's (Bolivia's 3rd largest city) water system was granted to a subsidiary of Bechtel, a US TNC, with an assured 16% annual profit rate enabled by concomitant rate increases. As the cost of water soared, an alliance of farmers, unions, and neighborhood groups organized meetings and marches against the privatization, culminating in an 8-day "water war" of protests and blockades. Local women, whose gender role makes them responsible for acquiring, storing, and distributing water, were protagonists in these confrontations. In April 2000 the government was forced to terminate Cochabamba's water contract (Olivera and Lewis 2004). A similar water war resulted in the expulsion of Suez from the Indigenous city of El Alto—outside the capital La Paz—in 2005. These mobilizations contributed to the election of Bolivia's first Indigenous president, Evo Morales, in 2009 (Achtenberg 2013).

In Buenos Aires, Argentina, Suez managed the private water supply as of 1993, leading to rising rates and poor service. After years of complaints, the government terminated the contract in 2006 and established a public water company, AySA, under a participatory ownership scheme, making it 90% owned by the state and 10% by the water company's workers' union. Worker cooperatives have also been established in Buenos Aires to involve residents of poor communities in decisionmaking around water system expansion (Lobina, Kishimoto, and Petitjean 2014).

Worker-Run Cooperatives

Worker-run cooperatives provide an alternative to neoliberal capitalism, akin to a "factory without bosses" (albeit still participating in capitalist markets). Distinguishing features of cooperatives include: shared vision and aspirations (solidarity); democratic governance (genuine participation); and possible surpluses (not profits), but the focus is on creating value for customers and reproducing workers' lives (not capital) (Co-operatives UK 2015). There are many types of cooperatives: farming, health, and industrial. Most famous is the Basque country's Mondragon, engaged in finance, construction and equipment production, retail, and education (Lafuente and Freundlich 2012). Argentina's worker-recovered companies—with 13,000 workers running over 300 companies bankrupted by the 2001–2002 economic crisis—offer another illustration of successful cooperatives, even as they operate within a larger capitalist world (Ozarow and Croucher 2014).

Perhaps the ideal way of protecting workers' rights and health is via collective arrangements for production, as exemplified by the "solidarity economy" (Allard, Davidson, and Matthaei 2008), based on worker co-management, involvement in organizing the labor process and making workplace decisions, coupled with popular participation via communal councils. An alternative economic system (outside of for-profits and state-owned companies), it includes both volunteer organizations and cooperatives, featuring self-help, reciprocity, and a social purpose. Women's membership in solidarity economy groups, such as Indigenous crafts producers in Bolivia, show that while insufficient for dealing with root causes of gender inequities and persistent gender-based wage gaps, the solidarity economy offers a productive strategy for challenging the labor neoliberalization that has cornered women into low-wage, poor condition jobs (Hillenkamp 2015).

> "Everything is now for sale. Even those areas of life that we once considered sacred like health and education, food and water and air and seeds and genes and a heritage. It is all now for sale."—Maude Barlow speaking at the Seattle International Forum on Globalization Teach-In, 1999

Social Movements Contesting Neoliberal Globalization

As these experiences show, governments can be influenced by pressure from below, though the struggles are arduous. A key question is whether social movements of recent years, such as the Arab Spring, Occupy Wall Street, and protests against austerity in Greece and Spain, provide the conditions for an alternative approach to the world order (and to health). The

Majority World has produced numerous social movements contesting the dominant order, leading to the election of governments going against the neoliberal grain, especially in Latin America's pink tide of the 2000s (see chapter 13). In Egypt and Tunisia, for example, the 2010–2011 uprisings aimed as much to undo the negative consequences of neoliberalism (including in the health arena) as to overthrow repressive political regimes (Sutcliffe 2012). But Euro-American and Saudi (corporate) interests quelled this resistance with a firm hand, helping envelop the entire region in sectarian and state violence, even as the revolution is unfinished (Prashad 2016).

Organized labor in LMICs is a key component of global social movement unionism, linking workplace, social, economic, and political forces in resistance against the negative effects of globalization (Bezuidenhout 2000). At the domestic level, labor unions have been instrumental in shaping government policies such as in South Africa, where the labor movement, in alliance with the African National Congress, helped dismantle many elements of apartheid (Ntshalintshali 2012). Networks, for instance StreetNet International, which consists of more than 30 unions, cooperatives, and associations across Africa, Asia, and Latin America, also bring a collective voice to advocacy on the rights of informal workers (e.g., street vendors during the 2014 World Cup in Brazil) (StreetNet International 2015).

The Occupy movement started with a small number of people, including health workers, protesting the oppressive power of corporate America as symbolized by Wall Street. Reaching across North America, Europe, and beyond, it is credited with popularizing the language of the 1% (of elites wielding economic power) versus the 99% (the majority of people). Today politicians and pundits of all stripes have been forced to discuss inequality (even as its underlying causes remain unaddressed) and the influence of wealth (inequality) on politics, while the struggle for higher minimum wages and the environmental movement have been re-energized (Levitin 2015).

Also indicating the level of discontent with the economic and political system is Spain's *Podemos*, which has transitioned from a popular movement to a new political party with an anti-austerity, pro–social welfare platform. As the Great Recession was unfolding, Spain's government imposed regressive labor reforms and large social spending cuts. Salaries declined by 10%, precarious work increased, and in 2013 unemployment reached 26%, double among young people. The youth-led *indignados* movement was born as a forum for questioning the legitimacy of the state and challenging the political claim that there are no alternatives. Protests were met with police repression but the movement endured, becoming the foundation of *Podemos* (Navarro 2015). *Podemos* has since become a legitimate political party engaged in an uphill battle for transformative change.

Globally, popular resistance to the IMF's role and influence appears to be growing. A study of *World Protests 2006–2013* found that of the 843 protests examined in 87 countries, the IMF was a target of 20% of the total, equally in richer and poorer countries. The IMF was widely challenged "for promoting a 'new Washington Consensus' that favors the interests of corporations, wealthy investors, and the financial sector," with many local protests opposing austerity measures, including cuts to public services, reductions in wages, regressive labor rights, and deteriorated working conditions, among other economic justice issues (Ortiz et al. 2013, p. 35).

CONCLUSION

Learning Points:

- Globalization has the potential both to benefit and harm population health, depending on who controls the flow of capital, labor, and knowledge, and who benefits and suffers.
- The features of neoliberal globalization—financialization, liberalization, unfair trade terms, investor privileges, illicit financial flows, debt crises and their policy consequences, labor market reorganization, and blatant disregard for the environment—are detrimental to public health and well-being and worsen health inequities.
- TNCs maximize profits by minimizing labor and production costs, threatening health through increased exploitation of workers, contamination of the environment, flouting of tax laws and labor, health, and safety regulations, and undemocratic political influence.

- Occupational safety and health is a critical and neglected area in global health.
- Community organizing and social justice movements can and have confronted undemocratic and unaccountable global financial and trade institutions and successfully pushed governments to take stronger stances in favor of public health and well-being.

The neoliberal globalization phase of capitalism, as defined in this chapter, is associated with unregulated markets and policies that favor growth and unfettered investment over social equity, profit over people and the environment, and "free trade" over "fair trade." Government protective and regulatory capacities have become weakened worldwide as global trade pacts have been pushed by corporate interests via the governments of dominant economies, with resultant downward pressure on health.

Neoliberal globalization affects health through major pathways and specific mechanisms, as follows. First, since the 1980s numerous LMICs have undergone structural adjustment reforms dictated by the World Bank and IMF, mandating reduced government expenditures on education and health, user fees for the poor, and decreased workplace, environment, and social protections, together exposing economies to the vicissitudes of an unjust global trade and financial system. Second, financial liberalization and currency speculation have led to economic crisis and cruel austerity policies in many countries. Meanwhile, capital flight and tax evasion by both domestic and foreign elites continue to rob countries of trillions of dollars of resources. Third, trade liberalization, including via the WTO and bilateral/regional trade and investment agreements, all have potentially deleterious effects on public health, reducing access to generic medications, privileging foreign investors over government decisionmaking, ratcheting down regulation of harmful products, food, and production processes, and privatizing essential services for public health (e.g., water). Fourth, TNCs play a particularly nefarious role in exacerbating neoliberal globalization's menace to health by imperiling workers (via inhumane pay, union busting, and hazardous working conditions) and by lobbying against, not complying with, or defying regulations intended to protect basic human rights, health, and the environment. Coupled with illicit financial flows, these tactics enable TNCs to fulfill their fiduciary responsibilities of maximizing profits to the detriment of well-being. Indeed, TNC profits are usually largest where governance is weakest and rife with disregard for economic, social, and cultural human rights.

Still, challenging the primacy of the neoliberal economic model is possible: social movements across the world have organized around health, environmental, and other concerns in order to resist and counter TNCs and the undemocratic decisions made by IFIs. A world with accountable governance, truly fair trade relationships, and enforced occupational health and safety standards can change health for the better. But, as we shall see in the next chapter, the contemporary capitalist world order—driving endless economic growth based on a nexus of exploitation, production, and consumption—is contaminating and depleting the world's natural resources, and provoking climate change, at such a pace that without significant transformation of the extant economic model, the Earth may become unlivable.

NOTE

1. For more on professionals and administrators in so-called contradictory class locations (or middle-class locations), see chapter 7. On the growing traction of social and economic arrangements that serve as alternatives to capitalism, see chapter 13.

REFERENCES

Achtenberg E. 2013. From water wars to water scarcity: Bolivia's cautionary tale. *Nacla*, June 5.

Ajayi SI and Ndikumana L. 2015. Scale, causes, and effects of capital flight from Africa. In Ajayi SI and Ndikumana L, Editors. *Capital Flight from Africa: Causes, Effects, and Policy Issues.* Oxford: Oxford University Press.

Al Jazeera. 2014. Deaths reported in China coal-mine explosion. *Al Jazeera*, November 27.

Allard J, Davidson C, and Matthaei J. 2008. *Solidarity Economy: Building Alternatives for People and Planet.* Chicago: Changemaker Publications.

Amnesty International. 2014. *'30 Years is too Long. to Get Justice'.* London: Amnesty International.

———. 2016. *"This is What We Die For": Human Rights Abuses in the Democratic Republic of Congo Power the Global Trade in Cobalt.* London: Amnesty International.

Armitage J. 2014. Big Tobacco puts countries on trial as concerns over TTIP deals mount. *The Independent,* October 21.

Baker BK. 2010. The impact of the International Monetary Fund's macroeconomic policies on the AIDS pandemic. *International Journal of Health Services* 40(2):347–363.

Barlow M. 2011. *Our Right to Water: A People's Guide to Implementing the UN's Recognition of the Right to Water and Sanitation.* Ottawa: Council of Canadians.

———. 2015. NAFTA's ISDS: Why Canada is one of the most sued countries in the world. *Global Justice Now,* October 23.

Basu N and Hu H. 2010. *Toxic Metals and Indigenous Peoples near the Marlin Mine in Western Guatemala: Potential Exposures and Impacts on Health.* Cambridge: Physicians for Human Rights.

Basu S, Stuckler D, Gonsalves G, and Lurie M. 2009. The production of consumption: Addressing the impact of mineral mining on tuberculosis in southern Africa. *Globalization and Health* 5:11.

Baum FE and Anaf JM. 2015. Transnational corporations and health: A research agenda. *International Journal of Health Services* 45(2):353–362.

Baum FE, Sanders DM, Fisher M, et al. 2016. Assessing the health impact of transnational corporations: Its importance and a framework. *Globalization and Health* 12(1).

Beall RF, Kuhn R, and Attaran A. 2015. Compulsory licensing often did not produce lower prices for antiretrovirals compared to international procurement. *Health Affairs* 34(3):493–501.

Benach J, Muntaner C, Solar O, et al. 2013. *Employment, Work, and Health Inequalities: A Global Perspective.* Barcelona: Icaria Editorial SA.

Benach J, Vives A, Amable M, et al. 2014. Precarious employment: Understanding an emerging social determinant of health. *Annual Review of Public Health* 35:229–253.

Bezuidenhout A. 2000. *Towards Global Social Movement Unionism? Trade Union Responses to Globalization in South Africa. Discussion Papers DP/115/2000.* Geneva: ILO.

Blue Planet Project. Our right to water. 2012. http://www.blueplanetproject.net/index.php/our-right-to-water/. Accessed September 4, 2015.

Blue Planet Project, the Council of Canadians, the Institute for Policy Studies, et al. 2014. *Debunking Eight Falsehoods by Pacific Rim Mining/OceanaGold in El Salvador.* International Allies against Mining in El Salvador.

Bohme SR. 2015. *Toxic Injustice: A Transnational History of Exposure and Struggle.* Oakland: University of California Press.

Bond P. 2004. The political roots of South Africa's cholera epidemic. In Fort M, Mercer M, and Gish O, Editors. *Sickness and Wealth: The Corporate Assault on Global Health.* Cambridge: South End Press.

Breman A and Shelton C. 2007. Structural adjustment programs and health. In Kawachi I and Wamala S, Editors. *Globalization and Health.* New York: Oxford University Press.

Brenner R. 2006. *The Economics of Global Turbulence: The Advanced Capitalist Economies from Long Boom to Long Downturn, 1945–2005.* London: Verso.

Bretton Woods Project. 2015. IMF moved on from structural adjustment? http://www.brettonwoodsproject.org/2015/02/imf-loans-conditions-increasing/. Accessed January 2, 2016.

Broughton E. 2005. The Bhopal disaster and its aftermath: A review. *Environmental Health* 4(1):6.

Bumann S, Hermes N, and Lensink R. 2013. Financial liberalization and economic growth: A meta-analysis. *Journal of International Money and Finance* 33:255–281.

Cajax CS, Berman H, Varcoe C, et al. 2014. Gold mining on Mayan-Mam territory: Social unravelling, discord and distress in the Western highlands of Guatemala. *Social Science and Medicine* 111:50–57.

Castleman B and Tweedale G. 2012. Turning the tide: The struggle for compensation for asbestos-related diseases and the banning of asbestos. In Sellers C and Melling J. *Dangerous Trade: Histories of Industrial Hazard across a Globalizing World.* Philadelphia: Temple University Press.

Chan J. 2015. *Politics in the Corridor of Dying: AIDS Activism and Global Health Governance.* Baltimore: Johns Hopkins University Press.

Chan M. 2008. Globalization and health. [New York]: Remarks at the United Nations General Assembly.

Chang H-J. 2002. *Kicking Away the Ladder: Development Strategy and Historical Perspective.* London: Anthem Press.

Chen MA. 2016. The informal economy: Recent trends, future directions. *NEW SOLUTIONS: A Journal of Environmental and Occupational Health Policy* 26(2):155–172.

Citizens Trade Campaign. 2015. The Trans-Pacific Partnership. http://www.citizenstrade.org/ctc/trade-policies/tpp-potential-trade-policy-problems/. Accessed September 7, 2015.

Clapp J and Dauvergne P. 2011. *Paths to a Green World: The Political Economy of the Global Environment, Second Edition.* Cambridge: MIT Press.

Collins M. 2015. The big bank bailout. *Forbes,* July 14.

Co-operatives UK. 2015. The co-operative economy 2015: an ownership agenda for Britain. http://www.

uk.coop/sites/default/files/uploads/attachments/co-op_economy_2015.pdf. Accessed July 25, 2015.
Cutler D, Deaton A, and Lleras-Muney A. 2006. The determinants of mortality. *Journal of Economic Perspectives* 20(3):97–120.
Damodaran S. 2015. The chimera of inclusive growth: Informality, poverty and inequality in India in the post-reform period. *Development and Change* 46(5):1213–1224.
Déneault A and Sacher W. 2012. *Paradis sous terre: Comment le Canada est devenu la plaque tournante de l'industrie minière mondiale.* Montréal: Ecosociété.
De Vogli R. 2011. Neoliberal globalisation and health in a time of economic crisis. *Social Theory and Health* 9(4):311–325.
De Vogli R and Owusu JT. 2015. The causes and health effects of the Great Recession: From neoliberalism to 'healthy de-growth'. *Critical Public Health* 25(1):15–31.
Diallo Y, Etienne A, and Mehran F. 2013. *Global Child Labour Trends 2008 to 2012.* Geneva: ILO.
Dijkstra G. 2011. The PRSP approach and the illusion of improved aid effectiveness: Lessons from Bolivia, Honduras and Nicaragua. *Development Policy Review* 29(s1):s110–s133.
Dollar D. 2001. Is globalization good for your health? *Bulletin of the World Health Organization* 79:827–833.
Easterly W. 2005. What did structural adjustment adjust?: The association of policies and growth with repeated IMF and World Bank adjustment loans. *Journal of Development Economics* 76(1):1–22.
Economist. 1992. Let them eat pollution. *Economist*, February 8 (7745).
ECPAT. 2016. Resources: Country monitoring reports. http://www.ecpat.net/resources#category-country-monitoring-reports. Accessed. February 3, 2016.
Epstein GA. 2005. Introduction: Financialization and the world economy. In Epstein GA, Editor. *Financialization and the World Economy.* Cheltenham, UK: Edward Elgar Publishing.
Escobar MAC, Veerman JL, Tollman SM, et al. 2013. Evidence that a tax on sugar sweetened beverages reduces the obesity rate: A meta-analysis. *BMC Public Health* 13:1072.
Extractive Industries Transparency Initiative. 2015. History of EITI. https://eiti.org/eiti/history. Accessed December 30, 2015.
FACT Coalition. 2015. Study: Offshore tax dodging by U.S. multinationals costs taxpayers $90 billion per year. http://thefactcoalition.org/study-offshore-tax-dodging-by-u-s-multinationals-costs-taxpayers-90-billion-per-year/. Accessed August 5, 2016.
Feachem R. 2001. Globalisation is good for your health, mostly. *British Medical Journal* 323:504–506.
Forman L and MacNaughton G. 2015. Moving theory into practice: Human rights impact assessment of intellectual property rights in trade agreements. *Journal of Human Rights Practice* 7(1):109–138.
Frank AL and Joshi TK. 2014. The global spread of asbestos. *Annals of Global Health* 80(4):257.
Freudenberg N. 2014. *Lethal but Legal: Corporations, Consumption, and Protecting Public Health.* New York: Oxford University Press.
Friedman M. 2006. In Simpson B, Producer, and Abbott J, Director. *The Corporation* [Film]. New York: Zeitgeist Films.
Gabble R and Kohler JC. 2014. To patent or not to patent? The case of Novartis' cancer drug Glivec in India. *Global Health* 10:3.
Gilmore AB, Fooks G, Drope J, et al. 2015. Exposing and addressing tobacco industry conduct in low-income and middle-income countries. *Lancet* 385(9972):1029–1043.
Gindin S. 2013. Puzzle or misreading? Stagnation, austerity and left politics. *The Bullet*, 920.
Glasgow S and Schrecker T. 2015. The double burden of neoliberalism? Noncommunicable disease policies and the global political economy of risk. *Health and Place* 34:279–286.
Global Exchange. 2015. Top reasons to oppose the WTO. http://www.globalexchange.org/resources/wto/oppose. Accessed December 29, 2015.
Goss S, Wade A, Skirvin JP, et al. 2013. *Effects of Unauthorized Immigration on the Actuarial Status of the Social Security Trust Funds. Actuarial Note No. 151.* Baltimore: Social Security Administration, Office of the Chief Actuary.
Government of Guatemala. 1983. Law on the marketing of breast-milk substitutes: *Guatemalan Presidential Decree 68–83.*
Groll E. 2013. The world's most powerful labor unions: From Tunisia to South Africa, where workers still rule. *Foreign Policy*, September 2.
Grossman E. 2015. Children are harvesting your food. Are they safe? http://civileats.com/2015/05/13/children-are-harvesting-your-food-are-they-safe/. Accessed September 7, 2015.
Harvey D. 2014. *Seventeen Contradictions and the End of Capitalism.* New York: Oxford University Press.
Hillenkamp I. 2015. Solidarity economy for development and women's emancipation: Lessons from Bolivia. *Development and Change* 46(5):1133–1158.
Hirst PQ, Thompson G, and Bromley S. 2009. *Globalization in Question, 3rd Edition.* Cambridge: Polity Press.

Hoddie M and Hartzell CA. 2014. Short-term pain, long-term gain? The effects of IMF economic reform programs on public health performance. *Social Science Quarterly* 95(4):1022–1042.

Human Rights Watch. 2014. *World Report 2014: Qatar. Events of 2013*. New York: Human Rights Watch.

———. 2015. Turkey: Mine disaster trial to open. https://www.hrw.org/news/2015/04/13/turkey-mine-disaster-trial-open. Accessed November 15, 2015.

IBFAN. 2014. *Breaking the Rules 2014: Evidence of Code Violations from Jan 2011 to Dec 2013. BTR: In Brief.* Penang: IBFAN.

Ifanti AA, Argyriou AA, Kalofonou FH, and Kalofonos HP. 2014. Physicians' brain drain in Greece: A perspective on the reasons why and how to address it. *Health Policy* 117(2):210–215.

Igumbor EU, Sanders D, Puoane TR, et al. 2012. "Big Food," the consumer food environment, health, and the policy response in South Africa. *PLoS Med* 9(7):e1001253.

ILO. 2010. *International Labour Migration: A Rights-Based Approach*. Geneva: ILO.

———. 2012. *ILO Global Estimate of Forced Labour: Results and methodology*. Geneva: ILO.

———. 2013a. *Global Employment Trends for Youth 2013: A Generation at Risk*. Geneva: ILO.

———. 2013b. *The Prevention of Occupational Diseases*. Geneva: International Programme on Safety and Health at Work and the Environment (SafeWork).

———. 2014. Labour migration: Facts and figures. http://www.ilo.org/global/about-the-ilo/newsroom/media-centre/issue-briefs/WCMS_239651/lang--en/index.htm. Accessed February 20, 2016.

———. 2015a. *World Employment and Social Outlook: Trends 2015*. Geneva: ILO.

———. 2015b. *World Report on Child Labour: Paving the way to decent work for young people 2015*. Geneva: ILO.

Imamura F, O'Connor L, Ye Z, et al. 2015. Consumption of sugar sweetened beverages, artificially sweetened beverages, and fruit juice and incidence of type 2 diabetes: systematic review, meta-analysis, and estimation of population attributable fraction. *BMJ* 351:h3576.

Institute for Global Labour and Human Rights. 2014. Rana Plaza: A look back, and forward. http://www.globallabourrights.org/alerts/rana-plaza-bangladesh-anniversary-a-look-back-and-forward. Accessed October 18, 2014.

International Trade Union Confederation. 2014. *The Case Against Qatar: Host of the FIFA 2022 World Cup. ITUC Special Report*. Brussels: International Trade Union Confederation.

Jafri A. 2015. Developing countries return empty handed from WTO's Nairobi Ministerial. http://focusweb.org/content/endwto-developing-countries-return-empty-handed-wto-s-nairobi-ministerial. Accessed December 19, 2015.

James D. 2015. Climate deception: Non-binding "targets" for climate, but binding rules on trade in services. *The Huffington Post*, December 4.

Jaworek M and Kuzel M. 2015. Transnational corporations in the world economy: Formation, development and present position. *Copernican Journal of Finance and Accounting* 4(1):55–70.

Jenkins R. 2004. Globalization, production, employment and poverty: Debates and evidence. *Journal of International Development* 16(1):1–12.

Kabeer N and Mahmud S. 2004. Globalization, gender and poverty: Bangladeshi women workers in export and local markets. *Journal of International Development* 16(1):93.

Kar D and Spanjers J. 2015. *Illicit Financial Flows from Developing Countries: 2004–2013*. Washington, DC: Global Financial Integrity.

Karanikolos M and Kentikelenis A. 2016. Health inequalities after austerity in Greece. *International Journal for Equity in Health* 15(83).

Karanikolos M, Mladovsky P, Cylus J, et al. 2013. Financial crisis, austerity, and health in Europe. *Lancet* 381(9874):1323–1331.

Kedir AM. 2015. Tax evasion and capital flight in Africa. In Ajayi SI and Ndikumana L, Editors. *Capital Flight from Africa*. Oxford: Oxford University Press

Kelsey J. 2015. Implications of the TiSA trade in health care services proposal for public health. https://awp.lu/data/international/18/analysis_en.pdf. Accessed February 15, 2016.

Kentikelenis A, Karanikolos M, Reeves A, et al. 2014. Greece's health crisis: From austerity to denialism. *Lancet* 383(9918):748–753.

Kentikelenis AE, Stubbs TH, and King LP. 2015. Structural adjustment and public spending on health: Evidence from IMF programs in low-income countries. *Social Science and Medicine* 126:169–176.

Khanna P. 2011. Making labour voices heard during an industrial crisis: Workers' struggles in the Bangladesh garment industry. *Labour, Capital and Society* 44(2):106–129.

Kilpatrick K. 2015. Taxing soda, saving lives: Mexico's surcharge on sugary drinks is the real thing. *Al Jazeera America*, August 19.

Kim I, Muntaner C, Vahid Shahidi F, et al. 2012. Welfare states, flexible employment, and health: A critical review. *Health Policy* 104(2):99–127.

Knox JH. 2014. *Transnational Corporations and Environmental Harm Statement. Side Event on Human Rights and Transnational Corporations, 11 March 2014.* Geneva: OHCHR.

Koivusalo M, Schrecker T, and Labonté R. 2009. Globalization and policy space for health and social determinants of health. In Labonté R, Schrecker T, Packer C, and Runnels V, Editors. *Globalization and Health: Pathways, Evidence and Policy.* New York: Routledge.

Koivusalo M. 2014. Policy space for health and trade and investment agreements. *Health Promotion International* 29:i29–i47.

Koivusalo M and Tritter J. 2014. "Trade creep" and implications of the Transatlantic Trade and Investment Partnership agreement for the United Kingdom National Health Service. *International Journal of Health Services* 44(1):93–111.

Kotz DM. 2015. *The Rise and Fall of Neoliberal Capitalism.* Cambridge: Harvard University Press.

Kyle MK and McGahan AM. 2012. Investments in pharmaceuticals before and after TRIPS. *Review of Economics and Statistics* 94(4):1157–1172.

Labonté R, Blouin C, and Forman L. 2009. Trade and health. In Kay A, Williams O, Editors. *Global Health Governance: Crisis, Institutions and Political Economy.* London: Palgrave Macmillan.

Labonté R, Mohindra KS, and Lencucha R. 2011. Framing international trade and chronic disease. *Globalization and Health* 7:21.

Labonté R, Schram A, and Ruckert A. 2016. The Trans-Pacific Partnership: Is it everything we feared for health? *International Journal of Health Policy and Management* 5(8):487496.

Labonté R and Schrecker T. 2007. Globalization and social determinants of health: The role of the global marketplace. *Globalization and Health* 3:6.

Labonté R, Schrecker T, Packer C, and Runnels V, Editors. 2009. *Globalization and Health: Pathways, Evidence and Policy.* New York: Routledge.

Lafuente JL and Freundlich F. 2012. The MONDRAGON Cooperative Experience: Humanity at Work. http://www.managementexchange.com/story/mondragon-cooperative-experience-humanity-work. Accessed July 25, 2015.

Lagarde C. 2014. *The IMF at 70: Making the Right Choices—Yesterday, Today, and Tomorrow.* Washington, DC: The IMF/World Bank Annual Meetings.

Levitin M. 2015. The triumph of Occupy Wall Street. *The Atlantic,* June 10.

Lindstrom B. 2010. Scaling back TRIPS-plus: An analysis of intellectual property provisions in trade agreements and implications for Asia and the Pacific. *New York University Journal of International Law and Politics* 42(3):917–980.

Lobina E, Kishimoto S, and Petitjean O. 2014. *Here to Stay: Water Remunicipalisation as a Global Trend.* Paris/Amsterdam: Public Services International Research Unit (PSIRU), Transnational Institute (TNI) and Multinational Observatory.

Lobstein T, Jackson-Leach R, Moodie ML, et al. 2015. Child and adolescent obesity: Part of a bigger picture. *Lancet* 385(9986):2510–2520.

London L. 2011. Human rights and health: Opportunities to advance rural occupational health. *International Journal of Occupational and Environmental Health* 17(1):80–92.

Lu JL. 2008. Occupational hazards and illnesses of Filipino women workers in export processing zones. *International Journal of Occupational Safety and Ergonomics* 14(3):333–342.

Lucchini RG and London L. 2014. Global occupational health: Current challenges and the need for urgent action. *Annals of Global Health* 80(4):251–256.

Lustig R. 2012. *Fat Chance: The Bitter Truth about Sugar.* London: Fourth Estate Ltd.

Masud T and Masud C, Directors. 2003. *A Kind of Childhood* [Film]. Xingu Films/Audiovision Production in association with TV Ontario.

McCallum JK. 2011. *Export Processing Zones: Comparative Data from China, Honduras, Nicaragua and South Africa.* Geneva: ILO.

Mezher M. 2015. WTO reviews India's trade policies, including drug patents, compulsory licensing. *Regulatory Affairs Professionals Society,* June 3.

Milanovic B. 2012. Global inequality recalculated and updated: The effect of new PPP estimates on global inequality and 2005 estimates. *The Journal of Economic Inequality* 10(1):1–18.

MiningWatch Canada. 2015. *In the National Interest? Criminalization of Land and Environment Defenders in the Americas.* Ottawa: MiningWatch Canada.

MiningWatch Canada and RAID. 2014. *Violence Ongoing at Barrick Mine in Tanzania: MiningWatch Canada and RAID (UK) Complete Human Rights Assessment.* Ottawa and Oxford: MiningWatch Canada and RAID.

Mishel L. 2012. *Unions, Inequality, and Faltering Middle-Class Wages. Issue brief #342.* Washington, DC: Economic Policy Institute.

Mitman G and Erickson P. 2010. Latex and blood: Science, markets, and American empire. *Radical History Review* 107:45–73.

Monteiro CA and Cannon G. 2012. The impact of transnational "Big Food" companies on the south: A view from Brazil. *PLoS Med* 9(7):e1001252.

Moyo J. 2015. Prepaid meters scupper gains made in accessing water in Africa. *Inter Press Service News Agency*, May 8.

Muižnieks N. 2013. Child labour in Europe: a persisting challenge. https://www.coe.int/et/web/commissioner/-/child-labour-in-europe-a-persisting-challen-1. Accessed August 4, 2016.

Mukherjee N and Krieckhaus J. 2011. Globalization and human well-being. *International Political Science Review* 33(2):150–170.

Murphy P. 2013. Shell, BASF agree to pay-out over Brazil chemical contamination. http://uk.reuters.com/article/shell-basf-payout-idUKL1N0C40IE20130312. Accessed January 1, 2016.

Navarro V. 2015. Report from Spain: The political contexts of the dismantling of the Spanish welfare state. *International Journal of Health Service* 45(3):405–414.

Navarro V and Muntaner C, Editors. 2014. *The Financial and Economic Crises and Their Impact on Health and Well Being*. Amityville, NY: Baywood Publishing Company, Inc.

Ndikumana L and Boyce JK. 2011. *Africa's Odious Debts: How Foreign Loans and Capital Flight Bled a Continent*. London: Zed Books.

Ndikumana L, Boyce JK, and Ndiaye AS. 2015. Capital flight from Africa: Measurement and drivers. In Ajayi SI and Ndikumana L, Editors. *Capital Flight from Africa*. Oxford: Oxford University Press.

Nestle M. 2015. *Soda Politics: Taking on Big Soda (and Winning)*. Oxford: Oxford University Press.

Neumayer E and De Soysa I. 2007. Globalisation, women's economic rights and forced labour. *The World Economy* 30:1510–1535.

Ngowi A, Mrema E, and Kishinhi S. 2016. Pesticide health and safety challenges facing informal sector workers: A case of small-scale agricultural workers in Tanzania. *NEW SOLUTIONS: A Journal of Environmental and Occupational Health Policy* 26(2):220–240.

NHS. 2014. Eating processed foods. http://www.nhs.uk/livewell/goodfood/pages/what-are-processed-foods.aspx. Accessed July 18, 2015.

Nkurunziza JD. 2015. Capital flight and poverty reduction in Africa. In Ajayi SI and Ndikumana L, Editors. *Capital Flight from Africa*. Oxford: Oxford University Press.

Nobel Media. 2014. The Nobel Peace Prize for 2014. http://www.nobelprize.org/nobel_prizes/peace/laureates/2014/press.html. Accessed January 13, 2016.

Ntshalintshali B. 2012. Preface. In Mosoetsa S and Williams M, Editors. *Labour in the Global South: Challenges and Alternatives for Workers*. Geneva: ILO.

Ocampo JA. 2013. *The Latin American Debt Crisis in Historical Perspective*. New York: Initiative for Policy Dialogue.

OECD. 2016. OECD Data. https://data.oecd.org/. Accessed January 2, 2016.

Ogunseitan OA. 2015. The asbestos paradox: Global gaps in the translational science of disease prevention. *Bulletin of the World Health Organization* 93:359–360.

O'Hara M. 2015. *Austerity Bites: A Journey to the Sharp End of Cuts in the UK*. Bristol: Policy Press.

Olivera O and Lewis T. 2004. *¡Cochabamba! Water War in Bolivia*. Cambridge: South End Press.

Olivet C and Villareal A. 2016. Who really won the legal battle between Philip Morris and Uruguay? *The Guardian*, July 28.

Ortiz I, Burke S, Berrada M, and Cortes H. 2013. *Initiative for Policy Dialogue and Friedrich-Ebert-Stiftung New York Working Paper 2013: World Protests 2006-2013*. New York: Columbia University.

Ottersen OP, Dasgupta J, Blouin C, et al. 2014. The political origins of health inequity: Prospects for change. *Lancet* 383(9917):630–667.

Oxfam International. 2015. *Africa: Rising for the Few, Oxfam Media Briefing*. Oxford: Oxfam.

Ozarow D and Croucher R. 2014. Workers' self-management, recovered companies and the sociology of work. *Sociology* 48(5):989–1006.

Padilla AJ. 2013. *Occupational Health and Safety of Agricultural Workers: ILO conventions and gaps*. Penang: Pesticide Action Network Asia and the Pacific.

Panitch L and Gindin S. 2012. *The Making of Global Capitalism: The Political Economy of American Empire*. New York: Verso Books.

Parayre C. 2006. World dumps toxic waste in Africa. http://health.iafrica.com/features/211720.htm. Accessed September 26, 2006.

Peabody JW. 1996. Economic reform and health sector policy: Lessons from structural adjustment programs. *Social Science and Medicine* 43(5):823–835.

Petras J and Veltmeyer H. 2014. *Extractive Imperialism in the Americas: Capitalism's New Frontier*. Neiden: Brill.

PHM, Medact, Medico International, et al. 2014. *Global Health Watch 4: An Alternative World Health Report*. London: Zed Books Ltd.

Piketty T. 2013. *Capital in the Twenty-first Century*. Cambridge: Harvard University Press.

Powell E. 2014. Recent trends in added sugar intake among U.S. children and adults from 1977 to 2010: Poster abstract presentation at The Obesity Society Annual Meeting, November 2–7. Boston: Obesity Society.

Prashad V. 2014. *The Poorer Nations: A Possible History of the Global South*. New York: Verso.

———. 2016. *The Death of the Nation and the Future of the Arab Revolution*. Berkeley: University of California Press.

PricewaterhouseCoopers. 2016. *Mine 2016: Slower, lower, weaker ... but not defeated*. Johannesburg: PricewaterhouseCoopers.

Public Citizen. 2015. About Public Citizen's global trade watch. http://www.citizen.org/Page.aspx?pid=3147. Accessed July 23, 2015.

Quinlan M and Sheldon P. 2011. The enforcement of minimum labour standards in an era of neo-liberal globalisation: An overview. *The Economic and Labour Relations Review* 22:5–31.

Rafferty Y. 2013. Child trafficking and commercial sexual exploitation: A review of promising prevention policies and programs. *American Journal of Orthopsychiatry* 83(4):559–575.

Rapley J. 2007. *Understanding Development: Theory and Practice in the Third World*. Boulder: Lynne Rienner Publishers.

Reeves A, McKee M, and Stuckler D. 2014. Economic suicides in the Great Recession in Europe and North America. *British Journal of Psychiatry* 205:246–247.

Roberts KM. 2014. *Changing Course in Latin America*. New York: Cambridge University Press.

Robinson WI. 2014. The fetishism of empire: A critical review of Panitch and Gindin's The Making of Global Capitalism. *Studies in Political Economy* 93:147–165.

Ruckert A, Labonté R, and Parker RH. 2015. Global healthcare policy and the austerity agenda. In Kuhlmann E, Blank RH, Bourgeault IL, and Wendt C, Editors. *The Palgrave International Handbook of Healthcare Policy and Governance*. London: Palgrave Macmillan.

Ruel MT, Garrett JL, Hawkes C, and Cohen MJ. 2010. The food, fuel, and financial crises affect the urban and rural poor disproportionately: A review of the evidence. *The Journal of Nutrition* 140(1):170S–176S.

Ruff K. 2012. Quebec and Canadian governments end their historic support of the asbestos industry. *International Journal of Occupational and Environmental Health* 18(4):263–267.

Russo G and Banda G. 2015. Re-thinking pharmaceutical production in Africa: Insights from the analysis of the local manufacturing dynamics in Mozambique and Zimbabwe. *Studies in Comparative International Development* 50(2):258–281.

Sachs JD. 2011. The global economy's corporate crime wave. *Project Syndicate*, April 30.

Saez E and Zucman G. 2014. *Wealth Inequality in the United States since 1913: Evidence from Capitalized Income Tax Data*. Cambridge: National Bureau of Economic Research.

SAPRIN [Structural Adjustment Participatory Review International Network]. 2002. *The Policy Roots of Economic Crisis and Poverty: A Multi-Country Participatory Assessment of Structural Adjustment*. Washington, DC: Structural Adjustment Participatory Review International Network.

Schrecker T, Editor. 2012. *The Ashgate Research Companion to the Globalization of Health*. Farnham: Ashgate Publishing, Ltd.

Schrecker T. 2014. The exterritorial reach of money: Global finance and social determinants of health. In Brown GW, Yamey G, and Wamala S, Editors. *The Handbook of Global Health Policy*. Hoboken: Wiley-Blackwell.

Schrecker T and Bambra C. 2015. *How Politics Makes Us Sick: Neoliberal Epidemics*. Basingstoke: Palgrave Macmillan.

Schrecker T and Labonté R. 2011. Globalization: The global marketplace and social determinants of health. In The Commission on Social Determinants of Health Knowledge Networks, Lee JH, and Sadana R, Editors. *Improving Equity in Health by Addressing Social Determinants*. Geneva: WHO.

Schrecker T, Labonté R, and De Vogli R. 2008. Globalisation and health: The need for a global vision. *Lancet* 372(9650):1670–1676.

Sengupta A. 2013. *Universal Health Coverage: Beyond Rhetoric. Occasional Paper No. 20*. Kingston: Municipal Services Project.

Serafini P. 2012. Juvenile prostitution in Brazil: An international call to action on female sex trafficking. *International Journal of Gynecology and Obstetrics* 118(2):89.

Shaffer ER and Brenner JE. 2009. A trade agreement's impact on access to generic drugs. *Health Affairs* 28(5):w957–w968.

———. 2014. *Public Health Comments – Public Interest Trade Advisory Committee Response to Federal Register Request for Comments*. San Francisco: Center for Policy Analysis on Trade and Health.

Shaikh A. 1990. Exploitation. In Eatwell J, Milgate M, and Newman P, Editors. *The New Palgrave: A Dictionary of Economic Theory and Doctrine*. London: The Macmillan Press.

Shandra CL, Shandra JM, and London B. 2011. World Bank structural adjustment, water, and sanitation: A cross-national analysis of child mortality in Sub-Saharan Africa. *Organization and Environment* 24(2):107–129.

Sikka P. 2011. Accounting for human rights: The challenge of globalization and foreign investment agreements. *Critical Perspectives on Accounting* 22(8):811–827.

Singh GM, Micha R, Khatibzadeh S, et al. 2015. Estimated global, regional, and national disease burdens related to sugar-sweetened beverage consumption in 2010. *Circulation* 132(8):639–666.

Siqueira CE. 2016. Does informal employment exist in the United States and other developed countries? *NEW SOLUTIONS: A Journal of Environmental and Occupational Health Policy* 26(2):337–339.

Smith KT, Martin HM, and Smith LM. 2014. Human trafficking: A global multi-billion dollar criminal industry. *International Journal of Public Law and Policy* 4(3):293–308.

Standing G. 2011. *The Precariat: The New Dangerous Class.* New York: Bloomsbury Academic.

Stiglitz J. 2002. *Globalization and its Discontents.* New York: W.W. Norton and Co.

StreetNet International. 2015. History. http://www.streetnet.org.za/show.php?id=19. Accessed January 6, 2016.

Stuckler D and Basu S. 2009. The International Monetary Fund's effects on global health: Before and after the 2008 financial crisis. *International Journal of Health Services* 39(4):771–781.

Stuckler D, Basu S, and McKee M. 2011. International Monetary Fund and aid displacement. *International Journal of Health Services* 41(1):67–76.

Stuckler D, McKee M, Ebrahim S, and Basu S. 2012. Manufacturing epidemics: The role of global producers in increased consumption of unhealthy commodities including processed foods, alcohol, and tobacco. *PLoS Medicine* 9(6):695.

Sutcliffe J. 2012. Labour movements in the global South: A prominent role in struggles against neoliberal globalisation? *Interface* 4(2):52–60.

Swinburn B, Kraak V, Rutter H, et al. 2015. Strengthening of accountability systems to create healthy food environments and reduce global obesity. *Lancet* 385(9986):2534–2545.

Takala J, Hämäläinen P, Saarela KL, et al. 2014. Global estimates of the burden of injury and illness at work in 2012. *Journal of Occupational and Environmental Hygiene* 11(5):326–337.

Tandon N. 2010. New agribusiness investments mean wholesale sell-out for women farmers. *Gender and Development* 18(3):503–514.

Tapia Granados JA. 2013. El libre comercio y la economía mundial según Ha-Joon Chang y Michael Spence [Free trade and the world economy according to Ha-Joon Chang and Michael Spence]. *Ensayos de Economía* 23(42):13–26.

Tapia Granados JA and Rodriguez JM. 2015. Health, economic crisis, and austerity: A comparison of Greece, Finland and Iceland. *Health Policy* 119:941–953.

Tax Justice Network. 2016. Capital Flight, Illicit Flows. http://www.taxjustice.net/topics/inequality-democracy/capital-flight-illicit-flows/. Accessed August 3, 2016.

Third World Network. 2015. Joint NGO statement: TRIPS council decision on extension of the transition period concerning pharmaceutical products. *TWN*, November 6.

't Hoen E, Berger J, Calmy A, and Moon S. 2011. Driving a decade of change: HIV/AIDS, patents and access to medicines for all. *Journal of the International AIDS Society* 14:15.

Thow AM and Hawkes C. 2009. The implications of trade liberalization for diet and health: A case study from Central America. *Globalization and Health* 5:5.

Toussaint E. 2013. The Euro crisis, contradictions between countries in the periphery and centre of the European Union. http://www.globalresearch.ca/the-euro-crisis-contradictions-between-countries-in-the-periphery-and-centre-of-the-european-union/5359408. Accessed July 30, 2016.

Toussaint E and Millet D. 2010. *Debt, the IMF, and the World Bank: Sixty Questions, Sixty Answers.* New York: Monthly Review Press.

Transnational Institute. 2015. Jakarta Court cancels world's biggest water privatisation after 18 year failure. *Transnational Institute* [press release], March 25.

UNCTAD. 2012. *Don't Blame the Physical Markets: Financialization is the Root Cause of Oil and Commodity Price Volatility. Policy Brief no. 25.* Geneva: UNCTAD.

———. 2015. *IIA Issues Note: Recent Trends in IIA and ISDS.* Geneva: UNCTAD.

UN-DESA [Department of Economic and Social Affairs of the UN]. 2013. *World Population Ageing 2013.* New York: UN-DESA.

UNDP. 1999. *Human Development Report 1999: Globalization with a Human Face.* New York: UNDP.

———. 2015. *Human Development Report 2015: Work for Human Development.* New York: UNDP.

UN Economic Commission for Africa. 2014. *Dynamic Industrial Policy in Africa: Economic Report on Africa.* Addis Ababa: UN Economic Commission for Africa.

UNEP. 2015. *Waste Crime - Waste Risks Gaps in Meeting the Global Waste Challenge: A Rapid Response Assessment.* Nairobi: UNEP.

UNFPA and UNICEF. 2010. *Women's and Children's Rights: Making the Connection*. New York: UNICEF.

UNODC. 2014. *Global Report on Trafficking in Persons*. New York: UN.

Victora CG, Bahl R, Barros AJ, et al. 2016. Breastfeeding in the 21st century: Epidemiology, mechanisms, and lifelong effect. *Lancet* 387(10017):475–490.

Walk Free Foundation. 2016. *The Global Slavery Index 2016*. Nedlands: Walk Free Foundation.

Wallach L and Woodall P. 2004. *Whose Trade Organization? A Comprehensive Guide to the WTO*. New York: The New Press.

Waning B, Diedrichsen E, and Moon S. 2010. A lifeline to treatment: The role of Indian generic manufacturers in supplying antiretroviral medicines to developing countries. *Journal of the International AIDS Society* 13:35.

Ward K and England K. 2007. *Neoliberalization: States, Networks, Peoples*. Malden: Blackwell Publishing.

Weisbrot M. 2015. Lessons from NAFTA for the TPP. *South-North Development Monitor*, October 16.

Weisbrot M, Baker D, Kraev E, and Chen J. 2002. The scorecard on globalization 1980–2000: Its consequences for economic and social well-being. *International Journal of Health Services* 32(2):229–253.

Weiss L. 2012. The myth of the neoliberal state. In Kyung-Sup C, Fine B, and Weiss L, Editors. *Developmental Politics in Transition: The Neoliberal Era and Beyond*. Basingstoke: Palgrave Macmillan.

WHO. 2004. *PRSPs: Their Significance for Health: Second Synthesis Report*. Geneva: WHO.

———. 2014. Protecting workers' health. http://www.who.int/mediacentre/factsheets/fs389/en/. Accessed December 17, 2015.

———. 2015. Fact sheet: Obesity and overweight. http://www.who.int/mediacentre/factsheets/fs311/en/. Accessed June 20, 2015.

———. 2016. Infants and young child feeding: Factsheet. http://www.who.int/mediacentre/factsheets/fs342/en/. Accessed July 26, 2016.

WHO and FAO. 2007. *Safe Preparation, Storage and Handling of Powdered Infant Formula: Guidelines*. Geneva: WHO.

WHO, UNICEF, and IBFAN. 2016. *Marketing of Breast-milk Substitutes: National Implementation of the International Code: Status Report 2016*. Geneva: WHO.

WHO, UNICEF, UNFPA, et al. 2014. *Trends in Maternal Mortality: 1990 to 2013*. Geneva: WHO.

Wilkinson R, Hannah E, and Scott J. 2014. The WTO in Bali: What MC9 means for the Doha development agenda and why it matters. *Third World Quarterly* 35(6):1032–1050.

Wise TA. 2015. Dumping responsibility on third world farmers yet again. *The Wire*, December 14.

Working Group on Mining and Human Rights in Latin America. 2014. *The Impact of Canadian Mining in Latin America and Canada's Responsibility: Executive Summary*. Washington, DC: Due Process of Law Foundation.

Wood EM. 1999. The politics of capitalism. *Monthly Review* 51(4).

World Bank. 2015a. Private participation in infrastructure database. http://ppi.worldbank.org/explore/ppi_exploreSector.aspx?sectorID=4. Accessed August 2, 2016.

———. 2015b. *Working to End Poverty in Latin America and the Caribbean Workers, Jobs, and Wages*. Washington, DC: World Bank.

———. 2015c. World Bank commodity price data. www.worldbank.org/commodities. Accessed December 15, 2015.

———. 2016a. *Migration and Remittances Factbook: Third Edition*. Washington, DC: World Bank.

———. 2016b. Social protection and labor. http://data.worldbank.org/topic/labor-and-social-protection. Accessed January 13, 2016.

WTO. 2001. *Declaration on the TRIPS Agreement and Public Health*. WT/MIN(01)/DEC/2. November 20, 2001.

———. 2013. *Final Statement by Bolivia, Cuba, Ecuador, Nicaragua, the Bolivarian Republic of Venezuela at the Ninth Ministerial Conference*. WT/MIN(13)/30. December 7, 2013.

———. 2015a. Anti-dumping, subsidies, safeguards: contingencies, etc. https://www.wto.org/english/thewto_e/whatis_e/tif_e/agrm8_e.htm. Accessed December 29, 2015.

———. 2015b. Dispute Settlement: Dispute DS495, Korea—Import Bans, and Testing and Certification Requirements for Radionuclides. https://www.wto.org/english/tratop_e/dispu_e/cases_e/ds495_e.htm. Accessed July 23, 2015.

———. 2015c. Regional trade agreements: Facts and figures. https://www.wto.org/english/tratop_e/region_e/regfac_e.htm. Accessed July 24, 2015.

———. 2016. Principles of the trading system. https://www.wto.org/english/thewto_e/whatis_e/tif_e/fact2_e.htm. Accessed January 16, 2016.

Zhukovsky M, Varaksin A, and Pakholkina O. 2014. Statistical analysis of observational study of the influence of radon and other risk factors on lung cancer incidence. *Radiation Protection Dosimetry* 160(1-3):108–111.

10

HEALTH AND THE ENVIRONMENT

Key Questions:

- How are health and environmental conditions inter-related?
- What are the major challenges involving health and the environment and how should they be addressed?

Worldwide environmental conditions have changed more rapidly in the past half-century than at any other time in human history, shaped and strained by economic, social, and military activities (McNeill 2000). The health consequences are multifarious. Increases in agricultural output have been accompanied by pollution from fertilizers and pesticides, excessive irrigation, deforestation, and soil and water depletion. Wars have displaced millions of people, with weapons producing dangerous radiation and chemical toxins. Manufacture of high-demand, disposable electronics and other consumer goods generates harmful heavy metals waste, often dumped in low-income countries (LICs). Oil drilling and spills threaten ecosystems, destroying bird and fish habitats. Mining denudes mountainsides of vegetation, provokes mudslides, and its by-products contaminate and deplete soil and water supplies of nearby communities. Cities concentrate both human and chemical waste, creating massive disposal problems. A cross-cutting issue that worsens many recognized pathways from environmental conditions to poor health is climate change—largely driven by the burning of fossil fuels—which contaminates and heats the earth's atmosphere, threatening the livability of the planet (Klein 2014).

Yet as scientists have amply demonstrated, environmental degradation—the contamination and depletion of natural resources—(and its harm to health) is not inevitable: it is provoked by a range of human pursuits, as just described, from industrial production to transportation and settlement patterns and the global capitalist system that underpins these activities. Looming as they seem, then, environmental health problems and their driving forces can also be mitigated—and even reversed—through concerted, collective efforts at community, national, and global levels as per a political economy framing.

When political economy focuses on ecology—the inter-relationship between living organisms and the environment—it becomes *political ecology*, which conceptualizes relations of power as central to environmental dynamics (Robbins 2012). A political ecology approach to health thus incorporates the economic, social, and political forces, actors, and institutions that shape *both* environmental change *and* health and disease patterns, as well as the relationship between them (King 2010). For further definitions see Box 10-1.

A political ecology of health framing helps us understand that while health-environment interactions are often highly circumscribed, in that water, soil, or air contamination have localized effects, these are also global issues that transcend particular places and borders in multiple ways (Hancock, Spady, and Soskolne 2015). To begin, the planet's biosphere is a

Box 10-1 Definitions

Natural Environment

- Physical, chemical, geological, and biological factors and processes external to people, though potentially of their making

Built Environment

- Human-made commercial, public (recreational facilities, housing, sewage systems, and transportation networks), and industrial buildings, dwellings, transportation, roads and other infrastructure, as well as policies relating to land use, zoning, and community design

Social Environment

- Conditions within which people live and work, as shaped by cultural, historical, social, economic, and political relations and factors

Environmental health

- Arena of research, monitoring, control, and assessment of the physical, chemical, geological, biological, and related factors external to a person and that can potentially affect health (does not typically cover factors related to the social and cultural environment)

Ecosystem

- System formed by the interaction of a community of organisms and their natural environment, usually geographically defined

Ecology

- Study of the relationships and interactions between living organisms and their environment

Political ecology

- The study of interacting social and ecological changes, focusing especially on issues of power and inequitable relations

Sources: Evans (2002); Prüss-Üstün and Corvalán (2006); Robbins (2012); WHO (2015c).

highly complex yet unified whole, and any local disturbances (e.g., pollution or deforestation) have truly global consequences. Oceanic currents, monsoons, hurricanes, and other hydrological and meteorological occurrences carry local pollutants (e.g., insecticides or heavy metals) to the farthest reaches of the earth (e.g., DDT is found in penguins in Antarctica and mercury in Pacific salmon).

Channeled through "natural" cycles, human (especially economic) activities amplify the global impact of many local events. On one level, factory production, agribusiness, and mining are increasingly controlled and influenced by transnational corporations (TNCs) that separate the points of production, consumption, and waste disposal: resources extracted or goods manufactured in one place, are bought, sold, and disposed of on global markets. Clothes, fruit, and electronics purchased in the United Kingdom, for example, are inextricably tied to chemical, pesticide, and mining waste from production processes in Cambodia, Colombia, and Mozambique. Meanwhile, the energy required to motor these industries and enable retail sales (including transportation of goods and consumers) has contaminating effects near Norwegian or Saudi Arabian refineries, as well as along production and transport routes. On another level, fossil fuel combustion everywhere provokes climate change, a truly global concern. On yet another level, not only do the causes and effects on health of environmental degradation cross borders, the problems have a worldwide reach, even as the benefits in terms of improved quality of life are shared unevenly. This also means that there is the possibility of mutual learning across settings to understand and address health and environment threats. Accordingly, while the effects of environmental problems on health are often acutely experienced via local air, water, and habitats, they are necessarily local, national, and global in their dimensions and solutions.

This chapter explores a range of pressing health-related environmental concerns facing communities and countries across the globe. We begin with a historical review of human interactions with the environment and the mounting impact on human health. Next we develop an explanatory framework for understanding the political, social, and economic forces that interact with and alter environmental conditions and the consequent human health implications. We then turn to the causes and effects on health of the overuse, misuse, and contamination of natural resources—air, water, land, forests, and living organisms—and the implications of these patterns for the built environment (the human-constructed infrastructure and surroundings where people live, work, and play). Following this overview, we apply a political ecology of health lens to the issue of climate change. Finally, we discuss an array of policies and practices—major and minor, incrementalist and transformative—at global, national, local, and individual levels that seek to address environmental health problems. We conclude with examples of social and environmental health justice and resistance movements making a difference around the world.

FRAMING ENVIRONMENTAL HEALTH PROBLEMS: THE MOTORS AND DRIVERS

Key Questions:

- How do different modes of production and consumption affect the environment and health?
- How does a political ecology of health approach frame the connections among capitalism, environmental health, and inequity?

Past Interaction of Humans with the Natural and Built Environments

Long-term survival for animal species, as well as humans, has historically depended on relations with other dimensions of the natural world, bearing both direct and indirect consequences for health. During most of the 150,000 years that *Homo sapiens* are known to have existed, they lived in hunter-gatherer societies—small nomadic communities that made tools and obtained food and supplies within the limits of their local environments, shifting locales as needed. Collective human efforts to control nature began some 10,000 to 15,000 years ago, as the domestication of plant and animal species initiated a gradual transition to agriculturalism. Stable settlements began several millennia later in the fertile crescent of the Middle East. Remarkably, for well over 90% of human history, humans minimally affected their surroundings (Krech, McNeill, and Merchant 2004).

The advent of agriculture transformed social and economic relations, with accompanying effects on the built and natural environments. As settlements grew, land productivity increased and crop surpluses were generated. Irrigation systems were devised along with other innovations, and more and more land was cleared.

Approximately 5,000 years ago cities arose, first in the Middle East and North Africa, then in Asia and the Americas, later in Europe. Gradually societies became stratified by wealth and power, and local chiefs began to fight over land and resources. To accumulate further wealth and as testament to their power, potentates, such as Roman emperors, captured rival groups as slave laborers, acquired new territories, built monuments, grand cities, and aqueducts to supply water. They obtained, transformed, and traded precious metals and minerals, generating dirty by-products of wood fires and smelter pollution. Where resource use was excessive (e.g., overgrazing of cedar trees by goats in ancient Lebanon), environmental degradation occurred.

By the Middle Ages (900–1500), extraction from quarries and mines had become an important source of commerce and wealth. With the growth of towns, the clearing of forests, and the development of small industries, particularly in Europe, the Middle East, and Asia, energy use began to rise, and mined coal became a necessary counterpart to wood burning (Hoffman 2014). The exploitation of natural resources accelerated during the transition from feudalism to capitalism and with the rise of colonialism. After European kingdoms were consolidated, monarchs—backed by noblemen and a growing merchant class—turned to more distant lands for resources, labor, wealth, and power. The military conquest and political subjugation of peoples across the Americas, Africa, Asia, and the Pacific was also an environmental occupation (Crosby 1987), involving forest clearing, mining and metallurgy (releasing plumes of lead and other contaminants), and the building of transport routes. These activities produced deleterious health effects on local populations and habitats and on millions of slaves and forced laborers.

While all civilizations—including ancient Chinese, Egyptian, Ethiopian, Greco-Roman, and Inca—subsumed nature to human needs, the scale and character of the European imperial enterprise made its environmental impact far larger. With the Industrial Revolution came vastly expanded energy demands and severe pollution, causing enormous environmental damage. Filthy emanations from factory smokestacks, spewing sulfur, chlorine, ammonia, and methane, blackened the air of countless towns and the lungs of their residents.

Urban and industrial waste proliferated with the rise of Europe's cities and factories. Previously, most edible garbage was used as animal feed, and human and animal dung were recycled as fertilizer or fuel. The few material goods no longer reusable were buried or burned, certainly sullying air and soil, but to a comparatively minor degree. With the industrial era, factory and food debris, excrement, and carcasses, rife with microorganisms and toxins, accumulated in city streets and improvised dumps, especially in immiserated areas. Waterways thick with industrial, human, and animal waste (in the 1800s the Thames River in London was infamously known as "Monster Soup") supplied drinking water to town dwellers and further downstream, causing innumerable deaths from ingestion of poisons and pathogens. The deadly mix of environmental degradation and dangerous occupational and living conditions across the industrial belt are echoed today across the Majority World.

The almost unfathomable magnitude of ecological change spawned by the Industrial Revolution has led scientists to argue that the post-1800 scale of the human imprint marks a new geologic era: the Anthropocene. Following the Holocene epoch, in which humanity evolved in relative environmental stability for 10,000 years after the last Ice Age, the Anthropocene is characterized by human-induced environmental changes that are provoking a perilous climatic imbalance (Waters et al. 2016).

Political Ecology of Health: How Imperialism, Production, and Consumption Patterns Shape Health and Environmental Degradation

Many cultural and social factors combine to influence the forces driving environmental change and its health consequences, but one stands out: global capitalism (Foster, Clark, and York 2011). Accelerating in the post-war consumer era, market- and profit-driven growth—accompanied by militarism and magnified by neoliberal globalization since the 1980s—has generated ever-growing demand for all sorts of goods, with little regard for the environmental resource depletion and contamination caused by extraction, production, energy generation, transport, use, and disposal. And herein lies the fundamental contradiction of our era. Even as the capitalist economic system is the main source of employment and livelihoods across the world, and has improved health and the quality of life (albeit highly inequitably and arguably only to a certain point), it is also the key driver of environmental degradation and associated illness, suffering, and death.

Enormous environmental changes were wrought by communist political systems as well, if under a capitalist world order. The Soviet economy was not primarily geared to individual consumption, instead serving state policies and politics (largely defined by Cold War competition with the West), but large-scale agricultural and industrial production in the USSR and the associated ecological/

environmental impact was as significant as that of Western economies.

As Soviet power waned in the 1980s, the capitalist model consolidated through accelerated economic integration and ever more globalized markets, privatization, growth of multinational firms, and a soaring financial sector (see chapter 9). The concomitant rise in the power of private corporate interests—at the expense of living and occupational conditions for the masses of workers, small farmers, and other vulnerable populations—has also translated into a privileging of capitalist needs over environmental protection at both national and global governance levels. Today the World Trade Organization (WTO) and regional trade and investment treaties, whose rules favor TNCs, are particularly responsible for putting "downward pressure on environmental standards" (Clapp and Dauvergne 2011, p. 139).

These features of capitalism and its neoliberal globalization phase also lengthen the distance between consumption and the consequences of production. Purchasers of cut-price electronic goods or clothing in, for example, Barcelona or Baltimore do not witness, or may not even contemplate, the human and environmental effects of production processes in Bangkok or Bangalore. Because social and environmental costs are externalized from production costs in a global market economy, consumer prices rarely reflect the costs of air pollution or chemical waste from garment factories, or water and forest contamination from mining the metallic ore coltan used for making cellphones.

As with other aspects of global health, the health-environment nexus reveals persistent and growing inequalities within and across countries: a political ecology framework lays bare the power asymmetries between rich and poor. On one level, environmental contamination, depletion, and climate change—involving ever-intensifying production, extraction, and consumption patterns—are heavily shaped by TNCs, government policies, and population demands of high-income countries (HICs), whereas those suffering the consequences are disproportionately located in low- and middle-income countries (LMICs). On another level, there is a hierarchy of environmental protection and exposure, with toxic pesticides banned in Europe and North America applied widely in the Global South—often by Northern-driven agribusiness—contaminating the food supply, water sources, and waste systems (UNEP 2015c). Likewise toxic waste mostly generated in/by HICs is routinely exported to low-income countries (LICs), with polluting and extractive industries increasingly located in LMICs (Clapp and Dauvergne 2011). Meanwhile, elites in HICs reap the profits, with counterparts in LMICs facilitating and also profiting from these arrangements. Though workers and consumers necessarily participate in this nexus, they do not control it or the global arrangements that sustain it, and the poorest benefit the least. Uneven control and use of resources are central to all of these processes, placing elites literally and figuratively in the driver's seat of the economic order and of resource contamination and depletion.

In sum, the high costs of environmental degradation and its health consequences are borne by those excluded from power and decisionmaking, even as the greatest advantages accrue to the more powerful—this constitutes what is called environmental injustice. Conversely, environmental justice refers to fairness in the distribution of and protection from environmental risk, including as it relates to human health and the participation of individuals and communities in the development and enforcement of protective measures (Brulle and Pellow 2006). Past and present, these circumstances have not gone unchallenged: 19th century social and political struggles against detrimental working and environmental circumstances served as important precursors to modern labor and environmental movements.

As presented in Figure 10-1, an understanding that human activity is at the core of environmental health problems does not imply a simple relationship. Instead, humans shape and are shaped by the forces driving the global economy, which place mounting pressure on the built and natural environments. In the sub-sections that follow, we discuss the main underlying forces identified in Figure 10-1: industrial production, the military-industrial complex, mining, energy extraction, and agribusiness.

Industrial Production and Toxic Agents

Since World War II, over 85,000 new chemicals have been manufactured and released into the environment, with almost 3,000 chemicals produced in

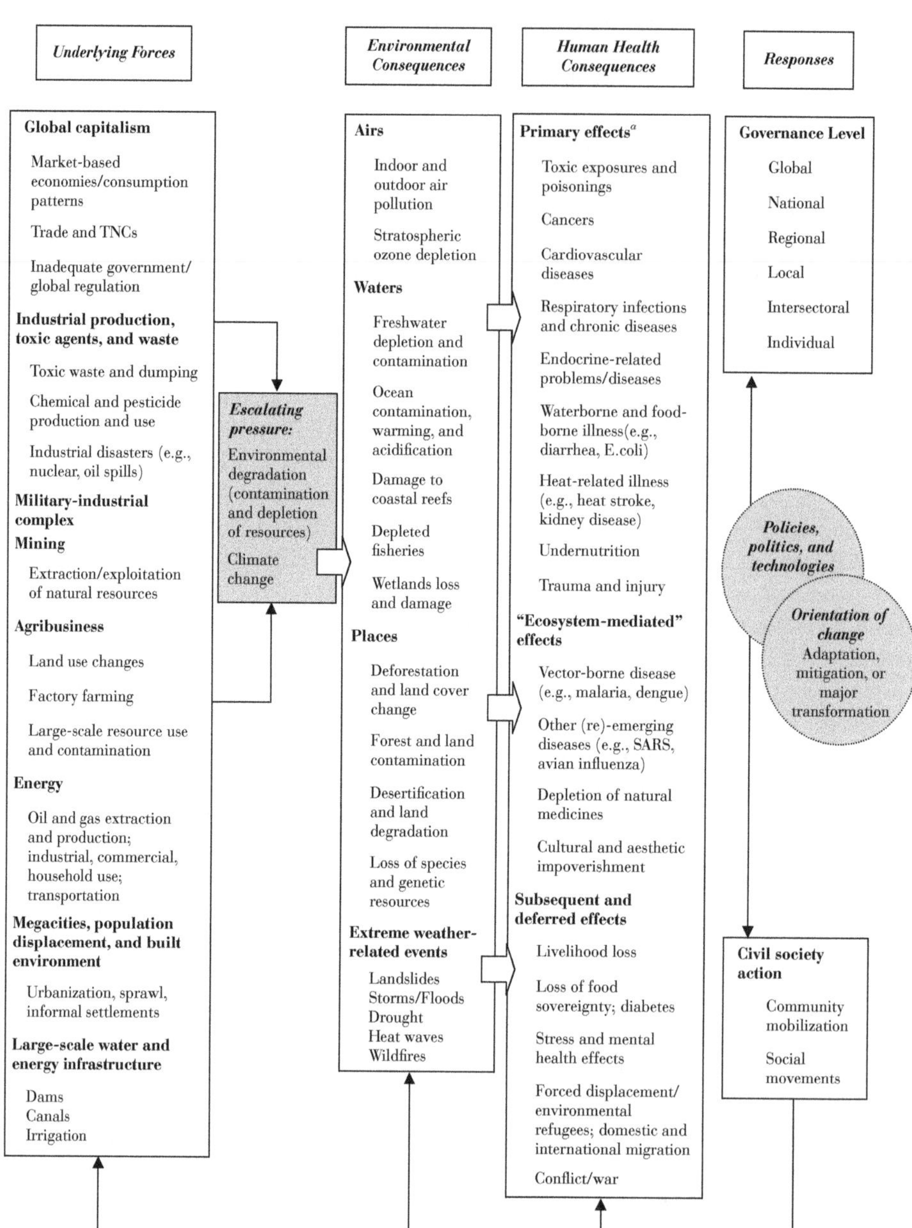

[a] Various primary health effects are also ecosystem-mediated and vice versa.

Underlying forces generate and combine with escalating pressure from environmental degradation and climate change, together leading to environmental consequences with a range of direct, ecosystem-mediated, and indirect health effects. These, in turn, engender greater or lesser responses from various governance levels, as well as civil society action (both potentially involving policies, politics, and technologies), which shape and are shaped by different orientations of change, including mitigation (reducing degradation), adaptation (altering social arrangements to adjust to environmental degradation and climate change), and major transformations (e.g., revolutionizing communities, regions, nations, and even the world order away from a capitalist growth model). The actions undertaken can influence both governance responses and affect the underlying forces, and/or environmental and human health conditions.

Figure 10-1: Political ecology of health: Determinants, effects, and responses.

Sources: Adapted extensively from WHO (2005); and UNEP (2007).

massive quantities (one million pounds or more annually) (Domínguez-Cortinas et al. 2013). The sheer magnitude of potentially dangerous substances makes testing for toxicity enormously complicated and expensive; where states take on this role, such as in Europe and North America, few chemicals have been subject to rigorous testing for dangers to health. When the US Toxic Substances Control Act (TSCA) was enacted in 1976, the powerful chemical industry ensured that 62,000 existing chemicals were "grandfathered" into the program without health or environmental impact assessments (Scruggs et al. 2014).[1] Even when harmful health effects of chemicals such as benzene have been demonstrated—and they have been banned or heavily restricted in one country—they may continue to be exported, used, and/or produced elsewhere, especially LMICs with few regulations (Sellers 2014). Indeed, enacting control measures for lead has been an uphill battle (Box 10-2).

Despite growing evidence, it can be difficult to establish precise causal connections between environmental exposures and health because effects may be indirect, delayed, and multifactorial. Moreover, epidemiology and toxicology are not well-equipped to trace the effects of long-term, low-level exposure to hazardous substances or the dangers posed by chemical interactions (Friis and Sellers 2014).

Military-Industrial Complex

The military-industrial complex is among the largest sources of environmental contamination, though secrecy means that comprehensive figures on the environmental impact of weapons research, production, and deployment are difficult to obtain. Undoubtedly, the permanent members of the UN Security Council—the United States, Russia (formerly the Soviet Union), China, France, and the United Kingdom—which are major producers of both conventional and nuclear weapons (see chapter 8), are largely to blame. Due to the testing, use, and storage of these weapons, military bases and proving

Box 10-2 Lead Contamination

Ambient levels of the toxic metal lead, widely used in an array of common products including paint, batteries, ammunition, X-ray shields, cosmetics, crayons, toys, pottery, cables, and gasoline (added to increase engine power), have risen markedly over the past century thanks to limited regulation and uneven enforcement. Ingested or inhaled via air, dust, soil, and water, lead causes increased blood pressure, cognitive deficits, and other neurodevelopmental problems (Grandjean and Landrigan 2014).

The toxicity of lead paint was recognized in the 1890s, but it took almost a century until mounting scientific evidence and accompanying activism regarding the dangers of lead exposure resulted in its wide abolition as a petrol and paint additive, initially in HICs (Dikshith 2013; Markowitz and Rosner 2014). There, manufacturing and workplace regulations have significantly reduced acute (occupational) lead poisoning, but in many LMICs, children, especially, are exposed to high lead levels in the soil and water due to waste from mines, and paint, smelting, and battery factories (Chatham-Stephens et al. 2014). Lead-related cognitive impairments are nearly 30 times higher where leaded gasoline is still used (in 2016 only Algeria, Yemen and Iraq) than where it has been phased out (Prüss-Üstün and Corvalán 2006).

Chronic, low-level lead exposure remains a significant public health issue, particularly among disadvantaged groups—those who live in substandard housing (where lead abatement has not been properly carried out) or near polluting industries or heavy traffic. In HICs, the most common sources of lead exposure among young children are ingested paint chips and water from corroded lead pipes. In LMICS, above all Southeast Asia, where most children affected by lead poisoning live, exposure routes are more varied, making it a far thornier abatement challenge (WHO 2014e).

grounds are major producers of toxic environmental waste and ionizing radiation (Rosenfeld and Feng 2011). On the Marshall Islands, a 1954 US hydrogen bomb test exposed thousands of people to radioactive chemicals, increasing thyroid cancer incidence for more than 60 years, and exiling islanders from their homes indefinitely (Westing 2008).

Elsewhere, a longtime US base in Vieques, Puerto Rico, shuttered in 2000 after a protracted social struggle, left behind a highly contaminated area (McCaffrey 2008). Today Vieques has among the top cancer rates in Puerto Rico, re-igniting activism to oblige the US Navy to pay for cleanup.

Around the world, US military bases have generated a toxic stew of polychlorinated biphenyls (PCBs), polycyclic aromatic hydrocarbons (PAHs), benzene, and other carcinogens at rates up to 1,000 times allowable limits, with adjacent populations experiencing soaring rates of leukemia, lung cancer, and other health problems. At Colorado's Rocky Mountain Arsenal, the dumping of over 100 toxic chemicals used in the production of nerve gas and pesticides has created "the most contaminated square mile on earth" (Westing 2008). Likewise, former Russian weapons factories (Table 10-1) are a source of extremely elevated incidence of cancer and other diseases.

Agribusiness

Approximately 40% of the world's land mass is dedicated to agriculture (FAO 2015), 75% of which is linked to agribusiness or large farms (Todhunter 2014). Globally, about 3.3 million tons of pesticides are used each year (Pimentel and Burgess 2014) in an expanding, self-perpetuating cycle of reliance and contamination. For example, extensive use in the United States of Monsanto Corporation's glyphosate herbicide (introduced as "Roundup" in the mid-1970s, and now considered a probable carcinogen) for multiple crops has led to highly pesticide-resistant weeds, leading to even further pesticide reliance (Union of Concerned Scientists 2013). As agribusiness has expanded in the Global South, glyphosate and other dangerous pesticides have been widely adopted because they are inexpensive and effective, at least in the short-term (Eastwood 2012).

Not only is agribusiness a prime driver of contamination, it is also responsible for resource depletion: agriculture is the single biggest user of water, accounting for 70% of world water consumption (other industries use 20%, and households consume just 10% of freshwater) (WWAP 2014). Hybridized high-yield seeds developed under Green Revolution schemes (see chapter 2) have displaced drought-resistant local varieties with water-guzzling crops, including on massive farms located in arid or semi-arid regions (such as central California). Maximizing crop output, in turn, is based on mega-sprinklers that waste enormous quantities of water through evaporation.

Agribusiness irrigation also depletes the water table and aquifers beneath, contaminating local soil and waterways, particularly affecting low-income, often Indigenous, rural populations and migrant workers. Additionally, pesticide formulation and application require large quantities of water and spread more contaminants than root-based irrigation systems that use soil as a filter. Pesticide runoff from, for example, the floriculture industry, makes its way into watersheds and water supplies, exposing nearby populations to harmful toxins (Breilh 2012).

As discussed in chapter 9, virtually all agribusiness jeopardizes the health of workers and nearby populations, even as it feeds rising global demand for year-round availability of (non-native) foods. To name but two examples: those administering pesticides frequently lack adequate protection, with policies and regulations unevenly implemented (Orozco, Cole, and Forbes 2009), resulting in at least 3.5 to 5 million poisonings and 250,000 fatalities each year (Marrs and Karalliedde 2012) atop the untold carcinogenic toll on farmers, child laborers, nearby residents, and consumers. Meat-processing, too, generates a range of contaminants in soil and groundwater, and abattoirs release allergens, toxic gases, ammonia, and pathogens, leading both workers and those living downwind to suffer from high rates of respiratory disease and other health problems (Gunderson 2015).

Mining

Mining is one of the most lucrative—and destructive—industries on earth. Beyond high occupational mortality and exploitation and brutal wars over mineral resource control (see chapters 8 and 9), mining operations typically leave behind a trail of environmental

Table 10-1 Selected Pollution Hotspots

Site Name and Location	Major Pollutants and Sources	Human Health Impact	Cleanup Status as of 2013
Dzerzhinsk, Russia	Chemicals, toxic by-products, lead, chemical weapons (was a Cold War era manufacturing site)	Contaminated water supplies, increased eye, lung, and kidney diseases and cancers; life expectancy up to 20 years lower than the national average in Russia	Some facility closedown and remediation
Agbogbloshie (Accra), Ghana	E-waste dumpsite for large electronics (i.e., refrigerators, microwaves, televisions); sheathed cable burned to recover copper	High levels of lead and other metals released into air and soil in proximity to homes, markets, and other public areas; an estimated 40,000–250,000 people at risk	Occupational safety training and e-waste recycling model being piloted to replace burning
Citarum River Basin (Bandung), Indonesia	Contaminated with lead, aluminum, and iron by industry and domestic sources	Contaminated drinking and irrigation water; affects 9 million people	15-year, US$3.5 billion plan by government for restoration
Matanza-Riachuelo River Basin, Argentina	Contaminated with toxic waste and sewage from 15,000 industries (one third from chemical manufacturers)	Diarrheal diseases, respiratory diseases, and cancers due to contaminated soil and drinking water	US$1 billion commitment for World Bank funded project on sanitation and abatement

Source: Blacksmith Institute and Green Cross Switzerland (2013).

devastation: hundreds of acres of open pits and stripped terrain; deadly mudslides (such as a November 2015 jade mine landslide in Myanmar killing 113 people, including nearby villagers); and seepage of heavy metals, cyanide, acids, and other toxic by-products into land and rivers, destroying forests and killing livestock and wildlife. Artisanal (informal) mining, which takes place on the outskirts of larger operations or when mining companies have abandoned sites, is notoriously unregulated and dangerous, harming miners and contaminating waterways (Armah et al. 2013).

Gold mining processes are particularly thirsty, requiring 30 tons of water per ounce of gold, and leaving behind toxic tailings. Restoring vegetation to mining areas is difficult because organic matter, nutrients, and water become either too acidic or too alkaline for plant growth. The local impact can be massive. In Kenya's Migori Gold Belt region, high concentrations of cadmium, lead, arsenic, and mercury have penetrated local water, soil, and the primary source of food—fish—from Lake Victoria (Ngure et al. 2014). Runoff from uranium mines in Namibia and South Africa, which have serviced nuclear power and atomic weapons industries since the 1950s, has devastated local environments and exposed miners and thousands of others to radiation (Scheele, Wilde-Ramsing, and de Haan 2011). Coal mining in India and across the world is a key cause of a range of lung ailments among miners and nearby populations due to high concentrations of particulate matter from extractive processes (Hota and Behera 2015).

Energy Extraction and Production

The extraction, refining, and distribution of nonrenewable fossil fuels plus production of biofuels, together making up almost four fifths of world energy consumption (oil-40%, natural gas-15%, coal-12%, and biofuels-12%) (International Energy Agency 2015), have a major impact on the environment and health well before the largest effect: combustion. From oil drilling underground and offshore, through refining into liquid fuels (gasoline and diesel), and transport over long distances via pipelines, trains, tankers, and trucks, there are multiple potential health hazards: spills, leaks, collision-related fires, and the burning of "excess" methane and other gases at oil wells, rigs, and refineries (Union of Concerned Scientists 2015) (Box 10-3). Nigeria has the world's highest rate of such gas flaring, with carbon emissions polluting air, surrounding forests, wetlands, and soil, in turn lowering agricultural productivity (Atuma and Ojeh 2013).

Coal mining is also linked to a range of environmental effects including the leaching of runoff into surface and groundwater and the ambient release of particulate matter and gases such as methane and sulfur dioxide (Bian et al. 2010). In addition to high occupational disease and death, residential proximity to coal mines is associated with increased heart and lung diseases, cancer, hypertension, and kidney disease (Hendryx and Ahern 2008).

Like oil, natural gas is extracted from underground deposits through drilling. While it is considered a cleaner energy source than oil and coal because it releases less carbon dioxide and particulates once burned, as with oil processing, natural gas processing plants flare gases, contributing to emissions associated with asthma, chronic bronchitis, cancers, and blood disorders (Davoudi et al. 2013). These emissions also contribute to ground-level ozone (i.e., smog), which damages respiratory systems and crops (David Suzuki Foundation 2014).

Box 10-3 Disastrous Consequences of Energy Extraction and Production

Oil spills, an all too frequent occurrence, can have grave health and environmental consequences. An April 2010 mega spill in the Gulf of Mexico began with an explosion on the Transocean Ltd. *Deepwater Horizon* offshore oil rig, killing 11 workers. Operating under multinational BP, the rig sank two days later, breaking a deep underwater well that started leaking oil. It took 87 days to install a containment cap to stop the leak. A record 210 million gallons of oil were discharged, putting the health of millions of Gulf Coast residents at risk through exposure to contaminated water, seafood, and beaches, plus air pollution generated by the cleanup process (Osofsky et al. 2012), as well as mental health consequences due to economic and social disruption (Palinkas 2012).

Nuclear energy production generates large quantities of hazardous radioactive waste with the potential for deadly disasters on a colossal scale. The Chernobyl (Ukraine, former Soviet Union) nuclear power plant explosion in 1986 killed 31 people instantly, and 50 people immediately after from high radiation exposure, with approximately 4,000 deaths documented subsequently. Deferred consequences have included elevated rates of cancer and congenital birth anomalies, with death estimates ranging up to 1 million. Likely 5 to 10 million people remain at elevated risk of cancer in Ukraine and surrounding Russia, Moldova, and Belarus (Pure Earth and Green Cross Switzerland 2015).

A quarter century later, the 2011 Fukushima nuclear disaster in Japan, following an earthquake-triggered tsunami, led to partial meltdown of the plant and release of over 1,000 tons of radioactive materials into groundwater and the Pacific Ocean and radiation into the air. The predicted long-term health effects include increased risk for cancers (especially thyroid, breast, and leukemia) and psychological consequences from relocation, displacement, and stigma for nearby populations (Hasegawa et al. 2015).

Production of biofuels, such as corn- or sugar-based ethanol, grew rapidly after 2000, less as an environmental strategy than as a cheaper substitute for oil at a time of rising prices. Not only is ethanol considered a climate change contributor (given the vast water and energy resources used to produce it), land-use competition with food crops has contributed to food shortages and price hikes, leading to loss of food sovereignty (self-determination in food and land policies) and food uprisings from Mauritania to Uzbekistan, the Philippines, and Italy in 2007–2008.

Renewable biogas entails fermentation of biodegradable waste (e.g., manure, solid waste) to form methane and carbon dioxide (CO_2), used for electricity and heating, and, compressed, as a fuel. Though biogas production has proliferated in Germany, India, China, and elsewhere (HLPE 2013), if not properly contained, the methane can explode, causing high greenhouse gas and toxic hydrogen sulfide emissions.

Even "clean" energy sources can have negative consequences. Hydroelectric power is a renewable energy source, but it depends on large dams that can cause ecological disturbances that reduce fish populations and raise exposure to waterborne and vector-borne diseases. Construction of large hydropower dams along the Mekong River, which runs through Cambodia, China, Laos, Myanmar, Thailand, and Vietnam, has reduced fish stocks and affected the food sovereignty of up to 67 million inhabitants (Ziegler et al. 2013). Approximately 40,000 large dam projects have displaced up to 80 million people in the past 60 years (International Rivers 2015), threatening the livelihoods of over 470 million people downstream (Richter et al. 2010).

Thanks to new technologies, and, until recently, rising commodity prices, "unconventional" oil and natural gas reservoirs previously too expensive to exploit have become profitable (and dirty) endeavors. For example, the conversion of raw bitumen from Canada's "tar sands" into crude oil requires chemical and heating processes that expose communities near strip-mining, drilling, and processing facilities to PAHs and benzene, linked to elevated cancer rates downstream. Methyl mercury and other toxic chemicals released from the tar sands accumulate in the food chain, posing a particular threat to nearby Indigenous communities who rely on hunting and fishing (National Resources Defense Council 2014).

Another technology, hydraulic fracturing (fracking), pumps vast quantities of water mixed with chemicals into shale rock deep underground to extract natural gas and oil. Not only does this process require up to 300 times more water than conventional gas extraction (water that becomes toxic), methane leaks into the ground and air both during and long after the extraction process (Kang et al. 2014). Fracking wells are increasingly associated with both earthquake risks and health problems, including contaminated water, reduced air quality, psychosocial stress, increased cardiac hospitalizations (Jemielita et al. 2015), and endocrine disrupting chemicals (EDCs) (Box 10-4).

In sum, the global fossil fuel-based economy imposes significant direct and indirect health consequences. The direct effects occur through energy extraction and production and its consumption counterpart—contamination caused by fossil fuel combustion, discussed under "Air Pollution." The burning of fossil fuels is also the driving force behind global climate change, linked to a range of indirect health effects.

Box 10-4 Endocrine Disrupting Chemicals

Endocrine disrupting chemicals (EDCs) are found in pesticides, thermal cash register receipts, detergents, cosmetics, plastics, food, and other household products. They imitate human and animal hormones, leading to adverse pregnancy and birth outcomes, neurobehavioral disorders in children, breast, prostate, and other endocrine-related cancers, and diabetes (Di Renzo et al. 2015). There are over 800 EDCs, mostly human-made. Because EDCs can alter hormonal production and responses, exposure is especially harmful during critical development periods such as in utero or during puberty. While some exposures lead to birth defects, many effects only manifest later in life (UNEP and WHO 2013).

Toxic Waste and Dumping

Common to all industry is the production of toxic waste. As industrialization has shifted eastward and southward from Western Europe and North America, contamination has followed. Across the world, over 200 million people are directly exposed to toxic pollution, with millions more indirectly affected (Blacksmith Institute and Green Cross Switzerland 2014). Over 95 million people in LMICs are exposed to the top six pollutants (lead, radionuclides, mercury, hexavalent chromium, pesticides, and cadmium) alone, a conservative estimate given that hundreds of thousands of toxic sites have yet to be assessed (Pure Earth and Green Cross Switzerland 2015). The world's 50 largest active dumpsites—half of which are known to contain hazardous waste—are primarily located in LMICs (D-Waste 2014). In older industrial settings, environmental struggles have compelled the cleanup of many contaminated sites, but rarely before disaster has struck.

In the United States, more than 450,000 brown fields—former industrial or commercial facilities—leak hazardous contaminants or pollutants into the environment, often in areas redeveloped for housing. In the 1970s, an environmental movement was galvanized after discovery that the Hooker Chemical Company had buried toxin-filled barrels near Niagara Falls several decades before, resulting in soaring birth defects and illnesses (Macey and Cannon 2007). The US government established a "Superfund" program in 1980 to monitor and clean up the most hazardous sites. Initially effective—with over 1,400 sites remediated (US Environmental Protection Agency 2014)—since 2000, Superfund has lost funding and momentum, as public and political pressure for monitoring and cleanup has declined.

Although many HICs have enacted stricter regulations, illegal toxic dumping continues in some locales. In southern Italy, the Camorra crime syndicate has been involved in decades-long illegal burying of toxic and nuclear waste near the city of Naples, leaving it to seep into ground and surface water and soil, and contaminate the air via burning and desiccation. In an area dubbed the "triangle of death" by epidemiologists, waste disposal in non-designated toxic dumps, such as cultivable areas, roads, and work sites, together with poor regional management of other urban and industrial waste, has been associated with elevated liver and lung cancer rates and congenital malformations (Senior and Mazza 2004; Triassi et al. 2015), killing at least 2,000 people. The situation was so dire that nearby US naval bases, themselves a prime source of toxins, carried out their own study in 2011 and now restrict personnel from consuming local produce and water (Mayr 2014). In 2014 the Italian government, which has long known of the problem, was finally pressured to begin cleaning up the sites and provide health screening to the local population, but it is doubtful that those responsible will ever be brought to justice.

With growing resistance to landfills in HICs, the problem has been displaced: exports of toxic industrial waste to LMICs are conservatively estimated at 8.5 million tons annually (UNEP 2011b). The 1989 Basel Convention on the Control of Transboundary Movements of Hazardous Wastes and their Disposal was designed to end such practices but has little enforcement capacity. Despite the much stronger 1991 Bamako Convention (in force since 1998) prohibiting the entry of hazardous, including radioactive, waste to Africa (UNEP 2015a), these imports continue. Among the main destinations of illegal hazardous waste are Ghana, Nigeria, and China, with many other African, Asian, and Eastern European countries serving as transit or final dumping points (UNEP 2015c).

A mounting problem is the estimated 50 million metric tons of e-waste generated annually (Khetriwal, Luepschen, and Kuehr 2013). Much of North America and Europe's "e-waste"—old computers, mobile phones, and other electronic equipment—is falsely labeled as second-hand goods to facilitate export and enable dumping in Chinese, Indian, and African landfills (UNEP 2015c). There, lead, mercury, cadmium, and other heavy metals and organic acids leach into soil and groundwater and expose waste pickers and local populations, including children, to dangerous toxins. Agbogbloshie, once a wetland in Accra, Ghana, is the world's largest e-waste dumping ground (Table 10-1).

Medical and pharmaceutical waste comprise another rising concern (WHO 2015a), with US hospitals generating 5 million tons of waste annually (about 25 pounds per hospital bed per day), the country's largest source of dioxin emissions (Blakemore 2015).

Approximately 20% of medical waste is considered hazardous (infectious, toxic, or radioactive).

HEALTH PROBLEMS AS ENVIRONMENTAL PROBLEMS AND VICE VERSA

Key Question:

- What are the most pressing issues at the nexus of health and the environment in the world? In your country? In your community?

None of us needs to go far to identify health-related environmental issues: the air we breathe, the water we drink, the food we eat, and our immediate surroundings may all pose health risks. As far back as the 5th century BCE, the famed physician Hippocrates observed the importance of "Airs, Waters, and Places" on disease patterns in ancient Greece; this same set of features frames our examination of key health problems linked to market-driven environmental degradation, including air pollution, and the overuse, misuse, and depletion of water, land, and forests, all interacting with the spaces and places where people work, play, and live. All told, environmental factors—unclean air, radiation (ultraviolet and ionizing), the hazards of built environments, occupational hazards, agricultural practices, climate change, chemical exposures, and inadequate water and sanitation—were responsible for 12.6 million deaths (23% of global deaths) in 2012 (Prüss-Ustün et al. 2016). For environmental exposure effects on child health see Box 10-5.

It is important to reiterate that the environment does not simply refer to natural resources (and their conservation) but also to the built environment, which directly affects health and facilitates or mitigates resource use and depletion. The built environment influences health via both indoor and outdoor (ambient) factors, for example, in relation to transportation, the safety and conditions of neighborhoods, access to water and sanitation, and the existence of green space. Built structures may generate health dangers through their very construction, such as via poor ventilation systems, use of toxic building materials, and inadequate structural protection against floods, landslides, storms, and other disasters (see chapter 8).

Box 10-5 Child Health and the Environment

The WHO attributes over one quarter of under-5 child mortality (nearly 2 million deaths per year) to environment-related causes, primarily in LMICs (Prüss-Ustün et al. 2016). Children's particular vulnerability stems from biological, developmental, and social factors. From a physiological perspective, children eat, breathe, and drink proportionately more than adults, thus taking in far higher concentrations of environmental toxins. Likelihood of toxin ingestion is heightened at young ages, when exploring children put their hands and sundry objects into their mouths. Small doses of certain toxins (such as lead, mercury, and pesticides) can cause permanent developmental abnormalities, ranging from learning disabilities to reproductive problems, endocrine disruption, cognitive deficits, and cancer (WHO and UNEP 2010). Poverty increases children's vulnerability and limits their resistance to environmental toxins due to immunological fragility (caused by nutritional deficiencies, repeat illnesses, and crowding, among other factors) and greater exposure, due to higher presence of contaminants in the soil, air, water, and foods in their social and neighborhood circumstances.

The annual impact of environmental conditions on child health includes (WHO 2014a):

- Acute respiratory infections from indoor air pollution, causing 1 million child deaths
- Lead exposure, causing approximately 600,000 cases of developmental disability
- Pesticide poisonings (1–5 million cases)
- Cancer deaths (up to 20% of all childhood cancers)

Airs

Outdoor Air Pollution

Air pollution is one of the most pervasive problems of modern societies, linked to industrial contamination, power plants, the cooling and heating of buildings, retail and household fuel use, and transport (including aircraft) exhaust. Outdoor air pollution was the underlying cause of an estimated 3.7 million premature deaths in 2012, almost 90% in LMICs (Figure 10-2). Of these premature deaths, 80% were due to coronary heart disease (CHD) and strokes, 14% to chronic obstructive pulmonary disease (COPD) or acute lower respiratory infections, and 6% to lung cancer (WHO 2014c).

Among the most infamous air pollution episodes was the December 1952 London Smog, which killed an estimated 4,000–10,000 people within just a week, mainly children, the elderly, and persons with underlying respiratory illnesses. The Smog became a potent political issue, resulting in some of the world's earliest emissions regulations (Bell and Davis 2001). Other industrial and vehicle-ridden cities, from Milano to Los Angeles, experienced similar smog crises, and the USSR's notorious air pollution was believed to rival that of Britain's Industrial Revolution.

Today, despite various measures, nearly 90% of city dwellers breathe unsafe air (WHO 2014b). The problem is worse in most LMICs due to: generally fewer controls on vehicular exhaust and factory smokestacks; primary reliance on incineration for waste disposal; unregulated burning of garbage and household fuels; little rail or alternative energy source-based public transport; and wide industrial use of inexpensive high sulfur fuels, such as brown coal. In recent years air pollution and respiratory disease rates have soared: a decade ago the World Health Organization (WHO) gauged that just breathing Mumbai's air was equivalent to smoking 2.5 packs of cigarettes per day.

The particulate matter (PM) in air pollution is linked to an array of acute and chronic health problems.[2] PM is a mixture of fine solid particles consisting of dirt, dust, mold, and aerosols formed from combustion by-products, for instance sulfur dioxide and nitrogen oxides, as well as pavement erosion from road traffic, abrasion of brakes and tires, and excavated mines (WHO EURO 2013). Health consequences of PM inhalation, especially PM2.5 (<2.5 microns diameter), include lung cancer, cardiopulmonary diseases, and aggravation of asthma and COPD. Soot (black carbon), comprising 5% to 15% of ambient PM, is among its deadliest components. Formed from the incomplete burning of fossil fuels and biomass (from agricultural and forest fires), soot is associated with excess all-cause and cardiovascular mortality and hospitalizations (WHO 2015d). Other air pollution constituents, such as ozone, aggravate upper respiratory ailments, including bronchitis. Diesel engine exhaust, now classified as a human carcinogen, is believed to cause 9,000 (6%) annual lung cancer deaths (Vermeulen et al. 2014), 27,000 heart attacks, and 21,000 overall deaths in the United States, with

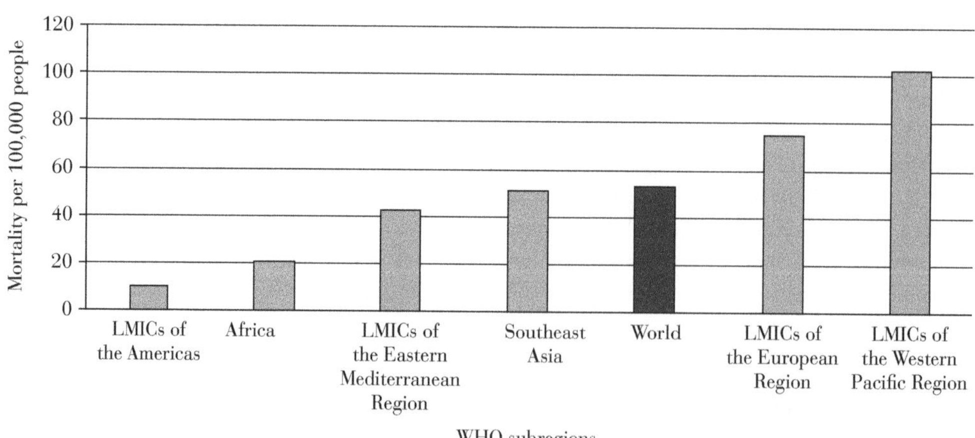

Figure 10-2: Ambient air pollution attributable deaths per 100,000 people, 2012.
Data Source: WHO (2015b).

analogous rates in France (Serrier et al. 2014). The same combustion processes generating air pollution also contribute to anthropogenic climate change, discussed ahead (Field et al. 2014).

Into the 1990s Mexico City was the world's most polluted city, largely due to the exhaust from over 5.5 million vehicles consuming some 50 million liters of petroleum every day (Calderón-Garcidueñas et al. 2015) and facilitated by an inversion layer trapping polluted air above the Mexico City Valley. Although air quality has improved in recent years thanks to removal of lead from gasoline, better public transportation, and relocation of factories and refineries, long-term exposure to PM in Mexico City remains a leading cause of premature mortality, including due to neurological effects starting in childhood (Caravanos et al. 2014). Certain mitigation policies have had unintended consequences: a mandatory weekday rest for every car increased rather than reduced the number of vehicles circulating because many people turned to taxis and mini-buses (not affected by restrictions) or acquired additional, often older and more polluting, cars to use on their primary vehicle's rest day.

At present the world's most polluted cities are in India and Pakistan, topped by New Delhi, whose 25 million inhabitants, especially children, face spiraling rates of upper and lower respiratory tract diseases (Mathew et al. 2015). Between 2010 and 2014 there was a 30% increase in acute respiratory infections in India (Central Bureau of Health Intelligence 2015), with an estimated 1.3 million excess deaths per year due to air pollution. India has the highest mortality rate from respiratory diseases in the world at 155 deaths per 100,000 people (WHO 2015b).

Record-breaking air pollution in China's cities, particularly in Hebei province, is likewise a byproduct of the country's rapid industrialization and urbanization, linked to significant respiratory deaths among the elderly (Zhou et al. 2015). According to a health-risk based air quality index, the pollution level in major Chinese cities is "very unhealthy" or "hazardous" 80% of days (Hu et al. 2015), provoking increasing numbers of "red alert" or "yellow alert" days in Beijing and other cities, forcing school closures and restrictions on construction, vehicles, and factory emissions.

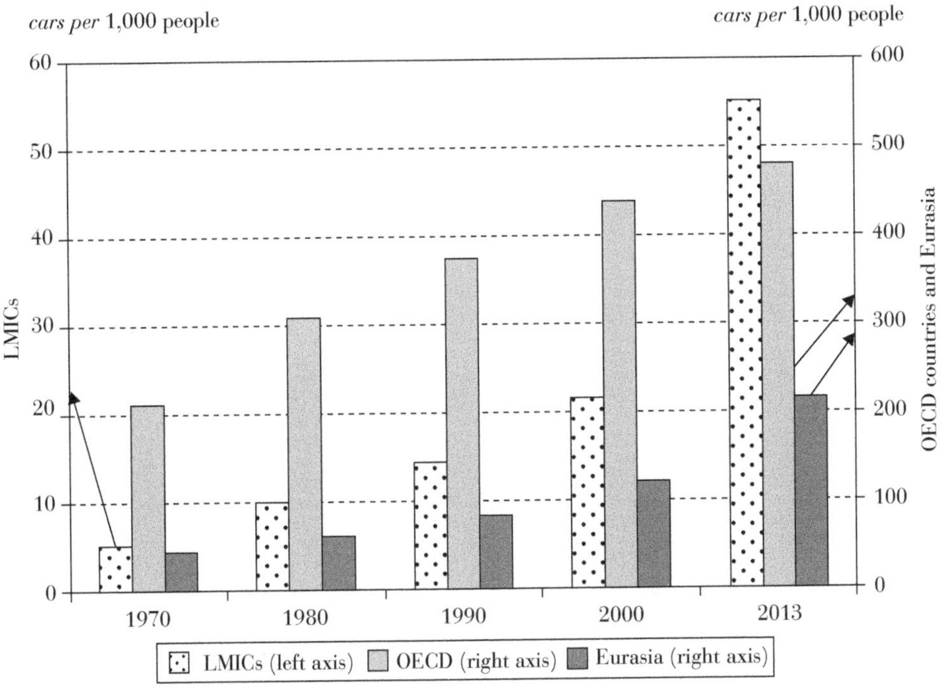

Figure 10-3: Passenger vehicles per 1,000 people by region, 1970–2013.
Source: Based on OPEC *World Oil Outlook* (2015).

Agricultural areas can also suffer from extreme smog and haze. In late 2015 illegal "slash and burn" techniques on Indonesia's Sumatra and Kalimantan islands—used to quickly clear land of vegetation and peat for new palm oil plantations—generated haze so severe (even reaching southern Thailand) that public institutions were forced to close and 500,000 respiratory illnesses were reported (Schecter and Wright 2015), with untold associated deaths. Deforestation accounts for over three fifths of Indonesia's greenhouse gas (GHG) emissions, more than vehicle and power plants together.

Although concentrated urban air pollution is worst in certain LMIC cities, it is important to note that per capita emissions of CO_2 and other air contaminants are far higher in HICs. With vehicle exhaust (together with industrial emissions) a dominant source of air contamination (WHO 2015d), transportation is a central factor. The per capita and total number of passenger vehicles has skyrocketed in recent years, with OECD countries leading but growth rates higher in LMICs (Figure 10-3 and Figure 10-4). In East and South Asia, there has been a three- to four-fold increase in the number of motor vehicles over the past two decades, with heavy reliance on highly polluting gasoline-based two-stroke engines (mopeds and three-wheelers) as well as ubiquitous minibuses for collective transport (Marcotullio, Cooper, and Lebel 2014).

Indoor Air Pollution

Each year, indoor air pollution is responsible for a staggering 4.3 million deaths: the main culprit is use of biomass fuels in poorly ventilated (open) cookstoves. In 2012, 60% of these premature deaths were due to CHD and strokes, 34% to COPD or acute lower respiratory infections, and 6% to lung cancer (WHO 2014d). Indoor air pollution also contributes to about 12% of outdoor combustion-derived PM (Smith et al. 2014b). Approximately three billion people use biomass, including animal dung, wood and logging waste, crop waste, or coal, as their main source of energy for cooking, heating, and repelling insects. Because biomass fuels do not burn completely, small particles and chemical contaminants are present in indoor smoke, causing inflammation of the eyes, airways, and lungs, impaired immune response, and leading to cardiovascular disease, asthma (Box 10-6), pneumonia, stroke, tuberculosis, and other illnesses. As well, carbon monoxide can cause fatal poisoning and reduces the oxygen-carrying capacity of the blood. Women, children, and the elderly in poor households are especially subject to inhalation of smoke and gases due to cooking and other social roles keeping them inside for long periods (WHO 2016).

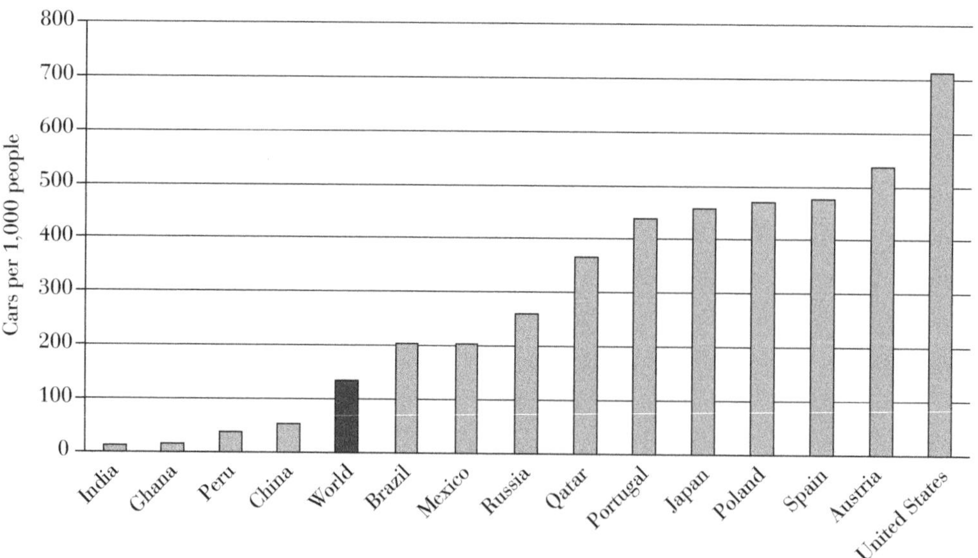

Figure 10-4: Passenger vehicles per 1,000 people in selected countries, 2011.
Source: Based on OPEC *World Oil Outlook* (2014).

Box 10-6 Asthma and Air Pollution

Airborne contaminants are associated with skyrocketing rates of asthma—chronic irritation and inflammation of the lung passages. Over 330 million people suffer from asthma, and associated deaths have reached over 340,000 annually. Most diagnosed cases are in HICs, particularly among low-income populations, but most asthma deaths occur in LMICs (WHO 2013).

Asthma has been linked to indoor allergens (such as cockroaches and domestic mites in bedding, carpets, and furniture), mold growth and dampness in homes, tobacco smoke (including prenatal and childhood exposure to second-hand smoke), chemical cleaning agents and irritants in homes and workplaces, desiccated rat feces where there is infrequent garbage collection, and the chemical irritants of outdoor air pollution (Global Asthma Network 2014).

Tables 10-2 to 10-4 provide examples of important agents of environmental health problems that enter the air, water, soil, food chain, and built environment, together with routes of human exposure, associated health and environmental consequences, and some of the underlying drivers.

Waters

Freshwater Depletion and Contamination

Freshwater—essential for fulfilling basic human needs, including hydration, food preparation,

Table 10-2 Agents of Environmental Health Problems and their Consequences: Air

Examples of Agents	• **Physical:** temperature, non-ionizing radiation, ionizing radiation • **Chemical:** PAHs, methane, nitrogen dioxide, carbon monoxide, benzene, asbestos, particulate matter, toxic metals (lead, arsenic, mercury, cadmium), ground-level ozone
Examples of Human Exposure	• Chemicals inhaled during home and building repairs • Household burning of biomass fuels, wood, and coal, especially exposing women, children, and the elderly • Occupational exposure of workers in mines and factories due to inadequate protection • Inhalation during outdoor activities • Use of electronics or medical devices emitting radiation (e.g., X-rays)
Environmental Effects	• Ambient air pollution • Indoor air pollution
Health Consequences	• **Morbidity:** respiratory impairments, cancer, mesothelioma, COPD, asthma, pneumonia, ocular damage, organ damage • **Mortality:** 3.7 million premature deaths/year attributed to ambient air pollution (88% in LMICs); 4.3 million deaths/year related to household air pollution; 46,000 deaths/year due to silicosis; 24,000 deaths/year due to asbestosis; 34,000 deaths/year due to mesothelioma
Underlying Forces	• Energy-industrial complex (public transport inadequacies, lax regulations on vehicle and industrial fossil fuel emissions, building standards, and air travel) • Household poverty

Data Sources: Agency for Toxic Substances and Disease Registry (2014); Friis (2012); Naghavi et al. (2015); WHO (2014c).

Table 10-3 Agents of Environmental Health Problems and their Consequences: Water

Examples of Agents	• **Physical:** temperature (heat) • **Biological:** pathogens (*Vibrio cholerae, Giardia lamblia, Cryptosporidium*); vectors (mosquitoes, ticks, fleas, flies) • **Chemical:** organochlorine and organophosphate pesticides; toxic metals
Examples of Human Exposure	• Ingestion of feces- or chemical-contaminated water • Ingestion of unfiltered water containing crustaceans • Consumption of contaminated fish • Proximity to vector reservoirs (stagnant water, forests, swamps, ditches) • Poor waste collection, overcrowded living conditions
Environmental Impact	• Contamination of ocean and freshwater • Depletion of freshwater supplies • Loss of marine life and biodiversity
Health Consequences	• **Morbidity:** waterborne diseases (cholera, giardia, Guinea Worm disease, diarrheal disease [58% water/sanitation-related]); vector-borne diseases (malaria, viral encephalitis, yellow fever, dengue, Zika, chikungunya, West Nile, hantavirus); poisonings; cancers; adverse reproductive health outcomes. • **Mortality:** 1.4 million deaths/year from inadequate clean water and sanitation access (842,000 deaths due to diarrhea) • **Livelihoods Losses:** Depletion/contamination of fish stocks affecting coastal populations
Underlying Forces	• Agribusiness practices (large-scale irrigation, fertilizer and pesticide use) • Insufficient and inequitable water and sanitation infrastructure • Industrial waste

Data Sources: Agency for Toxic Substances and Disease Registry (2014); Forouzanfar et al. (2015); Friis (2012); Prüss-Ustün et al. (2014); WHO (2014f); WWAP (2015).

and personal, home, and community hygiene—is plagued by intertwining problems of scarcity, unequal access, and contamination. Although two thirds of the earth's surface is water, just 1% is freshwater that is easily available for human use (97.5% is saline and 1.5%, while suitable for human consumption, is trapped in glaciers, ice, or inaccessible groundwater).

As discussed in chapter 7, one third of the world's population—2.4 billion people (UNICEF and WHO 2015)—faces some level of water shortage or inadequate sanitation facilities. Most persons lacking water and sanitation access are located in rural areas and growing peri-urban slums of LMICs, with particular water stress among internally displaced persons and refugees. In informal settlements, water service may be prohibitively expensive, nonexistent, or frequently interrupted due to shortages; in many rural areas, water and sanitation infrastructure is minimal. Yet industrial and agribusiness interests remain adept at capturing public water supplies at discounted rates, harming conservation efforts and equity (WWAP 2015).

Literally billions of people must use contaminated water to meet their daily survival needs, either from rivers, streams, lakes, and reservoirs or from rainwater accumulated in leftover industrial barrels laden with toxic chemicals. Ingestion of contaminated water and poor hygiene due to insufficient water availability can lead to: a variety of bacterial illnesses such as cholera, typhoid, and salmonella;

skin infections; cryptosporidium and other parasitic diseases; and foodborne pathogens (see chapter 6). Even households with access to some water may have to reuse it for multiple ends, inevitably leading to contamination. Moreover, people without household plumbing often resort to storing water in open containers, creating ideal breeding sites for disease-bearing mosquitoes.

Water- and sanitation-related diseases kill at least 1.4 million people each year (Forouzanfar et al. 2015). Hardest struck are infants and malnourished young children, more than 550,000 of whom die each year from diarrhea (90% attributable to contaminated water and lack of sanitation) (UNICEF 2015). As well, toxins entering water supplies from industrial and agricultural runoff can cause acute poisonings, reproductive health and neurobehavioral problems, and a variety of cancers.

Water and sewage access constitute a political problem of resource allocation rather than a technical one—after all, Roman aqueducts were built thousands of years ago, and modern engineering of waterworks and sanitation systems, and bacteriological monitoring, developed by 1900. In order to be safe for human consumption, water must undergo treatment and filtration (either at a plant or at the community/household level) and be routinely monitored for toxins and pathogens.

Ocean Water Contamination

The world's oceans are undergoing a "deadly trio" of changes: warming, acidification, and deoxygenation. Anthropogenic climate change is the main determinant of these changes (Burkett et al. 2014). The ocean absorbs one third of CO_2 emissions, accelerating acidification. Additionally, in the last 50 years, the ocean's oxygen level has declined due to warming and runoff from nitrogen and phosphorus in agricultural fertilizers, pesticides, livestock manure, industrial discharge, and sewage carried out to sea. These factors create "dead zones" where fish and other marine life can no longer thrive (Bijma et al. 2013), affecting food sovereignty and livelihoods for coastal communities.

While massive oil spills and nuclear disasters cause considerable contamination, everyday sources, including nutrient runoff and oil drippings from motor vehicles, are the source of 80% of ocean pollution (National Oceanic and Atmospheric Administration 2014). Toxic chemicals such as persistent organic pollutants (POPs) and, increasingly, nonbiodegradable plastics also make their way into oceans and fish stocks, traveling thousands of kilometers. For example, high POP levels among northern Canada's Inuit population, whose diet is based on fish and marine mammals, stem from these routes of contamination (Laird, Goncharov, and Chan 2013).

Places

Land Degradation (Changes in Land Use and Soil Erosion)

Arable land, which covers less than 10% of the earth's surface, has been grossly overworked in recent decades. Between 20,000 km^2 and 50,000 km^2 of soil is lost annually through degradation, with soil erosion rates up to six times higher in LMICs than HICs (Hester 2012). Land erosion stems from rising salinity levels due to deforestation and harmful agricultural practices such as overgrazing, poor irrigation, excess water use, overcultivation, and mono-crop production. The intensive use of chemical pesticides, defoliants, and synthetically produced nitrogen fertilizers—and associated toxic runoff from large-scale agribusiness—also plays a major role (Whitmee et al. 2015). Land degradation affects approximately 1.5 billion people, whose livelihoods depend upon farming and who may be subject to food shortages and forced migration (UNEP 2014a). In a cyclical relationship, "crop failure may lead desperate people to put further pressure on the land, resulting in a downward spiral of increasing poverty and further degradation" (Corvalán, Hales, and McMichael 2005, p. 11).

Deforestation

About 2 billion hectares (one third) of the earth's forests have been lost over the last 5,000 years, including 130 million hectares between 1990 and 2015. Intensive logging and the clear cutting of forests for construction materials, harvesting timber, charcoal fuel for domestic use, and the expansion of living and agricultural space have led to massive deforestation in recent decades (FAO 2016). Destructive forest fires—up to 90% of which are caused or exacerbated by illegal logging, poor planning, carelessness, drought, and inadequate fire fighting—have worsened the situation. This loss disproportionately affects LMICs, such as Haiti, which has lost over 80% of its original forest cover, leading to topsoil erosion, arable land shrinkage, and massive food insecurity (Swarup 2009).

Deforestation has many negative health and environmental effects, including displacement of disease-bearing insects, microclimate changes, release of GHGs, land degradation, disruption of animal habitats, and loss of biodiversity. Among other human health implications, unprecedented biodiversity loss (from pollution, over-exploitation, and destruction of natural habitats) alters ecosystems' ability to remove pollutants from air and water, increases risk of zoonotic disease spread, and diminishes pollination and pest control, as well as reducing sources of new medicines (Whitmee et al. 2015). In addition to contributing to up to half of malaria cases, deforestation has also led to new human-microbial interactions and the introduction (or reemergence) of Nipah virus and other diseases. Deforestation also jeopardizes health by worsening the effects of floods, landslides, tidal waves, and hurricanes.

Mangroves—biodiverse tropical forests located in coastal habitats—are also facing rapid destruction by conversion of land for agriculture (rice paddies and oil palm plantations), aquaculture (shrimp and fish farms), industrial development (tourism, canals, oil refineries, timber harvesting), and pollution (agricultural runoff, industrial waste, oil spills). The health implications are varied: mangroves serve as important carbon sinks; help maintain surrounding water quality by filtering out minerals, contaminants, and nutrients; and are an important local source of seafood. They also act as natural defenses against ecological disasters such as hurricanes and tsunamis (UNEP 2014b).

Consumption and Contamination

Household garbage disposal is illustrative of the interdependent relationship among the natural and built environments, social policies, patterns of consumption, and human health. North Americans generate the most household, institutional, and

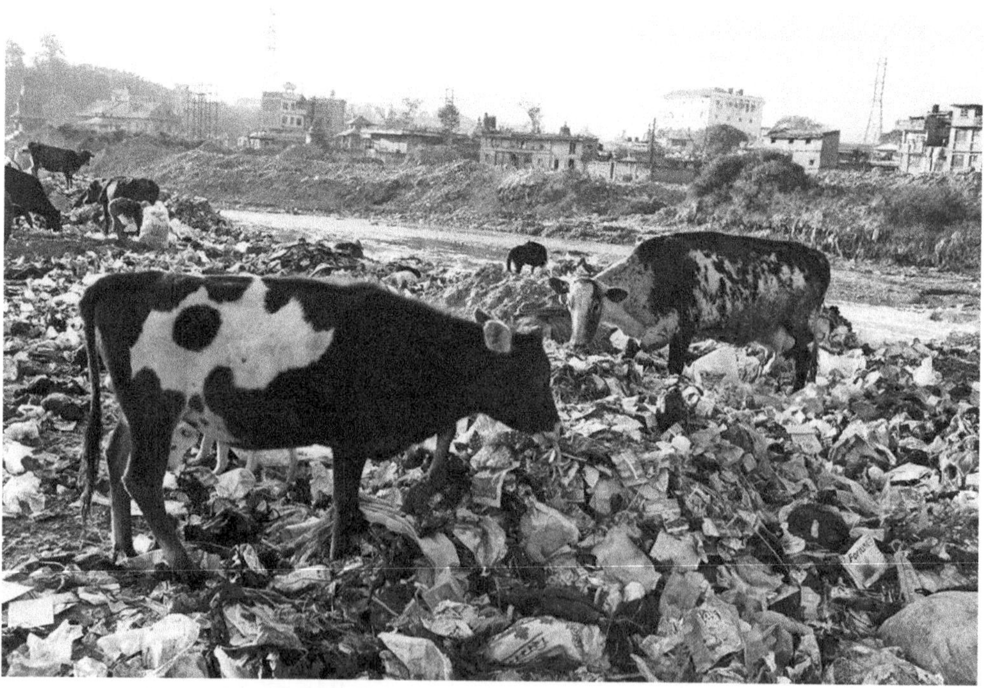

Figure 10-5: Garbage "pickers," Nepal.
Source: Photo courtesy of David Parker.

retail garbage—about 2.3 kg (5 pounds) per person per day, whereas sub-Saharan Africans generate less than 1 kg per person per day (UNEP 2015b). Additionally, 50% to 70% of solid waste in LMICs is organic compared with only 20% to 40% in HICs (UNEP 2015b). In terms of the European Union's (EU) waste generation, construction constitutes 33%; mining and quarrying 29%; manufacturing 11%; households 8.5%; waste collection, treatment, and disposal 7%; and water supply, sewage, and waste management 1.1% (Eurostat 2015).

In cities, garbage is typically collected by large, diesel-run trucks that contribute to air pollution and congestion. Garbage that is not composted, recycled, or burned ends up dumped either haphazardly or in large landfills (Figure 10-5). Landfills that are not well sealed may leak toxic metals (from batteries, electronics, and other manufactured products) and chemicals into the land and groundwater, endangering nearby human populations, destroying fish, bird, and plant habitats, and contaminating rivers and lakes. Landfills also generate methane (CH_4) and other gases, which

Table 10-4 Agents of Environmental Health Problems and their Consequences: Places

Examples of Agents	• **Physical:** temperature (heat), precipitation (patterns, acidity); radioactive waste (ionizing) • **Biological:** vectors (increase in larval breeding sites from deforestation) • **Chemical:** organochlorine and organophosphate pesticides; POPs (DDT, dioxin, PCBs); disinfection by-products (chloroform, bromate); benzene; formaldehyde
Examples of Human Exposure	• Exposure to insecticides, fungicides, herbicides via ingesting contaminated water, foods, and breastmilk • Bioaccumulation in wildlife and humans • Occupational exposure through production processes (e.g., production of pesticides, fertilizers, paper, plywood, clothing, household products)
Environmental Impact	• Land degradation • Soil contamination • Drought • Loss of arable land • Deforestation • Habitat destruction and loss of biodiversity
Health Consequences	• **Morbidity and mortality from pesticide use:** poisonings from pesticide exposure; nervous system effects; skin, kidney, liver damage; reproductive disorders; damaged immunological development; anemia; nose, eye, throat irritation; contribution to cancers • **Morbidity and mortality from deforestation:** malaria, Lyme disease • **Livelihood losses:** food insecurity, forced displacement, limited protection from landslides, floods, and hurricanes
Underlying Forces	• Agribusiness practices (land clearing, large-scale irrigation, use of fertilizers and pesticides) • Export of unsafe pesticides to LMICs • Inadequate regulation of logging • Consequences of spent fuel (nuclear, fossil)

Data Sources: Agency for Toxic Substances and Disease Registry (2014); FAO (2016); Friis (2012).

are fire risks, GHG contributors, and carcinogens. Despite staying in the atmosphere for a shorter time than CO_2, methane traps radiation more efficiently, making its long-term climate impact more than 25 times greater than that of CO_2 (US Environmental Protection Agency 2015).

Liquid sewage—industrial and household wastewater and human excreta—is also a significant contaminant. Without proper sewers and sewage plants to remove sludge and counter microbes, wastewater contaminates groundwater, rivers, and other potential drinking water sources. Even cities and towns with sewage systems may dump untreated liquid waste into waterways or the open ocean. Inadequate disposal of human excreta facilitates the fecal-oral transmission of pathogens. Pit latrines and dug sewers are often promoted as cheap alternatives to the longer-term (yet more cost-effective) commitment to building water and sewage systems, but the former, short-term solutions are more likely to result in groundwater contamination. In LMICs, 90% of wastewater is left untreated as it flows into rivers, lakes, and oceans (WWAP 2015).

CLIMATE CHANGE

Key Questions:

- What are the underlying causes of climate change?
- What are its health consequences?

Although ongoing contamination and depletion of resources pose the most serious long-term and continuous threats to human health, the problem of climate change has become a global environmental emergency. In this section we use a political ecology of health framework (Figure 10-1) to examine climate change—both a by-product of underlying forces and a factor exacerbating many forms of environmental degradation.

What Causes Climate Change?

In recent decades, the phenomenon of climate change has been splayed across the media, with doomsday predictions of the decreasing livability of the earth. While these predictions seemed improbable only a generation ago, today they already constitute lived experience for some (Baer and Singer 2009). Climate records date only from the 19th century, but geological evidence indicates that temperature rises over the last century have exceeded those of every other century in the last millennium, with 2001–2010 as the warmest decade on record (World Meteorological Organization 2014b). There is overwhelming scientific consensus from over 2,000 scientists in the 195-member country UN Intergovernmental Panel on Climate Change (IPCC)—that climate change (first and foremost warming) is taking place and that it is related to human activities, mainly the burning of fossil fuels.

The scientific consensus on the role of fossil fuel burning in climate change is an important initial step toward developing global responses, which have thus far been weak and slow. After all, powerful industrial interests—together with their political allies (and some scientists)—have long contested both the existence of climate change and the causative role of emissions, sponsoring a whole mini-industry of discredited climate change denialism (Oreskes and Conway 2010).

How has climate change happened? The earth is maintained at a habitable temperature by the "greenhouse effect," whereby naturally occurring GHGs trap the heat of the sun and raise the temperature of the atmosphere. However, this greenhouse effect has been magnified over recent centuries through the increased concentration of GHGs from human activity. Over the last 30 years, the earth's temperature is estimated to have risen by 1°C and is projected to rise by between 2°C and 10°C by 2100, in the absence of concerted efforts to control emissions (Field et al. 2014).

Global concentrations of the three main GHGs (carbon dioxide [CO_2], methane [CH_4], and nitrous oxide [N_2O]) have increased markedly since 1750 and now greatly exceed pre-industrial levels. Since 1970 alone, GHG emissions have increased by 75%. CO_2 is the single largest GHG contributor, at 76% (CH_4 accounts for 16%, N_2O for 6%, with 2% from other sources). Fossil fuel combustion accounts for almost two thirds of GHG emissions (industry 29%; heating and cooling buildings 18%; and transport 14%, with aircraft exhaust the fastest growing source). The remaining third comes from the extraction and production of fossil fuels, deforestation, agriculture (animal waste), and municipal waste and wastewater (Victor et al. 2014).

This means that in addition to significant locally based health problems caused by the extraction, processing, and burning of fossil fuels discussed earlier in this chapter, the GHG by-products of the global fossil fuel-based economy are a prime contributor to global climate change (Watts et al. 2015). Thus, while increased GHG emissions per capita are linked to many improvements in quality of life, from refrigeration to production and transport of foods and goods, its effects are also deadly.

Per Table 10-5, CO_2 emissions vary markedly by region. In 2012, non-OECD countries, with over 80% of the world's population, emitted 60% of worldwide CO_2 emissions, making per capita emissions 3.5 times higher in wealthier (OECD) than in poorer nations. The United States alone, with just 4.4% of the global population, consumes nearly 20% of the world's energy resources. The African continent, by contrast, comprises 16% of the world's population and accounts for a mere 3% of world energy consumption. Rapidly growing market economies—most notably China and India—are growing polluters due to industrial development, increased energy use for production and transportation, urbanization, and higher consumption stemming from income increases among urban middle and upper classes. Yet their per capita emissions levels trail those of HICs. For example, China surpassed the United States as the world's single biggest CO_2 polluter in 2008, but has just one third the per capita emissions. India, with 18% of the world's population, accounted for approximately 6% of global CO_2 emissions, whereas the United States, one fourth its size, generated 16%, an almost 10-fold difference (US Department of Energy 2016) (Figure 10-6).

It is important to note that population or population growth per se is *not* the driving force in fossil fuel emissions: instead it is industrial and market forces (mirroring world GDP growth) that frame production and consumption patterns and determine, at least in the short-term, atmospheric CO_2 concentration (Tapia Granados, Ionides, and Carpintero 2012). Of course, virtually every industry in every country releases GHGs, and most people use at least some manufactured products, travel in vehicles, and employ energy from the burning of fossil fuels. But contribution to the problem differs between countries—by level of marketization of the economy—and within countries, by income, geography, and other factors. Ultimately, climate change, like other problems connecting health and the environment, is deeply rooted in the capitalist system of production and consumption (Baer and Singer 2009; Klein 2014).

To illustrate the role of powerful players in the context of climate change, consider just one contributor to greenhouse emissions: motor vehicles. There are over 1.4 billion road vehicles (passenger and commercial) worldwide (OPEC 2014), with New Delhi and Beijing each adding over 1,400 new vehicles every day! The oil, automobile, and road construction industries wield enormous power and are formidable opponents of collective transport (e.g., subways and railroads) in the United States and

Table 10-5 World CO_2 Emissions (Billion Metric Tons) by Region, 1990–2012

Region	1990	2004	2012
North America	5.8	7	6.3
Europe	4.5	4.7	4.3
Japan and South Korea	1.3	1.7	1.9
Former Soviet Union	3.8	2.4	2.7
Asia and Oceania	5.3	9.5	14.9
Middle East	0.7	1.3	2.0
Africa	0.7	1.0	1.2
Central and South America	0.7	1.1	1.4
World	21.6	27.0	32.7

Data Source: US Department of Energy (2016).

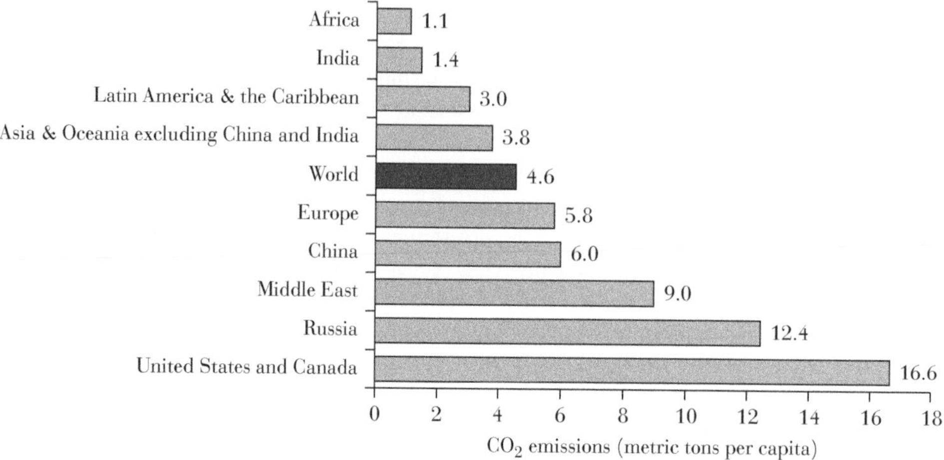

Figure 10-6: Per capita CO_2 emissions, selected countries and regions, 2012.
Data Sources: US Department of Energy (2016); UN (2015).

other places. As well, numerous features of the built environment—for instance unplanned and unregulated commercial, industrial, and urban growth—shape automobile overuse. Any long-term response will need to confront these power relationships.

Health Consequences of Climate Change

Notwithstanding scientific consensus that climate change is taking place and that human activity is driving it, there is considerable variability around the evidence linking climate change to particular environmental and health consequences on a global scale. Table 10-6 identifies key climate phenomena and summarizes the IPCC's projections on future changes based on current scientific knowledge. Effects of climate change include virtually certain changes, namely, warming surface temperatures and ocean warming and acidification, and likely changes, such as increased frequency of heat waves, melting polar icecaps and permafrost (in turn releasing trapped GHGs), rising sea levels, heavy precipitation, and droughts, affecting all settings albeit not equally (Field et al. 2014). These, in turn, have an array of demonstrated, likely, or probable health consequences.

How do we reconcile these uncertainties with action in the absence of definitive scientific findings? For instance, the IPCC reports that "there is low confidence in attributing drought changes to human influence" (Burkett et al. 2014, p. 189). Others document clear influences of anthropogenic climate change on major droughts from 2011 to 2013 in East Africa, New Zealand, and the United States. With such large implications for health and the possibility of unforeseen risks, the potential impact may be too ominous to await further substantiation (Whitmee et al. 2015). As scientists continue to study additional possible health effects of climate change, we would be wise to heed the precautionary principle (see Box 10-7)!

Like other environmental changes outlined in Figure 10-1, climate change has led to, and is likely to exacerbate, a range of human health problems, especially in places already burdened with climate-sensitive diseases (Luber and Lemery 2015). The relationship between climate change and health may be understood in terms of: (a) primary and direct consequences manifested through extreme weather and hazards including more intense (long-duration) heat waves, storms, and floods; (b) indirect or secondary consequences mediated through environmental and ecosystem change (e.g., disease vectors, lower harvest yields, air pollution, wildfires); and (c) more diffuse tertiary consequences mediated through economic and social disruptions (e.g., occupational and mental health effects and conflict due to food, water, and land shortages) (McMichael 2013; Smith et al. 2014a).

Table 10-6 Hierarchy of IPCC Projections of Changes in Climate-Related Phenomena for 2050–2100 and their Health Consequences

Phenomenon	Likelihood and Trend of Projected Change	Associated Human Health Consequences
• Warmer and/or more frequent hot days and nights • Fewer and/or less frequent cold days and nights • Ocean warming (increase) • Ocean acidification (increase)	Almost certain and uniform trend of change *(extremely likely or virtually certain)*[c]	• Increase in heat-related morbidity and mortality
• Longer and/or more frequent heat waves[a] • Heavy precipitation events[a] • More intense and/or longer droughts[a] • Extremely high sea level rise • Ocean deoxygenation	Probable with some regional differences in direction of change *(likely or very likely)*	• Greater food insecurity and undernutrition • Increased risk of food-, water-, and vector-borne diseases • Modest decrease in cold-related morbidity and mortality • Increased exposure to floods and storms • Disappearance of island states
• Floods (magnitude, frequency)[b] • Tropical cyclones (intensity, frequency)[b] • Monsoons[b] • Decline in water resources	Possible and plausible: precautionary approach needed, as awaiting verifiable scientific evidence may prove too late *(limited scientific consensus and/or unclear direction of change)*	• Forced migration due to land/ocean degradation, and sea level rise • Physical harm from collective violence due to environmental scarcity/degradation • Adverse mental health and psychosocial effects from displacement and violence

[a] Non-uniform trend of change but more regions increasing than decreasing.
[b] Direction of change varies by region or there is no clear trend.
[c] IPCC's language on likelihood and trends is in *italics*.
Sources: Burkett et al. (2014); Field et al. (2014); Levy and Patz (2015).

One of the primary and direct health consequences, and also where there is the strongest evidence tying climate change to health, is heat-related mortality (Watts et al. 2015). Both average temperatures and variability are important influences on human health, with key parameters being magnitude, duration, and speed of the temperature increase. Acute health consequences are heat exhaustion, heat rash, fainting, dehydration, heat stroke, and complications of pre-existing diseases such as heart, lung, and kidney disease, and diabetes; long-term effects include chronic kidney disease from repeated dehydration (Kjellstrom, Holmer, and Lemke 2009).

Anthropogenic climate change is estimated to have quadrupled extreme summer heat events

Box 10-7 Environmental Protection and Decisionmaking: EIA and the Precautionary Principle

Environmental Impact Assessment (EIA) is used to determine the effects of human activities on the environment (and on health). The purpose of this tool is to ensure that decisionmakers consider environmental effects before deciding whether to proceed with new projects. Since 1991 the World Bank—pushed by activist movements—has employed EIA as part of its funding approval process (Glasson, Therivel, and Chadwick 2013).

Another approach is the precautionary principle, which advocates preventive action to avoid or diminish scientifically plausible, but uncertain, health or environmental harms associated with human activities. The concept originated in Germany (from the idea of foresight) in the 1970s and became a tenet of the 1992 Rio Declaration (UNESCO 2005). Unlike EIA, the precautionary principle's burden of proof rests with the proponents of a new technology or activity. In 2014, several regional authorities within North America imposed moratoriums on fracking due to inadequate knowledge about long-term risks to health, water, and the environment; various European and North American governments have also invoked the precautionary principle to justify banning the plasticizer BPA from food-contact plastics because exposure potentially leads to cancer, neurological, and other health risks (Lofstedt 2014).

in Europe between 1999 and 2010 (Christidis et al. 2012), leading to 70,000 excess deaths during the 2003 European heat wave, including 15,000 in France. The 2010 Russian heat wave was similarly linked to an estimated 15,000 deaths. A 2015 heat wave with temperatures soaring to 49°C (120°F) killed approximately 2,500 people in India and 2,000 in Pakistan from heat stroke and dehydration.

Older people, infants, and young children—whose bodies are less able to thermoregulate—are particularly vulnerable to heat waves, as are those living alone, outdoor workers, indoor workers in buildings lacking cooling mechanisms, and people with chronic conditions, mental health problems, and disabilities. These conditions are worsened by poverty, which limits resources to mitigate heat stress, as demonstrated by higher mortality rates among lower socioeconomic groups across numerous heat waves (Basu 2015).

An important question is whether temperature increases could lead to a fall in *cold*-related mortality, globally a far larger share of temperature-related deaths than those attributable to heat. Alas, mounting evidence shows that moderate cold rather than extreme cold is the larger mortality culprit (Gasparrini et al. 2015), suggesting that climate change will only have a modest impact on reducing cold-related deaths (Dear and Wang 2015).

Another plausible, but not demonstrated, direct effect of climate change relates to storms and floods, whose direct health consequences consist of mortality due to drowning, injuries, and infectious diseases (see chapter 8). Though storms and floods have affected up to 3 billion people and killed 500,000 in recent decades, especially as populations and property have expanded into flood plains, the climate change connection remains uncertain (Smith et al. 2014a).

Turning to secondary, indirect consequences, the IPCC projects with very high confidence that climate change will lead to increases in food- and waterborne diseases, namely cholera and enteric bacteria and viruses, because changes in temperature and precipitation patterns affect the growth, survival, transmission, and virulence of pathogens (Smith et al. 2014a). In general, bacteria thrive in warmer temperatures (viruses preferring moderate temperatures). Additionally, heavy rainfall provoking sewage overflow and increased human and animal fecal waste runoff may contaminate surface water. By contrast, low rainfall and drought translate into a higher pathogen concentration of available water—particularly problematic where safe drinking water sources are scarce (El-Fadel et al. 2012). Diseases that may rise due to such changes include diarrhea. For example, in the next few decades, the incidence of diarrhea is projected to increase by about 13% in Northern India and globally by 8% to 11% (Moors et al. 2013).

The IPCC has medium confidence that increases in vector-borne diseases (e.g., malaria, dengue, tick-borne encephalitis, Lyme disease, chikungunya) transmitted by temperature-sensitive arthropods such as mosquitoes and ticks are related to climate change. Even modest warming may drive large increases in malaria and other vector-borne disease transmission, enhancing mosquito survival and reproduction, biting rates, pathogen proliferation, and extension of range into areas currently unaffected. Rain and stagnant water, meanwhile, create ideal breeding sites. Certain non-malarious regions, for instance the eastern highlands of Africa and the Andes, may begin to see seasonal epidemics as temperatures increase (Yu et al. 2015). Dengue has increased more than 30-fold in the past 50 years, largely due to climatic conditions more conducive to the *Aedes* mosquito (Bhatt et al. 2013).

The IPCC also predicts a number of indirect health effects of climate change on food sovereignty and nutrition. As discussed, anthropogenically caused ocean warming and acidification decrease availability of seafood, a key source of protein (McMichael 2013). Further likely consequences of continuing droughts are diminished agricultural output, food shortages, undernutrition, and loss of millions of hectares of arable land—and increased death and disease—in poor and already food-insecure areas (Smith et al. 2014a). In Niger, for instance, children born in drought years in the early 2000s were 72% more likely to be stunted (UNDP 2007), with similar effects in Kenya, especially in poor households (Grace et al. 2012).

There are also tertiary, more diffuse but potentially large-scale health effects of climate change, including livelihood loss, population displacement, and social conflict, with effects on physical and mental health due to heat waves, sea level rise, drought, and other phenomena (McMichael 2013; Watts et al. 2015). For example, storms and ensuing floods have profound effects on people's mental health, involving symptoms of depression, psychological distress, and anxiety. Similar mental health effects, plus undernutrition, respiratory illness, and increased maternal mortality, are reported in populations that are forcibly displaced due to harsh, sudden, or escalating environmental changes (Smith et al. 2014a).

A prime example is Syria, which between 2007 and 2010 experienced one of its worst droughts in history, arguably made more severe as a result of anthropogenic climate change. This was a likely stressor leading to the 2011 revolution and subsequent refugee crisis. As rural farmers struggled to grow their crops, the government encouraged agribusiness and export crops requiring heavy irrigation. Domestic production fell, food prices rose, and 1.5 million refugees fled to the cities in search of work. There they were packed in overcrowded slum settlements lacking basic services and faced unemployment, factors that generated political unrest (Kelley et al. 2015).

All told, WHO conservatively estimates that between 2030 and 2050, climate change will cause an *additional* 250,000 deaths per year via direct pathways (excluding economic and social conflict effects) (WHO 2014g). Crucially, all climate change-linked phenomena, whether virtually certain, probable, or potential, are far more likely to affect impoverished and marginalized people in the most fragile LMIC settings.

WHAT IS TO BE DONE?: MULTIPLE LEVELS OF CHANGE

Key Questions:

- Whose responsibility is it to address health problems linked to the environment? Is it consumers in HICs? TNCs? International organizations? Local or national governments?
- Does "reduce, reuse, and recycle" effectively address environmental degradation?
- What can be done to mitigate climate change and its impact on health?

Undoubtedly the consequences of environmental degradation and climate change go "beyond the lifetimes of politicians and business leaders" (Dauvergne 2014, p. 393). More importantly, tackling these issues will require significant changes to global economic production and consumption patterns... [and] governmental, corporate, and personal sacrifices" (ibid). Per a political ecology framing, the possible approaches to these problems are framed by different philosophical and political worldviews (Clapp and Dauvergne 2011):

Market Liberals: Proponents of "free markets" hold that "economic growth and high per capita incomes are essential for human welfare and the maintenance of sustainable development" (Clapp and Dauvergne 2011, p. 4) in the context of globalization. Advocates of market liberalism, such as the WTO and the World Business Council for Sustainable Development, reject the catastrophic urgency of environmental devastation and the call for precautionary policies, arguing that voluntary corporate efforts—together with market pressures and new technologies—will ultimately improve environmental management.

Institutionalists: Sharing market liberal assumptions regarding economic growth, trade, foreign investment, globalization, and technology, institutionalists focus on cooperation at global, state, and local levels. Institutionalists believe that improved global governance and consensus building offer effective means of addressing environmental problems. They see failures to reach or enforce international agreements as a principal reason for global environmental degradation. Institutionalists support the diffusion of knowledge and resources from HICs to LMICs, as well as cooperative action, to forestall further environmental deterioration.

Bioenvironmentalists: Emphasizing that humans—due to population growth and patterns of consumption—are depleting and abusing the planet's finite and fragile resources, bioenvironmentalists hold that the earth's capacity to sustain current levels of consumption has already been surpassed (see Box 10-8 for a way of measuring this). They view globalization as a negative force that fuels consumption and promotes environmentally destructive production processes in LMICs. Instead, they advocate limits on economic growth, curbs on immigration to HICs, individual approaches to lowering consumption, and family planning as key solutions to environmental degradation.

Social Greens: Social greens draw on radical social and economic theories that consider environmental problems to be inseparable from the capitalist system. Like bioenvironmentalists, social greens believe that there are physical limits to economic growth and that overconsumption is at least partially to blame. But for social greens the problem is systemic: the production and consumption logic that undergirds the capitalist world order, deeply rooted in historical processes and reproduction of inequality, is *the* driver of environmental crises. Rejecting bioenvironmentalist positions that population growth is at fault, social greens call for a complete overhaul of the global economic system, advocating the abandonment of industrial and capitalist life for self-reliant, equitable, small-scale economic communities.

Related to social greens is the *degrowth movement*, calling for a scaleback of the growth-oriented capitalist market model, and Indigenous Andean *Buen Vivir* philosophies, which espouse a way of life (and economic system) emphasizing ecological harmony, not exploitation and profiteering (see chapter 13 for further discussion).

Although elements of all of these worldviews are explored in the pages ahead, the market liberal approach is fundamentally at cross-purposes with addressing environmental degradation and climate change and so is covered minimally. Indeed, it is "market forces that are largely responsible for creating and deepening the crisis" (Klein 2014, p. 41). As we outline, the institutionalist approach, emphasizing global agreements on emissions, has gained ground but it, too, is constrained by corporate interests. National and local efforts influenced by institutionalists and bioenvironmentalists (and occasionally social greens) offer promise but remain insufficient. We will conclude with a survey of how social (green) movements around the world seek to address issues linking health and the environment (Brown and Zavestoski 2005).

The array of responses to environmental degradation is considerable, ranging from technological (e.g., lower-emission vehicles and solar energy devices), to behavioral (e.g., recycling and bicycling), policy-based (e.g., green planning), and political (e.g., pesticide regulation), and demonstrates that confronting environmental health problems demands attention at household, community, national, and international levels (Table 10-7). Each of these dimensions interacts with global health issues, either by: 1) tackling problems that are inherently global, such as health-related climate change, or involving transnational forces and actors, for instance around the movement of pesticides and toxic waste; or 2) engaging in solutions that entail policy learning back and forth and across borders.

Box 10-8 Ecological Footprint

A useful concept to assess the impact of human actions on the natural environment is the "ecological footprint" (EF), which translates human consumption of renewable natural resources into hectares of average biologically productive land required to sustain their use (Wackernagel and Rees 1996). There is considerable regional variation in the magnitude of EFs (Figure 10-7). Though the *global* average EF was 2.8 hectares per person in 2012, the average EF of someone in the United States was 8.2 hectares. By contrast, in Malawi, the average person's EF was 0.8 hectares (Global Footprint Network 2016). While offering a snapshot of the impact of human activity on the environment, EFs overlook the role of the larger economic system that shapes production and consumption patterns, limiting their utility (Blomqvist et al. 2013).

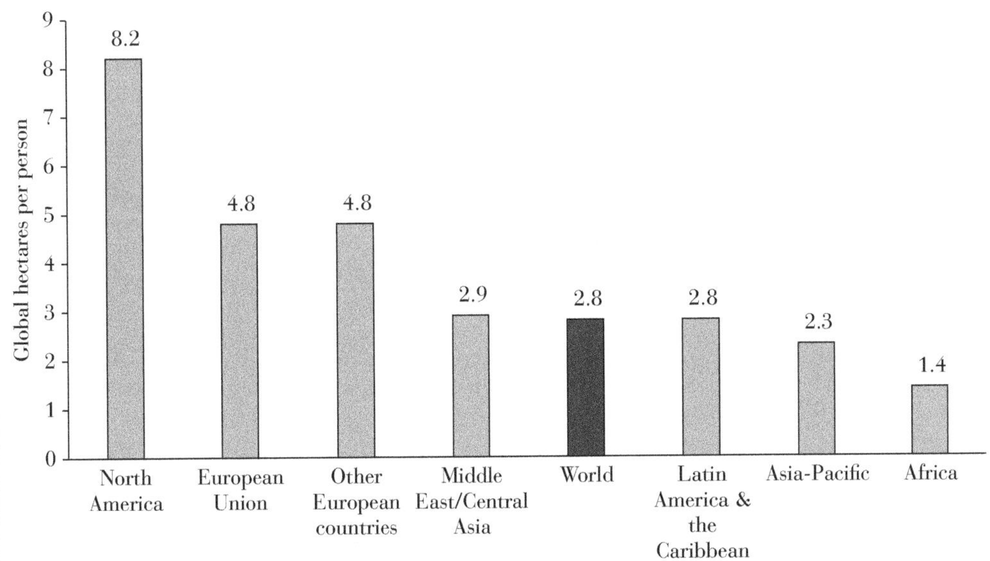

Figure 10-7: Ecological footprints: A global snapshot, 2012.
Data Source: © 2016 Global Footprint Network. National Footprint Accounts, 2016 Edition.

Global and Regional Responses

It was not until the 1960s that concern for the environment was transformed into a transcendent global issue, a transformation that took place within the context of social and political movements for economic justice, peace, and gender and racial equality. A pivotal moment was publication in the United States of Rachel Carson's *Silent Spring* (1962), which detailed how chemical pesticides entered the food chain, affecting flora, fauna, and human health. The book's focus on the effects of the insecticide DDT on birds led to DDT's ban in numerous countries. By the 1970s, local protests in India, Africa, and Latin America against the environmental effects of large-scale development projects garnered international attention, while social movements in Eastern and Western Europe protested the environmental implications of nuclear weapons production and warfare.

This worldwide environmental awakening spurred numerous international conferences, reports, and agreements (Box 10-9), reaching a crescendo in the 1990s, though concrete actions have lagged far behind concerted public and scientific attention.

Table 10-7 Actions to Confront Environment and Health Threats

Sphere of Action	Examples	Advantages	Disadvantages
Global and Regional	• CFC phaseout • Cap and trade • Kyoto Protocol • UN-REDD (carbon offsetting)	• Involves multiple actors • May have broad impact	• Operates within a "free" market paradigm • Targets are usually nonenforceable
National (Government) or Regional Authority (i.e., state, province)	• Environmental Impact Assessment • Regulations on pesticide and chemical use and disposal of hazardous waste • Incentives for organic agriculture; renewable energy sources • Fossil fuel use disincentives • Restoration of degraded land/forests • Carbon sequestration and carbon sinks • Green economy	• Involves legitimate body responsible for environmental standards, public health, and human rights • Can integrate environmental policies with health and livelihood needs and protection	• Sovereignty of national governments may be curtailed by WTO rules and regional trade agreements and treaties • Enforcement and legislative processes may lack transparency and legitimacy • Measures may generate inequities • Commitment to green economy may clash with vested interests in industries that contaminate and deplete resources
Local (Government or Community)—may also involve regional or national subsidies, policies, and incentives	• Local/urban agriculture • Public transport; cycling • Green cities • Waste recycling • Efficient lighting, heating, and cooling	• Generates high levels of public participation • Can address/plan for multiple issues at once	• Does not address large-scale industrial regulations and policies • May require national support/counterparts to succeed
Individual (Household/Behavioral)—may also involve subsidies and incentives by government (at all levels)	• Eco-friendly products and devices • Improved stoves, home insulation, ventilation • Rainwater collection • Composting	• Raises awareness • Helps mobilize and educate around environmental protection	• Diverts focus from structural issues • Individual behavior contributes but is not the prime motor of environmental degradation • May be costly and time consuming • Fails to address environmental injustice

Table 10-7 Continued

Sphere of Action	Examples	Advantages	Disadvantages
Environmental Justice Actors and Movements (Local, National, or Transnational)	• Lawsuits and protests against mining, energy, and agribusiness TNCs • Fossil fuel divestment • Indus Consortium • Kenya's Greenbelt Movement • Acción Ecológica • La Via Campesina • People's Health Movement	• Adopt a long-term outlook • Generate international solidarity • Provide a broad understanding of environment and health • Involve strong community and visible efforts at local level	• Gains may be slow • Activists may face violence and retribution • Hard to maintain adequate resources • Once gains are institutionalized (at local, national, or global levels), movements may disband
Technological Innovations (relevant to all spheres of action)	• Ecological building design • Water desalination • Renewable energy sources (e.g., geothermal, solar, wind) • Fuel-efficient vehicles and energy-efficient appliances	• Can make renewable energy more cost-efficient • Can be effective when employed with broader regulatory and redistributive measures	• Do not in and of themselves address equitable distribution and control of resources • May have high start-up costs • May improve access to some resources while contributing to depletion and contamination of others • Do not address root causes of environmental degradation and injustice

Major Climate Change Agreements

The 1997 Kyoto Protocol was the first core global agreement to address climate change. The initial commitment period required 36 HICs to reduce emissions of six GHGs by an average of 5% below 1990 levels between 2008 and 2012. The second period began in 2012 and requires countries to reduce GHG emissions by 18% below 1990 levels by 2020, but this round never entered into force because not enough countries ratified it (UNFCCC 2014).

The Kyoto Protocol is plagued by various shortcomings: emissions targets serve as quick fixes rather than long-term meaningful measures; the agreement promotes "flexible mechanisms" allowing the atmosphere to be commodified through market trade of emissions ("cap and trade" arrangements); and reporting/accountability mechanisms are too weak (PHM et al. 2011; Rosen 2015). While binding, the Kyoto Agreement's compliance system is risible: if a country fails to meet emission targets, it may make up the difference in the next compliance round, essentially "borrowing" from one period to the next indefinitely, with no consequences. Moreover, two of the biggest per capita polluters in the world, the United States and Canada, were uncooperative, at least until the leadup to the Paris 2015 (COP21) conference. Meanwhile, LMICs that ratified the Protocol, including India and China, were not required to

Box 10-9 Some Key International Environmental Conferences and Agreements and their Health Dimensions

Stockholm Conference (1972): For the first time, national governments reported on the state of their environments at a UN conference. Whereas HICs focused on preventing pollution, controlling "overpopulation," and conserving natural resources, LMICs expressed concern about widespread hunger, disease, poverty, and the environmental effects of growing industrialization. The conference sparked the founding of the UN Environment Programme (UNEP), which together with WHO began to document the relationship between environmental factors and human health.

The Rio Earth Summit (1992): The UN Framework Convention on Climate Change (UNFCCC) was agreed to in Rio de Janeiro, Brazil and ratified by 189 countries. It calls on parties to: "protect the climate system for the benefit of present and future generations of humankind, on the basis of equity and in accordance with their common but differentiated responsibilities and respective capabilities" with HICs playing a leading role (UN 1992).

Kyoto Protocol (1997): (see text).

Copenhagen Climate Change Conference (2009): One of the largest UN gatherings on climate change, its purpose was for member countries to agree to legally binding mitigation measures post-2012, a failure following days of unproductive negotiations.

World People's Conference on Climate Change and the Rights of Mother Earth (2010): After the disappointing outcome of Copenhagen, the city of Cochabamba, Bolivia hosted an alternate climate summit, bringing together government officials from 48 countries, together with upwards of 30,000 activists, civil society organization representatives, and scientists from over 100 countries. The conference produced a Universal Declaration on the Rights of Mother Earth and the *People's Agreement*, which, among other points, cites the incompatibility of capitalism and ecological harmony (World People's Conference 2011).

Rio+20 United Nations Conference on Sustainable Development (2012): This summit re-visited past political commitments and sought to build a global environmental policy agenda for the next 20 years, including establishing the new "Sustainable Development Goals" (UN 2011).

Paris Climate Change Conference (2015): (see text).

reduce their carbon emissions on the grounds that this could hinder economic progress.

Despite its limitations, many environmental activists believe Kyoto offered a promising step in the right direction, particularly influencing some EU countries (e.g., Germany and the United Kingdom) to adopt more ambitious targets to enable the EU to meet its commitments via burden-sharing. Ultimately, however, the Kyoto Protocol was flawed in that its very design impeded the possibility of effectively mitigating global climate change (Rosen 2015).

The highly anticipated COP21 meeting produced an agreement among 196 countries to limit global average temperature increases to below 2°C (aiming, without commitment, for a more ambitious 1.5°C limit). By late 2016, China and the United States—together producing 40% of global carbon emissions—along with dozens of other countries, had ratified the Paris agreement (enabling it to come into force). The agreement rests on intended nationally determined contributions (INDCs), emissions reduction targets for 2020 (renewed every 5 years thereafter) set entirely by individual nations on a voluntary basis with no penalties for noncompliance. In preparation for COP21, countries were asked to submit their INDCs, already revealing deficient goals (Bello

2015). The Paris agreement itself underscores the inadequacy of INDCs "to hold the increase in the global average temperature to below 2°C above pre-industrial levels," let alone to below 1.5°C (UNFCCC 2015).

Another contentious issue surrounds funding to support climate change mitigation (i.e., reducing emissions) and adaptation (i.e., societal efforts to cope with climate change consequences) in LICs. HIC pledges to raise US$100 billion per year by 2020 for a Green Climate Fund to help African states, small island LICs, and other vulnerable countries with mitigation and adaptation efforts (and eventual emissions reduction targets) have been slow to materialize (Bello 2015).

Though COP21 was hailed by institutionalists as a success, bioenvironmentalists and social greens disagreed. In the aftermath of the Paris gathering, former NASA scientist, James Hansen, world renowned for raising the climate change alarm in the 1980s, denounced the agreement as containing "no actions, just promises." He argued, "[a]s long as fossil fuels appear to be the cheapest fuels out there, they will continue to be burned" and that an across-the-board carbon tax is needed to avoid this cheap option (Mortimer 2015).

Other critics pointed out that, as with Kyoto, the agreement relies on ineffective market approaches to reducing emissions including cap and trade arrangements—whereby companies and governments that have achieved their emissions reduction targets can auction off their unused quota to larger polluters—and carbon offsetting, which provides credit for GHG reductions (e.g., via planting trees) that can be bought to compensate another party's emissions. To these critics, carbon offset projects such as UN-REDD crafted to curb deforestation in LICs, have at best made slow progress, and at worst perpetuated fraud and forced displacement (Pearse and Böhm 2014).

An ongoing geopolitical conundrum is where the balance of responsibility lies for addressing climate change. Because HICs have generated over 80% of historical carbon emissions—an even higher proportion under a consumption-based system of carbon accounting (whereby endpoint consumers are accountable for emissions from extraction, production, and transport)—pinning culpability on rapidly industrializing LMICs (especially China and India) is considered by some to be a form of carbon colonialism (Böhm 2015).

Other Environmental Treaties

There are over 500 multilateral environmental agreements (MEAs) that target environmental harms, including those aggravated by trade (Jaspers and Falkner 2013). In addition to the Basel and Bamako Conventions on transboundary movement and disposal of hazardous waste, key treaties are: the 1998 Rotterdam Convention calling for prior notification of international trade of hazardous pesticides and industrial chemicals; the 2001 Stockholm Convention, which aims to eliminate or restrict the production, use, and trade of POPs due to their harmful health effects; and the Montreal Protocol on Substances that Deplete the Ozone Layer (Box 10-10). MEAs have the potential to address many important global environmental health hazards but are unevenly regulated, often lacking robust oversight and compliance mechanisms (see also chapter 9).

National Level Responses and Efforts

The nation-state, with its broad purview over economic and industrial policy, land use, and social protection, is potentially the most important player in protecting the public from health consequences of environmental contamination and resource depletion.

As examined in chapter 9, the exigencies of market competition and enormous corporate power mean that governments privilege economic priorities and corporate interests over social and environmental needs, even in settings where democratic institutions and decisionmaking processes are marked by integrity and representativeness. Nonetheless, as we explore, there are also many instances of governments responding to collective demands to protect environmental health.

A growing number of governments are espousing a green economy as a means of boosting both the economy and social well-being through public investments, incentives, and other policies around public transport, renewable energy, sustainable technologies, and "green jobs" creation (Lee and Card 2012). Such institutionalist and

Box 10-10 Cooperating to Phase Out Chlorofluorocarbons: The Montreal Protocol

This landmark environmental cooperation effort involves the reduction of chlorofluorocarbons (CFCs) released into the atmosphere. Invented in 1928, CFCs quickly found broad industrial use as propellants (in aerosols), refrigerants, flame retardants (in insulation), and solvents. In 1974, three scientists (from Mexico, the Netherlands, and the United States) recognized that CFCs were drifting into the atmosphere and depleting the ozone layer, which provides a protective shield from the harmful effects of the sun's ultraviolet-B radiation (contributing to skin cancer, cataracts, decreased immunity, and lower plant productivity).

Efforts to reduce use of CFCs gained momentum in 1985 after a thinning of the ozone layer over a wide area (referred to as a "hole") was discovered over the Antarctic. The Montreal Protocol on Substances that Deplete the Ozone Layer was adopted in 1987, setting mandatory targets to reduce the production of human-made chlorines, including CFCs, halons, and other significant ozone-depleting substances. Within a decade, worldwide production and use of CFCs and other ozone-depleting chemicals was slashed by 95%.

The international effort to eliminate the use of CFCs is an environmental success story. There has been near-universal participation of countries and, following initial resistance, support from industry—due to the paced phase-out process and the development of alternative technologies. Moreover, because CFCs were produced by only 21 firms, enforcement was feasible (Clapp and Dauvergne 2011). In 2016 the Montreal Protocol was extended to cover a gradual phaseout of hydrofluorocarbons, which replaced CFCs but also contribute to global warming.

Notwithstanding the almost complete phase-out of CFCs, the ozone layer will likely not recover until 2050 (later in Antarctica) due to black-market trading, increasing air conditioning use, and because "old" CFC emissions are still drifting into the stratosphere (World Meteorological Organization 2014a). This makes Mother Earth akin to an ex-smoker.

bioenvironmentalist approaches—consistent with the UN's Sustainable Development Goals (see chapter 3) and led by "Green" political parties and politicians in many settings—advocate increasing efficiency, eliminating waste, and phasing out fossil fuel use. Unlike degrowth and *Buen Vivir*, however, the green economy seeks solutions within a market economy rather than challenging it.

Addressing Climate Change and Environmental Degradation

Atop the current environmental health agenda of many countries are mitigation, adaptation, and conservation policies around climate change. Mitigation refers to reducing GHG emissions through measures such as carbon sequestration (technology for capturing CO_2 from the atmosphere) and use of renewable energy sources (i.e., solar, wind, and geothermal, constituting 3% of global energy use [International Energy Agency 2015]). There are also major health co-benefits of mitigation independent of those relating to modifying climate risk. For example, emissions reductions will reduce air pollution and thus respiratory disease, and active transport (walking, biking) will likely lower rates of obesity, diabetes, cardiovascular disease, and cerebrovascular disease (Frumkin, Hess, and Luber 2015).

Tellingly, economic slowdown following the 2008 crisis (decreasing industrial and vehicular emissions in Europe and North America) has served as an unintended mitigation strategy; similarly, economic crisis in the 1990s compelled Cuba to develop alternatives to fossil fuels, pesticides, and food imports, turning it into an inadvertent carbon-neutral trailblazer.

Adaptation refers to lessening the risks and preparing for the adverse effects of climate change through measures including building regulations to withstand extreme weather events and installing defenses for low-lying coastal populations to protect against rising sea levels. Mitigation and adaptation are not mutually exclusive: measures such as wetlands restoration and reforestation contribute to both aims (VijayaVenkataRaman et al. 2012).

Important as is addressing fossil fuel-driven climate change, fully tackling environmental degradation and its health consequences requires comprehensive national environmental management and policy strategies that address the impact on livelihoods, especially in LMICs (Luginaah and Yanful 2009). In Brazil, for example, deforestation was reduced by 70% between 2005 and 2013 under pressure from civil society groups and social movements. A key player has been the Zero Deforestation campaign—a coalition formed in 2008 by Brazilian and international environmental, Indigenous, labor, human rights, and other groups that pressured the Brazilian government to take concerted action. These efforts achieved a beef and soy moratorium to slow industrial drivers of deforestation, putting the onus on businesses along the entire supply-chain. Additionally, the national government began bringing more land under the collective tenure of Indigenous peoples as of 2002, serving the dual purpose of ensuring Indigenous land rights and conservation (as most of the forest land has been preserved, reducing emissions from deforestation) (Boucher 2014).

Regulations, Standards, and Green Taxes

Environmental health protection involves numerous measures, ranging from elimination of hazardous materials and waste in industrial settings, to land conservation and zoning laws. Following protracted scientist-activist struggles, in the 1970s many governments began to pass legislation to regulate discharge of toxins in the air and water, protect endangered species, and limit the use of—and exposure to—hazardous substances in industrial settings and the built environment. Permanent agencies, such as the US Environmental Protection Agency (EPA, established in 1970) and counterparts elsewhere, set regulations and standards and are charged with enforcing the "polluter pays" principle. Enforcement ability waxes or wanes depending on budget allocations, reporting requirements, number and training of inspectors, and other activities affected by political decisions. One auspicious development is the EU's 2007 Registration, Evaluation and Authorisation of Chemicals program, which requires all companies to "identify and manage the [health and environmental] risks linked to the substances they manufacture and market in the EU" or face restrictions and substitutions (ECHA 2015).

More widely, the adoption of air pollution standards, introduction of unleaded gas and cleaner engines, and factory emissions controls have lowered pollution levels, especially in Europe and the Americas, with an important role for government enforcement (Phalen and Phalen 2012). For example, Chile's National Environmental Information System monitors air quality to inform environmental management and decisionmaking (Sistema Nacional de Información Ambiental 2015).

Other government measures include green taxes on carbon emissions, car purchases, household waste, groundwater withdrawal, and water pollutants and levies on industries, companies, and individuals. Measures range from Trinidad and Tobago's green sales tax to European countries' adoption of carbon and other eco-taxes to reduce air pollution and encourage more sustainable use of resources (European Commission 2015). Various regions are phasing out dirty industries such as coal plants. Green policies also involve subsidies and incentives to farmers to manage land more ecologically through carbon sinks and efficient irrigation (Clapp and Dauvergne 2011). All of these strategies can help to reduce waste and foster use of sustainable energy sources, but most underemphasize corporate accountability.

Corporate Accountability

The corporate sector has promoted market-based environmental protection through schemes to trade carbon emissions, "environmentally-friendly production processes" (for instance, making timber from sustainable sources), and voluntary corporate stewardship and transparency. Corporate social responsibility—the stated commitment made by businesses to enhance the public good (see chapter 9)—is portrayed as beneficial for the environment, but mostly it is good for marketing, public relations, and, ultimately, ensuring profits (Ameer and Othman 2012).

Voluntary agreements between industry and government have played a small role in some environmental policies, such as vehicle emissions standards and source reduction. For example, the World Resources Institute and World Business Council for Sustainable Development jointly developed the GHG Protocol, an international accounting tool used by governments and businesses (including 70% of Fortune 500 companies) to quantify emissions. However, in contrast to mandatory measures, these efforts have not achieved significant emissions reductions (Somanathan et al. 2014) because they lack enforcement and accountability mechanisms. Moreover, despite the self-serving publicity surrounding corporate social responsibility, the environmental repercussions of most past and present business activities remain unaddressed. In the end, as journalist Naomi Klein (2014, p. 41) contends, (environmental degradation and) climate change "detonates the ideological scaffolding on which [the] contemporary [world order] rests. A belief system that vilifies collective action and declares war on all corporate regulation and all things public simply cannot be reconciled with a problem that demands collective action on an unprecedented scale."

Waste Minimization and Recycling

Many national and municipal governments have implemented source reduction policies, which involve a change in production and packaging to reduce waste. Numerous cities in HICs and, increasingly, LMICs encourage or require recycling (through depots or regular collection) of reusable products, including paper, plastics, glass, metals, and organic waste, coupled in some cases with a monetary incentive or threat of fines. At least half of consumer waste is estimated to be recyclable, though municipal recycling rates are highly variable, ranging from 5% to 70% (UNEP 2015b).

Municipal recycling programs have also developed provisions for safely disposing of batteries, e-waste, and other hazardous materials, with varying effectiveness. More promising are European policies requiring electronics manufacturers to properly recycle their own products through "extended producer responsibility" policies. Switzerland, for example, has a longstanding collective "take-back" system for electronic products involving detoxification, shredding, and refining. However, much of this waste is still exported to LMICs (Khetriwal, Luepschen, and Kuehr 2013).

Sustainable Technologies and Energy Sources

Environmentally-friendly technologies, cleaner engines, and renewable energy sources offer some promising prospects to improve environmental health. Ecological building designs provide emissions-free cooling and heating, greatly reducing energy and water demands. Replacing biomass cooking and heating fuels (including agricultural residues and animal dung burned in inefficient stoves) with cleaner sources, such as electricity and kerosene—and better stoves—can reduce the production of black soot and other contaminants and improve the health of women, children, and the elderly exposed to high indoor air pollution. Improved living conditions and income generally enable the switch to safer fuels and stoves, but public policies are also necessary. For example, due to massive infrastructural growth, China currently has near-universal access to electricity, but one third of households continue to rely on biomass fuels because of electricity's high price (International Energy Agency 2015) and inadequate subsidies for lower-income populations.

Alternative energy sources also show promise. Geothermal energy comes from the heat of the earth's magma (the layer of molten rock below the earth's crust). Geothermal power plants tap into natural geothermal springs as either a direct energy source (from their hot water) or an indirect source (by capturing the steam they emit to power electric generators). Demonstrating the vast potential of this form of renewable energy (with increasingly competitive start-up costs), Iceland heats virtually all of its buildings and gets more than 50% of its domestic energy from geothermal sources (Union of Concerned Scientists 2014).

With solar power, energy from the sun is absorbed through panels that convert it to electricity or transfer it to storage places, such as batteries. Solar energy is also used directly, for example, to power water pumps providing potable water in remote communities.

Wind systems produce energy night and day. Wind is both efficient and far less costly than coal or nuclear energy. To date, wind power has not been widely used in LMICs due to topographic requisites and high start-up costs (which quickly dissipate through energy savings). Exceptionally, Uruguay's recent investments in wind, biomass cogeneration, and solar power enable it to obtain 55% of its energy from renewables (95% for electricity). This compares with 20% in Europe overall (Watts et al. 2015), 42% in Spain, where wind energy became the top electricity source in 2013 (Red Eléctrica de España 2013), and 100% on Denmark's Samso island.

Meanwhile, the problem of freshwater scarcity is being tackled through new desalination technologies in the Middle East that may prove useful for other settings, even as political and energy-use concerns persist. Israel, much of it desert, has long been in conflict over water access with neighboring Jordan and the Occupied Territories. Israel has exhausted its mountain aquifers and wrested control over Jordan River access from Palestinians in the West Bank, with Israeli authorities cutting off water supply and impeding the building of water infrastructure. Yet Israelis have access to at least thrice the daily water volume as Palestinians (Corradin 2016), and Israel's thirsty agriculture sector, accounting for almost 60% of water use—plus rising household consumption—has put ever greater pressure on freshwater supply (OECD and FAO 2012).

Having previously innovated parsimonious drip irrigation techniques, starting in 2007 Israel built the most efficient water treatment system in the world, able to recapture and reuse 86% of household water flowing into drains. New desalination plants were also developed, employing novel techniques to separate salt molecules from seawater to yield potable water (Jacobsen 2016). While Israel has cut desalination production costs by two thirds, energy use remains extremely high, roughly twice the cost of treating wastewater, although combined thermal power generation and desalination plants may make desalination more cost-effective in the future (WWAP 2014). Now supplying 55% of domestic water consumption through desalination, Israel's newfound freshwater surplus remains politically fraught, as Palestinians must purchase desalinated Israeli water despite having been dispossessed of their own water resources for decades (Hass 2014). Whether the Dead Sea-Red Sea pipeline venture—which includes plans for a massive shared desalination plant—is able to bring water justice to the region remains to be seen.

Technologies themselves, though potentially helpful, do not address the root causes of, or social inequities associated with, environmental problems (Trace 2016). Nevertheless, environmentally-friendly technologies can be highly effective when employed as part of political efforts that regulate industrial waste and emissions, subsidize public transportation rather than the auto industry, and redistribute income, enabling poor families to upgrade their housing conditions (e.g., through improved ventilation, stoves, and fuels) and water access.

Local Responses and Efforts

Even as national measures have wider reach, local jurisdictions can have considerable decisionmaking agency and enjoy public responsiveness, while potentially facing fewer market pressures.

Green Cities and Ecological Design

Cities are central to the global agenda of sustainability for several reasons. First, urbanization is accelerating: more than half the world's population lives in cities. Second, local government is closest to the population and usually the most effective at working with community organizations and movements—essential to many environmental health initiatives. Third, cities have massive carbon footprints (measured by GHG production): cities contribute almost 75% of GHGs—despite covering only 2% of global land mass—due to emissions from vehicular transportation, building heating and cooling, and electricity generation.

Because 40% of the world's energy consumption results from the construction and operation of commercial buildings and dwellings, ecological housing and "green" commercial buildings emphasize high-energy conservation, low water usage, and minimal need for cars due to accessible cycling and public transport infrastructure. Other ecological design features include solar energy, green roofs, organic gardens, grey water (recycled household and drainage water for watering gardens, sanitation, etc.), rainwater retrieval systems, high-efficiency natural gas furnaces, reused concrete in the foundation, and the installation of water-conserving taps, showerheads, and toilets. Notwithstanding its benefits, ecological design has not been widely implemented due to high up-front costs, complex logistics, and limited support from most municipal authorities.

Urban agriculture, meanwhile, has blossomed in recent years, touted for reducing transport costs, fuel emissions, and food waste (since fresh produce lasts longer), promoting healthier diets, ensuring food availability during distribution crises, and—via community gardens—helping build neighborhood solidarity and local engagement through the lifecourse. In environmental terms, urban green space absorbs stormwater, lessens urban heat in summertime, and enables food waste to be reused as compost (Royte 2015). Long a mainstay in LMICs—approximately 40% of African city-dwellers take part in urban agriculture, largely for economic reasons—some 15%-20% of worldwide food is produced in cities, involving 800 million people (Karanja and Njenga 2011).

Various other efforts harness the potential of cities to address environmental issues. The C40 network of over 80 large cities exchanges knowledge and experiences on climate mitigation and adaptation strategies related to renewable energy, waste management, transportation, building energy efficiency, and other urban planning measures. More transformationally, Transition Towns promote collective post-carbon strategies engaging entire communities (see chapter 13).

Green ecological design has enabled European cities to make noteworthy strides, limiting their carbon footprints to half the size of US cities. This also reflects the US's propensity to urban sprawl, less public transport, and higher energy consumption overall (Jones and Kammen 2014). Many green cities feature creative car-sharing schemes, as well as no drive-zones, physical barriers of all types (including placing trees in streets), and fewer parking lots.

Public Transport and Bicycling

An important element of urban ecology is the implementation of convenient, safe, low-pollution, affordable public transportation systems. European cities are well known for public investment in transport but so is, for example, Quito, Ecuador. Perhaps the best alternative to car-based transport is cycling, which—though both environmentally sustainable and health promoting—is often a missing link in urban transport planning. Local policies that promote cycling range from eco-taxes on car use to bike lanes, bike traffic signals, bike parking, employer/employee incentive schemes, and municipal bike-sharing systems (as in Bangkok, Barcelona, Beijing, Buenos Aires, Chicago, London, New York, Paris, Rio de Janeiro, San Francisco, Santiago, Taipei, Toronto, Vancouver, and Washington). Few nations encourage bicycle use as much as the Netherlands, where there are 18.7 million bicycles for 16.5 million people, Europe's highest per capita bicycle ownership. Bike lanes and paths (totaling 35,000 km compared with 110,000 km of streets and roads) enable the Dutch to make 27% of all trips by bicycle, 35% in Amsterdam (Miller et al. 2013).

In Helsinki, over 70% of all trips are made by public transit, walking, or cycling, indicating strong societal commitment (Thorpe 2015). Portland, Oregon (USA) is a viable green city, with a growth boundary, strong regional government, well-funded public transit, extensive parks and greenways, and minimum density legislation (City of Portland, Oregon 2014). These measures enabled carbon emissions reductions of 29% between 1990 and 2010; moreover, biweekly refuse collection reduced landfill waste by 40% (Sustainable Cities Institute 2014). But Portland is an exception for the carbon-hungry United States, where, for example, only 5% of commuting trips are made on public transit, 3% on foot, and under 1% by bicycle (McKenzie and Rapino 2011).

An increasing number of LMICs have contributed remarkable innovations to public transport, even as their carbon footprints grow. China has one of the world's most rapidly growing subway, magnetic levitation (maglev), and high speed rail networks. Shanghai's metro system, globally the longest, transports 3 billion riders annually. The latest development is a wide-bodied elevated electric bus (and platform stops) that straddles several lanes of traffic, enabling cars to pass through without halting traffic (albeit with safety concerns due to reduced driver visibility).

Curitiba, Brazil (population 1.8 million), a globally-recognized model of ecological planning, demonstrates some of the dilemmas of green policies in isolation. Since the 1970s, when longtime environmental plans to accommodate population growth were implemented, Curitiba has had among the world's most efficient and heavily used bus rapid transit systems, connecting above-ground buses through an integrated network of designated lanes to eliminate gridlock (Macedo 2013). Daily transport expenditures amount to approximately 10% of income of the 2.4 million daily users, lower than in many places. Yet Curitiba has the highest car-ownership rate in Brazil and low occupancy per vehicle (average of 1.4 persons per car) (de Freitas Miranda and Rodrigues da Silva 2012). Curitiba also has an extensive recycling system used by over two thirds of residents and appealing to children—green trucks with bells that circulate neighborhoods for weekly collection (UNEP 2009). However, Curitiba's efforts have paid far less attention to periurban areas: slums (*favelas*) are expanding (if less than elsewhere in Brazil), with few of these services available (Macedo 2013).

Community-Based Adaptation

Community-based adaptation (CBA) is the engagement of (typically) poor communities in reducing vulnerability and shaping locally relevant responses to climate change, often in ways that address other environmental, social, and economic problems (Forsyth 2013). For example, in the Himalayas, melting snow is a key water source but rising temperatures in recent years have accelerated springtime melting and evaporation, depleting water supplies and jeopardizing agriculture. One man's ingenuity has resolved this problem. Ladakh Engineer Chewang Norphel had the idea of building canals to divert melting water from natural glaciers into catchment areas that can store it in the summer and autumn, form it into artificial glaciers in the winter, and then melt it again in the spring when the community needs it most for irrigation (Vince 2014).

Small islands threatened with sea-level rise and extreme weather events have engaged in various CBA efforts, from a Maldives government cabinet meeting held underwater, to an intersectoral project in BoeBoe village, Solomon Islands, integrating traditional and scientific knowledge to project different sea level rise scenarios, enhance community awareness of potential coastal hazards, and enable adaptive management (Leon et al. 2015).

Consumer Efforts

In 1969, the largest US oil spill to that time sent 80,000 to 100,000 barrels of oil into the ocean off the Santa Barbara, California coast. Outraged citizens and political leaders were inspired to found Earth Day, which some consider the beginning of the environmental movement (Clarke and Hemphill 2002). Each April 22nd is marked across the world by reminders to carpool, recycle, and turn off unneeded lights. Yet virtually nobody mentions who was responsible for the oil spill—Unocal Union Oil Company (now merged with Chevron)—and most global Earth Day efforts focus on the individual and behavior change level, not on corporate regulation/accountability or on the need to transform the fossil fuel-driven economy.

To be sure, consumer efforts are a step toward addressing environmental depletion and contamination and may raise awareness among children and wide swaths of the citizenry. These measures include:

- Using eco-friendly and recycled products (cleaning solutions, bags, clothing, food, paper)
- Composting/home vegetable gardening/rainwater collection
- Expanding use of public transit, biking, walking
- Using reusable containers and coffee mugs
- Using energy efficient appliances, bulbs
- Using appliances during nonpeak hours
- Installing low-flush toilets
- Sealing cracks, installing new windows, insulation, roofs
- Lowering thermostats (in the winter) and water heater temperature
- Lowering or eliminating air conditioner use
- Ensuring better ventilation
- Employing solar cookers
- Limiting engine idling and auto use; using fuel-efficient vehicles

Of course, the consumer approach assumes that people have the time, access, resources, and education or desire to "change their lifestyles," and thus consumer efforts are far more relevant to middle- to high-income residents of middle- to high-income countries than to members of the working class or people in low-resource settings with far lower levels of consumption overall. When combined with municipal subsidies, producer and retailer taxes, and incentives, these measures can have wider reach. Some argue that if they serve to raise the social consciousness of the population, these approaches may lead to deeper change.

But there are real limits to what individual consumers can do in the absence of larger measures because: (a) individual level solutions do not affect structural determinants, including energy, industrial, and military production and waste processes that are based on a market logic that prioritizes profits over human and environmental health; and (b) consumers are seen as the agents of change, thereby encouraging more consumerism.

Instead, efforts to improve environmental health need to draw from multiple levels (local, national, global) of regulation and reduction of the overuse and misuse of natural resources and the built environment, and from the front lines of social struggles around these issues.

Environmental (Health) Justice and Resistance Movements

Leading up to the 2014 UN Climate Summit, international advocacy groups organized People's Climate Marches around the world to press for global action on climate change. Extraordinary in scale, over 2,500 events took place in 162 countries on September 21, 2014. In New York City alone, an estimated 400,000 people participated in the march, including then UN Secretary-General Ban Ki-moon. Other cities with major demonstrations were Bogotá, New Delhi, Istanbul, Johannesburg, Lagos, London, Paris, and Berlin, reflecting growing public recognition of the need for concerted societal commitment to address climate change.

Pope Francis entered into the fray with his unprecedented 2015 encyclical on climate change and environmental harm, stressing social injustice, particularly the interaction of environmental damage with global inequality and the suffering of the poor. He argued that "a true 'ecological debt' exists, especially between the Global North and Global South, connected to commercial imbalances with effects on the environment, and the disproportionate use of natural resources by certain countries over long periods of time" (Pope Francis 2015, *Laudato si'* para. 51). Pope Francis also denounced the global skewed distribution of power and a "system of commercial relations and ownership which is structurally perverse" (ibid, para. 52) calling for climate justice to be a spiritual beacon for our time.

A groundbreaking approach to activism is the environmental justice movement. At the confluence of grassroots civil rights and environmental struggles in the United States, the term *environmental racism* was coined in 1982 by Dr. Benjamin Chavis, amid the mobilization of African-American community and church leaders, politicians, and other civil rights groups against a chemical landfill slated for a majority African-American county in the state of North Carolina. In 1987 the United Church of Christ's Commission for Racial Justice published the study *Toxic Wastes and Race in the United States: A National Report on the Racial and Socio-Economic Characteristics of Communities of Hazardous Waste Sites*, which found that toxic waste facilities were over-represented in African-American and Latino communities (Bullard et al. 2008).

Since then, environmental justice activists, together with US and international scholar-allies, have monitored and mobilized against systematic environmental racism, tracking racial discrimination in the enforcement of environmental policies and regulations and pushing for government accountability in addressing environmental injustice. But in 22 years of existence, the US EPA's Office of Civil Rights has yet to make a single formal charge of discrimination, despite hundreds of extensively documented complaints (Lombardi, Buford, and Greene 2015). Most recently, the Black Lives Matter network, which "advocates for dignity, justice, and respect" in a US-based struggle against anti-Black racism, has called for reparations for environmental racism (The Movement for Black Lives 2016).

The aforementioned examples represent just a fraction of hundreds of health and environmental justice struggles of varying sizes (Magdoff and Foster 2011) that address the main determinants of environmental degradation laid out in the first part of this chapter. Here we discuss a sample of both lay and professional, occupationally-based, solidarity-oriented, Indigenous, gender-attuned, and other organizations, experiences, and movements that have raised awareness, brought abuses to justice, and spurred the development of policies to improve environmental (health) conditions at local, national, and transnational levels.

Conservation and Natural Resource Struggles

Chipko (meaning "to cling/embrace" in Hindi) began spontaneously in 1973 when Indian villagers, mainly women, began to hug trees that were destined to be cut down. In 1980, as a result of these actions, the government of Uttar Pradesh imposed a 15-year ban on logging in the Himalayan region. Chipko movements, which are based on Gandhi's principle of *satyagraha* (nonviolent resistance), are generally autonomous and have since extended to the protection of water and other resources (Menon 2009).

Indus Consortium is a partnership among rights-based organizations in 1,700 villages in the Indus River basin area of Pakistan working on socioeconomic and environmental projects, including emergency preparedness against annual monsoons and flooding (see chapter 8). Its objectives comprise raising awareness around the effects of climate change on rural riverine populations, advocating for agricultural policies that improve livelihoods of the poor, and fighting for safe drinking water and sanitation as well as fair access to water for small farmers whose needs are trumped by water-guzzling large landholders (Indus Consortium 2015).

Kenya's Greenbelt Movement, led by the late Wangari Maathai (2004 Nobel Peace Prize winner), combines women's empowerment with environmental projects. Local women help reforest by planting indigenous tree species, enabling small-scale farmers to become foresters. Through these efforts, women are able to earn income by selling seedlings, as well as reduce their likelihood of having to travel long distances to collect firewood, thus increasing their decisionmaking power. The Greenbelt Movement, active in Congo and other countries, also seeks to reduce migration from small communities to cities.

The Center for Environmental Concerns (CEC) in the Philippines was established by fishers, farmers, Indigenous peoples, women, urban poor, and professionals to defend common access to natural resources and healthy living and working environments. Nationally, CEC engages in policy advocacy for sound environmental protection and sustainability, and globally it participates in cross-cultural exchanges and solidarity initiatives on shared environmental concerns (Center for Environmental Concerns 2014).

Agriculture and Food Sovereignty

La Via Campesina, founded in 1993, is an international movement of hundreds of millions of peasants, small- and medium-sized producers, landless people, rural women, youth, Indigenous groups, and agricultural workers (see chapter 14). La Via Campesina works for: preservation of land, water, seeds, and other natural resources; sustainable agriculture; gender and equity; and fair economic relations. Its efforts around food sovereignty as an issue of economic and social justice—and an ethical and sustainable means of countering the degradation provoked by the rise of agribusiness export markets—make it as much (or more) an environmental health actor as many explicitly environmentally focused international agencies.

Lawsuits can also serve as a form of environmental health activism. When corporations subject communities to environmental injustice, social movements may seek distributional justice (questions around who gets to use environmental resources and for what purposes) and procedural justice (access to the decisionmaking process and the ability to act in the face of breached laws or injustices). Such lawsuits can lead to meaningful change in legalistic societies but are often just a slap on the wrist for perpetrators of environmental damage. Suits brought by Latin American and US lawyers on behalf of farm workers have garnered wide attention. Several involve the hazardous pesticide Nemagon, which was banned in the United States in the late 1970s but applied for years afterwards on US-owned banana plantations in Latin America, Asia, and Africa. Most notably, in 2002 TNCs Dow, Shell, and Dole were ordered to pay US$490 million in compensation to 583 Nicaraguan banana workers who were sterilized by Nemagon (Boix and Bohme 2012).

Challenging Energy, Mining, and Other Industrial Interests

Mobilization around fossil fuel divestment has been spearheaded by environmental organizations such as 350.org, which advocates carbon-free economies. Divestment entails getting rid of stocks, bonds, and other investments linked to fossil fuel industries (oil, coal, gas, etc.). Mirroring past divestment efforts against apartheid South Africa, these mostly HIC efforts seek to delegitimize and eventually eliminate the major GHG-emitting industries. As of mid-2016 there were over 500 institutions that had committed to divestment: 35 nongovernmental organizations (NGOs), 70 educational institutions, 79 city councils/municipalities, 127 philanthropic foundations (including the Rockefeller Brothers Fund and partial divestment by the Bill and Melinda Gates Foundation but none by the Wellcome Trust, which has £564 million invested in fossil fuel companies). Among others divesting are 142 faith-based organizations, several corporations (e.g., Guardian Media Group), and various professional associations and pension funds (e.g., Norway's parliament-ordered divestment from coal, over 30% of its holdings). The total amount divested is valued at over US$3 trillion (350.org 2016).

Going from global to local struggles, among the most horrific episodes of corporate impunity and state repression of popular mobilization to achieve environmental, social, and health justice is in Nigeria's Ogoniland region, where Shell Oil Company began drilling and polluting in the 1950s. The Indigenous Ogoni of the Niger Delta organized the Movement for the Survival of the Ogoni People (MOSOP) in 1990. Hundreds of thousands of people engaged in peaceful resistance against Shell's environmental degradation and exploitation and called for regional political autonomy, a share of oil profits, and environmental cleanup. Shell was forced out of Ogoniland in 1993, even as MOSOP members continued to decry Shell's inadequate remediation amidst ongoing repression and intimidation. In 1995 Nigeria's military government hanged MOSOP's leader—acclaimed writer Ken Saro-Wiwa—and eight other Ogoni activists on false murder charges (Henshaw 2015). To the present, the contamination effects of repeated oil spills has made the Niger Delta one of the world's most polluted locales, impeding farming and fishing and subjecting millions to toxic chemical-laced water (UNEP 2011a) and extreme poverty. Accused by the hanged activists' family members of conspiring with the Nigerian government to eliminate the MOSOP activists, Shell paid a paltry US$15.5 million in an out-of-court settlement in 2009; a landmark lawsuit brought against Shell in the United Kingdom by the Niger Delta's Bodo fishing community resulted in a 2015 US$84 million settlement (Hansia 2015). Symbolically important, these suits come nowhere close to UNEP's recommended US$1 billion needed to restore the area to health.

Also engaged in energy struggles is Acción Ecológica, founded in 1986 in Ecuador, which promotes the rights of nature, awareness on contamination, and environmental justice writ large. Working at the community level—through litigation, direct protest, and advocacy (Acción Ecológica 2015)—it has played an active role in the decades-long struggle against Chevron over contamination of the Ecuadorian Amazon. For nearly 30 years, Chevron (then Texaco) engaged in substandard methods to extract oil, with the Texaco-operated Trans-Ecuadorian pipeline spilling an estimated 19 million gallons into the rainforest. Although the company left the area in 1992 and litigation against the company began in 1993, health and environmental damages to the community have yet to be compensated and litigation continues (Kimerling 2013).

In the mining arena, solidarity-oriented MiningWatch Canada was founded in 1999 as a "public interest response" to industry and government failures to protect against "the threats to public health, water and air quality, fish and wildlife habitat and community [including economic and cultural] interests posed by irresponsible mineral policies and practices in Canada and around the world" (MiningWatch Canada 2015). In addition to pushing for corporate accountability, MiningWatch advocates for policies to reduce the human and environmental destruction stemming from mineral development. In 2015 MiningWatch was part of a civil society consortium with Costa Rican courts and community organizations that successfully stopped Infinito Gold from opening a gold mine.

Numerous other formal and informal groups seek environmental justice in the face of transnational mining interests. In 2011 Indonesian communities in Papua province increased their nonviolent protests against Freeport-McMoran Mining Corporation and the Indonesian government to demand inclusion in decisionmaking—one example from decades of struggle for Indigenous rights and autonomy in the region (Khoday and Perch 2012). Also in 2011, protests escalated against coal mining in Inner Mongolia, an autonomous region of northern China, where exposure to arsenic in water from mining pollution is linked to chronic skin problems and high cancer morbidity and mortality. The contamination issue is layered with ethnic tensions between Chinese investors seeing handsome profits while Inner Mongolian herdsmen experience grassland degradation, their animals dying due to contamination and from falling into abandoned open mining pits. The protests prompted the Chinese government to adopt more stringent environmental impact assessment guidelines (Liu, Liu, and Zhang 2014), though regulations remain weak.

Occasionally, due recognition is given to environmental justice activists. Phyllis Omido, the 2015 recipient of the Goldman Environmental Prize, brought attention to the toxic impact of a lead smelting plant in her community in Mombasa, Kenya. The fumes and acid wastewater creeping into freshwater led to child illnesses and miscarriages, killing farm animals and a worker at the plant. With the support of Human Rights Watch and the UN special rapporteur on toxic waste, Omido's leadership led to the closing of the plant in 2014. She has since established the NGO Center for Justice, Governance and Environmental Action to address other environmental justice issues in Kenya (Vives 2015).

Global Solidarity Around Environmental Health and Environmental Conflicts

Greenpeace began in 1971 in Vancouver to "bear witness" to US nuclear testing off the coast of Alaska. The publicity generated regarding the dangers nuclear testing posed to wildlife pressured the US government to suspend testing in that region and create a bird sanctuary. Greenpeace is often engaged in high-profile stunts to draw media attention, but the largest was not of its own making: in 1985, French secret agents bombed and sank the Greenpeace ship "The Rainbow Warrior" in Auckland, New Zealand, killing Dutch-Portuguese photographer Fernando Pereira who had joined the voyage to document the effects of nuclear testing for the world to see. French authorities believed that the bombing would prevent Greenpeace from witnessing and protesting French nuclear testing in the South Pacific, but it only galvanized the anti-nuclear movement. Today Greenpeace has approximately 2.8 million supporters and 41 offices around the world. Its victories have included successfully combating deforestation by one of the world's largest paper companies, and extending a 2008 moratorium on soy production in newly deforested areas of the Brazilian Amazon (Brindis 2014).

On a regional level, the Latin American Observatory of Environmental Conflicts (in Spanish, Observatorío Latinoamericano de Conflictos Ambientales [OLCA]) works with communities across the region facing environmental conflicts, advising on defense of environmental rights. OLCA investigates the corporate sources of environmental and health harms and promotes community mobilization for environmental justice.

The Health and Environment Alliance (HEAL) is a European group made up of 70 organizations with involvement of doctors, nurses, cancer groups, women's groups, nonprofit health insurers, environmental groups, and public health institutes. HEAL works to bring health concerns related to hazardous chemical and pesticide exposure, air quality, electromagnetic fields, and other issues to the attention of EU environmental policymaking bodies (Health and Environment Alliance 2015).

The People's Health Movement (PHM) promotes environmental health as a human right through efforts to reclaim knowledge and science for the public good and "end imperialist [and corporate] control of the earth's natural resources" (PHM 2012). Among its causes are a campaign for protecting the health of people and the environment from mining of gas and oil, carried out through a network of grassroots organizations from Sierra Leone, South Africa, Greece, the Philippines, Malaysia, Guatemala, El Salvador, Canada, the United States, and other countries; and a campaign on food sovereignty, which included 2013 protests in Mumbai together with the group Anna Adhikar Abhiyan (Right to Food, Maharashtra) against the government's policy of cash transfers instead of subsidized staples (PHM 2015).

CONCLUSION

Learning Points:

- Every society and economic order disrupts the environment to a greater or lesser extent. However, since the rise of global industrial capitalism in the 19th century, and especially in the last 50 years, environmental damage (and its health and ecosystem consequences) has been on a far larger scale than ever before.
- While all people are affected by unhealthy environmental conditions, impoverished and socially discriminated populations experience disproportionate morbidity and mortality arising from greater resource depletion and higher exposure to the hazardous by-products of resource extraction, energy use, manufacturing, waste dumping, and other industrial processes. They are also far more likely to be displaced due to environmental degradation and climate change effects.
- A critical concern of our time, climate change both results from and amplifies environmental degradation, with potentially drastic direct, indirect, and inequitable health and population effects, even as addressing climate change in isolation will not resolve all health problems linked to the environment.
- Environmental degradation and the means to redress it are simultaneously local and global: regional variations may be understood within the logic of global capitalism. Health professionals should think and act both locally and in solidarity transnationally with movements fighting environmental injustice.
- Ameliorating and preventing damage to the environment and to human health requires actions at household, community, national, and global levels to ensure passage of protective legislation and industrial regulation; social and political movements also play an essential role in raising awareness and realizing change.

Although many environmental health problems originate with a specific issue in a single locality, environmental degradation and its health consequences transcend place, affecting us all (McMichael 2013). We are now at a crucial crossroads. The solutions to our present environmental challenges are complex and difficult. They demand clever ideas, cooperation, and intense political struggle.

What are the best means of improving environmental health and reducing the impact of human activity on particular ecosystems and the globe as a whole? Undoubtedly, a single strategy is nonexistent. Addressing climate change alone is not enough. Certainly many community and individual actions play a vital educational role in raising consciousness, enabling resilience, and helping improve local environmental conditions (Whitmee et al. 2015). Nevertheless, the world economic order, production processes, and, fundamentally, questions of (unequal) political power and resources remain central to planetary health. Even the Pope has decried climate change, its link to corporate power and greed, and the worsening social injustice and global inequalities it is propagating.

Global capital plays the preeminent role: owners of national and transnational corporations and industries (and their political partners) are the largest producers and users of energy and resources, and, ultimately, the shapers of consumption, transport, and other factors in the use and abuse of the built and natural environments. Does this mean that industry should be regulated through incentives or penalties? Or are more revolutionary measures needed? Will prioritizing health and the environment return us to steady-state economies of "simple living," or will eco-building enable an integration of new technologies and environmental protection? And how will these changes affect and engage with the governance of societies?

A step in the right direction includes Sustainable Development Goal 3's call for reducing deaths and illnesses from hazardous chemicals and air, water, and soil pollution and contamination. However, for this measure to be more than symbolic, indicators need to be sharpened, concrete strategies developed, and pressure for reaching goals applied, with a key role for scientific and social movement advocacy.

While environmental health issues are momentous problems that may appear intractable, understanding the political and power dimensions is a critical first step to generating lasting change. Whether we frame climate change as the greatest potential threat to global health (Watts et al. 2015), root health and environmental problems in inadequate governance, excessive consumption and population, and the need for new technologies (Whitmee et al. 2015), or focus on the market forces that have led to the climate crisis (Klein 2014) has enormous bearing on what approaches are taken. Stopgap solutions may avert disaster in the short term, but constructive change in the long term will require vast transformations to the very foundations of our society. Of course, health- and environmentally-friendly decisionmaking capacity rest on economic and political sovereignty, accountability, and equity, struggles that are still in the making. Both current and future generations will need to wrestle with and address these vital issues.

NOTES

1. The TSCA was only reformed in 2016 with the Frank R. Lautenberg Chemical Safety for the 21st Century Act that mandates, for the first time, that the EPA review the safety of all chemicals that are available commercially. The effects of this reform remain to be seen (Environmental Defense Fund 2016).
2. Air pollution is also a primary factor in the formation of acid rain—precipitation carrying acidic compounds formed when air contaminants interact with water, oxygen, and other chemicals, harming forests, fish, and human health.

REFERENCES

350.org. 2016. Divestment commitments. http://gofossilfree.org/commitments/. Accessed February 4, 2016.

Acción Ecológica. 2015. Criminalización de defensores de la naturaleza. http://www.accionecologica.org/criminalizados. Accessed July 4, 2015.

Agency for Toxic Substances and Disease Registry. 2014. Substance Index for ToxFAQs. http://www.atsdr.cdc.gov/toxfaqs/index.asp. Accessed July 5, 2015.

Ameer R and Othman R. 2012. Sustainability practices and corporate financial performance: A study based on the top global corporations. *Journal of Business Ethics* 108(1):61–79.

Armah FA, Luginaah IN, Taabazuing J, and Odoi JO. 2013. Artisanal gold mining and surface water pollution in Ghana: Have the foreign invaders come to stay? *Environmental Justice* 6(3):94–102.

Atuma MI and Ojeh VN. 2013. Effect of gas flaring on soil and cassava productivity in Ebedei, Ukwuani local government area, Delta State, Nigeria. *Journal of Environmental Protection* 4(10):1054–1066.

Baer HA and Singer M. 2009. *Global Warming and the Political Ecology of Health: Emerging Crises and Systemic Solutions*. Walnut Creek: Left Coast Press.

Basu R. 2015. Disorders related to heat waves. In Levy B and Patz J, Editors. *Climate Change and Public Health*. New York: Oxford University Press.

Bell ML and Davis DL. 2001. Reassessment of the lethal London fog of 1952: Novel indicators of acute and chronic consequences of acute exposure to air pollution. *Environmental Health Perspectives* 109(Suppl 3):389–394.

Bello W. 2015. No climate deal is better than a bad one. *Foreign Policy in Focus*, December 2.

Bhatt S, Gething PW, Brady OJ, et al. 2013. The global distribution and burden of dengue. *Nature* 496(7446):504–507.

Bian Z, Inyang HI, Daniels JL, et al. 2010. Environmental issues from coal mining and their solutions. *Mining Science and Technology (China)* 20(2):215–223.

Bijma J, Pörtner H, Yesson C, and Rogers AD. 2013. Climate change and the oceans – what does the future hold? *Marine Pollution Bulletin* 74(2):495–505.

Blacksmith Institute and Green Cross Switzerland. 2013. *The World's Worst 2013: The Top Ten Toxic Threats: Cleanup, Progress, and Ongoing Challenges*. New York: Blacksmith Institute.

———. 2014. *Top Ten Countries turning the Corner on Toxic Pollution 2014*. New York: Blacksmith Institute.

Blakemore E. 2015. Ask a MacArthur genius: How are hospitals trashing the planet? *The Washington Post*, October 9.

Blomqvist L, Brook BW, Ellis EC, et al. 2013. Does the shoe fit? Real versus imagined ecological footprints. *PLoS Biology* 11(11):e1001700.

Böhm S. 2015. Why the Paris climate talks are doomed to failure, like all the others. *The Conversation US Pilot*, November 30.

Boix V and Bohme SR. 2012. Secrecy and justice in the ongoing saga of DBCP litigation. *International Journal of Occupational and Environmental Health* 18(2):154–161.

Boucher D. 2014. How Brazil has dramatically reduced tropical deforestation. *Solutions* 5(2):66–75.

Breilh J. 2012. Coping with environmental and health impacts in a floricultural region of Ecuador.

In Charron DF, Editor. *Ecohealth Research in Practice: Innovative Applications of an Ecosystem Approach to Health*. Ottawa: International Development Research Centre.

Brindis D. 2014. Good news from the Amazon: Soy moratorium renewed. http://www.greenpeace.org/usa/good-news-amazon-soy-moratorium-renewed/. Accessed August 20, 2015.

Brown P and Zavestoski S. 2005. Social movements in health: An introduction. In Brown P and Zavestoski S, Editors. *Social Movements in Health*. Oxford: Blackwell Publishing.

Brulle RJ and Pellow DN. 2006. Environmental justice: Human health and environmental inequalities. *Annual Review of Public Health* 27:103–124.

Bullard RD, Mohai P, Saha R, and Wright B. 2008. Toxic wastes and race at twenty: Why race still matters after all of these years. *Environmental Law* 38:371-411.

Burkett VR, Suarez AG, Bindi M, et al. 2014. Point of departure. In Field CB, Barros VR, Dokken DJ, et al., Editors. *Climate Change 2014: Impacts, Adaptation, and Vulnerability*. Cambridge: Cambridge University Press.

Calderón-Garcidueñas L, Kuleszab RJ, Dotyc RL, et al. 2015. Megacities air pollution problems: Mexico City Metropolitan Area critical issues on the central nervous system pediatric impact. *Environmental Research* 137:157–169.

Caravanos J, Dowling R, Téllez-Rojo M, et al. 2014. Blood lead levels in Mexico and pediatric burden of disease implications. *Annals of Global Health* 80(4):269–277.

Carson R. 1962. *Silent Spring*. Boston: Houghton Mifflin Company.

Center for Environmental Concerns. 2014. Helping communities address environmental challenges. http://www.cecphils.org/. Accessed November 18, 2015.

Central Bureau of Health Intelligence (Government of India). 2015. *National Health Profile 2015*. New Delhi: Central Bureau of Health Intelligence, Ministry of Health and Family Welfare.

Chatham-Stephens K, Caravanos J, Ericson B, et al. 2014. The pediatric burden of disease from lead exposure at toxic waste sites in low and middle income countries. *Environmental Research* 132:379–383.

Christidis N, Stott PA, Jones GS, et al. 2012. Human activity and anomalously warm seasons in Europe. *International Journal of Climatology* 32(2):225–239.

City of Portland, Oregon. 2014. PP&R by the Numbers 2014. http://www.portlandoregon.gov/parks/article/422533. Accessed June 15, 2015.

Clapp J and Dauvergne P. 2011. *Paths to a Green World: The Political Economy of the Global Environment, Second Edition*. Cambridge: MIT Press.

Clarke KC and Hemphill JJ. 2002. The Santa Barbara oil spill: A retrospective. *Yearbook of the Association of Pacific Coast Geographers* 64:157–162.

Corradin C. 2016. Israel: Water as a tool to dominate Palestinians. *Al Jazeera*, June 23.

Corvalán C, Hales S, and McMichael A. 2005. *Ecosystems and Human Well-Being: Health Synthesis. A Report of the Millennium Eco-System Assessment*. Geneva: WHO.

Crosby A. 1987. *Ecological Imperialism: The Biological Expansion of Europe 900-1900, 1st Edition*. Cambridge: Cambridge University Press.

Dauvergne P. 2014. Globalization and the environment. In Ravenhill J, Editor. *Global Political Economy, Fourth Edition*. Oxford: Oxford University Press.

David Suzuki Foundation. 2014. Natural gas. http://www.davidsuzuki.org/issues/climate-change/science/energy/natural-gas/. Accessed November 17, 2015.

Davoudi M, Rahimpour MR, Jokar SM, et al. 2013. The major sources of gas flaring and air contamination in the natural gas processing plants: A case study. *Journal of Natural Gas Science and Engineering* 13:7–19.

Dear K and Wang Z. 2015. Climate and health: Mortality attributable to heat and cold. *Lancet* 386(9991):320–322.

de Freitas Miranda H and Rodrigues da Silva AN. 2012. Benchmarking sustainable urban mobility: The case of Curitiba, Brazil. *Transport Policy* 21:141–151.

Dikshith TSS. 2013. *Hazardous Chemicals: Safety Management and Global Regulations*. Boca Raton: CRC Press.

Di Renzo GC, Conry JA, Blake J, et al. 2015. International Federation of Gynecology and Obstetrics opinion on reproductive health impacts of exposure to toxic environmental chemicals. *International Journal of Gynecology and Obstetrics* 131(3):219–225.

Domínguez-Cortinas G, Díaz-Barriga F, Martínez-Salinas RI, et al. 2013. Exposure to chemical mixtures in Mexican children: High-risk scenarios. *Environmental Science and Pollution Research International* 20(1):351–357.

Eastwood L. 2012. "Silent Spring": The reckless use of pesticides in modern agriculture. http://www.globalresearch.ca/silent-spring-the-reckless-use-of-pesticides-in-modern-agriculture/5315754. Accessed October 28, 2015.

ECHA [European Chemicals Agency]. 2015. Understanding REACH. http://echa.europa.eu/web/guest/regulations/reach/understanding-reach. Accessed December 5, 2015.

El-Fadel M, Ghanimeh S, Maroun R, and Alameddine I. 2012. Climate change and temperature rise: Implications on food-and water-borne diseases. *Science of the Total Environment* 437:15–21.

European Commission. 2015. Environment: Air quality standards. http://ec.europa.eu/environment/air/quality/standards.htm. Accessed November 18, 2015.

Eurostat. 2015. Generation of waste. http://ec.europa.eu/eurostat/web/waste/waste-generation-and-management. Accessed February 4, 2016.

Evans P. 2002. Introduction: Looking for agents of urban livability in a globalized political economy. In Evans P, Editor. *Livable Cities? Urban Struggles for Livelihood and Sustainability.* Berkeley: University of California Press.

FAO. 2015. FAOSTAT Database. http://faostat3.fao.org/home/E. Accessed November 13, 2015.

———. 2016. *State of the World's Forests 2016, Forests and Agriculture: Land-Use Challenges and Opportunities.* Rome: FAO.

Field CB, Barros VR, Dokken DJ, et al. 2014. *Climate Change 2014: Impacts, Adaptation, and Vulnerability.* Cambridge and New York: Cambridge University Press.

Forouzanfar MH, Alexander L, Anderson HR, et al. 2015. Global, regional, and national comparative risk assessment of 79 behavioural, environmental and occupational, and metabolic risks or clusters of risks in 188 countries, 1990–2013: A systematic analysis for the Global Burden of Disease Study 2013. *Lancet* 386(10010):2287–2323.

Forsyth T. 2013. Community-based adaptation: A review of past and future challenges. *Wiley Interdisciplinary Reviews: Climate Change* 4(5):439–446.

Foster JB, Clark B, and York R. 2011. *The Ecological Rift: Capitalism's War on the Earth.* New York: Monthly Review Press.

Friis RH. 2012. *Essentials of Environmental Health, Second Edition.* Sudbury: Jones & Bartlett Publishers.

Friis RH and Sellers T. 2014. Epidemiologic aspects of work. In Friis RH, Editor. *Epidemiology for Public Health Practice, 5th Edition.* Burlington: Jones & Bartlett Learning.

Frumkin H, Hess J, and Luber G. 2015. Public health policies and actions. In Levy B and Patz J, Editors. *Climate Change and Public Health.* New York: Oxford University Press.

Gasparrini A, Guo Y, Hashizume M, et al. 2015. Mortality risk attributable to high and low ambient temperature: A multicountry observational study. *Lancet* 386(9991):369–375.

Glasson J, Therivel R, and Chadwick A. 2013. *Introduction to Environmental Impact Assessment,* 4th Edition. London: Routledge.

Global Asthma Network. 2014. *The Global Asthma Report 2014.* Auckland, NZ: Global Asthma Network.

Global Footprint Network. 2016. *National Footprint Accounts, 2016 Edition.* Oakland: Global Footprint Network.

Grace K, Davenport F, Funk C, and Lerner AM. 2012. Child malnutrition and climate in sub-Saharan Africa: An analysis of recent trends in Kenya. *Applied Geography* 35(1-2):405–413.

Grandjean P and Landrigan PJ. 2014. Neurobehavioural effects of developmental toxicity. *Lancet Neurology* 13(3):330–338.

Gunderson R. 2015. Meat and inequality: Environmental health consequences of livestock agribusiness. In Emel J and Neo H, Editors. *Routledge Studies in Political Ecology: Political Ecologies of Meat.* Abingdon: Routledge.

Hancock T, Spady DW, and Soskolne CL, Editors. 2015. *Global Change and Public Health: Addressing the Ecological Determinants of Health.* Ottawa: Canadian Public Health Association.

Hansia F. 2015. Shell Pays Niger Delta Community $84 Million to Settle Pollution Claims. *CorpWatch,* February 5.

Hasegawa A, Tanigawa K, Ohtsuru A et al. 2015. Health effects of radiation and other health problems in the aftermath of nuclear accidents, with an emphasis on Fukushima. *Lancet* 386(9992):479–488.

Hass A. 2014. Otherwise occupied: The Israeli 'watergate' scandal: The facts about Palestinian water. *Haaretz,* February 16.

Health and Environment Alliance. 2015. About us. http://www.env-health.org/about-us/. Accessed October 30, 2015.

Hendryx M and Ahern MM. 2008. Relations between health indicators and residential proximity to coal mining in West Virginia. *American Journal of Public Health* 98(4):669.

Henshaw K. 2015. Enemy of Big Oil, Ken Saro-Wiwa showed power of resistance. *Green Left Weekly,* November 23.

Hester RE. 2012. *Soils and Food Security.* London: The Royal Society of Chemistry.

HLPE. 2013. *Biofuels and Food Security: A Report by the High Level Panel of Experts on Food Security and Nutrition of the Committee on World Food Security.* Rome: FAO.

Hoffman R. 2014. *An Environmental History of Medieval Europe*. Cambridge: Cambridge University Press.
Hota P and Behera B. 2015. Coal mining in Odisha: An analysis of impacts on agricultural production and human health. *The Extractive Industries and Society* 2(4):683–693.
Hu J, Ying Q, Wang Y, and Zhang H. 2015. Characterizing multi-pollutant air pollution in China: Comparison of three air quality indices. *Environment International* 84:17–25.
Indus Consortium. 2015. Indus Consortium for humanitarian, environmental, and development initiatives. http://www.indusconsortium.pk/. Accessed October 14, 2015.
International Energy Agency. 2015. *World Energy Outlook 2015*. Paris: International Energy Agency.
International Rivers. 2015. Human impacts of dams. http://www.internationalrivers.org/human-impacts-of-dams. Accessed July 7, 2015.
Jaspers N and Falkner R. 2013. International trade, the environment, and climate change. In Falkner R, Editor. *The Handbook of Global Climate and Environment Policy*. Chichester, UK: John Wiley & Sons.
Jemielita T, Gerton GL, Neidell M, et al. 2015. Unconventional gas and oil drilling is associated with increased hospital utilization rates. *PLoS One* 10(7):e0131093.
Jones C and Kammen DM. 2014. Spatial distribution of US household carbon footprints reveals suburbanization undermines greenhouse gas benefits of urban population density. *Environmental Science & Technology* 48(2):895–902.
Kang M, Kanno CM, Reid MC, et al. 2014. Direct measurements of methane emissions from abandoned oil and gas wells in Pennsylvania. *Proceedings of the National Academy of Sciences* 111(51):18173–18177.
Karanja N and Njenga M. 2011. Feeding the Cities. In *State of the World 2011: Innovations that Nourish the Planet*. Washington, DC: Worldwatch Institute.
Kelley CP, Mohtadi S, Cane MA, et al. 2015. Climate change in the Fertile Crescent and implications of the recent Syrian drought. *Proceedings of the National Academy of Sciences* 112(11):3241–3246.
Khetriwal DS, Luepschen C, and Kuehr R. 2013. *Solving the E-Waste Problem: An Interdisciplinary Compilation of International E-waste Research*. New York: United Nations University Press.
Khoday K and Perch L. 2012. *Green Equity: Environmental Justice for more Inclusive Growth*. Brasilia: International Policy Centre for Inclusive Growth.
Kimerling J. 2013. Lessons from the Chevron Ecuador Litigation: The Proposed Intervenors' Perspective. *Stanford Journal of Complex Litigation* 1(2):241–294.
King B. 2010. Political ecologies of health. *Progress in Human Geography* 34(1):38–55.
Kjellstrom T, Holmer I, and Lemke B. 2009. Workplace heat stress, health and productivity – an increasing challenge for low and middle-income countries during climate change. *Global Health Action* 2(1).
Klein N. 2014. *This Changes Everything: Capitalism vs. The Climate*. New York: Simon and Schuster.
Krech S, McNeill JR, and Merchant C. 2004. *Encyclopedia of World Environmental History Vol. 1-3*. London: Routledge.
Laird BD, Goncharov AB, and Chan HM. 2013. Body burden of metals and persistent organic pollutants among Inuit in the Canadian Arctic. *Environment International* 59:33–40.
Lee M and Card A. 2012. *A Green Industrial Revolution Climate Justice, Green Jobs and Sustainable Production in Canada*. Ottawa: Canadian Centre for Policy Alternatives.
Leon JX, Hardcastle J, James R, et al. 2015. Supporting local and traditional knowledge with science for adaptation to climate change: Lessons learned from participatory three-dimensional modeling in BoeBoe, Solomon Islands. *Coastal Management* 43(4):424–438.
Levy B and Patz J, Editors. 2015. *Climate Change and Public Health*. New York: Oxford University Press.
Liu L, Liu J, and Zhang Z. 2014. Environmental justice and sustainability impact assessment: In search of solutions to ethnic conflicts caused by coal mining in Inner Mongolia, China. *Sustainability* 6(12):8756–8774.
Lofstedt R. 2014. The precautionary principle in the EU: Why a formal review is long overdue. *Risk Management* 16(3):137–163.
Lombardi K, Buford T, and Greene R. 2015. Environmental racism persists, and the EPA is one reason why. *The Center for Public Integrity*, August 3.
Luber G and Lemery J. 2015. *Global Climate Change and Human Health: From Science to Practice*. San Francisco: Jossey-Bass.
Luginaah IN and Yanful EK. 2009. *Environment and Health in Sub-Saharan Africa: Managing an Emerging Crisis*. London: Springer.
Macedo J. 2013. Planning a sustainable city: The making of Curitiba, Brazil. *Journal of Planning History* 12(4):334–353.
Macey G and Cannon JZ. 2007. *Reclaiming the Land: Rethinking Superfund Institutions, Methods and Practices*. Berlin: Springer Science & Business Media.
Magdoff F and Foster JB. 2011. *What Every Environmentalist Needs to Know About Capitalism: A Citizen's Guide to Capitalism and the Environment*. New York: Monthly Review Press.

Marcotullio P, Cooper R, and Lebel L. 2014. Climate and urbanization. In Manton M and Stevenson LA, Editors. *Climate in Asia and the Pacific Security, Society and Sustainability*. New York: Springer Netherlands.

Markowitz G and Rosner D. 2014. *Lead Wars: The Politics of Science and the Fate of America's Children*. Berkeley: University of California Press.

Marrs TC and Karalliedde L. 2012. The toxicology of pesticides. Baker D, Karalliedde L, Murray V, et al, Editors. *Essentials of Toxicology for Health Protection: A Handbook for Field Professionals* (Second Edition). Oxford University Press.

Mathew J, Goyal R, Taneja KK, and Arora N. 2015. Air pollution and respiratory health of school children in industrial, commercial and residential areas of Delhi. *Air Quality, Atmosphere & Health* 8(4):421–427.

Mayr W. 2014. The Mafia's Deadly Garbage: Italy's Growing Toxic Waste Scandal. *Spiegel Online International*, January 16.

McCaffrey K. 2008. The struggle for environmental justice in Vieques, Puerto Rico. In Carruthers D, Editor. *Environmental Justice in Latin America: Problems, Promise, and Practice*. Cambridge, MA: MIT Press.

McKenzie B and Rapino M. 2011. *Commuting in the United States: 2009*. Buffalo: US Census Bureau.

McMichael AJ. 2013. Global health: Globalization, climate change, and human health. *NEJM* 368(14):1335–1343.

McNeill JR. 2000. *Something New Under the Sun: An Environmental History of the Twentieth-Century World (The Global Century Series)*. New York: WW Norton & Company.

Menon B. 2009. Social movements and the mass media. In Chandhoke N and Priyadarshi P, Editors. *Contemporary India: Economy, Society, Politics*. Delhi: Pearson.

Miller RE, Murphy RP, Neel WH, et al. 2013. ITE's bicycle tour of the Netherlands: Insights and perspectives. *Institute of Transportation Engineers, ITE Journal* 83(3):16–23.

Moors E, Singh T, Siderius C, et al. 2013. Climate change and waterborne diarrhoea in northern India: Impacts and adaptation strategies. *Science of the Total Environment* 468:S139–S151.

Mortimer C. 2015. COP21: James Hansen, the father of climate change awareness, claims Paris agreement is a 'fraud'. *The Independent*, December 14.

Naghavi M, Wang H, Lozano R, et al. 2015. Global, regional, and national age–sex specific all-cause and cause-specific mortality for 240 causes of death, 1990–2013: A systematic analysis for the global burden of disease study 2013. *Lancet* 385(9963):117–171.

National Oceanic and Atmospheric Administration. 2014. What is the biggest source of pollution in the ocean? http://oceanservice.noaa.gov/facts/pollution.html. Accessed April 22, 2015.

National Resources Defense Council. 2014. *Tar Sands Crude Oil: Health Effects of a Dirty and Destructive Fuel*. New York: National Resources Defense Council.

Ngure V, Davies T, Kinuthia G, et al. 2014. Concentration levels of potentially harmful elements from gold mining in Lake Victoria Region, Kenya: Environmental and health implications. *Journal of Geochemical Exploration* 144:511–516.

OECD and FAO. 2012. *OECD-FAO Agricultural Outlook 2012-2021*. Paris: OECD Publishing.

OPEC [Organization of the Petroleum Exporting Countries]. 2014. *World Oil Outlook 2014*. Vienna: OPEC.

———. 2015. *World Oil Outlook 2015*. Vienna: OPEC.

Oreskes N and Conway EM. 2010. *Merchants of Doubt: How a Handful of Scientists Obscured the Truth on Issues from Tobacco Smoke to Global Warming*. New York: Bloomsbury Press.

Orozco FA, Cole DC, Forbes G, et al. 2009. Monitoring adherence to the International Code of Conduct: Highly hazardous pesticides in central Andean agriculture and farmers' rights to health. *International Journal of Occupational and Environmental Health* 15:255–268.

Osofsky HM, Baxter-Kauf K, Hammer B, et al. 2012. Environmental justice and the BP Deepwater Horizon oil spill. *NYU Environmental Law Journal* 20:99–198.

Palinkas LA. 2012. A conceptual framework for understanding the mental health impacts of oil spills: Lessons from the Exxon Valdez oil spill. *Psychiatry* 75(3):203–222.

Pearse R and Böhm S. 2014. Ten reasons why carbon markets will not bring about radical emissions reduction. *Carbon Management* 5(4):325–337.

Phalen RF and Phalen RN. 2012. *Introduction to Air Pollution Science: A Public Health Perspective*. Burlington: Jones & Bartlett Publishers.

PHM. 2012. Defending people's health and our environment from extraction industries: Statement to the 3rd Assembly of the People's Health Movement. http://www.phmovement.org/sites/www.phmovement.org/files/Statement%20of%20the%20PHM%20Working%20Group%20to%20challenge%20extractive%20industries-1.pdf. Accessed July 8, 2015.

———. 2015. PHM Campaigns. http://www.phmovement.org/en/campaigns. Accessed July 8, 2015.

PHM, Global Equity Gauge Alliance, and Medact. 2011. *Global Health Watch 2011: An Alternative World Health Report.* London: Zed Books.

Pimentel D and Burgess M. 2014. Environmental and economic costs of the application of pesticides primarily in the United States. In Pimentel D and Peshin R, Editors. *Integrated Pest Management.* Dordrecht: Springer Science+Business Media.

Pope Francis. 2015. Encyclical Letter, *Laudato si'*, On Care for Our Common Home. http://w2.vatican.va/content/francesco/en/encyclicals/documents/papa-francesco_20150524_enciclica-laudato-si.html. Accessed July 5, 2015.

Prüss-Ustün A, Bartram J, Clasen T, et al. 2014. Burden of disease from inadequate water, sanitation and hygiene in low-and middle-income settings: A retrospective analysis of data from 145 countries. *Tropical Medicine & International Health* 19(8):894–905.

Prüss-Üstün A and Corvalán C. 2006. *Preventing Disease through Healthy Environments: Towards an Estimate of the Environmental Burden of Diseases.* Geneva: WHO.

Prüss-Ustün A, Wolf J, Corvalán C, et al. 2016. *Preventing Disease through Healthy Environments: A Global Assessment of the Burden of Disease from Environmental Risks.* Geneva: WHO.

Pure Earth and Green Cross Switzerland. 2015. *World's Worst Pollution Problems 2015.* New York: Pure Earth.

Red Eléctrica de España. 2013. *The Spanish Electricity System Preliminary Report 2013.* Madrid: Red Eléctrica de España.

Richter BD, Postel S, Revenga C, et al. 2010. Lost in development's shadow: The downstream human consequences of dams. *Water Alternatives* 3(2):14–42.

Robbins P. 2012. *Political Ecology: A Critical Introduction*, 2nd Edition. Malden: John Wiley & Sons Ltd.

Rosen AM. 2015. The wrong solution at the right time: The failure of the Kyoto Protocol on climate change. *Politics & Policy* 43(1):30–58.

Rosenfeld PE and Feng L. 2011. The United States military. In Rosenfeld PE and Feng L, Editors. *Risks of Hazardous Wastes.* Oxford: Elsevier Inc.

Royte E. 2015. Urban farming is booming, but what does it really yield. http://ensia.com/features/urban-agriculture-is-booming-but-what-does-it-really-yield/. Accessed August 9, 2016.

Schecter K and Wright E. 2015. Indonesia's burning problem: Putting a stop to slash and burn. *Foreign Affairs*, November 11.

Scheele F, Wilde-Ramsing J, and de Haan E. 2011. *Uranium from Africa: Mitigation of uranium mining impacts on society and environment by industry and governments.* Amsterdam: World Information Service on Energy (WISE) and Centre for Research on Multinational Corporations (SOMO).

Scruggs CE, Ortolano L, Schwarzman MR, and Wilson MP. 2014. The role of chemical policy in improving supply chain knowledge and product safety. *Journal of Environmental Studies and Sciences* 4(2):132–141.

Sellers C. 2014. From poison to carcinogen: Towards a global history of concerns about benzene. *Global Environment* 7(1):38–71.

Senior K and Mazza A. 2004. Italian "triangle of death" linked to waste crisis. *Lancet Oncology* 5(9):525–527.

Serrier H, Sultan-Taieb H, Luce D, and Bejean S. 2014. Estimating the social cost of respiratory cancer cases attributable to occupational exposures in France. *European Journal of Health Economics* 15(6):661–673.

Sistema Nacional de Información Ambiental. 2015. Aire. http://www.sinia.cl/1292/w3-propertyvalue-15480.html. Accessed November 18, 2015.

Smith KR, Bruce N, Balakrishnan K, et al. 2014b. Millions dead: How do we know and what does it mean? Methods used in the comparative risk assessment of household air pollution. *Annual Review of Public Health* 35:185–206.

Smith KR, Woodward A, Campbell-Lendrum D, et al. 2014a. Human health: Impacts, adaptation, and co-benefits. In Field CB et al. op. cit.

Somanathan E, Sterner T, Sugiyama T, et al. 2014. National and sub-national policies and institutions. In Edenhofer O, Pichs-Madruga R, Sokona Y et al., Editors. *Climate Change 2014: Mitigation of Climate Change.* Cambridge: Cambridge University Press.

Sustainable Cities Institute. 2014. Portland, Oregon. http://www.sustainablecitiesinstitute.org/cities/portland-oregon. Accessed April 5, 2015.

Swarup A. 2009. *Haiti: 'A Gathering Storm' Climate Change and Poverty.* Port-au-Prince: Oxfam International.

Tapia Granados JA, Ionides EL, and Carpintero O. 2012. Climate change and the world economy: Short-run determinants of atmospheric CO_2. *Environmental Science & Policy* 21:50–62.

The Movement for Black Lives. 2016. Reparations. https://policy.m4bl.org/reparations/. Accessed August 9, 2016.

Thorpe D. 2015. The city where 77% of journeys are by sustainable means. http://sustainablecitiescollective.com/david-thorpe/1034816/city-where-77-journeys-are-sustainable-means. Accessed June 15, 2015.

Todhunter C. 2014. How global agri-business destroys farming. http://www.globalresearch.ca/how-global-agri-business-destroys-farming/5384510. Accessed December 10, 2015.

Trace S. 2016. *Rethink, Retool, Reboot: Technology as if people and planet mattered.* Warwickshire: Practical Action Publishing.

Triassi M, Alfano R, Illario M, et al. 2015. Environmental pollution from illegal waste disposal and health effects: A review on the "triangle of death." *International Journal of Environmental Research and Public Health* 12:1216–1236.

UN. 1992. *United Nations Framework Convention on Climate Change.* New York: UN.

———. 2011. Rio +20 United Nations Conference on Sustainable Development. https://sustainabledevelopment.un.org/rio20. Accessed April 21, 2015.

———. 2015. *World Population Prospects, the 2015 Revision.* New York: UN.

UNDP. 2007. *Human Development Report 2007: Fighting Climate Change: Human Solidarity in a Divided World.* New York: UNDP.

UNEP. 2007. *Global Environment Outlook: Environment for Development, GEO 4.* Nairobi: UNEP.

———. 2009. *Sustainable Urban Planning in Brazil.* Nairobi: UNEP.

———. 2011a. *Environmental Assessment of Ogoniland.* Nairobi: UNEP.

———. 2011b. *Waste: Investing in Energy and Resource Efficiency.* Nairobi: UNEP.

———. 2014a. *Assessing Global Land Use: Balancing Consumption with Sustainable Supply.* Nairobi: UNEP.

———. 2014b. *The Importance of Mangroves to People: A Call to Action.* Cambridge: United Nations Environment Programme World Conservation Monitoring Centre.

———. 2015a. First conference of parties to the Bamako Convention. http://unep.org/delc/BamakoConvention/tabid/106390/Default.aspx. Accessed October 26, 2015.

———. 2015b. *Global Waste Management Outlook.* Nairobi: UNEP.

———. 2015c. *Waste Crime – Waste Risks Gaps in Meeting the Global Waste Challenge: A Rapid Response Assessment.* Nairobi: UNEP.

UNEP and WHO. 2013. *State of the Science of Endocrine Disrupting Chemicals – 2012.* Geneva: WHO.

UNESCO. 2005. *The Precautionary Principle: World Commission on the Ethics of Scientific Knowledge and Technology (COMEST).* Paris: UNESCO.

UNFCCC. 2014. Status of ratification of the Kyoto Protocol. http://unfccc.int/kyoto_protocol/status_of_ratification/items/2613.php. Accessed April 2, 2015.

———. 2015. *Adoption of the Paris Agreement.* Paris: UNFCCC.

UNICEF. 2015. *Committing to Child Survival: A Promise Renewed. Progress Report 2015.* New York: UNICEF.

UNICEF and WHO. 2015. *Progress on Sanitation and Drinking Water – 2015 Update and MDG Assessment.* Geneva: WHO.

Union of Concerned Scientists. 2013. *Policy Brief: The Rise of Superweeds—and What To Do About It.* Cambridge: Union of Concerned Scientists.

———. 2014. How geothermal energy works. http://www.ucsusa.org/clean_energy/our-energy-choices/renewable-energy/how-geothermal-energy-works.html#.V6i5rjX3iYM. Accessed August 8, 2016.

———. 2015. All about oil. http://www.ucsusa.org/clean-vehicles/all-about-oil#.VkECnr_YH3A. Accessed November 9, 2015.

US Department of Energy. 2016. International Energy Statistics. http://www.eia.gov/countries/data.cfm. Accessed June 24, 2016.

US Environmental Protection Agency. 2014. Superfund remedial annual accomplishments. http://www2.epa.gov/superfund/superfund-remedial-annual-accomplishments. Accessed October 28, 2015.

———. 2015. Overview of greenhouse gases. http://www3.epa.gov/climatechange/ghgemissions/gases/ch4.html. Accessed January 15, 2016.

Vermeulen R, Silverman DT, Garshick E, et al. 2014. Exposure-response estimates for diesel engine exhaust and lung cancer mortality based on data from three occupational cohorts. *Environmental Health Perspectives* 122(2):172–177.

Victor DG, Zhou D, Ahmed EHM, et al. 2014a. Introductory chapter. In Edenhofer O et al. op. cit.

VijayaVenkataRaman S, Iniyan S, and Goic R. 2012. A review of climate change, mitigation and adaptation. *Renewable and Sustainable Energy Reviews* 16(1):878–897.

Vince G. 2014. *Adventures in the Anthropocene: A Journey to the Heart of the Planet we Made.* New York: Random House.

Vives L. 2015. East African Environmental Activist Wins Major Prize. *Inter Press Service News Agency,* April 22.

Wackernagel M and Rees W. 1996. *Our Ecological Footprint: Reducing Human Impact on the Earth.* Gabriola Island: New Society Press.

Waters CN, Zalasiewicz J, Summerhayes C, et al. 2016. The Anthropocene is functionally and stratigraphically distinct from the Holocene. *Science* 351(6269):aad2622.

Watts N, Adger WN, Agnolucci P, et al. 2015. Health and climate change: policy responses to protect public health. *Lancet* 386(1006):1861–1914.

Westing A. 2008. The impact of war on the environment. In Levy BS and Sidel VW, Editors. *War and Public Health*. Oxford: Oxford University Press.

Whitmee S, Haines A, Beyrer C, et al. 2015. Safeguarding human health in the Anthropocene epoch: Report of The Rockefeller Foundation-Lancet Commission on planetary health. *Lancet* 386:1973–2028.

WHO. 2005. *Ecosystems and Human Well-Being: Health Synthesis. A Report of the Millennium Ecosystem Assessment*. Geneva: WHO.

———. 2013. Fact sheet: Asthma. http://www.who.int/mediacentre/factsheets/fs307/en/. Accessed March 26, 2015.

———. 2014a. 10 facts on children's environmental health. http://www.who.int/features/factfiles/children_environmental_health/en/. Accessed March 21, 2015.

———. 2014b. Air quality deteriorating in many of the world's cities. http://www.who.int/mediacentre/news/releases/2014/air-quality/en/. Accessed March 22, 2015.

———. 2014c. *Burden of Disease from Ambient Air Pollution for 2012*. Geneva: WHO.

———. 2014d. *Burden of Disease from Household Air Pollution for 2012*. Geneva: WHO.

———. 2014e. Fact sheet: Lead poisoning and health. http://www.who.int/mediacentre/factsheets/fs379/en/. Accessed March 24, 2015.

———. 2014f. Fact sheet: The top 10 causes of death. http://www.who.int/mediacentre/factsheets/fs310/en/. Accessed March 28, 2015.

———. 2014g. *Quantitative Risk Assessment of the Effects of Climate Change on Selected Causes of Death, 2030s and 2050s*. Geneva: World Health Organization.

———. 2015a. Fact sheet: Health-care waste. http://www.who.int/mediacentre/factsheets/fs253/en/. Accessed October 26, 2015.

———. 2015b. Global health observatory data repository. http://apps.who.int/gho/data/view.main.34300REG. Accessed March 24, 2015.

———. 2015c. Health topics: Environmental health. http://www.who.int/topics/environmental_health/en/. Accessed October 26, 2015.

———. 2015d. *Reducing Global Health Risks through Mitigation of Short-Lived Climate Pollutants. Scoping Report for Policymakers*. Geneva: WHO.

———. 2016. *Burning Opportunity: Clean Household Energy for Health, Sustainable Development, and Wellbeing of Women and Children*. Geneva: WHO.

WHO EURO. 2013. *Health Effects of Particulate Matter: Policy Implications for Countries in Eastern Europe, Caucasus and Central Asia*. Copenhagen: WHO EURO.

WHO and UNEP. 2010. *Healthy Environments for Healthy Children: Key Messages for Action*. Geneva: WHO.

World Meteorological Organization. 2014a. *Scientific Assessment of Ozone Depletion: 2014, World Meteorological Organization, Global Ozone Research and Monitoring Project—Report No. 55*. Geneva: WMO.

———. 2014b. *WMO Statement on the Status of the Global Climate in 2013*. Geneva: WMO.

World People's Conference [on Climate Change and the Rights of Mother Earth]. 2011. Press Release: Bolivia calls for urgent high level talks on cutting climate pollution. https://pwccc.wordpress.com/. Accessed November 29, 2015.

WWAP [United Nations World Water Assessment Programme]. 2014. *The United Nations World Water Development Report 2014: Water and Energy*. Paris: UNESCO.

———. 2015. *The United Nations World Water Development Report 2015: Water for a Sustainable World*. Paris: UNESCO.

Yu W, Mengersen K, Dale P, et al. 2015. Projecting future transmission of malaria under climate change scenarios: Challenges and research needs. *Critical Reviews in Environmental Science and Technology* 45(7):777–811.

Zhou M, He G, Liu Y, et al. 2015. The associations between ambient air pollution and adult respiratory mortality in 32 major Chinese cities, 2006–2010. *Environmental research* 137:278–286.

Ziegler AD, Petney TN, Grundy-Warr C, et al. 2013. Dams and disease triggers on the lower Mekong river. *PLoS Neglected Tropical Diseases* 7(6):e2166.

11

UNDERSTANDING AND ORGANIZING HEALTH CARE SYSTEMS

Key Questions:

- How do a society's values shape its health care system?
- How do different countries organize their health care systems and what are the current approaches to health reform?
- What are the main factors affecting the organization and delivery of care?

You have just been appointed national Minister of Health. Your country's health care system has been described as failing, hospi-centric, disease-focused, inadequately-funded, poor quality, and inequitable. Civil society activists, users of health care services, the local and international media, and bilateral and multilateral organizations have documented these failures. How do you begin thinking about the paths to remedy this situation and what approach will you take to reconstruct the health care system?

As discussed throughout this text, health derives not just from a society's health care system or particular health interventions, but from an array of interlocking political, social, economic, medical/public health, and cultural factors—including living, working, and environmental conditions, social and tax policies, the larger context of financial and trade regimes, the control of resources, and the distribution of wealth and power. Health care itself sometimes contributes to premature death and disability due to iatrogenic (literally, "doctor-generated") disease—medical errors, inappropriate or substandard medicines, and illnesses and disability resulting from medical treatment or neglect.

Yet health care systems are vital for a range of reasons, from promoting health and wellness to treatment of infections to trauma care and controlling chronic diseases. Even so, the most significant health sector measures—in terms of staving off disease and premature death at a population level—are not high visibility clinical and medical services, but rather preventive and primary health care as well as public health activities including regulation of housing, water supply and sanitation, food, medicines, transport safety, occupational health, and industrial pollutants. Despite mainstream views that do not adequately incorporate these and other societal factors into (public) health system decisionmaking, health personnel, researchers, and the public are increasingly recognizing the importance of intersectoral approaches to health—how health is shaped by and ought to be considered in all kinds of policies (see chapters 7 and 13).

A particularly important influence on health systems is medicalization (medicine's expanding purview into other arenas of life), and its current phase, biomedicalization, based on the dominant techno-scientific paradigm discussed in chapter 3 (Clarke et al. 2003). Through biomedicalization, societal issues (e.g., violence, anomie, obesity) are reinterpreted as medical problems, individualized and depoliticized, and subject to technical intervention. For example, the perceived inability of some schoolchildren to concentrate in class or conform to authority is too frequently diagnosed as "attention deficit hyperactivity disorder" (ADHD) to be controlled through physician-prescribed medication (especially, but not only, in North America). This approach decontextualizes children's behavior from: their household and neighborhood socioeconomic circumstances; access to safe shelter, healthy food, and responsive educational systems; the role of racism, classism, and gender stereotypes; and even developmental stage (most ADHD diagnoses are among younger children in the classroom).

Pervasive across social classes and most societies, and often framed in highly racialized and gendered ways, is "disease-mongering"—the "selling" and labeling of conditions such as pre-diabetes, prehypertension, prostate cancer, and expansive definitions of mood disorders—to create new markets for large-scale consumption of medical products and services. Such overdiagnosis, which burdens health systems and makes access to care harder for those with serious health needs, costs more than US$200 billion annually in the United States alone (Moynihan, Doust, and Henry 2012).

Indeed, Big Pharma, private insurance companies, medical real estate, medical supplies and equipment industries, and other private actors support, directly and indirectly, the crafting of research and social policies that favor their interests and maximize their profits, irrespective of human need. All told, the "medical-industrial complex" now constitutes almost one fifth of the US economy and a rapidly growing proportion of other high-income country (HIC) and some middle-income country (MIC) economies (Chernomas and Hudson 2013). At the same time, underdiagnosis in many low- and middle-income countries (LMICs) translates into inadequate care and preventable premature death (Bowry et al. 2015).

Adding one more ingredient to this mix, just as health care can be supportive and liberating, it can also be controlling and repressive. Perhaps most clearly evidenced in the medication and (coerced) hospitalization of people with mental illness, this dual/dialectic function is also at play in required doctor's notes for school and work absences. These latent social control dimensions of medicine, and the policing powers of public health and health systems (such as through quarantine, school vaccination, and workplace checkups), can create difficult dilemmas between protecting the public and individual rights. While not resolvable in any facile way, public trust, based on transparency and accountability, is an essential element in ensuring the legitimacy and functioning of public health systems and warrants far more attention in global health.

Lastly, like any other system, health care systems incorporate their own social dynamics of power. On one level they reflect larger societal asymmetries of power by wealth, race/ethnicity, sex/gender, social class, and other characteristics among a range of actors—the state, private sector, community, and civil society. On another level there are internal occupational divisions of labor (that operate at local/national levels in all countries) creating hierarchies among managers, physicians, nurses, support staff, technicians, and others. There are also power divisions based on the predominance of the medical model whereby physicians (seek to) wield power over, variably, nurses, midwives, and traditional healers. This scientific expertise-derived pecking order between those who "possess" knowledge and those deemed "ignorant" is commonly experienced in the asymmetry of the doctor–patient relationship, even as, paradoxically, it is the embodied patient who possesses knowledge that the physician is not trained to acquire (Waitzkin 1993).

To note, the hegemonic biomedical approach very much dominates global health, yet it is not the only model of healing. In all countries, and especially in LMICs other healing models based on longstanding empirical traditions, spirituality and cultural mores, and so-called alternative healing paradigms (ancestor worship, homeopathy, traditional Chinese medicine, Ayurveda, acupuncture, and so on) exist in parallel, and may be preferred, more effective, or the only accessible care (Menéndez 2003).

This chapter begins with an explanatory framework for the different kinds of health care systems and their principles, continuing with a historical analysis of various health care systems around the world. It then discusses two key health policy approaches—primary health care and universal health coverage—and presents a snapshot of health system reforms across the world. Finally it describes the building blocks of health care systems and the challenges they face. Although "Western" biomedical and various forms of traditional medicine operate simultaneously (and at times intersect), this chapter will focus primarily on Western medicine, while recognizing the problems of biomedical hegemony. An additional qualifier: the study of *health systems*, strictly speaking, takes into account the influence on health of a broad array of determinants. By contrast, this chapter focuses principally on *health care systems*, considering the societal factors that shape the contours of health care policy, organization, and delivery, but leaving discussion of the constellation of factors that produce health and ill health to other chapters.

What Is a Health Care System?

So how do health care systems—that is, "the combination of resources, organization, financing, and management that culminate in the delivery of health services to the population" (Roemer 1991, p. 31)—fit into the global health picture?

The organization of the health care system in each country is a reflection of its political trajectory, class dynamics, and societal ideals or values. As such, countries in which free market ideology dominates have health systems characterized by private delivery, even if much of the financing is public, whereas countries with a strong social democratic tradition and where social solidarity is deeply valued have primarily publicly funded and organized health care systems.

Health policy is also influenced by the political and economic order, nationally and internationally. The proliferation of bilateral, regional, and global trade agreements, which stipulate the opening of domestic markets and the removal of constraints on competition (defined to include the public provision of health and other social services), have increased markedly the power of transnational corporations (TNCs) to influence public policies. This development affects the ability of national governments to shape social, work, and policy environments, including the provision of health care services. Of course national governments, especially of more powerful countries, are shapers of (and party to) the global trade regime and specific agreements, and thus are themselves complicit in the larger capitalist system that impedes the realization of equitable health systems in the public domain. This chapter briefly addresses the impact of market ideology on recent health reforms; chapter 9 analyzes the role of trade agreements and globalization on health and health care systems, and chapter 12 explores the role of global health and development approaches on health care financing and organization.

Health care systems come in a great variety of sizes, forms, and levels of comprehensiveness and effectiveness. Milton Roemer's (1991) classic typology categorizes health systems according to a country's economic level and social and economic values, reflecting different relations among state, market, and family in capitalist societies. But even a political economy-oriented analysis that distinguishes societies by the extent of wealth and resource redistribution cannot be all encompassing. Each system is sui generis, and all except socialist systems (which themselves were/are not identical) have at least some mix of public and private delivery and financing. Still, as discussed ahead, certain prototypical health systems have developed over time and are useful to understanding the interrelationships among patients/population, providers, funding mechanisms, and government.

Within the structure of every government there is some entity, usually a ministry or department of health, which is the official agency charged with responsibilities relating to the health of the population. The ministry of health may be the dominant provider of health services, its main function may be to supervise and regulate the work of other organizations, or both.

Many countries have a formal health policy, sometimes enshrined in the national constitution together with the right to health or the entitlement to health care. This policy typically specifies the responsibilities assumed by the state for health. Health ministries may also have mission statements, for example:

> To promote health and wellbeing of Ethiopians through providing and regulating a comprehensive package of promotive, preventive, curative and rehabilitative health services of the highest possible quality in an equitable manner (Ethiopia, Ministry of Health 2012);

and

> The General Directorate of Health prepares public health policy and contributes to its

> implementation. It pursues four main objectives: to preserve and improve population health status, to protect the population from health threats, to guarantee the health system's quality, security, and equality in access, and to mobilize and coordinate partners (France, Ministère des Affaires Sociales et de la Santé 2016).

These statements suggest that health system missions transcend provision of health care services. In reality, however, health policy is usually focused on curative, medicalized care, underemphasizing community, preventive, and integrated services while privileging biomedical and behavioral models over a political economy of health approach (Raphael and Bryant 2010). Still, the missions remain relevant: regardless of the pragmatic efficiency of health systems, they also bear symbolic efficacy—that is the societal expectation that health services be available and delivered according to agreed upon terms. We must also remember that health systems play an under-recognized but vital role in alleviating pain and suffering and caring for the sick. Even as the latter goal is rarely and unevenly achieved (and often carried out by family members), it remains uniquely a health sector responsibility. The health system's (in)capacity to care for people who are sick, including the terminally ill, is highly revealing of health inequities within and between countries.

Although mission statements may resemble one another, the way in which different countries structure their health systems varies considerably. One common misconception is that most European countries have monolithic systems of "socialized medicine" under which a person need only appear on a clinic doorstep to be showered with free services. Equally erroneous is the widespread idea that LMICs generally have inadequate health systems. As with most stereotypes, neither of these images is accurate.

Classifying Health Care Systems: A Political Economy Approach

The clearest means of classifying health care systems is according to two variables: (1) the financing and delivery of health care services, and (2) whether each of these occurs in the public or private sector (Table 11-1). Financing is the means by which funds are collected to pay for health care services. This may be mostly through public revenues (taxes, social insurance funds, income from state-owned enterprises) or predominantly through private insurance, employers, and/or user fees at the point of delivery. Delivery is the means by which health care is provided. Under public delivery, hospitals and clinics are owned and operated by the state, with medical practitioners employed, contracted, or subsidized by the government. In a system of mostly private delivery, health care professionals, and

Table 11-1 Public vs. Private Financing and Delivery of Health Care Services

		Health Care Delivery	
Health Care Financing		**Public**	**Private**
	Public	(National Health Service) UK[a] Cuba Spain[a]	(National Health Insurance) South Korea Canada New Zealand[b] Thailand[b]
	Private/Mixed	N/A[c]	*Public/Private/Out-of-pocket mix* United States Guinea

[a]Currently undergoing privatization of delivery.

[b]Universal coverage, largely publicly financed, but mix of public/private delivery.

[c]There are no health care systems that are privately financed and publicly delivered.

Source: Adapted from (Roemer 1991).

Table 11-2 Evolution of Health Systems

Health System	Type 1: Private	Type 2: Pluralistic	Type 3: National Health Insurance	Type 4: National Health Service	Type 5: Socialized Health Service
Political and ideological values	Health care as an item of personal consumption	Health care as primarily a consumer good	Health care as an insured, guaranteed service	Health care as a state-supported service	Health care as a right and state-provided public service
Position of the physician	Solo entrepreneur	Solo entrepreneur and member of practitioner group	Private solo or group practice and/ or employed by hospitals	Private solo or group practice and/ or employed by hospitals	State employee
Ownership of facilities	Private	Private, not-for-profit, and public	Not-for-profit and public, some private	Mostly public	Entirely public
Source of financing	Private out-of-pocket payments	Mix of private, out-of-pocket, and public	Primarily public single-payer	Public monopsony	Public monopsony
Administration and regulation	Market	Market, some government	Government, some market	Government	Government
Prototype	Most countries until the 19th or 20th century	United States, Peru, Nigeria	France, Taiwan, Japan, Costa Rica	Italy, Sweden (de facto)	Former Soviet Union, Cuba

Sources: Adapted from Rodwin (1984); Field (1978).

the clinics, offices, and hospitals in which they work, operate as private entrepreneurs or businesses (usually not-for-profit in systems with public financing).

Few systems fit purely into a single category. For example, the health care system in Norway—which is largely publicly financed and delivered—has a small private sector, and the United States—where health care delivery is market-driven—is largely publicly financed (covering civil servants, senior citizens, people with disabilities, and certain low-income groups), and there are publicly delivered systems for Indigenous populations and veterans. Various countries, including Brazil and the United States, further publicly subsidize private health care through tax deductions and other incentives.

Although this typology offers a useful starting point for understanding the main organizational differences between health care systems, it does not explain *how* these differences materialized. As Vicente Navarro (1993, p. 11) argues, "we cannot understand . . . our health care system by looking [solely] at the actors and agents of its delivery . . . The economic and political order—capitalism—governs the financing and delivery of our health services." Accordingly, our political economy understanding of health care systems will revisit this approach, exploring the interplay of health care system features with:

- The political system and distribution of political power, wealth, and resources
- The ownership and social structure of the economy
- Historical attributes (e.g., the role of labor movements, the legacy of colonialism, the effects of structural adjustment policies)

We begin by considering the cultural and political values, organizational principles, quality, efficiency, and equity of health care systems. These factors and values—from free market tenets to mutual aid and community-driven preferences—shape whether health is viewed as a human right as opposed to a commodity or privilege. Although such values may not be explicitly stated in national health policy, the practices and principles of a health care system typically signal its underlying values and thus help explain its organization (Table 11-2).

PRINCIPLES OF HEALTH CARE SYSTEMS

Key Question:

- What basic principles (should) inform the variety of health care systems across both HICs and LMICs?

The principles (ideally) underpinning health care systems are straightforward, even as adherence to them may be challenging.

Universality

The extent to which a health care system is universal indicates the proportion of residents who have a legal right to obtain benefits and care. Scandinavian countries are viewed as models of universality in health care systems, as all legal residents have access to the same set of benefits. Yet even in universal systems, some groups may remain excluded, such as recently arrived immigrants and refugees, undocumented persons, and temporary laborers.

Accessibility

In a highly accessible health care system, all residents are equally able to obtain care in terms of geography, resource availability (e.g., the number of clinics or health professionals per capita), and financing mechanisms. Nonetheless, access may be impeded by multiple factors, from cost and inadequacy of transportation, to facility hours of operation, lost wages from work absence, and family care responsibilities. Sociocultural barriers include differences in language and healing beliefs between providers and patients, as well as provider discrimination based on race/ethnicity, class, disability, sex/gender, religion, and other factors.

Most countries have a skewed concentration of physicians, hospitals, laboratories, and equipment in urban areas. Globally 56% of rural populations lack health coverage, compared with 22% of urbanites, resulting in, for example, maternal mortality rates that are 2.5 times higher in rural than urban areas (Scheil-Adlung 2015). Also important to access is portability, which means that people can obtain care throughout the country and are not confined to one geographic location (salient to universal health care systems).

Equity

Health equity, discussed in chapter 7, is the absence of unjust, unfair, and avoidable differences in health according to socially-defined population groups. Health care system equity refers specifically to (Flores 2006):

- Equity in access to and utilization of health care services—financial, physical, organizational, or cultural accessibility
- Equity in resource allocation—e.g., by region or employment status
- Equity in the quality and delivery of services
- Equity in health outcomes

Inequities in health systems further exacerbate other societal inequities, as the poorest and most oppressed populations typically experience greater illness and premature mortality than those more privileged, albeit with less access to care. Ill health that is a result of health care system inequities may also generate further impoverishment and thus greater health inequities. This has been termed "the medical poverty trap" (Whitehead, Dahlgren, and Evans 2001).

Comprehensiveness

Comprehensiveness refers to the array and extent of necessary services that are publicly provided and/or covered through insurance mechanisms. Priority-setting seeks to determine what constitutes comprehensiveness in different political and cultural contexts, given variety in what counts as "medically necessary." Health care systems may not cover dental, vision, midwifery, abortion, or medications, for example, as per economic, religious, or inter-professional rationales. Though a foundational principle for many countries, comprehensiveness has been increasingly undermined, especially in countries lacking universal, single-tier health care systems. As discussed in chapter 12, the emphasis on cost-effectiveness and provision of a limited "basket" rather than a comprehensive range of services is a feature of current "universal health coverage" approaches backed by various global health actors (see ahead).

Affordability and Sustainability

A stable health care system must be affordable for both health care system users and society as a whole and sustainable over the long term. Affordability describes the extent to which the system can be financed through agreed upon means (taxes, premiums [monthly or annual payments for insurance], out-of-pocket payments, etc.), and how well it "fits" with social values. A system that is financially accessible, uses resources appropriately, and is societally acceptable is more likely to be sustainable in the long term.

Quality

Quality is a key determinant of health care service utilization, system productivity, and health outcomes. Quality can be based on perception (the notion that one set of practitioners is better than another) or more "objective" measures, for instance clinical outcomes of different procedures or types of providers. Some may consider wait times or so-called "hotel services," such as private hospital rooms with amenities, to be important indicators of quality health care. Persons who lack access cannot obtain services, but those who are dissatisfied with quality may refuse to use them. When provision of even minimal services is a struggle, the quality of health care may not be foremost in the minds of health planners and providers. However, accessibility and quality go hand in hand.

Methods of gauging quality include: asking patients to report on their experience of care (their level of satisfaction); measuring differences in type of care received by income, race/ethnicity, and geographic group; examining the availability and use of certain technologies and resources; and documenting the care received and tests performed, as well as the safety and effectiveness of care (Raleigh and Foot 2010). Health status and outcomes are critical measures of health care system quality, but they also depend on a range of societal factors.

Participation

The participation of citizens in the design, delivery, financing, and monitoring of health care systems may lead to increased equity and public responsiveness, ultimately enhancing satisfaction, quality, and utilization of services. Especially important for health care organization in LMICs is that "external actors" not usurp local and citizen-led efforts that define "the needs and priorities of communities" (Cape Town Statement 2014).

At the local level, participation needs to be considered in the context of national resources and equity to ensure that well-organized communities or those that have greater access to power do not absorb more resources than counterparts that are less able to articulate demands. Potentially a hallmark of democratic decisionmaking, participation must also be understood in the context of policymaking power, as participation may be more symbolic than substantive and lead to greater community-level responsibilities, or even cooptation, without quid pro quo benefits (Ruano,

Sebastián, and Hurtig 2014). Participation also unfolds in terms of social movement demands around public funding and quality, access, and equity of care.

Organizational Coherence, Health Promotion, and Intersectoral Cooperation

A well-integrated system enhances equity, limits duplication and waste in administrative functions, maximizes efficiency (that is, goods or services supplied at the lowest possible average total cost), and minimizes confusion on the part of providers and the public. By contrast, fragmented health services—those that are not comprehensive, responsive to needs, or integrated and coordinated at different levels, or fail to provide continuity of care—fall far short of achieving coherence. Likewise, segmented health care systems, which finance and deliver health care through separate subsystems that stratify the population by income, employment sector, and social group, are both inequitable and inefficient (WHO 2011a).

A crucial partner to health care system coherence is health promotion, which is not aimed narrowly at preventing disease but rather focuses on building and enhancing the larger societal conditions that foster good health (see chapter 13). As such, adequately addressing health concerns depends on intersectoralism—multiple sectors working in tandem, including urban planning, agriculture, labor, employment, housing, education, transportation, public safety, parks and recreation, and economic and trade policy, which all influence health outcomes.

In the next section we will see how historical processes and political and economic structures have culminated in the organization of health care systems. Class-based political parties, civil society organizations, trade unions, big business, economic elites, and social movements; how the economy is regulated; the extent to which states redistribute resources; historical legacies of colonialism; and state power vis-à-vis TNC interests and global financial policy—and their interaction—all have enormous bearing on the structure of health care systems.

HEALTH CARE SYSTEM ARCHETYPES

Key Questions:

- Which health care systems serve as organizational archetypes?
- What historical and political factors have led to different trajectories of health care system development?

Family members, local healers (from herbalists to faith-healers), and even "quack" practitioners have always cared for the sick, and religious institutions have a long tradition of providing charitable care. But an organized system to oversee the health care of large populations is a relatively recent development linked to the rise of the modern (capitalist) state and the professionalization and growing dominance of scientific medicine. In particular, industrialization, the rapid growth of cities, and the demands of imperial powers highlighted the need for a healthy labor force and military. By the 19th century, increasingly organized workers and city dwellers in many countries made claims on their governments to provide health care alongside other social services. Such services were extended in only highly circumscribed fashion to colonized populations. Amid these common pressures, a diversity of organizational arrangements emerged based upon the historical trajectories, political forces, economic interests, and social values of each setting.

As we cannot possibly trace the history and political economy of the health care systems of all countries, here we present several organizational archetypes (Germany, the United Kingdom, the former Soviet Union, China, and the US's market-driven "non-system"), comparing the circumstances of their development and their broader influence. Subsequently, we review a panorama of health care system reforms at the global level and worldwide; in chapter 13 we highlight a range of settings, especially LMICs (including Cuba, Costa Rica, and Sri Lanka), in which health care systems figure as only part of an array of equitable social investments that make these countries exemplars of "healthy societies."

Social Health Insurance: Germany

Germany's system of social insurance originated in the 1880s and provides one of the earliest examples of state-guaranteed health care coverage. The working class that formed during the late 18th and 19th century Industrial Revolution—when small tenant farmers were uprooted and forcibly transformed into factory laborers across much of Europe—sought protection against the vagaries of wage employment under capitalism. Workers began to form voluntary mutual-help groups, whose members agreed to make regular contributions to a common fund that would provide cash benefits in the event of sickness or unemployment.

These semi-autonomous health funds were organized along occupational, ethnic, religious, political, and geographic lines. Over time, thousands of voluntary funds were organized. The Prussian Parliament formalized the system into law in 1854, requiring regular contributions from workers to be matched by their employers. Three decades later, after orchestrating the unification of Germany, Chancellor Otto von Bismarck—faced with increasingly militant demands of organized labor and city dwellers—introduced a series of social insurance programs to protect vulnerable urban workers from the hazards of dangerous factories and life in unsanitary environments. The 1883 Sickness Insurance Act made sickness fund coverage obligatory for low-wage workers and established guidelines for regulation. The following year Bismarck introduced a law covering workers in case of industrial accidents, with all contributions made by employers. While industrialists decried the programs as unfair burdens, they effectively boosted worker productivity and profits. Bismarck's political strategy was to suppress social unrest and preempt the growing success of socialist parties through emphasis on "carrots" over repressive "sticks" (Sigerist 1943).

This was the dawn of the concept of social security, which has since spread to other countries in Europe, Latin America, Asia, and beyond. Whereas it took Germany over a century to legislate mandatory social health insurance coverage from its initial laws, Costa Rica realized this in 20 years by 1961, and South Korea in 26 years by 1989 (Carrin and James 2004). In Germany and elsewhere, social security protection was extended to "old age" pensions, disability, unemployment, maternity, death, and survivors' benefits, and children's allowances.

Despite the disruption of two world wars, the fascist Third Reich, the 1949–1990 division into two countries (under which all East Germans were covered by national health insurance) and reunification, Germany's decentralized system has proved extremely durable (Box 11-1). Today health insurance coverage is mandatory for all German citizens and residents, with 86% of the population covered by public, statutory health insurance via sickness funds, 11% by private health insurance (covering civil servants, higher income individuals opting out of statutory insurance, and, mostly, self-employed

Box 11-1 Basic Features of Germany's Social Insurance System

- Publicly funded social health insurance is compulsory for employees earning up to €54,900 (2015) and their dependents, financed through shared payroll (employer and employee) and income taxes; coverage for low-income and unemployed persons is government-subsidized.
- Health insurance is provided via more than 130 competing nonprofit, autonomous, nongovernmental health insurance plans—"sickness funds."
- Public, private nonprofit, and a growing number of private hospitals are reimbursed for patient care by sickness funds through a prospective system of diagnosis-related fees.
- Ambulatory care physicians, in solo or shared private practice, and organized in regional associations, are paid by capitation or fee-for-service, under negotiated rates.
- Patients are free to select any generalist or specialist physician.

Source: EU Commission (2013).

persons whose premiums skyrocket in late adulthood), and 3% by sector-specific funds (e.g., military) (Mossialos et al. 2016). The occupationally and geographically based sickness funds provide a comprehensive package of benefits, including drugs and appliances, basic dental care, paid sick leave, and, until recently, visits to health spas. Since 1993 there has been a separate mandatory long-term care insurance system. Almost one third of those covered by statutory insurance purchase supplementary insurance for additional benefits such as private hospital rooms. In 2015, public sources accounted for approximately 85% of health sector financing, with total health care spending at 11.1% of GDP (OECD 2016).

The sickness funds are nonprofit organizations. They do not provide medical care directly, instead functioning as financial intermediaries. Physicians in Germany work as private practitioners, either providing ambulatory care (medical services that do not require hospitalization) or working in hospitals. Hospital-based physicians are salaried by their hospitals (formerly public or nonprofit but increasingly private), which receive operating income by billing the sickness funds. Ambulatory care visits are paid on a mixed fee-for-service and capitation basis (i.e., physicians receive fees for each service, adhering to a list of allowed services by diagnosis; physicians who exceed a quarterly budget ceiling for their pool of patients are liable for the excess expenditures), as negotiated between sickness funds and doctors' associations.

The fragmented historical development of insurance schemes in various countries with national health insurance, like Germany, has led to the existence of separate plans for government employees, railroad workers, miners, sailors, and other groups. Many countries also maintain independent social security funds for agricultural workers and the self-employed. Such stratified and segmented systems, pervasive also in Latin America (Birn and Nervi 2015) and elsewhere, can generate large inequities among beneficiaries if left unregulated by the government. Nevertheless, a general consensus prevails in Europe and many other countries that health care is a societal responsibility, not a private one. Health care financing remains predominantly public, with delivery of services split between private and public arrangements.

National Health Service: United Kingdom

The United Kingdom has a long tradition of mutual aid societies and of government regulation of medical practice and the welfare of the poor. In 1804 England's "friendly societies" (which, like Germany's sickness funds, provided health coverage and other mutual assistance) had 1 million members, growing to 7 million by 1900. Some employers began to support these societies because they were good for business. As elsewhere, those who could afford to stayed away from hospitals, where the risk of death was higher.

By 1911, British Prime Minister Lloyd George's government was determined to make medical care more generally available to the poorest sectors of the population and passed the National Insurance Act. It mandated basic medical benefits and sickness compensation for workers earning, at that time, under £160/year, funded through tripartite contributions from workers, employers, and the state. Money was collected by the government and benefits were administered by "approved" societies, including a burgeoning number of competing private insurance companies that covered millions of women and other workers not invited to join friendly societies. Doctors were paid by capitation through local insurance committees made up of insured workers, doctors, and government officials. Although the number of people covered by social insurance doubled overnight, the reform did not cover dependents, specialist or hospital care, or large swaths of the population (Whiteside 2009).

While government insurance was popular, the increasingly chaotic and inadequate arrangements remained impermeable to reform. Two world wars and the Depression left large numbers of people unemployed and with growing medical needs—in 1938 only half the population was covered by the 1911 legislation. In 1942, the government-commissioned Beveridge Report recommended a broad social security package of state insurance to cover unemployment, ill health, old age, and widowhood as well as allowances to meet family needs. The report famously called for: "A comprehensive national health service [to] ensure that for every citizen there is available whatever medical treatment he requires, in whatever form he requires it" (Beveridge

1942, p. 158). In its subsequent proposal for a postwar national health service, the Ministry of Health reiterated William Beveridge's recommendation, emphasizing the need to "divorce the care of health from questions of personal means" (Ministry of Health of Great Britain 1944, p. 47).

The report's biggest contribution was to unify social policy across classes by proposing a single social insurance scheme for the whole nation, financed through income taxes. Basic protection—through a public and universal health service—against the hazards of illness and mortality and the vagaries of the economy was, like the vote, to be every citizen's birthright, meshing well with the population's social solidarity and rising expectations following years of Depression and wartime sacrifice.

A critical factor was the landslide Labor Party victory in 1945 (its first majority government), which ushered in sweeping welfare state reforms. An outgrowth of prior reforms and proposals, the plans for a National Health Service (NHS) still faced considerable opposition from the British Medical Association, which feared loss of physician autonomy and insisted on the right to private practice. For almost two years left-wing Minister of Health Aneurin Bevan waged an uphill battle against doctors and the Conservative Party, finally shepherding the NHS's launch in 1948, with a concession to doctors that they could remain in private practice rather than becoming salaried (Webster 2002). In short order, health insurance coverage was extended to the whole of the population, benefits were expanded, and hospitals were nationalized (in order to control their size, location, and operations). By no means was the NHS fully centralized: regional hospital boards were created, each centered in a university medical school, with hospital management committees overseeing nonteaching hospitals. County and borough councils were charged with community and environmental health services (Box 11-2).

Various other countries—such as Sweden, Spain (whose system is facing creeping privatization and cuts), and Chile (which underwent a major privatization reform in the 1980s, creating large inequities between public and private health care systems [Núñez and Chunhuei 2013])—adopted similar models.

In the 1980s, Conservative Prime Minister Margaret Thatcher's zealous pursuit of government downsizing and market ideology led to a major 1982 NHS reorganization (Scott-Samuel et al. 2014). However, the public's collective support for health care as a right forced her to defend the principle of universal access to health care regardless of ability to pay. Subsequent reforms created an "internal market," whereby, in a highly unpopular program, general practitioners (GPs) were encouraged to compete against one another as fundholders responsible for purchasing care for their patients (Light 2003). Starting in the late 1990s, Britain's New Labour government reversed some reforms, increased funding,

Box 11-2 Basic Features of the NHS[a]

- Comprehensive coverage for all residents.
- One system funded mostly through taxation (with structural differences under devolved local administrations in Northern Ireland, Scotland, and Wales).
- Mostly free at the point of service, although cost sharing is growing.
- The national government oversees primary care and delivery of most specialty and hospital care services through trusts, contracting to the private sector for some elective surgery.
- Hospital medical consultants (specialists) are generally employed in public hospitals.
- Independent GPs act as gatekeepers to specialized care and are paid via primary care trusts through a mix of capitation, salary, and fee-for-service methods.
- Other health professionals, including dentists, optometrists, and pharmacists, practice on a more independent commercial basis with few subsidies.

[a] Basic features up until 2012 Act; currently under reform.

reduced waiting times, and focused on primary care, while opening the door to further privatization, with often insidious competitive mechanisms increasing inequities in access (Toynbee 2007).

But "the most egregious act of vandalism" has been the 2012 Health and Social Care Act, imposed by the Conservative government that came into power in 2010 (and was reelected in 2015) (Pollock 2015a). The Act's confusing and extremely controversial reorganization of the NHS has wreaked havoc by abolishing primary health care trusts and Strategic (regional) Health Authorities, fragmenting the entire system. Most destructively, it has removed government responsibility for provision of care in England (but not the rest of the UK) and infused market forces via private administration and commercial contracting. These reforms were made in the name of cost-savings, even though the United Kingdom has long had one of the most efficient (and lowest per capita health spending) systems among 11 OECD countries (Davis et al. 2014). In recent years government health spending accounted for close to 80% of the total (OECD 2016), mostly funded by general taxes, with approximately 11% of the population holding private health insurance (King's Fund 2014).

Still, thus far, the NHS has managed to retain one of its key characteristics—a tax-based system, albeit with out-of-pocket payments growing to almost 15% of total health expenditures (OECD 2016). Ironically, the British Medical Association, once one of the NHS's fiercest opponents, has come out strongly in favor of a publicly-funded and provided NHS and of ending the market in health care (Pollock 2015b). The years ahead will prove pivotal as to whether the NHS will be reinstated or will wither (Owen 2014).

The uncertainty faced by the government following the June 2016 referendum calling for the UK's departure from the European Union (known as Brexit)—pitched in no small measure as enabling the freeing of funding to shore up the NHS—now appears to be replaced with a drive towards privatization of clinical services, as per the 2012 Act (Scott-Samuel 2016). Meanwhile Brexit is projected to jeopardize health and health care in multiple ways by: allowing Britain to scale back its environmental and public health protections; impeding intra-EU movement of health professionals, who have filled key staffing needs; provoking a loss of research funding and limiting public health cooperation; ending intra-EU health care treatment, and so on (McKenna 2016).

A Centrally Planned Health Care System: The Former Soviet Union

In contrast to the stepwise creation of health care systems in Germany and Britain, the Soviet system was born of radical change. The Bolshevik Revolution of 1917 defeated the monarchy and created a new government that was almost immediately faced with economic crisis and civil war. Soon after the Bolsheviks came to power, all private hospitals, clinics, and pharmacies were nationalized. In July 1918, the People's Commissariat of Health Protection was established as the central body in charge of the new nation's health care system and all aspects of public health—including medical and public health research, production of medicines, and health propaganda (promotion of healthy living)—with health commissar Nikolai Semashko at the helm until 1930.

Initially, the major issue in the Soviet Union was the control of epidemic diseases. Typhus infected tens of millions, and millions died. As Lenin famously declared in 1919, "Either socialism will defeat the louse, or the louse will defeat socialism." Accordingly, the Russian Communist Party set as its immediate tasks (Roemer 1991):

1. The implementation of broad sanitary measures such as the improvement of health conditions in residential areas (protection of soil, water, and air); the establishment of communal feeding based on scientific-hygienic principles; the organization of measures to prevent the outbreak and spread of contagious disease; and the enactment of sanitation legislation
2. The control of social diseases (e.g., tuberculosis [TB], venereal diseases, alcoholism)
3. The provision of accessible, free, and efficient medical and pharmaceutical services

Due to the territorial vastness and diversity of conditions, health commissariats were set up in a decentralized manner in each constituent republic. Under the new Constitution of 1923, and reaffirmed in 1936, the federal government established general rules for the protection of health, with uniform principles of Soviet medicine applied in all republics:

> The Soviet state acknowledges the right of every citizen of the USSR to obtain not only full medical attention, but also material assistance during illness, in old age or in invalidism at the expense of the state. Soviet mothers have the right to obtain the material assistance of the state during pregnancy, childbirth, and the rearing of their children. These rights are guaranteed by the Constitution of the USSR (1936, Article 120).

A distinctive feature of Soviet public health was strong central planning, involving the building of a massive intertwined network of health care facilities (hospitals, sanatoria, research institutions, as well as clinics and dispensaries) and the personnel to staff them. The national government projected the numbers of health workers needed and placed personnel accordingly, with tens of thousands of new doctors trained in the 1930s. Occupational health and community clinics, plus specialized TB, venereal disease, and cancer care dispensaries, were also prioritized to address the needs of industrial workers and city dwellers (Sigerist 1937). Local facilities made requests for equipment and personnel, which were forwarded up through the system; allocations of resources came from the top down (Box 11-3). Still, as in most countries, the health care system was marked by unequal quality across regions and remained underfunded, with coverage of the population prioritized over quality.

From the users' point of view, the system began at the local polyclinic, a multifunction health center located primarily in urban areas and industrial settings. Pregnant women, children, and workers attended distinct, specially staffed and equipped institutions. Rural areas had health posts staffed by paramedical personnel, initially *feldshers* (assistant doctors), and then mostly midwives and nurses. In rural areas community hospitals doubled as polyclinics. Patients with complex conditions could be referred up the system to district-level or larger hospitals. As elsewhere, specialized hospitals delivering increasingly complex services consumed growing portions of the health budget, which by the 1970s became more and more strained.

All personnel in the Soviet system were full-time government employees. Although private practice was strictly banned, persistent complaints about inefficiency and lack of service led to unofficial "moonlighting" by physicians during their off hours. With *glasnost* (openness) and *perestroika* (restructuring) in the late 1980s, a small amount of private practice was tolerated, and a few private clinics and fee-for-service practices operated openly in the larger cities.

The polyclinic-based system was adopted by other socialist countries—Cuba, North Korea, Vietnam, Poland, Czechoslovakia, among others—with greater or lesser fidelity depending on prevailing economic and social conditions.

The dissolution of the USSR and the creation of the Russian Federation in 1991 provoked large-scale privatization, and one of the world's most rapid and remarkable declines in GDP and in life expectancy (see chapter 3). This economic and social dismantling (which occurred to an equal or lesser extent in the former Soviet republics) resulted in major changes in the organization of the health care

Box 11-3 Basic Features of the (Former) Soviet Model

- Centrally planned and government operated facilities and service provision.
- Strong focus on prevention, occupational health, and community health.
- Doctors employed by the state, with medical training centrally planned.
- Comprehensive coverage—free of charge—for all citizens via extensive networks of facilities, starting with polyclinics in the local neighborhood or workplace (or community hospitals in rural areas) through to tertiary and specialty hospitals.
- Funded through general revenues (from state-owned enterprises).

system, including the opening of the private health care market.

The post-Soviet Russian Constitution retained the right to free medical care, but the public health care system met with severe budgetary constraints, even as oil and mineral revenues began to fill government coffers. A mandatory health insurance system based on payroll taxes was introduced in 1993, with shortages, long waiting times, and quality of care problems persisting, improving briefly, and then deteriorating once again (Rechel et al. 2013). There has been a significant loss of personnel, drug supplies, and equipment, especially outside Moscow and St. Petersburg, accompanied by burgeoning rates of both chronic (e.g., heart disease, cancer) and reemerging infectious diseases (e.g., HIV, TB, diphtheria, whooping cough). Access to services is considerably worse in rural than urban areas, and primary care services are underfunded compared with inpatient care (Popovich et al. 2011), though recent reforms have sought to improve access for vulnerable groups (Marten et al. 2014). Most health care services continue to be provided by the under-resourced public sector (supplemented significantly by under-the-table payments, further driving inequities in access), with a growing private sector covering elites and the middle class in major cities (Gordeev, Pavlova, and Groot 2014). Private spending constitutes over 52% of all health expenditures, 92% of which is paid out-of-pocket (WHO 2014a).

From Maoist Doctors to Market Socialist Hodgepodge: The People's Republic of China

With roughly one fifth of the world's population, China has become one of the world's most rapidly growing economic powers, following a century of dramatic political swings. The multi-millennia-long Imperial Period, which generally had a centralized bureaucratic state supported by an agrarian society, ended in 1911. As in many places, medical care in the 19th century was characterized by enormous pluralism, involving a range of traditional and spiritual practitioners, as well as Western missionaries who followed a mixed paradigm. During the ensuing Nationalist period under the Guomindang government, Western medicine made tentative steps into China via Christian missionaries and the Rockefeller Foundation, which starting in 1915 invested substantial sums in the Peking Union Medical College. Into the 1930s, the Foundation, assisted by the League of Nations Health Organisation, also operated a set of rural health clinics following social medicine precepts (Litsios 2005). Most of the population continued the long-standing practice of consulting multiple practitioners from various traditions, even as Western and traditional Chinese medicine adopted some of one another's precepts (Andrews 2014).

Meanwhile, pressured by Western powers, the Guomindang enlisted traditional medicine practitioners and trained them in public health to control pneumonic plague and other epidemic diseases, especially in urban areas. Under Japanese occupation (1937–1945), the internally-exiled Nationalist government pursued wartime medical and health measures, while the Communist Red Army was organizing public health and primary care services in its rural base areas and attempting a syncretization of Western and Chinese medicine (popularizing the former and scientizing the latter) (Yip 1995).

The successful revolution under Mao Zedong's forces and the establishment of the People's Republic of China in 1949 resulted in a period of cooperation with the Soviet Union lasting until 1960, with Soviet influence enduring for many years afterwards. Private property, including hospitals, was nationalized by the state, and rural land was redistributed to collectives of peasants, with rural public health continuing as before the revolution. Private medical practice was also phased out. Shanghai, for example, had 10,885 private physicians in 1950, reduced to zero in 1966. Chinese and Western medicine began to be unified, first via training Chinese practitioners in Western understandings, then the reverse. Amid Cold War tensions during the Korean War, the Chinese government—claiming US germ warfare attacks—launched patriotic hygiene campaigns to mobilize urbanites and educate the peasantry (Rogaski 2002).

During the Cultural Revolution from 1966 to 1976, formal medical education was halted, and physicians and professors were sent to do active labor in the countryside. In 1968 a system of "barefoot doctors"—local workers selected by their comrades and given several months of training—was created as China's first national network of practitioners serving the rural masses. These part-time medical workers earned regular work points for the time spent practicing medicine in lieu of laboring in the fields. In this way, accessible, low-cost, basic medical services were extended to 90% of villages and financed communally and by small family contributions. Though hailed as heroes domestically and helping shape the approach promulgated by the 1978 World Health Organization (WHO)-United Nations Children's Fund (UNICEF) International Conference on Primary Health Care, the barefoot doctors were not exactly purveyors of "one needle and a handful of herbs" as portrayed by government propaganda. Pressed for time and initially unsure of themselves, they employed Western medicines, vaccinations, and Chinese herbs and relied on the expertise of the urban doctors undergoing rural re-education (Gross 2016). As a result, while barefoot doctors played a role in the spread of Western medicine (and waning of Chinese medicine) in some semi-urban areas (Fang 2012), at bottom a new type of revolutionary medicine developed that was neither Chinese nor Western medicine, but was also not the revolutionary medicine the state imagined it was propounding (Gross 2016).

Enormous health gains were experienced in this period thanks to vast improvements in living and social conditions, including the new primary health care system. Between 1952 and 1982, life expectancy went from 35 to 68 years, infant mortality plunged from 250 to 40 deaths per 1,000 live births; and the overall population almost doubled to over a billion people.

After Mao's death in 1976, the policies of the Cultural Revolution were criticized and repudiated. In the 1980s China adopted a "socialist market economy" and increasingly participated in and was influenced by the World Bank, UNICEF, WHO, and other international agencies (having rejoined the UN and WHO in 1972). Medical schools reopened, the private practice of medicine was sanctioned, and the commune system was dismantled in favor of individual production. Once communes—the funding source for rural public health—were gone, no alternative financing scheme was put in place by the government. As a result, the rural population returned to paying for care out-of-pocket. With the barefoot doctor title officially abandoned, many stopped practicing, about half upgraded their skills and after passing qualifying exams opened private practices in rural areas, and the remainder became paramedical practitioners or hygienists.

By the early 1990s, cooperative medical schemes remained for only 5% of rural residents, with all others paying for medical services out-of-pocket. In the mid-1990s the Chinese government acknowledged that in poor rural areas, medical expenses could be ruinous to peasants with low incomes, and it began to renew rural medical schemes based on decentralized social insurance. Widespread discontent spurred the 2003 founding of a new Rural Cooperative Medical Scheme (RCMS), mostly government-funded with some individual and farmer collective contributions. RCMS insures over 800 million people, 98% of China's rural population, with 70% to 80% of inpatient spending reimbursed, but only for 20 "high-cost" conditions (Meng and Xu 2014).

Urban residents are served by two main insurance programs. One is the Urban Employee Basic Medical Insurance (UEBMI) for civil servants, and workers in state-owned, collective, and private enterprises, covering approximately 256 million people and financed by employer and employee contributions pooled at the municipal level. The other is the Urban Resident Basic Medical Insurance (URBMI) for those not working, such as children, students, the unemployed, the elderly, and people with disabilities; it serves 271 million people (Meng et al. 2015). Individual contributions make up a major portion of financing for URBMI, supplemented by some public funding. URBMI is less comprehensive than UEBMI, covering only hospitalization and severe illness (Qin, Pan, and Liu 2014), and 75% of inpatient billing. In 2007, a supplementary Medical Financial Assistance system was established to cover medical care for over 70 million people with severe disabilities and illnesses, and for elderly patients from low-income families (Marten et al. 2014).

China's aim to achieve universal coverage by 2020—atop its goals of increasing the scope of insurance benefit packages, strengthening primary care, implementing an essential medicines list, and improving public hospitals—has been marred by fragmentation across the various schemes with no universal way of accessing care. For example, the separation between rural and urban insurance schemes is problematic for the over 200 million migrant workers who lack job stability and are eligible to receive coverage only in rural areas (Qin, Pan, and Liu 2014) (Box 11-4).

Significantly changed from just a decade ago, China's health care system is plagued by numerous problems (Blumenthal and Hsiao 2015). Government-set medical fees are intentionally low to ensure affordability. Because prescribing and dispensing drugs is one of the few ways doctors can augment their incomes, they become pharmacists, leading the well-off to become over-medicated, and the poor unable to afford (regulated) medicines. A much repeated statistic (under-) estimates that 200,000 to 300,000 people die each year in China due to poor quality medicines. Meanwhile, privatized hospitals, with few regulatory controls, require and repeat a multitude of unnecessary, expensive tests followed by equally unnecessary procedures and surgeries, including caesarean sections, even as public health and prevention services have been squeezed by the pay-as-you-go system since most people do not recognize the value of paying for preventive services.

Despite rapid economic growth, public spending on health is relatively low, with out-of-pocket spending accounting for 34% of the total, especially burdensome for rural and low-income urban populations, whose insurance only covers a limited benefits package. Indeed, regional differences in health care spending and human resource distribution remain high (rural Chinese have half the doctors and spend twice as much of household income on health care compared with city dwellers), as are socioeconomic health inequities as measured by life expectancy, child mortality, and maternal mortality (Meng et al. 2015).

Market-Driven Health Care: The United States

It is difficult to speak of a health care system in the United States. Even after the passage of a major health reform law in 2010, the Patient Protection and Affordable Care Act (ACA), also known as "Obamacare," it is one of the world's most fragmented, bureaucratic, and inequitable examples of health services organization. Strikingly, despite delivering some of the world's most technologically advanced medicine, and being a leader in medical research, the United States ranks last out of 11 wealthy countries in terms of mortality amenable to medical care (Davis et al. 2014), infant mortality, and life expectancy at age 60. In addition to delivering poor outcomes, health care in the United States is far more expensive than in any other country. In 2015, US health care spending totaled a whopping US$3 trillion, US$9,451 per person, and 17% of its GDP compared with an OECD average of 9% (OECD 2016). The market-driven system in the United States generates inordinate waste on billing, marketing, administration, corruption, and profits. Overhead consumes 31% of US health spending, including 25.3% of hospital spending (Himmelstein et al. 2014).

Although 17 million people have gained insurance since the coverage expansion provisions of Obamacare went into effect in 2014, nearly 30 million US adults still have no health insurance at all (Congressional Budget Office 2015), and 31 million more are underinsured (Collins et al. 2015), together comprising approximately 40% of the adult population under age 65. The problems of coverage gaps, high out-of-pocket spending, and spiraling

Box 11-4 Basic Features of Health Care under China's "Market Socialism"

- Former "barefoot doctor" system abandoned, though more rural doctors now in practice.
- Three separate systems: better-resourced and organized urban worker system, with more comprehensive benefits; inadequately resourced systems for rural, urban unemployed, and low-income residents; migrant workers left out.
- Insufficient regulation of medical practice and pharmaceutical prescriptions.
- Large geographic inequities and high out-of-pocket expenditures, with inadequate public sector funding, exacerbated in rural areas by devolution of financing responsibilities to the lowest level of government.

costs—particularly for medications, with several new drugs costing more than US$100,000 per treatment course—persist, demonstrating the limits to a market-based system.

Notwithstanding over a century of political struggle, the United States is the only HIC that does not provide universal health insurance to its population. Analysts have ascribed the problem, variously, to: private interests (insurance, hospital, and pharmaceutical corporations and other businesses) with deep pockets and their armies of lobbyists; deep-seated individualist values (Quadagno 2004); and the absence of a labor party that mobilizes around working class needs (Hoffman 2003; Navarro 1989). Amid the misery of the 1930s Depression, national health insurance was excluded from social security legislation by a powerful alliance of insurance companies, business interests, physician groups, and hospital associations; legislative efforts were again defeated in the 1940s, 1970s, and 1990s, despite wide public support (Birn et al. 2003).

The US's largely private, employer-based health insurance system was cemented during World War II, when the mobilization of millions of soldiers left a shortage of workers, and the federal government encouraged companies to attract workers with insurance benefits (because wage and price controls precluded salary incentives). Unions subsequently incorporated these benefits into their bargaining packages. Meanwhile, insurance companies proliferated, becoming highly profitable.

Significant, if segmented, gains came in 1965 with government health plans for senior citizens and persons with low incomes, neither covered by workplace insurance. Medicare, a quasi–single-payer system, now serves 54 million people: those over 65 (regardless of income), people with end-stage renal disease, and persons under 65 who have permanent disabilities. Funded through taxes, monthly or annual insurance premiums, and out-of-pocket cost-sharing (deductibles and coinsurance), Medicare consists of medical (covering outpatient and preventive services) and hospital (covering inpatient acute care, short-term nursing care, and hospice) insurance plans, both based on private-sector delivery, plus optional outpatient prescription drug coverage. Medicare's privately-administered plans have inflated costs by US$280 billion since 1985 (Hellander et al. 2013). Medicare is one of the most popular social programs in the United States, after Social Security, and has been well-funded, in large part because it is universal, with rich and poor seniors in the same system. However, today its benefits are inadequate, leaving seniors with average out-of-pocket spending of US$4,500 annually.

A less well-funded government program, Medicaid, provides public insurance for low-income individuals, covering around 70 million people at some point during the year. With federal co-financing and broad guidelines, each state operates its own system, resulting in varying eligibility criteria, coverage, and quality. Although 70% of Medicaid beneficiaries are poor children and (primarily) working parents, including pregnant women (Salganicoff, Ranji, and Sobel 2015), most Medicaid spending is concentrated on the acute and long-term care needs of persons with disabilities and low-income senior citizens (Paradise 2015). A separate state-based health insurance program was established in 1997 for children (and in some states, parents) in low-income families above the poverty line who are not Medicaid-eligible. Federally subsidized, the program covers 8 million children, but long-term funding is not guaranteed.

Together, Medicare and Medicaid cover over one third of the population and account for almost half of US health care expenditures (the US colony/possession of Puerto Rico, with 60% of its population insured by these two programs, receives far lower reimbursement from the federal government than do the 50 states [Portela and Sommers 2015]). There are also public systems for veterans and Indigenous populations (and some prison inmates), and publicly-funded private insurance for members of Congress, government employees, and the military. Underfunded public hospitals, and community and free clinics are available in some cities. About half of working-age Americans have employer-based insurance (US Census Bureau 2014), and businesses providing coverage receive annual tax subsidies of nearly US$300 billion. Altogether, over 64% of US health expenditures are financed by taxes (Himmelstein and Woolhandler 2016), with over 20% financed out-of-pocket and the remainder by businesses. It is a myth that the United States has a privately funded health care system (Box 11-5).

In the 1990s, with health expenditures climbing to over 12% of GDP, "managed care" became a

Box 11-5 Basic Features of Health Care Financing and Delivery in the United States

- Almost two thirds publicly (taxpayer) financed, but overwhelmingly administered and delivered through the private sector.
- Private employer-based health insurance covers over half of the population, with significant public financing: employers receive tax subsidies for providing private health insurance (16% of tax-financed health expenditure).
- A quarter of employer-based insurance is for government employees whose coverage is publicly financed (10% of tax-financed health expenditure).
- Government-funded, albeit increasingly privately administered, system for the elderly and persons with disabilities (Medicare); separate public state-based systems for low-income groups (Medicaid, under mostly private administration); and publicly financed and delivered systems for Indigenous populations and veterans.
- Dominance of for-profit, market-driven health care via thousands of health plans, with a maze of incentives to purchase coverage (tax subsidies for employers and tax credits for individuals) and disincentives (penalties, high deductibles, and coinsurance) for patients to access care.
- Coverage increased through Obamacare's Medicaid expansion and subsidized private coverage, but 28.5 million remained uninsured in 2015, and employer-sponsored coverage is rapidly deteriorating.

popular strategy to control costs by shifting the financial risk of patients' use of services to providers and leaving patients to negotiate through an ever-changing set of restrictions and barriers to care. Private insurers profited by selectively enrolling healthier patients and requiring pre-authorization for many tests and treatments. But this experiment in cost control failed, and insurers switched to strategies like limiting choice of providers to a "narrow network" and making patients pay large deductibles and co-payments for care.

With the uninsured soaring to 50 million people by 2010, pressure mounted for an overhaul. That year, the ACA was signed into law as the largest reform to the health care system since the introduction of Medicare and Medicaid. The ACA mandates that individuals and employers (with over 50 employees) purchase health insurance, with financial penalties for noncompliance (DHHS 2015). It introduced health insurance exchanges—"online marketplaces" offering a range of subsidized (through tax credits) health insurance plans—for individuals and small businesses. The ACA also expanded Medicaid funding to cover all people under age 65 with income at or below 138% of the federal poverty level, superseding other eligibility criteria. Yet 19 of 50 states have rejected this provision for political reasons (governing parties reject the ACA's legitimacy even though the US Supreme Court ruled it constitutional) (KFF 2016a), leaving some 3 million low-income people with neither Medicaid nor subsidized coverage, disproportionately affecting poor, uninsured racial minorities (Garfield and Damico 2016).

The ACA includes various consumer protections aimed at preventing the most egregious health insurance abuses such as lifetime limits and "pre-existing condition" exclusions, and requires insurers to cover preventive services (without cost-sharing) and a package of "essential health benefits" (DHHS 2015). But insurers have been able to skirt the regulations by limiting access to providers and to costly medications (such as for HIV and other serious illnesses).

While the ACA has expanded coverage and enacted regulations and subsidies where they were lacking, nearly 10% of the US population remains uninsured and with very limited access to health services. Millions of undocumented immigrants are excluded from the ACA exchanges and Medicaid (Stutz and Baig 2014), and almost 500,000 legal immigrants lost coverage in 2015 due to requirements for additional documentation. A major problem is that deductibles are so high for ACA plans (e.g., US$10,000 for a family "bronze" plan and US$6,000 for a family "silver" plan) that coverage is "all but useless" (Pear 2015). Many new enrollees have now dropped out because they can no longer afford premiums or do not think the coverage is worth the cost. Meanwhile, insurance companies, finding the exchanges unprofitable, are pulling out of them.

Access to care is regulated by arcane contracts via 35 major insurers, each with dozens of subsidiaries and thousands of health plans (Schoen, Radley, and Collins 2015). Over 350,000 insurance company employees (and hundreds of thousands of other workers) (State Health Access Data Assistance Center 2013) govern which of the country's nearly 910,000 physicians and surgeons (KFF 2016b), and 5,700 hospitals can be accessed (American Hospital Association 2016). Uninsurance and underinsurance contribute to worse health outcomes for certain conditions (Dillman et al. 2014), rising costs (because delayed care leads to more complications) (Link and McKinlay 2010), and personal bankruptcies, half of which are due to medical debts (Khazan 2014).

Most importantly, even with increased public financing, the insurance industry's role in drafting the ACA has left the private sector in control of administering health coverage, not only for ACA health plans, but increasingly for traditionally publicly administered plans like Medicare and Medicaid (Chaufan 2015). Private insurance revenues are soaring, even (or especially) with premiums increasingly paid for by government. Out-of-pocket charges are skyrocketing, including for the approximately 150 million people with employment-based insurance (Congressional Budget Office 2015). In addition to copayments/coinsurance, spending ceilings, and barriers to providers, premiums have tripled since 2000, and deductibles have risen seven times faster than wages since 2000 (KFF and HRET 2014).

Indeed, health care after ACA remains an even more profitable capitalist enterprise than before, in part thanks to the half billion dollars spent by pharmaceutical and insurance firms on lobbying the US Congress each year. In 2010, the 10 largest health insurance companies collectively cleared US$12.7 billion in profits (not counting obscene CEO salaries and stock options) (Time Inc. 2010). In 2014, the largest health insurance company, UnitedHealth, made US$10.3 billion in profits on revenues of US$130.5 billion, a 7% increase from 2013 (Potter 2015). At the same time, from 2010 through 2013, overall US health care fraud resulted in US$19.2 billion in fines (Demko 2014), (mostly imposed on drug companies for illegal marketing tactics), with US$250 to US$500 billion in health care spending lost to corruption annually, involving every aspect of the health sector (Geyman 2015).

The majority of Americans have long supported a universal, single-tier health care system; however, conservative forces would like to see ACA repealed and eschew the notion of health care as a right. Though Obamacare has helped millions obtain health insurance and increases preventive coverage (Cohn 2014), it will not guarantee universality, and it entrenches a profit-based system. Ultimately, it won't fix the most "expensive, inequitable, and wasteful health system in the world" (Brill 2015).

In sum, the United States spends far more total and per capita than any other country: over double the OECD average of US$3,740 (in purchasing power parity). The US's enormous spending levels—driven by hundreds of billions of dollars of overhead, profiteering, duplication, and waste—are marked by a 26-fold increase in health care administrators (1970–2014), while the number of doctors has only tripled over that time (Himmelstein and Woolhandler 2014; Jiwani et al. 2014)! Ironically, what the United States spends per capita through public financing alone exceeds total average health spending in OECD countries, suggesting that a fully publicly administered and financed system eliminating private insurers and reducing administrative overhead would be much more efficient and far less expensive than the current arrangement (Sullivan 2013) (see chapter 12). Instead, health care provision in the United States remains highly inequitable. It offers the lowest quality and poorest outcomes at an aggregate level among peer countries and falls far short of meeting population needs (Mossialos et al. 2016).

Comparative Analysis, Redux

These various health care arrangements, from pluralistic, public-private patchwork systems like that of the United States and many LMICs to Bismarck's national health insurance, Beveridge's NHS, and socialized health care systems, such as the former USSR's, demonstrate considerable diversity in health care organization. There is one other prototype, known as the single-payer model, which will be discussed further in chapter 12. Typified by the health care systems of Canada and Taiwan (Cheng 2015), single-payer systems offer a hybrid of national health insurance and NHS, with the state (or in the case of Canada, provinces) serving as the sole public funder, and delivery of health services taking place in the private (most non–hospital-based doctors) and nonprofit (especially for hospitals and community health centers) sectors (Chaufan 2011).

It is important to stress that union density and effective social movements/political activism remain key determinants and predictors of both health and health care systems (Chernomas and Hudson 2013). Indeed, never in capitalist history has any regime, from Bismarck and Franklin Roosevelt's New Deal in the United States to governments of Scandinavia and South Korea (see ahead), ever implemented significant economic and social equity policies without some form of aggressive demands "from below." Both liberal and conservative governments may implement certain social security measures (Bismarck serving as a classic case) as a means to get elected, and undermine the more radical demands of unions and other (e.g., feminist, environmental) movements demanding change, without fundamentally reforming the social order.

PRIMARY HEALTH CARE, ITS RENEWAL, AND THE TURN TO UNIVERSAL HEALTH COVERAGE

Key Questions:

- What is a primary health care approach and what are its implications for health care system organization?
- How does UHC differ from PHC? What are the implications?

Primary Health Care

Primary health care (PHC) has been repeatedly demonstrated the most effective, equitable, and efficient component of health care and a policy and delivery model that can help address the social determinants of health in an integrated fashion (Kruk et al. 2010; Labonté et al. 2014; Ruano, Furler, and Shi 2015; Starfield, Shi, and Macinko 2005).

Though PHC and its variants—community-based care, social medicine, and basic health services—date back over a century, PHC gained global prominence with the joint WHO-UNICEF 1978 international primary health care conference held in Alma-Ata (Kazakhstan, former USSR). The *Declaration of Alma-Ata* represents a milestone in international consensus on priorities for health, with its reorientation of the narrow, increasingly medicalized approach characteristic of (international) health activity into an integrated political and technical health endeavor (Cueto 2004; Gillam 2008).

At the conference, WHO's then Director-General, Halfdan Mahler, challenged the 134 government delegations and 67 nongovernmental organizations (NGOs) present as follows (Mahler 1978):

> Are you ready to address yourselves seriously to the existing gap between the health "haves" and the health "have nots" and to adopt concrete measures to reduce it?
>
> . . .
>
> Are you ready to introduce, if necessary, radical changes in the existing health delivery system so that it properly supports primary health care as the overriding health priority?
>
> . . .
>
> Are you ready to make unequivocal political commitments to adopt primary health care and to mobilize international solidarity to attain the objectives of health for all by the year 2000?

The declaration itself remains both aspirational and concrete, as per the snapshots in Box 11-6.

The Alma-Ata declaration was a political statement as much as a call for primary health care services, and its focus on social inequality was

Box 11-6 Selections from the *Declaration of Alma-Ata*

I "Health... is a fundamental human right . . . the attainment of the highest possible level of health is a most important worldwide social goal whose realization requires the action of many other social and economic sectors in addition to the health sector.

II The existing gross inequality in the health status of the people particularly between developed and developing countries as well as within countries is politically, socially, and economically unacceptable and is, therefore, of common concern to all countries.

III Economic and social development, based on a New International Economic Order, is of basic importance to the fullest attainment of health for all and to the reduction of the gap between the health status of the developing and developed countries. The promotion and protection of the health of the people is essential to sustained economic and social development and contributes to a better quality of life and to world peace.

. . .

V Governments have a responsibility for the health of their people, which can be fulfilled only by the provision of adequate health and social measures.

VI Primary health care is essential health care based on practical, scientifically sound, and socially acceptable methods and technology made universally accessible to individuals and families in the community through their full participation and at a cost that the community and country can afford to maintain at every stage of their development in the spirit of self-reliance and self-determination.

VII Primary health care:

. . .

2. addresses the main health problems in the community, providing promotive, preventive, curative, and rehabilitative services accordingly;
3. includes at least . . . promotion of food supply and proper nutrition; an adequate supply of safe water and basic sanitation; maternal and child health care, including family planning; immunization against the major infectious diseases; prevention and control of locally endemic diseases; appropriate treatment of common diseases and injuries; and provision of essential drugs;

. . .

7. relies, at local and referral levels, on health workers, including physicians, nurses, midwives, auxiliaries, and community workers as applicable, as well as traditional practitioners as needed, suitably trained socially and technically to work as a health team and to respond to the expressed health needs of the community."

Source: WHO (1978).

groundbreaking for a specialized health agency (Werner and Sanders 1997). The consensus reached at Alma-Ata was confirmed in a resolution at the next (32nd) World Health Assembly (WHA) held in May 1979, transformed into a Global Strategy for "Health for All by the Year 2000," and endorsed by the UN General Assembly in 1981. However, as discussed in chapter 2, PHC soon faced political and ideological obstacles, and broadly-defined PHC was selectively dismantled into a technical shadow of its former comprehensive approach, especially through UNICEF's vertical campaigns for child survival.

Still, its basic contours endured—if unevenly and often only rhetorically—in the context of neoliberal cutbacks to health spending and a denuded understanding of PHC as the basic level of first-contact care with a provider. North Americans focused more on the continuity, coordination, and comprehensiveness of medical care provided by generalists than on the political dimensions of PHC. In Latin America, meanwhile, PHC was half-heartedly implemented under various authoritarian regimes and became known as "primitive health care" or "health care for the poor" (Breilh 1979; Testa 1988), even as community health efforts in some settings kept the spirit of PHC alive (Ramírez et al. 2011). By contrast, in some northern European countries and Iran, for example, PHC was taken on with enthusiasm.

PHC experienced a rebirth after 2000, strongly supported by civil society activists (including via the People's Health Charter [see chapter 14]) and progressive-minded governments (Barten, Rovere, and Espinoza 2010; PHM et al. 2014). After over a decade of neoliberal reforms, the Pan American Health Organization (PAHO) renewed its PHC strategy through the 2005 Declaration of Montevideo. Breaking with a health care for the poor approach, the declaration emphasized—among other principles—social inclusion, family and community participation, equity in health and health care access, intersectoral approaches, comprehensive, integrated, and appropriate health care, social solidarity, accountability, and the infusion of PHC principles throughout the health care system (Nervi 2008; PAHO 2007). While the obstacles to implementation are many, Latin America's return to democracy after decades of dictatorship has yielded participatory and inclusive PHC-based change, especially under recent left-leaning governments in many of the region's countries (discussed ahead). Indeed, PHC in its renewed guise offers the ideal means of integrating the societal determinants of health in public policy when applied as the "organizational strategy and underlying philosophy" of a health care system (Gilson, Doherty, and Loewenson 2011, p. 198).

The WHO reiterated its commitment to PHC in its 2008 *World Health Report*, affirming that the principles of PHC were just as valid as 30 years prior and important to realizing the Millennium Development Goals (MDGs) (WHO 2008a). The report also raised alarms about the negative impact of commercialized health systems on cost, efficiency, quality, safety, equity, and health overall. But activists and scholars have critiqued the WHO for its weak support for PHC, arguing that the MDGs, in ignoring broader determinants, were contrary to the spirit of Alma-Ata (Koivusalo and Baru 2008). Clearly, global commitment to PHC implementation is necessary, but WHO appears disinclined to provide leadership. The thrust of its 2008 report was far narrower than PAHO's, stressing the responsiveness and strengthening of health care systems and universal coverage, which, as we review next, comes with its own set of challenges.

Universal Health Coverage

One explanation for WHO's mild support for a renewed PHC is its more ringing endorsement of universal health coverage (UHC). This began with a 2005 World Health Assembly (WHA) resolution regarding prepaid pooling of resources to prevent catastrophic health expenditures and impoverishment (Sengupta 2013a), itself an outcropping of WHO's 2000-2002 Commission on Macroeconomics and Health. The Commission recommended public financing for private insurance and delivery of health care, reviving the discredited formula that poverty is chiefly a result of ill health rather than the other way around (Waitzkin 2003). (See chapter 12 for further discussion of this causal confusion.)

By 2010, after the onset of the Great Recession, with health care costs continuing to rise and many LMIC health care systems in disarray following decades of neglect and downsizing, the *World Health Report* conveyed WHO's full commitment to UHC, defined thus: ensuring that "all people have access to services and do not suffer financial hardship paying for them" (WHO 2010, p. 7). The World Bank endorsed UHC's aim of people having "access to the health care they need" without "falling into poverty due to illness" (World Bank 2014), but refrained from backing equity in access. WHO, for its part, while maintaining that UHC is "firmly based" in the the Alma-Ata declaration and the "Health for All" agenda (WHO 2016), has sidelined PHC and other integrated approaches to health even as it asserts that UHC is rooted in the fundamental human right to health. WHO Director-General Dr. Margaret Chan even grandly claimed:

> Universal health coverage is one of the most powerful social equalizers among all policy options. It is the ultimate expression of fairness. If public health has something that can help our troubled, out-of-balance world, it is this: growing evidence that well-functioning and inclusive health systems contribute to social cohesion, equity, and stability. They hold societies together and help reduce social tensions (Chan 2015).

On the surface, this latest global health policy trend seems unobjectionable and achievable (Reich et al. 2015). Who could oppose the appealing goal of extending health care coverage to entire populations? But the very ambiguity of the term *coverage* and the imprecision of the definition mask an approach that departs from (public) universal health care (or health care for all), because the term *coverage* typically refers to (private) insurance coverage. To illustrate, the Rockefeller Foundation (2009, p. 2), a key backer of the UHC goal, has recommended "models that harness the private health sector in the financing and provision of health services for poor people."

In making governments responsible for "ensur[ing] that all providers, public and private, operate appropriately and attend to patients' needs cost effectively and efficiently" (WHO 2010, p. xviii), UHC portends a departure from PHC's public, unified, comprehensive financing and delivery of care. WHO has called for improved tax collection, increased allocation of government budgets to the health sector (as well as development assistance financing), yet its inviting of market approaches that separate the purchaser and provider functions of health care systems will likely institutionalize inequity, despite pledges otherwise (Heredia et al. 2015). The potentially promising redistributive dimension of WHO's UHC call for innovative financing, especially through taxes levied on foreign currency transactions (WHO 2010), seems to have fallen by the wayside, although regressive "sin" taxes on alcohol, tobacco, and unhealthy food and beverages may have more traction.

Many UHC efforts (such as reforms in the United States and Mexico) involve multifaceted *financing* reforms that add coverage to some or most previously uninsured populations for some services ("packages of benefits"), but not necessarily for all needed services. In these proposals, the public sector either withdraws from provisioning altogether to become a manager and purveyor of funds or enters into a competitive relationship with an expanded, often for-profit, private sector, leading to further fragmentation. Through UHC, insurance companies gain access to public revenue streams (social security contributions and taxes) that finance contracts to provide a set of services to the previously uninsured. For their part, the newly insured, who are overwhelmingly economically precarious, may be required by law to contribute taxes, premiums, and user fees for their coverage, which may inadequately serve their needs. Moreover, formal sector financing mechanisms may exclude more vulnerable informal sector workers from coverage (Oxfam International 2013). As well, most UHC approaches do not call for funding via more equitable taxes—through which the rich would be contributing to risk pools directly or indirectly—but rather rely on cross-subsidies among uninsured populations and so-called charity or "free care" as part of providers' obligation to contribute "community benefit."

To be sure, universality is a key principle of health care systems, important to ensuring equity, social inclusion, and efficiency. It was certainly central to the Alma-Ata declaration, which advocated "health care based on practical, scientifically sound and socially acceptable methods and technology made universally accessible." For example, under the Canada Health Act (1984), which codified its national health insurance system, universality refers *both* to all residents being covered *and* to a single level of care for all.

As such, WHO's focus on universal *coverage*, without the guarantee of a uniform, solidarity-oriented, single-tiered, comprehensive set of services (characterizing PHC) is disconcerting. Stated differently, "if everyone has access to some health care benefits, but only a few have their cancer treatment covered, there is no universalism to speak of" (Martínez Franzoni and Sánchez-Ancochea 2016, p. 6). Nor can a health care system be considered universal when some people enjoy higher quality care or more resources than others, or where copayments impede access. Any policy that fragments more than it unifies or results in segmented financing or pools of beneficiaries inherently goes against universalism even if it is *called* universal.

If the state plays a central role in assuring funding for and access to a unified set of health care services and regulating quality, UHC may be helpful. As well, "progressive governments can try to privilege public systems" and equity (PHM et al. 2014, p. 81). But the core of UHC—adding new patient demand and a new revenue stream to profit-hungry insurers in a context of further fragmentation—makes this possibility extremely remote. Even solidarity-oriented UHC reforms in countries such as Brazil and Ecuador are contested by powerful private interests.

Another critique is that UHC does not adequately incorporate a social determinants of health perspective (Marmot 2013). For WHO's Director-General to assert that: "universal coverage is the single most powerful concept that public health has to offer" (Lancet [Editorial] 2012) belies WHO's articulated commitment to the social determinants of health and ignores its own ample evidence that social injustice—that is political, economic, and other societal inequities (among which lack of access to health care is but one aspect)—"is killing people on a grand scale" (WHO 2008b).

Despite these concerns, the WHO and World Bank successfully advocated for UHC to be enshrined in the post-MDG Sustainable Development Goals (SDGs) as a target under SDG 3 (Ensure healthy lives and promote well-being for all at all ages). UHC's promise was boiled down to: "Achieve universal health coverage, including financial risk protection, access to quality essential health-care services and access to safe, effective, quality and affordable essential medicines and vaccines for all." Alas, this SDG target reiterates WHO's concern with reducing financial risk due to health care spending but makes no reference to public provision or equitable financing.

In sum, aspiring language notwithstanding, UHC—unless explicitly focused on public health care system strengthening—is a misguided approach, justified by certain legitimate concerns around catastrophic health spending, but offering the likelihood of large-scale rapacious health care system penetration by—and channeling of resources to—private interests that reinforce health care system inequity and stratification. Unified and integrated national health care systems—which are based on health as a right rather than a commodity, pool resources across entire populations, and prevent impoverishment from catastrophic illness—offer the best prospects for equity and efficiency (even as quality has been threatened by resource starvation and privatization in recent decades) (Heredia et al. 2015). Why such systems are not at the heart of WHO's push for universality is puzzling indeed.

HEALTH CARE SYSTEM REFORM

Key Questions:

- What are the different forces driving health care reforms?
- What are the features of health care reform around the world?

In recent decades, many countries have undergone significant health care system reforms with five main characteristics, listed in Box 11-7. Some have been driven by rising expenditures, others by concerns over quality of care, and still others by pressures from international financial agencies. Two main (contradictory) trends have emerged in patterns of reform: one toward public administration and bona fide universality, and another toward privatization and market incentives under the umbrella of universal health coverage.

Reform in Stratified Systems: Latin America and the Caribbean

In many Latin American countries, the health sector has long been characterized by stratified health care arrangements. In countries as diverse as Argentina, Peru, and Guatemala, separate health insurance and social security schemes were founded in the early 20th century to cover broad and particular occupational groups (e.g., civil servants, formal sector workers, miners, railway workers, oil workers, industrial laborers) starting at different times. Strong labor movements in the region ensured that formally employed workers, including government functionaries, received publicly financed health coverage. Most of these schemes operate(d) publicly, with health workers—themselves government employees—working in public facilities. Wealthy

Box 11-7 Characteristics of Health Sector Reform

Regulation

- Policy changes (e.g., liberalization, public administration)
- Changes in regulatory structures

Financing

- User fees, insurance schemes, external financing mechanisms, taxes
- Community financing, social health insurance, unified public systems

Resource Allocation

- Comprehensiveness of services covered
- Management and supervisory arrangements
- Reforms in payment systems
- Efficiency reforms

Provision

- Nationalization, privatization, competition
- Quality improvement/use of evidence
- Primary health care
- Accountability/participation
- Decentralization

Access

- Population coverage
- Linguistic, geographic, cultural accessibility

Source: Adapted extensively from Gilson and Mills (1995) and Mills and Ranson (2012).

elites have long excluded themselves from public insurance schemes and paid for health services out-of-pocket or, increasingly, through private insurance. Those working outside the formal sector (e.g., agricultural workers, informal vendors, and day laborers) have typically been served by a resource-strapped set of public clinics and hospitals, almost always overcrowded, and often inaccessible to rural residents.

As such—with notable exceptions of Costa Rica and Cuba (discussed in chapter 13)—much of the region developed multi-tiered, segmented health care systems, with employment sector and level of wealth determining medical coverage, and leaving the large informal workforce and indigent populations to receive services in underfunded public facilities or pay out-of-pocket for private health care (Roemer 1964).

With deep cuts in public spending starting in the 1980s neoliberal onslaught, compounded by fragmentation and extreme inequities, huge swaths of the population had little or no access to health care. For example, in 2000 over 50% of Mexicans, especially poor, Indigenous, and rural residents, had no health insurance coverage and relied on public clinics of uneven quality, supplies, and staffing (Knaul et al. 2005). Meanwhile over half of health care expenditures occurred in the private sector, mostly covering a small elite.

By the 1990s, most Latin American countries embarked on extensive health sector reforms, many of which entailed privatization of both health and social security systems, as advised by the World Bank and other financial agencies (Armada, Muntaner, and Navarro 2001). These reforms enabled increased penetration of US-based private health insurance companies, especially catering to the lucrative managed care sector (Iriart, Merhy, and Waitzkin 2001).

Brazil's quarter-century old reform, though not able to withstand privatization altogether, has attempted to rectify inequities in health care access and financing, based on a publicly funded, integrated universal system (Elias and Cohn 2003; Lima et al. 2005). Drawing from the post-dictatorship 1988 Constitution's enshrining of health care as a universal right, Brazil operates a tax-funded unified health care system (SUS), free at the point of service for the entire population (Paim et al. 2011). This decentralized system, involving federal, state, and municipal governments in both management and financing, has sought to improve equity and created local decisionmaking councils and regional management roles to align health care system planning with needs (Fleury 2011). Today PHC is delivered through over 32,000 community-based family health teams, each consisting of a doctor, nurse, nurse technicians, and up to a dozen full-time community health workers, serving over 120 million people across the country. Even with SUS, problems and inequities persist, lately evidenced by a poorly managed dengue outbreak and the Zika virus crisis that surged in 2015–2016. Of course, vector-borne outbreaks are not only a function of health care access, but stem from poverty, inadequate sanitation, and other social conditions that facilitate the proliferation of mosquito breeding sites.

Provision of most tertiary care is contracted out to an increasingly expensive private sector, with private insurance—subsidized by the federal government even as SUS faces growing funding shortfalls—covering 25% of the population (though constituting over half of expenditures). Within SUS, the shortage of primary care doctors in the poorest and most rural areas compelled the Brazilian government in 2014 to contract over 14,000 doctors, mostly from Cuba, through the Mais Médicos program. This has met with both controversy and open arms in the almost one quarter of the population lacking physician access. Today Brazil's struggles against health care inequity are at a crossroads: political turmoil in 2016 (see chapter 14) portends the acceleration of SUS's privatization, elimination of guaranteed funding, and potential clawbacks of the right to health care, as well as the rights of women and of minorities.

Mexico's 2004 *Popular Health Insurance Program* (PHI) was established to cover the country's 50 million uninsured through voluntary health insurance coverage for a defined package of interventions (Frenk et al. 2006; Laurell 2007). However, instead of merging coverage for the uninsured population with the social security system, as did Brazil, Mexico's legislation created a new separate arrangement, atop an already highly segmented set of insurance systems for different population tranches: civil servants, private sector employees, and workers in particular industries. PHI is financed by state and federal governments, with premiums also paid by participating families (initially the lowest income quintile was exempt, now expanded to the two lowest quintiles) and delivered via contracts with both public and private providers.

In 2012, the Ministry of Health claimed that UHC had been achieved through incorporation of all persons previously uninsured (Knaul et al. 2012). But census and national survey data contradict this claim, indicating that between 25 and 30 million people remain uninsured including 10 million people in the poorest income quintile (Laurell 2015). Not only has private expenditure on health remained near its pre-reform level (48% of the total) (WHO 2014a) but PHI affiliates continue to pay proportionately more out-of-pocket than those covered by social security (Knaul et al. 2012), with out-of-pocket expenditures for the poorest groups barely declining (Laurell 2015).

Meanwhile, PHI covers just 20% of the services offered by the social security scheme. PHI's defined set of interventions exclude services related to common causes of mortality and morbidity such as complications from diabetes (Mexico's leading cause of death), cerebrovascular diseases, and trauma or burns due to accidents. Moreover, because PHI expansion has not been supplemented by new investments in infrastructure and human resources, many of the previous barriers to quality and access, especially in rural areas, persist. Regional disparities and inequitable and fragmented financing and coverage remain entrenched, and the populations who have historically benefited from—or been disadvantaged by—a segmented system remain the same as before the reform. To illustrate, those still uninsured and PHI affiliates access the same health care facilities but preference is now given to those with PHI, heightening discrimination toward the uninsured (Laurell 2015). In the end, establishing a true right to health care in Mexico will require ending fragmentation and duplication of services, and combating inequities in access, funding, and quality of care (López Arellano and López Moreno 2015).

Elsewhere in the region, reforms have been mixed (Giovanella et al. 2012). Colombia's famed "exemplary" (according to the World Bank) 1993 competition-oriented reform resulted in a virtual collapse of its social security-based health care system (Franco 2013). Peru amplified coverage through a fragmented system, and Uruguay created an integrated national health care system in 2008. Bolivia, Ecuador, and Venezuela have all moved to extend integrated PHC approaches through unified systems, but have been unable to eliminate inequities perpetuated through a costly private system (Heredia et al. 2015). Despite noteworthy political commitment, most Latin American countries face ongoing problems of stratified health care systems and large private health sectors, intensified amid recent economic and political volatility in various settings.

Post-Socialist Reform: Countries of the Former Soviet Bloc

With the breakup of the Soviet Union and the Soviet bloc in the early 1990s, Poland, Hungary, other Eastern European countries, and the newly independent republics of Eastern Europe and Central Asia, as well as Russia itself, were faced with depleted government resources. Health care systems had already begun to deteriorate in prior decades due to underinvestment, poor quality of care, corruption, and an overall shortage of resources (Barr and Field 1996).

Advised by IFI "experts," and shock-therapy economist turned development guru Jeffrey Sachs (see chapter 3), that privatization would help attract additional funds, and therefore provide a larger financial base from which to deliver care (World Bank 1993), most formerly socialist countries opened the health sector to private insurance and reinstituted private medical practice. While the principle of universality remained intact at a rhetorical level, market incentives generated parallel public–private systems of health care delivery, further weakening the public system and widening inequities (Balabanova et al. 2004).

As outlined earlier, Soviet and Soviet bloc health care systems were characterized by universal access to publicly-run health services, which contributed—as part of economic redistribution and vast improvements in literacy, nutrition, housing, and other social conditions—to a steep decline in communicable diseases and increased life expectancy. Since the 1980s, many former Soviet bloc countries experienced a reversal of these trends as social conditions deteriorated, with worsening infant mortality rates, a drastic increase in infectious diseases, particularly TB, and mounting stress-related ailments such as cardiovascular disease. Pensioners and low-income workers have faced the biggest barriers to health care access and utilization (see chapter 3).

Though the worst effects of the overall transition to capitalism have abated in some settings, former Soviet bloc health care systems rely heavily on the private sector and out-of-pocket payments, resulting in significant inequities (Rechel, Richardson, and McKee 2014).

Reform in "Emerging" Economies: South Korea, South Africa, and India

Some countries with fast-growing economies have pursued publicly financed, universal health care systems, while others have turned to market-based reforms.

South Korea's health care system was implemented in steps beginning in the late 1970s. A targeted basket of interventions steadily expanded until full implementation of national health insurance was reached in 1989. More recent reforms have subsumed hundreds of existing medical insurance funds into a single-payer system, more than halving administrative costs. These health reforms were enabled by a political environment conducive to change, greater economic resources due to rapid economic growth, and, especially, to increased democratic participation and extensive grassroots organizing, involving a coalition of farmers, progressive academics, unions, and civic groups.

As in other national health insurance systems, private hospitals and practitioners deliver over 90% of services in South Korea, with the public sector primarily responsible for public health campaigns. This has generated regional disparities, as proportionately more services are provided in urban than rural areas. Demonstrating an impressive commitment to national health insurance, the South Korean government increased public financing in 2000 (Jeong 2005) from 20.1% to 55.5% by 2008. Still, out-of-pocket payments average 34% of total healthcare expenditures and up to 5% of total household spending, among the highest in OECD countries (Lee and Shaw 2014). Moreover, the government has recently cut payments to providers, who in turn have recommended that fewer services be publicly covered, leading to higher patient payments for hospital care and certain procedures and technologies (Kwon 2011).

South Africa aims to implement a national health insurance system by 2026, building on efforts that began in 1994. The post-apartheid government, elected in 1994, made health care a universal right for the first time, starting with coverage for pregnant and breastfeeding women and children under 6. Within 2 years, primary health care services were provided free at the point of delivery to the entire population (Pillay 2001). Currently, the public sector is responsible for about 85% of the population, accounting for 44% of total health care expenditures, with the private sector accounting for 56% of expenditures but serving just 15% of the population. South Africa's private health sector includes multiple health insurance plans (90 organizations offering 311 different plans in 2013), which have experienced significant cost escalations in the past few years. Private hospital expenditures have soared, in 2012 constituting almost 30% of total private sector health expenditure (Day and Gray 2014).

Health sector reform in South Africa has involved decentralization of services from the national government to provincial governments and within provinces to health districts. The national government remains responsible for developing legislation and policies, whereas provincial governments are charged with providing primary and hospital care, and municipalities carry out environmental health measures (Government of South Africa 2004).

Despite advances made by the public sector—such as removal of user fees for primary care, expansion in the number of PHC facilities, introduction of community service requirements for a wide range of health professionals, and increased spending in the public sector (an annual average increase of 5.6% in real terms since 2002)—there remain sizeable inequities by region and social group. A decade ago per capita health funding was twice as high in some provinces as others, but since then inter-provincial per capita health spending inequities have been slashed by two thirds. However, there is still marked variation across the country's 52 health districts, with rural populations particularly jeopardized by less access to care than people living in urban areas or who are privately insured (Massyn et al. 2014). South Africa's health care system continues to face great challenges, including enormous social inequalities, HIV, and marginal living conditions for the majority of the population. Additionally, because the health care system increasingly relies on private sector delivery, an urban-based, curative care bias will likely worsen regional inequities in health spending (PHM et al. 2014).

Post-independence India sought to create a publicly funded health care system, focusing on facilities construction, training of health personnel, and direct delivery of services. However, the inadequately funded system fell short of providing accessible care to the majority of the population, particularly outside major cities, pushing people into a largely unorganized but extensive private medical sector. The public system experienced further erosion in the early 1990s, with the formal application of neoliberal economic policies. This led to institution of user fees and creeping privatization (Lister 2008).

With public sector spending on health just 1.4% of GDP (total health care spending is 4.7% of GDP) (WHO 2014a), and private health care—now increasingly driven by corporate chains—dominating both outpatient (80%) and inpatient (60%) spending, India has one of the most privatized (around 70%) and inequitable health care systems in the world (Sengupta 2013b). Since 2005, the Indian government has created both a National Health Mission, designed to strengthen public-sector health services, and several health insurance schemes—consolidated under Rashtiya Swasthiya Bima Yojana (RSBY)—to provide hospital care for the poor (covering certain designated occupations, the rural landless, and now a wider definition of people below the poverty line) with a defined set of benefits. These reforms were prompted by a number of factors: inadequacies of the grossly under-resourced public health care system; high out-of-pocket payments for private health care that further impoverished the poor; and popular pressure on the then newly elected government to expand social welfare programs (Rao et al. 2014; Shiva Kumar et al. 2011). With enrollment growing to 12%-13% of the urban and rural populations (prior claims cited twice this proportion), public funds for primary care (not covered by RSBY) are being squeezed. Though publicly funded, over 80% of RSBY monies are now channeled through health insurance schemes to contracted private providers, who are under-regulated (for example failing to report TB cases, resulting in non-treatment) and notoriously unethical (Sengupta 2013b).

The Central Government Health Scheme covers 3.6 million national government workers and dependents (Sarwal 2015), with around 35 million state government workers and private industry employees in a separate Employee State Insurance Scheme (Government of India 2012) that is sorely in need of reform (Duggal 2015). The approximately 10% of the population in the middle and upper economic strata spend most health rupees (perhaps half via growing commercial insurance coverage) (Growth Analysis 2013). Yet India's 900 million informal workers and working class population pay proportionately far more of their own income on health care, including the upwards of 150 million people enrolled in RSBY, who must nonetheless spend considerable sums out-of-pocket (Shahrawat and Rao 2012). A National Health Protection Scheme is planned for 2017, replacing RSBY with a scheme that envisions covering triple the expenses, but still only for inpatient care (Ministry of Health and Family Welfare 2016), likely further embedding poor quality, private delivery of care.

Reforms in High Income Countries

Western European countries, plus Canada, New Zealand, Japan, and Australia—constituting the majority of OECD nations where universal, publicly financed health care is standard—are facing similar concerns as LMICs, albeit with far more base resources for the health care sector, including larger per capita spending, greater infrastructure, and more personnel. Climbing health care expenditures (growing faster than GDP) in many HICs—though stagnating or even falling from 2010 to 2014—have been attributed to increased use of technology and pharmaceuticals, rises in non-communicable diseases (NCDs), inadequate regulation, provider incentives, and population aging.

Countries with national health care systems have historically operated under the principle that need must determine access to and coverage of care. Yet in many places inequitable access to care has persisted due to poor geographic distribution of health care services and barriers to care for undocumented immigrants (Cuadra 2012). Political and welfare state regimes (see chapter 7) have historically shaped the state's role in delivery of care and the extent of private providers, insurance, and out-of-pocket financing. Generally, countries with social democratic political parties in power or with strong collective social movements have given more emphasis to equity and public provision (Muntaner et al. 2011), with less such focus in more "liberal" regimes. For example, both Denmark and Switzerland have decentralized systems of care, but Denmark's is public and redistributive, while Switzerland's is organized via competing private insurers with little attention to issues of inequity (Mossialos et al. 2016).

In recent decades, rationalizing reforms have focused on regulating prices, instituting budget caps, and implementing cost-sharing measures. Because spending cuts met with public resistance, the next wave of reforms emphasized management and efficiency measures, including reduced length of hospital stays and increased competition among providers.

The 2008 financial crisis has generated far-reaching austerity policies in Euro-zone countries, especially in Southern Europe and the United Kingdom. Whereas growth in spending on health was on average 3.4% per year prior to the crisis, it fell to 0.6% on average between 2009 and 2013; in Greece and Ireland, health spending declined by 7.2% and 4%, respectively (OECD 2015), reflecting these countries' imposed fiscal austerity and post-2008 GDP declines.

Various countries, including those most affected by austerity measures, like Greece, Portugal, and Spain, introduced or increased user charges for health services to curb utilization and decrease costs (Karanikolos et al. 2013). In Greece, austerity policies have also cut physician and nurse salaries and triggered service cutbacks: out-of-pocket hospital payments reached over 52% in 2013 (Grigorakis et al. 2014), levels more typical of LMICs such as Bangladesh, Cambodia, and Laos (Kwon et al. 2012).

Thailand's National Health Security Scheme

Thailand broke with this trend of increasing user fees, creating in 2001 a new universal health scheme (initially known as "30 Baht Scheme," now called National Health Security Scheme [NHSS]) for poor and informal sector workers—about 48 million people or 75% of the population. The remainder of the population is covered either by Social Security or the Civil Servant Medical Benefit Scheme. The existing programs for low-income groups—which had uneven coverage, variable user fees, and left almost 17 million people uninsured—were folded into the NHSS, now offering comprehensive services, including for all HIV treatment. Within just a few years, most uninsured were covered, out-of-pocket payments declined, and in 2006 the 30-baht copayment was discontinued, together contributing to a 13%-30% decline in infant mortality (Gruber, Hendren, and Townsend 2014).

Although Thailand retains a multi-tiered system (with private insurance and a separate arrangement for medical tourists), access to care and responsiveness have increased without affecting quality overall. These favorable results stem in part from the wide swath of civil society, including informal workers, participating in the design and monitoring of the reform (Alfers and Lund 2012) and increased funding for public hospitals. Still, a huge gap in equity is that the substantial number of "non-Thais"—probably 5 to 6 million persons, both legal and nonlegal workers, many with significant care needs around TB and other health problems—are left out.

The Arab Spring and Health Care System Reform

Health care systems in Middle Eastern countries have faced the same privatization pressures as other LMICs, mixed with some efforts towards UHC. Though Egypt enjoyed a growing state-subsidized health care system in the 1950s and 1960s under "Arab socialism," it deteriorated by the 1970s with a turn to capitalism. This was followed by structural adjustment-linked underfunding and the beginnings of privatization and decentralization, with particularly detrimental effects on access to care for rural residents and informal workers. In the late 1990s, a PHC-based family health model sought to address fragmentation. Then, in 2007, in an unprecedented move, the Egyptian government decreed that its health insurance organization (serving more than 50% of the Egyptian population at this time) be transferred to a private holding company. While this action was deemed unconstitutional (Saleh et al. 2014), the Mubarak regime sought other paths to privatization. Health care justice was among the top demands of the Arab Spring protests, but the Egyptian government's efforts towards reaching UHC, largely based on private sector delivery, have done little to address this matter. Access to care remains highly inequitable, with the wealthy using twice as many services as the poor, who are spending a significantly greater proportion of household income on health care than the rich (Ministry of Health and Population Egypt et al. 2014).

In Syria, too, economic liberalization leading to job losses and health sector user fees generated widespread discontent and was a spark in the civil war that started in 2011 (Sen and al Faisal 2012). Syria's health care system has been decimated since then with public health efforts interrupted and water and sanitation systems in shambles. In Aleppo alone, targeted attacks have rendered most of the city's hospitals inoperative. Those remaining struggle to meet patient needs with scarce equipment, medicines, and human resources; about 95% of Aleppo's physicians have fled, or been killed or detained (Physicians for Human Rights 2015), a situation worsening on a daily basis.

In Tunisia, meanwhile, after post-independence growth in social protections and conditions, Cold War era authoritarianism combined with structural

Box 11-8 Political Economy of Ebola and Health Care System Crises in West Africa

The Ebola outbreak in West Africa in 2014–2015, with almost 30,000 cases and over 11,000 deaths, illustrates the long-term consequences of health infrastructure underfunding in sub-Saharan Africa. While the appearance and spread of Ebola (as discussed in chapter 6) was the fruition of a constellation of historical, ecological, political, and socio-cultural factors (Benton and Dionne 2015), the failure of health care systems exacerbated the spread of disease and contributed to the unprecedented number of Ebola fatalities. According to WHO officials, the health care systems in the most affected countries—Guinea, Liberia, and Sierra Leone—were unable to stem the outbreak for the following reasons: insufficient workforce; poor infrastructure and logistics; deficient health information and surveillance systems; inequity between public and private health sectors; inadequate pharmaceutical supply systems; and poorly financed, managed, and organized public health services (Kieny et al. 2014). In Liberia, this was compounded by lack of public trust, due to the legacy of a brutal civil war, repressive military, and corrupt politicians (Epstein 2014).

Left out of this analysis are the root causes of weak and poorly-financed health systems. Surely it is not lack of riches: although Liberia, Guinea, and Sierra Leone ranked 175, 179, and 183, respectively, out of 187 countries on the UN's 2014 Human Development Index, Liberia has the highest ratio of foreign direct investment to GDP in the world. The rapid expansion of Sierra Leone's nascent iron ore mining industry fueled economic growth of 20% in 2013, among the highest rates in the world. In 2010 its gold, diamond, and other mining interests contributed almost 60% of exports but only 8% of government revenue. In 2011, only one of the major transnational mining firms in the country was paying corporate income tax, and none of the top five was reporting profits despite the boom in mineral exports. TNC interests in "blood diamonds," "conflict timber," "land grabbing," and exploitation of minerals, palm oil, and rubber have left behind a trail of massive social and environmental damage (Sanders, Sengupta, and Scott 2015) even as the accompanying political pathologies and corporate greed—building on two centuries of imperial domination—go overlooked. In 2010, capital flight from Sierra Leone amounted to 524% (over 6 times!) of GDP, totaling over US$1,700 per person (Ndikumana, Boyce, and Ndiaye 2015), monies which could otherwise amply finance health and social infrastructure (see chapter 9). These current illicit financial outflows are atop decades of IMF and World Bank loan conditionalities, which have decimated public health infrastructure (Rowden 2014).

The population—and health systems—bear the brunt of these problems. More than 80% of Liberia's population lives on less than US$1/day and over half of Sierra Leoneans live in extreme poverty. The Ebola epidemic was aggravated by a missing health workforce: over half of doctors born in Liberia and Sierra Leone work in OECD countries (OECD 2010), and more than 500 of the region's health workers died from Ebola. The Ebola response only exacerbated the problem of domestic capacity—less than 2% of the US$3.3 billion sent to combat Ebola in Sierra Leone went to local health workers, the rest going to staff from donor countries, international NGOs, and international agencies (Maxmen 2015).

In short, the Ebola crisis is ultimately a symptom of a grossly unjust and exploitative global system in which private profiteering from natural resources, tax evasion, capital flight, corruption (also often involving government officials and foreign contractors), and continuing "brain robbery" (the term used by African ministers of health) (African Union 2002) flourish. The proposed governance "solutions" to such health crises, including stronger laws, intergovernmental coordination, and a global emergency unit, may allay the fears of rich countries but are unlikely to have much impact without addressing root causes (McInnes 2016; Sanders et al. 2015).

adjustment led to a significant ratcheting down of publicly provided care, leading to spiraling household contributions and a two-tiered system. After 2000, large-scale privatization in various sectors only accelerated health care deterioration and inequities, among the motivations for the 2010 Tunisian revolution that inspired and mobilized the Middle East region and far beyond. On a more optimistic note, there has been an increase in civil society advocacy and activism around health and social justice issues in Tunisia since then, though the struggle is uphill (PHM et al. 2014). While there have been efforts towards universal coverage, adequate protection from catastrophic health expenses and full population coverage have not been attained (Makhloufi, Ventelou, and Abu-Zaineh 2015) and further privatization is looming.

Reforms in sub-Saharan Africa (LICs)

In many of the lowest income countries, already fragile health sectors have been further eroded since the 1980s due to significant cutbacks in public sector spending under neoliberal market reforms heavily shaped by the World Bank and IMF's advice and loan conditionalities (Asakitikpi 2015). Almost all of the reforms resulted in lower health care access and a reduction in accountability mechanisms. Today over 80% of the rural population and 60% of urbanites lack health care entitlements, experiencing an extreme shortage of health care workers (Scheil-Adlung 2015).

The deleterious consequences of privatization were made more acute by civil conflict, significant brain drain of health personnel, and instances of corruption. The reforms were also coterminous with the (re)emergence of infectious diseases such as TB, malaria, and HIV, which are far better addressed through comprehensive, rights-based health care systems that are free at the point of care. Although billions of dollars have poured into the region over the past 10 to 15 years to address these and other health problems (see chapters 4, 6, and 12), most of these monies have gone into single-disease programs that have bypassed and further weakened health care systems (egregiously evident in the case of Ebola [Box 11-8]) and ignored the role of PHC (Lee 2012). The proliferation of donors and programs has resulted in bureaucratic confusion, duplication of existing activities, and distortion of priorities, in addition to incentivizing providers to meet donor targets rather than address actual need and impeding local participation in decisionmaking, all generating harmful and inequitable effects on marginalized populations (Barnes, Brown, and Harman 2014).

There are also hopeful signs across Africa. Rwanda, following its 1994 genocide (see chapter 8), has developed an effective intersectoral approach to health, involving community-based health insurance (with high enrollment, if inadequate funding, personnel, and national-level risk-pooling), a central role for community health workers, and a commitment to performance improvement, among other factors within and beyond the health sector. This complex set of features notably transcends the governance and intervention explanations to which health sector success is typically attributed (Sayinzoga and Bijlmakers 2016). On another front, the African Union adopted its first health strategy in 2007 (the African Health Strategy, 2007–2015), cataloguing the continent's various health care system ills, including poverty, underdevelopment, and underfunding, as well as the disruptive influence of structural adjustment and unfair trade practices (African Union 2007). In 2014 African Ministers of Health adopted a resolution to implement UHC by 2025 (noting the qualms outlined earlier).

BUILDING BLOCKS OF A HEALTH CARE SYSTEM

Key Questions:

- What are the building blocks of health care systems and how do they interrelate?
- How can the societal determinants of health be incorporated into the building of health care systems?

The basic building blocks of a health care system comprise—in addition to and drawing from the principles laid out at the beginning of this chapter—facilities, health care professionals and staff, and medicines and technologies, as well as the interface among these features and policymaking, information and research, training, regulation, financing and remuneration, and management (the latter two discussed in chapter 12).

Health care delivery is usually organized and distinguished by its level of specialization:

- *Primary care* (not to be confused with PHC): services offered to the population at the point of entry into the health care system (e.g., at a clinic, GP's office, or with another nonspecialist health care professional), ideally combining preventive, curative, household, and community aspects (and sometimes even providing social benefits). Polyclinics, a central health care system feature of the former USSR, various LMICs, and other countries, offer a range of generalist, specialty, and community-based services that effectively bridge primary and secondary care.
- *Secondary care*: standard inpatient services and specialist consultations, often on referral from primary care providers.
- *Tertiary care*: highly specialized services, such as neurosurgery or neonatal intensive care, available in hospitals equipped with advanced technology.

Facilities

Facilities refer to clinics, polyclinics, dispensaries, hospitals, nursing homes, health centers, pharmacies, medical schools, etc. Each health care system differs in its management of facilities and the private/public mix of financing. In recent years, with the growth of private health care markets and the adoption of ambulatory hospital care as a cost-cutting measure, free-standing specialized clinics have proliferated. Between 2000 and 2014 the number of hospital beds in OECD countries fell from an average of 5.5 per 1,000 population to 4.7 per 1,000 population, partly due to advances in ambulatory medical technologies as well as the pressure to reduce spending (OECD 2016). There are also numerous health care facilities and hospitals owned and operated by religious organizations (many dating from the colonial era in LMICs, or in Europe from the medieval Crusades), serving the general public but proscribing certain procedures (such as abortions).

Long-term care (LTC) (Box 11-9) is a burgeoning health care issue given worldwide increases in life expectancy. In Japan, characterized by its longevity, hospitals used to provide LTC, with almost half of inpatients over the age of 65 hospitalized for more than 6 months (Ikegami 2004). Given the huge cost implications, LTC insurance was introduced in Japan in 2000, although inadequate support to families and uncertain sustainability of services are ongoing problems (Tamiya et al. 2011).

Personnel

Health professionals personify the values and underlying goals of any health care system and normally serve as "gatekeepers" into the system. Responsiveness, effectiveness, and quality are often gauged by how people are treated by health personnel, globally (under-)estimated at 40 million professionals and 20 million support staff (GHWA and WHO 2013).

Physicians

Physicians are typically classified as "generalists" or "specialists." Generalists (also called GPs or family doctors) attend to a wide variety of acute problems and preventive needs, ideally through the continuous care of a stable set of patients in primary care settings. Specialists (e.g., thoracic surgeons, gastroenterologists, oncologists, cardiologists) usually practice in tertiary care hospitals and private offices, concentrating on a narrower set of ailments that require specialized knowledge and technical expertise. Human resource experts recommend that health care systems maintain parity between specialists and generalists. However, the lure of specialization, coupled with inadequate planning, means that many countries produce far too many specialists, causing shortages of generalists. For example, in the United States over 57% of doctors are specialists (Hing and Schapper 2012) compared with 31.8% in the United Kingdom (General Medical Council 2016) and 25% in Indonesia (WHO SEARO 2011).

In LMICs, government medical services and social security hospitals and clinics usually employ salaried physicians. In various countries newly-graduated physicians must undertake a period of full-time government service, generally in rural areas. Because of low wages in government health care systems across most LMICs, many physicians

Box 11-9 Long-Term Care Facilities and Hospices

LTC facilities and hospices are rarely considered a mainstay of health systems, but as populations age, the need for these facilities increases. By 2050, 2 billion people will be over the age of 65, with 85% of this number projected to be living in LMICs. In many countries, socio-cultural, economic, and demographic shifts mean that children or other relatives can no longer care for older family members as they have traditionally (Stuifbergen and Van Delden 2011). This has generated a greater need for LTC facilities and hospices for older populations, who may require complex, continuous health care.

While some countries have developed publicly funded and/or delivered LTC facilities and payment plans to replace informal caregivers (e.g., Germany), most do not have policies or plans in place to meet the needs of aging populations. This limits availability of LTC facilities, as well as regulation quality, accessibility, and affordability. An especially interesting LTC model has emerged in the Netherlands, where the Hogeway community enables people with severe dementia to live in an integrated village of houses, shops, and parks reminiscent of their younger years, yet protected from the outside world.

devote part of the day to public service and part to private practice. In some European countries, physicians similarly split their time among government service, private practice, and working for a private insurance plan.

Nurses

At both the primary care and hospital care levels, nurses play a crucial role. Yet in many LMICs there are fewer nurses than physicians. In some Latin American countries, where nursing may be considered a low-prestige, gendered occupation, the number of nurses is very low (e.g., Chile's density of nurses and midwives was 0.14 per 1,000 people in 2009, Bolivia's was 1.01 per 1000 in 2011) (WHO 2015). In the United States, the majority of physicians are male, and the majority of nurses female (US Census Bureau 2013; Young et al. 2013), whereas in the former Soviet Union most doctors and nurses were women. There is a relatively high ratio of nurses in the United States (9.8 per 1,000 persons) (World Bank 2015), but it recruits thousands of foreign nurses each year, particularly from the Philippines, which has less than half the nurse-population ratio (WHO 2015).

In some contexts, it may be difficult to distinguish the role of a nurse from that of a physician. Nurses, particularly nurse practitioners, may be better trained and assume more responsibility for patient care at a PHC level than some doctors, especially in medically underserved areas.

Other Health Professionals and Support Staff

There are many other types of health professionals, both licensed and unlicensed. Midwives practice in virtually every country, mostly as traditional practitioners, but a growing number of jurisdictions license and regulate them. In most LMICs, there is an extreme shortage of dentists, disproportionately affecting dental care access for poor and rural populations. Chiropractors are regulated in close to half of countries across all regions. There are an estimated 130,000 osteopathic practitioners in over 50 countries (Osteopathic International Alliance 2012). Other health professionals include psychologists, occupational therapists, nutritionists, and speech therapists, all of whom have important roles to play in the health care system yet may be scarce in LMICs. Physician assistants and nurse practitioners are trained to provide an array of primary care services. They are well established in some places but underused in most HICs.

In order for health care systems to run smoothly, there is also a great need for pharmacists, laboratory and equipment technicians, support staff, and medical auxiliaries. Technicians conduct laboratory tests and operate and maintain valuable health equipment (e.g., diagnostic equipment and infusion pumps). Pharmacists dispense, and sometimes prescribe, medicines. Physiotherapists provide essential rehabilitative services. Paramedics operate emergency medical services and ambulance services, stabilizing patients and transporting them to the hospital as rapidly and safely as possible. Administrative personnel and maintenance and cleaning staff provide crucial support services.

Community Health Workers

Numerous LMICs have long used community health workers (CHWs) as an effective means of strengthening health care systems. Locally based and selected, with a shorter training period than professionals, CHWs are ideally accountable first to their communities and supported by, if not always formally part of, health care systems (Lehmann and Sanders 2007). CHWs may be generalists—dealing with health promotion and prevention—or specialists focusing on, for example, sexual and reproductive health or TB. Following the Alma-Ata conference, various countries integrated traditional birth attendants into their maternal and child health programs.

Despite historic links to barefoot doctors and PHC ideas around social mobilization, the contemporary rationale for reliance on CHWs stems from their cost-effectiveness as a shortcut solution for the global shortage of health workers (GHWA and WHO 2010). Furthermore, CHWs are often women, who are expected to work voluntarily. With insufficient attention to undergirding health care systems, this vision of CHWs is bureaucratized and depoliticized, with their intersectoral and environmental activities watered down (PHM et al. 2014).

Traditional Healers

Traditional healing is widely employed across the world and is rapidly increasing in some countries due to population preferences or because many millions have limited access to biomedical care (WHO 2013). Only a few countries have made concerted efforts to integrate Indigenous medical practice with allopathic medicine. In India, public insurance schemes cover both allopathic doctors and practitioners of Ayurveda, yoga, naturopathy, Unani, Siddha, homeopathy and other Indigenous medical traditions (known as AYUSH in India, which has a dedicated Ministry). In China, persons may elect to receive traditional (herbal, acupuncture, moxibustion, etc.) or Western treatment or a blend of both. Various European health care systems have long included homeopathy, and private insurance companies increasingly cover complementary and alternative (or integrative) care, even as there are ongoing tensions between allopathy and naturopathy and other healing systems.

In Bolivia, a 2013 Traditional Medicine Law formally recognized Indigenous medicine, incorporating traditional healers into the national health care system (Babis 2014). Integrating Indigenous healers and Western doctors within the same health facility can help foster holistic care, but asymmetry of power may persist, leaving traditional healers delegitimized and uncompensated. The public, however, often finds community-based traditional healers easier to access, less discriminatory, and more consistent with their beliefs and worldview (Torri and Hollenberg 2013).

Training and Retention of the Health Workforce: The "Brain Drain" Problem

Close attention to training and recruitment of health personnel helps ensure appropriate supply, skills composition, standards, and quality, particularly for the public sector. In LICs, especially, a leading health care system problem is maldistribution and inadequate supply of doctors and nurses. The shortage of some 7.2 million health professionals is projected to grow to 13 or even 18 million by 2030, with 100 countries below the WHO threshold of 34.5 skilled health professionals per 10,000 people (GHWA and WHO 2013).

A key problem is "brain drain"—the emigration of skilled workers to another country. Health workforce migration is influenced by both push and pull factors. Some HICs recruit health professionals from LMICs as a human resource (and cost-savings) policy through direct campaigns, or indirectly by providing easy access to visas. On the push side: LMIC health workers are frequently underpaid (sometimes limited by public sector wage ceilings imposed by the IMF until 2007, and by other loan requirements); may lack continuing professional training; typically work in high-stress, understaffed, and under-resourced environments; and may experience high rates of absenteeism as both cause and result of the former (Nair and Webster 2013).

Even in countries without overall shortages, marginalized populations remain underserved, particularly in rural or remote regions, urban slums, and areas with high prevalence of certain ailments such as HIV. In some countries with shortages, trained health workers may be unemployed because there are no funded positions. Such absorption problems are often consequent to downsizing under recessions or financial crises. Indeed, post-2008 austerity policies in Greece have stimulated a huge physician outmigration, especially to Germany.

Notwithstanding renewed attention, the problem of migration of health workers from LMICs to HICs is longstanding: yet another way in which resources—such as capital and natural resources—flow from "South to North," with poorer countries essentially subsidizing wealthier nations (Navarro 1981). As such, LICs have in fact been "donors" of health aid rather than recipients, left struggling to maintain their health care workforce.

Four HICs—Canada, Australia, the United Kingdom, and the United States—account for 72% of foreign-born nurses and 69% of foreign-born doctors in the world (WHO 2012a), with India, Pakistan, and the Philippines the top sending countries. Outrageously, there are more doctors from sub-Saharan Africa working in the United States than the combined total of doctors in 34 African countries (Tankwanchi, Vermund, and Perkins 2015). Between 2001 and 2008 the number of new foreign trained nurses increased six-fold in Australia, four-fold in the USA and three-fold in Canada (OECD 2010). The Philippines alone has lost over 130,000 nurses to migration since 1997 (Romualdez Jr. et al. 2011).

Also troubling is the issue of "brain waste," where health professionals migrate to the Global North only to be faced with rigid licensing requirements and hiring barriers due to their lack of local work experience. Ironically many who form part of the brain drain end up unemployed or underemployed in low-skill jobs (Alam et al. 2015).

Some argue that the "export" of health workers is a deliberate policy by LMIC governments to increase remittances and obtain hard currency or services. In 2015 the Ugandan government sent over 250 doctors to work in Trinidad (with double the doctor-population ratio) in exchange for expertise in oil reserve development (Labonté et al. 2015). Certainly the families of health professional migrants benefit from remittances sent home by doctors and nurses practicing overseas. But in the Philippines, for example, some hospitals and clinics are left without staff after whole cohorts migrate, effectively shutting down services and denying care to local populations. The HIV pandemic (like the 2014–2015 Ebola outbreak) have posed a triple threat to the health workforce—increased workloads (more patients), emotional strain as a result of high patient mortality, and sickness and death (in part occupationally acquired) among workers themselves.

Seeking to address the problems surrounding health workforce migration, in 2010 the WHA unanimously adopted a Global Code of Practice on the International Recruitment of Health Personnel. However, this voluntary, unenforceable code has engendered little progress or awareness (Edge and Hoffman 2013), and physician migration from sub-Saharan Africa to the United States has continued. Most importantly, the code excludes the issue of financial compensation to countries that have experienced health personnel emigration (PHM et al. 2014).

A more promising response has arisen from some LMICs. In recent years China has hosted several thousand African students pursuing health degrees and has opened 4,500 additional spaces for African doctors and nurses to study in China into the future. China also conducted extensive on-the-ground training of over 10,000 local West African community health workers, nurses, and doctors to respond to Ebola, based on China's experience dealing with SARS (Forum on China-Africa Cooperation 2015).

Cuba, meanwhile, has for decades trained LMIC health workers both in Cuba and in situ. In 1999 the Cuban government founded the Latin American School of Medicine (ELAM) dedicated to increasing the number of LMIC doctors for underserved populations. Particularly intent on training those from minority and impoverished backgrounds, ELAM provides full scholarships on the condition that graduates return to practice in their home communities. To date, some 25,000 people from over 80 countries and dozens of ethnic backgrounds have graduated as physicians (ELAM 2016). Currently there are more than 20,000 students from almost 120 countries enrolled in medical faculties across Cuba. Over 200 US students from low-income and racial minority backgrounds have enrolled at ELAM (Remen and Bondi-Boyd 2013). Additionally, since the 1960s Cuba has sent more than 135,000 of its own doctors to work in over 100 LMICs, such as Angola, Nicaragua, Pakistan, South Africa, Venezuela, and Vietnam (and 256 doctors were deployed for the West African Ebola outbreak). This South–South health cooperation (including the founding of and collaboration with dozens of medical faculties in Africa and elsewhere) has been enabled by Cuba's large investment in physician training since the 1959 revolution (Feinsilver 1993; Kirk 2015). In 2014, for example, approximately 50,000 Cuban health personnel were working in over 60 countries, "a larger workforce than the Red Cross, Médecins Sans Frontières, and UNICEF, combined" (Huish 2014, p. 1).

Equipment, Diagnostics, and Technology

Proper equipment and supplies are essential to medical care. Basic supplies—for instance clean syringes, latex gloves, and disinfectant—can prevent many communicable diseases. Surgical items, sutures, and intravenous drips can turn potentially fatal procedures into lifesaving ones, as can asepsis and antibiotics. Advanced imaging equipment such as MRI machines may provide important information for diagnosis and treatment. Conversely, lack of accessible, affordable, and quality diagnostics (e.g., laboratories) leads to underdiagnosis or misdiagnosis in many LMICs.

Well-functioning and appropriate equipment is highly inequitably distributed: international market prices and patent protections make equipment prohibitively expensive. In some LICs, as much as 80% of medical equipment is furnished by donors, with only 30% used (e.g., before and after the 2010 Haiti earthquake [Dzwonczyk and Riha 2012]) due to malfunction, inadequate training, or insufficient or expensive spare parts and supplies (WHO 2011b), with further environmental burdens of disposal. Other efforts are more collaborative, for instance a program in The Gambia seeking to improve the availability and reliability of medical oxygen in health facilities through appropriate, cost-effective approaches that consider training and maintenance needs (Bradley et al. 2015).

Medical ingenuity in LMICs has also led to important South–North technology transfer, from Brazil's mass miniature radiographic screening in the 1930s, to the first successful heart transplant in South Africa in the 1960s, to contemporary examples of Botswana's solar hearing aids and Indian medical software innovations. There are also important solidarity efforts on the part of Engineering World Health volunteers who collaborate with LMIC partners in repairing equipment and multidirectional biomedical engineering innovation. Still, it is important for health personnel not to be seduced by technologies, particularly those that remain unregulated and unevaluated (PHM et al. 2014).

E-Health (and Telemedicine)

A potentially important tool to increase access to health care in rural areas and bridge the technology and equipment gap between HICs and LMICs is e-health—that is, medical communication and treatment using the Internet and other communications technologies. Telemedicine, one element of e-health, refers to the use of telecommunications (such as videoconferencing) for the provision of health services at a distance, increasingly between physicians and patients directly. For example, the Indian Space Research Organization connects 60 specialist hospitals with 306 rural hospitals using geostationary satellites, generating over 500,000 tele-consultations since 2001 (Indian Space Research Organization 2014).

Putative benefits of e-health include: increased knowledge base of health professionals and consultations with senior colleagues; improved access to specialist care for nonambulant patients and those in rural areas; empowerment of patients and families with Internet access; management of electronic health records leading to enhanced continuity of care; and greater efficiency in use of scarce resources, such as specialists and expensive medical equipment.

More recently, the use of mobile phone technologies (m-health) has been applied to patient tracking and clinical management, supply chain coordination, emergency care, data collection, and health information. In South Africa, over half of expectant mothers participate in an m-health system that monitors their clinic visits, distributes important information about prenatal care, and serves as a pregnancy information hotline. But many such projects are poorly planned and unsustainable (Ahmed et al. 2014).

Most HICs also use e-health to provide services to remote areas (for example in Canada's North or Australia's outback) or to enhance overall diffusion of specialized services (as in the United Kingdom and Sweden). MICs, too, have established e-health facilities at tertiary and regional hospitals to provide specialist support to generalists at district hospitals.

These developments notwithstanding, it is important not to overplay the advantages of e-health. It is a massive industry slated to be worth US$200 billion by 2020 and necessarily focuses on increasing market penetration and profit-making. Costs are high, and e-health savings claims are questionable (Congressional Budget Office 2008), not surprising given that health technology has been repeatedly ranked the most profitable corporate sector—with an estimated 21.6% net profit margin—besting even finance (Chen 2015).

Most of all, though useful to some degree for improving access and management, these technologies do not address underlying health care system and infrastructure inadequacies and inequities—not to mention the billions of people who lack adequate health services access.

Pharmaceuticals and the Political Economy of "Big Pharma"

The development over the past century of effective vaccines and drugs has contributed to significant health improvements, yet access to and affordability of medicines—as well as research and improved therapeutics for diseases of the most impoverished and discriminated populations in LMICs—constitute a pressing global health concern. WHO calls for essential medicines to be available in adequate amounts, at all times, of good quality, and at affordable prices, but an estimated 2 billion people (predominantly in LMICs) still lack access (Forman and MacNaughton 2015). For many households in both HICs and LMICs, expenditures on medicines are a growing share of health care expenses. In numerous LMICs, medicines comprise up to two thirds of total spending on health (Bigdeli, Peters, and Wagner 2014).

A variety of MICs have sizeable pharmaceutical production capacity, including India, China, Argentina, Mexico, Russia, Brazil, Cuba, Iran, Pakistan, Egypt, and Indonesia (Alfonso-Cristancho et al. 2015; WHO 2011c). India and China together supply approximately 80% of active pharmaceutical ingredients globally. Nonetheless, most LMICs must import a significant proportion of medicines. While India alone makes up 22% of the world's generic market (Kallummal and Bugalya 2012), much of the world is in the dubious hands of the pharmaceutical industry.

Big Pharma is big business: global sales were approximately US$1 trillion in 2014 (IMS 2014), with net profits for the top 11 earners reaching almost three quarters of a trillion dollars for the 2003–2012 decade (Hagopian 2015). Just four companies (Sanofi, Merck, Pfizer, and GlaxoSmithKline) control 80% of global vaccine revenues (Statista 2015). The largest 10 companies generated over US$420 billion in sales in 2013 (approximately 40% of the global total), with profit margins reaching 20%. Pfizer alone enjoyed a staggering 43% profit margin of US$22 billion (Anderson 2014); in 2015 Pfizer tried to relocate to Ireland (by buying an Irish company) as a shelter from US corporate taxes, which are triple Irish rates, but the US Treasury Department prohibited the move as part of a clampdown on tax avoidance.

Like other corporations, pharmaceutical companies are obliged to maximize profits for shareholders: this fiduciary role is in conflict with serving the public's needs. They engage in all sorts of unethical tactics, corporate crime, and corruption, including false advertising, illegal drug marketing, overpricing, biased research studies, suppression of unfavorable results and information on negative side effects, misleading package inserts, questionable marketing practices, and safety violations (Dukes, Braithwaite, and Moloney 2014; Lexchin 2012a).

In 2012, GlaxoSmithKline was fined US$490 million for bribery in China and US$3 billion in the United States for misbranding, kickbacks, overcharging, concealing study findings, and unlawfully promoting antidepressants to children and adolescents (having been fined US$3.4 billion in 2006 for prior violations). All told, between 2009 and 2015 US pharmaceutical industry financial penalties amounted to US$23.8 billion. To name just a few cases, Johnson & Johnson was fined US$2 billion for kickbacks and promoting unapproved psychiatric drugs in the United States, Teva was fined US$1.2 billion for monopoly practices, and Pfizer was fined US$2.3B, Abbott US$1.5B, Eli Lilly US$1.4B, and Merck almost US$1B, all for illegally promoting drugs (Almashat, Wolfe, and Carome 2016). Nevertheless, the fines barely cut into earnings, and profiteering tactics continue (Gøtzsche, Smith, and Rennie 2013).

This powerful industry is market-driven to the extreme, with companies determining what drugs to research and develop, where to distribute them, and how to set prices. Pharmaceuticals claim to price drugs in order to be able to invest in research and development (R&D) and bring drugs rapidly from laboratory through clinical trials and then to market. Yet these costs are heavily subsidized by public sector funding, with government grants underwriting much of the university-based research for new drug development (Stevens et al. 2011).

Moreover, pharmaceutical companies themselves carry out little research on original drugs. In recent years most newly approved drugs have been "copycat" (or "me-too") drugs, which have slight molecular variations from existing drugs and only marginal differences in efficacy (Prescrire International 2014). Another tactic is "evergreening"—obtaining separate patents for multiple attributes of a single drug—thereby extending patent protection. Pharmaceutical executives are handsomely rewarded for guiding such strategies, earning eight-figure salaries (nine figures when stock options are included) (Staton 2014).

Over half of drug revenues go straight to profits and marketing, involving aggressive sales representatives distributing free samples, direct-to-consumer advertising, ghost-written medical articles, professional journal advertisements, and physician gifts and incentives in HICs and, increasingly, LMICs (Gagnon and Lexchin 2008; Lexchin 2012b).

Since the 1990s, pharmaceutical companies have enjoyed enhanced global patent protection of 20 years thanks to World Trade Organization (WTO) enforcement of its 1995 Agreement on Trade-Related Aspects of Intellectual Property Rights (TRIPS; see chapter 9). Because of their ruthless campaigns against the production of generic drugs (e.g. to treat HIV in South Africa, cancer in Colombia, and so on), drug companies—bolstered by aggressive, ongoing US State Department interference and pressure on LMIC governments (Silverman 2016)—are among the most reprehensible global health players. Worldwide mobilization against the barriers to affordable medicines imposed by TRIPS forced WTO to adopt the 2001 Doha Declaration, which allows countries to circumvent patent protection to address pressing public health needs. But in practice these "flexibilities" are limited, complicated, and difficult to maneuver.

The profit-making imperative and patent protection system have led to a gap in funding for drug R&D for many ailments prevalent in LMICs. For example, after a 40-year hiatus, new TB drugs have only recently begun to be developed (and are astronomically priced). And from 2000 to 2011 only 4% of all new therapeutic products approved (and 1% of new chemical entities) were for neglected tropical diseases, although they account for 10% of the global burden of disease (Pedrique et al. 2013). Drug companies prioritize blockbuster drugs that mimic those already on the market—virility pills, multiple versions of antidepressants and antiallergy, arthritis, cholesterol, oncology and blood-pressure lowering medications—that generate high sales in HICs, while ignoring other needs.

Pharmaceutical companies have extremely limited interest in (the needs of) the lowest-income populations, compared with patients who have deeper pockets and more lucrative diseases. As the case of Ebola illustrates, market incentives determine which drugs Big Pharma develops and for whom. There have been over 30 documented Ebola outbreaks since 1976, mainly in sub-Saharan Africa, but serious vaccine and treatment development efforts only began with the most recent epidemic in 2014. It took international advocacy and what amounts to a huge public subsidy for Big Pharma, including a US$390 million commitment from GAVI, the Vaccine Alliance to purchase and roll out an Ebola vaccine (Bossche et al. 2015) (plus WHO's efforts to accelerate R&D), creating previously nonexistent incentives for pharmaceutical companies to begin to invest (virtually risk-free) in Ebola therapeutics.

As discussed in chapter 4, Big Pharma has a critical influence over global health organizations that commission development, and fund distribution, of pharmaceuticals and vaccines to LMICs, such as GAVI. MSF has long questioned the use of development aid by the United Kingdom and other countries to support GAVI, which in turn has provided funding to GlaxoSmithKline and Pfizer (Boseley 2013). Pharmaceutical companies also stand to profit considerably from expanded global financing prospects for NCDs and are actively shaping global NCD policy discussions (PHM et al. 2014).

A key question is: should donor countries subsidize for-profit pharmaceutical companies? Moreover, what does the move to subsidize the private sector say about the purported ability of the free market to embolden risk-takers and drive innovation when the pharmaceutical sector refuses to take risks without guaranteed profits? Rather than directly lining the pockets of Big Pharma to produce medicines and vaccines for diseases it routinely ignores, donor countries might instead support domestic (nonprofit) pharmaceutical R&D and manufacturing capacity in LMICs themselves. This would ensure sustainability, affordability, and protect LMICs from the rapaciousness of Big Pharma and the skewed global patent system (Karan and Pogge 2015).

In addition to problems stemming from exorbitant drug prices, the patent protection regime, and inadequate drug development for ailments of the poor is the issue of substandard medicines. An estimated 1% of medicines in HICs and 10% to 30% in LMICs are either falsified or substandard (Centers for Disease Control and Prevention 2014). Substandard medicines can cause serious harm: deterioration in clinical condition due to administration of non-therapeutic products or lower than expected dosages; death resulting from toxic preparations; and the development of resistance to a particular drug or class of drugs. Examples include: mold on antiretroviral drugs (found in Kenya in 2011) (Attaran et al. 2012); donations of inappropriate (expired, dumped, or useless) medicines especially in emergency responses (as reported in Mozambique, El Salvador, Aceh, and Sri Lanka [van Dijk, Dinant, and Jacobs 2011]); and medicines containing little to no active ingredient (e.g. antimalarial medicines in West and Central Africa in 2013–2014) (WHO 2014b). Better national regulatory mechanisms and enhanced public awareness of the dangers of adulterated and substandard medicines is key, but unless high quality medicines are made affordable and accessible, cheaper, poor quality drugs will remain attractive to producers and consumers alike. To be sure, Big Pharma is far less concerned with substandard quality than with counterfeit medicines—the trafficking of fake medicines that cut into their profits ('t Hoen and Pascual 2015).

In recent years WHO experts have proposed a set of strategies to address the inadequacies of existing drug development for LMICs: advance purchasing commitments, open source research, transferable IP rights, taxation, and patent pools (WHO 2012b). While UNITAID has thus far effectively used the latter (see chapter 4) and taxing Big Pharma profits may help in the short run, advance purchasing seems of questionable value, amounting to a subsidy to pharmaceutical companies for existing medicines rather than fostering new R&D (Birn and Lexchin 2011).

Most promising may be a return to accountable, nonprofit public sector drug development. Notable examples include Brazil's Butantan Institute and Biomanguinhos and Cuba's biotechnology sector, both of which have growing research and production capacity at a much lower cost (e.g., development of schistosomiasis, hepatitis B, and meningitis vaccines, diagnostics, cancer medicines, and other therapeutics) (Martins, Possas, and Homma 2015; Reid-Henry 2010). Indeed, innovation has historically been motivated by far more than profits and patents. The discoverers of two of the most enduring, important, and effective medicines—polio vaccine and penicillin—never sought patents. To note, penicillin's development and diffusion (like DDT's and that of many other disease control measures) was tied to military purposes. In order to meet military, civilian, and some international needs, US military leaders cooperatively pooled vital scientific information to accelerate industry penicillin production based on government process patents (Quinn 2013).

Health Policy and Planning

Health planning and policymaking is influenced by broad political, economic, social, medical, and cultural factors and by specific actors with a stake in certain issues or policies (Walt et al. 2008). Major players in health policy formation are: the state, through its (elected) leaders and civil servants; political parties; organized formations of health professionals; hospitals and other providers; commercial interests linked to health care; industry and employers; unions; the citizenry or other beneficiaries; and advocacy groups. External "stakeholders," including bilateral agencies (e.g., the US government through PEPFAR), philanthropies (e.g., the Bill and Melinda Gates Foundation), international financial institutions, and multilateral players (e.g., the Global Fund), may also exert significant direct or indirect pressure on priority-setting.

These and other entities may lobby for particular health campaigns or approaches, require government financial or in-kind support, and/or squeeze out other priorities, all with limited accountability (see chapters 3 and 12 for examples). Governments may also be bound to enact a range of regionally determined policies through membership in multilateral organizations, such as the African Union, EU, or UNASUR. Increasingly, trade and investment agreements (e.g., NAFTA) circumscribe the domestic policy space on issues such as pharmaceutical production, health promotion, and health care provision (see chapter 9).

Whereas policies are broad expressions of intent, the purpose of planning is to determine how, when, and where to employ resources to achieve policy goals most effectively. As with policymaking, decisions on who has access to health resources is also significantly influenced by who has the power to decide! In theory, effective planning involves consultation with various players within and outside the government, including the intended beneficiaries, as well as consideration for the resources that will be required. Resources may be financial, human (e.g., physicians, nurses, administrators), social (e.g., community involvement), infrastructure (e.g., medical equipment, clinics, hospitals, information systems), and consumable (e.g., medical supplies, pharmaceuticals). Determining how resources are planned for and allocated—and at what level of authority (Box 11-10)—has enormous equity implications. In countries as diverse as New Zealand (Sheridan et al. 2011) and Mozambique (Anselmi, Lagarde, and Hanson 2015), the poorest populations are not allocated sufficient or relevant resources based on need.

Health policy, planning, and resource allocation all lead to programs used by the public (e.g., maternal and child health services; health promotion campaigns). Because health programs do not function in a vacuum, a high degree of intersectoral cooperation is needed, which may be hampered where decisionmaking is spread among overlapping and competing authorities. A key concern remains how health policy and planning can better engage with the societal determinants of health.

Regulation

The issue of oversight and responsibility for health and medical services is vital, complex, and dependent on the particular political and economic context of each country. By definition and legal purview, the state should play the largest role in regulation regardless of whether health services are publicly delivered and financed, because market systems are notoriously poor at self-monitoring. Regulatory processes employ both sanctions and incentives, and are fundamentally political given that they influence the (bureaucratic) power and resources (and, potentially, profits) of the institutions involved.

The main purposes of (government-led) health care system regulation, all but the last germane to both market-driven and decommodified health care systems, are (Mills and Ranson 2012):

- *Protecting public safety and improving health*: legislating standards of training and care; approving drugs and devices; and monitoring safety
- *Designing and overseeing payment and remuneration systems:* regulating reimbursement mechanisms and salary negotiation processes; setting fair charges for medicines, physicians, and laboratory visits (where relevant)
- *Ensuring quality*: licensing and ongoing quality control of practitioners, facilities, and health plans (where present)
- *Enhancing access and equity*: ensuring fair and needs-based distribution of practitioners, facilities, and technologies
- *Correcting market failures* (where health services are market-based): planning where and by whom various services are offered and controlling prices of medical care and medication

Box 11-10 Decentralization and District Health Systems

Since the 1980s, many countries have introduced public sector decentralization reforms, including the decentralization of health services. Decentralization entails the transfer of authority and responsibility for health services delivery (planning, resource allocation, procurement, etc.) to subnational levels of government—municipalities, districts, and provinces—or to parastatal agencies and private contractors. Under decentralization, the national government typically retains broad policymaking and financing responsibilities, with the latter sometimes devolved to the local level. Because centralized systems can be bureaucratic, rigid, and unresponsive to local population needs, decentralization has been promoted as a strategy to achieve greater equity, efficiency, participation, intersectoral collaboration, and accountability (Mills 1994).

WHO's normative model of District Health Systems has been useful to countries seeking to develop, manage, and strengthen health care provision at the district level (usually encompassing 100,000–300,000 people) in terms of: integrating primary and community health care centers, and district hospitals at the secondary level; implementing referral and cross-referral systems; and managing health teams and community health workers, as per Alma-Ata principles.

Much of the pressure to decentralize has come from bilateral and multilateral financial and development agencies. Although decentralization has been hailed as cost-effective and democratic, it has faced numerous problems and yielded mixed results in health care system performance (Mitchell and Bossert 2010). Some governments have been unwilling to delegate real decisionmaking or spending powers to lower level authorities. As well, in various settings there is delayed disbursement of funds from central to local governments, little preparation or training for decentralization, and local management capacity is lacking. Most importantly, decentralization has often taken place simultaneous to considerable budget cuts and health care privatization. This has meant placing more responsibility on the shoulders of local authorities without allocating sufficient resources or policymaking ability to carry out these functions (Birn, Zimmerman, and Garfield 2000; Frumence et al. 2014). Denmark and Canada, among other countries, have revisited decentralization arrangements to address equity concerns (Mossialos et al. 2016).

While the protective, equity-enhancing, bureaucratic, efficiency, and quality roles of regulation are relevant to all settings, global and bilateral agreements on trade in services increasingly impinge on these national-level regulatory functions (see chapter 9).

CONCLUSION

Learning Points:

- Health care systems are shaped by values and principles, historical trajectories, and political factors in each society.
- PHC is central to the development of equitable health systems, offering the possibility of integrating societal determinants of health approaches into health care systems and ministries.
- UHC may extend protection against catastrophic health care expenditures, but unless enbedded within a comprehensive, public health care system, is likely to generate or entrench health care system inequities, stratification, inefficiencies, and profiteering.
- Biomedically based systems are dominant—but not the only approach to health care (and health care systems themselves are a crucial albeit not the sole determinant of health).

- Health care systems across the world are affected by interconnected forces and pressures, including corporate profiteering (especially, though not exclusively, by pharmaceutical and insurance companies and for-profit hospital systems), corruption, and brain drain.

As we have seen, many factors must be taken into account when analyzing health care systems. The main features of a health care system (delivery, financing, management, organization) cannot be considered in purely technocratic terms: values, principles, the interests of particular parties, historical precedent, unions, grassroots and social movements, and persistent class struggles are all fundamental influences on health care systems. The United States shows a disturbing example of how undemocratic political processes act against the interests and demands of the majority of the population who favor national health insurance (Turiano et al. 2009), whereas countries such as Norway or South Korea demonstrate how inclusive political processes can enhance health services coverage.

With the pervasiveness of neoliberal capitalist ideologies, in recent years many countries—both LMICs and HICs—have turned to private sector provision of health care, including through the seemingly progressive idea of UHC. Such shifts can exacerbate inequities in access to services and health outcomes and open the door to profit-making on the backs of the poor. At the same time, a growing number of countries recognize the role of PHC-driven publicly funded systems in the efficient, just, and equitable distribution of health care services, and defend existing publicly-run health care systems or are developing them anew.

REFERENCES

African Union. 2002. Decisions of the Seventy-Sixth Ordinary Session of the OAU Council of Ministers/Eleventh Ordinary Session of the AEC. CM/Dec. 671–680.

———. 2007. African health strategy, 2007–2015. http://www.nepad.org/system/files/AFRICA_HEALTH_STRATEGY%28health%29.pdf. Accessed July 5, 2015.

Ahmed T, Lucas H, Khan AS, et al. 2014. eHealth and mHealth initiatives in Bangladesh: A scoping study. *BMC Health Services Research* 14:260.

Alam N, Merry L, Mainul Islam M, and Cortijo C. 2015. International health professional migration and brain waste: A situation of double-jeopardy. *Open Journal of Preventive Medicine* 5(3):128–131.

Alfers L and Lund F. 2012. Participatory policy making: Lessons from Thailand's universal coverage scheme. *WIEGO Policy Brief (Social Protection)* 11:1–6.

Alfonso-Cristancho R, Andia T, Barbosa T, and Watanabe JH. 2015. Definition and classification of generic drugs across the world. *Applied Health Economics and Health Policy* 13(1):5–11.

Almashat S, Wolfe SM, and Carome M. 2016. *Twenty-Five Years of Pharmaceutical Industry Criminal and Civil Penalties: 1991 Through 2015 (Chart Book).* Washington, DC: Public Citizen.

American Hospital Association. 2016. Fast facts on US hospitals. http://www.aha.org/research/rc/stat-studies/fast-facts.shtml. Accessed August 9, 2016.

Anderson R. 2014. Pharmaceutical industry gets high on fat profits. *BBC News*, November 6.

Andrews B. 2014. *The Making of Modern Chinese Medicine, 1860–1960.* Vancouver: University of British Columbia Press.

Anselmi L, Lagarde M, and Hanson K. 2015. Going beyond horizontal equity: An analysis of health expenditure allocation across geographic areas in Mozambique. *Social Science & Medicine* 130:216–224.

Armada F, Muntaner C, and Navarro V. 2001. Health and social security reforms in Latin America: The convergence of the World Health Organization, the World Bank, and transnational corporations. *International Journal of Health Services* 31(4):729–768.

Asakitikpi A. 2015. Health policy reform in sub-Sarahan Africa. In Kuhlmann E, Blank RH, Bourgeault IL, and Wendt C, Editors. *The Palgrave International Handbook of Healthcare Policy and Governance.* Basingstoke: Palgave MacMillan.

Attaran A, Barry D, Basheer S, et al. 2012. How to achieve international action on falsified and substandard medicines. *BMJ* 345:e7381.

Babis D. 2014. The role of civil society organizations in the institutionalization of Indigenous medicine in Bolivia. *Social Science and Medicine* 123:287–294.

Balabanova D, McKee M, Pomerleau J, et al. 2004. Health service utilization in the Former Soviet Union: Evidence from eight countries. *Health Services Research* 39(6 Pt 2):1927–1950.

Barnes A, Brown GW, and Harman S. 2014. *Global Politics of Health Reform in Africa: Performance, Participation, and Policy.* Basingstoke: Palgrave Macmillan.

Barr DA and Field MG. 1996. The current state of health care in the Former Soviet Union: Implications for health care policy and reform. *American Journal of Public Health* 86(3):307–312.

Barten F, Rovere M, and Espinoza E. 2010. *Salud Para Todos: Una Meta Posible.* San Salvador, El Salvador: Ministerio de Salud Publica y Asistencia Social Pueblos Movilizados y Gobiernos Comprometidos.

Benton A and Dionne KY. 2015. International political economy and the 2014 West African Ebola outbreak. *African Studies Review* 58(01):223–236.

Beveridge W. 1942. *Social Insurance and Allied Services: American Edition.* New York: The Macmillan Company, Inter-departmental Committee on Social Insurance and Allied Services.

Bigdeli M, Peters DH, and Wagner AK. 2014. *Medicines in Health Systems: Advancing Access, Affordability and Appropriate Use.* Geneva: WHO.

Birn A-E, Brown T, Fee E, and Lear W. 2003. Struggles for national health reform in the United States. *American Journal of Public Health* 93(1):86–91.

Birn A-E and Lexchin J. 2011. Beyond patents: The GAVI Alliance, AMCs and improving immunization coverage through public sector vaccine production in the global south. *Human Vaccines* 7(3):291–292.

Birn A-E and Nervi L. 2015. Political roots of the struggle for health justice in Latin America. *Lancet* 385(9974):1174–1175.

Birn A-E, Zimmerman S, and Garfield R. 2000. To decentralize or not to decentralize, is that the question? Nicaraguan health policy under structural adjustment in the 1990s. *International Journal of Health Services* 30(1):111–128.

Blumenthal D and Hsiao W. 2015. Lessons from the East—China's rapidly evolving health care system. *New England Journal of Medicine* 372(14):1281–1285.

Boseley S. 2013. Aid for vaccines is subsidising Big Pharma, doctors claim. *The Guardian*, February 4.

Bossche GV, Malvolti S, Nguyen A, et al. 2015. *Ebola Update: Report to the Board 2-3 December 2015.* Geneva: Gavi, the Vaccine Alliance.

Bowry AD, Lewey J, Dugani SB, and Choudhry NK. 2015. The burden of cardiovascular disease in low-and middle-income countries: Epidemiology and management. *Canadian Journal of Cardiology* 31(9):1151–1159.

Bradley BD, Chow S, Nyassi E, et al. 2015. A retrospective analysis of oxygen concentrator maintenance needs and costs in a low-resource setting: Experience from The Gambia. *Health and Technology* 4(4):319–328.

Breilh J. 1979. Community medicine under imperialism: A new medical police? *International Journal of Health Services* 9(1):5–24.

Brill S. 2015. *America's Bitter Pill: Money, Politics, Backroom Deals, and the Fight to Fix Our Broken Healthcare System.* New York: Random House.

Cape Town Statement. 2014. Third Global Symposium on Health Systems Research Cape Town, South Africa. http://healthsystemsglobal.org/Portals/0/files/Cape-Town-Statement.pdf. Accessed July 5, 2015.

Carrin G and James C. 2004. *Reaching Universal Coverage via Social Health Insurance: Key Design Features in the Transition Period.* Discussion Paper 2. Geneva: WHO.

Centers for Disease Control and Prevention. 2014. Counterfeit drugs. http://www.cdc.gov/features/counterfeitdrugs/. Accessed May 1, 2015.

Chan M. 2015. Keynote address at the ministerial meeting on universal health coverage: The post-2015 challenge. http://www.who.int/dg/speeches/2015/singapore-uhc/en/. Accessed March 2, 2015.

Chaufan C. 2011. Influence of policy on health care for families. In Craft-Rosenberg MJ, Editor. *Encyclopedia of Family Health.* Newbury Park, CA: SAGE Publications.

———. 2015. Why do Americans still need single-payer health care after major health reform? *International Journal of Health Services* 45(1):149–160.

Chen L. 2015. The most profitable industries in 2016. *Forbes*, December 21.

Cheng TM. 2015. Reflections on the 20th anniversary of Taiwan's single-payer national health insurance system. *Health Affairs* 34(3):502–510.

Chernomas R and Hudson I. 2013. *To Live and Die in America: Class, Power, Health and Healthcare.* London: Pluto Press.

Clarke AE, Shim JK, Mamo L, et al. 2003. Biomedicalization: Technoscientific transformations of health, illness, and U.S. biomedicine. *American Sociological Review* 68(2):161–194.

Cohn J. 2014. 7 charts that prove Obamacare is working. *New Republic*, September 29.

Collins SR, Rasmussen PW, Beutel S, and Doty MM. 2015. *The Problem of Underinsurance and How Rising Deductibles Will Make It Worse—Findings from the Commonwealth Fund Biennial Health Insurance Survey.* New York: The Commonwealth Fund.

Congressional Budget Office. 2008. *Evidence on the Costs and Benefits of Health Information Technology.* Washington, DC: Congressional Budget Office.

———. 2015. *Insurance Coverage Provisions of the Affordable Care Act—CBO's March 2015 Baseline.* Washington, DC: Congressional Budget Office.

Cuadra CB. 2012. Right of access to health care for undocumented migrants in EU: A comparative study of national policies. *European Journal of Public Health* 22(2):267–271.

Cueto M. 2004. The origins of primary health care and selective primary health care. *American Journal of Public Health* 94(11):1864–1874.

Damrongplasit K and Melnick GA. 2009. Early results from Thailand's 30 Baht health reform: Something to smile about. *Health Affairs* 28(3):w457–w466.

Davis K, Stremikis K, Schoen C, and Squires D. 2014. *Mirror, Mirror on the Wall, 2014 update: How the Performance of the U.S. Health Care System Compares Internationally.* New York: The Commonwealth Fund.

Day C and Gray A. 2014. Health and Related Indicators. In Padarath A, English R, Editors. *South Africa Health Review 2013/14.* Durban: Health Systems Trust.

Demko P. 2014. Healthcare fraud investigations recover $4.3B in FY 2013. *Modern Healthcare,* February 26.

DHHS [Department of Health and Human Services]. 2015. Key features of the Affordable Care Act by year. http://www.hhs.gov/healthcare/facts/timeline/timeline-text.html. Accessed April 28, 2015.

Dillman J, Mancas B, Jacoby M, and Ruth-Sahd L. 2014. A review of the literature: Differences in outcomes for uninsured versus insured critically ill patients: Opportunities and challenges for critical care nurses as the Patient Protection and Affordable Care Act begins open enrollment for all Americans. *Dimensions of Critical Care Nursing* 33(1):8–14.

Duggal R. 2015. Saving the employees' state insurance scheme. *Economic and Political Weekly* 50(17):25.

Dukes G, Braithwaite J, and Moloney JP. 2014. *Pharmaceuticals, Corporate Crime and Public Health.* Cheltenham: Edward Elgar Publishing.

Dzwonczyk R and Riha C. 2012. Medical equipment donations in Haiti: Flaws in the donation process. *Revista Panamericana de Salud Pública* 31(4):345–348.

Edge JS and Hoffman SJ. 2013. Empirical impact evaluation of the WHO global code of practice on the international recruitment of health personnel in Australia, Canada, UK and USA. *Globalization and Health* 9(1):60.

ELAM [Escuela Latinoamericana de Medicina]. 2016. Historia de la ELAM. http://instituciones.sld.cu/elam/historia-de-la-elam/. Accessed July 10, 2016.

Elias PEM and Cohn A. 2003. Health reform in Brazil: Lessons to consider. *American Journal of Public Health* 93(1):44–48.

Epstein H. 2014. Ebola in Liberia: An epidemic of rumors. *New York Review of Books* 61(20):91.

Ethiopia, Ministry of Health. 2012. Vision, Mission, and Objective. www.moh.gov.et/visionmission. Accessed August 10, 2016.

EU Commission. 2013. *Your Social Security Rights in Germany.* Brussels: European Commission.

Fang X. 2012. *Barefoot Doctors and Western Medicine in China.* Rochester: University of Rochester Press.

Feinsilver JM. 1993. *Healing the Masses: Cuban Health Politics at Home and Abroad.* Berkeley: University of California Press.

Field MG. 1978. *Comparative Health Systems: Differentiation and Convergence.* Rockville: National Center for Health Services Research.

Fleury S. 2011. Brazil's health-care reform: Social movements and civil society. *Lancet* 377(9779):1724–1725.

Flores W. 2006. *Equity and Health Sector Reform in Latin America and the Carribbean, from 1995 to 2005: Approaches and Limitations.* Report Commissioned by the International Society for Equity in Health—Chapter of the Americas.

Forman L and MacNaughton G. 2015. Moving theory into practice: Human rights impact assessment of intellectual property rights in trade agreements. *Journal of Human Rights Practice* 7(1):109–138.

Forum on China-Africa Cooperation. 2015. China trains over 10,000 Ebola medical staff for West Africa. http://www.focac.org/eng/zt/1_1_1/t1235617.htm. Accessed August 10, 2016.

France, Ministère des Affaires Sociales et de la Santé. 2016. Direction Générale de la Santé (DGS). http://social-sante.gouv.fr/ministere/organisation/directions/article/dgs-direction-generale-de-la-sante. Accessed September 23, 2016.

Franco S. 2013. Entre los negocios y los derechos. *Revista Cubana de Salud Pública* 39:268–284.

Frenk J, González-Pier E, Gómez-Dantés O, et al. 2006. Comprehensive reform to improve health system performance in Mexico. *Lancet* 368(9546):1524–1534.

Frumence G, Nyamhanga T, Mwangu M, and Hurtig AK. 2014. The dependency on central government funding of decentralised health systems: Experiences of the challenges and coping strategies in the Kongwa District, Tanzania. *BMC Health Services Research* 14(1):39.

Gagnon MA and Lexchin J. 2008. The cost of pushing pills: A new estimate of pharmaceutical promotion expenditures in the United States. *PLoS Medicine* 5(1):e1.

Garfield R and Damico A. 2016. *The Coverage Gap: Uninsured Poor Adults in States that Do Not Expand Medicaid – An Update.* Menlo Park: Kaiser Family Foundation.

General Medical Council. 2016. List of Registered Medical Practitioners – statistics. http://www.gmc-uk.org/doctors/register/search_stats.asp. Accessed August 11, 2016.

Geyman J. 2015. Growing Bureaucracy and Fraud in US Health Care. *Huffington Post*, December 12.

GHWA [Global Health Workforce Alliance] and WHO. 2010. *Global Experience Of Community Health Workers for Delivery of Health Related Millennium Development Goals: A Systematic Review, Country Case Studies, and Recommendations for Integration into National Health Systems.* Geneva: GHWA.

———. 2013. *A Universal Truth: No Health Without a Workforce.* Geneva: GHWA.

Gillam S. 2008. Is the Declaration of Alma Ata still relevant to primary health care? *BMJ* 336(7643):536–538.

Gilson L, Doherty J, and Loewenson R. 2011. Challenging inequity through health systems. In Commission on Social Determinants of Health Knowledge Networks, Lee JH, and Sadana R, Editors. *Improving Equity in Health by Addressing Social Determinants.* Geneva: WHO.

Gilson L and Mills A. 1995. Health sector reforms in sub-Saharan Africa: Lessons from the last ten years. In Berman PA, Editor. *Health Sector Reform in Developing Countries: Making Health Development Sustainable.* Boston: Harvard University Press.

Giovanella L, Feo O, Faria M, and Toba S, Editors. 2012. *Sistemas de Salud en Suramérica.* Río de Janeiro: Instituto Suramericano de Gobierno en Salud.

Gordeev VS, Pavlova M, and Groot W. 2014. Informal payments for health care services in Russia: Old issue in new realities. *Health Economics, Policy and Law* 9(01):25–48.

Gøtzsche PC, Smith R, and Rennie D. 2013. *Deadly Medicines and Organised Crime: How Big Pharma Has Corrupted Healthcare.* London: Radcliffe Publishing.

Government of India. 2012. Employees state insurance scheme. http://www.archive.india.gov.in/spotlight/spotlight_archive.php?id=18. Accessed May 29, 2015.

Government of South Africa. 2004. *Strategic Priorities for the National Health System: 2004–2009.* Pretoria: Department of Health.

Grigorakis N, Floros C, Tsangari H, and Tsoukatos E. 2014. *The Effect of Out of Pocket Payments on the Income of Hospitalized Patients: Evidence from Greece.* 7th Annual Conference of the EuroMed Academy of Business: The Future of Entrepreneurship, September 18-19. Kristiansand: EuroMed Research Business Institute.

Gross M. 2016. *Farewell to the God of Plague: Chairman Mao's Campaign to Deworm China.* Oakland: University of California Press.

Growth Analysis. 2013. *India's Healthcare System–Overview and Quality Improvements.* Östersund: Swedish Agency for Growth Policy Analysis.

Gruber J, Hendren N, and Townsend RM. 2014. The great equalizer: Health care access and infant mortality in Thailand. *American Economic Journal: Applied Economics* 6(1):91–107.

Hagopian J. 2015. The evils of big pharma exposed. *Centre for Research on Globalization*, January 18.

Hellander I, Himmelstein DU, and Woolhandler S. 2013. Medicare overpayments to private plans, 1985–2012: Shifting seniors to private plans has already cost Medicare US $282.6 Billion. *International Journal of Health Services* 43(2):305–319.

Heredia N, Laurell AC, Feo O, et al. 2015. The right to health: What model for Latin America? *Lancet* 385(9975):e34–e37.

Himmelstein DU, Jun M, Busse R, et al. 2014. A comparison of hospital administrative costs in eight nations: US costs exceed all others by far. *Health Affairs* 33(9):1586–1594.

Himmelstein DU and Woolhandler S. 2014. Analysis of the Census Bureau's Annual March Current Population Survey for 2014 [unpublished].

———. 2016. The current and projected taxpayer shares of US health costs. *American Journal of Public Health* 106(3):449–452.

Hing E and Schappert SM. 2012. Generalist and specialty physicians: Supply and access, 2009–2010. *NCHS Data Brief* No.105.

Hoffman B. 2003. Health care reform and social movements in the United States. *American Journal of Public Health* 93(1):75–86.

Huish R. 2014. Why does Cuba 'care' so much? Understanding the epistemology of solidarity in global health outreach. *Public Health Ethics* 7(3):261–276.

Ikegami N. 2004. Japan's health care system: Containing costs and attempting reform. *Health Affairs* 23(3):26–35.

IMS Institute for Health Informatics. 2014. *Global Outlook for Medicines Through 2018*. Parsippany: IMS Institute for Healthcare Informatics.

Indian Space Research Organization. 2014. Tele-Medicine. http://www.isro.gov.in/applications/tele-medicine. Accessed May 2, 2015.

Iriart C, Merhy EE, and Waitzkin H. 2001. Managed care in Latin America: The new common sense in health policy reform. *Social Science and Medicine* 52(8):1243–1253.

Jeong H-S. 2005. Health care reform and change in public–private mix of financing: A Korean case. *Health Policy* 74(2):133–145.

Jiwani A, Himmelstein D, Woolhandler S, and Kahn JG. 2014. Billing and insurance-related administrative costs in United States' health care: Synthesis of micro-costing evidence. *BMC health services research* 14(1):556.

KFF [Kaiser Family Foundation]. 2016a. Status of State Action on the Medicaid Expansion Decision. kff.org/health-reform/state-indicator/state-activity-around-expanding-medicaid-under-the-affordable-care-act/. Accessed August 9, 2016.

———. 2016b. Total professionally active physicians. http://kff.org/other/state-indicator/total-active-physicians/. Accessed August 9, 2016.

KFF and HRET [Health Research and Educational Trust]. 2014. Web briefing for media: 2014 Kaiser/HRET employer health benefits survey. https://kaiserfamilyfoundation.files.wordpress.com/2014/09/ehbs-final-slide-deck-for-web.pdf. Accessed July 8, 2015.

Kallummal M and Bugalya K. 2012. *India's Trade in Pharmaceutical Sector: Some Insights*. New Delhi: Centre for WTO Studies.

Karan A and Pogge T. 2015. Ebola and the need for restructuring pharmaceutical incentives. *Journal of Global Health* 5(1):010303.

Karanikolos M, Mladovsky P, Cylus J, et al. 2013. Financial crisis, austerity, and health in Europe. *Lancet* 381(9874):1323–1331.

Khazan O. 2014. Why Americans are drowning in medical debt. *The Atlantic*, October 8.

Kieny MP, Evans DB, Schmets G, and Kadandale S. 2014. Health-system resilience: Reflections on the Ebola crisis in western Africa. *Bulletin of the World Health Organization* 92:850.

King's Fund. 2014. *Commission on the Future of Health and Social Care in England: The UK private health market*. London: The King's Fund.

Kirk JM. 2015. *Healthcare without Borders: Understanding Cuban Medical Internationalism*. Gainsville, FL: University Press of Florida.

Knaul FM, Arreola H, Mendez O, and Miranda M. 2005. *Preventing Impoverishment, Promoting Equity and Preventing Households from Financial Crisis: Health Insurance through Institutional Reform in Mexico*. Arenal Tepepan, México: Fundación Mexicana para la Salud.

Knaul FM, González-Pier E, Gómez-Dantés O, et al. 2012. The quest for universal health coverage: Achieving social protection for all in Mexico. *Lancet* 380(9849):1259–1279.

Koivusalo M and Baru R. 2008. Global social policy forum, introduction: Reclaiming primary health care - why does Alma Ata still matter? Or can we still speak of the relevance of Alma Ata? *Global Social Policy* 8(2):147–148.

Kruk ME, Porignon D, Rockers PC, and Van Lerberghe W. 2010. The contribution of primary care to health and health systems in low- and middle-income countries: A critical review of major primary care initiatives. *Social Science and Medicine* 70(6):904–911.

Kwon S. 2011. *Health Care Reform in Korea: Key Challenges*. IMF Conference, October 3. Tokyo: IMF.

Kwon S, Meng Q-Y, Tangcharoensathien V, et al. 2012. *Direct Household Payments for Health Services in Asia and the Pacific: Impacts and Policy Options*. Geneva: WHO Asia Pacific Observatory on Health Systems and Policies.

Labonté R, Attaran A, Bourgeault I, et al. 2015. Trading health for oil? Uganda should not export its health workers. *Lancet* 385(9970):e13.

Labonté R, Sanders D, Packer C, and Schaay N. 2014. Is the Alma Ata vision of comprehensive primary health care viable? Findings from an international project. *Global Health Action* 7:24997.

Lancet [Editorial]. 2012. The struggle for universal health coverage. *Lancet* 380(9845):859.

Laurell AC. 2007. Health system reform in Mexico: A critical review. *International Journal of Health Services* 37(3):515–535.

———. 2015. The Mexican popular health insurance: Myths and realities. *International Journal of Health Services* 45:105–125.

Lee MM. 2012. Vertical aid externalities: Evidence from the case of PEPFAR. https://ncgg.princeton.edu/IPES/2012/papers/S215_rm1.pdf. Accessed 5 July 2015.

Lee WY and Shaw I. 2014. The impact of out-of-pocket payments on health care inequity: The case of national health insurance in South Korea. *International Journal of Environmental Research and Public Health* 11(7):7304–7318.

Lehmann U and Sanders D. 2007. *Community Health Workers: What Do We Know About Them? The State of the Evidence on Programmes, Activities, Costs and Impact on Health Outcomes of Using Community Health Workers.* Geneva: WHO.

Lexchin J. 2012a. Social responsibility and marketing of drugs in developing countries: A goal or an oxymoron. In Forman J and Kohler JC, Editors. *Access to Medicines as a Human Right: Implications for Pharmaceutical Industry Responsibility.* Toronto: University of Toronto Press.

———. 2012b. Those who have the gold make the evidence: How the pharmaceutical industry biases the results of clinical trials of medications. *Science and Engineering Ethics* 18:247–261.

Light D. 2003. Universal health care: Lessons from the British experience. *American Journal of Public Health* 93(1):25–30.

Lima NT, Gerschman S, Edler FC, and Suárez JM, Editors. 2005. *Saúde e democracia: História e Perspectivas do SUS.* Rio de Janeiro: Fiocruz.

Link CL and McKinlay JB. 2010. Only half the problem is being addressed: Underinsurance is as big a problem as uninsurance. *International Journal of Health Services: Planning, Administration, Evaluation* 40(3):507–523.

Lister J. 2008. *WHO Commission on Social Determinants of Health: Globalization and health systems change. Globalization and Health Knowledge Network: Research Papers.* Ottawa: Institute of Population Health.

Litsios S. 2005. Selskar Gunn and China: The Rockefeller Foundation's "other" approach to public health. *Bulletin of the History of Medicine* 79(2):295–318.

López Arellano O and López Moreno S. 2015. *Derecho a la salud en México.* México: Universidad Autónoma Metropolitana-Xochimilco.

Mahler H. 1978. Speech at the opening ceremony. International Conference on Primary Health Care, September 6–12. Alma-Ata, Kazakhstan (USSR former): WHO.

Makhloufi K, Ventelou B, and Abu-Zaineh M. 2015. Have health insurance reforms in Tunisia attained their intended objectives?. *International Journal of Health Economics and Management* 15(1):29–51.

Marmot M. 2013. Universal health coverage and social determinants of health. *Lancet* 382(9900):1227–1228.

Marten R, McIntyre D, Travassos C, Shishkin S, et al. 2014. An assessment of progress towards universal health coverage in Brazil, Russia, India, China, and South Africa (BRICS). *Lancet* 384 (9960):2164–2171.

Martínez Franzoni and Sánchez-Ancochea. 2016. *The Quest for Universal Social Policy in the South: Actors, Ideas and Architectures.* Cambridge: Cambridge University Press.

Martins R de M, Possas C de A, and Homma A. 2015. Historical review of clinical vaccine studies at Oswaldo Cruz Institute and Oswaldo Cruz Foundation - technological development issues. *Memórias do Instituto Oswaldo Cruz* 110(1):114–124.

Massyn N, Day C, Peer N, et al. 2014. *District Health Barometer, 2013/14.* Durban: Health Systems Trust.

Maxmen A. 2015. Frontline health workers were sidelined in $3.3bn fight against Ebola. *Newsweek*, May 19.

McInnes C. 2016. Crisis! What crisis? Global health and the 2014–15 West African Ebola outbreak. *Third World Quarterly* 37(3):380–400.

McKenna H. 2016. *Five Big Issues for Health and Social Care After the Brexit Vote.* London: The King's Fund.

Menéndez E. 2003. Modelos de atención de los padecimientos: de exclusiones teóricas y articulaciones prácticas. *Ciencia & Saude Coletiva* 8(1):185–207.

Meng Q and Xu K. 2014. Progress and challenges of the rural cooperative medical scheme in China. *Bulletin of the World Health Organization* 92:447–451.

Meng Q, Yang H, Chen W, et al. 2015. People's Republic of China: Health system review. *Health Systems in Transition* 5(7):1–217.

Mills A. 1994. Decentralization and accountability in the health sector from an international perspective: What are the choices? *Public Administration and Development* 14(3):281–292.

Mills AJ and Ranson MK. 2012. The design of health systems. In Merson MH, Black RE, and Mills AJ, Editors. *Global Health: Diseases, Programs, Systems and Policies.* Third Edition. Burlington, MA: Jones & Bartlett Publishers.

Ministry of Health and Family Welfare. 2016. Shri Shripad Yesso Naik: Need to reach out to unreached populations and meet their healthcare needs. http://pib.nic.in/newsite/PrintRelease.aspx?relid=145282. Accessed August 9, 2016.

Ministry of Health of Great Britain, and Department of Health for Scotland. 1944. *A National Health Service.* London, HMSO. Cmnd 6502.

Ministry of Health and Population Egypt, Partnership for Maternal, Newborn & Child Health, WHO, et al. 2014. *Success Factors for Women's and Children's Health: Egypt.* Geneva: WHO.

Mitchell A and Bossert TJ. 2010. Decentralisation, governance and health-system performance: 'Where you stand depends on where you sit.' *Development Policy Review* 28(6): 669–691.

Mossialos E, Wenzl M, Osborn R, and Anderson C. 2016. *International Profiles of Health Care Systems, 2015.* New York: The Commonwealth Fund.

Moynihan R, Doust J, and Henry D. 2012. Preventing overdiagnosis: How to stop harming the healthy. *BMJ* 344:e3502.

Muntaner C, Borrell C, Ng E, et al. 2011. Review article: Politics, welfare regimes, and population health: Controversies and evidence. *Sociology of Health & Illness* 33(6):946–964.

Nair M and Webster P. 2013. Health professionals' migration in emerging market economies: Patterns, causes and possible solutions. *Journal of Public Health* 35(1):157–163.

Navarro V. 1981. The underdevelopment of health or the health of underdevelopment: An analysis of the distribution of human health resources in Latin America. In Navarro V, Editor. *Imperialism, Health and Medicine.* Farmingdale: Baywood Publishing Company.

———. 1989. Why some countries have national health insurance, others have national health services, and the U.S. has neither. *Social Science and Medicine* 28(9):887–898.

———. 1993. *Dangerous to Your Health: Capitalism in Health Care.* New York: Monthly Review Press.

Ndikumana L, Boyce JK, and Ndiaye AS. 2015. Capital flight from Africa: Measurement and drivers. In Ajayi SI and Ndikumana L, Editors. *Capital Flight from Africa: Causes, Effects, and Policy Issues.* Oxford: Oxford University Press.

Nervi L. 2008. *Alma Ata y la Renovación de la Atención Primaria de la Salud*: Encuentro Regional "Retos para la Revitalización de la APS en las Américas," September 22-25. Las Palmas: Comité Regional de Promoción de la Salud Comunitaria.

Núñez A and Chunhuei C. 2013. Equity in health care utilization in Chile. *International Journal for Equity in Health* 12:58.

OECD. 2010. International migration of health workers: Improving international co-operation to address the global health workforce crisis. http://www.who.int/hrh/resources/oecd-who_policy_brief_en.pdf. Accessed March 7, 2015.

———. 2015. *Health at a Glance 2015: OECD Indicators.* Paris: OECD.

———. 2016. OECD Health Statistics 2016. http://stats.oecd.org/Index.aspx?DataSetCode=HEALTH_STAT. Accessed August 10, 2016.

Osteopathic International Alliance. 2012. *History and Current Context of the Osteopathic Profession.* Chicago: OIA.

Owen D. 2014. *The Health of the Nation: NHS in Peril.* London: Methuen.

Oxfam International. 2013. Universal Health Coverage: Why health insurance schemes are leaving the poor behind. www.oxfam.org/en/policy/universal-health-coverage. Accessed June 20, 2014.

PAHO. 2007. *Renewing Primary Health Care in the Americas: A Position Paper of the Pan American Health Organization/World Health Organization.* Washington, DC: PAHO.

Paim J, Travassos C, Almeida C, et al. 2011. The Brazilian health system: History, advances, and challenges. *Lancet* 377(9779):1788–1797.

Paradise J. 2015. *Medicaid Moving Forward.* Menlo Park: Kaiser Family Foundation.

Pear R. 2015. Many say high deductibles make their health law insurance all but useless. *New York Times,* November 14.

Pedrique B, Strub-Wourgaft N, Some C, et al. 2013. The drug and vaccine landscape for neglected diseases (2000–11): A systematic assessment. *Lancet Global Health* 1(6):e371–e379.

PHM, Medact, Medico International, et al. 2014. *Global Health Watch 4: An Alternative World Health Report.* London: Zed Books Ltd.

Physicians for Human Rights. 2015. *Aleppo Abandoned: A Case Study on Health Care in Syria.* New York: Physicians for Human Rights.

Pillay Y. 2001. The impact of South Africa's new constitution on the organization of health services in the post-apartheid era. *Journal of Health Politics, Policy and Law* 26(4):747–766.

Pollock A. 2015a. Will politicians be architects or destroyers of the NHS? *Lancet* 385(9974):1171–1172.

———. 2015b. British Medical Association backs bill to reinstate NHS. http://www.pnhp.org/news/2015/may/british-medical-association-backs-bill-to-reinstate-nhs. Accessed July 6, 2015.

Popovich L, Potapchik E, Shishkin S, et al. 2011. Russian Federation: Health system review. *Health Systems in Transition* 13(7):1–190.

Portela M and Sommers BD. 2015. On the outskirts of national health reform: A comparative assessment of health insurance and access to care in Puerto Rico and the United States. *Milbank Quarterly* 93(3):584–608.

Potter W. 2015. Health insurers watch profits soar as they dump small business customers. *Center for Public Integrity*, January 26.

Prescrire International. 2014. New drugs and indications in 2013: Little real progress but regulatory authorities take some positive steps. *Prescrire International* 34(364):132–136.

Qin X, Pan J, and Liu GG. 2014. Does participating in health insurance benefit the migrant workers in China? An empirical investigation. *China Economic Review* 30: 263–278.

Quadagno J. 2004. Why the United States has no national health insurance: Stakeholder mobilization against the welfare state, 1945–1996. *Journal of Health and Social Behavior* 45(extra issue):25–44.

Quinn R. 2013. Rethinking antibiotic research and development: World War II and the penicillin collaborative. *American Journal of Public Health* 103:426–434.

Raleigh VS and Foot C. 2010. *Getting the Measure of Quality: Opportunities and Challenges*. London: The Kings Fund.

Ramírez NA, Ruiz JP, Romero RV, and Labonté R. 2011. Comprehensive primary health care in South America: Contexts, achievements and policy implications. *Cadernos de Saúde Pública* 27(10):1875–1890.

Rao KD, Petrosyan V, Araujo ED, and McIntyre D. 2014. Progress towards universal health coverage in BRICS: Translating economic growth into better health. *Bulletin of the World Health Organization* 92:429–435.

Raphael D and Bryant T. 2010. The political economy of public health: Public health concerns in Canada, the U.S., U.K., Norway, and Sweden. In Bryant T, Raphael D, and Rioux M, Editors. *Staying Alive: Critical Perspectives on Health, Illness, and Health Care*, 2nd edition. Toronto: Canadian Scholars' Press.

Rechel B, Richardson E, and McKee M. 2014. *Trends in Health Systems in the Former Soviet Countries*. Copenhagen: The European Observatory on Health Systems and Policy.

Rechel B, Roberts B, Richardson E, et al. 2013. Health and health systems in the Commonwealth of Independent States. *Lancet* 381(9872):1145–1155.

Reich MR, Harris J, Ikegami N, et al. 2015. Moving towards universal health coverage: Lessons from 11 country studies. *Lancet* 387:811–816.

Reid-Henry SM. 2010. *The Cuban Cure: Reason and Resistance in Global Science*. Chicago: University of Chicago Press.

Remen R and Bondi-Boyd B. 2013. Doctors across blockades: American medical students in Cuba. In Birn AE and Brown TM, Editors. *Comrades in Health: US Health Internationalists, Abroad and at Home*. New Brunswick, NJ: Rutgers University Press.

Rockefeller Foundation. 2009. *Transforming Health Systems Initiative: Strategic Overview*. New York: Rockefeller Foundation.

Rodwin VG. 1984. *The Health Planning Predicament: France, Quebec, England, and the United States*. Berkeley: University of California Press.

Roemer MI. 1964. Medical care and social class in Latin America. *The Milbank Memorial Fund Quarterly* 42(3):54–64.

———. 1991. *National Health Systems of the World. Vol. 1: The Countries*. Oxford: Oxford University Press.

Rogaski R. 2002. Nature, annihilation, and modernity: China's Korean War germ-warfare experience reconsidered. *The Journal of Asian Studies* 61(2):381–415.

Romualdez Jr. AG, de la Rosa JFE, Flavier JDA, et al. 2011. The Philippines health system review. *Health Systems in Transition* 1(2):1–129.

Rowden R. 2014. West Africa's Financial Immune Deficiency. *Foreign Policy*, October 30.

Ruano AL, Furler J, and Shi L. 2015. Interventions in primary care and their contributions to improving equity in health. *International Journal for Equity in Health* 14(1):153.

Ruano AL, Sebastián MS, and Hurtig AK. 2014. The process of social participation in primary health care: The case of Palencia, Guatemala. *Health Expectations* 17(1):93–103.

Saleh SS, Alameddine MS, Natafgi NM, et al. 2014. The path towards universal health coverage in the Arab uprising countries Tunisia, Egypt, Libya, and Yemen. *Lancet* 383(9914):368–381.

Salganicoff A, Ranji U, and Sobel L. 2015. Medicaid at 50: Marking a milestone for women's health. *Women's Health Issues* 25(3):198.

Sanders D, McCoy D, Legge D, et al. 2015. Social and political remedies needed for the Ebola tragedy. *Lancet* 386(9995):738.

Sanders D, Sengupta A, and Scott VE. 2015. Ebola epidemic exposes the pathology of the global economic and political system. *International Journal of Health Services* 45(4):643–656.

Sarwal R. 2015. Reforming central government health scheme into a 'Universal Health Coverage' model. *The National Medical Journal of India* 28(1):e1–e9.

Sayinzoga F and Bijlmakers L. 2016. Drivers of improved health sector performance in Rwanda: A qualitative view from within. *BMC Health Services Research* 16(1).

Scheil-Adlung X, Editor. 2015. *Global Evidence on Inequities in Rural Health Protection: New Data on Rural Deficits in Health Coverage for 174 Countries.* Geneva: ILO Social Protection Department.

Schoen C, Radley D, and Collins SR. 2015. *State Trends in the Cost of Employer Health Insurance Coverage, 2003-2013.* New York: The Commonwealth Fund.

Scott-Samuel A. 2016. Tory plans for NHS privatisation released during parliamentary recess. *BMJ blogs*, August 5.

Scott-Samuel A, Bambra C, Collins C, et al. 2014. The impact of Thatcherism on health and well-being in Britain. *International Journal of Health Services* 44(1):53–71.

Sen K and al Faisal W. 2012. Syria neoliberal reforms in health sector financing: Embedding unequal access? *Social Medicine* 6(3):171–182.

Sengupta A. 2013a. *Universal Health Coverage: Beyond Rhetoric. Occasional Paper No. 20.* Kingston: Municipal Services Project.

———. 2013b. *Universal Health Care in India: Making it Public, Making it a Reality. Occasional Paper No. 19.* Kingston: Municipal Services Project.

Shahrawat R and Rao KD. 2012. Insured yet vulnerable: Out-of-pocket payments and India's poor. *Health Policy and Planning* 27(3):213–221.

Sheridan NF, Kenealy TW, Connolly MJ, et al. 2011. Health equity in the New Zealand health care system: A national survey. *International Journal for Equity in Health* 10:45.

Shiva Kumar AK, Chen LC, Choudhry M, et al. 2011. Financing health care for all: Challenges and opportunities. *Lancet* 377:668–679.

Sigerist HE. 1937. *Socialized Medicine in the Soviet Union.* New York: W. W. Norton & Co.

———. 1943. From Bismarck to Beveridge: Developments and trends in social security legislation. *Bulletin of the History of Medicine* 13(4):365–388.

Silverman E. 2016. State Department accused of interfering with efforts for affordable medicines. *STAT*, July 25.

Starfield B, Shi L, and Macinko J. 2005. Contribution of primary care to health systems and health. *Milbank Quarterly* 83(3):457–502.

State Health Access Data Assistance Center. 2013. *State-Level Trends in Employer-Sponsored Health Insurance.* Minneapolis: University of Minnesota.

Statista. 2015. Top 10 pharmaceutical companies based on global vaccine revenue market share in 2013 and 2020. http://www.statista.com/statistics/348702/leading-global-pharmaceutical-companies-by-vaccine-market-share/. Accessed May 13, 2015.

Staton T. 2014. 15 Highest-paid biopharma CEOs of 2013. *FiercePharma.* http://www.fiercepharma.com/special-reports/15-highest-paid-biopharma-ceos-2013. Accessed May 13, 2015.

Stevens AJ, Jensen JJ, Wyller K, et al. 2011. The role of public-sector research in the discovery of drugs and vaccines. *NEJM* 364(6):535–541.

Stuifbergen MC and Van Delden JJM. 2011. Filial obligations to elderly parents: A duty to care? *Medicine, Health Care and Philosophy* 14(1):63–71.

Stutz M and Baig A. 2014. International examples of undocumented immigration and the Affordable Care Act. *Journal of Immigrant and Minority Health* 16(4):765–768.

Sullivan K. 2013. How to think clearly about Medicare administrative costs: Data sources and measurement. *Journal of Health Politics, Policy and Law* 38(3):479–504.

't Hoen E and Pascual F. 2015. Viewpoint: Counterfeit medicines and substandard medicines: Different problems requiring different solutions. *Journal of Public Health Policy* 36(4):384–389.

Tamiya N, Noguchi H, Nishi A, et al. 2011. Population ageing and wellbeing: Lessons from Japan's long-term care insurance policy. *Lancet* 378(9797):1183–1192.

Tankwanchi ABS, Vermund SH, and Perkins DD. 2015. Monitoring sub-Saharan African physician migration and recruitment post-adoption of the WHO Code of Practice: Temporal and geographic patterns in the United States. *PLoS ONE* 10(4):e0124734.

Testa M. 1988. Atención ¿Primaria o primitiva? De Salud. In *Segundas Jornadas de Atención Primaria de la Salud.* Buenos Aires: Asociación de Médicos Residentes del Hospital de Niños Ricardo Gutiérrez.

Time Inc. 2010. Fortune 500 2010. http://fortune.com/fortune500/2010/. Accessed June 25, 2015.

Torri MC and Hollenberg D. 2013. Indigenous traditional medicine and intercultural healthcare in Bolivia: A case study from the Potosi region. *Journal of Community Health Nursing* 30(4):216–229.

Toynbee P. 2007. NHS: The Blair years. *BMJ* 334(7602):1030–1031.

Turiano L, Anderson M, Jailer T, et al. 2009. Health-care reform and the right to health in the USA. *Lancet* 374(9705):1887.

U.S. Census Bureau. 2013. *Men in Nursing Occupations American Community Survey Highlight Report.* Washington, DC: U.S. Census Bureau.

———. 2014. Income, poverty and health insurance coverage in the United States: 2013. http://census.gov/newsroom/press-releases/2014/cb14-169.html. Accessed July 8, 2015.

van Dijk D, Dinant GJ, and Jacobs JA. 2011. Inappropriate drug donations: What has happened since the 1999 WHO guidelines? *Education for health* 24(2):462.

Waitzkin H. 1993. *The Politics of Medical Encounters: How Patients and Doctors Deal with Social Problems.* New Haven, CT: Yale University Press.

———. 2003. Report of the WHO Commission on Macroeconomics and Health: A summary and critique. *Lancet* 361(9356):523–526.

Walt G, Shiffman J, Schneider H, et al. 2008. 'Doing' health policy analysis: Methodological and conceptual reflections and challenges. *Health Policy and Planning* 23(5):308–317.

Webster C. 2002. *The National Health Service: A Political History,* 2nd Edition. Oxford: Oxford University Press.

Werner D and Sanders D. 1997. Alma-Ata and the institutionalization of primary health care. In *Questioning the Solution: The Politics of Primary Health Care and Child Survival.* Palo Alto, CA: HealthWrights.

Whitehead M, Dahlgren G, and Evans T. 2001. Equity and health sector reforms: Can low-income countries escape the medical poverty trap? *Lancet* 358(9284):833–836.

Whiteside N. 2009. *Social Protection in Britain 1900–1950 and Welfare State Development: the Case of Health Insurance.* Coventry: University of Warwick.

WHO. 1978. *Declaration of Alma-Ata.* International Conference on Primary Health Care, September 6-12. Alma-Ata, Kazakhstan (USSR former): WHO.

———. 2008a. *World Health Report, 2008: Primary Health Care, Now More Than Ever Before.* Geneva: WHO.

———. 2008b. *Closing the Gap in a Generation: Health Equity Through Action on the Social Determinants of Health. Final Report of the Commission on Social Determinants of Health.* Geneva: WHO.

———. 2010. *World Health Report. Health Systems Financing: The Path to Universal Coverage.* Geneva: WHO.

———. 2011a. *Health Systems Strengthening Glossary.* Geneva: WHO.

———. 2011b. *Medical Device Donations: Considerations for Solicitation and Provision.* Geneva: WHO.

———. 2011c. *Local Production and Access to Medicines in Low- and Middle-Income Countries: A Literature Review and Critical Analysis.* Geneva.

———. 2012a. The health workforce: Advances in responding to shortages and migration, and in preparing for emerging needs. Report by the Secretariat EB132/23. Geneva: WHO.

———. 2012b. *Research and Development to Meet Health Needs in Developing Countries: Strengthening Global Financing and Coordination.* Geneva: WHO.

———. 2013. *WHO Traditional Medicine Strategy: 2014–2023.* Geneva: WHO.

———. 2014a. Global Health Expenditure Database. http://apps.who.int/nha/database/Select/Indicators/en. Accessed April 23, 2015.

———. 2014b. Information Exchange System Drug Alert No. 131, Falsified antimalarial medicines in west and central Africa. http://www.who.int/medicines/publications/drugalerts/Alert_131_antimalarials_essential_drugs_programme_pre_final.pdf. Accessed May 1, 2015.

———. 2015. Global Health Observatory Data Repository. http://apps.who.int/gho/data/node.main.A1444?lang=en&showonly=HWF. Accessed July 5, 2015.

———. 2016. What is universal coverage? http://www.who.int/health_financing/universal_coverage_definition/en/. Accessed August 9, 2016.

WHO SEARO. 2011. *Human Resources for Health Country Profile: Indonesia.* New Delhi: WHO SEARO.

World Bank. 1993. *World Development Report 1993: Investing in Health.* Washington, DC: World Bank.

———. 2014. Universal health coverage overview. http://www.worldbank.org/en/topic/universalhealthcoverage/overview. Accessed February 12, 2014.

———. 2015. World Development Indicators. http://data.worldbank.org/indicator/SH.MED.NUMW.P3. Accessed April 30, 2015.

Yip KC. 1995. *Health and national reconstruction in nationalist China: The Development of Modern Health Services, 1928-1937.* No. 50. Association for Asian Studies.

Young A, Chaudhry HJ, Thomas JV, and Dugan M. 2013. A Census of Actively Licensed Physicians in the United States, 2012. *Journal of Medical Regulation* 99(2):11–24.

12

HEALTH ECONOMICS AND THE POLITICS OF HEALTH FINANCING

Key Questions:

- What is the relationship between health and the economy?
- How is health care system organization linked to financing and management?
- What are the different approaches to health economics and what does each emphasize?
- Where does global health (and development assistance) fit into this picture?

Health and the economy are intertwined in multiple ways. On one level, the health sector has become one of the world's largest industries, and how it is financed has enormous bearing on national and domiciliary economies. At a household level, ill health and health care spending can lead to impoverishment, although poverty causes more ill health than vice versa. Both global and national health policymaking are concerned with determining how much and how to allocate health care spending—ideally efficiently, effectively, and equitably—in order to achieve health-related goals. But there are different political and economic approaches to reaching these ends. Moreover, as we will see, greater health care spending does not automatically engender better health: there are diminishing returns after a certain point, and even low per capita health care spending can yield positive health outcomes depending on how monies are spent and how other dimensions of the economy and society are organized.

Many argue that a growing economy necessarily improves living conditions and health, but the evidence is mixed depending on when, where, and how economic growth takes place and on how wealth is distributed (Deaton 2013). Previous chapters showed that gross domestic product (GDP) growth often exacerbates inequalities and may even jeopardize social conditions unless economic gains are extensively redistributed. Even in low-income countries (LICs), where economic growth may be necessary to ensure basic access to water and sanitation, education, housing, public health, nutrition, and other necessities, there is no guarantee that the fruits of growth will be channeled to these ends or remain in the country. Nigeria, for instance, enjoyed booming growth of over 6% per year over the past decade thanks to its oil sector (Trade Economics 2015), and GDP per capita rose to PPP$5,423 per capita in 2014, leading the World Bank to categorize it (controversially) as a lower-middle income country in 2016. Yet high levels of capital flight and tax evasion, enormous wealth concentration, and pervasive domestic corruption and political mismanagement have impeded growth from being collectively allocated and equitably invested in public infrastructure and social services (Pringle et al. 2012).

Indeed, growth and productivity gains under a neoliberal capitalist system frequently come at the expense of health, evidenced by the ratcheting down of environmental regulations, work conditions, social protections, corporate taxes, government social spending, and wages, all to maximize profits. Consequently, the importance of growth is increasingly contested: according to this line of reasoning, degrowth (and such Indigenous variants as Andean *Buen Vivir*; see chapter 13) is good for health because it reduces environmental degradation and uses resources in a more economical, balanced, and ethical fashion.

The pages ahead offer a road map to understanding health economics and financing from the contrasting perspectives of mainstream and social justice-oriented economics. First, we offer an overview and critique of key tenets of health economics, turning next to health care system financing and management. Then we analyze the aims, assumptions, and uses of cost analyses. Subsequently, we turn to the role of the dominant global health agencies and actors in shaping market approaches to health in low- and middle-income countries (LMICs) and in health financing. Last, we discuss alternative framings of investing for health equity.

Health Economics: A Snapshot

Global spending on health is immense but inequitable. This over US$6.5 trillion industry, including both public and private spending (WHO 2012), totals around 9% of world GDP, but masks a wide range of spending across the globe (Table 12-1). For example, per capita health expenditure for 2014 was over US$9,000 in Norway, Switzerland, and the United States, whereas the Central African Republic, Democratic Republic of Congo (DRC), and Madagascar each spent less than US$20 per capita on health (WHO 2015a). Yet across the world, between 20% and 40% of total expenditure is wasted through, among other factors, overpriced and inappropriately used medicines and services, fraud, and corruption (WHO 2010).

How should these concerns be addressed? Mainstream health economics focuses on:

> the allocation of resources between various health-promoting activities; the quantity of resources used in health service delivery; the organization, funding, and behavior of health services institutions and providers; the efficiency with which resources are used for health purposes; and the effects of disease and health interventions on individuals, households, and society (Mills 1997, p. 964).

Political economy and related critical approaches to health economics are similarly concerned with efficient and effective use of resources but consider questions of equity and social justice central to understanding how health and the economy interact and how health care systems should be financed and organized. Critical approaches underscore that equity does not preclude efficiency—indeed, as elaborated upon ahead, efficiency and equity can be mutually achieved.

Whereas orthodox health economics proposes various (technocratic) measures to address deficient health care delivery, for instance introducing private

Table 12-1 Spending on Health: Examples of the Extent of Inequities (in US$), 2014

Total global expenditure on health (2012)	$6.5 trillion
Per capita expenditure globally	$1,058
WHO estimate of minimum needed expenditure per capita (2012)	$44
Country with highest per capita expenditure	Switzerland ($9,674)
Country with lowest per capita expenditure	Madagascar ($14)
Number of WHO member countries spending less than $50 per capita	25

Data Sources: WHO (2012); WHO (2015a).

management systems, a political economy of health approach focuses on underlying forces:

- Grossly inequitable distribution of power and resources within and across countries
- Profiteering by corporations, including those linked to health care, such as insurance companies and pharmaceuticals (which paradoxically benefit from enormous public subsidies while creating inequities in health care access)
- A global neoliberal capitalist system representing the interests of transnational corporations (TNCs) and wealthy elites and marked by global TNC penetration, exploitative resource extraction, unfair terms of trade, labor oppression, financialization, tax evasion, capital flight, and corruption. These activities impoverish and oppress the majority of the world's population, especially those in LMICs, and compel disinvestment in social services including health, education, and housing.

As such, critical political economists seek solutions that go beyond symptoms, supporting the role of social and political movements struggling for health care as a right instead of a commodity; contesting the private sector's role in health care financing and provision; regulating TNCs and global capital to diminish rampant exploitation and illicit financial flows; and even advocating redistributive revolution—all solutions that could enhance *both* equity and efficiency.

Worldwide, health economics is playing a growing role in health care system planning and program implementation but also in overall economic considerations. Both national governments and international agencies have zeroed in on health care spending in the context of economic crises. While many economists regard health (and associated spending) largely in terms of targeted prevention and medical treatment, others understand health as subject to a range of influences, including education, medical care and public health, safe housing and employment, water and sanitation, environmental protection, as well as the global economic context framing domestic policies around these issues (Loewenson and Gilson 2012). A health economics lens can illuminate global health care spending and decisionmaking, yet it is crucial to remember the distinction between societal spending on health—which involves the intertwined and dynamic societal determinants of health—and spending on health care, just one, albeit important, determinant of health. Above all, allocating resources for health, both within and well beyond the health sector, is not a neutral technocratic exercise but one that is profoundly political.

The World Bank and other proponents of orthodox (neoclassical) health economics have historically supported targeted low-cost interventions for LMICs (Jamison et al. 2013), though not for high-income countries (HICs). This advice is based on evidence of health improvements measured by declines in specific disease rates, including those affecting infant and child mortality. According to this approach, allocation decisions must prioritize resources and interventions that have the greatest impact at the lowest cost because health resources are considered to be scarce.

Proponents of health and social justice approaches, by contrast, argue that technical cost analyses favor short-term, narrowly focused approaches to health improvement rather than overall health gains in the long run. Instead, progressive health economists stress the importance of comprehensive means of improving health that integrate primary health care (PHC)-oriented universal health care systems with social and political investment and redistribution of wealth, power, and other societal resources on a broad scale.

Ideally, health economics can help assess the fairness and equity of health-oriented investments, though these concerns often remain at a rhetorical level. Even the most technically elaborate economic analyses of health policies are not neutral but rather based on value judgments and decisions.

Indeed, health care system priority-setting and resource allocation are heavily influenced by both social objectives and political factors (Khayatzadeh-Mahani, Fotaki, and Harvey 2013). This is true in the context of resource allocation for HIV programs in Malawi, where donor interests are highly influential (Jenniskens et al. 2012), or among decentralized health authorities in Sweden, where local politics and historical patterns influence resource allocation based on nationally adopted principles of human dignity, need, and solidarity, in addition to cost-efficiency (Sabik and Lie 2008). A further problem with standard priority-setting mechanisms is that most reflect Western values and are applied with little regard for local historical, cultural, and political contexts.

ECONOMIC APPROACHES TO PUBLIC HEALTH AND MEDICAL SPENDING

Key Questions:

- What are the underlying assumptions of markets?
- How does health care differ from other goods/services?
- Why are markets incapable of equitably providing health services?

As evidenced by ancient engineering feats such as Roman and Incan aqueducts, recognition of the merits of health investment is far from new. By the 19th century the terrible working and living conditions created by the Industrial Revolution awakened a renewed rationale for societal spending on health. Although merchants, manufacturers, and colonial authorities were averse to paying for water, sanitation, and housing upgrades, gradually some employers recognized the health of workers, particularly skilled laborers, as a productivity input. Meanwhile, unionized workers and their allies fought for rights such as factory safety, workers' compensation, prohibition on child labor, and an 8-hour workday, launching ongoing struggles for occupational health.[1] By 1900, political pressure mounted for public investment to improve public health conditions in the workplace and community (and to stave off unrest [see chapter 1]), and in many settings the state was pushed to take on responsibility for health care provision (see chapter 11).

Today, notwithstanding the recognized value to society of (preventive and primary) health care services, and the role therein of public policy and planning, the most orthodox health economists portray health care system organization largely as the fruition of consumer choices, seeing government involvement as distorting market "efficiencies."

Neoclassical economic theory holds that the price of a good or service is determined by demand for that good/service (i.e., how many people are willing and able to pay for it), as well as its supply (the amount produced/that exists): because many goods are finite, the market provides a forum for consumers to compete for them. This school of thought argues that the extent of scarcity of an item, combined with the level of competition, determines its price. In particular, when supply is limited and demand climbs, the price of a product is driven up. As the price climbs, people begin to be "priced out" of the market—meaning they no longer desire (or cannot afford) the product at that price. Conversely, as a product becomes more abundant, its price falls, stimulating demand among those who previously deemed the product too expensive, with excess supply then leading demand to fall. Eventually, equilibrium is reached among supply, demand, and price.

But health problems are special: they threaten life and limb, and can cause pain and dysfunction. Alleviating these problems is not simply a question of choice. For this reason, the demand for health care is highly inelastic (that is, not dependent on manipulation of supply, but based on bona fide need) and often extraordinarily time sensitive, all factors distinguishing health care from other kinds of economic activities.[2] Consequently, the classic supply and demand curve—whereby the relationship between supply and demand is mediated by price—does not apply to health care (Table 12-2). Instead, suppliers (providers, principally doctors and facilities) have the capacity to create their own demand, so that as supply goes up so does demand, though still constrained by ability and willingness to pay at an individual or societal level.

In economic terms, the health sector is one where "producer sovereignty" (provider decisionmaking autonomy) can overshadow "consumer sovereignty." In addition to the special nature of health care in terms of human vulnerability, health care providers have far greater information and decisionmaking capacity (services are ordered by health personnel, not patients) than do consumers. The complexity—and time-consuming character—of acquiring medical knowledge makes consumer sovereignty untenable. The neoclassical solution is for doctors to serve as agents for their patients' consumption of health care services, assuming either perfect symmetry of interests or that patients can and will reject the agent's

Table 12-2 How the Health Care Sector Differs from Markets

Typical Market Assumptions	Using Health Care Services
Buyers and sellers freely enter and exit the market at any time, based on personal preferences.	Most people use health care services due to an emergency, to a chronic condition that requires long-term care, or to comply with school, workplace, or government regulations.
	Health care providers usually decide what services are needed and when they should be discontinued.
Buyers use personal resources to purchase goods and services.	Governments, employers, or privately-run insurance companies are often the main purchasers of health care services, with consumers paying indirectly through taxes, premiums, and/or coinsurance (or directly out of pocket).
Buyers are free to choose which good/service they wish to purchase, if any.	Health plans typically provide limited choice to "buyers" (with private insurance also restricting choice). In many places there is little choice in health care services or providers.
	Consumers may prioritize accessibility and availability of health services over choice of services or providers.
	Health decisions may be made for the patient by health care providers or by family members.
Buyers and sellers have equal access to information from which to make rational decisions.	Due to asymmetric information between providers and consumers, patients are often unaware of which health good/service is needed, if any, or which is most effective or cost-effective. Conversely, patients may not always disclose vital health information to providers.

advice when their interests differ. Physicians may prioritize professional status and earnings, making for a complicated and imperfect agency relationship that fails to adequately represent patient interests. For the patient, it is difficult to reject medical opinion or obtain different advice under circumstances of stress and pain and when there are serious consequences for health and well-being. Auto mechanics also have information advantages over customers, but the consequences of rejecting advice may involve taking public transport, learning how to do repairs yourself, or buying a new car. These are not trivial choices, but you may yet drive another day with mind and body intact.

What Makes Health Care Different from Markets?

Health care operates on a different basis from the more familiar market of goods and services for a variety of reasons. First, for personal medical care especially, the patient (i.e., the consumer) cannot control when or how he/she will spend money on care. Whereas, say, a schoolbag can be purchased now or postponed, with minimal import (not a life and death matter), an injury or illness may require immediate health care services. Once the decision has been made by, or for, a person to enter the health care system, that person is no longer in charge of most subsequent decisions. Physicians maintain control over medical decisions due to specialized knowledge and legal privilege through licensure (with decisions increasingly mediated by health plan restrictions and incentives). Decisions regarding diagnostic tests, surgery, medicines, return visits, and many other costly "purchases," are either heavily influenced by the recommendations of a physician (or other practitioner), or are made directly by the physician, not the patient. Moreover, the choice of grade, size, quality, or cost per item, usually available to the consumer in a market economy, is also absent.

Second, not only are patients essentially powerless to control expenditures, they are far less aware of medical needs. In contrast to markets, health care includes a structural asymmetry of knowledge among the parties (Arrow 1963). Still, direct consumer pharmaceutical marketing seeks to redress this imbalance to generate demand (Iriart, Franco, and Mehry 2011), and Internet access potentially empowers (wealthier) people (with the caveat that some information may be dangerous).

Third, when the money spent or allocated by the physician is from a government program or insurance company, this may lead physicians to overuse or underuse services depending on the administrative or payment structure. Under fee-for-service arrangements, wherein clinical decisions are separate from financial considerations, physicians have little incentive to economize. In fact, they may overprescribe to maximize income, generating unnecessary surgery, tests, and use of drugs that are often not only ineffective but iatrogenic (harmful to health). Doctors working for "managed care" systems (see chapter 11), by contrast, tend to underserve, leaving "customers" without the health care they need.

Still, under privately-driven systems like that of the United States, maximizing income only determines part of utilization; much is based on the physician prerogative of maintaining status and practice standards) among fellow physicians (and avoiding malpractice suits). In a classic study, US heart attack patients were almost eight times as likely to undergo coronary artery bypass surgery compared with their Canadian counterparts, without any difference in long-term outcomes (Tu et al. 1997). In addition, the inpatient cost for a bypass in the United States was twice as high as in Canada (Eisenberg et al. 2005). However, because likely frightened and uninformed patients do not know what they need, and their agents (doctors) recognize this, doctors act in accordance with professional practice standards rather than medical need per se. This helps explain wildly differing rates of utilization (and costs) both within the United States and between the United States and other countries.

Meanwhile, private sector insurers seek to minimize the "medical loss ratio" (what insurance companies define, quite literally, as the potential profits lost when medical care is actually delivered) rather than reduce administrative costs and profits. Health professional decisionmaking is also compromised by growing conflicts of interest (Iacobucci 2013), such as doctors directly benefiting from prescribing particular medications (Herman 2015) or by ordering services (e.g., if the doctor owns shares in a diagnostic clinic) (Gawande 2015; Snepp 2012).

Insurance companies argue that they are subject to "moral hazard" in the form of a limitless demand for health care (Gladwell 2005; Pauly 1968); the patient does not worry about generating health expenditures because it "doesn't cost me anything." While this idea is popular in economics circles, it is a myth. Unlike in other sectors, more health care does not provide automatic gratification, though its end results may do so. Certainly medical care can ameliorate illness and provide comfort and understanding to the sick. Yet medicine remains painful, unpleasant, stressful, scary, and downright dangerous, and few people needlessly demand care.

In order for market economics to apply even partially to the health sector, virtually everyone in a given society would have to suffer from Munchausen's syndrome—the feigning of symptoms in order to garner medical attention—and have the wherewithal to repeatedly purchase services. The view that health care system users create boundless demand for health care unless somehow reigned in is faulty, even as elites generally demand more services than the working class.

Providers—and the economic interests often surrounding them—influence most decisions about what constitutes disease and the use of health care services, including norms and inducements regarding routine preventive care and advice on when symptoms require medical attention. Doctors, framed by health system principles and incentives, thereby generate most of the demand for health care. Instituting free, comprehensive universal health care systems is thus not likely to cause overspending: evidence from Taiwan and Canada's single-payer health care system affirms this (Cheng 2015; Lu and Hsiao 2003; Starfield 2010). In sum, moral hazard is on the producer side not the consumer side. Supply-side (financial) incentives to oversupply or misallocate health care services helps explain why almost two thirds of urban Chinese women deliver by C-section (Feng et al. 2012), whereas Canada's single-payer health care system has fewer unnecessary procedures and lower administrative costs than the United States (Pozen and Cutler 2010).

There are many ways in which insurers can limit and deny access to health care services: by making premiums (monthly or annual payments made to a health scheme for coverage) unaffordable; by forcing those with pre-existing conditions to pay more while offering the young and well cheaper premiums; by requiring high patient copayments; by imposing large deductibles (paid out-of-pocket before insurance kicks in); by setting annual or lifetime ceilings on coverage; and by providing only limited benefits in terms of type and volume of services (Vargas et al. 2010).

Fourth, varying amounts of money charged for health care services may go to purposes having no health benefit. Some medical procedures are patently useless; others positively perilous. If unnecessary diagnostic services, surgeries, and other interventions were reduced, resources would be freed up, such as for expanding public health, dental, or vision care.

Moreover, high incomes, fancy facilities, premiums for malpractice insurance, corruption and profits, error, inefficiency, incentives for profitable but "no-value" care, and large bureaucracies all absorb substantial amounts of health sector monies across countries (Jorgensen 2013). Nowhere is wasteful spending more apparent than in the United States, where overhead and administration reach close to one third of hospital health expenditures (Himmelstein et al. 2014), and the practice of "defensive medicine" to avoid potential accusations of malpractice leads to a surfeit of diagnostic and therapeutic procedures, amounting to 2.4% of total health care spending (Mello et al. 2010). All told, excess spending in the United States—including from unnecessary services, excess administrative costs, missed prevention, exhorbitantly high prices, and corruption—totals over US$760 billion each year (Evans 2013).

Fifth, money is not the only consideration when analyzing health care services. Health (or its absence) underpins virtually every human activity and is thus different from almost all other goods or services. It may be far better *not* to need health care services than to need them. Sixth, health care services reflect the characteristics and values of particular societies (see chapter 11). As such, the use of health resources is shaped more by political and cultural factors than by "rational" allocation based on consumer decisions or by classic market forces.

Ultimately, the most compelling argument as to why health should not be viewed in market terms is that most people around the world deem health to be a universal human right that should not be determined by an individual's ability to pay or by market forces (PHM et al. 2014). Framing health as a marketable good based on supply and demand undermines this right. If access to health care is viewed as a human right, then it should be funded as a public good.

Because of the insuperable problems with providing health care services through market systems, most countries have—to a greater or lesser degree—turned to regulation and nonmarket provision of health services for effectiveness and efficiency reasons and as a means of protecting health as a public good (or human right). Nonetheless, the dominant global health actors continue to encourage private delivery of health services, especially in LICs where donors play a predominant role in health financing.

HEALTH CARE FINANCING REDUX

Key Questions:

- How are decisions regarding health financing made?
- What are the health financing challenges particular to countries of different income (GDP per capita) levels?
- What is the role of international agencies in shaping health care system financing policies?

Health Care Spending

Many international analyses of health care systems—such as those carried out by the Organisation for Economic Co-operation and Development (OECD)—begin by comparing how much countries spend on health care services. While dramatic differences may be found, it does not necessarily follow that the higher the percentage of GDP spent on health care the better the health status of a population. This results from several factors:

1. The distribution of health resources may not relate to need. According to the "inverse care law," as proposed by British general practitioner and prolific health care analyst Julian Tudor Hart (1971, p. 405), "The availability of good

medical care tends to vary inversely with the need for it in the population served. This . . . operates more completely where medical care is most exposed to market forces, and less so where such exposure is reduced." In most countries, even where there is universal coverage, care is more accessible (geographically, culturally, financially) for the wealthy than for poorer populations, who are typically most in need. In highly redistributive welfare states, this problem may be corrected through systems of targeting within universal programs, as per Marx's dictum, "to each according to need, from each according to ability."
2. Equitable access to resources such as clean water, housing, sanitation, education, wealth, decent work conditions, social security, and a host of other societal factors also affect health (see chapter 7).
3. Medical care (spending) does not reduce (and may even worsen) overall inequalities in wealth and power (which correlate with health status).

Yet health care spending remains a leading policy concern in most countries. In many LMICs health care is under-funded, whereas there has been a spiraling proportion of GDP spent on health care in many HICs (due to privatization, underregulation, and greater use of increasingly expensive technology and pharmaceuticals). OECD countries spent an average of 9% of GDP on health care in 2015 (down 0.6% from 2009, following austerity cuts)—with outlier US spending exceeding 17% (OECD 2016)—while LMICs spend around 5.8% (World Bank 2015).

One frequently cited factor in increased health care spending in HICs (and increasingly in LMICs) is population aging. At the aggregate level, older people use more health care than do younger, given the accumulation of chronic diseases over time, greater likelihood of dying, and concentration of health care expenditures in the months leading up to death (Hyun, Kang, and Lee 2015). At the margins, however, it is patterns of medical technology utilization—more diagnostic tests, more interventions—if not necessarily the extra needs of the elderly, that is driving spending increases (Zweifel, Felder, and Meiers 1999). For this reason, focusing on regulating unnecessary utilization of technology and private profiteering, together with compressing the period of morbidity prior to death, may well be the key to resolving health care spending crises (Fries, Bruce, and Chakravarty 2011).

In some LICs, the percentage of GDP spent on health care may appear to be relatively high, though the per capita expenditure is extremely low, such as in Burundi, which spends 8% of GDP on health but only US$22 per capita (World Bank 2015). As well, the relatively high cost of drugs and medical equipment may be squeezing out spending on PHC. This problem has worsened in recent years due to WTO-enforced patent regimes (see chapter 9) and the high cost of HIV, cancer, and tuberculosis (TB) diagnostics and drugs, among other factors.

At the same time, various LMICs have achieved *Good Health at Low Cost* (Balabanova et al. 2013; Halstead, Walsh, and Warren 1985; Riley 2008). The most widely cited examples of favorable population health outcomes notwithstanding relatively low spending include Sri Lanka, Cuba, Costa Rica, and the state of Kerala in India, all discussed in chapter 13. Aggregate numbers also hide differences between population groups, as explored in chapters 5 and 7, so it remains essential to examine within-society inequities in health care spending and outcomes.

As shown in Table 12-3, despite Cuba's GDP and health expenditure per capita being much lower than those of the United States, the two countries have similar health indicators, though neither as good as Iceland's. According to spending comparisons alone, some may find Cuba's good health outcomes hard to understand (surely it is not just the sun and sea!). By now readers are sufficiently versed in a political economy of health explanation to recognize that "good health at low cost" derives from concerted attention to the societal determinants of health well beyond but still including public, equitable (and efficient), universal health care systems.

Not only does increased health sector spending not necessarily lead to better health, at the extreme, excessive spending on health care services may prevent societies from marshaling resources to other key determinants of health, such as adequate housing and occupational health measures.

Additionally, even in universal single-payer health care systems, not all services (e.g., pharmaceuticals, dental care) or residents (e.g., migrant and undocumented workers, new immigrants) are publicly covered. However, universal public systems generally

Table 12-3 Comparison of Health Indicators: Cuba, the United States, and Iceland, 2014

Health Indicator	Cuba	United States	Iceland
GDP per capita (PPP international $)[a]	$20,649	$54,399	$43,993
Health expenditure as % of GDP	11%	17%	9%
Health expenditure per capita (PPP international $)[a]	$2,475	$9,403	$3,882
Life expectancy at birth (years)	79.4	78.9	82.1
Infant mortality rate (infant deaths/1,000 live births)	4.1	5.7	1.6
Physicians per 1,000 people (2010–2012)	6.7	2.5	3.5
Nurses and midwives per 1,000 people (2010–2012)	9.1	9.8 (2005)	15.6

[a] Purchasing Power Parity in international dollars. See http://www.who.int/choice/costs/ppp/en/index.html.

Data Sources: WHO (2015a); World Bank (2015).

reduce both private expenditure on health care services and aggregate costs, because they employ price controls, the purchasing power of the state, and have lower administrative overhead, yielding less spending per person overall (Chernomas and Hudson 2013).

As per Table 12-4, most countries with the lowest private proportion of total health care expenditures have (had) universal, national health insurance or national health service systems.

Private health care expenditures encompass both out-of-pocket payments and private health insurance. LMICs comprise less than 10% of the worldwide private health insurance market, with an accelerating trend especially in Asia and Eastern Europe (Drechsler and Jütting 2010). In many countries, out-of-pocket expenditures dwarf private health insurance spending. In India, for instance, out-of-pocket expenditures make up over 62% of expenditure on health care (WHO 2014a). A significant part of this expenditure is considered "distressed health care financing" because it pushes families to sell household assets, borrow money, and seek contributions from relatives and friends to meet health care needs (Joe 2014).

As total private expenditures increase, those with the fewest disposable resources suffer disproportionately. An increasing dominance of private health care expenditures usually exacerbates social

Table 12-4 Private (Including Out-of-Pocket) Expenditures as % of Total Health Care Spending in Selected Countries, 2014

Private Expenditures as % of Total Health Care Spending	Countries
70%–80%	Cambodia, Georgia, Haiti, Uganda, Venezuela
60%–69%	Afghanistan, Comoros, Guatemala, Indonesia, Morocco
50%–59%	Guinea, Iran, Paraguay, South Africa, United States
40%–49%	Botswana, China, Mexico, Russia, South Korea
30%–39%	Dominican Republic, Gambia, Greece, Jordan, Serbia
20%–29%	Bhutan, Canada, Colombia, Poland, Saudi Arabia
10%–19%	New Zealand, Sweden, Thailand, Timor-Leste, United Kingdom
<10%	Cuba, Samoa, San Marino, Seychelles, Solomon Islands

Data Source: WHO (2014a).

inequalities in health, and may provoke increases in preventable illnesses as people are forced to postpone needed health care.

Health Care Financing

Health care financing is a crucial element of health care systems and entails three dimensions: revenue collection, pooling, and purchasing (including provider payment mechanisms) (McIntyre and Kutzin 2011). All financing systems are shaped by both domestic and global economic contexts, and, especially, political values and parties in power. Programmatic needs, technological advances, demography, and epidemiology all play a role. There are five main channels for financing health services:

1. *General tax revenues*: corporate, personal, and consumption (across-the-board, on luxury goods, and specific to tobacco, alcohol, gambling, etc.) taxes collected by national, regional and local governments;
2. *Social security/social insurance*: compulsory contributions via payroll and similar taxes to cover the groups paying into these systems;
3. *Private/voluntary insurance*: privately purchased coverage from private companies through or by employers, by individuals, or via certain community health financing schemes;
4. *International ("donor") funding*: reimbursable loans and nonreimbursable bi-/multilateral grants, and philanthropy/charity, particularly to LICs, usually for specific disease programs, or, infrequently, as health sector-wide approaches (SWAps; see chapter 3); and
5. *Private/household/out-of-pocket payments*: including fee-for-service payments (sometimes a sliding fee based on household income), premiums, deductibles, copayments (a set fee per visit), or coinsurance (a percentage of the total cost of care, such as a period of hospitalization), or the full cost of health services provided.

Overall fiscal mechanisms (government revenue-raising and spending patterns), including personal and corporate income taxes and redistribution through transfers (see chapter 7), are central to equity in health care access.

Different types of health care system financing yield different levels of progressivity (fairness): (a) financing through general taxation is most fair, especially when generated from progressive income taxes (tax rates that increase as earnings rise), not taxes on basic goods and services; (b) depending on how contribution rates are established, social security-based health insurance can be more regressive than general taxation if there are income ceilings on contribution requirements (i.e., the wealthy only have to contribute based on a portion of their earnings), and/or if there is a flat premium, rather than an income-scaled premium, and/or significant copayments are required; (c) private, voluntary health insurance is more regressive than mandatory health insurance because "risk" is usually evaluated at the individual rather than the community or societal level—with higher premiums and other out-of-pocket contributions charged to people with an increased "risk" of illness or death—leading the sick to pay more than the healthy; (d) donor funding may be progressive or regressive, depending on the terms. It is also unpredictable, and may be both undemocratic (donors define the agenda) and unsustainable (see ahead and chapter 3); and (e) out-of-pocket payments are the most regressive form of health financing, as people with the lowest incomes generally have the highest health care costs (McIntyre and Kutzin 2011) and pay more proportionate to their incomes (or even in absolute terms) than the wealthy.

Health care financing that is more progressive generally leads to more equitable health care systems, as pooling mechanisms cover increasing swaths of the population (i.e., all residents are covered by social security) and fewer persons face impoverishment as a result of health care expenditures (Box 12-1). Inadequate health care financing, conversely, pushes up to 100 million people into poverty, with even more annually facing "financial catastrophe" (WHO 2010), a prime motivator for the current universal health coverage (UHC—see chapter 11) push. In the United States, for example, the share of household income spent on health care has been rapidly increasing (Blumberg et al. 2014), with health care debt the leading cause of personal bankruptcy (Emami 2010). Nevertheless, according to this calculus, only

Box 12-1 Two Sides of Turkey's Experiences with Changes in Health Care Financing

In 1961 the Turkish government called for the "socialization of health services" through community-oriented PHC, but this policy was never fully implemented, leaving millions of informal workers and the poor without entitlement to the state health insurance system. Following decades of cutbacks and World Bank loans, the Turkish government launched its Health Transformation Program (HTP) in 2003, aiming to address the country's poor health outcomes compared with other OECD countries, increase the number of health personnel, and unify the fragmented health financing mechanisms contributing to inequity and inefficiency. A prime objective of the HTP was to consolidate Turkey's multiple insurance plans into a single purchaser of health care services and expand benefits, as well as strengthen the public health sector and upgrade information systems (Atun 2015).

In 2008 the HTP expanded to include free and universal PHC and emergency and intensive care. This significantly increased access to health insurance for the poor, with coverage going from approximately 70% of the population in 2002 to near universality by 2013. The HTP, together with improvements in women's education and other social factors (Jelamschi and De Ver Dye 2010), helped drive infant mortality down from 26.5 per 1,000 in 2003 to 11.6 per 1,000 in 2015 (WHO 2015a).

But this narrative tells only one side of the story. Although public financing rose to 77% of total health care expenditures in 2015 (OECD 2016), the HTP has enabled and encouraged growing privatization of health care delivery. The number of private hospitals has doubled since 2000 to over one third of the total, mostly serving outpatients, for whom the private sector receives higher reimbursements (and consumes a growing share of the health care budget) than does the public sector. As well, despite declining out-of-pocket expenditures overall, financing remains regressive and inequitable, with the poorest quintile of households paying more of their income on health care than the wealthiest (Ökem and Çakar 2015).

In recent years, a further dimension of health care injustice involves access to care for Turkey's refugee and immigrant populations. While the almost 3 million Syrian refugees in Turkey have the right to free health care, in practice the vast majority—who reside outside refugee camps—have highly limited access to health care (European Commission 2016). Meanwhile, immigrants are considered tourists and charged steep fees to access care. Given current political turmoil, the prospects for returning to community-oriented PHC are not bright.

a fraction of global poverty, conservatively estimated at 3.2 billion people living under $3/day (2005 PPP) (World Bank 2015) can be attributed to catastrophic health care costs per se.

The Health Insurance Model

Health insurance in one form or another has been around for centuries. In the Middle Ages, guilds and other groups began mutual aid societies to help one another through periods of ill health and injury that prevented wage earning. By the late 19th century these "friendly societies" became common throughout industrializing settings and among immigrants to the Americas. In various countries, these societies became the backbone of national health care systems. In the United States, where struggles around national health insurance were more protracted, private companies began to offer health insurance as a profit-making enterprise, and the government encouraged employers to include insurance as a workplace rather than a citizenship benefit (see chapter 11).

Insurance plans promise to fund health care as need arises, but "need" and "fund" are increasingly contested notions. Private insurance companies may override doctors' decisions and may fund only a portion of care. In public systems, decisions must be made, ideally in consultation with the public, about what services should be provided. Health insurers seek to predict the occurrence of certain health events based on the illness, disability, or mortality patterns of large pools of individuals. When many people pay premiums or taxes into a common pool, covering the needs of contributors, this is known as *risk pooling*. The risk pool becomes larger as more households participate; when 100% of households are included in an insurance scheme, it is universal (WHO 2014b). Single-payer, universal health insurance provided by the state covers all legal residents in one pool (usually after a waiting period), but private sector risk-pooling mechanisms often exclude those who are most in need of care and coverage.

Private insurers may choose who they will cover, or may decide to provide only limited benefits (known as risk selection). Public health insurance programs, by contrast, do not engage in individual risk selection and are therefore far more equitable. Still, in countries with universal coverage or where health insurance is obligatory, not all governments implement a public insurance plan. Instead they may regulate the private insurance industry or contract delivery of services to private providers, ideally requiring uniform premiums for a package of benefits, regardless of risk. In such circumstances insurance companies may skirt regulation by: offering high deductible options requiring enrollees to pay for most care; raising everybody's rates; increasing copayments; or limiting access to certain providers.

In the private health insurance industry, premiums or benefits may be adjusted based on age, family size, and so on—except where the law requires the application of community rating (where age, occupation, or prior health conditions cannot be used to individually rate risk). This practice seeks to limit "cherry picking" the young and healthy while excluding others, or charging higher premiums to unhealthy or elderly persons. Based on past data, the insurer averages individual risks over the entire pool of policyholders to come up with the expected number of payouts in any time period. The amount each individual should contribute to the insurance scheme is then calculated, factoring in administration, marketing, and, of course, profits.

To discourage excessive use, and purportedly to save money for all taxpayers, policyholders, or health plan members, private insurers (and some governments) require some form of cost-sharing such as a copayment for each visit. The insurer may also place limits on certain types of claims, or only insure for limited periods of time with frequent renewability requirements for coverage.

Among the most perverse trends of recent years is medical tourism (Box 12-2), which saves money for HIC governments and private insurance companies while generating funds for LMIC health care systems even as it embeds inequities.

Another approach is community-based health insurance, which arose in the wake of the 1978 Alma-Ata primary health care conference, and which brings together geographic, ethnic, or occupational groups into small nonprofit, insurance schemes. These schemes have been growing across Africa in the absence of widespread and good quality public provision of health services. Community-based health insurance offers financial protection against health care costs in countries without other forms of social insurance, but it does not distribute health financing equitably across the population, and has faced problems of low enrollment, leaving out the poorest groups, and having no accountability framework (De Allegri et al. 2009).

US and Canadian Health Financing Models Compared

Various health economists have assessed the difference between single-payer public health insurance (employed in Canada) and multiple-payer private–public insurance (United States) in terms of equity and efficiency. Despite claims that single-payer systems are more costly, comprehensive reviews have found government-sponsored, unified coverage considerably less expensive and more successful at containing costs than multiple-payer arrangements (Morra et al. 2011). Single-payer systems are also considered more egalitarian, as everyone has the same access to services, independent of ability to pay (Gorey et al. 2015; Starfield 2010).

Longitudinal patterns of health care spending in the United States and Canada enable a useful comparison that correlates neatly with policy and institutional changes. In 1970, health care expenditure as a

Box 12-2 Medical Tourism

"Medical tourism," sometimes called "health tourism," involves patients (mostly from HICs) traveling mostly to LMICs expressly to receive health care services ranging from surgery to dental work. Medical tourism to LMICs, rather than to HICs, is a relatively new phenomenon. For example, between 2000 and 2010, the United Kingdom went from being a net importer of medical tourists to being a net exporter (Hanefeld et al. 2013). Medical tourism attracts foreign currency to LMICs and saves anywhere from 25% to 90% of costs to patients from countries where out-of-pocket costs for private or elective services are high or where people lack adequate insurance coverage (e.g., the United States). Private insurance companies in HICs may cover medical tourism to cut their costs, and some HIC governments implicitly favor—or even subsidize—care-seeking abroad as a savings measure, to deliver specialized services not offered domestically, and to reduce waiting lists (Snyder et al. 2013). A related practice is diagnostic tourism, whereby interpretation of medical results is outsourced from HICs to lower paid doctors in LMICs located in different time zones (e.g., after-hours clinics in the United States transmit X-rays electronically to pathologists working during daytime hours in India, rather than hiring overtime staff).

A burgeoning number of countries, including Lithuania, Argentina, South Africa, Turkey, India, Israel, Jordan, Singapore, Thailand, South Korea, and Barbados—receiving an estimated 7 million medical tourists per year—participate in this US$10–30 billion market (KPMG 2014). The Malaysian government promotes health tourism as a fast-growing sector, and Thailand has hospitals just for foreigners (many from elsewhere in East and Southeast Asia) accredited by US boards. One of the largest medical tourism destinations is India (Chanda 2013), accounting for almost US$4 billion in 2014 (KPMG 2014). Direct and online marketing of medical tourism, also covering travel information, is increasingly common. Some countries offer specialty services, such as Cuba's treatment for retinitis pigmentosa (night blindness). Hungary, Brazil, and Costa Rica are top cosmetic surgery destinations. In small Caribbean countries, the growing medical tourism industry has attracted diasporic health workers to return home to practice, potentially exacerbating brain drain from other LMICs. Medical tourism investments sometimes offer new training opportunities, but these can be skewed to the needs of medical tourists rather than the local population (Snyder et al. 2015).

Although beneficial to some, medical tourism distorts already fragile LMIC health care systems, with particular damage to primary care and services for the poor. In expanding the private sector, medical tourism draws resources (e.g., expensive technologies) and health professionals (through higher remuneration) away from the public sector, already evident in India, Malaysia, and Thailand (Chen and Flood 2013). Even when the public sector benefits from medical tourism revenues, two-tiered systems are usually created, with foreign patients treated in separate (better) wards with dedicated facilities, equipment, and health professionals. In the end, medical tourism is a paradoxical example of how health care policies pursued to address deficiencies of HICs jeopardize health care service resources in LMICs.

percentage of GDP was 6% for both countries (with Canada just shifting from a multiple-payer, US-style arrangement to a single-payer system); by 2014, health expenditures comprised 17.5% of GDP in the United States compared with 10.9% in Canada (Figure 12-1). Per capita health care spending in Canada is now approximately 60% of US spending (i.e., US$5,626 per capita in Canada versus US$9,451 in the United States) (OECD 2016). This stems from far higher administrative costs and the difficulty regulating the US's "fragmented mix of public and private insurance coverage and out-of-pocket payment. [In Canada]

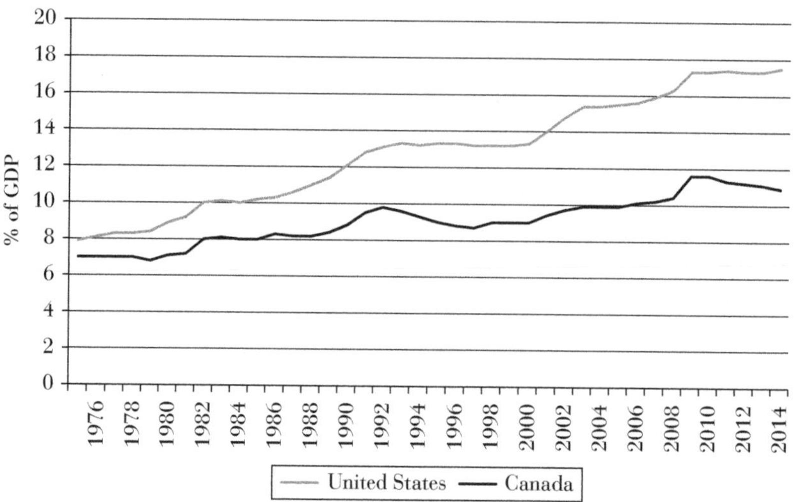

Figure 12-1: Health care expenditures as percent of GDP in the United States and Canada, 1975–2014.
Data Sources: Graph inspired by David Himmelstein and Stephanie Woolhandler; data from Centers for Medicare and Medicaid Services (2015) and Canadian Institute for Health Information (2015).

Consolidation of expenditures in the hands of a single payer made possible the control" of escalating costs (Evans 2007, p. 8). The other key difference relates to significant sums going to marketing and profits in the United States.

Indeed, the extent to which there has been an increase in Canada's health care spending from 6% to 10.9% of GDP is related to the continued role of the private market: only 70% of the health care spending is publicly controlled. The public sector—in terms of hospital and physician spending—has remained relatively stable as a percentage of GDP over the past 40 years, whereas private spending (e.g., insurance, out-of-pocket costs, drugs, and ancillary services) has been increasing (Canadian Institute for Health Information 2015).

In sum, publicly funded, single-payer systems are more efficient, effective, and accessible and thus do a better, if less than perfect, job of providing for the health care needs of their populations (Table 12-5). Lower overall spending and greater equity (and outcomes) are due to better regulation, less duplication, greater access, and higher quality care (Seidman 2015).

Out-of-Pocket Financing: User Fees in Africa

In the late 1980s, in the midst of debt crises and structural adjustment reforms in LMICs (see chapters 2 and 9), World Bank analysts began to promote user fees as a cost-recovery/cost-sharing mechanism for chronically underfunded health care systems. The Bank's 1987 report, *Financing Health Services in Developing Countries: An Agenda for Reform*, argued that people were willing to pay for health care and that free services impeded government revenue collection. The same year the report became a pillar of the Bamako Initiative, adopted in 1987 by African Ministers of Health across 33 countries to expand PHC access in a time of severe health services cutbacks. (The Initiative also called for community financing and participation and a donor-assisted revolving fund to help pay for health worker salaries and essential drugs.)

The Bank asserted that market-level user fees would generate needed health care system revenues, improving access, efficiency, and quality of care. In addition, resources would shift from expensive inpatient treatment to more affordable primary care services (World Bank 1987). If patients paid for services, according to this reasoning, they would use health resources more rationally.

It turned out that the Bank's report was based more on ideology than evidence. Although it recommended that user fees be accompanied by vouchers or exemptions for the poorest populations, both in-house and external reviews showed that fees resulted in significant barriers to care (Lagarde and Palmer 2011; Russell

Table 12-5 Organization and Effects of Single-Payer versus Multiple-Payer Health Care Systems

Public Single-Payer	Multiple-Payer, Privately-Driven
• Raises funds, administers claims, and shares costs across the population more efficiently and equitably • One authority with an incentive and the capacity to contain costs • No marketing expenses • No need to estimate risks to establish differentiated premiums • No profits paid to owners/shareholders	• Overhead costs can be upwards of 10 times higher among private insurers compared to a public, single payer • Administrative costs up to three times higher in the United States compared with Canada • The larger the share of private health care financing, the more difficult it is to control expenditures (e.g., for-profit hospitals are up to 10% more expensive than nonprofit hospitals) • Employer-provided health insurance is a disincentive for labor mobility and hence negatively affects the allocation of labor • As the cost of health insurance increases, so do costs to employers who provide health insurance, resulting in fewer salary increases, cuts in benefits, decreased employment levels, and more costs passed on to employees through higher premiums and copayments and greater limits on coverage • Premiums for those with chronic conditions are typically larger—placing a higher financial burden on the sick • For-profit hospitals provide minimal care for the poor, leaving public and nonprofit facilities with a disproportionate financial responsibility

Sources: Adapted from Sepehri and Chernomas (2004); Gusmano and Rodwin (2015).

and Gilson 1997). The Bamako Initiative ended up harming the very people it aimed to support—poor, rural populations. For example, when Burkina Faso eliminated user fees for children under 5, access doubled, and both utilization and equity improved markedly (Ridde, Haddad, and Heinmüller 2013).

Numerous governments, NGOs, and advocacy groups called for abolition of user fees in LMICs (PHM et al. 2005; Robert and Ridde 2013). Yet for years World Bank analysts continued to argue that free services do not "constitute the most promising approach to meeting the needs of disadvantaged population groups" (Gwatkin 2005, p. 9). Only after more than two decades evidencing relentless suffering among the poor of LMICs did the World Bank finally recant its position on user fees (Rowden 2013).

Remuneration

Remuneration of health workers typically comprises a sizeable portion of total health care expenditures—on average over one third: 38% in HICs and 29% in LICs (Hernández-Peña et al. 2013). Levels of remuneration affect the number and mix of health workers in each country, with personal care workers paid the least and doctors the most, with a wide span of salary inequities within and across countries (Tijdens, de Vries, and Steinmetz 2013).

Most health workers are salaried, but physicians function under a variety of payment mechanisms, more so in HICs and private systems than in public systems and in LMICs, where salaries are more the norm. Under fee-for-service, doctors bill patients, private health plans, or the government, with a clear

Table 12-6 Provider Remuneration Mechanisms

Remuneration Mechanism	Description	Benefits	Limitations
Fee-for-service	Physician/facility is reimbursed by the government, patient, or insurance plan for each service performed	Remuneration closely linked to provider output	Inflationary, with incentives for unnecessary treatment
Capitation	Provider is paid (by the government, insurance plan, etc.) a set fee per patient over a set period of time, regardless of actual volume of services provided	Administratively simple; predictable expenditures	Encourages selection of young, healthy patients; incentive to enroll excessive numbers of patients and underserve them; may include a "gag clause" (doctors barred from discussing treatment options not covered by the insurance plan); precarious balance of neglect and prevention
Per case	A flat fee is charged per illness episode (e.g., for a hospital stay)	Encourages minimal use of resources	May lead to misrepresentation of diagnosis in order to generate higher payment
Salary/global budget	Annual wages or budget for total work performed	Simplest to administer and budget; no perverse incentives	Potential loss of productivity (though evidence is unclear)
Mixed	Combination of the above mechanisms	Mixed, depending on system	Mixed, depending on system

Source: Adapted from Glaser (1993).

advantage to maximizing patient visits and services. Under capitation, a physician is paid according to the number of patients in their practice, not by the number of services performed. As such, there is a clear incentive to minimize return visits and patient contact perceived as unnecessary. Most countries use a mix of salary, fee-for-service, and capitation systems (Table 12-6).

Healthcare facilities may be financed in a number of ways including:

- Global budgets (annual)
- Retrospective fee-for-service reimbursement
- All-payer (the same retrospective fee-for-service negotiated for all facilities/insurers)
- Per diem (prospective payment, amount set in advance, adjusted for severity of case)
- Per case/stay (prospective payment, amount set in advance, adjusted for severity of case)
- Private fund raising and donations
- Mixed payment systems

Remuneration mechanisms have a large influence on the (dis-)incentives to provide care and also affect overall system costs, quality, access, and equity.

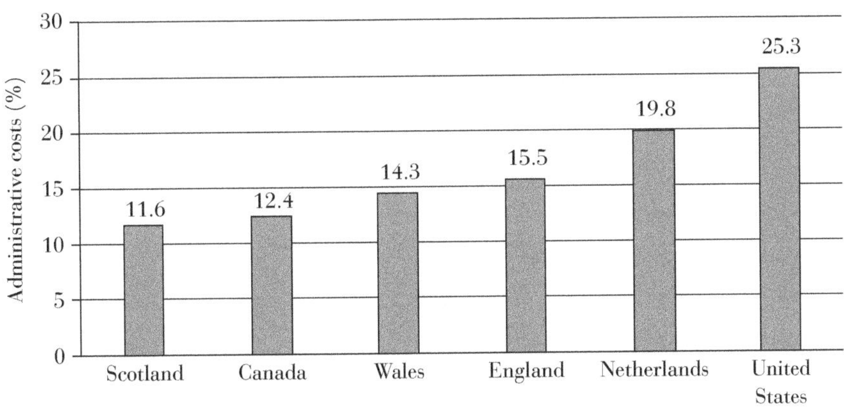

Figure 12-2: Administrative costs as a percent of total hospital costs in selected countries.
Data Source: Himmelstein et al. (2014).

Management

Good health care system management is necessary in all countries and at every level and critical to: determining priorities and projecting future needs; allocating and monitoring use of resources; establishing needs in terms of human and physical resources, including health workers, infrastructure, transport, maintenance, technology, and equipment; developing and implementing policy and programmatic strategies; and evaluating system performance.

Health care system management also plays an important role in creating a supportive work environment, health worker recruitment (right number of health workers, in the right places, performing needed services), retention, training, and appraisal of performance of health workers.

Key to health care management is the use of information: integrating health information systems (which focus on discrete health indicators such as antenatal visits and infant mortality rates) with management information systems (which focus on tracking funds, staff, equipment, activities, achievement of goals, etc.). Despite its importance, management remains one of the most challenging aspects of health care delivery. In many settings, management is compromised by insufficient resources, lack of adequate delegation to make decisions, and no clear direction from regional or national authorities. In resource-constrained health care systems, providing adequate training and funds for administrative purposes may not be seen as high a priority compared with ensuring sufficient numbers of frontline health care workers and other resources. As a result, both management and service delivery may suffer.

Countries with significant private sector spending tend to face greater management problems due to duplication of functions and inequitable resource distribution. For example, in South Africa, although most of the population uses public health services, 46% of all generalists and 56% of specialists serve the 15% of the population insured in the private sector (Ashmore 2013). While such discrepancies may be partially addressed through improved management, major policy questions regarding health care system organization and budgetary allocations are political rather than managerial decisions: a central consideration is that countries with multiple social security and private insurance arrangements tend to spend excessively on administration (Figure 12-2).

COST ANALYSES OF HEALTH SECTOR INTERVENTIONS

Key Questions:

- What are cost-effectiveness analysis and cost–benefit analysis?
- Why are they used and how do they differ?
- What are their respective limitations?

For specific health problems, orthodox health economists attempt to calculate how to accomplish a better outcome for the same cost, the same outcome at a lower cost, or, a better outcome at a lower cost. Even as cost analyses can be useful, these tools are accompanied by ideological assumptions around how decisions are or should be made, what kinds of evidence and values should be taken into account, and how success should be gauged.

Cost–Benefit Analysis

Typically those responsible for planning and financing any project want to know the return that they may expect on their investment. Economists frequently use the concept of marginal returns—the magnitude of the benefit that will accrue from a given additional expenditure—for decisionmaking purposes. Implicit in their decisionmaking is the idea that costs and benefits can be measured, or at least estimated and projected.

At the simplest level, cost–benefit analysis (CBA) is an accounting mechanism that calculates the benefits of a particular activity, its costs, and whether the benefits outweigh the costs (i.e., Benefits − Costs = Net Benefits). If the net benefits exceed zero, then the activity is deemed worth carrying out. It all sounds simple enough. The complexity arises when trying to decide what should count as costs and benefits, and how to take into account future amounts in addition to current ones. The most problematic issue of all is trying to set a monetary equivalent to the value of a life.

Calculating future costs and savings according to standard business investment models is central to CBA. Future benefits must be "discounted" by a certain percentage because one euro or yuan is valued more highly today than the same amount next year due to inflation and to the opportunity costs from not investing in another arena. The value of benefits and costs after discounting is called the net present value. As per CBA, only if the net present value of future benefits and costs is positive should a project or intervention be carried out.

According to CBA, measures that avert future costs altogether seem the best way to spend on health. Despite their merit, paradoxically, these investments are all but invisible to the public because nothing happens. Parents do not notice when their child does not get diarrhea, diphtheria, or diabetes, nor do they recognize that money was saved as a result. However, even this concern is dwarfed by the issue of how both costs and benefits are calculated.

The World Health Organization's (WHO's) 1967–1980 smallpox eradication campaign (see chapter 2)—estimated to have cost over US$300 million in 1980 dollars, nearly US$1 billion today—is widely cited to be the best global health investment ever made, as gauged by CBA. D.A. Henderson, the smallpox campaign's late director, calculated that eradication of smallpox saves more than US$1 billion every year, indefinitely, in reduced productivity losses and medical costs (Henderson 2009), augmented by savings from averted deaths and disability.

While sounding incontrovertible, this CBA overlooks the fact that targeted smallpox spending displaced other investments in health by WHO, donors, and, especially, participating governments, including basic infrastructure, nutrition, and water/sanitation, which could have yielded even more savings over time. Additionally, Henderson's CBA did not parse who spent, and who benefits, from what and where: the LICs where smallpox was endemic paid approximately two thirds of total campaign costs, but most of the benefits are reaped by affluent countries where productivity gains and costs of routine smallpox vaccination and medical care for patients is far higher. As former Director-General of WHO Halfdan Mahler argued, these cost-savings "will have a punch-line only if the governments of these countries decide to plough back the money they have saved into other activities for attaining world health" (WHO 1980, p. XII).

It is important to note that CBA shows impressive results when focused on narrow, vertical interventions, such as oral rehydration therapy, implemented over short time frames. However, interventions that are much broader in scope, for instance education or housing, typically do not provide immediate gains due to large start-up costs and diffused effects. Over the long term, social investments yield vastly greater benefits (see chapters 3 and 13). As these investments increase, many health problems—particularly those attributable to poverty—decline, but they are usually undervalued by CBA, which favors current savings over future savings. Moreover, although interventions also depend on the prior existence of facilities, trained personnel, and other related infrastructure, these factors are difficult to account for and often not included in cost–benefit calculations.

Yet CBA might still be useful for larger, long-term policymaking if societal investments are adequately incorporated. Indeed, in one of its earliest applications in 1873, Max von Pettenkofer, Munich's municipal health officer, attempted to demonstrate "the value of health to a city" through a rational economic calculation. Seeking to understand why London's death rate was so much lower than Munich's, he found that the difference was not due to superior medical care or hospitals but, rather, stemmed from London's better water and sanitation, housing, and nutritional conditions. Pettenkofer then carried out a CBA to measure the value of investing to improve Munich's poor health status. Valuing health in terms of lost earnings due to sickness, he found that Munich's population had 3.4 million days of sickness per year resulting in 3.4 million florins lost annually due to work absences. Interpreting the city's failure to invest in public health as a feudal tax that impeded economic growth, Pettenkoffer estimated that an investment in municipal health would see gains far outstripping the costs. He calculated that a reduction in work absences based on improved water supply and sewage systems would save almost 350,000 florins per year, equivalent to the profits from investing 7 million florins (at returns of 5%). Pettenkofer concluded that spending 7 million florins in taxes on a comprehensive water and sewerage system was thus a sound investment:

> It is not a matter of indifference if, in a city, the dwellings of the poor become infested with typhoid and cholera but is a threat to the health of the richest people also. This is true for all contagious or communicable diseases. Whenever causes of disease cannot be removed or kept away from the individual, the citizens must stand together and accept taxation according to their ability.
>
> When a city provides good sewerage, good water supplies, good and clean streets, good institutions for food control, slaughter houses and other indispensable and vital necessities, it creates institutions from which all benefit, both rich and poor. The rich have to pay the bill and the poor cannot contribute anything; yet the rich draw considerable advantages from the fact that such institutions benefit the poor also (Pettenkofer 1941, p. 48).

Ethical Considerations

Although cost analyses are usually presented as value neutral, any evaluation method has ideological assumptions and implications. The first assumption is that trade-offs must be made when setting policies regarding health because there are only finite resources available for investment. The limited resources argument can serve as a rationale for restricting spending on the broader determinants of health, which, as discussed, yield gains over longer periods of time. A second crucial ethical dimension germane to CBAs in particular is the need to put a monetary value on human life and well-being in order to quantify the benefits and the costs of a specific activity or intervention.

Valuations of life typically take into account an individual's earning potential at the time of death or disability, placing the highest value on the life of a middle-aged man (assumed most likely to be productively employed). In the 1970s US health economist Dorothy Rice proposed that the monetary value of human life increased until the age of 60, at which point it began to decline. Additionally, due to their higher salaries, men at their "most valuable" were deemed to be worth almost 70% more than women at their "most valuable" (Max et al. 2004).

Rice's influential calculations were based on problematic suppositions regarding who is worth what. In many HIC settings, women and racial/ethnic minority populations earn less on average than men of European descent and are typically evaluated as having less "value" or monetary worth than white men. Given the lower earning power of women, working class, racialized, and LMIC populations, CBAs may value life at lower levels for these groups.

There are other ways of calculating the monetary value of life. For example, "opportunity costs" assess what investment possibility is lost because money is spent on a particular intervention. Once again, this determination varies by who is making the judgment. Cost utility analysis is a variant of CBA, which uses outcome measures based on people's preferences (gauged through surveys, focus groups, etc.) rather than monetary amounts.

Asking people their "willingness to pay" through surveys (or, in litigious societies, via lawsuit outcomes) prompts basic questions such as: whose willingness? And paying for what? Not only are these questions challenging to measure, the information is flawed because healthy people may undervalue relatively low cost, life-extending preventive care whereas people in ill health may value expensive, curative care, even if to less effect. Further, individual choices may not coincide with societal choices, and are mediated by social class, race/ethnicity, gender, experience, and age (Martín-Fernández et al. 2013).

The inherent problems of assigning concrete monetary values to life, health, and suffering has led health economists and policymakers to consider cost-effectiveness analysis (CEA), which does not require such explicit valuations.

Cost-Effectiveness Analysis

In CEA, the desired health outcome is established a priori and the attainment of the outcome is measured via: (1) a comparison of two or more interventions of the same cost and their respective health outcomes; or (2) a comparison of several interventions with the same outcome to determine variation in the cost of the interventions (also known as cost minimization). In other words, CEA overcomes the problem of monetizing health outcomes by evaluating interventions or activities against one another. Either spending or the desired effects remain constant, and different routes to achieving these ends are compared.

Illustrating the application of CEA, Table 12-7 presents comparisons of different health-related services and interventions in terms of cost per averted DALY (disability-adjusted life year—see chapter 5 for details). Some interventions, such as expanding childhood vaccination coverage, have a very low cost per DALY saved; others, for example bypass surgery, have a very high cost. Following from these calculations, it appears more cost-effective to focus limited resources on childhood immunization, given the relatively greater savings accrued. A general maximum cut-off point for CEA designated by the World Bank is US$150 per DALY averted in LICs (or US$25 per DALY as "highly attractive") (Shillcutt et al. 2009). Of course, this, like any, level is arbitrary and depends on a country's epidemiological profile and health needs, political and social preferences, and public health infrastructure. We must also recall that DALYs may calculate illness and death at different levels for different groups, skewing results from this and other built-in assumptions.

Moreover, much depends on the way costs are calculated: not all inputs may be considered, including health care system and personnel costs, electricity for refrigerating vaccines, transport costs, and so on. As well, CEA cannot be used to compare extremely dissimilar programs.

Most importantly, these estimates do not consider the larger social impact or effectiveness over time. In-house piped water supply and sewer connections, for example, exceed the US$150 per DALY CEA cut-off by a factor of at least four, whereas household treatment with chlorination *without infrastructure investment* (at a tiny fraction of the cost per DALY of in-house piped water!) appears far more cost-effective. Yet the valuation of water infrastructure does not cover the time, energy, and physical strain of carrying water over long distances, the advantages of increased water access for food preparation and personal hygiene, or the gained/lost opportunities for school attendance by children (usually girls) charged with this responsibility, and the potential salutary/disease effects of these factors over time. Further, CEAs typically overemphasize initial infrastructure costs rather than appropriately spreading these out over the lifespan of the infrastructure (Haller, Hutton, and Bartram 2007). A "social CBA," by contrast, seeks to take into account broad, long-term livelihood advantages such as school completion and the time saved from not collecting water (Pond, Pedley, and Edwards 2011).

Most saliently, CEA, like CBA, rarely addresses the societal determinants of health, not least social security systems (including medical care), which despite high investment have wide public support and a far larger impact (and diffuse indirect effects) on health outcomes than do specific health care interventions.

In sum the limitations of cost analyses include:

- Only the direct costs of the service or intervention are evaluated. The time or cost to the recipient and the role of infrastructural and social inputs are typically excluded.
- Evaluations are carried out for individual interventions related to individual ailments, but not for activities that have effects in many arenas or for joint efforts that may have synergistic effects (i.e., housing and educational improvements). For example, the multiple

Table 12-7 Using Cost-Effectiveness Analysis to Determine Health Priorities

Service or Intervention	Cost per DALY Averted (current US$)
School-based control of schistosomiasis and soil-transmitted helminthiases, global estimate (WHO 2011)	14
Expanding child immunization for vaccine-preventable diseases, global estimate (WHO 2011)	10–20
Provision of long acting insecticide-treated bednets to protect against malaria, overall LMIC estimate (Pulkki-Brännström et al. 2012)	17
Vitamin A orange maize fortification, Zambia (HarvestPlus 2014)	24
Increasing excise tax on tobacco products (by 60%), high mortality Southeast Asian countries (Ortegón et al. 2012)	87
HPV vaccination, Chad (Kim et al. 2013)	
- Cost per dose (subsidized by GAVI, the Vaccine Alliance):	
US.55	<100
US$5	600
US$26.75	2,800
HPV vaccination, Honduras (Molina Aguilar et al. 2015)	
- Cost per dose (negotiated through PAHO Revolving Fund):	
US$13.45	926
Preventing mother-to-child-transmission of HIV, Malawi (Fasawe et al. 2013)	37–69 (depending on prophylaxis and treatment regimen)
Community-based maternal-newborn package (95% coverage): prenatal care, skilled birth attendance, medical care for pre-eclampsia, postpartum hemorrhage, pneumonia, tetanus, sepsis, age, and neonatal emergency care, Latin America (Valencia-Mendoza et al. 2011)	186
Neonatal intensive care unit, Mexico (Profit et al. 2010)	
- Gestational age: 24–26 weeks	1,200
27–29 weeks	650
30–33 weeks	240
Household water treatment (chlorination at point of use), high mortality sub-Saharan Africa (Haller, Hutton, and Bartram 2007)	20
In-house piped water supply and sewage connection, high mortality sub-Saharan Africa (Haller, Hutton, and Bartram 2007)	687
Coronary artery bypass grafting (bypass surgery) in "high-risk" patients (i.e., with co-morbidities), global estimate (Jamison et al. 2006)	>25,000

benefits of environmental cleanup for reducing cancer and respiratory disease rates, and increasing exercise and overall well-being, are not part of standard CBA/CEA calculations.

- They are decontextualized—it is assumed that if the results are "positive" the activity should be undertaken, without accounting for equity or other contextual factors.

In the end, "using simple technical criteria to plan solutions to complex public health problems" (Berman 1982, p. 1054), while a seemingly logical and convenient approach to health planning, is marred by numerous shortcomings.

Equity versus Efficiency: Trade-off or False Dichotomy?

Mainstream economic analyses focus on costs in relation to effectiveness and efficiency and usually sidestep the importance of equity. Indeed, there is believed to be an inevitable equity–efficiency tradeoff in economic decisionmaking in general, and in health care system financing and delivery in particular (Hsiao and Heller 2007).

A focus on equity implies that (re)distribution of resources must prioritize those who are worst off, and that health goods and services must be distributed primarily according to need. However, orthodox economic evaluations of health care implicitly favor efficiency over equity because market mechanisms are notoriously poor at equitably distributing resources. As well, in the case of LICs that are highly indebted, health care system structuring and financing is heavily influenced by international financial institutions (IFIs) (see chapters 3 and 9), which have historically paid little more than rhetorical attention to issues of equity.

Yet even many mainstream analysts agree that because of the problems of market failure (the inability of the market to adequately supply and distribute goods) in health and other social sectors, equity might need to be considered over efficiency whenever marginalized populations have little access to welfare-enhancing activities (Bourguignon, Ferreira, and Walton 2007; Collier and Dercon 2006).

As per chapter 7, reducing inequities in health necessitates a fair distribution of societal resources and power. But this is not necessarily at the expense of efficiency. Indeed, equitably addressing the societal determinants of health can pay for itself by generating a more educated, healthy, and productive population, a lesson learned in many HIC and various LMIC settings. Nevertheless, donors either argue that equity-oriented approaches are too costly for LICs or evaluate equity narrowly in terms of access to particular interventions (BMGF 2015).

A variant on the equity-efficiency question is whether health care system goals should emphasize average health gains or health equity (Reidpath et al. 2012). But this dichotomy is misconstrued: greater health equity almost invariably engenders health gains, but the reverse is not always true. In global health priority-setting, overall health gains (such as child mortality declines) often take precedence over questions of equity. Yet aggregate health gains may be at the expense of equity, marking rapid improvements among the better-off and stagnation or deterioration among poorer groups. In the end, any tradeoffs that seek to pit equity against either efficiency or overall health improvements are fallacious: the more useful challenge is developing an efficient health care system that is also equitable (*and* leads to overall health gains).

MARKET APPROACHES TO HEALTH IN LMICS

Key Question:

- What do market approaches to health services in LMICs entail and why are they being promoted?

The 1993 World Development Report

In 1993 the World Bank issued its first health-oriented World Development Report (WDR), titled *Investing in Health*. The report argued that in LMICs private health providers are "often more technically efficient than the public sector and offer a service that is perceived to be of higher quality" and more accountable (World Bank 1993, p. 4). Moreover, it coopted a social justice position (Birn, Nervi, and Siqueira 2016) by deceptively arguing: "The main problem with universal government financing is that it subsidizes the wealthy, who could afford to pay for their own services, and thus leaves fewer government resources for the poor" (World Bank 1993, p. 11). In reality, except in the case of total tax evasion by the wealthy, publicly funded, universal services (especially, but not only, when income taxes are progressive) are more equitable than public-private financing because they enable redistribution of resources.

The 1993 WDR recommended that LMICs adopt a "basket" of cost-effective interventions—valued at US$12 and US$21.50 per capita per year for LICs and middle-income countries, respectively—as a top public health priority. The basic basket covered immunization, sick-child care, school health services, family planning, prenatal and delivery care, TB treatment, control of sexually-transmitted infections, and HIV prevention. Left out of the "minimal package of essential clinical services" were treatments for diabetes, mental illness, and other chronic conditions, emergency medical care for adults, and broader public health measures, such as housing improvements and water supply/sanitation (the latter, the report recommended, could be purveyed by the private sector) (World Bank 1993).

Activists, advocates, and many policymakers denounced the prescriptions in the 1993 WDR for: their narrow assessment of health and health interventions based almost exclusively on in-house studies; defining health as a private responsibility and health care as a private good; failing to recognize the ongoing deleterious effects of World Bank structural adjustment policies on health care systems; and for disregarding the responsibility of governments in protecting health as a human right (Laurell and López Arellano 1996; Pfeiffer and Chapman 2010; Waitzkin, Jasso-Aguilar, and Iriart 2007). These critiques proved prescient.

The 1993 WDR's recommended privatization reforms did little to strengthen health care services, instead contributing to increased health care system inequities. In spite of overwhelming evidence that private health services delivery reduces access to care, especially among the marginalized (Waitzkin and Jasso-Aguilar 2015), the World Bank has continued to encourage privatization through its policies and publications, for example, its 2007 business manual entitled, *Establishing Private Health Care Facilities in Developing Countries: A Guide for Medical Entrepreneurs*. Similarly the World Bank's International Finance Corporation's "Health in Africa" initiative, aimed at injecting capital into the private health care sector, has been heavily critiqued for increasing inequity in access while promoting expensive private sector health facilities in Chad, Nigeria, and South Africa (Marriott and Hamer 2014).

Health as Productivity: The WHO Commission on Macroeconomics and Health

In 2000, the WHO established the Commission on Macroeconomics and Health (CMH), to "assess the place of health in global economic development." The Commission's report, *Macroeconomics and Health: Investing in Health for Economic Development*, proposed that donors partner with LMICs to invest in health as a means of increasing global economic development, productivity, and investment prospects (WHO 2001). The report's title echoed the 1993 WDR, conveying "a double meaning—investing to improve health, economic productivity, and poverty; and investing capital, especially private capital, as a route to private profit in the health sector" (Waitzkin 2003, p. 523).

The CMH justified this approach based on the following findings: (a) countries with lower infant mortality rates experienced higher economic growth; (b) improved health resulted in higher per capita income; (c) countries with a long life expectancy invested more in education and had higher personal savings rates; and (d) personal spending on health was disproportionately shouldered by the most economically marginalized groups, resulting in further impoverishment. Out-of-pocket or catastrophic health care spending was estimated to impoverish approximately 100 million people every year, with an additional 150 million pushed into significant financial hardship (WHO 2001). Yet the Commission left out the much larger causal directionality in the association between poverty and ill health; that is, poverty generates far more ill health than the other way around (see chapter 7).

The CMH found that economic losses associated with excess or preventable disease led to reductions in market income, labor productivity, longevity, and psychological well-being. It argued that "Increased investments in health . . . would translate into hundreds of billions of dollars per year of increased income in the low-income countries" (WHO 2001, p. 16), preventing some 8 million deaths annually from HIV and AIDS, malaria, TB, childhood infections, maternal and perinatal conditions, tobacco-related illnesses, and micronutrient deficiencies, as well as reducing fertility.

To achieve these objectives the report proposed sizeable increases in health sector spending—from an average of US$13 per person in LICs to a minimum of US$30 to US$40 per person per year—for specific, cost-effective interventions combined with a restructured health delivery system, co-financed by donors and LICs. Notwithstanding its ambitious mandate, the CMH had almost nothing to say about the factors influencing health outside of health care services per se, including global trade and financial regimes, organization of the production process, wealth distribution, and living and working conditions, which arguably comprise the most fundamental "macroeconomics and health" issues.

Instead, it built upon the focused health care services reform approaches laid out in the 1993 WDR, such as public sector management improvement, a publicly financed basket of technical health interventions for the poor (but private financing for others), and combined public–private provision of services, including encouragement for consumer prepayment of services, provider competition, and public financing for private insurance and delivery of health care.

The Commission's report largely continued along previous cost-effective, pro-private market paths for health improvement established by leading donors over prior decades (Katz 2004), and the supply-side interventions it has inspired have proved equivocal at best (Hanson 2011).

An accompanying effort is the Disease Control Priorities Project (DCP2)—a bible of cost-effective interventions to "reduce the burden" of dozens of diseases and health problems. This project, jointly sponsored by the World Bank, the WHO, the US National Institutes of Health, and the Bill and Melinda Gates Foundation (BMGF), originated alongside the World Bank's 1993 WDR, employing CEA as the basis of recommendations to LMICs for reducing the "burden of disease" (see chapter 5). The three editions of the DCP justify the disease-control approach in almost identical terms as the CMH: health is a key precursor of productivity, education, and investment, which together generate economic growth. Ill health, by contrast, impedes these factors, thereby preventing growth (Jamison et al. 2006). In sum, although public health advocates and scholars have cogently argued that: (a) health should be conceptualized as a right in and of itself, not just as a potential drain or boost to the economy; and (b) that CEA should only be used after the most pressing needs have been met (PHM et al. 2005), the CMH and DCP have recycled the ideology of controlling individual diseases (particularly those that jeopardize economic growth) through cost-effective measures: this is the conventional mantra of major donors and technocrats involved in global health policymaking.

Global Health 2035

Fast forward to 2013 when *The Lancet* published Global Health 2035, by a commission chaired by economists Lawrence Summers and Dean Jamison, both former World Bank officials who were intimately involved in the creation of the 1993 WDR and invited to build on its legacy (Jamison et al. 2013). Funded primarily by the BMGF and the Norwegian Agency for Development Cooperation, the commission's objective was to re-examine the case for investing in health and develop a global roadmap to accelerate progress towards an optimistic "grand convergence": reducing the burden of infections and reproductive, maternal, newborn, and child health disorders in LMICs with high mortality down to current levels in Chile, China, Costa Rica, and Cuba. However, the commission's report is devoid of understanding of how the historical trajectory or political economy of these countries has shaped their health outcomes.

The Commission proposes three convergence goals to be achieved by 2035: under-5 mortality lower than 16/1,000 live births; fewer than 8 HIV deaths/100,000 people; and under 4 TB deaths/100,000. An accompanying investment framework advocates for UHC via "progressive universalism." This means providing the poor with an essential package of cost-effective services, eventually graduating to a "larger benefit package," all enabled by economic growth and technological innovations. These prescriptions, drawing from ever more sophisticated health metrics, are remarkably similar to the failed IFI approaches since the 1980s and raise the same problems regarding: inequities (which the report glosses over and which are masked by population-wide goals); who decides what is essential; and why there should be separate, scaled-down policies for the poor instead of equal and comprehensive services for all based on the right to health. Global Health 2035 also underplays such critical issues as the role of the pharmaceutical patent regime and the part played by the International Monetary Fund (IMF) and the Alliance for a Green Revolution in Africa in undermining small farmers' livelihoods and rural nutrition, which are key to improving maternal and child health (Dionisio 2014). Indeed, Global Health 2035 all but ignores the societal determinants of health, only broaching taxation of tobacco, alcohol, and sugar (framed as key to addressing risk factors), and the reduction of fossil fuel subsidies (a fine start, to be sure, but a small step in terms of addressing climate change and environmental degradation [see chapter 10]). In the end, the Global 2035 report "puts all its trust in high growth and technology, with no role for redistributive justice" (Qadeer and Baru 2016, p. 768).

THE ROLE OF INTERNATIONAL AGENCIES IN HEALTH CARE FINANCING

Key Question:

- What activities do international agencies finance in health and why?

As discussed in prior chapters, IFIs and other international agencies play an important direct and indirect role in policymaking in many LMICs. They participate in financing health care reforms (e.g., via "results-based financing" which rewards for quality and quantity of services delivered), significantly so in countries that rely heavily on development assistance (Table 12-8). Countries most affected are those with the lowest GDP per capita and the highest rates of illicit financial flows, including tax evasion, which otherwise could likely finance domestic health needs. In 2014, external resources contributed 45% of total health expenditure or more in Burundi, Central African Republic, Gambia, Lesotho, Liberia, Malawi, Micronesia, Mozambique, Niue, Rwanda, Solomon Islands, and Vanuatu (WHO 2014a). The external debt levels for most of these countries range from 16% to 59% of GDP (World Bank 2015). At the same time, many of them experience soaring illicit financial flows: for example, in 2010 capital flight was 215% (over triple!) the size of GDP in Mozambique (Ajayi and Ndikumana 2015).

Official development assistance (ODA) makes up a large percentage of national health care budgets in some LICs, but health aid is not a top bilateral or multilateral aid priority for most donor nations. In 2014, only 17% of all ODA went to general health (e.g., services, disease control, infrastructure), population policies and reproductive health, and water and sanitation (OECD 2015). Still, development assistance for health (DAH)—which also includes corporate and philanthropic as well as non OECD country donors— has grown considerably over the past two decades, increasing from US$6.8 billion in 1990 to US$36.4 billion by 2015, with over one third going to countries in sub-Saharan Africa (IHME 2016). The US government provided 36% of all DAH in 2015. In terms of how funds were channeled, just four entities—the World Bank; the BMGF; the US government; and the Global Fund—accounted for 40% of global health financing in 2015 (IHME 2016). Most of these monies have been directed to specific disease initiatives, with considerable agenda-driving implications for recipient countries (Biesma et al. 2009; Vassall and Martínez-Álvarez 2011).

The largest donor agencies have significant influence on national and international health

Table 12-8 GDP, Debt, Health Expenditures, and Donor Funding in Selected Countries (2014)

	Low-income		Lower-middle income		Upper-middle income	
	Burkina Faso	Nepal	P. New Guinea	Cameroon	Albania	Peru
Population (millions)	17.6	28.2	7.5	22.8	2.9	31
GDP per capita (PPP international $)	$1,626	$2,382	$2,865	$2,983	$11,167	$12,047
% GDP spent on health	5%	6%	4%	4%	6%	5%
External resources for health as % of total health expenditure	25%	13%	21%	11%	1%	1%
External debt as % of GDP	20%	20%	124%	17%	60%	33%

priorities due to their global reach, matching grant strategies that require recipient countries to co-finance many activities through personnel allocations, substantial financing and in-kind support, and agenda-setting capacity. Moreover, the scale of programs may require governments to absorb large amounts of funding and implement programs at high speed (Vassall and Martínez-Álvarez 2011), fracturing weak health sectors and diverting them from core health system activities (Nervi 2014) (see chapter 3).

Overall, DAH is currently focused 30% on HIV (US$10.8B), 28% on maternal, neonatal, and child health (US$10.1B), 6% on malaria (US$2.3B), 3% on TB (US$1.2B), with far less going to noncommunicable diseases 1.3% (US$475M) (IHME 2016). As reviewed in other chapters, disease initiatives rely on reductionist technology-based tools such as antiretroviral drugs (ARVs), bednets, vaccines, and nutritional supplements, without concomitant attention to living, working, and environmental conditions that shape, and would enhance, the effectiveness of these tools (Storeng 2014). While HIV and AIDS have undoubtedly had a devastating impact on individuals, families, and communities, especially in sub-Saharan Africa—and scaling up ARV treatment has helped millions stay alive—many other health problems of extreme poverty are left out of most DAH efforts, as are environmentally and occupationally related diseases, and sanitary infrastructure. These problems cannot be solved with ready technical tools, though improving living and working conditions, and ensuring comprehensive PHC access, would make a significant difference.

Even donors admit that without basic health system strengthening, vaccines and medicines have little hope of reaching populations in need. Yet few donors have interest in such long-term investments. Indeed, a paltry 7% of DAH (US$ 2.7B) (IHME 2016) goes to health sector support, including SWAps, which aim to reduce fragmentation of donor efforts but have garnered little participation (Natuzzi and Novotny 2014).

The narrowly disease-based targeting by DAH has both bureaucratic and ideological dimensions. Donor criteria typically require that discrete targets be met within a specified period to rationalize the appropriate spending of monies and demonstrate measurable outcomes (McCoy et al. 2013) according to business-like metrics captured in quarterly or annual reports. Therefore for bureaucratic reasons, donors tend to favor short-term cost-effective interventions that can meet targets more readily. A prime example is PEPFAR, which uses efficiency and effectiveness criteria based on four core interventions: prevention of mother-to-child transmission of HIV; antiretroviral therapy; condoms; and voluntary medical male circumcision (Birx 2014). Notably, countries in Africa that received PEPFAR assistance showed worse outcomes for neonatal mortality than those not PEPFAR-funded, suggesting that PEPFAR's vertical focus had a negative impact on health care system capacity (Lee and Izama 2015). Moreover, funding focused on individual diseases may be both unsustainable and displace domestic investment in health care systems and other needs (Collins et al. 2012).

The ideological dimensions of the reductionist approach derive from the dominant belief that health problems can be resolved technically with little regard for political and economic underpinnings and processes. Conceptualizing health problems otherwise would, of course, require the current arrangements of financial and political power to be upended. Impeding such potential threats to vested interests helps drive the search for ever more (often misguided) magic bullets to address the problems of the Majority World, from new therapeutics to micro-financing.

Though the pervasive technical targeting approach is under mounting fire for disregarding poverty and the underlying determinants of health and for underfunding health system strengthening (The Conversation 2014), to date it remains the principal channel for DAH.

CONTRASTING APPROACHES TO INVESTING *FOR* HEALTH (AND HEALTH EQUITY)

Key Question:

- How do mainstream and social justice approaches to health economics compare and contrast, and what are the implications of each?

Neoliberal Health Economics and LMICs

Most of the concepts of health economics were developed in HICs over the past half-century, after these societies had already undergone major improvements in living and working conditions and established greater or lesser variants of the welfare state (Mills 2014). But in countries where many basic needs remain unmet, these principles may not fit, especially where they have been imposed by donor agencies. Arguably, universal coverage of certain cost-effective interventions can be an efficient means of improving selected health indicators and may increase equity if the interventions are targeted to the populations with the worst health indicators (Giedion, Alfonso, and Díaz 2013). However, in many LMICs, cost analyses often lead to short-term responses to larger problems: a band-aid approach to disease control that does not address the underlying conditions that foster illness. In this context, targeted interventions may not provide the lasting outcomes desired, particularly when other issues that affect health are left unaddressed as would be the case in any setting. Indeed, in terms of the ingredients and challenges for promoting equitable health and health care, HICs and LMICs share far more than is usually portrayed, from the need for broad societal investments to the damaging effects of corruption (Box 12-3).

Moreover, investments in societal determinants of health—such as clean water provision—may be initially costly, but their long service life and broad utility can make them very (cost-)beneficial/effective from a health standpoint—if the effects and

Box 12-3 Corruption in the Health Sector

In 2013 World Bank President Jim Kim named corruption "Public Enemy No. 1" (Yukhananov 2013). Corruption in health care systems occurs when suppliers, public officials, providers, insurers, or patients take health care resources for personal or private institutional gain. This may take place via: bribery, kickbacks, or extortion; favoritism, nepotism, and misuse of high level positions; irregular billing or claims; procurement or sale of adulterated or knowingly substandard drugs and supplies; conflicts of interest among researchers, purchasers, suppliers, and providers; misuse of diagnostic technologies and unnecessary treatment; refusal to provide needed services; diversion of resources; profiteering from denial of needed care (particularly in the private insurance sector); misrepresentation of treatments that are not covered to obtain reimbursement (e.g., cosmetic nose surgery billed to insurers as deviated-septum repairs) (NHCAA 2015); recruitment of public sector patients to be treated in the private sector or illegally using public facilities and resources for treatments and services not covered by the public system; and embezzlement of funds, medicines, and medical devices (Hussmann 2011).

Annually, 10% to 25% of public spending on health (e.g, procurement for medicines, equipment, and infrastructure) is lost to corruption, with most individual HICs losing US$12–23 billion (WHO 2010). The problem of corruption is even higher in privatized health care systems that rely heavily on private providers and suppliers, and out-of-pocket expenditures. In LMICs, up to 80% of the population has experienced corruption in the health sector (Holmberg and Rothstein 2011), with petty bribery common at all levels.

Corruption takes many forms, from hundreds of billions of dollars in over-billing and fraud (Gee and Button 2014) and illegal practices by Big Pharma (see chapter 11) in the United States, to informal payments made to physicians in Eastern Europe (Holmberg and Rothstein 2011), falsified malaria drugs across Asia and Africa (Nayyar et al. 2012), bribery in India (Jain, Nundy, and Abbasi 2014), and stolen equipment and drugs in Tanzania (Holmberg and Rothstein 2011).

International agencies cite corruption in LICs as an important health care system problem, arguing that close monitoring of ODA can circumvent corrupt practices and ensure that health aid reaches target populations (Michaud, Kates, and Oum 2015). Yet the scale of corruption is often much greater in HICs than in LICs, even though HICs are barely covered in international corruption reports. The United States, for example, is marked by extensive fraud: up to half a trillion dollars are lost annually due to corruption in the health care sector (Geyman 2015).

benefits are calculated out across 5 years, 10 years, or even a generation. The problem is that long-term investments are usually underrated by CBA/CEA and their adherents, who are looking for fast returns on investment. Yet as discussed in chapter 3, integrated and sustained investment in social conditions, health infrastructure, and redistribution were used systematically and effectively to improve health outcomes in HICs.

International (health) financing agencies usually expect or require LMICs to use CEA in order to prioritize the allotment of (scarce) health resources. (This assumes that there are no other means to increase these resources, for example through addressing unfair terms of trade, capital flight, tax evasion, corruption, and debt.) Much of this guidance and pressure comes from leading bilateral and multilateral institutions, among them the World Bank and the Global Fund, in the form of loan or grant conditions and certain recommendations aimed at LMICs and based on neoliberal capitalist ideology (see chapter 9). Nevertheless many of the countries that have attained a high health status themselves reject CEA when planning for and allocating health care resources.

Back to the bigger picture, the politics of health and development economics and financing writ large, are particularly salient in the context of the transition from the Millennium Development Goals (MDGs) to the Sustainable Development Goals (SDGs) (see chapter 3). While the MDGs were largely financed by development aid and debt forgiveness, the SDGs require countries to self-finance their development

Table 12-9 Neoliberal and Social Justice Approaches to Health Compared

Neoliberal Capitalist Approach to Health	Social Justice/Human Rights Approach to Health
Assumptions	
• Health is seen instrumentally as either a wasted resource or an input to economic growth.	• Health is a social right, undergirded by equitable and sustainable use and distribution of resources.
• Health results from health care services and individual behavior changes.	• Health results from meeting broad social needs, including health care services.
Key Features	
• Addresses symptoms of health problems	• Addresses root causes of health problems
• Short-term focus	• Long-term focus
• Promotes cost-effective interventions delivered through health care services and "magic bullets"	• Promotes public infrastructure and collective social policies and regulations to meet basic needs, improve living conditions, and decrease inequities
• Emphasizes mixed public and private financing and delivery of care, with little regard for equity and out-of-pocket spending by the poor (based on advice, loans, and conditionalities from international agencies)	• Emphasizes redistributive economic justice enabling public and equitable funding for health, together with fair terms of trade, curbing of tax evasion, corruption, and capital flight
• Maintains the status quo of concentrated wealth and power	• Calls for an equitable international social and economic order
• Focuses on individual responsibility and tends to blame "victims" for their ill health	• Focuses on structural poverty, inequality, and violence, and seeks to redress systemic imbalances of power and resources

Source: Adapted from Katz (2004, p. 756).

and encourage resource mobilization from the private sector, bringing multifarious problems (WHO 2015b), as we have amply seen. A much fairer and accountable channel for private sector funding of the SDGs—targeting illicit financial flows and ensuring efficient and fair taxation of TNCs and domestic elites—was proposed at the 2015 Financing for Development conference in Addis Ababa, but large donor countries blocked any formal mechanisms to enable this possibility.

A Viable Alternative: Investing for Health and Health Equity through Social and Redistributive Approaches

As examined elsewhere in this textbook, donor-led investment in narrowly framed cost-effective interventions—and policies emphasizing private sector insurance schemes as the best means of achieving universal coverage—are not the sole path to health. Societies that embrace social justice approaches and address the broad determinants of health (typically with little or no donor involvement) have achieved far more than the gains projected by mainstream health economists following neoliberal capitalist logic. These two approaches to health are compared in Table 12-9.

Are governments capable of implementing a social justice approach to health? Good health is clearly in the interest of individuals and families, but it is also in the best interest of governments to minimize the societal costs and effects of ill health, disability, and premature death. Not only does this offer a powerful rationale for publicly funded preventive, curative, and rehabilitative health care, it provides a justification for sustained investment in the societal determinants of health and health equity, which in turn are central to overall well-being. To note, the responsibility of governments to improve tax collection and purvey services efficiently can align well with social justice approaches, drawing from public demands and democratically accountable political systems.

To be sure, social, political, and redistributive approaches to health do not negate certain gains realized from targeted cost-effective interventions. But for long-term improvements, especially in health equity—such as those achieved in muscular social welfare states—far more than decontextualized interventions are needed.

CONCLUSION

Learning Points:

- Understanding the economic dimensions of health care systems involves analysis of how the state-market-household nexus operates in terms of health care financing and spending, and consideration of the politics of DAH.
- Public, universal (single-payer) health care systems are fairer, more effective, and less costly than systems that embrace private competition.
- The principal tools of orthodox health economics—cost analyses emphasizing efficiency over equity—are guided by a set of principles that prioritize short-term, narrowly focused, and technical priority-setting, based on the values of technocrats, elites, and other dominant political and economic actors.
- As many countries are moving towards UHC, the different health care financing models adopted will have a great bearing on both equity and efficiency.
- Orthodox health economics approaches increasingly influence global and domestic health policymaking, yet there are also heterodox social justice-oriented approaches pursued by various countries.
- The relationship between health care spending and health outcomes is complex, mediated by health system equity and influenced by the broader determinants of health.

When all is said and done, do countries that spend more on health care obtain better health outcomes? Not necessarily!

Plotting annual health care expenditures per capita against life expectancy shows that there is a general correlation between health care spending and health outcomes (Figure 12-3). However, above approximately US$300–US$500 per capita, health care expenditures do not result in a predictable relationship between additional resources devoted to health services and life expectancy. For example, in 2014 Germany spent over five times as much on health care per capita as Costa Rica, with virtually no difference in life expectancy.

Likewise, Preston curves, which plot GDP per capita against life expectancy, find a strong positive relationship between the two variables, but only up to a certain point, after which the relationship

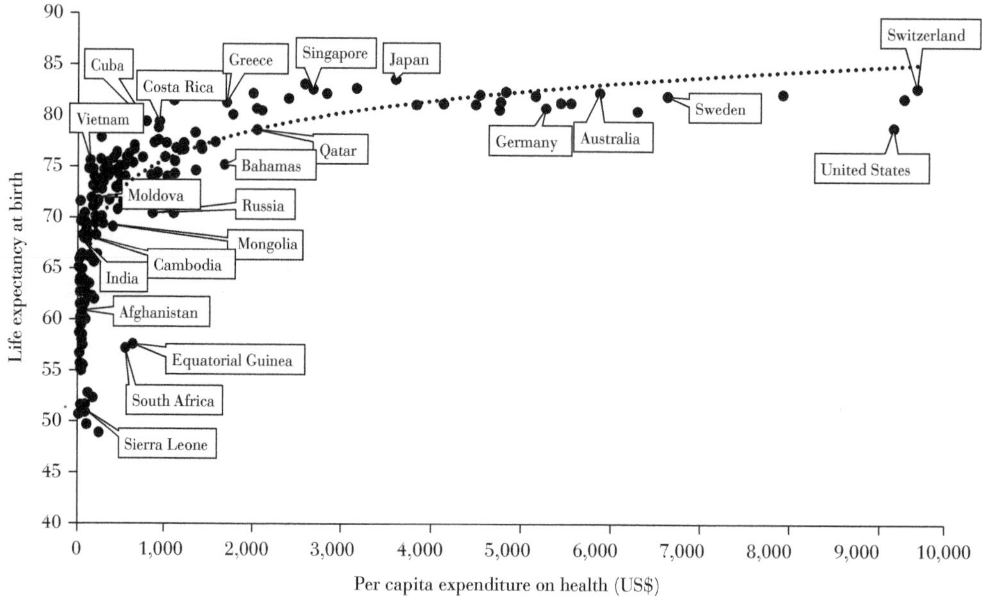

Figure 12-3: The Preston Curve applied to health spending: Annual health care expenditures per capita and life expectancy at birth, 2014 (180 countries).
Data Sources: WHO (2016); World Bank (2015b).

flattens out and there are diminishing or even negative returns. This may be best explained by the way a country's resources are spent and distributed—that is, how social and political values shape priorities, matters that orthodox health economists fail to take into account. Ultimately, inequality of power and resources, not low GDP per capita, remains the leading impediment to health and health equity.

It is important to reiterate that although resources are not limitless, their scarcity may be overstated or misstated. In HICs, much of the activity in the bloated financial sector is "socially useless" (Cassidy 2010), that is, oriented to profiteering rather than to broad societal investments. If these resources were directed to collective needs rather than private greed, there would be more than enough money to sustain social security programs, national health care systems, and many other societal determinants of health. In that sense, austerity budgets are a deliberate policy approach, not a necessity. In LMICs, scarcity is also often manufactured. Limited resources are largely a function of the global and domestic political and economic arrangements examined in prior chapters: capital flight, tax evasion, unfair terms of trade, extreme wealth concentration, and corruption all undermine government capacity to capture revenues and harness them to social well-being.

Mainstream health economists have been particularly puzzled by the seeming paradox of good health outcomes at low levels of GDP per capita, leading them to ask: do these settings enjoy good health outcomes because of especially efficacious expenditure on health care (e.g., effective management and cost-analysis-based allocation of technical resources) (Novignon, Olakojo, and Nonvignon 2012; Savedoff 2007)? Perhaps these economists are not asking the right question. After all, health interventions and economic growth do not offer sufficient explanations for these examples of health success. As discussed next in chapter 13, the making of healthy societies has more to do with broad redistribution of power and resources (including public health and health care spending) than with narrowly defined health care efficiency valuations.

NOTES

1. To this day nonunionized workers, whether in HICs or LMICs have few, if any, such protections. In recent years, unionized workers have also seen job security and safety eroded under austerity policies (see chapter 9).
2. Only insofar as expenditures on health serve to eliminate inconsequential symptoms or to enhance social status (e.g., through cosmetic surgery) may they be considered a form of consumption equivalent to the purchase of any other commodity.

REFERENCES

Ajayi SI and Ndikumana L, Editors. 2015. *Capital Flight from Africa: Causes, Effects, and Policy Issues.* Oxford: Oxford University Press.

Arrow KJ. 1963. Uncertainty and the welfare economics of medical care. *The American Economic Review* 53(5):941–973.

Ashmore J. 2013. 'Going private': A qualitative comparison of medical specialists' job satisfaction in the public and private sectors of South Africa. *Human Resources for Health* 11:1.

Atun R. 2015. Transforming Turkey's health system—Lessons for universal coverage. *New England Journal of Medicine* 373(14):1285–1289.

Balabanova D, Mills A, Conteh L, et al. 2013. Good Health at Low Cost 25 years on: Lessons for the future of health systems strengthening. *Lancet* 381(9883):2118–2133.

Berman PA. 1982. Selective primary health care: Is efficient sufficient? *Social Science and Medicine* 16(10):1054–1059.

Biesma RG, Brugha R, Harmer A, et al. 2009. The effects of global health initiatives on country health systems: A review of the evidence from HIV/AIDS control. *Health Policy and Planning* 24(4):239–252.

Birn A-E, Nervi L, and Siqueira E. 2016. Neoliberalism Redux: The Global Health Policy Agenda and the Politics of Cooptation in Latin America and Beyond. *Development and Change* 47(4):734–759.

Birx D. 2014. Delivering an AIDS free generation. Presentation to the Kaiser Family Foundation Town Hall Forum, 23 June, 2014.

Blumberg LJ, Waidmann TA, Blavin F, and Roth J. 2014. Trends in health care financial burdens, 2001 to 2009. *Milbank Quarterly* 92(1):88–113.

BMGF. 2015. Gates Annual Letter. http://www.gatesnotes.com/2015-annual-letter?page=0&lang=en. Accessed August 13, 2016.

Bourguignon F, Ferreira FH, and Walton M. 2007. Equity, efficiency and inequality traps: A research agenda. *Journal of Economic Inequality* 5(2):235–256.

Canadian Institute for Health Information. 2015. *National Health Expenditure Trends, 1975 to 2015.* Ottawa: Canadian Institute for Health Information.

Cassidy J. 2010. What good is Wall Street? *New Yorker,* November 29.

Centers for Medicare and Medicaid Services. 2015. National health expenditure data: Historical. http://www.cms.gov/Research-Statistics-Data-and-Systems/Statistics-Trends-and-Reports/NationalHealthExpendData/nationalHealthAccountsHistorical.html. Accessed June 24, 2016.

Chanda R. 2013. Medical value travel in India: Prospects and challenges. In Labonté R, Runnels V, Packer C, and Deonandan R, Editors. *Travelling Well: Essays in Medical Tourism.* Ottawa: Institute of Population Health, University of Ottawa.

Chen YYB and Flood CM. 2013. Medical tourism's impact on health care equity and access in low- and middle-income countries: Making the case for regulation. *Journal of Law, Medicine, & Ethics* 41(1):286–300.

Cheng TM. 2015. Reflections on the 20th anniversary of Taiwan's single-payer national health insurance system. *Health Affairs* 34(3):502–510.

Chernomas R and Hudson I. 2013. *To Live and Die in America: Class, Power, Health and Healthcare.* London: Pluto Press.

Collier P and Dercon S. 2006. Review article: The complementarities of poverty reduction, equity and growth: A perspective on the *World Development Report 2006. Economic Development and Cultural Change* 55(1):223–236.

Collins C, Isbell M, Sohn A, and Klindera K. 2012. Four principles for expanding PEPFAR's role as a vital force in US health diplomacy abroad. *Health Affairs* 31(7):1578–1584.

De Allegri M, Sauderborn R, Kouyate B, and Flessa S. 2009. Community health insurance in sub-Saharan Africa: What operational difficulties hamper their successful development? *Tropical Medicine and International Health* 14(5):586–596.

Deaton A. 2013. *The Great Escape: Health, Wealth, and the Origins of Inequality.* Princeton: Princeton University Press.

Dionisio D. 2014. Inside views: Global Health 2035 Report: Flawed projections. http://www.ip-watch.org/2014/01/23/

global-health-2035-report-flawed-projections/. Accessed July 11, 2015.

Drechsler D and Jütting JP. 2010. Six regions, one story. In Preker AS, Zweifel P and Schellekens OP, Editors. *Global Marketplace for Private Health Insurance: Strength in Numbers*. Washington, DC: The World Bank.

Eisenberg MJ, Filion KB, Azoulay A, et al. 2005. Outcomes and cost of coronary artery bypass graft surgery in the United States and Canada. *Archives of Internal Medicine* 165(13):1506–1513.

Emami S. 2010. *Consumer Over-Indebtedness and Health Care Costs: How to Approach the Question from a Global Perspective*. Geneva: WHO.

European Commission. 2016. *Turkey: Refugee Crisis, ECHO Factsheet*. Brussels: Humanitarian Aid and Civil Protection.

Evans RG. 2007. *Economic Myths and Political Realities: The Inequality Agenda and the Sustainability of Medicare*. Vancouver: Centre for Health Services and Policy Research, University of British Columbia.

———. 2013. Waste, economists and American healthcare. *Healthcare Policy* 9(2):12.

Fasawe O, Avila C, Shaffer N, et al. 2013. Cost-Effectiveness analysis of option B+ for HIV prevention and treatment of mothers and children in Malawi. *PLoS ONE* 8(3):e57778.

Feng XL, Xu L, Guo Y, and Ronsmans C. 2012. Factors influencing rising caesarean section rates in China between 1988 and 2008. *Bulletin of the World Health Organization* 90(1):30–39A.

Fries JF, Bruce B, and Chakravarty E. 2011. Compression of morbidity 1980–2011: A focused review of paradigms and progress. *Journal of Aging Research* 2011:261702.

Gawande A. 2015. Overkill. *New Yorker*, May 11.

Gee J and Button M. 2014. *The Financial Cost of Healthcare Fraud 2014: What Data from Around the World Shows*. London: BDO LLP.

Geyman J. 2015. Growing Bureaucracy and Fraud in US Health Care. *Huffington Post*, December 12.

Giedion U, Alfonso EA, and Díaz Y. 2013. *The Impact of Universal Coverage Schemes in the Developing World: A Review of the Existing Evidence*. Washington, DC: The World Bank.

Gladwell M. 2005. The moral hazard myth: The bad idea behind our failed healthcare system. *The New Yorker*, August 29.

Glaser WA. 1993. How expenditure caps and expenditure targets really work. *The Milbank Quarterly* 71(1):97–127.

Gorey KM, Richter NL, Luginaah IN, et al. 2015. Breast cancer among women living in poverty: Better care in Canada than in the United States. *Social Work Research* 39(2):107–118.

Gusmano MK and Rodwin VG. 2015. Comparative health systems. In Knickman JR and Kovner AR, Editors. *Jonas and Kovner's Health Care Delivery in the United States, 11th Edition*. New York: Springer Publishing Company.

Gwatkin DR. 2005. Are free government health services the best way to reach the poor? In Preker AS and Langenbrunner JC, Editors. *Spending Wisely: Buying Health Services for the Poor*. Washington, DC: The World Bank.

Haller L, Hutton G, and Bartram J. 2007. Estimating the costs and health benefits of water and sanitation improvements at global level. *Journal of Water and Health* 5(4):467–480.

Halstead SB, Walsh JA, and Warren KS, Editors. 1985. *Good Health at Low Cost*. A Rockefeller Foundation Conference Report. New York: Rockefeller Foundation.

Hanefeld J, Horsfall D, Lunt N, and Smith R. 2013. Medical tourism: A cost or benefit to the NHS? *PLoS ONE* 8(10):E70406.

Hanson K. 2011. Delivering health services: Incentives and information in supply-side innovations. In Smith RD and Hanson K, Editors. *Health Systems in Low- and Middle-Income Countries: An Economic and Policy Perspective*. New York: Oxford University Press.

Hart JT. 1971. The inverse care law. *Lancet* 297(7696): 405–412.

HarvestPlus. 2014. *Biofortification Progress Briefs*. Washington, DC: International Food Policy Research Institute.

Henderson DA. 2009. *Smallpox - the Death of a Disease: The Inside Story of Eradicating a Worldwide Killer*. Amherst, NY: Prometheus Books.

Herman B. 2015. Drugmakers funnel payments to high-prescribing doctors. *Modern Healthcare*, May 23.

Hernández-Peña P, Poullier JP, Van Mosseveld CJM, et al. 2013. Health worker remuneration in WHO Member States. *Bulletin of the World Health Organization* 91:808–815.

Himmelstein DU, Jun M, Busse R, et al. 2014. A comparison of hospital administrative costs in eight nations: US costs exceed all others by far. *Health Affairs* 33(9):1586–1594.

Holmberg S and Rothstein B. 2011. Dying of corruption. *Health Economics, Policy and Law* 6:529–547.

Hsiao W and Heller PS. 2007. *What Should Macroeconomists Know about Health Care Policy?* Washington, DC: International Monetary Fund.

Hussmann K. 2011. *Addressing Corruption in the Health Sector.* Bergen, NO: U4 Anti-Corruption Resource Centre.

Hyun KR, Kang S, and Lee S. 2015. Population aging and healthcare expenditure in Korea. *Health Economics* [Epub ahead of print].

Iacobucci G. 2013. More than a third of GPs on commissioning groups have conflicts of interest, BMJ investigation shows. *BMJ* 346:f1569.

IHME. 2016. *Financing Global Health 2015: Development Assistance Steady on the Path to New Global Goals.* Seattle: IHME.

Iriart C, Franco T, and Merhy EE. 2011. The creation of the health consumer: Challenges on health sector regulation after managed care era. *Globalization and Health* 7:2.

Jain A, Nundy S, and Abbasi K. 2014. Corruption: Medicine's dirty open secret. *BMJ* 348:g4184.

Jamison DT, Breman JG, Measham AR, et al, Editors. 2006. *Disease Control Priorities in Developing Countries, Second Edition.* Washington, DC: The World Bank; New York: Oxford University Press.

Jamison DT, Summers LH, Alleyne G, et al. 2013. Global health 2035: A world converging within a generation. *Lancet* 382(9908):1898–1955.

Jelamschi L and De Ver Dye T. 2010. *Decline in the Under 5 Mortality Rate (U5MR) in Turkey: A Case Study.* New York: UNICEF.

Jenniskens F, Tiendrebeogo G, Coolen A, et al. 2012. How countries cope with competing demands and expectations: Perspectives of different stakeholders on priority setting and resource allocation for health in the era of HIV and AIDS. *BMC Public Health* 12(1):1071.

Joe W. 2014. Distressed financing of household out-of-pocket health care payments in India: Incidence and correlates. *Health Policy and Planning* 30(6):728–741.

Jorgensen PD. 2013. Pharmaceuticals, political money, and public policy: A theoretical and empirical agenda. *Journal of Law, Medicine & Ethics* 41(3):561–570.

Katz A. 2004. The Sachs report: Investing in health for economic development—or increasing the size of the crumbs from the rich man's table? Part I. *International Journal of Health Services* 34(4):751–773.

Khayatzadeh-Mahani A, Fotaki M, and Harvey G. 2013. Priority setting and implementation in a centralized health system: A case study of Kerman province in Iran. *Health Policy and Planning* 28(5):480–494.

Kim JJ, Campos NG, O'Shea M, et al. 2013. Model-based impact and cost-effectiveness of cervical cancer prevention in sub-Saharan Africa. *Vaccine* 31:F60–F72.

KPMG. 2014. Medical value travel in India: FICCI Heal Conference. https://www.kpmg.com/IN/en/IssuesAndInsights/ArticlesPublications/Documents/KPMG-FICCI-Heal-Sep2014.pdf. Accessed May 20, 2015.

Lagarde M and Palmer N. 2011. The impact of user fees on access to health services in low and middle-income countries. *Cochrane Database System Review* (4):CD009094.

Laurell AC and López Arellano O. 1996. Market commodities and poor relief: The World Bank proposal for health. *International Journal of Health Services* 26(1):1–18.

Lee MM and Izama MP. 2015. Aid externalities: Evidence from PEPFAR in Africa. *World Development* 67:281–294.

Loewenson R and Gilson L. 2012. The health system and wider social determinants of health. In Smith RD and Hanson K, Editors. *Health Systems in Low-and Middle-Income Countries: An Economic and Policy Perspective.* New York: Oxford University Press.

Lu JFR and Hsiao W. 2003. Does Universal Health Insurance Make Health Care Unaffordable? Lessons from Taiwan. *Health Affairs* 22(3):77–78.

Marriott A and Hamer J. 2014. *Investing for the Few: The IFC's Health in Africa Initiative.* Oxford: Oxfam International.

Martín-Fernández J, del Cura-González MI, Rodríguez-Martínez G, et al. 2013. Economic valuation of health care services in public health systems: A study about Willingness to Pay (WTP) for nursing consultations. *PloS One* 8(4):e62840.

Max W, Rice DP, Sung H-Y, and Michel M. 2004. Valuing human life: Estimating the present value of lifetime earnings, 2000. *Economic Studies and Related Methods.* http://escholarship.org/uc/item/82d0550k. Accessed August 13, 2016.

McCoy D, Jensen N, Kranzer K, et al. 2013. Methodological and policy limitations of quantifying the saving of lives: A case study of the Global Fund's approach. *PLoS Medicine* 10(9):e1001522.

McIntyre D and Kutzin J. 2011. Revenue collection and pooling arrangements in financing. In Smith RD and Hanson K, Editors. *Health Systems in Low- and Middle-Income Countries: An Economic and Policy Perspective.* New York: Oxford University Press.

Mello MM, Chandra A, Gawande AA, and Studdert DM. 2010. National costs of the medical liability system. *Health Affairs* 29(9):1569–1577.

Michaud J, Kates J, and Oum S. 2015. *Corruption and Global Health: Summary of a Policy Roundtable.* Menlo Park: Kaiser Family Foundation.

Mills A. 1997. Leopard or chameleon? The changing character of international health economics. *Tropical Medicine and International Health* 2(10):963–977.

———. 2014. Reflections on the development of health economics in low-and middle-income countries. *Proceedings of the Royal Society B* 281(1789).

Molina Aguilar IB, Otilia Mendoza L, García O, et al. 2015. Cost-effectiveness analysis of the introduction of the human papillomavirus vaccine in Honduras. *Vaccine* 33:A167–A173.

Morra D, Nicholson S, Levinson W, et al. 2011. US physician practices versus Canadians: Spending nearly four times as much money interacting with payers. *Health Affairs* 30(8):1443–1450.

Natuzzi ES and Novotny T. 2014. Sector wide approaches in health care: Do they work? *Global Health Governance* 8(1):77–95.

Nayyar G, Breman JG, Newton PN, and Herrington J. 2012. Poor-quality antimalarial drugs in southeast Asia and sub-Saharan Africa. *Lancet Infectious Diseases* 12(6):488–496.

Nervi L. 2014. Easier Said than Done (in Global Health): A Glimpse at Nonfinancial Challenges in International Cooperation. http://www.peah.it/2014/02/easier-said-than-done-in-global-health-a-glimpse-at-nonfinancial-challenges-in-international-cooperation/. Accessed July 22, 2015.

NHCAA [National Health Care Anti-Fraud Association]. 2015. The challenge of health care fraud. http://www.nhcaa.org/resources/health-care-anti-fraud-resources/the-challenge-of-health-care-fraud.aspx. Accessed July 18, 2015.

Novignon J, Olakojo SA, and Nonvignon J. 2012. The effects of public and private health care expenditure on health status in sub-Saharan Africa: New evidence from panel data analysis. *Health Economics Review* 2(1):1–8.

OECD. 2015. Query Wizard for International Development Statistics (QWIDS). http://stats.oecd.org/qwids/. Accessed February 13, 2015.

———. 2016. OECD Health Statistics 2016. http://stats.oecd.org/Index.aspx?DataSetCode=HEALTH_STAT. Accessed August 10, 2016.

Ökem ZG and Çakar M. 2015. What have health care reforms achieved in Turkey? An appraisal of the "Health Transformation Programme". *Health Policy* 119(9):1153–1163.

Ortegón M, Lim S, Chisholm D, and Mendis S. 2012. Cost effectiveness of strategies to combat cardiovascular disease, diabetes, and tobacco use in sub-Saharan Africa and South East Asia: Mathematical modelling study. *BMJ* 344:e607.

Pauly M. 1968. The economics of moral hazard: Comment. *American Economic Review* 58(3):531–537.

Pettenkofer MJ von. 1941. *The Value of Health to a City: Two Lectures Delivered in 1873*. Translated by HE Sigerist. Baltimore: Johns Hopkins University Press.

Pfeiffer J and Chapman R. 2010. Anthropological perspectives on structural adjustment and public health. *Annual Review of Anthropology* 39:149–165.

PHM, Medact, and Global Equity Gauge Alliance. 2005. *Global Health Watch 2005–2006: An Alternative World Health Report.* London: Zed Books Ltd.

PHM, Medact, Medico International, et al. 2014. *Global Health Watch 4: An Alternative World Health Report.* London: Zed Books Ltd.

Pond K, Pedley S, and Edwards C. 2011. Background. In Cameron J, Hunter P, Jagals P and Pond K, Editors. *Valuing Water, Valuing Livelihoods Guidance on Social Cost-Benefit Analysis of Drinking-water Interventions, with Special Reference to Small Community Water Supplies.* WHO: Geneva.

Pozen A and Cutler DM. 2010. Medical spending differences in the United States and Canada: The role of prices, procedures, and administrative expenses inquiry. *Inquiry: The Journal of Health Care Organization, Provision, and Financing* 47(2):124–134.

Pringle JD and Cole DC. 2012. The Nigerian lead poisoning epidemic: The role of neoliberal globalization and challenges for humanitarian ethics. In Abu-Sada C, Editor. *Dilemmas, Challenges, and Ethics of Humanitarian Action: Reflections on MSF's Perception Project.* Montreal: McGill-Queen's University Press.

Profit J, Lee D, Zupancic JA, et al. 2010. Clinical benefits, costs, and cost-effectiveness of neonatal intensive care in Mexico. *PLoS Medicine* 7(12):1506.

Pulkki-Brännström A-M, Wolff C, Brännström N and Skordis-Worrall J. 2012. Cost and cost effectiveness of long-lasting insecticide-treated bed nets - a model-based analysis. *Cost Effectiveness and Resource Allocation* 10(5):10–1186.

Qadeer I and Baru R. 2016. Shrinking spaces for the 'public'in contemporary public health. *Development and Change* 47(4):760–781.

Reidpath DD, Olafsdottir AE, Pokhrel S, and Allotey P. 2012. The fallacy of the equity-efficiency trade off: Rethinking the efficient health system. *BMC Public Health* 12(Suppl 1):S3.

Ridde V, Haddad S, and Heinmüller R. 2013. Improving equity by removing healthcare fees for children in Burkina Faso. *Journal of Epidemiology and Community Health* 67:751–757.

Riley JC. 2008. *Low Income, Social Growth, and Good Health: A History of Twelve Countries*. Berkeley: University of California Press.

Robert E and Ridde V. 2013. Global health actors no longer in favor of user fees: A documentary study. *Globalization and Health* 9:29.

Rowden R. 2013. The ghosts of user fees past: Exploring accountability for victims of a 30-year economic policy mistake. *Health and Human Rights* 15(1):175–185.

Russell S and Gilson L. 1997. User fee policies to promote health service access for the poor: A wolf in sheep's clothing? *International Journal of Health Services* 27(2):359–379.

Sabik LM and Lie RK. 2008. Priority setting in health care: Lessons from the experiences of eight countries. *International Journal for Equity in Health* 7:4.

Savedoff WD. 2007. What should a country spend on health care? *Health Affairs* 26(4):962–970.

Seidman L. 2015. The Affordable Care Act versus Medicare for All. *Journal of Health Politics, Policy and Law* 40(4):909–919.

Sepehri A and Chernomas R. 2004. Is the Canadian health care system fiscally sustainable? *International Journal of Health Services* 34(2):229–243.

Shillcutt MSD, Walker DG, Goodman CA, and Mills AJ. 2009. Cost effectiveness in low-and middle-income countries. *Pharmacoeconomics* 27(11):903–917.

Snepp F. 2012. Doctor-run physical therapy clinics scrutinized. *NBC Los Angeles*, June 6.

Snyder J, Crooks VA, Johnston R, and Kingsbury P. 2013. Beyond sun, sand, and stitches: Assigning responsibility for the harms of medical tourism. *Bioethics* 27(5):233–242.

Snyder J, Crooks VA, Johnston R, et al. 2015. Medical tourism's impacts on health worker migration in the Caribbean: Five examples and their implications for global justice. *Global Health Action* 8:27348.

Starfield B. 2010. Reinventing primary care: Lessons from Canada for the United States. *Health Affairs* 29(5):1030–1036.

Storeng KT. 2014. The GAVI Alliance and the 'Gates approach' to health system strengthening. *Global Public Health* 9(8):865–879.

The Conversation. 2014. We can't hope to solve global ills without action against poverty. https://theconversation.com/we-cant-hope-to-solve-global-ills-without-action-against-poverty-35278. Accessed July 11, 2015.

Tijdens K, De Vries DH, and Steinmetz S. 2013. Health workforce remuneration: comparing wage levels, ranking, and dispersion of 16 occupational groups in 20 countries. *Human Resources for Health* 11:11.

Trade Economics. 2015. Nigeria GDP annual growth rate. http://www.tradingeconomics.com/nigeria/gdp-growth-annual. Accessed July 22, 2015.

Tu JV, Naylor CD, Pashos CL, et al. 1997. Use of cardiac procedures and outcomes in elderly patients with myocardial infarction in the United States and Canada. *New England Journal of Medicine* 336(21):1500–1505.

Valencia-Mendoza A, Danese-dlSantos LG, Sosa-Rubí SG, and Aracena-Genao B. 2011. Costo-efectividad de prácticas en salud pública: Revisión bibliográfica de las intervenciones de la Iniciativa Mesoamericana de Salud. *Salud Pública de México* 53:S375–S385.

Vargas I, Vazquez ML, Mogollon-Perez AS, and Unger J-P. 2010. Barriers of access to care in a managed competition model: Lessons from Colombia. *BMC Health Services Research* 10(1):297.

Vassall A and Martínez-Álvarez M. 2011. The health system and external financing. In Smith RD and Hanson K, Editors. *Health Systems in Low- and Middle-Income Countries: An Economic and Policy Perspective*. New York: Oxford University Press.

Waitzkin H. 2003. Report of the WHO Commission on Macroeconomics and Health: A summary and critique. *Lancet* 361(9356):523–526.

Waitzkin H and Jasso-Aguilar R. 2015. Empire, health, and health care: Perspectives at the end of empire as we have known it. *Annual Review of Sociology* 41:271–290.

Waitzkin H, Jasso-Aguilar R, and Iriart C. 2007. Privatization of health services in less developed countries: An empirical response to the proposals of the World Bank and Wharton School. *International Journal of Health Services* 37(2):205–227.

WHO. 1980. *The Work of WHO 1978-1979: Biennial Report of the Director-General to the World Health Assembly and to the United Nations*. Geneva: WHO.

———. 2001. *Macroeconomics and Health: Investing in Health for Economic Development. Report of the Commission on Macroeconomics and Health*. Geneva: WHO.

WHO. 2010. *World Health Report 2010*. Geneva: WHO.

———. 2011. *Helminth Control in School-Age Children: A Guide for Managers of Control Programmes*. Geneva: WHO.

———. 2012. Spending on health: A global overview. http://www.who.int/mediacentre/factsheets/fs319/en/. Accessed November 1, 2014.

———. 2014a. Global Health Expenditure Database. http://apps.who.int/nha/database/Select/Indicators/en. Accessed August 12, 2016.

———. 2014b. What is universal health coverage? http://www.who.int/features/qa/universal_health_coverage/en/. Accessed July 4, 2015.

———. 2015a. Global Health Observatory Data Repository. http://www.who.int/gho/en/. Accessed July 17, 2015.

———. 2015b. *Health in 2015: from MDGs, to SDGs*. Geneva: WHO.

World Bank. 1987. *Financing Health Services in Developing Countries: An Agenda for Reform*. Washington, DC: World Bank.

———. 1993. *World Development Report 1993: Investing in Health*. New York: Oxford University Press for the World Bank.

———. 2015. World Development Indicators. http://data.worldbank.org. Accessed July 18, 2015.

Yukhananov A. 2013. World Bank president calls corruption 'Public Enemy No. 1.' *Reuters*, December 19.

Zweifel P, Felder S, and Meiers M. 1999. Aging of population and health care expenditure: A red herring? *Health Economics* 8(6):485–496.

13

BUILDING HEALTHY SOCIETIES

From Ideas to Action

Key Questions:

- What makes for a healthy society?
- How do global health policies and activities aid or impede the building of healthy societies?

In 1970 Dr. Salvador Allende, the newly-elected socialist President of Chile, ambitiously laid out his goals in his inaugural speech:

> Only by advancing along this path of basic transformations in the political and economic fields will we be able to draw ever nearer to the ideals that are our objective:
>
> To create a new society . . . without having to resort to exploitation. . . .
>
> To create a society that guarantees each family—every man, woman and child—rights, securities, freedom, hope and other basic guarantees. We aim to have all the people filled with a sense of their being called upon to build a new nation which will also mean the construction of more beautiful, more prosperous, more dignified and freer lives for all (Allende 2000, p. 61).

Four years later, Samora Machel, a trained nurse and soon-to-be first President of independent Mozambique, marked the tenth anniversary of the beginning of the armed struggle against Portuguese colonialism with a speech linking health to political expectations:

> Any center of ours, whether a school or a health center . . . in addition to its specific task, must also spread our political approach towards a new life as part of its work; it must itself be a model of the new society we are constructing and of the new social relations between people (Machel 1974).

In prior chapters, we critically examined the history and political economy of global health and development aid, key contemporary players and activities in these areas, and global profiles of morbidity and mortality. We also explored the structural forces and array of factors—from militarism and conflict to: global trade and investment regimes, corporate power, and relations between social groups; social policies, labor protections, migration, health, and the environment; and neighborhood conditions—that shape health patterns both within and across countries. Now we turn to the hopeful arena of building healthy societies.

In contrast to the aspirations of Allende and Machel, dominant global health donors, actors, and associated global health initiatives and PPPs prioritize technical magic bullets usually at the expense of integrated and comprehensive approaches to well-being. Allende and Machel, both health professionals whose lives were tragically cut short, proposed that healthy societies required: social and economic security and justice to protect the vulnerable from exploitation; freedom of expression and opportunities for full participation in civic life; and universal and equitably distributed services, including water, sanitation, education, shelter, and health care.

This chapter explores how, and under what conditions, the goals espoused by these leaders may be realized, drawing on key issues raised in chapter 7. In gauging success in global health, we begin by contrasting disease-control approaches and broad-reaching societal efforts aimed at addressing the underlying causes of ill health. We also review hybrid approaches that target poor groups with social interventions absent larger political and social change. Then we focus on the makings of healthy societies in practice—highlighting efforts in a range of municipalities, regions, and countries. The last section revisits healthy public policy from the angles of health promotion, healthy cities, and emerging alternative frameworks. Many of the societal case studies that we use in this chapter (as elsewhere) are from low- and middle-income countries (LMICs), revealing widely relevant lessons. By focusing on societal change through a lens of critical political economy, these approaches provide a counterbalance to mainstream efforts in global health.

What Constitutes Success in Global Health?

Defining and identifying success in global health—and, ideally, reproducing the conditions of success—comprise a key global health preoccupation. Global health progress is typically measured in terms of disease control and eradication achievements, number of cases prevented, infant mortality declines, and improvements in life expectancy (Birn 2009; Hay and McHugh 2014). Many global and transnational actors seek to contribute to such progress.

Dominant global health efforts focus on donor aid as a catalyst for better outcomes, as clocked by these metrics (Sachs 2015). Bill and Melinda Gates's 2015 annual letter, for example, suggests that targeted approaches are all that is needed. They make a "bold bet"—that the lives of people living in poor countries will improve faster from now until 2030 than ever before. Offering a smorgasbord of health predictions, they wager that child mortality will be halved because almost all countries will implement vaccination against diarrhea and pneumonia and better sanitation will be achieved "through simple actions like hand-washing as well as innovations like new toilets designed especially for poor places." They are also betting on eradication of a slew of diseases: polio, guinea worm, onchocerciasis, lymphatic filariasis, and blinding trachoma (BMGF 2015).

Other development specialists cite the concept of global public goods as a rationale for addressing global health and development needs, suggesting that self-interested parties are more likely to participate if they see gains for their own, as well as collective, interests (Birdsall and Diofasi 2015). The basic idea is that everyone will enjoy advantages from spending and attention to public goods (i.e., if air is cleaner, all will benefit, and one group's enjoyment of this benefit will not impinge on another's) and nobody can be excluded, offering at least the potential to improve some global health inequalities (Hunter and Dawson 2011).

Yet both of these stances disregard the central role of power and resource inequalities across multiple axes (class, race/ethnicity, income-level of country, sex/gender, etc.) in determining the distribution of health and well-being. Indeed, celebrating that over 10% of global spending on official development assistance has gone to global public goods (and advocating for more), such as "encourag[ing] private production and marketing of a pneumococcal vaccine" in low-income countries (LICs) (Birdsall and Diofasi 2015) is hardly the stuff of collective action to reduce inequalities! Instead this suggested approach exacerbates inequalities by transferring public monies to the already unfathomably profitable pharmaceutical sector and entrenching their (market) position in LICs.

Although donor aid—especially solidarity-oriented aid (see chapter 14)—can be helpful under particular circumstances, alternative strategies, for instance socially just rules around trade and financial transactions, may offer a far more sustainable approach to human welfare (Gottiniaux et al. 2015).

There are a number of ways in which success in global health can be gauged, some more narrowly focused than others. Take, for example, a cataract surgery program, such as Cuba's Misión Milagro (Operation Miracle) or Canada's Operation Eyesight.

At a purely technical level, success may be measured by the number of cataract surgeries performed in an LMIC by a team of doctors and nurses from a high-income country (HIC) (or, in the case of Cuba and Tunisia, another LMIC). It can certainly be argued that in a country with a significant backlog of cataracts that require removal, even a handful of operations are beneficial. Continuing with this example, a more important indicator of success might be how many local professionals have been trained by the team to provide cataract surgeries going forward. At another level, success might be appraised by the team's efforts to campaign for adherence to the World Health Organization's (WHO's) Global Code of Practice on the International Recruitment of Health Personnel so that HICs refrain from recruiting LMIC ophthalmologists.

At yet another level, success could be clocked by the team's participation not only in providing surgery, but in country-to-country solidarity exchanges or in advocating, as health professionals, for an equitable trade and development system, whereby LMICs are not subject to cycles of debt crises and international financial institution (IFI) conditionalities, foreign direct investment squeezing out farmers and domestic industries, capital flight, and tax evasion (and accompanying domestic corruption), so that there are more resources in public coffers to fund health worker training and retention and comprehensive health care systems.

The latter activities do not preclude the initial medical mission to provide cataract surgery—in fact such missions may spark consciousness of global health inequities. But a critical political economy approach to global health argues for going beyond the charity model of providing cataract surgery to pursue a deeper understanding of, and activism around, the larger determinants of health inequity and health needs. The ultimate goal, of course, is to prevent premature death and disability, alleviate suffering, and improve living conditions to allow all people to thrive, equitably and over the long term.

In sum, success in global health may best be measured in terms of the field's ability to integrate political economy, human rights, and collective health approaches with public health's technical tools to benefit health and health equity.

VERTICAL HEALTH PROGRAMS AND GLOBAL HEALTH INTERVENTIONS: SUCCESSES AND LIMITATIONS

Key Questions:

- What are the characteristics of targeted interventions?
- How might they be enhanced?

As outlined in chapters 1 and 2, the first generation of international disease campaigns was launched a century ago by various colonial authorities and the Rockefeller Foundation, mostly based on narrowly framed interventions. WHO later championed such technology-based campaigns against yaws, malaria, smallpox, and then polio and other diseases; the United Nations (UN) Children's Fund's (UNICEF's) child survival campaigns, too, involved a collection of disease-specific and technically-oriented initiatives. Based on a defined target of eradicating a single disease, just two efforts have achieved these aims: in 1980 via WHO's smallpox eradication campaign, and some 20 years later through the Global Rinderpest Eradication Programme against this viral cattle disease, led by the UN's Food and Agriculture Organization and World Organization for Animal Health (FAO 2011).

Attempts to eliminate malaria, however, have proved thornier. Before DDT (insecticide) spraying was introduced in the mid-1940s, early 20th century efforts focused on reducing larval breeding sites of the *Anopheles* mosquito vector through swamp drainage, use of larvicidal fish, and the spraying of larvicidal oils. Together with housing and sanitation improvements—such as screened windows (to keep mosquitoes out) and piped water and sewage (to diminish the use of water receptacles, thereby eliminating breeding sites)—these measures enabled malaria's disappearance from North America and Europe. When the WHO inaugurated its Global Malaria Eradication Programme in 1955, such multipronged methods were ignored in favor of an almost exclusive focus on DDT. Within a few years, an estimated 1 billion people were no longer threatened by malaria. But by the mid-1960s, both donors and endemic countries lost interest in funding the campaign and there was growing resentment toward its vertical (top-down) structure. Moreover, DDT was increasingly met with both mosquito resistance and mounting concerns over its damaging environmental effects. By 1969, eradication was abandoned in favor of control.

Yet as global health historian Randall Packard (2007) has argued, it was not mosquito or human resistance that doomed the malaria campaign, but its technologically focused mentality. The several dozen places that reached eradication included only HICs, a few islands (with geographic advantages), and socialist countries, largely in the Eastern bloc. All shared an understanding of and commitment to addressing malaria as inextricably linked to living conditions, agricultural practices, and other societal factors. Elsewhere, as discussed in chapter 6, malaria rates crept up again, reaching crisis proportions by the 1990s. Despite this lesson, the technical approach to global health was not buried, but routinely resurrected, first through the massive smallpox eradication campaign (not unproblematically; see chapter 2), and again through more recent global health initiatives. Each of these has been marred by a limited ability to transcend the malaria campaign's flaw of overlooking the social fabric, even as past malaria efforts demonstrate the (enhanced) effectiveness of integrating technical with socio-political approaches.

Which Interventions Work, According to Whom, and What Is the Evidence?

Notwithstanding its disputed record, the narrowly-focused technical approach is usually given the benefit of the doubt. The US Institute of Medicine (2009, p. 33) argues that "progress in health over the last half-century can mostly be attributed to the creation, dissemination, and adoption of interventions to improve health," to which the US has "contributed greatly." Not only is the question of *who* is responsible for health successes debatable, but deciding on the metrics is contested (e.g., what if mortality from one cause declines but from another rises . . .?). There are also differing views around the importance of time frames, cost-effectiveness, and the context of success. One of the recurring dilemmas, articulated early on by the Rockefeller Foundation, is whether global health needs new research (and what kind) or whether "public health can be improved by making better use of the resources we have in our grasp" (Jasny et al. 2014, p. 1256). As an example, should existing clean water and sanitation systems that have proved effective for over a century in HICs be extended to low-income populations across the world or would, as the BMGF (2014) proposes, "development of radically new sanitation technologies as well as markets for new sanitation products and services" in LMICs be preferable?

One highly-publicized approach, *Millions Saved*, developed by the Washington think tank Center for Global Development, seeks to identify "proven successes in global health" (Levine et al. 2007). In several iterations, "proven" successful cases have been selected according to: scale (mostly national); importance (as per disease burden); measurable impact (on population health); and duration (at least 5 years); with special attention paid to cost-effective programs; and, added in 2016, global relevance and equity improvements (Glassman and Temin 2016).

Of the dozens of cases submitted for consideration by several hundred global health experts, twenty success stories were identified in the initial 2004 and 2007 rounds, almost all based on biomedical approaches to underscore the authors' claim that overall social and economic betterment was unnecessary in at least half the instances of global health success identified. The cases selected include the eradication of smallpox, HIV prevention in Thailand, tuberculosis (TB) control in China, reduction of tobacco use in Poland, and measles elimination in southern Africa.

Key ingredients of success were named as (Levine et al. 2007):

- Predictable and adequate funding
- Political leadership
- Affordable technologies
- Technical consensus about the appropriate biomedical or public health approach
- Use and sharing of quality information
- Effective health delivery and management
- In certain cases, community participation and NGO involvement

Yet in minimizing the salience of the broader environment, the analysis was left wanting. For instance, the durability of successful national TB control in

China has been jeopardized by poor coverage in rural areas, high multidrug-resistant TB in low-income groups, and rampant profiteering from hospitalization fees (Wei et al. 2014), all reflecting inequitable and worsening social conditions.

Similarly, while the *Millions Saved* report notes that there were just 117 measles cases in southern Africa in 2000, this rose to 667 by 2005, and in 2009–2011 there were almost 145,000 confirmed measles cases (Shibeshi et al. 2014). Although this increase may have resulted from factors not present during the period under study, it demonstrates that even when effective vaccine technology is available, diseases remain subject to the larger political, social, and economic context, encompassing issues including labor migration, deteriorating health care systems, economic crises, and civil wars.

At bottom, in its quest to focus on interventions, *Millions Saved* sidesteps the social and political aspects of the highlighted stories of success. For example, "saving mothers' lives in Sri Lanka" (cited in the earlier rounds)—entailing a 90% reduction in maternal mortality since the 1950s—is attributed to a universal, free health care system with extensive rural coverage, trained midwives, good data for decisionmaking, and targeted efforts to marginalized groups. These are all undoubtedly important factors. What is missing is the *context* of these policies—what enabled them, what sustained them, and what other measures accompanied them (see ahead).

The 2016 round of 18 cases adds monitoring and evaluation and effective delivery systems as hallmarks of success and appears to expand the focus beyond the prior mostly disease-specific, vertical approaches. New cases cover broader social investments such as health system strengthening (e.g., Brazil's family health program—see chapter 11), regulatory public health policies (e.g., a comprehensive motorbike helmet law in Vietnam), and even redistributive approaches that affect the social determinants of health (SDOH) (e.g., cash transfers in South Africa; see ahead).

Still, the authors continue to stress that:

> In each success story, solid evidence . . . strongly suggests that health improvements are attributable to the specific program or policy of interest rather than other factors, such as economic growth or social improvements (CGD 2016).

Identifying what *Millions Saved* underplays, that is, expansive social improvements integrated with specific public health efforts—rather than carved away from them—is precisely the aim of this chapter.

Evaluating the Evidence

Another approach for assessing the success of interventions is employed by the Abdul Latif Jameel Poverty Action Lab (J-PAL) at the Massachusetts Institute of Technology. J-PAL tries to replicate randomized controlled trials (RCTs[1]), what it calls "randomized evaluations," of poverty reduction interventions, many with a health focus, in order to assess their effectiveness. The aim is to promote the "scaling up"—that is, taking a project from pilot to wide application—of interventions that demonstrate evidence of success (J-PAL 2015).

Economist Esther Duflo, a co-founder of J-PAL, sees the potential of, for example, randomized evaluations that identify which incentives will make poor farmers seek to increase crop output or what kind of regulations will improve teacher attendance—often a predictor of children's school attendance (Chernomas and Hudson 2016). This work focuses on acute problems that may be tweaked through better information and micro-level interventions.

There are certainly valid arguments for vigorously evaluating health and development efforts. Indeed, a randomized study by Duflo's group showed that microfinance programs, long hailed by IFIs, had almost no impact on health or other key development indicators (Banerjee, Karlan, and Zinman 2015). Yet the promise and perils of larger societal policies and changes, which may not be aimed directly at health or social development outcomes despite deeply affecting them, remain unexamined by this approach. If structural adjustment programs had been subject to RCTs (prior to widespread implementation) to investigate their impact in both economic and social (including health) realms, arguably millions of premature deaths and untold misery would have been averted (whether ethics approval would have been obtained is doubtful!). Crucially, the more positive examples of healthy societies explored in this chapter are not

RCT material, for they represent decades of struggle and rest on political factors that cannot be randomized or decontextualized, even as particular policies may have broader relevance. For this reason randomized evaluations may be best suited to demonstrating the futility of identifying development panaceas through generalizable (and assumption-ridden) poverty-alleviation interventions.

To take a current popular example, the community-led total sanitation (CLTS) movement, backed by the World Bank, UNICEF, and various international NGOs, responds to longstanding critiques of development programs lacking community involvement and control (Setiawan and Parry 2011). The accompanying rationale is that responsibility for building latrines rests with the community, using their own resources, and based on behavioral change from an outside trigger—in this case a process of shaming residents who engage in outdoor defecation to convince them to clean up their act (PHM et al. 2014). Some of the sparse RCT evidence on CLTS shows no decrease in diarrheal illness but claims positive results in terms of latrine hygiene and access, with associated child health improvements including decreased stunting and lower diarrheal mortality (Alzua et al. 2015). Another CLTS study in East Java, Indonesia, showed only minimally higher latrine construction in treatment versus control areas (Cameron, Shah, and Olivia 2013).

Yet the assertion of lasting and effective behavior change requiring no subsidies is rife with assumptions: as with most RCTs, follow-up is short—based on just 1 or 2 years—so sustainability remains an unknown. Moreover, the notion that all that poor rural communities need is an outside impetus and knowledge is patronizing and problematic, given that lack of local resources—linked to a host of local, national, and global factors (see chapters 7 and 9)—remains the major impediment to rural sanitation and water access. Lastly, the assumption that latrines are the only viable (or evaluable) alternative for addressing rural sanitation (Luby 2014) begs the question of why communities should not aspire to more permanent forms of sanitation as opposed to second class variants.

A related assumption on individual behaviors is that people will place greater value on items they purchase compared with those they receive free of charge. This was the ideology put forth by "social marketing" gurus at the World Bank, who for many years insisted that health enhancing goods, such as insecticide-treated bednets (or clean cookstoves), should be sold as commodities rather than distributed for free because people would "value" and use them more (World Bank 2008). Yet studies in Kenya and elsewhere show that *willingness* to pay for bednets is more a reflection of *ability* to pay than of valuation or actual health need (Cohen and Dupas 2010), and that free distribution increases coverage more rapidly and equitably than cost-sharing schemes (Ahmed et al. 2011).

In the case of J-PAL's and Duflo's work—echoed in the World Bank's behavioral economics approach to development (Fine et al. 2016)—the underlying conviction is that the poor can lead better lives without changes to social and political structures and without addressing the root causes of poverty and inequity: all that is needed is for poor people to modify their own behavior. As such, the reason people are poor or unhealthy is not relevant: all that matters is applying RCTs, whose results make it "easier for the poor to make the right decisions" (Chernomas and Hudson 2016, p. 33). Employed in this way, RCTs may identify the most efficacious among several interventions (worth "scaling up"), but they limit the kinds of interventions evaluated and, critically, assume that the micro-level is independent of the societal context in which decisions take place (Reddy 2012).

On the aim of "scaling up" more generally, a prime concern is "absorptive capacity"—whether authorities in other regions and at higher levels (beyond the pilot program) are able to effectively utilize mandated programs and resources according to donor criteria and rules (Kapilashrami and Hanefeld 2014; Mangham and Hanson 2010). The very metaphor of "scaling up"—evoking a single person climbing a vertical structure—implies a narrow and dangerous form of social service delivery. A more politically contextualized metaphor might be "building stairs, bridges, and foundations," suggesting that programs are protected, solid, and connected to the larger community. A national, public, social well-being system could be the embodiment of such a metaphor (Krieger 2008), but, metaphorically or literally, this kind of model is not at the heart of mainstream development efforts.

Conditional Cash Transfers and other "Pro-Poor" Approaches

In recent years, as once touted microfinance efforts have proved inadequate to alleviate poverty (Roodman 2012) or downright exploitative (Bateman 2010), other so-called "pro-poor" approaches have taken center stage in addressing the lead Millennium (and now, Sustainable) Development Goal of "eradicat[ing] extreme poverty" (World Bank 2015a). Prime among these are cash transfer programs, entailing government provision of supplementary income to low-income (means-tested) households through *conditional* cash transfers (CCTs). CCTs require recipients to fulfill certain obligations, such as ensuring children's regular school attendance and up-to-date vaccinations, and, in the case of India, requiring young women to remain unmarried until the age of 18 (as an effort to curb early marriage) (Krishnan et al. 2014).

Two pioneering CCT programs are Mexico's *Oportunidades* (established in 1997, initially as *Progresa*) and Brazil's *Bolsa Familia* (2003). Focused on intergenerational social investment, and often providing essential livelihood support especially to poor women and children (Kabeer, Piza, and Taylor 2012), CCTs presume a patently gendered responsibility for fulfilling conditions (Gideon 2014).

Proliferating first through Latin America, transfer programs are employed in many African, Middle Eastern, and Asian countries, as well as New York City. Cash transfer programs have been financed by development banks and bilateral agencies, and promoted by the UN Development Programme (UNDP) and the India-Brazil-South Africa Dialogue Forum. In 2013, the World Bank was supporting 58 CCT programs in 30 countries plus 84 non-conditional programs in 47 countries (World Bank 2013). This financial support has played an important role in the wide uptake of cash-transfer programs (Martínez Franzoni and Voorend 2011).

Mexico's *Oportunidades* (since 2014 replaced by *Prospera*), covered 6.1 million families by 2014 (21% of the population) (World Bank 2015b), focusing on education, health, and nutrition. In its initial formulation, the program was means-tested, with eligibility determined by household demographic and socioeconomic characteristics (e.g., number of children, household connection to running water) (Coady, Martinelli, and Parker 2013). It consisted of a guaranteed package of primary care services (covering 27 basic services) and monthly cash transfers distributed to female heads of households with primary-school children. The program provided micronutrient-fortified milk-based supplements to children 6 to 23 months old, underweight 2- to 4-year-olds, and pregnant and lactating mothers. Cash transfer support was later extended to older school children, plus youths under 20 eligible for vocational education scholarships (Martínez Martínez 2012). The conditions for receiving these benefits included obligatory primary care visits to monitor children's growth, prenatal and postpartum visits for pregnant women, and children's regular attendance at school (Leroy et al. 2008).

Several randomized studies have found a positive impact on child health from participation in *Oportunidades,* such as cognitive improvements, fewer behavioral problems, height advantages (Fernald, Gertler, and Neufeld 2009), and better overall dietary intake for children in CCT households compared with control groups (Ramírez-Silva et al. 2013). These results mirror overall cash transfer experiences in Latin America, demonstrating improved nutrition and access to health care for young children (Owusu-Addo and Cross 2014).

Although CCT advocates celebrate these results, cautionaries are warranted. Certainly recipients are responsive to incentives, but there is no guarantee of adequate quality of services (historically an impediment to their use). Additionally, pitting renewable income supplements that rest on poor women fulfilling obligations (and losing decisionmaking autonomy) against social security entitlements for the non-poor can be politically and ethically fraught (Handl and Spronk 2015). In the end, culpabilizing dispossessed women for the ill health of their families (as per the victim-blaming model discussed in chapter 3) and burdening them with improving their own life-choices to help themselves and advance development offer a dismal antidote to the business-as-usual neoliberal social and economic policies Mexico is intent on pursuing (Wilson 2015).

Indeed, Mexico's poverty results are far less sanguine than the measured health outcomes. *Oportunidades*, in combination with other social programs—including *Seguro Popular* to extend health insurance coverage (see chapter 11), the

PROCAMPO rural agricultural development program, and the National Crusade Against Hunger—have had little impact on poverty reduction. Between 1992 and 2012 the proportion of people living in poverty and extreme poverty in Mexico fell by less than 2% (Laurell 2015), and in recent years the number of poor people has increased, a countertrend to most Latin American countries (Godoy 2015). These findings highlight both programmatic shortcomings—most notably lack of job creation for program "graduates"—and the state's regressive social spending, lack of new resources invested in health and education (improved quality and availability of schools and health centers have not sufficiently accompanied social programs), and mismanagement (Teichman 2016). For instance, PROCAMPO was intended to support small-scale farmers but has instead largely served agribusiness interests (Godoy 2015).

While maintaining eligibility criteria and programs, *Prospera* has more recently sought to address the employment vacuum, albeit indirectly, through job counseling and training, microfinance lending, scholarships for post-secondary education, and connecting beneficiaries to other social programs supporting rural development (SEDESOL 2015). But these strategies rely on existing federal programs, and in the health arena, for example, there is little evidence of new resources allocated for improving quality of care above routine maintenance of existing health unit services (García Miramón 2015). It remains to be seen whether *Prospera* is able to address the multi-dimensional aspects of poverty.

Bolsa Familia by contrast, covering 14 million families (26% of the population) (World Bank 2015b), was from the beginning nested within a range of programs launched by the Workers' Party under former Brazilian President Luiz Inácio Lula da Silva's *Fome Zero* (Zero Hunger) initiative in 2003, from 2011 called *Brasil Sem Miséria* (Brazil without Extreme Poverty). First, all low-income families with children under age 18 are eligible. Monthly cash transfers are made to female heads of households, with similar requirements as in Mexico for regular school attendance and health checkups for children and pregnant women (Paes-Sousa and Vaitsman 2014). A counterpart to CCTs, *Brasil Sem Miséria* includes a Food Purchasing Program (PAA), supporting family farming, and the National School Feeding Program (PNAE), with approximately 43 million daily student beneficiaries. At least 30% of PNAE's budget goes to purchasing food from small farmers, as per PAA objectives (Swensson 2015). As well, the synergy between *Bolsa Familia* and Brazil's simultaneous expansion of primary health care (PHC) coverage enabled accelerated infant mortality reductions, especially in the country's poorest northeast region (Guanais 2013). Other measures, such as an increase in the minimum salary, have bolstered *Bolsa Familia's* poverty reduction achievements: all told, in just over a decade, approximately 36 million Brazilians have been lifted out of poverty (Governo Federal Brasil 2014). Still, despite modest gains in formal sector employment, *Bolsa Familia* has not transcended the predominance of informal work (Bohn et al. 2014), a problem it was not designed to address.

Brazil's integrated social investment approach has stimulated previously disenfranchised groups to generate greater claims on the state (moreso in the face of mammoth government spending to host the 2014 World Cup and 2016 Olympics). To note, in the past three Brazilian elections all major candidates expressed support for *Bolsa Familia* (Zucco 2015), which amounts to under 0.6% of gross domestic product (GDP) (Governo Federal Brasil 2015) and up to 2.5% of government spending. Even so, resources for *Bolsa Familia* derived more from state oil revenues (now declining) than from improved fiscal (taxation) justice. A crucial question going forward is how social protections, plus the enhanced gender and racial equity rights of recent years, can be made into permanent elements of a strengthened welfare state amid raised public expectations—a tall order given current political and economic turmoil. Powerful interests only begrudgingly back CCTs to forestall "more aggressive distributive measures" (Teichman 2016, p. 49), and in Brazil these forces may withdraw support in the wake of the 2016 politically orchestrated impeachment that removed the President and her party from power.

Indeed, because of the importance of the political context in which cash transfers are implemented, it is problematic to regard this as a "one-size-fits-all" technical intervention. Whether transfers are considered short-term charitable measures or long-term entitlements makes for very different policies and approaches. Many CCT programs draw from the economic rationale that people's behaviors can be influenced through financial incentives (Adato, Roopnaraine, and Becker 2011) and that improvements in "human capital" provide a way out of poverty (Ulrichs and Roelen 2012). While investments in health and education can certainly enhance social conditions, behavioral assumptions ignore the basis of poverty and social exclusion in the first place—that is, what systemic local (e.g., housing and sanitation), regional or national (e.g., access to land, education, employment generation), and international conditions and policies (e.g., unfair trade and investment agreements, corporate taxation policy) provoke or exacerbate poverty (Fine et al. 2016). Moreover, "informal employment, with its low income and precarious nature, remains the most prevalent income-generating source for those served by CCT programs" (Teichman 2016, p. 59).

Without addressing the underlying causes of poverty—and without secure forms of employment (enabling a stable exit from poverty) and short of inscribing the redistributive mechanism of transfers as a right—politicians, voters, and donors may tire of long-term targeted programs, and they can disappear with a change in administrations (Lomeli 2008). As well, financial incentives for school and clinic attendance are no substitute for improving the quality and accessibility of education (and employment opportunities) and health care.

"If we are serious about ending poverty, we have to be serious about ending the system that creates poverty by robbing the poor of their economic wealth, livelihoods, and incomes. Before we can make poverty history, we need to get the history of poverty right. It's not about how much wealthy nations can give so much as how much less they can take." (Shiva 2005)

A key debate is whether cash transfers need to be conditional; after all, transfers to the wealthy, for example via tolerance of evaded taxes placed in semi-legal shelters and havens, are rarely subject to scrutiny! Imposing conditions on recipients of cash transfers also mirrors the quid pro quo of IFI conditionalities in its paternalism and intrusion over domestic decisionmaking. In addition to being patronizing and placing primary onus on poor women, monitoring conditions is costly and bureaucratically cumbersome. Most important, many transfer programs are achieving their goals without such onerous requirements: notable improvements in child health have been reached via *un*conditional cash transfers in Ecuador (Fernald and Hidrobo 2011), Uruguay (Amarante et al. 2011), and South Africa (DFID 2011). Even where conditional transfers have yielded positive health outcomes, as with Mexico's *Oportunidades*, there is no consensus as to whether such results are attributable to conditionality per se (Martínez Franzoni and Voorend 2011).

From a methodological perspective, a pro-poor approach assumes that one is able to identify who "the poor" are. Yet poor and marginalized populations are by definition hard to reach, often living in remote or unstable areas, with precarious housing conditions, sometimes moving from place to place, and frequently not captured in social services registries or surveys. In many countries, the most socially excluded groups, including refugees and undocumented workers, may not have proof of identity, nationality, or residence and may fear deportation, discrimination, or punishment (see chapter 7), and thus are unlikely to sign up for government programs that might jeopardize their status.

In Mexico, even *Oportunidades's* elaborate targeting mechanism has excluded most remote Indigenous households (arguably the country's poorest group), who are left out of national censuses and have little access to schools and health services (Ulrichs and Roelen 2012). Were these households to receive cash transfers, whether they would manage to meet the conditions, given lack of access to most basic social services, remains questionable.

Another concern around transfers relates to eligibility criteria. Whereas Brazil relies on self-reported income, Mexico uses proxy measures to limit perceived fudging. South Africa's current programs seek to deal with post-apartheid inequities among racial groups and between rich and poor, but with distinct eligibility groups. The government's means-tested (but not conditional) social grants focus on the "deserving poor" (Leubolt 2014), defined as low-income seniors, children, and people living with disabilities. Moreover unlike Latin American variants, it makes no assumptions about household structure, providing support to the primary caregiver of poor children regardless of familial relations. Yet even expanded, South Africa's targeting mechanism excludes large numbers of unemployed persons, mostly men (estimated to be at least 25% of the workforce). In combination with better labor market conditions, Brazil's implementation of multiple social programs reduced inequities significantly more than South Africa's focus on the "deserving poor" (dos Santos 2015).

To be sure, many policymakers view cash transfers as politically appealing (Teichman 2016). Nonetheless, whether conditional or not, cash transfers do not address (and may even obscure) the need for broad entitlements—such as social security protections and PHC-based public universal health care systems—and act instead as a politically palatable form of undoing the deleterious effects of decades of neoliberal macroeconomic policies (Bello 2011) (see chapter 9). In the end, the underlying assumption of these approaches is that poor people, not poverty, are the problem.

Why critique pro-poor policies that seemingly benefit the poor? Unequal societies and exploitative conditions create poverty, and poverty reflects highly skewed access to power and material resources at community and transnational levels. Preferable, then, might be social policies that are not pro-poor, but rather anti-poverty and that reduce societal inequalities, which in turn require political struggle to challenge the asymmetrical power of vested local, national, global interests in the status quo. The campaign for a "basic income grant" in South Africa does just that, proposing a monthly cash payment to all individuals based on national citizenship, as opposed to focused policies for the "dependent" or "deserving poor." It portends a new ethics of "rightful shares" owed to the "rightful owners" of a collective national wealth, not based on a wage-labor logic of distribution but on due claims on the commons (Ferguson 2015). While attractive philosophically, the country's looming austerity budget suggests that such distribution of national wealth would amount to little more than crumbs, hardly the basis of anti-poverty social policy transformation (Bond 2015).

Still, transfers as universal rights have played a key role (along with progressive taxation) in reducing child (and senior) poverty rates in HICs and some LMICs (e.g., Uruguay), especially where there has been ample investment in health and education. France, for example, has a longstanding system of progressive taxation, unemployment pay, earned income tax credits, and an array of social services and child benefits, including universal free or subsidized daycare and preschool. These measures have enabled it to reduce its high child poverty of almost 28% by three quarters, almost reaching Scandinavian levels. Various countries, for instance Hungary, the United Kingdom, and New Zealand, have followed suit, with Ireland reducing its child poverty rate in 2013 from 40% to under 10% through similar mechanisms. But other OECD members, such as the United States and Mexico, have achieved little redistribution of market income (UNICEF Office of Research 2014).

This varied evidence suggests that there is a need to look far more critically at what constitutes success in global health. Differential effects (e.g., rural–urban, citizens–migrants, elites–workers–peasants) must be assessed. Long-term effects (far beyond 5-year success rates) and opportunity costs of targeted programs in the absence of societal approaches also warrant further scrutiny. Most importantly, the decontextualization of global health success leads to an inadequate understanding of what measures work and under what conditions. It is both shortsighted and unscientific to separate narrowly evaluated policy and technical successes from the larger societal and political environments that shape the distribution of power and resources (including access to technical resources) and enable health improvement in an integrated fashion. What if, for a change, we asked what makes for a healthy society instead of what makes for a global health success?

HEALTHY SOCIETIES: CASE STUDIES

Key Questions:

- What enables some societies to be healthier than others?
- How do HIC and LMIC healthy society efforts compare and contrast?

As discussed throughout this text, the determinants of and pathways to health and disease are complex. Health cannot be adequately addressed through unidimensional interventions, even when effective medicines and vaccines are available, nor by focusing solely on the choices of individuals. How societies are organized—politically, economically, socially, culturally—are fundamental to health. The largest set of arguably healthier societies are high-income, industrialized nations that have integrated improvements in economic, working, and living conditions with extensive social and health services. However, these countries do not provide uniform levels of protection and health; they vary based on the structures of power and distribution of resources, the particular policies pursued, and the paths taken to fulfill these policies (level of benefits and coverage; whether programs are universal, etc.). And, strikingly, there are some significantly redistributive LMIC welfare states—with accompanying strong population health performance, comparable to those of much wealthier settings—a vivid illustration of how the divvying up, and not just the level, of resources really matters.

Chapter 7 classifies a variety of capitalist industrial workforce-based welfare states: liberal (minimum safety-net oriented); wage earner (employment-based benefits); conservative-corporatist (benefits based on religious, geographic, or union affiliation and family status); and the most generous citizenship rights-oriented social democratic welfare states. The health implications may be understood as deriving from the state's various policy mechanisms (e.g., taxes and transfers) that affect poverty and well-being (Beckfield et al. 2015). In the case of LMICs, it is important to take into account that formal sector wage-earner-based economic growth is not a necessary precursor to welfare states (i.e., universal social policies can be constructed in the absence of high formal employment) (Martínez Franzoni and Sánchez-Ancochea 2013a). Here we detail the making of these healthy societies.

HIC Welfare States

Generally, HICs with egalitarian and redistributive welfare states based on universal social rights (e.g., Denmark, Finland, Iceland, Norway, and Sweden) have better population health outcomes than those that are employment-based (e.g., New Zealand), conservative-corporatist (e.g., Italy), or liberal welfare states (e.g., Ireland), where protections are based on often tightly targeted policies that may come and go with different administrations. What accounts for good (and differential) health in these countries?

Overall, social democratic regimes (with long tenure)—those with leftist and egalitarian political traditions—are associated with better societal health due to universal social welfare policies and generous provisions (Muntaner et al. 2011). These include key features of the most comprehensive welfare states: progressive taxation, redistribution of resources, public provision of services, and broad social safety nets—social assistance for the vulnerable, family benefits (e.g., paid parental leave for all new parents), pensions and "old age" security, health services, housing or income support, unemployment subsidies, and other benefits provided universally or as necessary. Collectively, these measures have a strong tendency to improve the health of the entire population, not just beneficiaries. Health spending by the state is also related positively to some health indicators, though it becomes increasingly less important past a certain level (Bergqvist, Åberg Yngwe, and Lundberg 2013).

Sweden, in particular, has a long history of addressing the societal determinants of health under the leadership of the Swedish Social Democratic Party, which was in power starting in 1932 and for much of the 20th century. Sweden's welfare state, launched during the Great Depression and amplified after World War II, involves deep public investment in universal education, health care, and other social services, strong regulations, and active labor market policies, amid union activism and societal mobilization for social justice (Burström 2003), resulting in one of the lowest levels of inequality (Gini coefficient[2] of 0.20 in 1980) in the world and impressive (especially maternal and child) health indicators (Table 13-1).

While the country's almost century-long commitment to both fiscal and social justice has endured through several neoliberal administrations, the center-right coalition in power from 2006 to 2014 presided over a retrogression. Sweden's 2014 Human Development Index moved it from 6th to 14th place in world rankings and its Gini coefficient climbed to 0.27 (UNDP 2015), still far better than most countries but a worrisome deterioration regardless. Like Canada and other countries that have seen conservative political shifts in recent years, Sweden has

Table 13-1 Health and Social Indicators for Selected Welfare States, 2015

Country	Infant mortality/1,000 live births	Under-5 mortality/1,000 live births	Maternal mortality/ 100,000 live births	Life expectancy at birth	Gini coefficient (2012)
Denmark	2.9	3.5	6	80.5	0.29
Norway	2.0	2.6	5	81.8	0.26
Sweden	2.4	3.0	4	82.0	0.27
United Kingdom	3.5	4.2	9	81.1	0.33
Uruguay	8.7	10.1	15	77.0	0.42

Data Sources: WHO (2015a); World Bank (2015c).

experienced both significant increases in inequality (Burström 2015) and concomitant declines in child well-being (Pickett and Wilkinson 2015).

In comprehensive welfare states, resources are pooled and services provided based on need—rather than ability to pay—with significant cross-subsidization deriving from the principles of universalism and solidarity (Buendía 2015). Such comprehensive approaches (where universality may be even more important than generosity [Ferrarini, Nelson, and Sjöberg 2014]), rather than technical interventions applied in isolation, have a broad impact. Some features of welfare states are so powerful that they at least partially transcend political regimes, as in the case of Sweden, and become part of the value structure—ideological fabric—of a society that endures regardless of which party is in power. That said, the welfare state is the object of ongoing political contestation, with, for example, how Europe is addressing the migrant crisis exposing important cleavages in its underpinnings. Moreover, even the redistributive policies of the most solidarity-minded welfare states are insufficient to addressing enduring facets of oppression, including unequal power and the legacy and ongoing effects of discrimination and exploitation (Young 2011).

LMIC Healthy Society Exemplars: Costa Rica, Sri Lanka, Uruguay, Cuba, and Kerala State, India

Unlike the countries mentioned in the previous section, Costa Rica, Cuba, Sri Lanka, Uruguay, and Kerala State, India are LMIC settings. While there are many differences among them, they share two interlocking features: concerted public investment in social well-being and significantly better health outcomes than generally expected given their income or "development" level (i.e., GDP per capita; Table 13-2), such as sustained mortality declines and other health indicator improvements. Not fitting neatly into the welfare state categories developed for HICs, they may be considered, in the case of Costa Rica, Sri Lanka, and Uruguay, state protectionist (Martínez Franzoni 2008) and in Cuba and Kerala, socialist. Together they provide bona fide models for the level of social protection that can be achieved in low-income settings.

Costa Rica

Costa Rica, with a population of almost 5 million people, is perhaps best known for its lack of armed forces, burgeoning ecotourism industry, and universal health care system. On 1 December 1948, after a brutal civil war, President José Figueres announced the disbandment of the armed forces—the country has been at peace with itself and its neighbors ever since. With almost no domestic expenditure on arms or the military (albeit receiving US subsidies during the Cold War), resources have been freed up for other government functions, especially the provision of social services: education, social security, health, nutrition, and environmental protection.

Costa Rica's economy was traditionally based on export of primary products, mainly bananas and coffee. Like most LMIC economies, it was dependent

Table 13-2 Data on Selected Determinants of Health and Mortality Rates for Three LMICs and the United States

	Costa Rica	Cuba	Sri Lanka	United States
Infant mortality/1,000 live births (2015)	8.5	4.0	8.4	5.6
Under-5 mortality/1,000 live births (2015)	9.7	5.5	9.8	6.5
Maternal mortality /100,000 live births (2013)	38	80	29	29
Life expectancy at birth (2014)	79.4	79.4	74.8	78.9
% population using improved drinking water sources (2015)	97	95	96	99
% population using improved sanitation facilities (2015)	95	93	95	100
Gross primary school enrollment rate (2008–2014)	100	98	98	98
Total adult literacy rate (2005–2013)	97	100	91	ND
Health expenditure per capita (US$, 2014)	$970	$817	$127	$9,403
GDP per capita (PPP international $, 2014)	$14,973	$20,649	$11,195	$54,399
Gini coefficient (2013)	0.49	ND	0.39	0.41

Data Sources: UNDP (2015); UNICEF and WHO (2015); WHO (2015a); WHO (2015b); World Bank (2015c).

on fluctuating commodity prices set by international markets. Unlike others, however, Costa Rica set the foundations in the 1940s for what by the late 1970s would become a comprehensive welfare state. With Cuba, it leads Latin America with the highest scope of universal protections and government services (Martínez Franzoni and Sánchez-Ancochea 2013b).

Although the economic crisis of the 1980s led to severe recession in Costa Rica, the government (with considerable foreign assistance) continued to invest in specialized employment generation (most prominently pharmaceutical and other high tech industries that benefited from the country's high level of education), social services, and the public health sector—particularly PHC—enabling sustained improvements in infant mortality and health status (Mesa-Lago 1985; Morgan 1987). Also notable is that favorable health indicators have been achieved with modest health spending compared with other countries. Today, Costa Ricans (together with Cubans) enjoy the longest life expectancy in the Americas after Canadians.

To what can one ascribe Costa Rica's health gains? First, its mandatory social insurance system, launched in 1941, began with the lowest paid blue-collar workers, over time incorporating higher paid workers until universality was reached, from the bottom up. As well, a single fund was created so—unlike in other Latin American countries—there was no segmentation by industry. Expanding coverage thus enjoyed wide public support. By the 1970s, when the wealthy were mandated to contribute payroll taxes into social insurance, a unified set of high-quality benefits covered the entire population (although because doctors were not prohibited from practicing privately, elites paid for privileged medical access without going through the social security system) (Martínez Franzoni and Sánchez-Ancochea 2013b). In terms of organization of health services, several features of the system stand out, including: public provision (rather than services contracted out to the private sector); a single public insurer; no purchaser–provider split or autonomy for hospital managers; integration into a single system; and user involvement in the management of services (Unger et al. 2007).

Other factors are also key. In the 1970s, a special fund was created for the poorest groups previously excluded from Costa Rica's social policies. The fund both targeted particular needs, such as nutrition, health, pensions, and other income support, and integrated these efforts into existing programs to avoid duplication and ensure fairness and support across the population. Wide backing for social entitlements helped Costa Rica partially resist neoliberal reforms when its economy faltered (i.e., fending off privatization of social service provision), although the quality and funding for some services deteriorated markedly at this time (Seligson and Martínez Franzoni 2009). Emphasis on the principles of collectivism and worker solidarity, and the state's prioritization of human development (with high levels of literacy, employment generation, and women's insertion in the paid labor force)—all part of Costa Rica's long tradition of social protection—helped cushion it against the worst hardships of recent economic crises (Martínez Franzoni and Sánchez-Ancochea 2013b). Still, since the 1990s the education and health care systems have faced deterioration in both quality and equity, with creeping privatization and out-of-pocket spending and the entry of for-profit insurance corporations.

Costa Rica maintains a mythic status, even pledging to become carbon-neutral by 2021, but its integration into the Central America Free Trade Agreement means that preserving domestically honed social policies will become increasingly difficult.

Sri Lanka

Sri Lanka has also been widely cited for its good health status (Halstead, Walsh, and Warren 1985; Pathmanathan et al. 2003). Infant mortality, at 8.4 per 1,000 live births, is the lowest in South Asia and ranks among the best in LMICs, and the country has a relatively high life expectancy of 75 years at birth. The maternal mortality ratio, 29 deaths per 100,000 live births (a 90% reduction since the 1950s), is identical to the US's (WHO 2015c) (Table 13-2). More Sri Lankan residents have access to safe drinking water (89%) and sanitation (85%) (UNICEF 2012) than in most other LMICs; and antenatal coverage and births with skilled attendants are remarkably high at 99% (WHO 2015c), with about 90% of births taking place in public facilities (Sri Lanka 2012). This is all carried out with health care spending of US$127 per capita (US$71 in government spending, and US$56 in private spending) for 2014 (WHO 2015b).

The UNDP, WHO, and various other global and domestic agencies proudly attribute these achievements to district-level health services within a free national health care system, involving comprehensive reach of prenatal and childbirth services provided by publicly trained midwives, integration of family planning into the maternal health program, targeted outreach to marginalized groups, and a well-functioning health information system (Levine et al. 2007; UNDP 2005; WHO 2007).

But without understanding the historical and political context of Sri Lanka's achievements, it is difficult to fathom how and why these policies came about and what factors might jeopardize their durability. Starting in the 1930s, when Britain highlighted Ceylon (its former name) as an exemplary colony (Jayasuriya 2000), Sri Lanka has been marked by extensive and multi-layered social well-being policies. These include: universal right to vote (1931); free education (1945); high levels of female literacy (reaching 96%); provision of subsidized rice (1940s–1970s); land reform; economic security measures; and well-developed water and sanitation systems (Balakrishnan 1985). From 1951 Sri Lanka has had a publicly-funded, free (in Sinhalese evoking the notion of freedom rather than free of charge) health care system based on the principles of equity and efficiency with no user fees, protecting against illness-induced impoverishment in conjunction with overall health care justice.

Mainstream interpretations point to Sri Lanka's efforts as the fruition of "political will," an oft-cited but ill-defined and curiously depoliticized term (Birn 2009). Instead, integral to Sri Lanka's record have been the political values and social struggles of organized trade unions and a strong socialist movement since the 1930s (starting before independence from Britain in 1948) that compelled conservative parties to adopt many progressive policies even before the socialist alliance came to power in the 1960s and 1970s (Herring 1987).

Sri Lanka's approach to health and social policy persisted through decades of civil war and troubling discriminatory policies against Tamil-speaking minorities. The war resulted in 40,000 to over

100,000 deaths (the number is highly contested) and large numbers of injuries, several hundred thousand refugees and displaced persons, and extensive infrastructure destruction. Understanding why Sri Lanka's social welfare system endured through this period may provide lessons for other conflict situations. Certainly public investment in social welfare has historically been supported by the majority of Sri Lanka's population since long before the civil war escalated in 1983 (Meegama 1986). Furthermore, demand for social services remained high—even in northeastern Sri Lanka where the war was concentrated—and education, health, and other social services, though weakened, continued to be supported by all parties (Sivarajah 2007).

In many ways, the toll of three decades of neoliberal cutbacks has been as damaging to health as the effects of war in the North and East of the country. Childhood undernutrition and stunting are persistently high, particularly among the poorest groups and despite overall economic growth (Rannan-Eliya et al. 2013). Social services remain nominally universal but have deteriorated considerably in terms of equity and public funding (Skanthakumar 2013), which may erode prior gains. Sri Lanka's health care system, while still public and free at the point of service, has been increasingly displaced by a parallel private sector (Govindaraj et al. 2014): there has been substantial growth in private hospital beds (Amarasinghe et al. 2015), and private spending constitutes 44% of total health expenditures (WHO 2015b), though the government has stepped up public spending since the war ended (Kadirgamar 2015). As well, Sri Lanka's overall health statistics mask inequities by class, region, and ethnicity, with higher infant and maternal mortality rates in rural provinces, and among ethnic minorities and plantation workers (Jayaweera et al. 2007). Moreover, even as women's secondary school enrollment rates are among the world's highest, and approximately 10% more women attend university than men, gender equity has stagnated. Women's unemployment rate is twice that of men, and women face considerable workplace discrimination (Gunewardena 2015). Also exacerbating the gender gap, women's political representation remains low, including compared with virtually all other South Asian countries: Sri Lankan women hold under 6% of parliamentary seats (Joshi 2015).

In sum, the longstanding political underpinnings of Sri Lanka's healthy society reflect broader claims on the state launched with universal suffrage in the 1930s that continued through struggles for wide-ranging collective social policies. However, reliance on achievements in one or two areas, such as women's and girls' education and the public health system (whose quality and equity are under threat by private sector competition), may be insufficient to maintain Sri Lanka's healthy society legacy.

Uruguay

Various countries have sought to augment social protection and reduce inequality in the wake of political and economic crises. Following a harsh dictatorship in the 1970s and 1980s, Uruguay was able to build on its welfare state tradition and reduce the infant mortality rate by half, from 20 deaths per 1,000 live births to the current 8.7 per 1,000 (Table 13-1).

After a sustained economic crisis and inadequate resources for social services in the early 2000s, Uruguay's newly elected social democratic government implemented a national Plan to Address the Social Emergency (PANES) in 2005. When PANES took effect, one third of the population lived in poverty and/or were without stable employment; over half of all children were born into poverty; 10% of Uruguayans had no health care coverage; and over 50% of workers lacked social security benefits.

In the 2005–2007 period, PANES provided the poorest households (8% of the population, half of whom were categorized as indigent) with a monthly stipend; furnished nutritional support, health promotion activities, and sanitation improvements; provided assistance to people living on the streets; and funded housing upgrades in informal settlements. A year after it was initiated, PANES had reached 80,000 households. Within 2 years, the country's rate of extreme poverty was cut by more than half. By the end of 2007, school attendance had significantly increased and child labor decreased for those aged 6 to 13 years old (Amarante, Burdín, and Vigorito 2007). PANES's unrestricted, unconditional cash transfers were associated with a 15% reduction in low birthweight babies, markedly improving birth outcomes (Amarante et al. 2011).

In 2008 Uruguay began implementing a new tripartite Social Equity Plan (PE). First, tax reform simplified the tax code, improved collection, and made tax rates fairer and more progressive, with the wealthy paying the highest tax rate (Martorano 2014). A second measure also deepened redistribution toward families with children by shoring up the existing contributory family allowance system (originating in 1943) through general revenues. The PE has tripled or quadrupled the family allowance in real terms, with payment partially contingent on children attending school (Pribble and Huber 2011). This transformation of PANES into a family wage, in parallel with the contributory family allowance system, included a much wider target, starting with 20% of the population and aiming to cover over half the country's 500,000 children by 2009 (Borgia 2008).

PE's third component was the 2008 creation of the Integrated National Health System (SNIS), which has sought to unify Uruguay's segmented and fragmented health care financing and delivery system, as well as incorporate previously excluded groups. The National Health Care Fund has streamlined health insurance financing into a single public financing pool, covering *both* the existing social security system for civil servants, formal sector workers, their respective families, and retirees (most of whom were covered by nonprofit insurance companies), *and* informal workers, the unemployed, and indigent populations, who previously could access services only at government facilities (Fernández Galeano and Benia 2014). Mandating health insurance for children and teenagers, SNIS is financed through payroll taxes, premiums, and government subsidies (Fuentes 2013). Although the private sector has not been eliminated, there is greater equity between the 500,000 newly insured low-income beneficiaries and those who have long obtained services through nonprofit insurance companies (Pribble 2013). Private providers are now more likely to take public patients, as fees between the two systems are similar (with private copayments somewhat higher) (Martínez Franzoni and Sánchez-Ancochea 2016). A small number of wealthy persons are insured through for-profit companies not covered by the reform.

Overall, in the course of a decade these policies—together with employment and wage increases—have resulted in a 5-point increase towards equality as measured by the Gini coefficient (Antía et al. 2013) and have given the Uruguayan public greater confidence to make claims on the state to improve social conditions.

While some of these improvements were related to overall economic recovery, Uruguay's dual focus of strengthening welfare protection through family stipends and an increased minimum wage (OCDE/CEPAL 2014), combined with targeted support for the most vulnerable, has helped the country return to its position as one of the *least unequal* countries in Latin America, with associated benefits for health and well-being. Uruguay has also taken bold, if controversial, positions on other health and social issues, such as decriminalizing marijuana to stave off gang violence and a harm-reduction approach to abortion (amid abortion's equivocal criminalized status), enabling the proportion of maternal deaths due to unsafe abortions to drop from 47% to zero in the space of a decade (Chung 2016).

Cuba

Cuba is a socialist country whose commitment to redistributive policies was forged following its 1959 revolution, at the height of the Cold War. Building on social security and child health services that reached only part of the population, the revolution spurred nationalization of productive assets and extended broad social welfare protections to all Cubans. Under Fidel Castro's almost half-century rule, the government prioritized universal social services—water, sanitation, housing, health, and education—plus full employment (Mesa-Lago 2012), leading to a marked decline in social inequality (Box 13-1).

Starting with rural health services in the most remote and underserved areas, Cuba soon developed an integrated network of polyclinics at the primary level, with corresponding secondary and tertiary care facilities, all providing free, universal, high quality care, and featuring both popular participation and intersectoral action (Birn and Nervi 2015). Although half the physicians fled the country after the revolution, a large-scale medical training effort ensured sufficient staff, with a near quadrupling of per capita physicians by the late 1980s and a concomitant 67% infant mortality decline (Farber 2011).

Box 13-1 Factors Contributing to the Success of Cuba's Social Services

Even a World Bank review admitted that Cuba's success derived at least partially from the following (with various points representing the *opposite* of standard World Bank advice):

1. The public sector is dominant and health is a government priority.
2. Cuba's social policy objectives have remained unchanged since 1960.
3. Government spends a relatively large part of the GDP on health, and health spending remained high even during the mid-1990s crisis, at the expense of defense spending.
4. Cuba has demonstrated a notable capacity to mobilize the population, and community participation is well-ensured.
5. Policies are based on comprehensive monitoring and evaluation, and quality data.

Source: Adapted from Erikson, Lord, and Wolf (2002), cited in de Vos, de Ceukelaire, and van der Stuyft (2006, p. 1609).

The impact of Cuba's socialist redistributive and collective policies for population health are palpable in its positive health outcomes (Pagliccia and Álvarez Pérez 2012). As per Table 13-2, Cuba's infant and under-5 mortality rates are lower than those of the United States, which spends significantly more per capita on health and whose GDP per capita (PPP) is almost three times higher than Cuba's. In its latest integrated health and societal determinants success, in 2015 Cuba became the first country in the world to have eliminated mother-to-child-transmission of HIV and syphilis.

Indeed, Cuba has managed to thrive despite a US economic and foreign policy embargo since the 1960s and still in place as of mid-2016, tightened in 1992 to include food and medicine (violating UN policy). Facing these challenges, Cuba instituted food rationing prioritizing children, pregnant women, and the elderly, ensuring stable low mortality rates in those groups (Garfield 2000). Adaptive policies were also evident during the "special period in peacetime"—when Cuba was plunged into severe economic crisis and oil shortages following the end of Soviet subsidies. In the early 1990s the average daily intake dropped to 1,863 calories and 46g of protein per person, 74% and 61%, respectively, of recognized basic needs (Cruz and Medina 2003). Remarkably, infant and child mortality did not increase during this period, and life expectancy continued to rise (Borowy 2013). At least from a general public health perspective, the US embargo appears to have failed (Drain and Barry 2010).

Even so, poverty rates increased and historical social inequalities by race, gender, geographic region, and age were exacerbated (Veiga and Bello 2015). Cuba also experienced an epidemic of optic neuropathy, mostly in men, likely due to acute nutritional deficiencies (Ordúñez-García et al. 1996) structured by the rationing system, in which adult men were fed last.

On another front, creatively responding to fuel scarcity, the Cuban government purchased and subsidized the sale of almost 1 million Chinese bicycles, transforming health and transport in major towns and cities and helping reduce road traffic fatalities, air pollution, and cardiovascular disease (Borowy 2013). Food production was similarly revolutionized. Prior to the early 1990s, most Cuban cities depended on rural agriculture and food imports. To combat shortages, Cuba's Ministry of Agriculture created the world's first public urban agriculture program, coordinating: access to land; research; new supply stores with tools and agricultural inputs for small farmers and urban residents; technical support; and markets, both with and without state price controls (Koont 2009). Chemical pesticides were banned within city limits, leading gardeners to use organic fertilizers. By 1995, the food shortage was largely overcome, and Cuba became a global leader in urban and sustainable agriculture, enjoying food sovereignty and transnational agro-ecological solidarity. By 2003, urban gardens produced 60% of vegetables consumed in Cuba (90% in Havana), generating over 300,000 jobs (Gürcan 2014). Together, these measures are, incidentally, leading Cuba's transformation toward a carbon-neutral economy.

Cuba's healthy society efforts extend far beyond its borders. Its longstanding engagement in health diplomacy (see chapters 11 and 14) involves sending doctors in solidarity to countries in crisis or where impoverished populations face physician shortages (including Eritrea, Haiti, Honduras, Niger, South Africa, and Ebola-affected countries) and hosting thousands of low-income and ethnic minority students from across the world to receive medical education based on a pledge to return to serve their communities (Feinsilver 2010; Kirk 2015). The Barrio Adentro exchange of doctors for oil with Venezuela (see ahead) helped Cuba return to more solid economic footing while supporting the needs of Venezuela's urban poor. However, some connect Cuba's medical internationalism with a decline in quality of care and availability of specialists (Farber 2011).

With Fidel Castro's ceding of power to his brother Raúl in 2008, the restoration of diplomatic relations with the United States in 2014, and signs of Cuba's opening to the global market portending further change, for now, at least, its population still enjoys the health legacy of over five decades of socialism.

Kerala State, India

Another setting with a long healthy society arc is Kerala. Home to over 33 million people, the southern state of Kerala is among the poorest in India, with a per capita income of less than US$1,500 (Government of India 2016). Yet Kerala has had consistently good health and social outcomes (Table 13-3), achieving a female life expectancy of 76.3 years in 2012 (Lekshmi et al. 2014).

The reasons behind these outcomes are multifaceted, but most agree that the long history of organized political struggle for social and economic rights is central. Voter turnout is high, and much of the population is engaged in civic activity. Kerala is one of the few places in the world where a communist party has been repeatedly elected to power in democratic elections. Since 1957, the state has intermittently been run by the (Marxist) Communist Party of India. Given broad support for redistributive measures, even non-communist governments have pursued them, if with less vigor.

Kerala's success shares several key characteristics with countries like Costa Rica and the island of Mauritius: state-sponsored social services; widely-improved access to education well beyond the upper class (castes); subsidized staple foods; localized decisionmaking and planning; land reform; and large social investments in health, sanitation, infrastructure, and housing (Franke and Chasin 1992; Oommen 2014; Parayil 1996).

Kerala's accomplishments have a substantial gender dimension: over a century of investment in girls' education, impressive levels of women's political participation (e.g., through the People's Campaign for Decentralized Planning, initiated in 1996), high rates of women's employment, and a relatively late age at first marriage, factors residing at the confluence of political mobilization and particular historical features, such as matrilineal kinship. For example, although son preference—expressed through high rates of aborting female fetuses—is a grave problem across India, Kerala, exceptionally, has a female–male ratio of 1,084:1,000 compared with 940:1,000 for India (Oommen 2014).

Table 13-3 Selected Population Indicators, Kerala and India

	Kerala	India
Life expectancy at birth (2011)	76	67
Infant mortality rate (2013)	12/1,000	42/1,000
Maternal mortality ratio (2013)	66/100,000	178/100,000
Female literacy rate (2011)	92%	65%
Human Development Index (2011)	0. 625	0. 504

Data Sources: Ministry of Health and Family Welfare, India (2014); Suryanarayana, Agrawal, and Seeta Prabhu (2011); Susuman, Lougue, and Battala (2016).

Despite its historic success, Kerala—and its social solidarity measures—have been under assault in recent decades amid privatization pressures, rising inequality, and public spending cuts (Raman 2009). Reduced employment opportunities have led to high levels of out-migration among educated youth, and growing economic dependency on remittances, also contributing to inequality (Balakrishnan 2015). Mounting privatization of health care across India has undermined Kerala's public and egalitarian service provision, with the poor spending proportionately more out-of-pocket on health care than the well-off (Thresia 2013). Environmental protection, employment security (especially for Indigenous peoples), and gender-based violence prevention, among other SDOH, are also suffering. Still, analyzing and disseminating the elements of Kerala's long-term achievements, while weighing current challenges to these achievements, can serve as a useful step towards preserving them.

These examples illustrate that even in resource-constrained settings, welfare states with comprehensive approaches can, in the medium term, bring about large health and social justice gains. They also highlight the role of civic involvement in governing processes, another key aspect of health-promoting societies. Yet simultaneously, given pressures on redistributive social spending in recent decades, the welfare state architecture across the world sorely needs renewal, especially in regards to solidarity (Filgueira 2014). These challenges are being confronted by several efforts in Latin America.

Latin American Social Medicine in Action

Three recent examples in Porto Alegre and Belo Horizonte, Brazil, Mexico City, and Venezuela, of innovative social interventions that focus on systemic changes have their roots in Latin American Social Medicine (LASM), a movement almost a century old that was inspired by the ideas of Rudolf Virchow of Germany and Salvador Allende of Chile (see chapter 3).

LASM is based on the "economic, political, subjective, and social determinants of the health-disease-care process of human collectivities" (Tajer 2003, p. 2023). After World War II, and accelerating in subsequent decades, LASM became an important regional movement, as institutionalized in various schools of public health in Chile, Brazil, and elsewhere—and particularly through the work of committed health professionals who organized nationally and regionally to fight for better health—even as the region was swept by authoritarian regimes. Waitzkin and his colleagues (2001, pp. 1599–1600) found:

> Social medicine in Latin America has emerged as a sometimes dangerous but very productive field of work. A focus on the social origins of illness and early death inherently challenges the relationships of economic and political power in Latin America. As a result, participation in social medicine has led to suffering and even death for some of the movement's most talented and productive adherents.

Regionwide, the organizational expression of LASM is the *Asociación Latinoamericana de Medicina Social* (ALAMES), established in 1984 (Box 13-2).

Mexico City, Mexico

In recent years LASM principles have helped shape health and social policies in various Latin American settings, such as El Salvador, which has sought to implement community-based PHC, and, notably, in Mexico City. Despite the 2000 federal election of a right-wing party that extended neoliberal policies nationally, Mexico City elected a social democratic government that implemented comprehensive and redistributive policies to address inequities among social and geographic groups. The city's 2000–2006 Integrated Territorial Social Program drew from four tenets: the right of the municipal population to social benefits; large-scale, universal social programs; progressive income taxes; and a collective focus (Laurell 2008). The poorest sectors of the city were targeted first, en route to universality. The program's components included housing and neighborhood renewal, scholarships for children of single mothers, free breakfast in public schools, economic aid for people with disabilities, subsidies to small peri-urban farmers, and pensions and health care for senior citizens.

A second program targeted those without health insurance and provided free health care and

Box 13-2 ALAMES's Guiding Principles and Key Aspects of its Political Agenda

Principles:

- Health is a prized asset of human beings; for health to be a reality requires a radical defense of life and well-being.
- Health is a human and social right and a public good; the state has a duty to guarantee it and society has the responsibility to demand it.
- Health must be detached from the logic of the marketplace.
- Addressing health inequities is an ethical imperative; it involves changes in the social, economic, political, environmental, and cultural determinants of health and the recognition of diverse health needs.

Political Agenda:

- Demand social policies that affect the structural determinants of health.
- Ensure worker health and defend and build upon the rights of workers.
- Demand the consolidation of universal and free health care systems.
- Defend the right to health in the face of war, militarization, and violence.
- Demand that health inequality be eliminated with urgent and diverse public programs (prevention, protection, education, curative, and rehabilitative assistance), and organization and management of health services that expands social participation and responds to claims on the state.
- Promote alliances for a radical defense of life among movements working for the rights to health, water, food security and land, the environment, and gender equality, and the rights of Indigenous and African-origin populations, among others.

Source: Torres Tovar (2007). Courtesy of *Social Medicine/Medicina Social.*

pharmaceuticals to families, enrolling 95% of eligible families by mid-2006. Resource allocation was transformed to emphasize equity, with service delivery based on PHC. To fund these programs, the city government applied a range of measures to eliminate corruption, tax evasion, and waste, including reduction in salaries of top officials (Jasso-Aguilar and Waitzkin 2015).

These measures, which have continued under subsequent left-wing coalition governments (Gobierno de México D.F. 2015), have contributed to reductions in infectious and nutrition-related deaths, maternal mortality, and AIDS mortality. However, as throughout Mexico, the rate of chronic diseases has increased, in the context of, for example, NAFTA's food transnational corporation (TNC) invasion and shifts in dietary patterns (see chapters 7 and 9), bringing new challenges for local governments.

Participatory Budgeting in Porto Alegre and Belo Horizonte, Brazil

Porto Alegre, Brazil offers another example of collective action based on social medicine principles. In 1989, the city began a novel participatory budgeting (PB) process that allows citizens to set priorities for a significant proportion of municipal resources. PB is based on four principles: "redirecting public resources for the benefit of the poorest; creating a new relationship between municipalities and citizens (i.e., a new form of governance); rebuilding social ties and social interest; and inventing a new democratic culture and promoting active citizenship" (Lieberherr 2003, p. 1). In essence, PB embraces both representative and participatory democracy principles.

Most analysts of the Porto Alegre experiment have praised its inclusiveness of a wide array of citizen groups—in particular poor populations and women (Marquetti, Schonerwald da Silva, and Campbell 2012). Between 10% and 15% of the annual budget is subject to the PB process (Wampler 2012), which has benefited the citizens of Porto Alegre in a number of ways. In the first 10 years (1989–1999) more than US$700 million was invested in public works, largely for the provision of water and sanitation. Spending on social services, including health, education, housing, and welfare, quadrupled in a decade, and school dropout rates decreased by approximately 85%. As well, 30 km of roads were paved annually in the poorest neighborhoods, and there was a 50% increase in tax revenues (Wagle and Shah 2003). Between 1989 and 2001, access to water services increased from 95% to 99% and sewage system access increased from 70% to 83%. Although seemingly modest improvements, these services reached the most marginalized areas where populations had been waiting the longest for access (Marquetti, Schonerwald da Silva, and Campbell 2012).

PB was instituted in Belo Horizonte, one of Brazil's top 5 largest cities, in 1993. By 2008, US$170 million had been invested in 1,000 public works projects: schools, health care clinics, sports and cultural facilities, leisure space, social housing, and infrastructure (such as drainage canals to reduce flooding), with over 6,600 housing units approved for low-income families. In 2006, the city implemented "digital participatory budgeting" to expand channels for involvement. Over 150 "digital inclusion centers" (housed in municipal facilities, schools, and community Internet hubs) were made available to those without Internet access, expanding PB participation (Prefeitura Municipal de Belo Horizonte 2009).

Projects have reached the poorest communities within the city and outlying communities and *favelas* (informal settlements), advancing the argument that PB can be a vehicle for social justice. Cities in Brazil employing PB strengthened civil society and reduced infant mortality (Touchton and Wampler 2014), albeit amid occasional conflicts between community priorities and those of professional groups. Literally tens of thousands of people shape local public policy through involvement in PBs in each of these cities (with some participants as entrenched as politicians), but it is important to remember that PBs are able to address only some health determinants. Structural inequalities in wealth and power, gender-based violence, and persistent racial discrimination deeply affect Brazilian society even as both local programs, such as PB, and national policies—which pulled almost 40 million people out of poverty—improved conditions following the election of several Workers' Party governments starting in 2003. These policies, while not going far enough for the working poor who constitute the majority of Brazil's population, risk being dismantled with another political party, of dubious legitimacy, now in power.

Misión Barrio Adentro, Venezuela

One of the best recent examples of LASM as a global health endeavor is Venezuela's *Misión Barrio Adentro*, an alternative model to neoliberal health reforms. In the early 2000s President Hugo Chávez (deceased 2013) initiated a series of reforms, launched by a new 1999 constitution declaring: health to be a human right guaranteed by the state; that the health system should be publicly funded with free health care at the point of delivery; and that health promotion and prevention should be prioritized (Muntaner et al. 2006). *Misión Barrio Adentro* was founded as a community–national–international mechanism to meet these constitutional obligations.

Inaugurated in 2003 at the behest of the mayor and constituents of one of the capital Caracas's poorest neighborhoods (*barrios*) who were fed up with broken government promises to provide health care and Venezuelan doctors' refusal to serve them, *Misión Barrio Adentro* turned the principles of global health cooperation upside down. Rather than an international agency selecting the activity and setting the terms of cooperation, community-level committees—extended throughout the country—have hosted over 14,000 Cuban doctors and dentists to live in their neighborhoods and serve as their practitioners following a principle of solidarity (at a popular level) and exchange (at the level of the state—i.e., Cuban doctors for Venezuelan oil) rather than aid (Jardim 2005). These doctors are not privileged short-term consultants, but rather eat and sleep in the same shantytown dwellings where they practice.

The bona fide bottom-up approach of *Barrio Adentro* emphasizes participatory democracy and management, covering a wide scope including housing, education, employment, and neighborhood improvement. In barely a decade, over 3,200 popular health clinics were built in poor neighborhoods that had never enjoyed such attention to their (health) needs. Access to primary care doubled, reaching near universality, and over 530 million medical consultations have been carried out under the program (Walker 2015). In 2010 Venezuela's Bolivarian government began an ambitious program to train its own community physicians and reduce dependence on foreign doctors. By March 2015 almost 19,000 Venezuelan physicians had graduated with degrees in Integral Community Medicine and begun working with *Barrio Adentro* (MPPS 2015). Crucial challenges, particularly given ongoing political and economic turbulence, involve the need to integrate *Barrio Adentro* with the existing state public health system (the two operate in parallel) and to fund community health workers who currently work as volunteers (Cooper 2015).

The enormously popular *Barrio Adentro* program has been associated with a reduction in infant mortality from 16.8 deaths per 1,000 live births in 2003 to 12.9 deaths per 1,000 births in 2013, with under-5 mortality declining from 19.7 per 1,000 to 14.9 per 1,000 (UNICEF 2013). Simultaneously, between 2003 and 2011, the population living in poverty went from 54% to 27% of households and the Gini index fell remarkably from 0.48 to 0.39 (Weisbrot and Johnston 2012). There have also been significant increases in preschool and primary school attendance, and access to post-secondary education, among other indicators (Muntaner et al. 2013).

As one woman from Catia, a large slum in Caracas, noted:

> I think it is something great, really the best thing that has happened here in Venezuela . . . Barrio Adentro is a good way of doing things because the services are actually in the [neighbor]'hoods supporting people who truly need them . . . Never before had we seen a doctor come to a barrio to provide care. And we have learned a lot—at least in terms of organizing ourselves as a community. We are helping one another and our neighbors (Catia resident, 2005).

These national, state, and municipal examples reveal a number of common threads. First, grassroots organizing and bottom-up representation in the political process are key to making the voices of poor and marginalized groups heard. Second, collective commitment to social justice and equity and comprehensive approaches are critical to ensuring a healthy population. Finally, a vital strategy to achieve such a commitment is social action, especially important amid destabilization and undermining of Latin America's "pink tide" gains of recent years. Such action is sometimes easier to achieve at the local level, as shown in the next section.

HEALTHY PUBLIC POLICY: HEALTH PROMOTION, HEALTHY CITIES, AND EMERGING FRAMEWORKS

Key Questions:

- What are the most effective avenues to health promotion?
- How might "alternative" frameworks contribute to promoting health?

Health Promotion

Health is experienced "by people within the settings of their everyday life; where they learn, work, play, and love" (WHO 1986, p. 3). But, as per chapter 7, the determinants of health exist and are produced and reproduced at global and structural, societal and national levels, as well as in the community and household. Responding to this reality, a global health conference was held in Canada in 1986 to build on the principles of the *Declaration of Alma-Ata* (see chapters 2 and 11). The document adopted, the *Ottawa Charter*, envisioned health promotion as "the process of enabling people to increase control over, and to improve, their health" (WHO 1986, p. 1). The Charter outlined eight fundamental prerequisites for health—peace, shelter, education, food, income, a stable ecosystem, sustainable resources, and social justice and equity—with five action areas for reaching Alma-Ata's goal of "health for all" by 2000:

1. *Creating supportive environments*: conserving natural resources and creating working and living conditions that promote health
2. *Strengthening community action*: ensuring communities are in control of matters affecting their health and are able to voice their opinions and concerns
3. *Developing personal skills*: increasing the opportunities for people to make healthy choices through education and action
4. *Reorienting health services*: moving health systems beyond curative care toward prevention and overall health promotion, in a culturally sensitive manner
5. *Building healthy public policy*: ensuring that health is a component of policy development in all government sectors

Health promotion, unlike public health or global health, is focused on creating and maintaining healthy societies based on societal strengths, not on disease prevention per se. As such, health promoters must be knowledgeable about the economic, social, and political underpinnings of health to even start asking how the prerequisites for health can be addressed. This means that instead of tackling health as a technical problem, health promoters need to identify and address both the determinants of health linked to living conditions—including, food, water, shelter, and livelihoods—and those connected to broader societal matters that shape access to these resources: peace; class, race/ethnicity, and gender relations; the distribution of power; workplace and environmental conditions; and the larger global political and economic order influencing patterns of (in)equity and social (in)justice.

Building on the Ottawa Charter, WHO has sponsored a series of international health promotion meetings and declarations. The 2005 *Bangkok Charter for Health Promotion in a Globalized World* emphasized health promotion as national and civil society priorities and its centrality to the global development agenda. Like the subsequent *Adelaide Statement on Health in All Policies (HiAP)* (WHO 2010a), it advocated a whole-of-government approach, with many sectors collaborating to promote health. The Bangkok Charter cited the impact of corporations on health, wealth distribution, and the determinants of health, arguing that the private sector should be responsible for complying with national and international regulations that promote and protect health, including environmental and safe workplace standards. Although it recognized the importance of global governance for reducing the negative health impact of trade, the Charter did not directly address the role of the WTO and investment agreements on health and public health policies.

Indeed, despite the documented negative effects of debt, unfair trade, TNCs, and international financial agency policies (such as loan conditionalities) on health and well-being in both LMICs and HICs (see chapter 9), most health promotion research and practice pays little attention to these issues (Yanful and Jackson 2012). One important global effort that serves as an exception is the Framework Convention on Tobacco Control (Box 13-3).

The 2013 *Helsinki Statement on HiAP*, developed at the 8th Global Conference on Health Promotion in Finland, reaffirmed that addressing health inequities requires action across public policy sectors (well beyond health). The Helsinki statement underscored that "equity in health is an expression of social justice" (WHO 2013a), bolstered by WHO Director General Dr. Margaret Chan's argument that "the formulation of health policies must be protected from distortion by commercial or vested interests" (WHO 2013b). However, civil society groups, led by the People's Health Movement, held that the Helsinki Statement's action plan was too mild and pragmatic and for the first time issued a counter-statement and a call to action declaring, "we hold that the translation of capitalist values into political power is overwhelmingly responsible for the inequalities in health faced by poor and marginalized peoples" (PHM 2013) (Box 13-4).

This radical statement reflects the notion that health promotion should aim to reduce health inequities rather than only focus on raising average population health (Rice 2011) through politically-oriented approaches covering numerous SDOH.

But although the health promotion field purports to address personal, local, and global determinants of health together, in practice much health promotion has been coopted, focusing at the level of individual volition—for example, persuading people to quit smoking, reduce drug and alcohol use, modify their diet, practice safer sex, improve personal

Box 13-3 Wherefore International Efforts? Promise and Limitations of the Framework Convention on Tobacco Control

Tobacco use accounts for about 6 million deaths each year (WHO 2016)—more than the mortality attributed to HIV (1.1 million), TB (1.5 million), and maternal deaths (303,000) combined. To address tobacco-related disease, the WHO Framework Convention on Tobacco Control (FCTC), was approved by the World Health Assembly in 2003, and to mid-2016 179 governments (plus the EU) were FCTC parties. The first and only global health treaty of its kind, the FCTC, in effect since 2005, sets out price, tax, and regulatory measures to reduce demand for tobacco, involving product packaging, education, and elimination of tobacco advertising, promotion, and sponsorship. Core measures include halting the illicit trade in tobacco and sales to minors and offering economically viable alternatives for tobacco farmers.

Many countries face steep challenges in implementing the FCTC: political interference from the tobacco industry around regulation; little interest beyond the health sector; and insufficient technical and financial resources for public awareness, cessation programs, testing and regulating tobacco products, researching changes in prevalence and economic impact, and control of illicit trade (WHO 2012).

The struggle to stem tobacco use shows that even with significant evidence and consensus at hand, challenging powerful corporate forces and their government allies is no simple task. Trade and investment agreements further augment corporate power at a global level. Tobacco companies have tried to counter national tobacco control measures by covering the legal costs of WTO members willing to challenge tobacco policies of other member countries through the WTO dispute settlement process (Martin 2013); bilateral trade agreements and their investor-state dispute settlement mechanisms also undermine the FCTC, as with Philip Morris's lawsuit against Uruguay (see chapter 9).

Given the deep pockets and many legal tools at the disposal of Big Tobacco and other TNCs, taking a substance-by-substance approach (akin to disease-by-disease eradication) to controlling the harms of transfats, alcohol, sugar, and other products will prove an uphill battle. Moreover, it does not address the power asymmetries undergirding the marketing and sale of all harmful products. Legal and regulatory strategies that turn the tables—putting the onus on corporations to demonstrate that their production processes and products are safe—would be a veritable boon to global health.

hygiene, and increase their physical activity (Kahan et al. 2014). This is evidenced by burgeoning personal health education workshops, social marketing and media campaigns, and government efforts in recent decades, which rarely address advocacy or action regarding the larger political and economic context of health—even when there is rhetorical recognition that structural inequalities affect health (Duncan et al. 2015).

Undoubtedly some individually-focused interventions may affect health positively, for instance reduced HIV transmission due to condom use or better personal hygiene to reduce spread of diarrhea. However, viewed from a critical political economy perspective, behaviorally oriented health promotion efforts *alone* have little long-term effect because they do not adequately address the structural influences on health or health inequities (also see chapters 3 and 7). Likewise, intermediate level measures linked to health promotion, such as regulating transfat content, taxing harmful products, or reducing the availability of sugary beverages in or near schools can only go so far. This makes the narrowly conceived behavioral approach a poor avenue for reducing inequities and achieving health for all, not surprising given its ideological compatibility

Box 13-4 Promoting Health for All and Social Justice in the Era of Global Capitalism: A Call to Action by the People's Health Movement at the 8th Global Conference on Health Promotion (2013)

1. "That Health in All Policies be established as a high priority within the WHO so as to enable it to work across sectors and in particular where there are conflicting interests and priorities, such as trade and investment policies.
2. That member states strengthen WHO's leadership role in health to enable it to legitimately guide the work by all international and multilateral institutions, particularly in the UN system and in the World Bank, World Trade Organization and International Monetary Fund.
3. That member states commit more "assessed contributions" to WHO instead of "voluntary contributions." . . . [The] latter is a way for member countries to influence WHO programs . . . [allowing] rich countries . . . [to use] this mechanism to bias WHO's work toward transnational corporate (especially pharmaceutical, agriculture, chemical, food, alcohol, soda, military and extractive industries) positions . . . over public health.
4. WHO should put in place effective and comprehensive systems to identify and manage individual and institutional conflicts of interest. Such transparency is essential to identifying, addressing and minimizing risks posed by conflicts of interest caused by close interaction between companies and public sector decisionmakers and institutions.
5. That member States that govern global bodies, including the UN, World Bank, World Trade Organization, International Monetary Fund and similar institutions, democratize governance of those bodies, in order to rebalance social considerations alongside the economic and political conditions that shape population health.
6. That governments and international institutions regulate financial, commercial, labour, and resource depletion and contamination practices, including elimination of tax evasion, to ensure sustainable health, environmental and social well-being, including worker protection; and to respect, protect and fulfill health equity and health-related human rights.
7. That all governments . . . give priority to people's health over corporate profits through transparent processes that involve all branches of government concerned. . . .
8. That governments, with the support of public interest civil society, ensure participation in policymaking and processes related to the Health in All Policies approach, through community-led, democratic processes based on equitable gender, racial, and religious/cultural, and social class representation. . . .
9. That WHO implement and be accountable for equity-based, publicly provided and publicly financed systems for social protection and health that address the social, political, economic, environmental and behavioural determinants of health [and] focus on reducing health inequities.
10. That governments [prioritize] the implementation and enforcement of progressive income taxes, fair corporate taxes, wealth taxes and the elimination of tax evasion including appropriate international tax mechanisms to control global speculation, to finance action on the social determinants of health and health in all policies initiatives. . . .
11. That governments and international bodies regulate finance capital, reduce its dominance of the global economy and protect health and social well-being from financial crises.
12. That governments, WHO, and other UN organisations utilise impact assessments on health, well-being and environment to document the ways in which unregulated and unaccountable transnational corporations and financial institutions constitute barriers to Health for All.
13. That governments ensure that health considerations are a top priority in the negotiation of international trade and investment agreements. . . .

14. That donors remove conditionalities for development assistance for health, and thereby recognise aid as part of an equal partnership among countries of varied income levels under human rights principles.
15. That all Health in All Policies efforts work to mitigate climate change, resource depletion and contamination, and other environmental concerns that are crucial to human health.
16. That governments change the mechanisms through which the present intellectual property regime promotes the interests and profits of TNCs and the countries which benefit from their exports, with the abolishment of the TRIPS agreement being an absolute priority; and facilitate the worldwide development and equitable sharing of expertise, technologies and scientific data as global public goods.
17. . . . develop . . . international treaties that promote good health and address the social determinants of health . . . and work with the ILO to ensure decent working conditions and standards across the world."

Source: PHM (2013).

with neoliberal worldviews (Baum and Fisher 2014; Duncan et al. 2015).

Those most likely to benefit from mainstream approaches to health promotion are advantaged groups who have the social and economic resources to act on these messages. This limited reach threatens to amplify health inequities (Buchanan 2000), as seen in the case of smoking cessation campaigns. While these campaigns are widely touted for drastically reducing overall rates of tobacco use, smoking cessation has occurred unevenly by social and economic group, leading to marked inequities in smoking rates within countries (Hill et al. 2014). For example, 50% of Canadians smoked in 1965, dropping to 19.3% of the overall population in 2013, following increased smoking restrictions, tobacco taxes, and behavioral campaigns. However, among Indigenous populations, up to 60% are smokers (Statistics Canada 2015).

As discussed in chapter 7, the interplay of brutal settler colonialism, dispossession of land and livelihood, oppression through residential schools and child welfare policies, and centuries-long government maltreatment combine in complex ways to make smoking cessation and other public health campaigns all but irrelevant to many Indigenous people. The roots of smoking, alcohol, and substance ab/use thus need to be recognized and addressed in historical context. To illustrate, when Indigenous soldiers returned from fighting with the Canadian military in WWII, having taken up social drinking alongside other soldiers, they were not celebrated like their non-Indigenous counterparts (Gaffen 1985; Lackenbauer and Mantle 2007). Enjoying neither housing nor educational benefits, and not legally allowed to drink in a bar, they returned to communities with few job opportunities, their service ignored, and many turned to smoking, alcohol, and substance use as a salve to isolation and a response to societal rejection (Thompson and Genosko 2009; Valverde 1998), even as alcohol consumption continued to be criminalized (Maxwell 2011).

Certainly various countries (e.g., Brazil and Sweden) have sought to infuse the Ottawa Charter's principles of health promotion (specifically equity, community action, and primary care-oriented health systems) into social policies that extend far beyond the health sector. However, the current global campaign for universal health coverage in LMICs, with its focus on health care services and insurance provision (see chapter 11), is poised to jeopardize recent gains in the embrace of health promotion (Coe and de Beyer 2014).

When health promotion engages citizens, advocates for transformative policies, focuses on the broad determinants of health, and uses multi-faceted strategies, as exemplified by HiAP and the healthy cities movement (reviewed ahead), it works for everyone. Notwithstanding support for HiAP, health ministries typically lack leverage to shape other government departments, not to mention global economic policies, trade treaties, and so on, which have major health implications. Still, progressive voices in the field consistently argue for health promotion efforts that incorporate the social, environmental, and behavioral determinants of health and also take on commercial and political determinants of health (Kickbusch 2012). Many press for health promoters to serve as advocates for policies that move beyond individual lifestyle change (Alvaro et al. 2011) to support social protection and health-related rights in the midst of global economic changes (Caldbick et al. 2014).

Healthy Cities/Settings Program and Transition Towns

The Healthy Cities Program (HCP) (expanded to cover non-urban settings, islands, schools, etc.) is an innovative health promotion initiative that uses public policy and institutional incentives to improve "the physical, social, economic and spiritual dimensions of urban development . . . in the home, the school, the workplace, the city and other places or 'settings' where people live and work" (WHO EURO 2003, p. 11). Originating with public health physician and Green Party leader Trevor Hancock (2002), the HCP movement began in Toronto, Canada in 1984, and HCP initiatives were implemented in many European cities soon thereafter (Tsouros 2015). Today the WHO European Healthy Cities Network consists of almost 100 cities in 30 countries. Cities commit to 5-year "phases," each with a set of priorities such as supportive environments, healthy urban design, or the current priority of participatory governance (WHO EURO 2015). While consciousness of health equity and social determinants of health is visible in local level policies, most cities do not collect adequate data to discern the impact of equity-oriented action (Ritsatakis, Ostergren, and Webster 2015)—a reminder of the need to collect SDOH-related data, discussed in chapter 5.

HCP is also enhancing local health planning in various LMICs. In the early 1990s in Bogotá, Colombia, a city marred by violence and inequality, municipal authorities worked together on an overarching healthy city plan entailing: increased lighting in public areas; higher parking fees to reduce traffic; better public transit and car-free days; "women only" evenings to encourage women to walk in the city center; improved sanitation and water services; and stricter enforcement of bar hours. In order to increase citizen participation in, and acceptance of, the proposed changes, street performers and artists were hired to promote a culture of respect, and incentives for supportive participation were instituted. From 1993 to 2014, traffic fatalities declined from 1,300 per year to 606 per year, homicide rates dropped from 80 per 100,000 to 17.3 per 100,000, and the bus rapid transport system went from serving 30,000 to more than 2 million passengers per day (Gobierno de Bogotá 2015; Hidalgo 2015; Semana 2015). In 7 years, bicycle-only lanes were expanded to cover over 300 km, with the number of cyclists increasing by about 40% annually (Global Research Network on Urban Health Equity 2010). Not to be outdone, another Colombian city, Medellín, has transformed itself from the narco-terror capital of the world to winning the *Wall Street Journal*'s "city of the year" title in 2013, with improvements in public transport and social inclusion through citizen participation in urban management.

Iran's model HCP, launched in 1990 and formalized through the creation of a National Coordination Council for Healthy Cities and Healthy Villages (NCCHCHV) in 1996, builds on the country's long urban planning tradition. Its healthy cities network incorporates the ministries of health, information, culture, labor, housing and urban development, education, industry, power, environment, and welfare, as well as the mayor of Tehran (Mohammadi 2010). Outcomes include: increased green space and urban agriculture; improved drinking water and sanitation; mental health promotion; and community engagement. Tehran was also one of few cities that pilot-tested WHO's Urban Health Equity Assessment and Response Tool, which helps policy-makers assess urban health inequities and identify action steps by sector (WHO 2010b). In addition, the NCCHCHV has stimulated national and regional authorities to implement an HiAP approach to address health and health inequities and inform policies in areas such as child nutrition and hazardous employment conditions (Khayatzadeh-Mahani et al. 2015).

As reviewed in chapter 10, a variety of local environmental initiatives (e.g., green cities) also show promise for overall urban health improvement. Originating in the United Kingdom in 2004, the practice-oriented Transition Towns movement promotes concrete local strategies to recreate communities for a post-carbon, post-energy intensive world as an alternative paradigm to the hegemonic model of development. Transition Towns in places as distinct as Brazil and Australia foster micro-revolutions in areas including community agriculture, cooperative food production, and time banks for shared work, with the benefits of improving social solidarity and collective well-being. These strategies help create supportive environments, an important area of action outlined in the *Ottawa Charter* (Poland, Dooris, and Haluza-Delay 2011). The movement has expanded into a Transition Network of over 470 local initiatives around the world.

Viewed from a critical political economy perspective, healthy cities and transition towns that develop effective local measures, from alternative transport to organic food production and universal social services (Corburn 2015), are nonetheless limited in their ability to address, for example, global trade, austerity policies, conflict, and global environmental pressures. Despite these limitations, healthy cities and transition towns have considerable potential to galvanize local communities, especially in conjunction with social redistribution efforts at higher political/administrative levels.

Emerging Alternative Paradigms/Frameworks

Buen Vivir (Living Well or Collective Well-Being)

A contemporary development from Latin America, *Buen Vivir,* questions and reframes conventional assumptions about "growth" and "development" and their links to well-being, instead calling for a new paradigm of "living well" within existing resources and in harmony with the natural environment. These efforts have circulated within Latin America, moving from the local to the national, and are enshrined in the Constitutions of Ecuador (2008) and Bolivia (2009) (Jackson et al. 2013). Participatory governance around watershed management in Ecuador's Tungurahua province, based on the principles of *Buen Vivir,* provided a model for its inclusion in the constitution and galavanized global alliances in support of *Buen Vivir* as an alternative to neoliberal globalization (Kauffman and Martin 2014).

Interestingly, Indigenous tradition offers an important contribution precisely because constructs of "development" or "progress" are virtually absent from Indigenous culture. Because *Buen Vivir* sees living well in terms that do not align with modern-day patterns of production and consumption, or accumulation of material wealth as an indicator of well-being, degrowth (explored ahead) may well become a consequence of *Buen Vivir,* if not necessarily an objective (Gudynas 2015).

With Evo Morales's election in 2006 as the majority Indigenous country's first Indigenous leader, Bolivia's leftist government sought to integrate its challenge to neoliberalism and mainstream development approaches with long-suppressed Indigenous knowledge and traditions (Rice 2012). Its health policies, for example, reflect the complementarity between *Vivir Bien* (its Spanish name in Bolivia) and the societal determination of health (see chapter 7), as reflected in collective values such as solidarity, dignity, gender and social equity, and social justice (Gudynas 2015). Integrating an array of Indigenous ideas around living in harmony with nature, in a virtuous "land without evil," and finding the path to a noble life, Bolivia's pluralistic commitment is evidenced in the Family, Community and Intercultural Health policy, guided by community participation, intersectoral action, and respect for Indigenous cultures and traditional medicine as a means of achieving a universal health care system (PHM et al. 2014).

While incorporating *Buen Vivir* into national constitutions is encouraging, the entrenchment of economic growth as the vehicle to development (and redistribution) remains. Bolivia has not escaped its economic dependence on extractive resources, leading to a collision between economic interests and the constitutional protection of Indigenous lands (Kröger and Lalander 2016). Still Morales's nationalization of oil and gas reserves has been tethered to collective well-being: profits go to a range of social benefits, even as exploitation continues.

In Ecuador, *Buen Vivir,* known by the *kichwa* concept *sumac kawsay* appears more as a set of rights than as guiding principles or ethics. Remarkably, the rights of nature, like Buen Vivir principles, are inscribed in the constitution (Villalba 2013). One effort invoking these ideas to limit resource extraction was launched in 2007 by the Ecuadorian government to protect the Yasuní National Park from oil exploitation in exchange for pledges from governments, multilateral organizations, civil society groups, and private donors of US$3.6 billion over 13 years to offset part of the foregone revenues. The Yasuní-ITT Initiative would have conserved the area's rich biodiversity, preserved the homes of Indigenous groups, avoided vast deforestation, and prevented the release of at least 400 million metric tons of CO_2 into the atmosphere, helping mitigate climate change (Vallejo et al. 2015). Unfortunately, the initiative was abandoned by the Ecuadorian government in 2013 due to insufficient international backing. Oil extraction and mining have recently expanded, albeit with government assurances of greater sharing of profits. This has the potential for reducing inequality but as yet the tensions between relying on growth to enable social investment and living in harmony with nature based on existing economic levels has not been transcended through *Buen Vivir* approaches.

Degrowth (versus Sustainable Development)

Philosophies that contest capitalism's growth model such as "small is beautiful" (Meadows et al. 1972; Schumacher 1973) are hardly new, but since the early 2000s, the idea of degrowth has (re-)emerged (Demaria et al. 2013; Martinez-Alier et al. 2010). In addition to its skepticism of an ever-expanding production and consumption paradigm, degrowth[3]—like *Buen Vivir*, Buddhist economics (Linn 2015), and solidarity economy models (Matthaei [forthcoming])—is critical of "sustainable development."

The concept of sustainable development (see chapter 3) suggests a consciousness around channeling growth in a manner that protects social well-being and the environment. But Martinez-Alier et al. (2010) argue that sustainable development is an oxymoron because it implies that growth is not the problem as long as it is "greener," more efficient, and less harmful to the environment. But each of these elements is questionable: gains in efficiency have largely been outweighed by overall increases in production; and green shifts from energy-intensive industries to service industries typically involve off-loading resource-intensive production or waste to other countries, which shoulder the environmental burdens (Victor 2010) (see chapters 9 and 10).

Thus, degrowth:

> challenges the consensus on growth in parliamentary politics, in business, in the bulk of the labour movement and in the social imaginary. Rather than accepting a fake consensus (such as the need to grow in order to pay the debts, or sustainable development, or climate change discourse . . .) where everyone is supposedly in the same boat, degrowth gives visibility to the contradictions and the conflicts at different scales (Demaria et al. 2013, p. 210).

Nevertheless, degrowth does not necessarily argue for decreasing GDP or negative growth. Rather, it calls for a paradigm shift that replaces the objective of growth with one of hovering around a steady level (Missoni 2015). The shift in values includes emphasis on quality over quantity and productivity, on cooperation over competition, and on solidarity over individualism (Martinez-Alier et al. 2010).

Why is degrowth relevant for health? Some argue that economic growth is a necessary precursor for health, though this is hotly debated (see chapters 3 and 12). Described earlier in the chapter, the "special period" in Cuba resulted in nearly a decade of negative economic growth and provides some insights into degrowth and its potential impact on health, through Cuba's experiences of, for example, urban agriculture and greater reliance on bicycle transport. Of course, in the case of Cuba degrowth was not a policy choice, but the result of geopolitical circumstances. Furthermore, the struggle of many Cubans in the face of food and medicine shortages cannot be downplayed. Still, this example of adapting to fewer resources and implementing health-promoting policies, while maintaining life expectancy levels and even achieving health gains, shows that growth is not a necessary prerequisite for health.

Similarly, in Kerala economic development and high growth rates were not the foundations of success in health and social outcomes: in the 1970s and 1980s, per capita growth was slow or even negative. Yet predicted social well-being declines did not materialize. Instead, as of the early 2000s, it was increased growth rates—combined with public sector spending cuts—that triggered these problems. Moreover, expansion of technology and communications sectors, where wages are high compared to stagnant wages in other industries, has led to increases in income inequality (Oommen 2014).

A degrowth approach might also entail greater attention to prevention and health promotion to reduce expensive curative care, and in general, a more conscious use of health care resources. Beyond the health care sector, a degrowth framework has the potential for improving environmental and societal determinants of health through, for example, a shorter work week, which would lead to less air pollution, a reduction in consumption and emissions, and a shift of time and spending toward low carbon intensity activities (Gough 2015; Missoni 2015).

It is important to stress that the degrowth movement is not only focused on excessive consumerism or wasteful lifestyles at the individual level. Similar to the limitations of individually-focused health promotion, Missoni (2015, p. 446) argues that it is "improbable that post-growth alternatives to the current economic system can be built solely on the promotion of change in individual behaviors and on initiatives at community level, without concomitant supportive policies at national and global level[s]."

Although *Buen Vivir* and degrowth alternatives are still in their infancy, they may help build long-term change by raising consciousness about the feasibility and fairness (and environmental viability) of steady-state resource use and a shift in paradigms (or the world order) emphasizing equity over growth. These examples suggest that micro-revolutions ignited by collective action can improve social solidarity and begin to address population well-being.

CONCLUSION: THE MAKING OF HEALTHY SOCIETIES

Learning Points:

- Key ingredients for healthy societies moving toward greater health and social justice include:
  - Universal and public provision of social services combined with policies addressing racial, gender, and class inequities
  - Subsidized clean water, sanitation, nutrition, housing, and education
  - Expanded services to rural and marginalized urban areas and groups
  - Wide-ranging social protections
  - Strong regulation of work and environmental conditions
  - Redistribution of power and control over resources in the context of larger anti-oppression struggles
  - Effective regulation of transnational and national private and corporate interests to make them publicly accountable
- Narrow interventions and technical quick fixes (whether disease and behavioral campaigns or cash transfers) that ignore the underlying political and societal determinants of health are limited in scope, reversible, and often exacerbate existing inequalities. Yet when integrated into broadly redistributive and accountable societal efforts, such technical approaches can help contribute to permanent health improvement.
- Global health success may best be gauged by *how* and *how well* health inequities have been addressed and reduced within and between countries.
- Various LMICs that have made concerted investments in social welfare have seen extraordinary gains in health conditions. In several settings (e.g., Costa Rica and Mexico City), SDOH-oriented welfare policies have been implemented *despite* neoliberal pressures.
- Bona fide health promotion efforts require attention to the SDOH at grassroots, municipal, national, and global levels.
- Alternative routes to building healthy societies have (re-)emerged in recent years that incorporate the inter-relations among community and societal health, environmental harmony, and the transformation of the global political economy order.

As argued here, unless local and global social, political, and economic realities are taken into account, prescriptive, narrowly conceived interventions yield little overall health betterment in the long run, and may be more harmful than helpful. Even as more funding is injected into global health, a growing chorus of critics, and some insiders, agree that most existing global health approaches contribute little to the building of healthy societies. As these observers lament, mainstream approaches privilege donor criteria over local needs, favor technical over integrated efforts, and focus more on disease control and making the poor "responsible" than on fostering circumstances (including at the global level around, for example, issues of TNC exploitation and illicit financial outflows) conducive to health and social justice (Baum and Fisher 2014). Moments of crisis should not lead us to despair, however. Renewed worldwide mobilization around collective well-being demonstrates that conditions can improve, given concerted political struggle.

As this chapter shows, countries, regions, and cities with strong trajectories of social action and citizen participation advocating for bona fide equity and collective and redistributive policies have launched and effectively sustained long-term health and social well-being improvements regardless of the level of GDP per capita. This counters the neoliberal capitalist claim that governments ought to be left on the sidelines while the private sector leads. Indeed, healthy societies require that there be a greater, not a smaller, governmental role in social policymaking and implementation, as long as governments represent broad collective interests.

What then is the role of global health? How can people and organizations involved in this arena positively influence long-term, integrated actions to improve health and well-being? These issues will be explored in the next, and final, chapter of this textbook.

NOTES

1. RCTs are considered the "gold standard" of medical study designs. A typical RCT has a control group and a treatment group, intended to be highly comparable. In conventional clinical RCTs testing the efficacy of, for example, a new medication for controlling high blood pressure, the control group receives a placebo or an existing drug, whereas the treatment group receives the test drug. Because the two groups are alike according to a range of characteristics (age, occupation, sex/gender, ethnicity/race, SES, locality, etc.), differences in outcomes between the two groups are ascribed to the respective treatments (Gordis 2014). J-PAL seeks RCT-like conditions, but instead of dealing with discrete measures in relatively controlled clinical contexts, it is testing health, education, and poverty relief interventions in complex social settings.
2. The Gini coefficient assesses the degree of income inequality within a country, with 0 representing a perfectly equal society in which everyone has the same income and 1 a society skewed in the other direction, with a small group earning all income and the rest of the population earning nothing. However, the Gini does not include wealth or the value of non-income social transfers, making it an incomplete measure of economic inequality.
3. Variants of degrowth include the steady-state economy, elaborated by Herman Daly (also see www.steadystate.org). De-development, Sara Roy's characterization of occupied Palestine's economy, has been taken up more aspirationally by Jason Hickel, among others.

REFERENCES

Adato M, Roopnaraine T, and Becker E. 2011. Understanding use of health services in conditional cash transfer programs: Insights from qualitative research in Latin America and Turkey. *Social Science & Medicine* 72(12):1921–1919.

Ahmed SM, Hossain S, Kabir MM, and Roy S. 2011. Free distribution of insecticidal bed nets improves possession and preferential use by households and is equitable: Findings from two cross-sectional surveys in thirteen malaria endemic districts of Bangladesh. *Malaria Journal* 10:357.

Allende S. 2000. Inaugural address in the national stadium, Santiago November 5, 1970. In Allende Gossens S, Cockcroft JD, and Canning J, Editors. *Salvador Allende Reader.* Melbourne: Ocean Press.

Alvaro C, Jackson LA, Kirk S, et al. 2011. Moving Canadian governmental policies beyond a focus on individual lifestyle: Some insights from complexity and critical theories. *Health Promotion International* 26(1):91–99.

Alzua ML, Pickering AJ, Djebbari H, et al. 2015. *Final Report: Impact Evaluation of Community-Led Total Sanitation (CLTS) in Rural Mali.* New York: UNICEF.

Amarante V, Burdín G, and Vigorito A. 2007. *Evaluación cuantitativa del impacto del PANES.* Montevideo: Instituto de Economía, Facultad de Ciencias Económicas, Universidad de la República.

Amarante V, Manacorda M, Miguel E, and Vigorito A. 2011. *Do Cash Transfers Improve Birth Outcomes? Evidence from Matched Vital Statistics, Social Security and Program Data. CEP Discussion Paper No 1106.*

London: Centre for Economic Performance, London School of Economics and Political Science.

Amarasinghe S, Alwis SD, Saleem S, et al. 2015. *Private Health Sector Review 2012*. Colombo: Institute for Health Policy.

Antía F, Castillo M, Fuentes G, and Midaglia C. 2013. La renovación del sistema de protección uruguayo: El desafío de superar la dualización. *Revista Uruguaya de Ciencia Política* 22(2):171–194.

Balakrishnan N. 1985. Sri Lanka as a welfare state: An overview. *Economic Review* 11(4&5):45–53.

Balakrishnan P. 2015. Kerala and the rest of India. *Economic & Political Weekly* 50(2):35.

Banerjee A, Karlan D, and Zinman J. 2015. Six randomized evaluations of microcredit: Introduction and further steps. *American Economic Journal: Applied Economics* 7(1):1–21.

Bateman M. 2010. *Why Doesn't Microfinance Work? The Destructive Rise of Local Neoliberalism*. London: Zed Books Ltd.

Baum F and Fisher M. 2014. Why behavioural health promotion endures despite its failure to reduce health inequities. *Sociology of Health & Illness* 36(2):213–225.

Beckfield J, Bambra C, Eikemo TA, et al. 2015. An institutional theory of welfare state effects on the distribution of population health. *Social Theory and Health* 13(3/4):227–244.

Bello W. 2011. The Conditional Cash Transfer debate and the coalition against the poor. http://focusweb.org/content/conditional-cash-transfer-debate-and-coalition-against-poor. Accessed October 14, 2015.

Bergqvist K, Åberg Yngwe M, and Lundberg O. 2013. Understanding the role of welfare state characteristics for health and inequalities – an analytical review. *BMC Public Health* 13:1234.

BMGF. 2014. Water, Sanitation & Hygiene: Strategy Overview. http://www.gatesfoundation.org/What-We-Do/Global-Development/Water-Sanitation-and-Hygiene. Accessed August 24, 2014.

———. 2015. 2015 Gates Annual Letter. http://www.gatesnotes.com/2015-annual-letter?page=0&lang=en. Accessed June 23, 2015.

Birdsall N and Diofasi A. 2015. *Global Public Goods for Development: How Much and What For*. Washington, DC: Center for Global Development.

Birn A-E. 2009. The stages of international (global) health: Histories of success or successes of history? *Global Public Health* 4(1):50–68.

Birn A-E and Nervi L. 2015. Political roots of the struggle for health justice in Latin America. *Lancet* 385:1174–1175.

Bohn S, Fernandes Veiga LF, Da Dalt S, et al. 2014. Can conditional cash transfer programs generate equality of opportunity in highly unequal societies? Evidence from Brazil. *Revista De Sociologia e Política* 22(51):111–133.

Bond P. 2015. Bretton Woods Institution narratives about inequality and economic vulnerability on the eve of South African austerity. *International Journal of Health Services* 45(3):415–442.

Borgia F. 2008. Health in Uruguay: Progress and challenges in the right to health care three years after the first progressive government. *Social Medicine/Medicina Social* 3(2):110–125.

Borowy I. 2013. Degrowth and public health in Cuba: Lessons from the past? *Journal of Cleaner Production* 38:17–26.

Buchanan DR. 2000. *An Ethic for Health Promotion*. New York: Oxford University Press.

Buendía L. 2015. Expansion and retrenchment of the Swedish welfare state: A long-term approach. *International Journal of Health Services* 45(2):226–245.

Burström B. 2003. Social differentials in the decline of infant mortality in Sweden in the twentieth century: The impact of politics and policy. *International Journal of Health Services* 33(4):723–741.

———. 2015. Sweden—Recent changes in welfare state arrangements. *International Journal of Health Services* 45(1):87–104.

Caldbick S, Labonte R, Mohindra K, and Ruckert A. 2014. Globalization and the rise of precarious employment: The new frontier for workplace health promotion. *Global Health Promotion* 21(2):23–31.

Cameron L, Shah M, and Olivia S. 2013. *Impact Evaluation of a Large-Scale Rural Sanitation Project in Indonesia. Policy Research Working Paper 6360*. Washington, DC: World Bank.

Catia resident. 2005. Interviewed by René M. Guerra Salazar in Caracas, Venezuela, August.

CGD [Center for Global Development]. 2016. FAQ. http://millionssaved.cgdev.org/frequently-asked-questions. Accessed March 31, 2016.

Chernomas R and Hudson I. 2016. *Economics in the Twenty-First Century: A Critical Perspective*. Toronto: University of Toronto Press.

Chung C. 2016. How Uruguay made it easier to have a safe abortion. *News Deeply*, August 10.

Coady D, Martinelli C, and Parker SW. 2013. Information and participation in social programs. *World Bank Economic Review* 27(1):149–170.

Coe G and de Beyer J. 2014. The imperative for health promotion in universal health coverage. *Global Health: Science and Practice* 2(1):10–22.

Cohen J and Dupas P. 2010. Free distribution or cost-sharing? Evidence from a randomized malaria prevention experiment. *Quarterly Journal of Economics* 125(1):1–45.

Cooper A. 2015. What does health activism mean in Venezuela's Barrio Adentro program? Understanding community health work in political and cultural context. *Annals of Anthropological Practice* 39(1):58–72.

Corburn J. 2015. *Healthy Cities.* London: Routledge.

Cruz MC and Medina RS. 2003. *Agriculture in the City: A Key to Sustainability in Havana, Cuba.* Kingston, JM: Ian Randle.

Demaria F, Schneider F, Sekulova F, and Martinez-Alier J. 2013. What is degrowth? From an activist slogan to a social movement. *Environmental Values* 22(2):191–215.

de Vos P, de Ceukelaire W, and van der Stuyft P. 2006. Colombia and Cuba, contrasting models in Latin America's health sector reform. *Tropical Medicine and International Health* 11(10):1604–1612.

DFID [Department for International Development]. 2011. *Cash Transfers Evidence Paper: Policy Division 2011.* London: DFID.

dos Santos MPG. 2015. Income security systems in comparative perspective: Brazil and South Africa. In Ribeiro GL, Dwyer T, Borges A, and Viola E, Editors. *Social, Political and Cultural Challenges of the BRICS.* Sao Paulo: ANPOCS.

Drain PK and Barry M. 2010. 50 years of U.S. embargo: Cuba's health consequences and lessons. *Science* 328(5978):572–573.

Duncan P, Bertolozzi MR, Cowley S, et al. 2015. "Health for All" in England and Brazil? *International Journal of Health Services* 45(3):545–563.

Erikson D, Lord A, and Wolf P. 2002. *Cuba's Social Services: A Review of Education, Health and Sanitation.* Washington, DC: World Bank.

FAO [Food and Agriculture Organization of the United Nations]. 2011. Rinderpest eradicated - what next? http://www.fao.org/news/story/en/item/80894/icode/. Accessed August 15, 2015.

Farber S. 2011. *Cuba Since the Revolution of 1959: A Critical Assessment.* Chicago: Haymarket Books.

Feinsilver J. 2010. Cuban health politics at home and abroad. *Socialist Register* 46: 216–239.

Ferguson J. 2015. *Give a Man a Fish: Reflections on the New Politics of Distribution.* Durham, NC: Duke University Press.

Fernald LCH, Gertler PJ, and Neufeld LM. 2009. 10-year effect of oportunidades, Mexico's conditional cash transfer programme, on child growth, cognition, language, and behaviour: A longitudinal follow-up study. *Lancet* 374(9706):1997–2005.

Fernald LCH and Hidrobo M. 2011. Effect of Ecuador's cash transfer program (bono de desarrollo humano) on child development in infants and toddlers: A randomized effectiveness trial. *Social Science & Medicine* 72(9):1437–1446.

Fernández Galeano M and Benia W. 2014. Salud. In *Nuestro tiempo: Libro de los bicentenarios.* Montevideo: Comisión del Bicentenario.

Ferrarini T, Nelson K, and Sjöberg O. 2014. Decomposing the effect of social policies on population health and inequalities: An empirical example of unemployment benefits. *Scandinavian Journal of Public Health* 42(7):635–642.

Filgueira F. 2014. *Towards a universal social protection model in Latin America.* Santiago: CEPAL.

Fine B, Johnston D, Santos AC, and Waeyenberge E. 2016. Nudging or fudging: The World Development Report 2015. *Development and Change* 47(4):640–663.

Franke RW and Chasin BH. 1992. Kerala State, India: Radical reform as development. *International Journal of Health Services* 22(1):139–156.

Fuentes G. 2013. *La creación del Sistema Nacional Integrado de Salud en Uruguay (2005-2012): Impulso reformista y freno de puntos y actores de veto.* PhD [dissertation]. Madrid: Instituto Universitario de Investigación Ortega y Gasset.

Gaffen F. 1985. *Forgotten Soldiers.* Penticton, BC: Theytus Books.

García Miramón F. 2015. *PROSPERA: Reglas de Operación 2015.* México D.F.: Centro de Investigación Económica y Presupuestaria.

Garfield R. 2000. The public health impact of sanctions: Contrasting responses of Iraq and Cuba. *Middle East Report* 215:16–19.

Gideon J. 2014. *Gender, Globalization, and Health in a Latin American Context.* New York: Palgrave Macmillan.

Glassman A and Temin M. 2016. *Millions Saved: New Cases of Proven Success in Global Health.* Washington, DC: Center for Global Development.

Global Research Network on Urban Health Equity [GRNUHE]. 2010. *Improving Urban Health Equity through Action on the Social and Environmental Determinants of Health: Final Report.* London: GRNUHE.

Gobierno de Bogotá 2015. ¿Porqué en Bogotá no ceden las cifras en muertes violentas? http://www.gobiernobogota.gov.co/prensa/93-noticias/1379-porque-en-bogota-no-ceden-las-cifras-en-muertes-violentas-2. Accessed June 12, 2015.

Gobierno de México D.F. 2015. Sistema nacional de programas de combate a la pobreza: Distrito Federal. http://www.programassociales.mx/?page_id=28&st=9. Accessed July 20, 2015.

Godoy E. 2015. Mexico's *Anti-Poverty Programmes Are Losing the Battle. Inter Press Service News Agency,* August 5.

Gordis L. 2014. *Epidemiology,* 5th Edition. Philadelphia: Elsevier Saunders.

Gottiniaux P, Munevar D, Sanabria A, and Toussaint E. 2015. *World Debt Figures 2015.* Liège: Committee for the Abolition of Third World Debt.

Gough I. 2015. Can growth be green? *International Journal of Health Services* 45(3) 443–452.

Government of India. 2016. State wise data. http://www.esopb.gov.in/static/PDF/GSDP/Statewise-Data/state%20wise%20data.pdf. Accessed August 16, 2016.

Governo Federal Brasil. 2014. Brazil lifts 36 million out of extreme poverty and hits UN target for child mortality. http://www.brasil.gov.br/centro-aberto-de-midia/news/brazil-lifts-36-million-out-of-extreme-poverty-and-hits-un-target-for-child-mortality. Accessed October 24, 2015.

———. 2015. Bolsa Família tem grande alcance social com baixo custo fiscal, aponta relatório do FMI. http://www.brasil.gov.br/cidadania-e-justica/2015/05/bolsa-familia-tem-grande-alcance-social-com-baixo-custo-fiscal-aponta-relatorio-do-fmi. Accessed October 24, 2015.

Govindaraj R, Navaratne K, Cavagnero E, and Seshadri SR. 2014. *Health Care in Sri Lanka: What Can the Private Health Sector Offer?* Washington, DC: World Bank.

Guanais FC. 2013. The combined effects of the expansion of primary health care and conditional cash transfers on infant mortality in Brazil, 1998-2010. *American Journal of Public Health* 103(11):2000–2006.

Gudynas E. 2015. Buen Vivir. In D'Alisa G, Demaria F, and Kallis G, Editors. *Degrowth: A Vocabulary for a New Era*. New York: Routledge.

Gunewardena D. 2015. *Why aren't Sri Lankan Women Translating their Educational Gains into Workforce Advantages?* Washington, DC: Brookings Institution.

Gürcan EC. 2014. Cuban agriculture and food sovereignty beyond civil-society-centric and globalist paradigms. *Latin American Perspectives* 41(4):129–146.

Halstead SB, Walsh JA, and Warren KS, Editors. 1985. *Good Health at Low Cost*. A Rockefeller Foundation Conference Report. New York: Rockefeller Foundation.

Hancock T. 2002. Indicators of environmental health in the urban setting. *Canadian Journal of Public Health* 93(Supp 1):S45–S51.

Handl M and Spronk S. 2015. With strings attached. *Jacobin* 19.

Hay SI and McHugh G. 2014. Measuring progress in global health. *Transactions of The Royal Society of Tropical Medicine and Hygiene* 108(9):521–522.

Herring RJ. 1987. Economic liberalisation policies in Sri Lanka: International pressures, constraints and supports. *Economic and Political Weekly* 22(8):325–333.

Hidalgo D. 2015. After 15 years of moving people, here's what Bogotá's BRT should do next. *The City Fix*, December 4.

Hill S, Amos A, Clifford D, and Platt S. 2014. Impact of tobacco control interventions on socioeconomic inequalities in smoking: Review of the evidence. *Tobacco Control* 23(e2):e89–e97.

Hunter D and Dawson A. 2011. Is there a need for global health ethics? For and against. In Benatar S and Brock G, Editors. *Global Health and Global Health Ethics*. Cambridge: Cambridge University Press.

Institute of Medicine. 2009. *The US Commitment to Global Health: Recommendations for the Public and Private Sectors*. Washington, DC: The National Academies Press.

Jackson SF, Birn A-E, Fawcett SB, et al. 2013. Synergy for health equity: Integrating health promotion and social determinants of health approaches in and beyond the Americas. *Revista Panamericana de Salud Pública* 34(6):473–480.

Jardim C. 2005. Prevention and solidarity: Democratizing health in Venezuela. *Monthly Review* 56(8):35–39.

Jasny B, Roberts L, Enserink M, and Smith O. 2014. What works. *Science* 345(6202):1256–1257.

Jasso-Aguilar R and Waitzkin H. 2015. Resisting the imperial order and building an alternative future in medicine and public health. *Monthly Review* 67(3):130.

Jayasuriya L. 2000. *Welfarism and Politics in Sri Lanka, Experience of a Third World Welfare State*. Perth: University of Western Australia.

Jayaweera S, Wijemanne H, Wanasundera L, Vitarana KM. 2007. *Gender Dimensions of the Millennium Development Goals in Sri Lanka*. Colombo: Centre for Women's Research.

Joshi DK. 2015. The inclusion of excluded majorities in South Asian parliaments: Women, youth, and the working class. *Journal of Asian and African Studies* 50(2):223–238.

J-PAL [Abdul Latif Jameel Poverty Action Lab]. 2015. About J-PAL. http://www.povertyactionlab.org/about-j-pal. Accessed June 21, 2015.

Kabeer N, Piza C, and Taylor L. 2012. *What are the Economic Impacts of Conditional Cash Transfer Programmes? A Systematic Review of the Evidence. Technical Report*. London: EPPI-Centre, Social Science Research Unit, Institute of Education, University of London.

Kadirgamar A. 2015. Progressive facets of the 2016 budget. *Daily News*, December 18.

Kahan S, Gielen AC, Fagan PJ, and Green LW, Editors. 2014. *Health Behavior Change in Populations*. Baltimore: Johns Hopkins University Press.

Kapilashrami A and Hanefeld J. 2014. Meaningful change or more of the same? The Global Fund's new funding model and the politics of HIV scale-up. *Global Public Health* 9(1-2):160–175.

Kauffman CM and Martin PL. 2014. Scaling up Buen Vivir: Globalizing local environmental governance from Ecuador. *Global Environmental Politics* 14(1):40–58.

Khayatzadeh-Mahani A, Sedoghi Z, Mehrolhassani MH, and Yazdi-Feyzabadi V. 2015. How Health in All Policies are developed and implemented in a developing country? A case study of a HiAP initiative in Iran. *Health Promotion International* [Epub ahead of print].

Kickbusch I. 2012. Addressing the interface of the political and commercial determinants of health. *Health Promotion International* 27(4):427–428.

Kirk JM. 2015. *Healthcare without Borders: Understanding Cuban Medical Internationalism*. Gainsville: University Press of Florida.

Koont S. 2009. The urban agriculture of Havana. *Monthly Review* 60(1):63–72.

Krieger N. 2008. Proximal, distal, and the politics of causation: What's level got to do with it? *American Journal of Public Health* 98(2):221–230.

Krishnan A, Amarchand R, Byass P, et al. 2014. "No one says 'no' to money" – a mixed methods approach for evaluating conditional cash transfer schemes to improve girl children's status in Haryana, India. *International Journal for Equity in Health* 13(1):11.

Kröger M and Lalander R. 2016. Ethno-territorial rights and the resource extraction boom in Latin America: do constitutions matter? *Third World Quarterly* 37(4):682–702.

Lackenbauer PW and Mantle CL. 2007. *Aboriginal Peoples and the Canadian Military: Historical Perspectives*. Kingston, ON: Canadian Defence Academy Press.

Laurell AC. 2008. Health reform in Mexico City, 2000-2006. *Social Medicine* 3(2):145–157.

———. 2015. Three decades of neoliberalism in Mexico: The destruction of society. *International Journal of Health Services* 45(2):246–264.

Lekshmi S, Mohanta GP, Revikumar KG, and Manna PK. 2014. Developments and emerging issues in public and private health care systems of Kerala. *International Journal of Pharmacy and Pharmaceutical Sciences* 6(Suppl 2):92–98.

Leroy JL, García-Guerra A, García R, et al. 2008. The oportunidades program increases the linear growth of children enrolled at young ages in urban Mexico. *Journal of Nutrition* 138(4):793–798.

Leubolt B. 2014. *Social policies and redistribution in South Africa. Working Paper No. 25*. Geneva: International Labour Office Global Labour University.

Levine R and What Works Working Group. 2007. *Case Studies in Global Health: Millions Saved*. Boston: Jones and Bartlett.

Lieberherr F. 2003. Participatory budgets: A tool for a participatory democracy. *Urban News* 7. Bern: *Swiss Agency for Development and Cooperation*.

Linn V. 2015. *The Buddha on Wall Street: What's Wrong with Capitalism and What We Can Do about It*. Cambridge: Windhorse Publications.

Lomeli EV. 2008. Conditional cash transfers as social policy in Latin America: An assessment of their contributions and limitations. *Annual Review of Sociology* 34:475–499.

Luby S. 2014. Is targeting access to sanitation enough? *Lancet Global Health* 2(11):e619–e620.

Machel S. 1974. *Estabelecer o Poder Popular Para Servir as Massas*. Maputo, MZ: Instituto Nacional do Livro e o Disco.

Mangham LJ and Hanson K. 2010. Scaling up in international health: What are the key issues? *Health Policy and Planning* 25(2):81–96.

Marquetti A, Schonerwald da Silva C, and Campbell A. 2012. Participatory economic democracy in action: Participatory budgeting in Porto Alegre, 1989–2004. *Review of Radical Political Economics* 44(1):62–81.

Martin A. 2013. Philip Morris Leads Plain Packs Battle in Global Trade Arena. *Bloomberg Business*, August 22.

Martínez-Alier J, Pascual U, Vivien F, and Zaccai E. 2010. Sustainable de-growth: Mapping the context, criticisms and future prospects of an emergent paradigm. *Ecological Economics* 69(9):1741–1747.

Martínez Franzoni J. 2008. *Domesticar la Incertidumbre en América Latina: Mercado Laboral, Política Social y Familias*. San José: Universidad de Costa Rica, Instituto de Investigaciones Sociales.

Martínez Franzoni J and Sánchez-Ancochea D. 2013a. Can Latin American production regimes complement universalistic welfare regimes?: Implications from the Costa Rican case. *Latin American Research Review* 48(2):148–174.

———. 2013b. *Good Jobs and Social Services: How Costa Rica Achieved the Elusive Double Incorporation*. New York: Palgrave Macmillan.

———. 2016. *The Quest for Universal Social Policy in the South: Actors, Ideas and Architectures*. Cambridge: Cambridge University Press.

Martínez Franzoni J and Voorend K. 2011. Actors and ideas behind CCTs in Chile, Costa Rica and El Salvador. *Global Social Policy* 11(2-3):279–298.

Martínez Martínez OA. 2012. Efectos de las becas educativas del programa Oportunidades sobre la asistencia escolar: El caso de la zona urbana del noreste de México. *Desarrollo y Sociedad* 69:99–131.

Martorano B. 2014. The impact of Uruguay's 2007 tax reform on equity and efficiency. *Development Policy Review* 32(6):701–714.

Matthaei J. [Forthcoming]. *From Inequality to Solidarity: Co-Creating a New Economics for the 21st Century*. Amherst, MA: Union for Radical Political Economics.

Maxwell K. 2011. *Making History Heal: Settler-Colonialism and Urban Indigenous Healing in Ontario, 1970s-2010*. PhD [dissertation]. Toronto: Dalla Lana School of Public Health, University of Toronto.

Meadows DH, Meadows DL, Randers J, and Behrens WW. 1972. *The Limits to Growth: A Report for the Club of Rome's Project on the Predicament of Mankind.* New York: Universe Books.

Meegama SA. 1986. *The Mortality Transition in Sri Lanka.* New York: United Nations.

Mesa-Lago C. 1985. Health care in Costa Rica: Boom and crisis. *Social Science and Medicine* 21(1):13–21.

———. 2012. *Sistemas de protección social en América Latina y el Caribe: Cuba.* Santiago: CEPAL.

Ministry of Health and Family Welfare, India. 2014. *Annual Report 2013-14.* New Dehi: Ministry of Health and Family Welfare.

Missoni E. 2015. Degrowth and health: Local action should be linked to global policies and governance for health. *Sustainability Science* 10(3):439–450.

Mohammadi H. 2010. *Citizen Participation in Urban Planning and Management: The case of Iran, Shiraz city, Saadi community.* Kassel, DE: Kassel University Press.

Morgan LM. 1987. Health without wealth? Costa Rica's health system under economic crisis. *Journal of Public Health Policy* 8(1):86–105.

MPPS. 2015. Se incrementa en Venezuela la matrícula de médicos comunitarios. http://www.mppeuct.gob.ve/actualidad/noticias/se-incrementa-en-venezuela-la-matricula-de-medicos-comunitarios. Accessed October 25, 2015.

Muntaner C, Benach J, Victor MP, et al. 2013. Egalitarian policies and social determinants of health in Bolivarian Venezuela. *International Journal of Health Services* 43(3):537–549.

Muntaner C, Borrell C, Ng E, et al. 2011. Politics, welfare regimes, and population health: Controversies and evidence. *Sociology of Health & Illness* 33(6):946–964.

Muntaner C, Guerra Salazar RM, Benach J, and Armada F. 2006. Venezuela's Barrio Adentro: An alternative to neoliberalism in health care. *International Journal of Health Services* 36(4):803–811.

OCDE/CEPAL. 2014. *Estudio Multi-Dimensional de Uruguay: Volumen 1. Evaluación Inicial.* Paris: OECD.

Ordúñez-García PO, Nieto FJ, Espinosa-Brito AD, and Caballero B. 1996. Cuban epidemic neuropathy, 1991 to 1994: History repeats itself a century after the "amblyopia of the blockade." *American Journal of Public Health* 86(5):738–743.

Oommen MA. 2014. Growth, inequality and well-being: Revisiting fifty years of Kerala's development trajectory. *Journal of South Asian Development* 9(2):173–205.

Owusu-Addo E and Cross R. 2014. The impact of conditional cash transfers on child health in low- and middle-income countries: A systematic review. *International Journal of Public Health* 59(4):609–618.

Packard RM. 2007. *The Making of a Tropical Disease: A Short History of Malaria.* Baltimore: Johns Hopkins University Press.

Paes-Sousa R and Vaitsman J. 2014. The zero hunger and Brazil without extreme poverty programs: A step forward in Brazilian social protection policy. *Ciência & Saúde Coletiva* 19(11):4351–4360.

Pagliccia N and Álvarez Pérez A. 2012. The Cuban experience in public health: Does political will have a role? *International Journal of Health Services* 42(1):77–94.

Parayil G. 1996. The "Kerala model" of development: Development and sustainability in the Third World. *Third World Quarterly* 17(5):941–957.

Pathmanathan I, Liljestrand J, Martins JM, et al. 2003. *Investing in Maternal Health: Learning from Malaysia and Sri Lanka.* Washington, DC: The World Bank.

PHM. 2013. Promoting Health for All and Social Justice in the Era of Global Capitalism: A call to action by the People's Health Movement at the 8th Global Conference on Health Promotion Helsinki, Finland – 14 June. http://www.phmovement.org/sites/www.phmovement.org/files/PHMStatementat8GCHP-PromotingHealthforAllandSocialJusticev_FINAL25July.pdf. Accessed August 15, 2015.

PHM, Medact, Medico International, et al. 2014. *Global Health Watch 4: An Alternative World Health Report.* London: Zed Books Ltd.

Pickett KE and Wilkinson RG. 2015. The ethical and policy implications of research on income inequality and child well-being. *Pediatrics* 135(Supplement 2):S39–S47.

Poland B, Dooris M, and Haluza-Delay R. 2011. Securing 'supportive environments' for health in the face of ecosystem collapse: Meeting the triple threat with a sociology of creative transformation. *Health Promotion International* 26:ii202–ii215.

Prefeitura Municipal de Belo Horizonte. 2009. *Participatory Budgeting in Belo Horizonte: Fifteen Years 1993-2008 Report.* Belo Horizonte: Prefeitura Municipal de Belo Horizonte.

Pribble J. 2013. *Welfare and Party Politics in Latin America.* Cambridge: Cambridge University Press.

Pribble J and Huber E. 2011. Social policy and redistribution: Chile and Uruguay. In Levitsky S and Roberts KM, Editors. *The Resurgence of the Latin American Left.* Baltimore: Johns Hopkins University Press.

Raman KR. 2009. Asian Development Bank, policy conditionalities and the social democratic governance: Kerala Model under pressure? *Review of International Political Economy* 16(2):284–308.

Ramírez-Silva I, Rivera JA, Leroy JL, and Neufeld LM. 2013. The Oportunidades program's fortified food supplement, but not improvements in the home diet, increased the intake of key micronutrients in rural Mexican children aged 12-59 months. *The Journal of Nutrition* 143(5):656–663.

Rannan-Eliya RP, Hossain MM, Anuranga C, et al. 2013. Trends and determinants of childhood stunting and underweight in Sri Lanka. *Ceylon Medical Journal* 58:10–18.

Reddy S. 2012. Randomise this! On poor economics. *Review of Agrarian Studies* 2(2):63.

Rice R. 2012. *The New Politics of Protest: Indigenous Mobilization in Latin America's Neoliberal Era.* Tucson: University of Arizona Press.

Rice W. 2011. *Health Promotion through an Equity Lens: Approaches, Problems and Solutions.* Toronto: The Wellesley Institute.

Ritsatakis A, Ostergren P-O, and Webster P. 2015. Tackling the social determinants of inequalities in health during Phase V of the Healthy Cities Project in Europe. *Health Promotion International* 30(S1):i45–i53.

Roodman D. 2012. *Due Diligence: An Impertinent Inquiry into Microfinance.* Washington, DC: Center for Global Development.

Sachs JD. 2015. *The Age of Sustainable Development.* New York: Columbia University Press.

Schumacher EF. 1973. *Small Is Beautiful: A Study of Economics As If People Mattered.* New York: Harper Perennial.

SEDESOL. 2015. Componentes. https://www.prospera.gob.mx/swb/es/PROSPERA2015/Componentes. Accessed October 23, 2015.

Seligson M and Martínez Franzoni J. 2009. Limits to Costa rican heterodoxy: What has changed in "paradise?" In Mainwaring S and Scully T, Editors. *The Politics of Democratic Governability in Latin America: Clues and Lessons.* Palo Alto, CA: Stanford University Press.

Semana. 2015. En Bogotá hay 50 muertes cada mes por accidentes de tránsito. *Semana*, May 27.

Setiawan E and Parry J. 2011. Engaging with government to scale-up community-based total sanitation in Indonesia: Proceedings of the 35th WEDC International Conference, UK: Loughborough University.

Shibeshi ME, Masresha BG, Smit SB, et al. 2014. Measles resurgence in southern Africa: Challenges to measles elimination. *Vaccine* 32(16):1798–1807.

Shiva V. 2005. New emperors, old clothes. *The Ecologist*, July 1.

Sivarajah N. 2007. *War and Health in Northern Sri Lanka: How Did the People Survive? Professor Chellathurai Sivagnanasundram Inaugural Memorial Lecture.* Jaffna, SR: University of Jaffna.

Skanthakumar B. 2013. *Growth with Inequality: The Political Economy of Neoliberalism in Sri Lanka.* Country Report 2013. Kathmandu: South Asia Alliance for Poverty Eradication (SAAPE).

Sri Lanka. 2012. *National Policy on Maternal and Child Health.* Colombo: Ministry of Health.

Statistics Canada. 2015. Smokers, by sex, provinces and territories (Percent). http://www.statcan.gc.ca/tables-tableaux/sum-som/l01/cst01/health74b-eng.htm. Accessed April 5, 2015.

Suryanarayana MH, Agrawal A, and Seeta Prabhu K. 2011. *Inequality-adjusted Human Development Index for India's States: 2011.* New Delhi: UNDP India.

Susuman AS, Lougue S, and Battala M. 2016. Female literacy, fertility decline and life expectancy in Kerala, India: An analysis from census of India 2011. *Journal of Asian and African Studies* 51(1):32–42.

Swensson LFJ. 2015. *Institutional Procurement of Food from Smallholder Farmers: The Case of Brazil.* Rome: FAO.

Tajer D. 2003. Latin American social medicine: Roots, development during the 1990s, and current challenges. *American Journal of Public Health* 93(12):2023–2027.

Teichman JA. 2016. *The Politics of Inclusive Development: Policy, State Capacity, and Coalition Building.* New York: Palgrave Macmillan.

Thompson S and Genosko G. 2009. *Punched Drunk: Alcohol, Surveillance, and the LCBO: 1927-75.* Black Point, NS: Fernwood Publishers.

Thresia CU. 2013. The privatization and commodification of the welfare state: Rising private sector and falling 'good health at low cost': Health challenges in China, Sri Lanka, and Indian State of Kerala. *International Journal of Health Services* 43(1):31–48.

Torres Tovar M. 2007. ALAMES: Organizational expression of social medicine in Latin America. *Social Medicine* 2(3):125–130.

Touchton M and Wampler B. 2014. Improving social well-being through new democratic institutions. *Comparative Political Studies* 47(10):1442–1469.

Tsouros AD. 2015. Twenty-seven years of the WHO European Healthy Cities movement: A sustainable movement for change and innovation at the local level. *Health Promotion International* 30(S1):i3–i7.

Ulrichs M and Roelen K. 2012. *Equal Opportunities for All? A Critical Analysis of Mexico's Oportunidades. Institute of Development Studies Working Paper 413.* Brighton, UK: Institute of Development.

UNDP. 2005. *Human Development Report 2005: International Development at a Crossroads: Aid, Trade and Security in an Unequal World.* New York: UNDP.

———. 2015. *Human Development Report 2015: Work for Human Development.* New York: UNDP.

Unger J-P, de Paepe P, Buitrón R, and Soors W. 2007. Costa Rica: Achievements of a heterodox health policy. *American Journal of Public Health* 98(4):636–643.

UNICEF. 2012. Briefing sheet: water, sanitation, and hygiene. http://www.unicef.org/srilanka/2012_SL_Fast_Facts_WASH.pdf. Accessed October 24, 2015.

———. 2013. UNICEF data: Monitoring the situation of children and women. http://data.unicef.org/

child-mortality/under-five.html. Accessed April 5, 2015.
UNICEF Office of Research. 2014. *Children of the Recession: The Impact of the Economic Crisis on Child Well-Being in Rich Countries, Innocenti Report Card 12.* Florence: UNICEF.
UNICEF and WHO. 2015. *Progress on Sanitation and Drinking Water – 2015 Update and MDG Assessment.* Geneva: WHO.
Vallejo MC, Burbano R, Falconí F, and Larrea C. 2015. Leaving oil underground in Ecuador: The Yasuní-ITT initiative from a multi-criteria perspective. *Ecological Economics* 109(Complete):175–185.
Valverde M. 1998. The Liquor of Government and the Government of Liquor. In *Diseases of the Will. Alcohol and the Dilemmas of Freedom.* Cambridge: Cambridge University Press.
Veiga R and Bello W. 2015. Cuba necesita modernizar su política social: Entrevista a Mayra Espina. http://cubaposible.net/articulos/cuba-necesita-modernizar-su-politica-social-2-aa5-3-23-5-3. Accessed July 20, 2015.
Victor P. 2010. Questioning economic growth. *Nature* 468:370–371.
Villalba U. 2013. Buen vivir vs development: A paradigm shift in the Andes? *Third World Quarterly* 34(8):1427–1442.
Wagle S and Shah P. 2003. Case study 2—Porto Alegre, Brazil: Participatory approaches in budgeting and public expenditure management. *Social Development Notes* Note no. 71.
Waitzkin H, Iriart C, Estrada A, and Lamadrid S. 2001. Social medicine then and now: Lessons from Latin America. *American Journal of Public Health* 91(10):1592–1601.
Walker C. 2015. *Venezuela's Health Care Revolution.* Halifax, NS: Fernwood Publishing.
Wampler B. 2012. Participation, representation, and social justice: Using participatory governance to transform representative democracy. *Polity* 44(4):666–682.
Wei X, Zou G, Walley J, et al. 2014. China tuberculosis policy at crucial crossroads: Comparing the practice of different hospital and tuberculosis control collaboration models using survey data. *PLoS ONE* 9(3):e90596.
Weisbrot M, and Johnston J. 2012. *Venezuela's economic recovery: Is it sustainable?* Washington, DC: Center for Economic and Policy Research.
WHO. 1986. *Ottawa Charter for Health Promotion: First International Conference on Health Promotion.* Geneva: WHO.
———. 2007. *Report of the External Review of Maternal and Newborn Health Sri Lanka.* Colombo: WHO.
———. 2010a. *Adelaide Statement on Health in All Policies.* Geneva: WHO.
———. 2010b. *Urban HEART: Urban Health Equity Assessment and Response Tool.* Geneva: WHO.
———. 2012. *Global Progress Report on Implementation of the WHO Framework Convention on Tobacco Control.* Geneva: WHO.
———. 2013a. The 8th Global Conference on Health Promotion, Helsinki, Finland, 10-14 June 2013: The Helsinki Statement on Health in All Policies. http://www.who.int/healthpromotion/conferences/8gchp/statement_2013/en/. Accessed June 15, 2015.
———. 2013b. Opening address at the 8th Global Conference on Health Promotion Helsinki, Finland 10 June 2013.
———. 2015a. Global Health Observatory data repository. http://www.who.int/gho/database/en/. Accessed June 9, 2015.
———. 2015b. Global Health Expenditure Database. http://apps.who.int/nha/database. Accessed September 18, 2015.
———. 2015c. *World Health Statistics 2015.* Geneva: WHO.
———. 2016. Tobacco: Factsheet. http://www.who.int/mediacentre/factsheets/fs339/en/. August 16, 2016.
WHO EURO. 2003. *Healthy Cities around the World: An Overview of the Healthy Cities Movement in the Six WHO Regions.* International Healthy Cities Conference, Belfast, Northern Ireland. Copenhagen.
———. 2015. WHO European Healthy Cities Network. http://www.euro.who.int/en/health-topics/environment-and-health/urban-health/activities/healthy-cities/who-european-healthy-cities-network. Accessed June 15, 2015.
Wilson TD. 2015. Mexico's rural poor and targeted educational and health programs. *Human Organization* 74(3):207–216.
World Bank. 2008. Reaching the poor with health services, Tanzania: Social marketing for malaria prevention. Washington, DC: World Bank.
———. 2013. World Bank Support to Social Safety Nets. http://www.worldbank.org/en/results/2013/04/11/world-bank-support-to-social-safety-nets. Accessed June 12, 2015.
———. 2015a. *A Measured Approach to Ending Poverty and Boosting Shared Prosperity: Concepts, Data, and the Twin Goals.* Policy Research Report. Washington, DC.
———. 2015b. *The State of Social Safety Nets 2015.* Washington, DC: World Bank.
———. 2015c. World Development Indicators. http://data.worldbank.org/. Accessed June 9, 2015.
Yanful B and Jackson S. 2012. Effectiveness of health promotion strategies. In Juvinya D and Arroyo H, Editors. *Health promotion, 25 years later.* Catalonia: Documenta Universitaria.
Young IM. 2011. *Justice and the Politics of Difference.* Princeton University Press.
Zucco CJ. 2015. The impacts of conditional cash transfers in four presidential elections (2002–2014). *Brazilian Political Science Review* 9(1):135–149.

14

TOWARDS A SOCIAL JUSTICE APPROACH TO GLOBAL HEALTH

We hope that reading this book will have stimulated you to think anew about the prospects and dilemmas of global health. Ideally, the analyses and arguments presented will have sparked your desire to become involved—or transform your involvement—in addressing the challenges of this arena. We also invite you to "decenter" your own role. After all, the bulk of what is considered "global" health activity—though perhaps in dialogue with transnational practices and agendas—is carried out by local health personnel, government policymakers, community organizers, health promoters, laboratory technicians, mothers, traditional birth attendants, parasitologists, and innumerable others, often with very limited resources and inadequate remuneration or recognition for their work.

De-centering your role means not privileging your personal interests and aspirations; rather, it entails figuring out where and how your participation can be useful based on your knowledge, abilities, and inclinations in the context of pressing global health issues. Given your experience and potential to contribute, what is the appropriate geographical or organizational setting for your engagement and activism? Pushing this further, what alternatives to international experiences might powerfully contribute to improving global health justice, considering the constraints and possibilities of the political economy order? What should you know and learn about the local, national, and global contexts of your potential activities and work and the related ethical and ideological implications? What kinds of sources should you consult? These are all questions that anyone contemplating paid or volunteer work in global health should reflect on, whether at home or transnationally (Ventres and Fort 2014).

As we have seen, contradictions abound in the field of global health. Much global health activity remains premised on a one-way diffusionist model of funding, professionals, and agenda-setting from high-income countries (HICs) to low- and middle-income countries (LMICs). Yet past and present, such a unidirectional framing of ideas, resources, and expertise is both simplistic and erroneous (Ventres and Gusoff 2014). Without LMICs there would be no HICs. The profits extracted from labor and natural resources in Europe's African, American, and Asian colonies (and via post-colonial Euro-American imperialism) enabled industrialization and helped finance generous welfare states, contributing to better, if unequal, health in HICs. But LMICs, barring elites, have benefited far less. (In conducive contexts, a confluence of unions and social movements have struggled for broad social protections. LMIC welfare states have invariably evolved on a shoestring, some creatively and equitably so, others in more beleaguered fashion.) Similarly, far more health professionals from LMICs go to work in HICs than vice versa, as part of the "brain drain" in which LMICs paradoxically (but consistent with past experience) heavily subsidize HICs (see chapter 11).

There are also countless, albeit little touted, public health policies and innovations from LMICs that have shaped developments in HICs. This frames, for instance, how a child rights approach to health, pioneered by Uruguay in the 1930s, moved onto the international agenda (Birn 2017); such a circulation of influences also helps explain the community health movement's appearance in the United States in the 1960s, drawing from prior efforts in South Africa (Geiger 2013) and the enduring African community health worker (CHW) model for New York City's efforts. Similarly, the United Kingdom has been inspired by Brazil's family health strategy to better integrate CHWs into its primary care system (Johnson et al. 2013). In addition, a significant portion of global health activity takes place outside of HICs' ambit altogether. Across non-metropolitan centers, cooperation ranges from Latin American sanitary treaties and mutual public health policy sharing starting in the late 19th century—renewed more recently under UNASUR—to the Group of 77's challenging of neo-imperialism (sparked by the 1955 Bandung conference) leading to mutual aid arrangements outside the Cold War blocs, among other initiatives (see chapters 1 and 2).

Undoubtedly, there are various ways of thinking about work in global health. Some consider it a learning adventure: well-meaning health professionals and students typically from HICs travel to low-income countries (LICs) in hopes of alleviating health problems. Others regard global health as providing humanitarian and technical assistance during times of civil conflict or ecological disaster. Still others see it in terms of mutual cooperation aimed at improving health and social conditions, whether via international agencies and nongovernmental organizations (NGOs), between LMICs, or among networks of health workers, organizations, and professionals.

From a critical political economy viewpoint, global health work involves a lifelong commitment to transformative social change. In implementing this perspective, students, health professionals, and community actors may collaborate in solidarity (i.e., mutual support based on shared values) actions toward improving health and social justice, whether at home or abroad (Hanson 2010). Integrating technical, personal, social, institutional, and political approaches is feasible, if an ongoing and uphill challenge, as witnessed in a variety of "healthy societies" (see chapter 13).

In this chapter we lay out a committed and hopeful activist approach to global health—neither based upon naïve optimism that fails to question structural inequities nor on cynical realism that views systemic injustices as inevitable and intractable. Instead, we draw from the notion of "critical hope," based on the ideas of Brazilian educator-philosopher-activist Paulo Freire (1992), pushing us to think realistically and critically about the possibilities for transformative change and how it can be achieved through long-term collective struggle. Using this premise as a guide, we explore how to move beyond mainstream approaches to foster a truly equitable form of global health based on solidarity with oppressed peoples. We do not purport to have the answers—but present an array of activities that heed the spirit of health and social justice.

We thus invite readers to navigate the complex world of global health from a critical perspective and consider engaging in global health work that seeks bona fide social justice. This chapter begins by recapping key aspects of the dominant models, challenges, and points of inspiration in global health discussed throughout this textbook. Next, we highlight solidarity-oriented approaches based on humility and commitment to political values that contest oppression and aim to transform societies so that power and resources, and control over them, are truly equitably shared. Throughout we showcase locales, organizations, and movements that draw from critical hope to address global health problems "at home and abroad." We wrap up by reviewing the challenges, possibilities, and limits of global health work from individual and organizational perspectives, bearing in mind the larger constellation of forces and interests examined in previous chapters.

RECAPPING THE GLOBAL HEALTH ARENA: DOMINANT APPROACHES, ONGOING CHALLENGES, AND POINTS OF INSPIRATION

Key Questions:

- What are the limitations of dominant (mainstream) approaches to international health in the past and global health today?
- What inspiring efforts have emerged that address global health's ongoing challenges and serve as alternatives to mainstream approaches?

Dominant Approaches

Global health today remains deeply marked by international health's historical trajectory. As discussed in chapter 1, starting circa 1500 leading European powers ventured "overseas" to explore, settle, exploit, convert, colonize, "civilize," and profit from peoples and lands of less powerful societies. Millions of people were forced into slavery, indentured servitude, and other forms of involuntary migration/labor and worked under oppressive and dangerous conditions on plantations, in extractive industries, and, later, in factories and sweatshops. Colonial health and tropical medicine played a central part in the imperial enterprise, whether protecting soldiers and settlers to enable colonial expansion, increasing worker productivity, staving off epidemics to safeguard trade and investment, reinforcing political, economic, and social stratification, "saving" subjugated populations on religious and "civilizing" grounds, or attenuating social uprisings.

For example, in the 19th century Britain's Army Medical Service prided itself on bringing "sanitary science to India, stopping the ravages of cholera and improving the whole conditions there" (Harrison 1994, p. 227), even as its primary mission was to protect the health of British soldiers and colonists; any benefit to the local population was secondary. Moreover, many of India's health problems—ascribed to local cultural and racial deficiencies—were in fact created by the British through conquest and colonialism's commercial ventures, such as agricultural practices that "disrupted traditional systems of drainage exposing huge tracts of the country to the ravages of malaria and waterborne disease" (ibid).

In a related vein, the part played by Protestant and Catholic medical missionaries in disseminating Western medicine to European colonies in Latin America, Asia, and Africa has been hailed by some: to this day, across Africa many hospitals are run by missionaries, providing care that might not otherwise be available. Yet the missionary project historically facilitated imperialist exploitation and extraction, as exemplified in colonial Belgian Congo (today the Democratic Republic of Congo [DRC]), which had one of the world's most extensive networks of missionary hospitals (Lyons 2002) and among the richest mineral deposits—making the country simultaneously vastly wealthy and indescribably poor.

As former colonies gained independence in the 19th and 20th centuries, asymmetrical power relations in the realms of trade, global politics, and other arenas persisted, albeit under a new guise. At the end of World War II, both continued imperialism and decolonization movements influenced the new United Nations (UN) and World Health Organization (WHO). The emerging post-war world (health) order was also shaped by Cold War geopolitical relations among so-called First (capitalist bloc), Second (communist bloc), and Third (non-aligned) World countries and accompanying ideologies of development (chapter 2). WHO initially built upon the legacies of the Rockefeller Foundation, pursuing disease eradication programs (e.g., against yaws, malaria, and smallpox), in the 1970s turning to a contrasting approach of primary health care (PHC) underpinned by the non-aligned countries' demands for a New International Economic Order.

The WHO's role at the fulcrum of international health waned in the 1980s as dominant bilateral players, particularly the United States (as part of its larger pullback from the UN), withheld significant financial support in disagreement with WHO's advocacy of affordable essential medicines and of restraining the marketing of breastmilk alternatives (both actions defying corporate interests). This took place in the context of an ideological realigning of the world order under neoliberal globalization, forcing a circumscribed and pro-corporate role for the public sector and a concomitant (re-)entry of private (and philanthropic) actors. At the end of the Cold War, international health was rebaptized as global health to evoke the field's unified enterprise, yet many of the dilemmas and arrangements of the past have persisted (chapter 2).

While those involved in global health today might (smugly) distance themselves from past prejudices and practices, it is important to bear in mind that self-interested agendas still pervade, accompany, and motivate a range of the field's current activities, such as controlling feared epidemics from crossing the globe (e.g., the US-led, 50-member Global Health Security Agenda, which envisions a "world safe and secure from global health threats posed by infectious diseases" [GHSA 2016]) and pursuing strategic alliances (e.g., PEPFAR's focus countries). Indeed, the foreign policy agendas of many leading powers unabashedly frame health as vital national security and economic concerns, employing this dual rationale to justify involvement in health-related multilateral decisionmaking bodies and the use of activities and negotiations around health as a diplomatic tool (see chapters 3 and 4).

Even as the "soft power" of health diplomacy is flaunted by both traditional donors and emerging players as an effective alternative to more aggressive foreign policy, there is inadequate transparency around spending and its consequences. For instance, the largest donor, the United States, annually spends roughly US$10 billion on global health, yet there is insufficient coordination, accountability, and timely reporting around these efforts (Post and Glassman 2016).

In the economic domain, global health is playing a renewed role in market expansion, advancing commercial interests (Big Pharma, Big Food, etc.) over public health needs. Meanwhile, the palpable and cumulative effects of global capitalism (especially in its neoliberal form; see chapter 9) on health inequity and social injustice are problems sidestepped by dominant global health actors.

For these reasons, some wonder whether contemporary approaches to global health—including those that express profound moral sentiments in favor of reducing poverty and improving health in LMICs—represent a neocolonialist mode (Horton 2013), whereby "solutions" emanate from powerful interests and are imposed on subordinate countries and groups, all the while protecting profitable global arrangements. This "white man's burden," as per the phrase popularized by British imperial poet Rudyard Kipling, supposes that aid stems from generosity and responsibility on the part of imperial donors—who disregard the past and present exploitation of subjugated economies and peoples.

Nowadays, global health actors have proliferated to encompass multilateral and bilateral aid agencies, international financial institutions (IFIs), regional organizations, military actors, NGOs, humanitarian and religious agencies, research initiatives, foundations, think tanks, advocacy groups, social and political movements, public-private partnerships (PPPs), and business interests (see chapter 4). Particularly influential are a growing array of private and philanthropic actors active in global health, which embrace social entrepreneurship (Lim and Chia 2016), venture investment, and profit-oriented business models to addressing development and global health problems, an ideology embodied in the term "philanthrocapitalism" (Wilson 2015).

Indeed, mainstream global health efforts increasingly draw from social enterprise strategies to "brand" their programs (distinguish them from others; create a niche; show how they are "unique") and "perfect the pitch" (to launch and obtain funding for new ideas and promote existing programs) (Cruikshank, Clark, and Bartlett 2014). As well, market approaches to health favoring private sector health care delivery, in places as varied as the United States, India, South Africa, and Mexico (see chapter 11), presume greater efficiency despite evidence otherwise. Market models also favor priority-setting driven by cost analyses that demonstrate a "bang for the buck" for specific interventions over the short term, while rejecting broad social investments that are conducive to health and health equity over the long term and may ultimately be far more effective and efficient (see chapter 12).

Another dominant feature of contemporary global health is its relentless biomedical and behavioral bias, notwithstanding ample evidence of the shortcomings of bio-behavioral understandings of health and well-being. As explored in chapter 3, these models emphasize biology, genetics, and biomedical interventions (e.g., medications and insecticide-spraying) and lifestyle factors (e.g., diet, smoking, and physical activity). Both models focus on the individual as the basis for health improvement, underplaying the role of societal politics, power, and social relations, all central to a critical political economy of health approach.

As just one of countless illustrations of the entrenchment of bio-behavioral approaches, to mark World Diabetes Day on November 15, 2015, then UN Secretary General Ban Ki-moon stated: "There is much all of us can do to minimize our risk of getting the disease and, even if we do get it, to live long and healthy lives with it," suggesting, for example, that "anyone who can stand instead of sit, walks a little bit more each day and is generally more active should do so." He also urged that health facilities "expand care for diabetes" and that the private sector "improve the availability and affordability of healthier products and essential medicines" (UN 2015). Yet he disregarded the factors a critical political economy approach considers crucial: the role of trade treaties enabling global penetration of transnational corporations (TNCs) that disrupt dietary patterns; fossil fuel dominance that leads to unhealthy urban air quality; inadequate tax revenues (due to illicit financial flows) impeding investment in safe neighborhoods, daycare, clean water access, and public transport; and the propagation of "flexible" work under neoliberal globalization, leading to unpredictable work schedules, multiple jobs, and long commutes (as per chapters 7, 9, and 10); all interacting together with still other factors to impede exercise.

Bio-behavioral and market approaches are also ubiquitous in vertical disease programs—global health's dominant modus operandi that entails attacking diseases one by one. Numerous analysts have critiqued such initiatives for not addressing the underlying political, economic, and social determinants of health or the need to strengthen infrastructure and PHC (Forman 2016; Gopinathan et al. 2015). In addition, excessive reliance on technical tools, effective as they may be under controlled conditions, is highly problematic when the tool becomes the end in itself, to be clocked rather than integrated into broad socio-political approaches (Adams 2013).

Disease initiatives can cause significant distortions in health systems. As health care workers are drawn away from primary care to receive training for and staff disease-specific programs, their former positions often remain unfilled (Keugoung et al. 2011; Pfeiffer et al. 2008). Furthermore, health professionals in LMICs may be overseen by outside "experts" or consultants who impose their own values and tools and negate, or even denigrate, the importance and utility of local knowledge and the existing organization of social and medical services.

Disease programs may be so narrowly focused that they overlook, or fail to treat, people who present with problems not directly related to the campaign in question (Harper and Parker 2014). Moreover, the focus on a few diseases comes at the expense of other primary care concerns, including routine immunization. India's eradication of polio, for instance, took place amid decreasing overall child immunization coverage and high rates of other vaccine-preventable diseases such as pneumonia—the number one cause of child mortality in the country (Laxminarayan and Ganguly 2011).

At its most extreme, the vertical approach can justify neglect in such obvious determinants of health as clean water access, adequate nutrition, and decent housing (not to mention the underlying factors of uneven power and resource control). For instance, elevating polio eradication above other approaches and health goals, former President of Nigeria, Goodluck Jonathan went so far as to declare:

> One thing I promise the Nigerian child, and also the Nigerian father and mother, is that if we cannot solve all the health problems in this country now, one thing this present administration is committed to is to eradicate polio by 2015 (Global Polio Eradication Initiative 2012).

It is both galling and unacceptable that in a country as oil-rich as Nigeria, polio eradication has served as an excuse for inaction in other areas (perhaps harming the polio campaign itself, evidenced by resurgence of wild poliovirus cases in 2016).

Because mainstream donor agencies typically follow corporate-style governance objectives that prioritize short-term, efficient activities to demonstrate success, they tend to favor narrowly targeted, cost-effective, measurable interventions (and associated supportive research [Box 14-1]) that quickly show results according to specified criteria. For example, donor-funded mass drug delivery for neglected tropical diseases—such as lymphatic filariasis and schistosomiasis (see chapter 6)—is frequently portrayed as hugely successful by local implementers and global advocates because shedding light on its shortcomings might affect future funding. In reality, uptake is often suboptimal due to poor consideration of context and structural factors that affect adherence to treatment (Parker and Allen 2014).

In sum, "the longer we isolate public health's technical aspects from its political and social aspects, the longer technical interventions will squeeze out one side of the mortality balloon only to find it inflated elsewhere" (Birn 2005, p. 519). Yet global health initiatives sponsored by the likes of the Global Fund,

Box 14-1 Global Health Research and its Ethical Dimensions

This textbook draws from a gamut of global health research findings; here we examine a few central issues around the production, ethical quandaries, and political dimensions of global research in health. The scope of research in the global health arena ranges from tracking longstanding and emerging patterns of mortality and morbidity to discovering and distributing effective, accessible, and affordable preventives and treatments for the leading causes of illness, disability, and death; and identifying and addressing the societal determinants of health (SDOH) and disease patterns and their (in)equitable distribution (see chapters 6–7). These areas of course interact. As discussed, understanding and remedying the underlying causes of health inequities perforce rests on relevant data collection, which in turn reflects larger political struggles around how populations are counted and how information is shared and used (see chapter 5).

Scientific research plays a vital role in global health, especially when it involves ethical, non-exploitative collaborations and when both research agendas and discoveries are integrated with policies aimed at enhancing equity and addressing SDOH. Alas, this goal is rarely met: the private sector funds half of all global health research and development (R&D) (Chakma et al. 2014)—a trend that will likely continue. Expectations of favorable returns on investments in this more than quarter trillion dollar industry means that research disproportionately attends to the places/people generating the greatest profits, thereby excluding most LMIC inhabitants and many in HICs.

In the 1990s, the Commission on Health Research for Development adopted the term "10/90 gap" to signal that the health needs of 90% of the global population were being addressed by only 10% of the world's health research monies. This gap entails (Pang 2011):

1. "Imbalances," reflecting who wields power and whose interests are privileged in setting and realizing research agendas, leading to:
    - Barriers to setting priorities and accessing the benefits of health research, particularly for LMIC populations (e.g., between 1975 and 2004 only 1.3% of new drugs developed were for "tropical" diseases, and today 75% of LMIC-targeted health research funding goes to just three diseases: HIV, TB, and malaria)
    - Limited research spending on chronic diseases, violence, and road traffic injuries in LMICs
    - More research on developing new technologies (e.g., new vaccines) than on better access to existing interventions (e.g., antibiotics or clean water) or on SDOH (e.g., how living and working conditions interact with disease processes)
    - Almost no research on the political economy (and world order) factors underlying multiple diseases (most research assumes a bio-behavioral model of disease control)
2. Improved LMIC research capacity (e.g., around HIV), but continued lags (in contexts with limited resources, research infrastructure, and posts for scientists)
3. Inadequate research accountability and problematic ethics:
    - Growing clinical research taking place in India, South Africa, and China, among other LMIC settings (motivated by lower costs and large numbers of potential participants), often under the auspices of private companies or PPPs
    - Unethical research practices (e.g., illegal and/or unsafe testing of unproven therapies)
4. Weak knowledge translation (connecting research/evidence to health policy/practice)
5. Inadequate governance of global health research, especially with many new players pursuing their own agendas, mainly disease-specific interests

This is not to say that LMICs lack research capacity—to the contrary, given constraints, there has been remarkable research production in various MICs and some LICs (see chapter 11). To name just two examples, past and present: Brazilian physician-bacteriologist Carlos

Chagas's identification of American trypanosomiasis, its etiology, and carrier insect in 1909—an unprecedented discovery of all links in the epidemiological chain by a single person; and Chinese chemist Youyou Tu's isolation of artemisinin, extracted from a traditional herbal medicine plant, for the treatment of malaria, earning her a 2015 Nobel prize in medicine.

Nonetheless, the imbalance of research funding, capacity, and infrastructure between HICs and LMICs persists. A growing number of North–South (and some South–South) research and training partnerships have emerged to address this issue. Reciprocal North–South research efforts are typically fragmented and underfunded compared with university backing and donor support for biomedical research (Pinto et al. 2014). In some places, such as Rwanda, research partnerships and exchanges must have government approval and assurances of non-extractive research (Chu et al. 2014). Other arrangements, although promising on paper, perpetuate uneven power relations (Moyi Okwaro and Geissler 2015; Smith, Hunt, and Master 2014). Many institutions in LMICs are unable to effectively partake in joint research, and HIC participants and priorities often dominate partnerships and publications. Each year thousands of HIC health researchers receive grants to carry out studies in LMICs, but it is virtually unheard of for a scientific team from, for instance, India or Senegal to be funded to investigate health problems in, say, Canada or France. Of course, resident researchers in some LMICs may be as well-trained as many foreigners (and frequently poached by HICs), and are almost universally more knowledgeable about the local situation.

But "research imperialism" is only one side of the coin. The US's 1980 Bayh-Dole Act granted permission to federally funded researchers to patent and license inventions, generating rising conflicts of interest between the pharmaceutical industry and university-based researchers (Liang and Mackey 2010). This has also fostered "academic capitalism," whereby universities articulate missions of global health equity and innovation while profit-seeking from global health (Merson 2015)—patenting research, attracting resources (often with directives) and contracts from the private sector—making them bound to donors and potentially exploiting LMIC partners (Cantwell and Kauppinen 2014).

The Ethics and Politics of Global Health Research

Another key concern connected to global health research is ethical conduct, an issue only systematically addressed as of the mid-20th century. Following revelation of the atrocities of Nazi human medical experiments before and during World War II, the Nuremberg Code of 1947 established the requirement for voluntary consent by all human medical research subjects. Subsequently, codes of research ethics have been promoted by various professional groups, based on the principle of informed consent and individual decisionmaking autonomy.

Yet even as these codes were developed, harmful research continued. Among the most infamous cases was the Tuskegee Syphilis Study, conducted by the US Public Health Service (USPHS) between 1932 and 1972 on over 400 poor African-American men in the US state of Alabama who had been diagnosed with syphilis. The recruited men believed they were receiving treatment but in fact were never appropriately treated, even once penicillin became the standard syphilis cure following World War II. The study resulted in at least 40 deaths and a gross health and ethical violation (Gamble 1997; Reverby 2009). After the study was uncovered, the US government enacted more stringent regulations and control over research involving human subjects, beginning with the 1974 establishment of a National Commission for the Protection of Human Subjects.

More recently, historian Susan Reverby uncovered an international arm of the syphilis study, supported by the Pan American Sanitary Bureau and the Guatemalan government. From 1946 to 1948, USPHS researchers intentionally infected more than 1,300 Guatemalan prison inmates, psychiatric patients, sex workers, and soldiers with syphilis—without participant consent—to test the efficacy of penicillin (Reverby 2011). Following a US government apology, and the Guatemalan government's declaration of the experiments as "crimes against humanity," the Presidential Commission for the Study of Bioethical Issues (2011) concluded that the scientists involved in this research violated the ethical standards of the time, going to great lengths to keep their experiments secret while still obtaining funding from high level authorities who should have halted the research. Almost 800 of the former research subjects and their families are pursuing legal action and demanding compensation in both the United States and Guatemala, with no resolution to date (Reverby 2016). The United States was hardly the only powerful entity sponsoring ethically fraught research; for example, in the 1950s, a dangerous and largely ineffectual trypanosomiasis vaccine made by a French pharmaceutical company was the basis of a coercive campaign in multiple African colonies (see chapter 1).

Seeking to prevent such violations, ethical guidelines have been produced by the World Medical Association (Helsinki Declaration, revised in 2013), the Council for International Organizations of Medical Sciences (most recent biomedical revision 2016, epidemiology revision in 2009), UNESCO's World Commission on the Ethics of Scientific Knowledge and Technology (1997), and the African Union (2003 Protocol to the African Charter on Human and Peoples' Rights on the Rights of Women in Africa), as well as by many national health ministries.

Yet ethical concerns abound. The proportion of clinical trials conducted in LMICs rose from 10% in 1991 to 62% in 2010, in part because in 2008 the US Food and Drug Administration withdrew its compliance with the Helsinki Declaration and its restrictions around placebo use, post-study treatment access, public disclosures, and compensation for study-related harms (Burgess and Pretorius 2012). Moreover, rising costs and restrictions on R&D in HICs have made it increasingly attractive for pharmaceutical companies to conduct drug trials in locales where expenses are low, the length of the trial may be reduced, and administrative oversight is relatively lax (though regulatory and ethical restrictions have begun to tighten in many LMICs). Rates of certain diseases (e.g., HIV) are higher in LMICs than HICs, making it easier to reach required study sample sizes and lowering costs (Okonta 2014), important considerations to be sure, also for publicly-funded research. But "offshoring" has turned LMIC-based research into an attractive "cheap bargain" for a profit-maximizing industry that spends US$80–90 billion annually on clinical trials (Durisch and Gex 2013). As such, issues of adequate ethical oversight and study monitoring, including ensuring informed consent, are critical (PHM et al. 2014): arguably there should be stringent justification for conducting pharmaceutical trials in LMICs, especially when only a fraction of the local population might benefit from the results, and study sponsors leave little or nothing behind in terms of health system infrastructure or access to medications.

In the mid-1990s, a series of US government and UNAIDS-funded experiments focused in sub-Saharan Africa sought to determine whether there were less expensive ways than established HIC standards of in utero AZT administration to reduce vertical transmission of HIV. Half of the 12,000 pregnant women participants received AZT in varying dosages and for varying lengths of time, and half received an inert placebo. When the study came to light, critics demanded that it be halted on ethical grounds, given existing evidence of AZT's efficacy (albeit with a different regimen) and arguing that hundreds of babies would needlessly contract HIV (Lurie and Wolfe 1997). Although considered a question of equipoise by the US National Institutes of Health and Centers for Disease Control and Prevention, which sponsored the research—they argued employing placebos was the only way to obtain quick, inexpensive, reliable results and most of the women would not have had AZT access outside of the trial (Varmus and Satcher 1997)—subsequent studies were compelled to discontinue use of placebos.

Private pharmaceutical companies continue to operate similarly unethical overseas clinical trials, subject to less public oversight. For example, a mid-1990s study carried out by Pfizer on a meningitis drug in Nigeria—amid a government-MSF treatment campaign—failed to obtain ethical clearance or informed consent, taking advantage of the desperation of the local population and abandoning the community after the trial was over despite the ongoing epidemic (Okonta 2014). As recently as 2010, a schizophrenia drug trial conducted by Merck in several LMICs withdrew all current treatments—replacing them with either the study drug or a placebo—jeopardizing the health and well-being of both research subjects and their communities (Durisch and Gex 2013).

The main mechanisms for applying ethical guidelines are ethical research committees (ECs) or institutional review boards (IRBs), which decide if the proposed research violates the rights of subjects. Problems abound: ECs may be composed of fellow researchers who are more sympathetic to researchers than the rights of subjects; in small institutions, committee members may be collaborators with proposal authors; EC members may not be adequately trained; ECs may lack representatives of the subjects' background; or they may be thousands of miles away from the context of the research (Durisch and Gex 2013). Whether in HICs or LMICs, ECs often neither consider Indigenous ethics around community governance nor reflect Indigenous conceptions of health or promote self-determination. Moreover, many communities never benefit from the research (Minaya and Roque 2015).

Furthermore, IRBs in various LMICs are overwhelmed by the number of applications they are asked to review, a reality that some foreign companies abuse to conduct research without appropriate oversight (PHM et al. 2014). EC approval, though important in terms of patient protection, may become just another way for HIC private market actors to penetrate LMICs.

The practice of compensating study participants may also compromise informed consent in poor communities (in HICs and LMICs alike), serving as an inducement to participate (Snyder 2012). Trials may constitute the only way patients can access treatment for their conditions and thus can exploit their vulnerability (Wemos Foundation 2010). Additionally, some trials offer only limited and unsustainable access to interventions after clinical trials end: either drugs and devices become exorbitantly expensive or the country regulatory authority does not approve them. The importance of protecting the rights of the "researched" extends to taking into account the power differential between researchers and those researched, language differences, literacy levels, the impact of patriarchy on women participants' ability to provide truly informed consent, and other matters (PHM et al. 2014).

Important as are issues of locally grounded, equitably directed, ethical research, they remain insufficient to address the principal global health problems. As attention to global health research mounts, it is high time that critical political economy of health questions become priorities (Kickbusch 2016). Ongoing research—and application of findings—around the impact of skewed political, social, and economic power across the world (Hanefeld 2016), as well as how some countries have struggled to challenge these lopsided power relations, is crucial. One approach might entail research on the building of healthy societies, especially regarding how some LMICs have fruitfully integrated public health with equitable investments in housing, education, neighborhoods, and secure employment, undergirded by overall efforts at fair societal distribution of power and resources.

This is not merely a question of adding a few more variables and continuing prior lines of research. To begin there must be "political articulation of an issue, and collective mobilization based on such an articulation" (Askheim, Heggen, and Engebretsen 2016, p. 117), deriving from the reality that global health is a contested field, with contrasting ideologies shaping distinct research questions and resultant policies and practical approaches.

PEPFAR, and the Gates Foundation (chapters 4, 11, and 13) continue to operate on this premise.

Ongoing Challenges

Amplifying the constraints of dominant approaches to global health are a set of ongoing challenges raised throughout the text. One issue has to do with global governance for health, an arena that offers the potential to improve the coordination, representativeness, and fairness of current global health and development institutional and decisionmaking arrangements. However, the proliferation and penetration into the global health arena of powerful non-state actors, especially corporations and large philanthropies, poses a threat to democratic governance of WHO and global health writ large, perpetuating donor-driven agendas that have been repeatedly critiqued by the G-77, the Paris Declaration, public interest NGOs, social movements, and many others (see chapters 2–4). Rather than uncritically celebrating the infusion of funds into global health over recent years, it is essential to ask why these monies are being invested and how they are shaping global health activities.

A political economy approach also helps to identify, at a theoretical level, variables that influence health and health inequities and to translate them into data that are collected and monitored in support of efforts to modify and transform global, national, and local policies to enhance health equity. Many countries lack adequate civil registration systems to collect vital statistics (foremost, births and deaths), there is uneven quality of population health data collected through censuses and surveys, and major deficiencies in cause of death (especially in LICs) and morbidity data (globally). To be sure, data collection is more than a technical exercise or challenge. It is permeated by political and ideological agendas around generation of and access to data: identifying and addressing health inequities is circumscribed by what (and who) is counted and not counted, who controls information, and how it is disseminated (see chapter 5).

Likewise, mapping the distribution of morbidity and mortality is both a technical and political activity. One challenge is tracking patterns by setting and over the lifecourse, as we do in chapter 6, and health concerns that are specific to or pronounced in particular groups, including women, men, LGBTQIA, people living with disabilities, and Indigenous populations.

Another challenge is transcending the traditional dichotomy of communicable versus noncommunicable (chronic) diseases, which explains little about the conditions that produce disease or even the very nature of communicability or chronicity. Instead, we employ a political economy of disease typology: diseases of marginalization and deprivation (e.g., diarrhea, malaria, and respiratory infections); diseases of modernization and work (e.g., cardiovascular disease, cancer, and road traffic deaths and injury); diseases of both marginalization and modernization (e.g., diabetes, tuberculosis, and HIV); and diseases of emerging (global) social and economic patterns (e.g., Zika and influenza). Rather than distinguishing between chronic and infectious diseases—a misleading divisory line since some chronic diseases are infectious (e.g., cervical cancer due to human papillomavirus [HPV]) and vice versa (e.g., HIV and tuberculosis [TB]) and because there is much shared underlying etiology across these categories—our typology relates patterns of disease, disability, and death to the larger political economy order that spans countries of different income levels and development trajectories.

Related to this is how the global health arena addresses the SDOH and health inequities, beyond a rhetorical or superficial level. We grapple with this issue in chapter 7, using SDOH to operationalize chapter 3's critical political economy of global health framework. We examine how health and disease are produced (determined) at multiple, co existing levels: historical, social, economic, and political contexts (including colonialism, the trade and production regime, the distribution of wealth, and class, race, and gender-based power arrangements and social structures); societal governance and social policies (democratic processes, welfare state regimes, conditions related to migration, poverty, education, work, environment, and public health); and living conditions (neighborhood, housing, and nutrition). For example, we show the interaction between particular agents of disease and death—be they chemical exposures, microbes, weapons, narcotics, or unhealthy foods and beverages—and the societal circumstances that shape differential exposure to them and their varied consequences based on class and occupation, gender, race/ethnicity, work and neighborhood factors, and governance and policy contexts. Drawing from eco-social theory, we explore how these synchronous levels and the intersectionality of SDOH over the lifecourse lead to the embodiment of health and illness in individuals and manifest in patterns of health inequities.

Here we stress both between-country *and* within-country inequities—for example, the enormous and enduring health inequities between dominant and Indigenous populations in country after country, linked to historical and ongoing internal colonization—and how societal factors shape health at every level, from discriminatory power structures to social policies, resource access, daily living conditions, and ultimately evidenced in shorter, sicker lives for Indigenous groups worldwide.

Public health and health care systems are important SDOH and their absence can contribute to global health problems. Certainly the global community's neglect of health care system investment in the face of high-profile disease campaigns is reprehensible. Moreover, though health care systems are largely a national concern governed by domestic politics, they remain heavily influenced by the larger world order, whether due to loan conditionalities requiring reduced public spending, trade and investment treaties favoring privatization of social services, or illicit financial outflows depleting national treasuries (see chapters 3, 9, and 11).

Global health activities may also be directly responsible for health care system deficiencies. A notable illustration: global health initiatives are typically siloed from health care systems, facilitating donor monitoring and evaluation while fragmenting policies and diverting resources, infrastructure, and personnel. In most HICs, by contrast, disease control campaigns are integrated into primary care and overall health care systems, averting these problems. Global health donors whose activities weaken health systems arguably should be held accountable for this problem.

Another challenge has to do with generations of global health policy prescriptions for health care reform (see chapter 12), which have often had the effect of decreasing accessibility, quality, affordability, equity, coherence, and comprehensiveness. The latest reform flavor advocated by the World Bank, WHO, and the Rockefeller Foundation, among others, is universal health coverage (UHC). UHC sounds promising but addresses only the question of coverage, not the other principles listed here, and indeed may exacerbate them, for example, by only offering a reduced package of services, lowering quality by introducing competing private providers, and further fragmenting and stratifying coverage.

This points to an overarching concern around the dominant global health arena's cooptation of social justice-oriented concepts (invoking social justice principles without practicing them or infusing them into research and work), such as gender empowerment, community participation, sustainability, equity, and so on (and even solidarity and political economy). In this context, the long struggle for universal health systems—that is, unified, accessible, equitable, and high quality publicly financed, national health systems—has been coopted and distilled into a market-oriented approach that expands population coverage (and insurance revenues) without the elements integral to the full meaning of universal health care (Birn, Nervi, and Siqueira 2016). In sum, a social justice approach to global health also rests on vigilance around "mainstreaming" of progressive ideas—and being alert to their appropriation, with prior intent changed.

Among the most widely shared, if at times contentious, rationales for global health relates to the humanitarian impulse to address health under crisis situations. Many people are drawn into this field through desire to provide first-hand assistance (clinical, logistical, advocacy, organizing) to deal with the health consequences of ecologic disasters, food insecurity and famine, violence and war, and complex humanitarian emergencies in conflict and/or politically unstable settings, such as the plight of soaring refugee and displaced populations. Although to some it is unthinkable to critique humanitarianism, others argue that humanitarian assistance (e.g. food aid and war relief) ought to be subject to a political economy analysis to examine the extent to which aid agencies (inadvertently) contribute to the proliferation of humanitarian emergencies by enabling governments and corporate interests to continue "business as usual" (including promoting and profiting from militarism) and by not sufficiently advocating for transforming the conditions that lead to war and other crises in the first place.

As novelist Teju Cole (2012) remarks on this controversial point:

> there is much more to doing good work than 'making a difference.' There is the principle of first do no harm. There is the idea that those who are being helped ought to be consulted over the matters that concern them . . . [and that beyond the immediate urgency of] hungry mouths, child soldiers, or raped civilians, there are more complex and more widespread problems. There are serious problems of governance, of infrastructure, of democracy, and of law and order. These problems are neither

> simple in themselves nor are they reducible to slogans. Such problems are both intricate and intensely local.

This is certainly a tall order for humanitarian workers who are already sacrificing much, but perhaps a fitting quid pro quo for witnessing and mitigating the suffering of others.

Moving to the environmental domain, while the issue of climate change has belatedly captured mounting global attention, there has not been concomitant concern with the even larger problems of environmental degradation: resource depletion and the contamination of the air we breathe, the water we drink, the food we eat, and the places where we live. These, in turn, lead to direct and indirect health effects: cardiovascular disease, respiratory infections, cancers, waterborne diseases, loss of food sovereignty, and even forced population displacement (Birn et al. 2015). A challenge going forward is how the global health community will analyze and address the link between the environment and health issues and the associated underlying forces including: global capitalism and market-based, consumption-driven economies; industrial production; and polluting industries such as energy, mining, and agribusiness.

The greatest underlying global health challenge of our era is, of course, the role of the current political economy order: the neoliberal phase of global capitalism (see chapter 9). The pathways that tie neoliberal globalization to patterns of ill health and death are complex and at times seem so unfathomable that they cannot be tackled. But the centrality and impact on health of the features of the contemporary world order, from structural adjustment programs in LMICs following the 1980s debt crisis to the post-2008 financial crisis austerity agendas in HICs—and from trade and investment agreements to corporate power and tax abuse—is undeniable (Schrecker 2016). In particular, global health actors are insufficiently attentive to documenting, decrying, and redressing the extraordinarily deleterious impact of TNC-controlled extractive, food, and manufacturing sectors. Bolstered by neoliberal globalization, TNCs, national elites, and their government allies have ratcheted down environmental regulations, consumer protections, labor standards, and occupational safety and health, aggravating precarious and dangerous work conditions across the world, social and economic inequality, and civil strife.

Health and human rights approaches offer some prospects for addressing these issues (Box 14-2), but the challenges remain gargantuan.

Points of Inspiration

As we send this edition of the textbook to press—amid a global refugee crisis, repression and seemingly intractable wars in the Middle East and Central Africa, political volatility across Latin America, spikes in xenophobia and racism in Europe and North America, repressive economic policies and militarism in which corporate elites and powerful countries have a heavy hand, and yawning inequities within South and East Asia and across the world—there appear to be countless reasons for dismay. But the tendency to despair might be kept at bay by notable examples of health and social justice activism under equally or even more challenging historical moments. Presuming that many readers are relatively young and undoubtedly energetic, we hope you will take inspiration from examples highlighted here (and drawing especially from chapters 9, 10, and 13) pointing to the importance of persistence in the fight for health justice.

Throughout the text we have incorporated experiences of movements and organizations struggling for global health and social justice. For instance, in chapter 7 we explore various Health in All Policies approaches to achieving health equity (ensuring that health and health inequity are tackled through every dimension of societal decisionmaking). Examples include Scotland's radical critique of neoliberal macroeconomic policy buttressed by government protagonism around redistributive measures, and an informal Mombasa (Kenya) settlement's intersectoral commitment to reducing child malnutrition and inequity by engaging with health care, education, agriculture, gender, child and social development, and water constituencies, creating a national model for Kenya.

In chapter 9 we profile various ongoing social movements, organizational, and governmental struggles against neoliberal globalization. These efforts include: resistance to water privatization in Bolivia and Indonesia; public-interest NGOs in Canada fighting to ban asbestos, and global-level efforts against unethical

Box 14-2 Health and Human Rights

The health and human rights movement arose in the early 1990s in response to the AIDS epidemic. Calling for broad structural issues—such as poverty, discrimination, and accessible health care systems—to be addressed in order to curb the spread of HIV, health and human rights advocates sought to transcend dominant biomedical and behavioral approaches to the epidemic. Health and human rights, according to its progenitors, are linked via three pathways (Mann et al. 1999): (1) Health affects human rights—health policies and programs can respect or violate people's rights in their design and implementation; (2) Human rights affect health—violations to human rights can have devastating, even fatal, effects with both short- and long-term consequences; conversely, upholding human rights can improve health; and (3) There is a synergistic relationship between health and human rights: the protection and promotion of one is not only related to the protection and promotion of the other, but dependent upon it.

In recent years, there has been increasing incorporation of a human rights-based approach "into the implementation of policies, programs, projects, and other health-related interventions with a view to enhancing effectiveness" (Hunt, Yamin, and Bustreo 2015, p. 1). This operationalization of the principles outlined in human rights treaties and declarations (and the WHO Constitution) as applied to health and its determinants—bolstered by advocacy for and monitoring of governmental responsibility for assuring these rights (Gruskin and Tarantola 2013)—offers a useful framing of health and social justice values. However, these treaties are not universally ratified, and enforceability rests largely at the national level, with few repercussions when they are not enforced. Where international human rights treaties are ratified and/or included in domestic constitutions *and* there are effective and willing judiciaries, social justice movements—together with political parties representative of worker and peasant interests, and political systems that do not privilege moneyed interests over others—play a key role in the realization of rights (Schuftan, Turiano, and Shukla 2009).

The main international reference document on the right to health is Article 12 of the International Covenant on Economic, Social, and Cultural Rights. The UN's General Comment 14 (2000) interprets Article 12's articulation of the "right of everyone to the enjoyment of the highest attainable standard of physical and mental health" as encompassing both the right to health care and rights to underlying determinants of health including water, basic sanitation, food, housing, and safe and fair working environments. States have the duty to respect, protect, and fulfill these rights, allowing for a *progressive* realization (i.e., incremental steps) of some of these rights if limited resources affect the ability and speed at which rights can be realized. An important caveat is that resource constraints do not justify taking *regressive* measures in the realization of rights.

Table 14-1 summarizes certain government and international obligations on the right to health outlined in General Comment 14. Minimum core obligations of the right to health should be guaranteed by states irrespective of resource constraints (i.e., progressive realization is not enough) (Forman et al. 2013). General Comment 14 also outlines which state actions (or inactions) can be considered violations of the right to health. Violating the obligation to respect may occur through discriminatory denial of access to health services. Violation of the obligation to protect may transpire through failure to adequately regulate corporations, such as mining and energy TNCs, so as to prevent them from harming health via environmental degradation. Violation of the obligation to fulfill could stem from failing to implement a national health policy that ensures the right to health for all or from misallocating public resources in a way that jeopardizes socially excluded groups.

Table 14-1 **Summary of State Obligations with Respect to the Right to Health**

Obligations	State Measures
Minimum national core obligations	• Ensure at a minimum, provision and realization of these core obligations: - Non-discriminatory access to health care facilities, goods, and services, including for socially excluded groups - Access to nutritional and safe food and freedom from hunger - Safe drinking water and basic sanitation - Basic shelter and housing - Access to essential medicines as defined in the WHO Action Programme on Essential Drugs - Equitable distribution of health care resources - National public health strategy with right to health indicators and benchmarks
Selected international obligations	• Respect the right to health in other countries and prevent third party violations via legal or political measures. • Ensure that international agreements do not negatively affect the right to health. • Ensure that lending policies and agreements, and structural adjustment programs of IFIs (IMF, World Bank, regional development banks) are in accordance with protecting the right to health.

Source: General Comment 14 (2000)

While General Comment 14 interprets the right to health as comprising a range of SDOH, many other health-related rights have significant health and health equity consequences without falling within the purview of the right to health. These include: the right to education, an adequate standard of living, social security, civil participation, the benefits of scientific progress, and protection from all forms of violence and discrimination (see chapter 7).

Emerging social rights jurisprudence in South Africa and various Latin American countries is showing that on one hand health rights are increasingly enforceable, and on the other, the use of litigation as a means for realizing rights necessitates careful evaluation to ensure that unequal access to justice does not exclude people who most need their social and economic rights claims addressed (Yamin 2011).

Litigation is not the only channel for promoting human rights at the domestic policy level. Notwithstanding political instability, since 2000 Nepal has implemented explicit rights-based maternal and child policies around safe abortion, neonatal health, paid maternal leave, and gender equality (Bustreo et al. 2013). In 2015 Nepal adopted its first democratic Constitution, which recognizes the right to free basic health services, and equal access to health care, clean drinking water and sanitation, safe motherhood, and reproductive health, as well as health, social, economic, and other rights of socially excluded groups including *Dalits* (the most excluded and discriminated group based on Nepal's centuries-old caste system), Indigenous persons, people with disabilities, and sexual and gender minorities (Simkhada et al. 2015). Though ongoing challenges remain, infusion of human rights principles into Nepalese social policy, influenced by international declarations (e.g., 1978 *Declaration of Alma Ata*) and social movements, has contributed to improvements in women's and children's health, with infant mortality halved from 59.6 to 29.4 per 1,000 live births between 2000 and 2015 (WHO 2016).

Human rights approaches, when anchored by broad social and political movements, can be well aligned to the political economy perspective portrayed in this book. Humanitarian organizations such as Oxfam International and CARE also integrate rights-based approaches into their work through concepts of "dignity," "injustice," "sustainable livelihoods," and "non-discrimination" (Gruskin, Bogecho, and Ferguson 2010).

Yet global health actors also risk distilling the "right to health" into a "right to health care" because improvements in the broad determinants of health may be harder to realize than the right to health care (Health and Human Rights Journal 2015). In some domains, the right to health care has been further interpreted to signify access to a particular package of biomedical technologies. Important as are access to diagnostic tools, surgery, medicines, and other treatments (Weigel et al. 2013), they constitute just one component of the right to health and ought not push out health-related economic and social rights.

Some critique health and human rights approaches for drawing heavily from Western concepts based on individual rights rather than collective needs. Others express concerns around the cooptation of human rights by mainstream development actors, including corporate interests (e.g., via the UN's Global Compact—see chapter 3). In the end, there is a certain dilemma to invoking health as a right without attention to the politics of the distribution of power and resources, returning us to the origins of health and human rights approaches.

TNC marketing of infant formula; plus experiences of Brazilian and Indian governments challenging monopolistic patent regimes. We also cover political movements contesting austerity, the alternative of worker-run cooperatives, and worker activism against corporate impunity.

Not all such efforts reach a felicitous outcome and advances may be tenuous. Brazil's 1988 Constitutional guarantee of the right to health care (see chapter 11) grew out of decades of struggle against dictatorship: in recent decades Brazil has built a national health care system widely admired in LMICs, combatted poverty through cash transfers (see chapter 13), and enhanced rights based on gender and race. However, this has taken place in the context of a capitalist, highly unequal society with entrenched elite interests unwilling to cede financial and social power. As resources for social programs began to dry up, particularly after the collapse of oil prices in 2014, the unmet expectations of the population led to mounting protests, fueled by soaring costs of living and accusations of political corruption. Capitalizing on the unrest, elites eager to dismantle the public health care system and other social entitlements orchestrated a dubious impeachment of the President. As soon as it could, the new government began attacking the health care system, claiming that the Constitutional right to health was too expensive to fulfill. That a health care system that took years to build could begin to be dismantled in a matter of days points to the centrality not just of public policies but of the overall political and economic order: Brazil's long struggles fell short of achieving a profound political transformation. The crisis may yet serve as an opportunity, but it is too early to know what shape this might take.

Some more sanguine experiences are emerging around protecting health from global environmental degradation and contamination (see chapter 10). These occur at multiple levels of change: global and regional responses such as agreements banning harmful chemicals and treaties controlling export and disposal of hazardous waste; national environmental regulations (e.g., limiting deforestation) and standards (e.g., air quality); and local energy conservation efforts. Perhaps portending the greatest transformation are a wide range of environmental justice actors and movements: mobilization to conserve natural resources (e.g., Pakistan's Indus Consortium), preserve food sovereignty (e.g., La Via Campesina), confront mining and oil TNCs contaminating local environments and committing human rights violations (e.g., in Indonesia, Ecuador, and Nigeria and via MiningWatch Canada), protest weak government environmental protections, and pressure large academic, government, and private entities to divest from fossil fuels (e.g., 350.org movement).

Most importantly, chapter 13 showcases the making of healthy societies across diverse settings. Prime illustrations are the integrated political, social, and public health approaches of high-income welfare states, such as Sweden, and the even more remarkable LMIC exemplars of Costa Rica, Cuba, Uruguay, Sri Lanka, and Kerala state, India. In these places, decades-long political and social struggles have led to widely-embraced public, universal, and inclusive policies around education, health, work, and well-being. Some of these settings have sought to upend social and political power structures, others have been engaged in more gradual transformations, and various are pursuing post-industrial, more environmentally sound economic policies. The envy of some far wealthier societies, LMIC welfare states remain fragile, subject to both domestic constraints and global political and economic pressures.

Another point of departure for progressive health efforts is health promotion (articulated in the 1986 Ottawa Charter) espousing a social justice and participatory approach to addressing the factors underlying health. These ideas have inspired Health in All Policies and Healthy Cities efforts, characterized by green space, urban agriculture, improved water and sanitation, and accessible public transport—in locales as varied as Bogotá and Tehran. We also cover the viability of alternative paradigms of *Buen Vivir* and degrowth for generating healthy and environmentally harmonious societies.

In addition, we cover social medicine-inspired efforts that demonstrate how progressive taxation, universal social programs, and entitlements prioritizing the most oppressed groups (Mexico City), and run by community-level social policy committees (*Misión Barrio Adentro* in Venezuela) can improve the health and well-being of socially excluded groups. The latter draws from social justice forms of South–South collaboration—that is, when LMICs with shared political and social values cooperate symmetrically with one another—as an alternative to dominant patterns of aid (Box 14-3).

Box 14-3 Social Justice-Oriented South-South Health Diplomacy and Cooperation

Although most global health efforts have long reflected and entrenched dominant political and economic interests, contrasting health and social justice-oriented approaches also have a considerable historical trajectory. A notable past example was the medical solidarity provided by health worker brigades from around the world to democratic forces fighting fascism during the 1930s Spanish Civil War (Lear 2013). In the 1950s and 1960s Third World countries took on this mantle through the non-aligned movement challenging neocolonialism in aid, demanding "respect for national sovereignty," and calling for a New International Economic Order, an idea embedded in the 1978 Alma-Ata declaration (see chapter 2).

More recent attention to South–South cooperation (SSC) as a form of "soft power" health diplomacy does not always evoke the social justice dimensions of these earlier examples. Indeed, focus on the role of so-called BRICS countries (Brazil, Russia, India, China, South Africa), highlights the geographic (and income level) provenance of these "emerging" donors (Bliss 2013) more than the nature of their engagement. A frequent assumption, often advanced by BRICS countries themselves, is that SSC differs in form and orientation from North–South cooperation (NSC) by its very "Southern-ness" (Harmer and Buse 2014), that is, entailing the interactions of formerly colonized, dominated, or "underdeveloped" countries that operate on a non-imperial, non-hierarchical, ethical basis (Cabral, Russo, and Weinstock 2014).

Though societies with common histories of oppression may be better able to identify and address their own population health problems, without having to enter into the unequal power relationships inherent to North–South cooperation, this contention should not be taken at face value (Bond and Garcia 2015). There are also self-interested motives with SSC apparent in, for instance, Chinese and Brazilian oil, mining, and construction interests in Africa, South and Southeast Asia, and Latin America: these need to be scrutinized when assessing the true nature of SSC health projects.

Both countries have pursued mainstream *and* solidarity-oriented SSC. China sent medical teams to decolonized Algeria and in support of Nyerere's African socialist efforts in Tanzania as far back as the 1960s (see chapter 2), even as its current cooperation goes hand in hand with primary resource extraction. Brazil's structural cooperation approach has involved capacity-building, health systems support, and "horizontal" dialogue and decisionmaking with national and international counterparts, particularly within Latin America and in Portuguese-speaking countries in sub-Saharan Africa (Ferreira et al. 2016). Dozens of projects in Africa—many led by Fiocruz, Brazil's famed national health research and training institute—range from training programs for physicians and other health care personnel (e.g., lab technicians) to technical support for HIV, TB, and malaria programs, donation of HIV drugs, and establishment of an ARV factory in Mozambique (Santana 2011; Roa and Silva 2015). While Brazil has sought to challenge the dominant political order framing aid—prioritizing the interests and needs of LMICs and refraining from incorporating conditionalities into its own aid—its aggressive economic interests in African mining, construction, and other industries operate parallel to health diplomacy (Garcia and Kato 2015; Ventura 2013), just as is the case with NSC. Nonetheless within Latin America, Brazil's leadership in UNASUR around disease surveillance, health human resources policy, universal health systems development, access to medications, and policy cooperation around SDOH and health promotion (e.g., unified regional deliberations with WHO) has been carried out on more equal footing (Buss and Ferreira 2011).

To distinguish South–South cooperation that is truly social justice-oriented, guided by shared political values around social rights, shared power, redistribution, and solidarity with social and political movements toward health equity, the notion of social justice-oriented SSC (SJSSC, [Birn, Muntaner, and Afzal 2016]) implies a departure from prevailing models of international cooperation. These more solidarity-inspired forms of global health diplomacy, which contest the dominant, self-interested, and "realist" geopolitical-economic forces propelling the field, emerged particularly in Latin America (Riggirozzi 2015). A confluence of factors enabled this development: the (re-)election over the past decades of progressive and social democratic parties on welfare regime-building and social rights platforms (Fleury 2010; Mahmood and Muntaner 2013), coupled with economic growth based on rising oil prices in certain MICs, such as Brazil and Venezuela (growth that has now stalled, and in conjunction with political turmoil, is putting the future of these efforts in jeopardy). In sub-Saharan Africa, too, growing interest in health diplomacy stresses regional unity, an ethic of liberation, and equitable forms of development, though new possibilities of SSC suggest the need for vigilance around a "disguised role of private actors" (Loewenson, Modisenyane, and Pearcey 2014, p. 1).

Cuba is one of the most longstanding and active proponents of bilateral and triangular SJSSC (and arguably the most consistently solidarity-oriented): since the 1960s over 135,000 Cuban medical professionals have served abroad in South Africa, Haiti, Pakistan (after the disastrous 2005 earthquake), Angola, Guatemala, Bolivia, Sierra Leone (2014–2015 Ebola response), and many other countries. Remarkably, all of this has been carried out with minimal financial resources given Cuba's small economy. Like any such program, Cuba's health cooperation offers political advantages (Feinsilver 2010). Yet most countries it has helped, including Haiti, provide no payment or quid pro quo for services (Beldarraín Chaple 2006), even as more recent examples of thousands of Cuban medical personnel working in Venezuela and Brazil have been in exchange for oil and currency (in the context of recent decades of economic difficulties in Cuba). Cuba's placement of doctors "where no doctor has gone before" has made a significant impact in communities around the world (Huish 2013). This is complemented by Cuba's health care workforce training effort at Havana's Latin American School of Medicine, which has granted full scholarships to students of low-income backgrounds from over 80 LMICs and the United States (see chapters 11 and 13).

Despite often purveying similar forms of cooperation as NSC and SSC in terms of health personnel training, human resources, health care equipment and infrastructure, distribution of medication, and surgical interventions, SJSSC also places greater emphasis on PHC and international policy activism (such as against monopolistic patent protections).

Moreover, SJSSC differs from mainstream development assistance for health on at least three counts: first, it decreases dependence on aid channels from HICs and multilateral agencies, which constrain sovereignty by attaching conditions to receipt of aid. SJSSC does not dictate unilaterally the terms of health and development cooperation, instead responding to national and local demands for equity and drawing from a strong emphasis on social rights, involving legal obligations and constitutional protections for health-related human rights and local participatory democracy in areas including public provision of PHC (Medicus Mundi 2010). Aid is a priori invited on equal terms: with power and resource differentials between donor and recipient much reduced, aid is turned into genuine horizontal cooperation or exchange. Second, much SJSSC aid seeks to be transformative, for example in building social infrastructure, training PHC practitioners, and working hand in hand with government agencies to create lasting and equitable means of addressing essential needs. Third, even while sometimes convening international partners through "triangular" cooperation, many of these efforts are community based: not only are priorities defined through local agenda-setting, but local populations are integral to shaping cooperative activities through their ideas, labor, and decisionmaking.

There are also examples of social-justice oriented NSC, including organizations working in transnational solidarity (e.g., the Hesperian Foundation, which produces multilingual PHC-oriented guides for community health workers and activists around the world) and Scandinavian countries that historically supported PHC efforts. A prime illustration derives from Nicaragua in the 1980s. After the 1979 Sandinista revolution ousted the longtime dictatorial Somoza dynasty, USAID, the IMF, the World Bank, and the Inter-American Development Bank pulled out to protest the country's new leftist administration (which subsequently won [and later lost] democratic elections). Even as US-backed rebels were waging a destructive civil war against the Sandinista government, cooperation from Sweden, among other countries, supported the hallmark expansion of PHC units across the country (White and Dijkstra 2003).

A SOCIAL JUSTICE APPROACH TO PRACTICING GLOBAL HEALTH: INDIVIDUALS, ORGANIZATIONS, AND THE LOGIC OF THE WORLD ORDER

Key Questions:

- How can global health efforts contribute to social justice and address the roots of health inequities?
- What are the connections among personal motivations, institutional goals, and the geopolitical context of global health?
- What alternatives to mainstream global health help foster bona fide cooperation in terms of shared social justice values?

> The secret to change is to focus all your energy not on fighting the old, but on building the new.
>
> —Socrates
>
> First they ignore you, then they laugh at you, then they fight you, then you win.
>
> —Mahatma Gandhi

A society's model of justice determines how resources and burdens are allocated and, hence, whether the population's health is protected via individual responsibility (market justice) or—fundamentally countering this approach—through collective action (social justice) (Beauchamp 1976). Transposed to the world order, (neoliberal) capitalist ideology holds that the market pursuit of profits under capitalism, locally and globally, is the engine of human well-being. Counterposing this stance is equitably allocating resources according to need (Reid-Henry 2016). But "just giv[ing] money to the poor" (Hanlon, Barrientos, and Hulme 2010) to tackle extreme povery and attenuate economic inequality does not go far enough.

Indeed, social justice moves well beyond distribution of resources according to moral fairness or even ensuring rights and opportunities. As political philosopher Iris Marion Young (2011, p. 16) has argued, "The concepts of domination and oppression, rather than the concept of distribution, should be the starting point for a conception of social justice" because of the centrality of processes (not only certain end results, such as income distribution) and the rules, relations, and institutional contexts in which distribution occurs. This means that it is not enough to guarantee rights or access to material goods as per a distributive paradigm, but that transforming the relations of power among social groups and the institutional arrangements in which power is wielded are central to pursuing and achieving social justice.

Health and social justice-oriented beliefs, movements, and activities have been explored throughout this textbook. Here we consolidate discussion of these efforts based on individual aspirations, organizational aims, and the possibilities of the world order. It is important to note that most global health training programs focus on mainstream, largely technical approaches, often paying only minor attention to the political economy and social justice perspectives presented here. We invite students to encourage their current or prospective institutions to cover (or require!) critical political economy of global health framings and approaches in courses (or better yet make critical political economy central to global health training), so that they do not finish their academic careers thinking that health aid provided via donor organizations is THE solution to global and local health problems and health inequity.

Social justice approaches do not exclude dominant global health research, interventions, institutional roles, or humanitarian impulses, but they imply that each of these be carried out in an entirely different way, one that places the struggle against oppression at the heart of solidarity efforts, putting the needs of the majority of people, and those most vulnerable, first (Biehl and Petryna 2013).

As emphasized in various chapters, the struggle for health and social justice rests on collective action by citizens, governments, civil society organizations, social movements, and international agencies representing and responding to the needs of workers, peasants, Indigenous and racially-discriminated groups, children, youth, LGBTQIA, the elderly, people with disabilities, women in the home, community, and workplace, and people lacking homes and adequate income—against the concentrated power of social and economic elites, corporate and financial interests, and their political associates. Striving politically—at local, national, and transnational levels—for equitable distribution of power and resources and fair rules governing these arrangements are thus central to human progress everywhere.

As we have discussed, in mainstream global health approaches "experts" go to look, see, learn, provide some technical assistance, and then leave. By contrast, a transformative approach to global health, drawing from the principles of introspection, humility, solidarity, and commitment to health and social justice, incorporates the following elements:

1. As full an understanding as possible of the socioeconomic, cultural, and political contexts and the implications for health, SDOH, and health care services
2. A willingness to learn from local communities and local experts
3. A nonjudgmental attitude to local problems
4. A commitment to share and learn from expertise in ways that empower local people and contribute to lasting change
5. Solidarity work, which, without necessarily involving travel or "assistance" per se, may be extremely useful
6. Incorporating social justice movement building into one's work

As well, those involved in global health endeavors are encouraged to remain conscious of historical patterns and legacies, not so much because people link their ongoing oppression to the distant past but because the present conditions and realities of making a living endured by the majority of the global population (and the actions of most health and development actors) are molded by historical trajectories, from the colonial period to the Cold War and decolonization, to the more recent experience of neoliberal reforms. Indeed, those currently working in global health need to continuously bear in mind the troubling possibility that even the most well-meaning and well-informed global health efforts may perpetuate inequalities in power (and thus unintentionally contribute to health inequities) (Hanson, Harms, and Plamondon 2011). People who seek to participate in solidarity-oriented work need to be able to recognize these patterns in order to begin to break with them (Ventres and Gusoff 2014).

It is also important to be cognizant of the potentially high personal costs of speaking out, that is, articulating social justice-oriented transformative positions or being involved in organizations that challenge mainstream global health. These costs may include institutional isolation, missed funding and work opportunities, public humiliation, or in extreme cases under authoritarian and repressive regimes, incarceration or worse (Birn and Brown 2013). Paying such a high price is not common, even as it is possible: working with supportive movements and organizations (e.g., the Asociación Latinoamericana de Medicina Social [ALAMES]; see chapter 13) can help shield individuals from the gravest dangers.

In sum, how can people concerned with global health and social justice reconcile the larger world order with the reality of practicing global health day-to-day in an organization? Approaches include:

- Working with/for an organization in whose long-term vision and modus operandi you believe

Many progressive-minded agencies are listed in chapter 4. For example, Doctors for Global Health goes only where it is invited, and uses the concepts of "health as reconciliation" and "anti-colonization" as its guiding principles when setting up cooperative projects in marginalized communities (Smith, Kasper, and Holtz 2013) (Box 14-4).

- Working from within a mainstream well-established organization, pushing it toward more socially just global health approaches and practices

Those who work for mainline agencies can play an important role in advocating that their employers: practice symmetrical and pro-equity agenda-setting; abide by their articulated missions; and vocally decry the deleterious health effects of larger political economy forces, such as militarism and harmful investment agreements. Crucially, civil society alone cannot be responsible for ensuring that public and humanitarian institutions fulfill their missions and eschew conflicts of interest. Those working in UN and other multilateral or bilateral agencies or at universities (especially well-funded HIC institutions) arguably have a special obligation to serve the public given their privileged positions. For instance, the struggle against unaccountable private sector actors at WHO has been spearheaded by current and former WHO employees, together with public-interest civil society activists and researchers (Velásquez and Alas 2016).

- Acting in solidarity with a social-justice movement to transform ideologies and practices related to global health, locally and in the larger political economy order

For decades, grassroots movements worldwide have been tackling the negative consequences of neoliberal globalization with the support of committed transnational allies. La Via Campesina, representing 200 million peasants, agricultural workers, and smallholders from over 160 organizations in almost 75 countries, explicitly challenges corporate ownership and control of land, water, seeds, livestock, and biodiversity. As a vigorous voice for food sovereignty, it has been one of the most effective movements in favor of social justice for producers and against the incursion of agribusiness across the world.

In another vein, street medic groups have a long history of supporting movements that seek to transform power dynamics locally and globally, from civil rights movements to the Arab Spring (Nakad 2016). Doctors for the 99% and National Nurses United are coalitions whose members have

Box 14-4 Health Solidarity in El Salvador

The small Central American country of El Salvador suffered a brutal civil conflict from 1980 to 1992, a war largely fueled by the US's support of an oppressive government. The "scorched earth" policy of the Salvadoran military resulted in 80,000 deaths, and produced one million refugees and innumerable tortured and "disappeared" persons in a country of only 6 million people. Massive aerial bombardment and use of napalm caused severe deforestation. The Salvadoran government was responsible for grievous violations of human rights, including murderous attacks on cleric advocates of liberation theology calling for social justice for the oppressed (among those assassinated was Catholic Archbishop Arnulfo Romero). During the conflict, the health budget was cut in half and many health posts were abandoned. NGO-trained CHWs became the backbone of health care, covering approximately one third of the country. However, after the Peace Accords were signed in 1992, with the health care system in shambles, the Ministry of Health refused to hire these workers, arguing that they were communists and had been part of the insurgency (Smith-Nonini 2010).

In the mid-1990s, Doctors for Global Health (DGH) was invited by several communities in the rural region of Morazán—which had experienced extreme violence and devastation—to work with them in addressing the underlying causes of ill health. Following the principles of a community-based grassroots approach and accompaniment (working directly and in solidarity with local communities), DGH responded to the issues and projects prioritized by the community: construction of a bridge to reduce deaths from river crossings, nutrition, soil conservation, community gardens, rehabilitation, women's rights, early childhood education, childhood preventive care, and veterinary, dental, and medical care. Clinics were built, and local health care providers now work in the area.

Since 1995, DGH has grown from a small informal group working in northeast El Salvador to a formal member-supported NGO with volunteers working together with communities in their struggles for social justice and human dignity in Guatemala, Chiapas and Oaxaca (Mexico), Uganda, Peru, Burundi, and the United States. A Salvadoran NGO was also created, Doctors for the Right to Health, which continues to work to improve the lives of the rural poor (Smith, Kasper, and Holtz 2013).

El Salvador has recently made gains in delivering comprehensive PHC, enabling maternal mortality reductions, high use of prenatal care, and declines in child and infant mortality (PHM et al. 2014). Under the remarkable leadership of Dr. María Isabel Rodríguez, the former Minister of Health under a progressive, if beleaguered, administration, El Salvador advanced a rights-based approach to health and promoted "health sovereignty" in international cooperation to ensure nationally-defined agendas for health equity (Rodríguez 2009). Yet 25 years later, and notwithstanding DGH's ongoing solidarity, the effects of civil war and societal divisions are still felt in terms of inequality, violence, and health and social infrastructure deficiencies, especially in rural areas.

provided care and worked in solidarity with the Occupy movement, among other mobilizations. Similarly, Greece's citizen-run social health clinics sprang up following mass austerity measures in 2011 that cut access to health care services; the clinics benefit from volunteer medics and international solidarity.

Inspiring as they are, these endeavors face many challenges. Although many social movements are engaged in reforming trade, aid, and debt servitude, well-established organizations usually have more resources and access to power than do social movements and can serve as influential and "respectable" advocates for change. An important caveat is that as social movements grow they may be forced to seek more stable funding. For example, the Informal Settlement Network (ISN), organized by a "bottom-up agglomeration" of urban poor groups in South Africa, addresses lack of decent housing in the context of rapidly growing settlements on the periphery of towns and cities. ISN has a local base in Durban and is also part of a global movement—the Federation of the Urban and Rural Poor (FEDUP) and Shack/Slum Dwellers International (SDI). In recent years SDI has accepted funding from several large philanthropies (e.g., Gates and Mott foundations), and while its advocacy for land and proper housing for the poor has continued, the bottom-up approach representing the demands of the urban poor is dissipating. This experience suggests a need for continuous renewal of activism.

To note, the three approaches outlined above are not mutually exclusive: you may work for a mainline organization *and* be active in a social movement, and also volunteer with a social-rights-based NGO. All are valid ways of contributing to health and social justice. That said, as you contemplate your potential or actual role in global health, it is essential to recognize the possibilities and limits of your own participation and aspirations based on critical political economy analysis. In this sense, global health may be conceived of as operating at three levels:

1. Motivations and involvement of individuals
2. Missions and actions of organizations
3. Logic and structures of the world order

The three levels operate simultaneously, but each is constrained by the next level. Individual motivations or institutional missions may conflict with the logic of global capitalism, and the impact of individuals and institutions is limited by the world order. Carried out together, efforts at each level can help in larger struggles to transform market capitalism into a world order based on a shared commitment to equitably protecting human well-being and reducing oppression according to truly democratic governance. Though individual actions by themselves cannot transcend the world order, they can contribute to changing it, in part through the formation of organizations and movements that challenge its logic and power (Box 14-5).

Individual Level: Motivations, Training, and Work Experience

Motivations

Global health encompasses a wide array of activities, from working within agencies to social and political activism "at home and transnationally" outlined ahead. Although clinical work is often highlighted

Box 14-5 Inspiring Individuals: Dr. Denis Mukwege

Translating a political economy of health approach into action can take the form of dedicated research, advocacy, teaching, and political engagement, or arise from the powerful realities of daily work. As an illustration, DRC-based gynecological surgeon Denis Mukwege has long focused on improving childbirth conditions for Congolese women to lower maternal mortality and prevent and treat the debilitating problem of obstetric fistulae. After the outbreak of the Second Congo War (see chapter 8), his hospital began to receive numerous patients who had been subject to horrific sexual violence. He and his team have treated some 40,000 women and girls who were raped and sexually brutalized, also offering legal, psychological, and social assistance. But Dr. Mukwege, the recipient of multiple human rights awards and other honors, has done far more. Risking his own life, he has become a spokesperson on the responsibility both of all Congolese men to combat sexual violence and of the international community to end the mineral-resource driven war in Eastern DRC (Right Livelihood Award 2013). As a result, Dr. Mukwege faced an assassination attempt in which his bodyguard was killed. This reveals the potential dangers of embedding medical work in a political economy framework, considered incendiary in many quarters and engendering various kinds of professional and political hostility.

in the imaginary and visual imagery of the field, working as a doctor, nurse, or medical technician is not the sole avenue to a meaningful contribution. Community organizing, social mobilization, health promotion, policy development, laboratory and social science investigation, economic analysis of the impact of trade treaties, and epidemiological research are all key roles that need to be filled, domestically and internationally.

For those with limited experience, there may be numerous personal reasons for wanting to partake in global health work: research and professional opportunities, idealism around changing the world and helping the world's poor, learning from abroad, and humanitarianism motivated by charitable or religious values. While the desire to be of service on some level may seem laudable, validating overseas engagement based on generosity and "helping" people is illusory, especially when "help" has not been sought and when it does not address the factors shaping the presumed need for help (Tiessen and Huish 2014). Key questions students and others should ask themselves include (Pinto and Upshur 2009): Is the proposed global health effort feasible, necessary, sustainable, and justified? What are the viable local or transnational alternatives? What are the benefits and who will gain from them? What are the costs and risks (e.g. impact on inequities) and who will bear them? What do you hope to bring home and how will you share these learnings?

People who undertake health-related work or volunteer experience in another country—that is, those in the privileged position to travel abroad—may be surprised to discover that the greatest benefit is to themselves. Countless medical relief trips run every year by well-meaning organizations are nothing more than "global health tourism" or "voluntourism." Such trips are usually financed by the participants themselves, who may pay large sums of money for the chance to sew up wounds in the Amazon (complete with rainforest river cruises on the weekend), treat exotic diseases in the jungles of Rwanda (with side tours to see silver back gorillas), or distribute eyeglasses to Tibetan refugees in the foothills of the Himalayas (with the possibility of an audience with the Dalai Lama).

Exciting as these opportunities may be, it is important to recognize that international placements can put an enormous burden on settings with already stretched resources. Health workers in LMIC programs and institutions are typically given little or no compensation for acting as supervisors or trainers for those from overseas. Such expeditions often do more harm than good, leaving behind no capacity for follow-up and applying "band-aids" to deep problems and ultimately justifying the political status quo (McLennan 2014). In addition, outsiders may disrupt social services by bringing in short-term treatments and solutions that are not available once they leave (Lasker 2016).

Residents of HICs may not typically consider people working in their home country, year after year, as taking part in global health: clearly the perspective and relative contribution of those engaged in a lifetime of work differs greatly from those of outsiders flying in and out. Likewise, many health and social justice actors in the Majority World may not view their work in terms of global health, as this is predominantly an HIC term. It is equally important for HIC nationals working in LMICs to recognize that they are in a position of power and need to be very careful not to abuse this power. Foreigners and transnationals enjoy relative wealth, advanced education, the possibility to leave (the country or community), and the luxury to challenge decisions without jeopardizing their livelihoods, as well as organizational access to resources and influence over policymaking. All of these factors shape the interactions of transnational and foreign health professionals and students with government offices, communities, local health workers, leaders, and educators.

Pinto and Upshur (2009) outline four core ethical principles for persons entering the global health field. The first is introspection, beginning with articulating your positionality and personal motivations, and contemplating the potential impact of your global health involvement. Whether you are embarking on or redirecting your career in global health, excessive idealism, overconfidence (in your tools, role, abilities, or approach), and ignorance about the realities of global health politics and power can be impediments and even cause grave damage to local populations.

A second core ethical principle is humility. It is commonplace for people from HICs to display ethnocentrism, paternalism, or condescension toward people from LMICs (prejudices they may not recognize in themselves). Students might assume that they can provide some benefit to a community without knowing the setting, understanding the political, cultural, and economic history, social dynamics, language, or the role and limits of outside organizations (Gupta and Farmer 2005; Ventres and Fort 2014). Local inhabitants and health practitioners invariably know their context better than anyone and have thought profoundly about the best ways to approach problems. Keeping an open and humble mind is essential to foreigners' appropriate involvement (Ventres and Gusoff 2014). For clinicians, this also means understanding the broad political and social context of prevention and treatment, not simply the biomedical encounter (Gupta and Farmer 2005).

Next is fostering solidarity, including "developing a sensitivity to the suffering of others and working to prevent their marginalization" (Pinto and Upshur 2009, p. 9). Solidarity means establishing on-going relationships and exchanges, supporting local movements in their struggles and aspirations, not superimposing your or your organization's ideas of community needs. As the People's Heath Movement (PHM) argues, "true solidarity exists when citizens of the community are mobilized, when capacity building of local organizations and strengthened links within civil society occurs, and when attempts are made to bridge power imbalances between the wealthy and the poor" (ibid).

The last in the quartet of ethical principles outlined by Pinto and Upshur (2009) is social justice, recalling its earlier framing in terms of contesting oppression and societal asymmetries of power and resources, addressing inequity, working extensively in solidarity with communities and responding to their priorities, and understanding the nature of global political and economic forces, such as militarism and corporate power.

Social justice approaches may also draw from the notion articulated by practitioners of liberation theology in Latin America: a "preferential option for the poor" (Gutiérrez 1973), that is, solidarity with, and giving voice to, oppressed people in their struggles for justice, re-cast by DGH co-founder Lanny Smith (et al. 2013) as "liberation medicine." In addition, Gupta and Farmer (2005) emphasize the importance of continued engagement with global health struggles wherever you are located, a point we will expand upon ahead. Accordingly, international placements should not be voyeuristic episodes to see "how the majority lives" but bestow a continuing responsibility to work through advocacy, activism, education, and other solidarity measures, recognizing how (and mobilizing around) the policies of powerful HICs (and lead global health actors) affect the health and health inequities of populations across the world.

Of course many readers likely have sophisticated understandings of how social change works and recognize that there are numerous ways to be involved in global health through activism and solidarity (Hanson 2015). At whatever degree of experience and level of involvement, appreciation of the political and economic underpinnings of global health is pivotal to making you more informed and your work more effective. Such understanding, we hope, may also move you to challenge the forces that produce and reproduce local, national, and international inequalities as part of the uphill struggle against global social injustice.

Knowledge, Training, and Work Experience

Though many people who consider themselves global health professionals and activists have entered the field circuitously, a common question for young professionals is when or whether to invest time and resources in formal training in global health. This could involve pursuing a master's of public health (or global health) to acquire specific skills, a doctorate in anthropology or social epidemiology to deepen research abilities, courses in community planning or political organizing, or a degree in economics to be able to understand the world trade regime, financialization trends, and how these affect health in both HICs and LMICs.

Among the best ways for neophytes to become exposed to social justice and global health efforts is through the courses (e.g., on trade, PHC and political economy of health, equity and health rights, and movement building) run by the International People's Health University (IPHU) in dozens of countries across South Asia, Africa, Europe, the Americas, the Middle East, and the Pacific. The IPHU "aims to contribute to 'health for all' by strengthening people's health movements around the globe, by organizing and resourcing learning, sharing and planning opportunities for people's health activists, particularly from Third World countries." The IPHU also "sponsors research into the barriers to Health for All and strategies to support the people's struggle for health" (IPHU 2016).

More formal academic global health training from a critical perspective exists in various settings. Brazil's National School of Public Health, based in Rio de Janeiro, has foci in social program implementation and environmental health and justice. In Mexico City, the Universidad Autónoma Metropolitana offers a master's degree in social medicine and publishes *Revista Salud Problema*, highlighting health-disease processes from a critical perspective. Similarly, the Centre of Social Medicine and Community Health at Jawaharlal Nehru University in New Delhi analyzes health needs and interventions in the context of structural constraints. At Johns Hopkins Bloomberg School of Public Health (Baltimore, USA), jointly with Pompeu Fabra University in Barcelona, a range of courses examine the political economy of social inequalities and their consequences for health, and the impact of financial, economic, and political crisis on health. South Africa's University of the Western Cape School of Public Health trains policymakers and implementers "whose practice is based on research, influenced by informed and active communities, and implemented with a commitment to equity, social justice and human dignity" (UWC 2013). Courses (and sometimes programs) at the Universities of Saskatchewan (e.g., on global health and social inequalities), Bologna (Centro Studi e Ricerche in Salute Internazionale e Interculturale), Oslo, Thammasat (Thailand), British Columbia, Washington, Sussex, and Harvard, among others, marshaled by committed faculty involved in progressive transnational movements, are similarly illuminating.

Many of these classroom experiences incorporate health advocacy, activism, and alliance-building components. At the same time, some of the most useful training for the key (health justice) solidarity activities of monitoring, witnessing, and speaking out take place through apprenticeship or participation in activism itself, as discussed in the next section of the chapter. You might also contemplate how university and other training venues can help bridge the academic–activist divide by studying health activism (historically, in policy terms, or as a participant-observer) or working with and helping forge alliances, such as the student-led Universities Allied for Essential Medicines, which works to improve accessibility and affordability of medicines globally.

Likewise, spending time learning about grassroots organizing (e.g., at the Highlander Research and Education Center in the Appalachian mountains of Tennessee, USA) and research methods for social change (e.g., at the Center for Social Well Being in the Peruvian Andes; and political economy and activist-oriented Centre for Civil Society at the University of KwaZuluNatal, South Africa) can provide the building blocks for lifelong organizing skills and collective action. Staying informed via news, advocacy platforms, and social media outlets that provide in-depth political and social coverage is also indispensable (Box 14-6).

It is important to be conscious, nonetheless, of the cooptation of progressive language and the hypocrisy that may surround it. Remarkably, some authors and academic institutions invoke issues around politics, power, and privilege in global health without considering the role of global capitalism as the overarching political economy context (Ooms 2015; Shiffman 2014). Others may promote "safe spaces" for discussion of social justice and critical political economy perspectives, shamefully hiding or ghettoizing these debates. Conversely, holding such conversations in the open may lead to deeper understanding and underscore the contradictions around mainstream global health activities that characterize much academic work in this area.

One of the most important dimensions of being an effective global health justice advocate and practitioner is communication: speaking local languages is essential. A good start is learning one or more important regional languages such as Arabic, Swahili, Hindi-Urdu, French, Russian, Spanish, or Mandarin. In most LMICs, this still limits communication to dominant social and cultural groups. While mastering local languages is not always feasible, at the very least, it is important to acknowledge that a great deal will be missed without knowing the language. Many English speakers are accustomed to communicating in their native tongue wherever they go, yet over half the world's population is bilingual. For those whose work takes place internationally or involves people from many different places, language skills are an imperative companion to being historically, culturally, and politically aware.

Box 14-6 Alternative Media/Activist Outlets

A small sample of independent, critically-minded news and activist sources (to be expanded with your own suggestions from other places/languages):

Zimbabwe-based
EQUINET: http://www.equinetafrica.org/newsletter/current
Kenya/Senegal-based
Pambazuka News: http://www.pambazuka.net/en/
India-based
The Economic and Political Weekly: http://www.epw.in/about-us.html
Vikalp: http://www.vikalp.ind.in/
Malaysia-based
Third World Resurgence magazine: http://www.twn.my/title2/resurgence/twr.htm
Australia-based
Green Left Weekly: https://www.greenleft.org.au/node/60698
Latin America-based
La Izquierda Diario (network of news outlets in Venezuela, Bolivia, Argentina, Chile, Uruguay, Brazil, Mexico, United States, Germany, France, Spain): http://www.laizquierdadiario.com/Red-Internacional/
Argentina-based
Resumen Latinoamericano: http://www.resumenlatinoamericano.org
Canada-based
Socialist Project: http://www.socialistproject.ca/
briarpatch magazine: http://briarpatchmagazine.com/issues
rabble.ca: http://rabble.ca/
UK-based
Open Democracy: https://www.opendemocracy.net/
US-based
Democracy Now: http://www.democracynow.org
Portside: https://portside.org
Real News: http://therealnews.com/t2/index.php

Every country has laws and regulations governing the practice of different types of health professionals. Students who find themselves in clinical settings in another country should not expect to examine patients, prescribe medicines, or engage in any other clinical activity that they would not legally be allowed to do at home. This dictum, however, may be defied by HIC students who see LMICs as a training ground to hone their skills. Licensed health professionals, too, frequently violate this rule, assuming that their training is equivalent or superior to that of local clinicians. Not only is practicing without a local license illegal, it may be dangerous: different treatment standards in each country mean that outsiders cannot presume that what they have been trained to do is appropriate (Hanson, Harms, and Plamondon 2011).

As well, those trained or acculturated in Western biomedicine often overlook the many Indigenous practices, including acupuncture, Ayurveda, and homeopathy that have been adopted and accepted as complementary or superior to biomedicine for various health problems. Persistent ethnocentric attitudes can result in failure to appreciate local understandings of disease and ill health. This goes well beyond issues of cultural sensitivity. As discussed in chapters 3 and 11, the Western biomedical model has conceptual and practical limitations and biases—it is individualistic, mechanistic, invasive, generally ignores holistic understandings and the societal context of health, can do little for many chronic conditions, frequently represents profit-making interests, can be dangerous/lead to iatrogenic disease (see chapter 6)—and thus should be avoided in many instances.

When traditional healing and biomedicine cooperate as equal partners based on mutual respect, they can be complementary. For example, Jambihuasi, a community-based clinic in Otavalo, Ecuador founded in 1984 by Quichua traditional healers and biomedically-trained Quichua health professionals, takes a patient-led approach. Those attending the clinic can choose either or both traditional and biomedical services, and healers from each of these traditions communicate closely around patient care (Bouchard 2009).

In addition to understanding local traditions and needs, any person interested in global health needs to be tolerant, self-critical, a good listener, patient, able to work with people in diverse fields and with varied backgrounds, broad-minded, modest, and have or be able to develop expertise that is relevant. Ultimately, the contribution of global health workers and, by extension, the programs they support, depends as much on understanding broad sociopolitical issues as on possessing particular technical skills. Decentered solidarity actions, abroad and at home, are perhaps the most effective approach of all.

Nevertheless, we all ought to consider that admonishments, thoughtful approaches, and well-intentioned efforts still do not remove—and may even exacerbate—the incongruities of engaging in international work in the context of personal, organizational, and global power asymmetries. Reminding ourselves of this reality through continual reflexivity and "critical consciousness" (Freire 1970) is thus a crucial aspect of global health justice efforts.

Organizational Level: Missions and Actions

Because many readers of this text are or will go on to become global health advocates/activists, and/or work or volunteer in this area, a few words of advice may be warranted around how individuals and organizations inter-relate. The term *organization* serves as a broad umbrella encompassing a gamut of actors of all shapes and sizes that are valuable and intersect in different ways, from small-scale grassroots activities to established local groups, medium and large-sized regional and national entities—both longstanding and more recent—and global and transnational agencies and movements. Involvement at personal, professional, and political levels can be considered a continuum with overlapping elements and categories, but generally moving from one's own advocacy to institutional efforts and acting in solidarity with and for movements that can be global in scale.

When deciding on an organization to work or volunteer for, one should learn as much as possible, formally and informally, about the entity's mission and funding sources, its past and current activities, and the larger context of its role. For example, during the Cold War many social-justice committed US Peace Corps volunteers in LMICs did not realize that they were often perceived by local residents to be part of the US's (particularly the Central Intelligence Agency's) response to the "communist threat."

In a similar vein, reflecting on his role as a graduate student consulting with the Aga Khan Foundation in post-USSR Tajikistan in the mid-1990s, physician-anthropologist Salmaan Keshavjee learned that his health and development work was part of a larger trend to foster civil society as a neoliberal alternative to the strong state that marked the Soviet era:

> . . . after spending time in Badakhshan, I realized that the rise of NGOs as major regional and global development actors, a social apparatus hitherto unknown in the Soviet world, was no accident. Their rise was linked to profound changes in economic and political thinking . . . which combined neoliberal economics and, at least on paper, a commitment to liberal democratic theory and good governance (Keshavjee 2014, pp. 6–7).

Analyzing such political and ideological tentacles is a complex endeavor. On one level, US foreign policy goals and global health efforts, most prominently PEPFAR (see chapter 4), should not be considered "strange bedfellows." After all, US global security concerns and the "political capital" garnered through funding HIV control, as well as (at least initially) the commercial interests of Big Pharma, fit together well with this program. Yet on another level, even as former US President George W. Bush's (and his successor US President Barack Obama's) PEPFAR billions are consistent with US strategic priorities, they also represent the culmination of years of struggle for access to ARVs and health equity on the part of local movements such as South Africa's Treatment Action Campaign, transnational activist efforts including Health GAP, and by committed WHO leaders and staff members, who campaigned for global AIDS treatment access in the early 2000s before adequate funding was allocated (Messac and Prabhu 2013).

By pursuing such questions, a critical political economy (of health) perspective can be infused into almost any work or activist setting. Though challenging an organization or movement to be true to its mission, better define its goals, or demonstrate how it is publicly accountable can potentially imperil both the challenger and the entity, it is one of the most important means of effectuating equitable global health change both at home and abroad.

At the very least, consulting the International Aid Transparency Initiative, which tracks information on aid spending of over 400 organizations around the world, might be helpful. The watchdog organization Charity Navigator gauges the quality of organizations based on a number of financial, spending, and transparency criteria. For example, Partners In Health receives a high rating due to its accountability, transparency, and large proportion of resources spent on programs versus administrative and fundraising activities.

Of course, organizations (anthropomorphically speaking) want to survive. Thus, NGOs, government agencies, and consulting firms write grant proposals and bid on contracts for things that they know how to do, or hope to learn to do, for which funding is available, and for which they can demonstrate success so they can seek further funding.

Herein lies the yoke of short-term, narrowly technical, measurable interventions that characterize mainstream global health and often impede social justice approaches. Even organizations that act in solidarity with local knowledge and social justice priorities can be severely constrained by the funding milieu. In that sense, helping an organization to find alternative funding sources or ways of working (i.e., via committed volunteers), especially sources that are locally accountable, can make all the difference.

But it is also important not to let governments and international agencies and their staff members eschew responsibility, given that they (are meant to) serve the public interest, and have a role to play, together with local and transnational movements, in both calling for and supporting policies that move countries toward greater social justice. Voting, advocating, and struggling for public support for long-term equitable policies, services, and politics, at every level, from within and outside organizations, are thus vital activities.

Some individuals, perhaps due to frustrations with other organizations or motivated by unfilled needs, decide to establish their own NGO. While sounding appealing, it is important to decenter one's own desires and consider, for example, why an international NGO is preferable to a local organization—such as Jamkhed's Comprehensive Rural Health Project, operating in Maharashtra state, India since 1970 (Arole and Arole 1994)—or advocating for public efforts, and what other avenues might be pursued.

The proliferation of thousands of small and large NGOs operating at local, national, and transnational levels has had numerous negative consequences, including duplication of efforts, the draining of enormous logistical and administrative resources, and lack of sustainability. Moreover, NGOs often become dependent on funding and interests of larger donors, turning them into unwitting interlocutors or implementers of dominant priorities (Pfeiffer 2003) and displacing social movements (Roy 2004).

Rather than founding a new organization, you might consider participating and helping form coalitions and networks of existing organizations and political movements that pressure for universal access to water, health care, education, and other basic human needs, against gender-based violence (Box 14-7), ethnic, racial, and caste-based discrimination (e.g., the Dalit Movement in India), against illicit financial flows (e.g. the Global Alliance for Tax Justice), for worldwide labor standards and occupational health protections (e.g., Institute for Global Labour and Human Rights), SDOH-grounded fair trade (Hanson et al. 2012), and so on. For instance, the Third World Network, based in Penang, Malaysia, with offices in Kuala Lumpur, Geneva, Montevideo, and Accra, and affiliates in various other LMIC settings, is an

Box 14-7 Challenging Gender Norms to Address Gender-Based Violence and HIV Prevention

For decades, women's movements have been calling for action on the unacceptably high rates of gender-based violence (GBV) (Michau et al. 2015). Challenging the status quo of harmful gender norms requires engagement of multiple actors and actions, including government commitment to intersectoral policies that address women's political, social, and economic subordination (García-Moreno et al. 2015b), so that both the practice of GBV and the larger context shaping this harmful behavior are addressed (see chapter 7).

In Spain, for example, following a broad 2006 national GBV awareness and prevention plan involving social services, the judicial system, and the media, the health care system began training providers to identify GBV and provide psychosocial and post-rape care for sexual assault survivors. Two critical components of the health system protocol are addressing gender-based discrimination among providers themselves, and emphasizing providers' role in connecting women with other services (such as housing and legal services) in order to prevent further abuse (García-Moreno et al. 2015a).

Increasingly, GBV prevention programs engage boys and men to critically reflect on masculinity (i.e., norms and behaviors associated with manhood) in order to raise awareness and transform beliefs and practices toward gender-equitable relationships (Casto and Messner 2016; Jewkes, Flood, and Lang 2015). Gender equity and GBV prevention approaches have also been adopted in some HIV prevention programs. The South African organization Sonke, for example, delivers "One Man Can" workshops to guide men and boys through analysis and discussion of how masculinity is embedded in gender ideologies in their families and communities, as well as in historical and contemporary race and class relations in South African society. Sonke's workshops have helped increase men's support for women's rights and equitable gender relations, transforming both HIV and GBV prevention (Dworkin et al. 2013).

The challenges ahead rest on consolidating integrated anti-GBV efforts and extending them to every society where GBV remains a problem.

independent, non-profit research and activist network that effectively focuses attention on trade, development, health, and other social and political issues that affect the lives and livelihoods of the majority of people in LMICs.

National and transnational alliances against militarism (see chapter 8), or for binding codes of conduct to hold TNCs accountable for their practices, or the Tobin tax—a proposed levy on cross-border currency transactions that would be channeled to environmental and human needs—also have great potential for improving global health (equity). A particularly effective network is Help Age International, which works with some 180 partners across over 65 countries to support healthier, more dignified lives of older persons. In most instances, building on existing social justice efforts is likely to be more effective and sustainable than founding new organizations.

Another approach has to do with monitoring and holding to account the actions and policies of government and international organizations. ActionAid International, based in South Africa, is a social auditing group that works with communities to hold governments accountable on a range of issues such as food and land rights, women's rights, democratic governance, and climate change. Its counterpart ActionAid USA monitors TNC tax evasion, shedding light on the injustice of lost tax revenues for health, education, and other social sectors in LMICs. India's Centre for Health and Social Justice also carries out social auditing; its health-related work includes gauging community participation in policymaking and the realization of health rights. PHM, meanwhile, sponsors WHO Watch and PAHO Watch activities, which monitor the governing bodies of global health's designated multilateral agencies and report publicly on policy debates, agenda-setting, and budgetary decisions to make these agencies accountable to broad constituencies well beyond the usual insider "stakeholders." In different ways, these monitoring organizations serve as both ends and means for health advocacy and activism.

How can we ensure that the global health projects/programs we participate in further the goals of solidarity and social justice in health? Good intentions are insufficient: also needed is political economy analysis of the profusion of bilateral and multilateral aid agencies and the international and local NGOs they support. All are ostensibly working to improve the health of local residents, yet they often work at cross-purposes with population needs or in competition with one another. From Nicaragua to Mozambique, the aid milieu has proved problematic, leading to hierarchies of inclusion and exclusion within and beyond the health care sector (see chapters 2, 3, 4, and 12).

As analyzed by Health Alliance International (HAI) medical anthropologist James Pfeiffer (2003, pp. 725–726):

> The Mozambique experience reveals that the deluge of NGOs and their expatriate workers over the last decade has fragmented the local health system, undermined local control of health programs, and contributed to growing local social inequality. Since national health system salaries plummeted over the same period as a result of structural adjustment, health workers became vulnerable to financial favors offered by NGOs seeking to promote their projects in turf struggles with other agencies ... The multiplicity of competing organizations that duplicate program support, create parallel projects, pull health service workers away from routine duties, and disrupt planning processes has generated concern for both donors and recipients ...
>
> In this engagement, the exercise of power by wealthy donors over their target populations, including local health workers, is laid bare and the disempowerment of public sector services by international agencies is most visible.... In addition to their expatriate staff, agencies usually employ small armies of 'nationals,' from trained health professionals and office workers to drivers and guards.... paid far more than their counterparts in the public sector.

Whether knowingly or inadvertently exacerbating these problems, global health organizations and expatriate personnel should ensure that they do not contribute to poaching of health professionals, fragmenting of services, or skewing of priorities but rather assist in strengthening the host country's organization and delivery of services and activities on its own terms.

A key to equitable and transformative global health work, either by individuals or organizations, is sustained commitment to a specific population

Box 14-8 Health Alliance International: *Cooperantes* Working in Solidarity to Create Healthy Societies

The global health groups that have most contributed to the making of healthy societies are those that adhere to principles of solidarity and "horizontal" cooperation for the long haul. Over the past three decades, members of Health Alliance International (HAI), mostly from the United States, have worked to promote public health and social justice in Mozambique, with a shared commitment to local and national goals of strengthening public infrastructure and the country's health system.

Following Mozambique's independence in 1975, the Ministry of Health (MOH) developed a comprehensive national plan to rapidly extend health care to its rural population, despite scarce human and financial resources—with only 40 physicians for 11 million people. In the late 1970s numerous foreign physicians and public health advocates moved to Mozambique to support the new socialist government's ambitious PHC plans. As *cooperantes*, they worked as MOH employees paid at local rates and accountable to local authorities. Though widely supported by the public, the country's social programs were soon undermined by a 14-year proxy war backed by South Africa's apartheid government. Health infrastructure and personnel became military targets.

In 1987, heeding a request from the Mozambican government, a group of US *cooperantes* came together to form the Mozambique Health Committee (later HAI) to support the rebuilding of severely damaged health infrastructure. In the 1980s and 1990s, HAI provided technical assistance and material support to the MOH, strengthening primary care provision in the central provinces of Manica and Sofala. By this time, the country was faced with new threats to the health system, including structural adjustment programs and privatization.

Starting in 2003, Mozambique's MOH was one of the first in Africa to initiate a national HIV treatment program, with HAI a strong partner in this effort ever since. Mozambique experienced a large influx of foreign aid, stretching the MOH's management capacity and already inadequate workforce, motivating HAI's move into the realm of advocacy. One key advocacy effort has been leading development of an International NGO Code of Conduct for Health System Strengthening that calls on NGOs to support, not usurp, MOH health sector leadership. Adhering to the Code, HAI's integration of its efforts around health system strengthening, immunization, and HIV, TB, and malaria treatment into Mozambique's government-purveyed PHC system serves as an important counterexample to the prevailing model of NGOs competing against or displacing publicly provided health services. Yet since HAI—which has expanded its work to Côte d'Ivoire, East Timor, and Sudan—began accepting US donor funding, it has faced mounting dilemmas around ensuring organizational survival while maintaining its solidarity-based principles (Gloyd, Pfeiffer, and Johnson 2013).

or country. HAI, for example, has been working in Mozambique for decades, maintaining its support through war, political strife, government change, structural adjustment pressures, and funding challenges (Box 14-8). This contrasts considerably with donors that pursue high-profile efforts and do little to work in solidarity with national or local needs.

Box 14-9 presents critical questions any individual or organization should consider before embarking on transformative global health work. A cardinal rule for global health work is the same as it is for medicine: *primum non nocere*—first do no harm. Organizations and individuals involved in global health must be prepared to shed their own prejudices and opinions, work together with organizations and people from the host country as true partners, and understand that the appropriate role of outside groups is supportive and subsidiary to what national and local health and social justice movements wish to achieve.

For instance, consider the role of outsiders versus local efforts in the situation of military regimes that infiltrate the health sector. In 2015 in Myanmar, health care workers protested the appointment of military officers without health expertise to the Ministry of Health. The protest, called the Black Ribbon Movement, also spurred parallel protests against militarization of other sectors, such as education. Although the movement did not achieve removal of current military officers, the Minister of Health promised no additional military appointments (Palatino 2015). What might foreigners do in solidarity with this important effort? Joining it would be inappropriate or potentially dangerous. Supporting from afar, talking over the situation with students and colleagues, and participating in a solidarity campaign might all provide important succor to Black Ribbon, while recognizing that the movement remains very much national.

Indeed, even the most sensitive, solidarity-minded, noble, and knowledgeable persons and organizations cannot transcend the larger context—or world order—of oppression and unequal power, recognizing that leadership on these questions is important at every level of society. For this reason, working collectively based on shared values

Box 14-9 Key Questions Individuals and Organizations Should Consider in Carrying Out Global Health Projects

- How are the country, population, and activity selected? For what purpose?
- How are problems conceptualized by local residents, policymakers, and global health workers?
- What are the central political, economic, and social issues locally and nationally (and what historical factors are at play)?
- Who defines the agenda for work and how are priorities selected? How have similar activities been carried out in the past?
- What is the approach to cooperation? Is it technical, environmental, political, social, or a mixture? How are ethical issues taken into account?
- Is this a one-time intervention or is it sustained over time? What are its longer-term social and environmental effects?
- How is the program funded and over what time frame? To what extent might national or local health systems and priorities (and other institutions) be distorted by the program?
- What are the benefits and drawbacks for the communities, organizations, and health workers participating in the initiative?
- How will power differentials between players be identified and mitigated?
- Is the program tackling the SDOH? In what ways?
- How is the program evaluated, by whom, and when? (What constitutes success? Who decides?)
- What is the potential for the program to do harm to or jeopardize local participants or implementing organizations? What are the short- and long-term responsibilities of cooperating organizations?
- How is the activity linked to transformative change? What is the role of ongoing transnational solidarity in this effort?

around health and social justice—as illustrated in the innumerable current acts undertaken every day by various groups and movements that create the micro-revolutions that pre-figure and contribute to larger changes—is so important. But this involves more than tweaking at the margins, notwithstanding enormous good will (Panter-Brick, Eggerman, and Tomlinson 2014). Addressing the structures of power, at every level and from every angle far beyond global health, per se, has the potential to be truly transformative.

The Logic of the World Order: Movements, Local and Transnational, and their Relation to Global Health

Over 100 years ago, the socialist philosopher and revolutionary Rosa Luxemburg posed the question of whether reform (change from within) was useful and possible or whether it impeded revolution (change from without). Her espousal of the latter position, leading to her participation in the Berlin revolution, cost her her life in 1919 when she was captured by German authorities and tortured to death. The "reform versus revolution" question continues to be evoked today. Davidson Gwatkin, a prominent advisor on health and poverty to the World Bank, has argued, "The health of the world's poor would be best served by a series of revolutions that bring into power national leaderships that are centrally concerned about the well-being of disadvantaged groups within their borders" (Yamey 2007, p. 1558). The World Bank, however, has long supported private enterprise, not socialist revolution, as the formula for progress. How might this paradox be reconciled?

Today, many regard the reform versus revolution dichotomy to be false or at least exaggerated, instead viewing transformative reforms—especially the creation or resurrection of social justice-based welfare states with universal rights to safe housing, employment, neighborhoods, environmental conditions, water and sanitation, education, health care, and nondiscrimination—together with a robust and equitable reorientation of power and decisionmaking to combat multiple forms of oppression, as the scaffolding of structural change.

Returning to the previous example, as an alternative to more revolutionary calls for the World Bank's elimination, reform might be pursued to ensure that it democratically represents not only all countries but people of distinct social classes, racial and ethnic groups, genders, and other dimensions of social, economic, and political power. In this way, the World Bank would become a people's bank, rather than a bank representing elite interests. Pushing this point further, every multilateral or UN agency might be reformed through such policies, enabling priority-setting and scientific expertise to be grounded and integrated into larger anti-oppression efforts.

How might democratization change the World Bank? The widespread misery caused by its loan and development packages could be addressed not through tinkering with loan programs or symbolic debt forgiveness, but through: total and unconditional debt cancellation; abolition of loan conditionalities; payment of reparations for centuries of enslavement, plundering, and exploitation; and the creation of reverse conditionalities (i.e., no loan would be approved unless it decreased a country's Gini coefficient, increased access to water or education, and fostered equitable power over decisionmaking, etc.), as decided through genuinely democratic and accountable governance processes (Jubilee Debt Campaign 2014). While this may seem like wishful thinking, Jubilee, Centre Europe Tiers Monde, and other public interest civil society groups call for IFIs to be completely revamped and become responsible lenders, a Sisyphean challenge, to be sure, but not a hopeless one.

Another key group that straddles reform and revolution particularly in relation to global health is PHM. Founded by health workers in 2000 in Bangladesh, PHM has become an international movement with national counterparts, struggling for health as a human right in the context of global solidarity (Figure 14-1). Its *People's Charter for Health* has been translated into dozens of languages and endorsed by thousands of people and organizations across the world, becoming the "most widely endorsed consensus document on health since the Alma Ata Declaration" (PHM 2016). PHM employs a political economy of health analysis as a call for multilevel action to collectively tackle the broad determinants of health in order to achieve Alma-Ata's vision of "health for all." For PHM (2016):

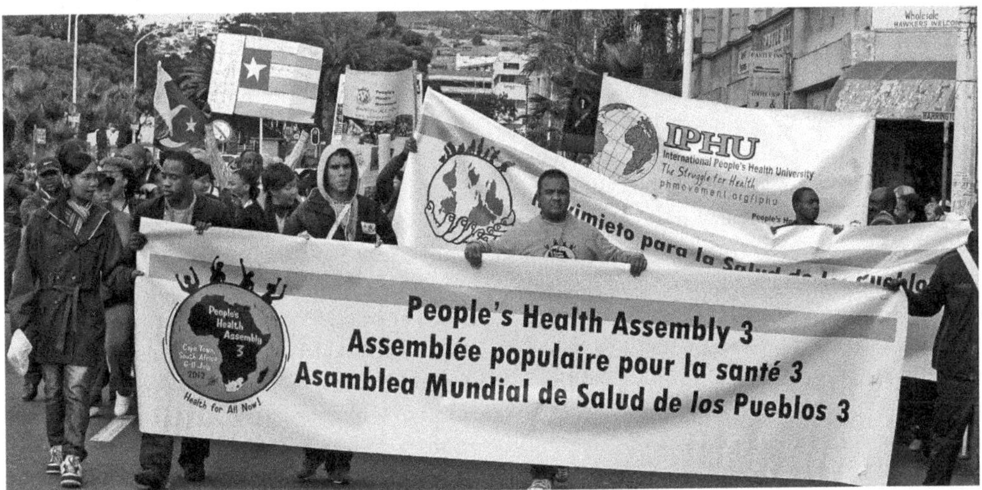

Figure 14-1 People's Health Assembly, Cape Town, South Africa, July 2012.
Source: PHM (2012).

> Equity, ecologically-sustainable development and peace are at the heart of [their] vision of a better world - a world in which a healthy life for all is a reality; a world that respects, appreciates and celebrates all life and diversity; a world that enables the flowering of people's talents and abilities to enrich each other; a world in which people's voices guide the decisions that shape our lives.

PHM is also involved with the activist organizations Medact, Medico International, Third World Network, Health Action International, and ALAMES in bringing together hundreds of health practitioners, scholars, and advocates to produce the triennial *Global Health Watch: An Alternative World Health Report*. In four editions to date, the report has critically assessed the state of global health and the current paradigm of development and provided an alternative array of achievable solutions for "a society that is more just, more equal and more humane" (PHM et al. 2014, p. 1).

So, too, might you see your own work in global health as a micro-transformation en route to improving the determinants of health at each level of the political economy of global health framework explored in this book. Should you find yourself working—or advocating for change—within an organization that follows "business as usual" in global health, your efforts, together with those of colleagues and supporters, could help reform the organization in a variety of ways. For example, as an epidemiologist employed by an international disease surveillance agency, you might insist that surveys of HIV prevalence include variables regarding living and work conditions, food sovereignty, and wealth and social stratification. Or if you live in an HIC, you may decide that your efforts will be more effective through activism with a transnational movement that calls for changes in trade and investment rules, challenges foreign aid strategies that further entrench power imbalances, or defends occupational health conditions worldwide.

How might such activism be harnessed to transform the field? Individual motivations of social justice and shared well-being are a good start but they are not enough. Pushing organizations to improve the accountability and equity of their actions is also important, yet still not enough. Understanding the nature and structures of power and oppression, and how the skewed distribution of political, social, and economic resources affects the determinants of health and well-being—alongside participating in committed efforts to upend the concentration of power and resources—are fundamental to improving global health equity and social justice.

Practicing Global Health "At Home and Transnationally"

Global health can also be practiced without a passport: in many ways, working to transform the "foreign" policies of powerful HIC governments, which have tremendous sway over the rules and arrangements of the global order, may have a far greater impact than working in another country. Not only is activism at home (for those based in HICs) among the best forms of solidarity with progressive social movements transnationally, but educating fellow residents/citizens and organizing for socially just change can profoundly influence the underlying determinants of global health inequity. This entails both visible and behind-the-scenes activism:

- Helping build mass movements at home that practice health and social justice and struggle for political transformation domestically and globally (Stedile 2002) by participating through supportive campaigns, logistical help, collecting funds and supplies, providing needed information and advocacy; and informing the public of HICs about the damages caused by their governments' economic policies, foreign aid, and military policies
- Participating in struggles for: truly equitable systems of trade and investment; solidarity cooperation; ensuring systems of fair and adequate taxation and redistribution; ending illicit financial flows; strengthening domestic and transnational regulations and protections; and other forms of "mobilizing against global capital" (Labonté 2013, p. 2159)
- Campaigning against financialization (promulgated by IFIs, private banks, and insurance corporations)
- Working to eliminate patent protections that limit access to needed drugs and devices

- Organizing against harmful and exploitative TNC practices
- Working to change HIC health care system and training policies to prevent poaching of professionals from other countries
- Forming truly collaborative partnerships with colleagues and students around the world involved in global health and social justice research and activities
- Mobilizing around "global health" issues at home—for example, against classist, gender-based, and racist violence and institutionalized discrimination; in favor of just societies that prioritize the needs of all oppressed populations including migrants and refugees; for equitable and adequate financing of and access to public medical care, housing, employment, quality education, and other entitlements; and for radically democratic forms of societal decisionmaking
- Struggling against past and present human rights violations at home—against Indigenous and other oppressed populations (Box 14-10)—by law enforcement and other public institutions
- Working to combat climate change and environmental degradation by fighting for stronger standards—and enforcement mechanisms—on reduction of greenhouse gas emissions, extractive industries, industrial pollution, and production and export of toxic substances
- Working to reform international organizations (beginning with WHO) so they represent the interests of people, not corporations, and are true to their public mandates
- Fighting domestically and transnationally to protect workers from labor that is exploitative,

Box 14-10 Indigenous Movements Influencing the Societal Determinants of Health

Across the world, Indigenous movements have made concerted efforts to protect the well-being, cultural traditions, and livelihoods of their communities with broad (though not necessarily intended) repercussions for health, including for the larger society. Some efforts combine local acts of sabotage and engagement with state institutions, such as the Khmu resistance to Chinese-owned rubber concessions in Northern Laos (McAllister 2015); other movements struggle against corporate impunity from environmental damages, among them the decades-long battle of the Movement for the Survival of the Ogoni People in Nigeria against Shell Oil Company (see chapter 10).

In Canada, *Idle No More* sprang into motion in 2012 in response to attacks on Indigenous sovereignty and the weakening of environmental regulations by the conservative government then in power, allowing industrial projects—including pipelines and mining expansion in Western Canada (mega-mines and tar sands; see chapter 10)—to proceed without community input, water and ecosystem protections, or environmental assessments. Starting from the province of Saskatchewan, the grassroots *Idle No More* movement—brainchild of three local Indigenous women, Jessica Gordon, Sylvia McAdam, and Nina Wilson, plus white settler ally Sheelah McLean (Caven 2013)—took a range of actions to protest the dismantling of environmental protection. These consisted of: Indigenous leaders going on hunger strikes, rallies, teach-ins around the "historical and contemporary context of colonialism," the blockading of roads and railways, and flash-mob style traditional dance performances in public areas (Idle No More 2016). *Idle No More* soon gained support from trade unions, students, and other groups across Canada, inspiring and standing in solidarity with movements in the United States, Ukraine, New Zealand, and beyond (Klein 2014). While not aimed at protecting health per se, this struggle to protect Indigenous rights to water and to traditional ways of life has enormous resonance for the SDOH, from historical legacies of oppression, to land and resource protections, and the right to self-determination.

hazardous, and precarious and to improve occupational health and safety

Many people, not only those at the beginning of their careers, may not recognize that participating in global health struggles without leaving home may be far more significant than going abroad under the auspices of a humanitarian agency. While not appearing as exciting as an international experience, these efforts have the potential to effectively address the root causes of ill health across the world (Labonté 2013), leave less of a carbon footprint, and may waste fewer local resources than a stint overseas. For example a 2015–2016 campaign bringing together environmental organizations, consumer watchdogs, and scientists, with the transnational support of millions of people from home bases around the world, successfully pressured the EU (in the face of an army of corporate lobbyists) to ban Monsanto's herbicide Roundup, a probable carcinogen.

Various activist organizations and movements that take on corporate impunity for unethical, unhealthy, and illegal behavior have had a dramatic impact in the political sphere and in global health, for instance: the Global Campaign to Dismantle Corporate Power; US-based Corporate Accountability International, which has a campaign to stop TNC junk food marketing to children; and the European Coalition for Corporate Justice, whose work focuses on TNCs and their excesses, including in relation to the UN's uncritical embracing of corporate interests in the realization of the SDGs.

Undoubtedly, as discussed in various chapters, public-interest civil society organizations, social movements, and the activists and advocates involved in these, such as IBFAN, Acción Ecológica, Treatment Action Campaign, and 50 Years is Enough, have played a critical part in ongoing struggles to make governments transparent, representative, and accountable for equitable policies protective of people's needs. They have also pressed multilateral organizations to act in—and trade treaties adhere to—the interests of human well-being, not the private sector, and regulators to keep toxins out of food supplies and the environment, among other recent mobilizations. These efforts are hugely important, worthwhile, and necessary.

Yet the growing emphasis on social justice-oriented advocacy and activism has led to reliance on civil society as a principal realm where transformative change will occur. Not only has this resulted in the sometime lumping of public interest groups with philanthropies and TNCs (as has played out at WHO around its problematic framework for interacting with nonstate actors [Lhotská and Gupta 2016]; see chapter 4), but such reliance can let local, national, and international civil servants, large organizations, and academics off the hook in terms of battling inequity and fighting for health justice. Public interest groups and social movements can be extremely influential—and involve incredibly committed and formidable, if often exhausted, individuals—but they are also fragile, usually lacking the resources, access, legitimacy, permanence, and even protection from repression that academic, national, and international organizations possess. Just obtaining information and entrée to decision-making fora consumes tremendous energy, before substantive issues are even broached. For these reasons, action around—and courageous stances for—health and social justice need to happen on every level and at every kind of institution, not just via civil society efforts.

As a reminder of the importance of using institutional platforms to speak out, we turn to Dr. Mary Travis Bassett, the New York City Health Commissioner, who spent several decades as a physician-scholar-activist in Zimbabwe. She brought back to the United States new understandings of the challenges of collective struggles for health and the insight that notwithstanding the enormous poverty generated under structural adjustment that she witnessed, researched, and sought to address in Zimbabwe, she never saw worse health conditions than in Harlem Hospital—in one of the poorest and most racially oppressed parts of New York City. These experiences have moved Dr. Bassett to use her stage as Health Commissioner to invest in mapping racial, economic, and social inequities across neighborhoods to marshal resources to concretely implement Health in All Policies. In the wake of brutal police force violence and racism across the United States, she has publicly asked:

> Should health professionals be accountable not only for caring for individual black patients but also for fighting the racism—both institutional and interpersonal—that contributes to

> poor health in the first place? Should we work harder to ensure that black lives matter. . . .? In terms of broader advocacy, some physicians and trainees may choose to participate in peaceful demonstrations; some may write editorials or lead "teach-ins"; others may engage their representatives to demand change in law, policy, and practice. Rightfully or not, medical professionals often have a societal status that gives our voices greater credibility. . . . (Bassett 2015, pp. 1085–1087).

CONCLUSION: WHAT IS TO BE DONE?

Learning Points:

- While mainstream approaches dominate the global health field, there are also inspirational approaches to global health's ongoing challenges, including social justice-oriented South–South cooperation, social and environmental movements operating locally and transnationally, and social auditing to hold governments, corporations, and non-state actors publicly accountable.
- Engaging in social justice approaches to global health requires critical self-reflection and decentering one's role, desires, and expectations, as well as understanding the profoundly political underpinnings of most global health action.
- Working toward health and social justice globally rests on solidarity and sustained commitment with local, national, and transnational organizations and movements that represent the needs of ordinary people rather than donors or TNCs.
- Participation in organizations—whether grassroots endeavors, large humanitarian entities, government agencies, or transnational social movements—can spark important micro-level changes, as part of larger uphill struggles essential to the making of healthy societies.
- Transformative work in global health involves a critical understanding and commitment to challenging the world political and economic order so as to improve the SDOH and build more equitable and socially just societies.
- Some of the most effective social action for global health justice can be done from home and in solidarity with movements elsewhere, on issues ranging from corporate impunity, to harmful military and foreign policy, inadequate and under-enforced worker and environmental regulations, and illicit financial flows.

At this point it is useful to revisit the three levels at which global health work can be conceptualized: individual actions and motivations, organizational missions and interventions, and the logic and structures of the world order. It is not uncommon to become frustrated that your own heartfelt motivations and hard work are not changing the public health reality in a marginalized community. Yet given the complexity of political, social, and economic forces that affect health at local, national, and global levels, this is to be expected. On the other hand, your own work, and that of the organizations and networks in which you participate, can also influence the logic of the world order, whether by fighting for comprehensive welfare states that go beyond redistribution and enable a just sharing of political and social power, for fair rules of international trade and finance, or for local and global political accountability. This kind of activity requires long-term commitment and patience, as change usually occurs slowly. That said, being part of such an effort is the most human, humane, and social justice and human rights-infused endeavor imaginable.

Ultimately, the global health community should be:

> a catalyst, a world health conscience behind national change, and, when requested, a helper giving visible expression to progressive ideas and decisions within national social policies. . . . this means the end of well-intentioned international technical paternalism in health and its replacement by an era of [global] collaboration and cooperation (WHO 1976, pp. 80–81).

Before or while reading this textbook, you might have asked: who could possibly critique global health actors and actions—a heartwarming domain involving committed advocates, specialized practitioners, and glamorous celebrities (Kapoor 2013)? Yet, as we have seen, global health and development activities are not neutral, technical endeavors but embedded in larger political structures and considerations. This helps explains the presence of institutions and activities within the ambit of global health that: squeeze out local priorities; come with conditions; interfere with democratic processes; increase inequity and social injustice; and perpetuate dependency and power differentials, while legitimating neoliberal capitalism. Paradoxically, mainstream health aid often violates the "do no harm" ethic despite the typically good intentions of the individuals and agencies participating. To put it differently, imagine if public health in your own community or country were influenced by, or dependent on, the charity of an international philanthropist, the interests of TNCs, the whims of a famous rock star, or the strategic foreign policy priorities of another country, paying little heed to locally defined needs.

As Paulo Freire (1978, p. 8) put it:

> Authentic help—this can never be said enough—is that in which all who are involved help each other, growing together in the common effort of understanding the reality they seek to transform. Only such a practice, in which those who give help and those who are helped simultaneously help each other, is the only kind in which the act of helping is not distorted into the dominance of those who help over those who are helped.

Above all, as the authors of this textbook, we believe that naïveté, willful ignorance, or rhetorical cooptation of global health are unacceptable. We find that continuous learning about—and engaging with to the extent possible—micro-level everyday acts, national policies and struggles, and the geopolitics and economic imperatives shaping global health are essential.

We agree with activists that responsibility for—and civil courage around—speaking out at injustice is vital and that global health actors of all kinds and at all levels share in this responsibility. Certainly this is the case within academia, where research and evidence produced on global health typically sidesteps discussion of capitalism, oppression, and injustice, instead reflecting the priorities of powerful funding agencies (and global health itself is increasingly viewed as a profitable realm, including for patentable interventions). This is also a responsibility shared by government and UN agencies, where—despite mandates for equity and openness—secretive, non-transparent processes enable private actors to squeeze out the public interest.

Recognizing the need to challenge global health power helps us decenter our own work and view it as subsidiary to larger movements for health and social justice. The solidarity we strive for is not channeled through one avenue; we seek to contribute on multiple levels based on our skills and expertise, always bearing in mind long-term and transformative goals. As slain US civil rights leader Martin Luther King Jr. powerfully put it, "the arc of the moral universe is long, but it bends towards justice" (King, Jr. 1965).

In this sense, global health and social justice activism can serve as both a rallying cry and a brick in building solidarity movements across stages of change—from decrying unjust political and social systems, to reforming them, radically altering them, and building from anew, all with contextualized rationales at particular moments in time.

The activities and campaigns we have covered here, causing smaller and greater ripples both within the health realm and outside it suggest how global health might be better practiced well into the 21st century. This chapter, and the book as a whole, also propose that a critical political economy approach cognizant of the structural factors, arrangements, and rules generating poor health and enormous inequities, is valuable—or rather invaluable—for reflection, a keen appreciation of, and action on these issues (ultimately for purposes of transforming society—praxis, in Freire's terms). Individual and institutional motivations and principles to combat all forms of oppression, discrimination, exploitation, and harm at an interpersonal and organizational level are necessary to improve global health justice. But they are not sufficient. Understanding how to make global health transformative for the majority of humanity beset by the unfair distribution of local and global resources and social and political power—and associated ill health and premature death—requires a further set of conceptual and analytic tools and perspectives that are not often taught in global health programs or to health professionals.

It is our hope that this book will serve as a primer for such understanding and help inspire readers' lifelong commitment to equitable engagement in global health as a social justice endeavor. Now it is up to you to harness your imagination, drive, commitment, persistence, knowledge, and skills to bettering and transforming global health in solidarity with the struggles of billions of people.

REFERENCES

Adams V. 2013. Evidence-based global public health: Subjects, profits, erasures. In Biehl J and Petryna A, Editors. *When People Come First: Critical Studies in Global Health.* Princeton, NJ: Princeton University Press.

Arole MR and Arole R. 1994. *Jamkhed: A Comprehensive Rural Health Project.* London: Macmillan.

Askheim C, Heggen K, and Engebretsen E. 2016. Politics and power in global health: The constituting role of conflicts. *International Journal of Health Policy and Management* 5(2):117–119.

Bassett MT. 2015. #BlackLivesMatter—A challenge to the medical and public health communities. *New England Journal of Medicine* 372(12):1085–1087.

Beauchamp D. 1976. Public health as social justice. *Inquiry* 13(1):3–14.

Beldarraín Chaple E. 2006. Public health in Cuba and its international experience (1959-2005). *História, Ciências, Saúde – Manguinhos* 13(3):709–716.

Biehl J and Petryna A, Editors. 2013. *When People Come First: Critical Studies In Global Health.* Princeton, NJ: Princeton University Press.

Birn A-E. 2005. Gates's grandest challenge: Transcending technology as public health ideology. *Lancet* 366(9484):514–519.

———. 2017. Little agenda-setters: Uruguay's International Institute for the Protection of Childhood and rights approaches to child health, 1920s-1940s. *Journal of Social History of Medicine and Health* [in Chinese] 2:1 [forthcoming].

Birn A-E, Aguilera M, Brisbois B, and Holtz TH. 2015. Why addressing climate change is not enough. *Huffington Post Blog,* December 25.

Birn A-E and Brown TM, Editors. 2013. *Comrades in Health: U.S. Health Internationalists, Abroad and at Home.* New Brunswick, NJ: Rutgers University Press.

Birn A-E, Muntaner C, and Afzal. 2016. La cooperación sur-sur en salud en América Latina: ¿aporte a la justicia social o continuidad de padrones dominantes de la asistencia norte-sur? [Unpublished manuscript]

Birn A-E, Nervi L, and Siqueira E. 2016. Neoliberalism redux: The global health policy agenda and the politics of cooptation in Latin America and beyond. *Development and Change* 47(4):734–759.

Bliss K, Editor. 2013. *The Changing Landscape of Global Health Diplomacy.* Washington, DC: CSIS Global Health Policy Center.

Bond P and Garcia A, Editors. 2015. *BRICS: An Anti-Capitalist Critique.* London: Pluto Press.

Bouchard L. 2009. The awakening of collaboration between Quichua healers and psychiatrists in the Andes. In Incayawar M, Wintrob R, Bouchard L, and Bartocci G, Editors. *Psychiatrists and Traditional Healers: Unwitting Partners in Global Mental Health.* Hoboken, NJ: John Wiley & Sons, Ltd.

Burgess LJ and Pretorius D. 2012. FDA abandons the Declaration of Helsinki: The effect on the ethics of clinical trial conduct in South Africa and other developing countries. *South African Journal of Bioethics and Law* 5(2):87–90.

Buss PM and Ferreira JR. 2011. Cooperação e integração regional em saúde na América do Sul: a contribuição da Unasul-Saúde. *Ciência & Saúde Coletiva, 16*(6), 2699–711.

Bustreo F, Hunt P, Gruskin S, et al. 2013. *Women's and Children's Health: Evidence of Impact of Human Rights.* Geneva: WHO.

Cabral L, Russo G, and Weinstock J. 2014. Brazil and the shifting consensus on development co-operation: Salutary diversions from the 'aid-effectiveness' trail? *Development Policy Review* 32(2):179–202.

Cantwell B and Kauppinen I, Editors. 2014. *Academic Capitalism in the Age of Globalization.* Baltimore: Johns Hopkins University Press.

Casto J and Messner LA. 2016. *Gender-based Violence Initiative Synthesis Report.* Arlington: Strengthening High Impact Interventions for an AIDS-free Generation (AIDSFree) Project.

Caven F. 2013. Being Idle No More: The Women Behind the Movement. https://www.culturalsurvival.org/publications/cultural-survival-quarterly/being-idle-no-more-women-behind-movement. Accessed June 8, 2016.

Chakma J, Sun GH, Steinberg JD, et al. 2014. Asia's ascent—global trends in biomedical R&D expenditures. *New England Journal of Medicine* 370(1):3–6.

Chu KM, Jayaraman S, Kyamanywa P, and Ntakiyiruta G. 2014. Building research capacity in Africa: Equity and global health collaborations. *PLoS Medicine* 11(3):e1001612.

Cole T. 2012. The White-Savior Industrial Complex. *The Atlantic,* March 21.

Cruikshank LW, Clark C, and Bartlett R. 2014. *Fundraising for Global Health Social Enterprises: Lessons from the Field.* Durham: Center for the Advancement of Social Entrepreuneurship.

Durisch P and Gex M. 2013. *Clinical Trials: Human Guinea - Pigs on the Cheap.* Zurich: Déclaration de Berne.

Dworkin SL, Hatcher AM, Colvin C, and Peacock D. 2013. Impact of a gender-transformative HIV and antiviolence program on gender ideologies and masculinities in two rural, South African communities. *Men and Masculinities* 16(2):181–202.

Feinsilver J. 2010. Fifty years of Cuba's medical diplomacy: From idealism to pragmatism. *Cuban Studies* 41:85–104.

Ferreira JR, Hoirisch C, Fonseca LE, and Buss PM. 2016. International cooperation in health: The case of Fiocruz. *História, Ciências, Saúde-Manguinhos* 23(2):267–276.

Fleury S. 2010. What kind of social protection for what kind of democracy? The dilemmas of social inclusion in Latin America. *Social Medicine* 5(1):34–49.

Forman L. 2016. The ghost is the machine: How can we visibilize the unseen norms and power of global health? *International Journal of Health Policy and Management* 5(3):197–199.

Forman L, Ooms G, Chapman A, et al. 2013. What could a strengthened right to health bring to the post-2015 health development agenda?: Interrogating the role of the minimum core concept in advancing essential global health needs. *BMC International Health and Human Rights* 13(48).

Freire P. 1970. *Pedagogy of the Oppressed.* New York: Continuum.

———. 1978. *Cartas a Guiné-Bissau. Registros de uma Experiencia em Processo.* Rio de Janeiro: Ed Paz e Terra.

———. 1992. *Pedagogy of Hope: Reliving Pedagogy of the Oppressed.* London: Bloomsbury.

Gamble V. 1997. Under the shadow of Tuskegee: African Americans and health care. *American Journal of Public Health* 87(11):1773–1778.

Garcia A and Kato K. 2015. The story of the hunter or hunted? Brazil's role in Angola and Mozambique. In Bond P and Garcia A, Editors. *BRICS: An Anti-Capitalist Critique.* London: Pluto Press.

García-Moreno C, Hegarty K, d'Oliveira AFL, et al. 2015a. The health-systems response to violence against women. *Lancet* 385(9977):1567–1579.

García-Moreno C, Zimmerman C, Morris-Gehring A, et al. 2015b. Addressing violence against women: A call to action. *Lancet* 385(9978):1685–1695.

Geiger HJ. 2013. Contesting racism and innovating community health centers: Approaches on two continents. In Birn A-E and Brown TM, Editors. *Comrades in Health: U.S. Health Internationalists, Abroad and at Home.* New Brunswick, NJ: Rutgers University Press.

General Comment 14 [Committee on Economic, Social and Cultural Rights, 22nd session]. 2000. *The Right to the Highest Attainable Standard of Health – Article 12 of the International Covenant on Economic, Social and Cultural Rights (CESCR)* (E/C.12/2000/4). Geneva: United Nations Economic and Social Council.

GHSA. 2016. About. https://ghsagenda.org/about.html. Accessed June 2, 2016.

Global Polio Eradication Initiative. 2012. What are people saying about polio eradication? http://www.polioeradication.org/Aboutus/Peoplearesaying.aspx#sthash.UgJgsWPz.dpuf. Accessed June 2, 2016.

Gloyd S, Pfeiffer J, and Johnson W. 2013. Cooperantes, solidarity, and the fight for health in Mozambique. In Birn A-E and Brown TM, Editors. *Comrades in Health: U.S. Health Internationalists, Abroad and at Home.* New Brunswick, NJ: Rutgers University Press.

Gopinathan U, Watts N, Hougendobler D, et al. 2015. Conceptual and institutional gaps: Understanding how the WHO can become a more effective cross-sectoral collaborator. *Globalization and Health* 11(1).

Gruskin S, Bogecho D, and Ferguson L. 2010. Rights-based approaches' to health policies and programs: Articulations, ambiguities, and assessment. *Journal of Public Health Policy* 31(2):129–145.

Gruskin S and Tarantola D. 2013. Bringing human rights into public health. In Grodin MA, Tarantola D, Annas GJ, and Gruskin S, Editors. *Health and Human Rights in a Changing World.* New York: Routledge.

Gupta R and Farmer PE. 2005. International electives: Maximizing the opportunity to learn and contribute. *Medscape General Medicine* 7(2):78.

Gutiérrez G. 1973. *A Theology of Liberation.* Maryknoll, NY: Orbis Books.

Hanefeld J. 2016. Advancing global health – the need for (better) social science. *International Journal of Health Policy and Management* 5(4):279–281.

Hanlon J, Barrientos A, and Hulme D. 2010. *Just Give Money to the Poor: The Development Revolution from the Global South.* Sterling, VA: Kumarian Press.

Hanson L. 2010. Global citizenship, global health, and the internationalization of curriculum: A study of transformative potential. *Journal of Studies in International Education* 14(1):70–88.

———. 2015. Experiences of creating internationalized curricula through global health programs at the University of Saskatchewan. In Green W and Whitsed C, Editors. *Critical Perspectives on Internationalising the Curriculum in Disciplines.* Dordrecht, NL: SensePublishers.

Hanson L, Harms S, and Plamondon K. 2011. Undergraduate international medical electives: Some ethical and pedagogical considerations. *Journal of Studies in International Education* 15(2):171–185.

Hanson L, Terstappen V, Bacon CM, et al. 2012. Gender, health, and Fairtrade: Insights from a research-action programme in Nicaragua. *Development in Practice* 22(2):164–179.

Harmer A and Buse K. 2014. The BRICS: A paradigm shift in global health? *Contemporary Politics* 2:127–145.

Harper I and Parker M. 2014. The politics and anti-politics of infectious disease control. *Medical Anthropology* 33(3):198–205.

Harrison M. 1994. *Public Health in British India: Anglo-Indian Preventive Medicine, 1859–1914.* Cambridge: Cambridge University Press.

Health and Human Rights Journal. 2015. Special issue: Evidence of the impact of human rights-based approaches to health. *Health and Human Rights* 17(2):1–179.

Horton R. 2013. Offline: Is global health neocolonialist?. *Lancet* 382(9906):1690.

Huish R. 2013. *Where No Doctor Has Gone Before: Cuba's Place in the Global Health Landscape.* Waterloo, ON: Wilfrid Laurier University Press.

Hunt P, Yamin AE, and Bustreo F. 2015. Making the case: What is the evidence of impact of applying human rights-based approaches to health? *Health and Human Rights Journal* 2(17):1–9.

Idle No More. 2016. http://www.idlenomore.ca/. Accessed June 8, 2016.

IPHU. 2016. Welcome to IPHU website! http://www.iphu.org/. Accessed June 2, 2016.

Jewkes R, Flood M, and Lang J. 2015. From work with men and boys to changes of social norms and reduction of inequities in gender relations: A conceptual shift in prevention of violence against women and girls. *Lancet* 385(9977):1580–1589.

Johnson CD, Noyes J, Haines A, et al. 2013. Learning from the Brazilian community health worker model in North Wales. *Globalization and Health* 9(1).

Jubilee Debt Campaign. 2014. Election 2015: How to avert a new debt crisis. http://jubileedebt.org.uk/reports-briefings/briefing/election-2015-avert-new-debt-crisis. Accessed June 7, 2016.

Kapoor I. 2013. *Celebrity Humanitarianism: The Ideology of Global Charity.* Abingdon, UK: Routledge.

Keshavjee S. 2014. *Blind Spot: How Neoliberalism Infiltrated Global Health.* Oakland: University of California Press.

Keugoung B, Macq J, Buvé A, et al. 2011. The interface between health systems and vertical programmes in Francophone Africa: The managers' perceptions. *Tropical Medicine & International Health* 16(4):478–485.

Kickbusch I. 2016. Politics or technocracy – what next for global health? *International Journal of Health Policy and Management* 5(3):201–204.

King, ML. Jr. 1965. "How long? Not long." Selma to Montgomery march. March 25, 1965, Montgomery, AL.

Klein N. 2014. *This Changes Everything: Capitalism vs. The Climate.* New York: Simon and Schuster.

Labonté R. 2013. Health activism in a globalising era: Lessons past for efforts future. *Lancet* 381(9884):2158–2159.

Lasker JN. 2016. *Hoping to Help: The Promises and Pitfalls of Global Health Volunteering.* Ithaca, NY: Cornell University Press.

Laxminarayan R and Ganguly NK. 2011. India's vaccine deficit: Why more than half of Indian children are not fully immunized, and what can—and should—be done. *Health Affairs* 30(6):1096–1103.

Lear WJ. 2013. American medical support for Spanish democracy, 1936-1938. In Birn A-E and Brown TM, Editors. *Comrades in Health: U.S. Health Internationalists, Abroad and at Home.* New Brunswick, NJ: Rutgers University Press.

Lhotská L and Gupta A. 2016. Whose health?: The crucial negotiations for the World Health Organization's future. *Asia & the Pacific Policy Society*, May 19.

Liang BA and Mackey T. 2010. Confronting conflict: Addressing institutional conflicts of interest in academic medical centers. *American Journal of Law & Medicine* 36(1):136–187.

Lim YW and Chia A. 2016. Social entrepreneurship: Improving global health. *JAMA* 315(22):2393–2394.

Loewenson R, Modisenyane M, and Pearcey M. 2014. African perspectives in global health diplomacy. *Journal of Health Diplomacy* 1(2).

Lurie P and Wolfe SM. 1997. Unethical trials of intervention to reduce perinatal transmission of the human immunodeficiency virus in developing countries. *New England Journal of Medicine* 337(12):853–856.

Lyons M. 2002. *The Colonial Disease: A Social History of Sleeping Sickness in Northern Zaire, 1900-1940.* Cambridge: Cambridge University Press.

Mahmood Q and Muntaner C. 2013. Politics, class actors, and health sector reform in Brazil and Venezuela. *Global Health Promotion* 20(1):59–67.

Mann J, Gruskin S, Grodin MA, and Annas GJ, Editors. 1999. *Health and Human Rights: A Reader.* New York: Routledge.

McAllister KE. 2015. Rubber, rights and resistance: The evolution of local struggles against a Chinese rubber concession in Northern Laos. *Journal of Peasant Studies* 42(3-4):817–837.

McLennan S. 2014. Medical voluntourism in Honduras: 'Helping' the poor? *Progress in Development Studies* 14(2):163–179.

Medicus Mundi. 2010. *La Participación Social en Salud: El Reto de Pasar del Discurso a la Práctica Marco Legal, Estratégico y de Políticas Públicas que dan Énfasis en los Procesos de Participación e Incidencia Social Existente en los Sistemas Públicos de Salud de la Región Centroamericana.* Ministerio de Asuntos Exteriores y de Cooperación/Medicus Mundi/AECID.

Merson M. 2015. Why should North Carolinians care about global health? *The Herald-Sun*, July 15.

Messac L and Prabhu K. 2013. Redefining the possible: The global AIDS response. In Farmer P, Kim JY, Kleinman A, and Basilico M, Editors. *Reimagining Global Health an Introduction.* Oakland: University of California Press.

Michau L, Horn J, Bank A, Dutt M, and Zimmerman C. 2015. Prevention of violence against women and girls: Lessons from practice. *Lancet* 385(9978):1672–1684.

Minaya G and Roque J. 2015. Ethical problems in health research with indigenous or originary peoples in Peru. *Journal of Community Genetics* 6(3):201–206.

Moyi Okwaro F and Geissler PW. 2015. In/dependent collaborations: Perceptions and experiences of African scientists in transnational HIV research. *Medical Anthropology Quarterly* 29(4):492–511.

Nakad J. 2016. Care for where there is no justice: The modern history of street medics and how they support social movements. *Hesperian Health Guides Blog*, January 6.

Okonta PI. 2014. Ethics of clinical trials in Nigeria. *Nigerian Medical Journal* 55(3):188.

Ooms G. 2015. Navigating between stealth advocacy and unconscious dogmatism: The challenge of researching the norms, politics and power of global health. *International Journal of Health Policy and Management* 4(10):641.

Palatino M. 2015. Myanmar's ribbon movements challenge militarization. *The Diplomat*, October 10.

Pang T. 2011. Global health research: Changing the agenda. In Benatar S and Brock G, Editors. *Global Health and Global Health Ethics.* Cambridge: Cambridge University Press.

Panter-Brick C, Eggerman M, and Tomlinson M. 2014. How might global health master deadly sins and strive for greater virtues? *Global Health Action* 7(10).

Parker M and Allen T. 2014. De-politicizing parasites: Reflections on attempts to control the control of neglected tropical diseases. *Medical Anthropology* 33(3):223–239.

Pfeiffer J. 2003. International NGOs and primary health care in Mozambique: The need for a new model of collaboration. *Social Science and Medicine* 56(4):725–738.

Pfeiffer J, Johnson W, Fort M, et al. 2008. Strengthening health systems in poor countries: A code of conduct for nongovernmental organizations. *American Journal of Public Health* 98(12), 2134–2140.

PHM. 2012. The final Cape Town call to action. http://www.phmovement.org/en/pha3/final_cape_town_call_to_action. Accessed June 8, 2016.

———. 2016. People's Health Movement. http://www.phmovement.org/en. Accessed June 8, 2016.

PHM, Medact, Medico International, et al. 2014. *Global Health Watch 4: An Alternative World Health Report.* London: Zed Books Ltd.

Pinto AD, Cole DC, ter Kuile A, et al. 2014. A case study of global health at the university: Implications for research and action. *Global Health Action* 7:24526.

Pinto AD and Upshur REG. 2009. Global health ethics for students. *Developing World Bioethics* 9(1):1–10.

Post L and Glassman A. 2016. Six ways the next US President can do better on global health. http://www.cgdev.org/blog/six-ways-next-us-president-can-do-better-global-health. Accessed September 17, 2016.

Presidential Commission for the Study of Bioethical Issues. 2011. *"Ethically Impossible" STD Research in Guatemala from 1946 to 1948.* Washington, DC.

Reid-Henry S. 2016. Just global health? *Development and Change* 47(4):712–733.

Reverby SM. 2009. *Examining Tuskegee: The Infamous Syphilis Study and its Legacy.* Chapel Hill: University of North Carolina Press.

———. 2011. "Normal exposure" and inoculation syphilis: A PHS "Tuskegee" doctor in Guatemala, 1946–1948. *Journal of Policy History* 23(1):6–28.

———. 2016. Restorative justice and restorative history for the sexually transmitted disease inoculation experiments in Guatemala. *American Journal of Public Health* 106(7):1163–1164.

Riggirozzi P. 2015. Regionalism, activism, and rights: New opportunities for health diplomacy in South America. *Review of International Studies* 41(2):407–428.

Right Livelihood Award. 2013. Denis Mukwege. http://www.rightlivelihood.org/mukwege.html. Accessed June 2, 2016.

Roa AC and Silva FRB. 2015. Fiocruz as an actor in Brazilian foreign relations in the context of the Community of Portuguese-Speaking Countries: An untold story. *História, Ciências, Saúde-Manguinhos* 22(1):153–169.

Rodríguez MI. 2009. *Construyendo la esperanza: estrategias y recomendaciones en salud 2009–2014*. San Salvador: Ministerio de Salud de El Salvador.

Roy A. 2004. Help that hinders. *Le Monde Diplomatique*. November. http://mondediplo.com/2004/11/16roy. Accessed June 8, 2016.

Santana JP. 2011. Um olhar sobre a Cooperação Sul-Sul em Saúde. *Ciência & Saúde Coletiva* 16(6):2993–3002.

Schrecker T. 2016. 'Neoliberal epidemics' and public health: Sometimes the world is less complicated than it appears. *Critical Public Health* 26(5):477–480.

Schuftan C, Turiano L, and Shukla A. 2009. The right to health: A People's Health Movement perspective and case study. In Clapham A and Robinson M, Editors. *Realizing the Right to Health Swiss Human Rights Book Vol. 3*. Zurich: Rüffer & Rub.

Shiffman J. 2014. Knowledge, moral claims and the exercise of power in global health. *International Journal of Health Policy and Management* 3(6):297–299.

Simkhada P, Regmi PR, Pant PR, et al. 2015. Stipulating citizen's fundamental right to healthcare: Inference from the Constitution of Federal Republic of Nepal 2015. *Nepal Journal of Epidemiology* 5(4):516–517.

Smith E, Hunt MR, and Master Z. 2014. Authorship ethics in global health research partnerships between researchers from low-medium income and high income countries. *BMC Medical Ethics* 15(42).

Smith L, Kasper J, and Holtz TH. 2013. Applying liberation medicine and accompanying communities in their struggles for health and social justice. In Birn A-E and Brown TM, Editors. *Comrades in Health: U.S. Health Internationalists, Abroad and at Home*. New Brunswick, NJ: Rutgers University Press.

Smith-Nonini S. 2010. *Healing the Body Politic: El Salvador's Popular Struggle for Health Rights from Civil War to Neoliberal Peace*. New Brunswick: Rutgers University Press.

Snyder J. 2012. Exploitations and their complications: The necessity of identifying the multiple forms of exploitation in pharmaceutical trials. *Bioethics* 26(5):251–258.

Stedile JP. 2002. A movement of movements: Landless battalions. *New Left Review* 15:77–104.

Tiessen R and Huish R, Editors. 2014. *Globetrotting or Global Citizenship?: Perils and Potential of International Experiential Learning*. Toronto: University of Toronto Press.

UN. 2015. Secretary-General, in Message for World Diabetes Day, Says People Must Take Steps towards Healthy Lives, while Governments Create Conditions to Stem Disease. http://www.un.org/press/en/2015/sgsm17320.doc.htm. Accessed June 2, 2016.

University of Western Cape. 2013. About the School of Public Health. https://www.uwc.ac.za/Faculties/CHS/soph/Pages/About-Us.aspx. Accessed June 2, 2016.

Varmus H and Satcher D. 1997. Ethical complexities of conducting research in developing countries. *New England Journal of Medicine* 337(14):1003–1005.

Velásquez G and Alas M. 2016. The slow shipwreck of the World Health Organization? *Third World Network*, May 19.

Ventres WB and Fort MP. 2014. Eyes wide open: An essay on developing an engaged awareness in global medicine and public health. *BMC International Health and Human Rights* 14(29).

Ventres W and Gusoff G. 2014. Poverty blindness: Exploring the diagnosis and treatment of an epidemic condition. *Journal of Health Care for the Poor and Underserved* 25(1):52–62.

Ventura D. 2013. Public health and Brazilian foreign policy. *SUR International Journal On Human Rights* 10(19):95–113.

Weigel J, Basilico M, Kerry V, et al. 2013. Global health priorities for the early twenty-first century. In Farmer P, Kim JY, Kleinman A, and Basilico M, Editors. *Reimagining Global Health an Introduction*. Oakland: University of California Press.

Wemos Foundation. 2010. *The Globalization of Clinical Trials: Testimonies from Human Subjects*. Amsterdam: Wemos Foundation.

White HN and Dijkstra AG. 2003. Aid, debt and dependence: Programme aid in Nicaragua. In *Programme Aid and Development: Beyond Conditionality*. London: Routledge.

WHO. 1976. *Introducing WHO*. Geneva: WHO.

———. 2016. Global Health Observatory Data Repository. http://apps.who.int/gho/data/node.imr. Accessed June 2, 2016.

Wilson J. 2015. The village that turned to gold: A parable of philanthrocapitalism. *Development and Change* 47(1):3–28.

Yamey G, on Behalf of the Interviewees. 2007. Which single intervention would do the most to improve the health of those living on less than $1 per day? *PLoS Medicine* 4(10):1557–1560.

Yamin AE. 2011. Power, suffering, and courts: Reflections on promoting health rights through judicialization. In Yamin AE and Gloppen S, Editors. *Litigating Health Rights: Can Courts Bring More Justice to Health?* Cambridge, MA: Harvard University Press.

Young IM. 2011. *Justice and the Politics of Difference*. Princeton: Princeton University Press.

INDEX